Mohs Micrographic Surgery

Keyvan Nouri
Editor

Mohs Micrographic Surgery

Springer

Editor
Keyvan Nouri, M.D.
Department of Dermatology
and Cutaneous Surgery
University of Miami
Leonard M. Miller School of Medicine
Miami, FL
USA

Sylvester Comprehensive Cancer Center
University of Miami Hospital and Clinics
Miami, FL
USA

ISBN 978-1-4471-2151-0 e-ISBN 978-1-4471-2152-7
DOI 10.1007/978-1-4471-2152-7
Springer London Dordrecht Heidelberg New York

British Library Cataloguing in Publication Data
A catalogue record for this book is available from the British Library

Library of Congress Control Number: 2011944218

Printed on acid-free paper

Springer is part of Springer Science+Business Media (www.springer.com)

Foreword

The incidence of skin cancers is rising annually. Non-melanoma skin cancers (NMSC) constitute a large majority of all skin cancers, with more than 3,500,00 new cases reported in the United States per year. There has been a noticeable rise in NMSCs among the immunosuppressed population such as transplant patients, HIV/AIDS patients etc.

The technique of Mohs micrographic surgery was invented by Frederic E. Mohs while he was working as a cancer research assistant during his medical school in the early 1930s. His observation that the microscopic details of the tissue were retained upon an intratumoral injection of 20% zinc chloride, led to the genesis of the idea of excising cancer under microscopic control.

Later in 1953, Dr. Mohs demonstrated the fresh tissue technique while performing Mohs on a basal cell carcinoma (BCC) on the eyelid. A 5-year cure rate of 100% using the fresh-tissue technique to excise eyelid carcinomas was reported in 1969. Wide acceptance of the fresh-tissue technique increased substantially and has become a very popular method in the United States. It is considered the technique of choice and standard of care for NMSCs with certain criteria due to the fact that it provides the highest cure rate and maximal tissue conservation with smallest possible defect. Mohs Surgery has been used for NMSCs, some forms of melanoma and other rare cutaneous tumors.

Mohs Micrographic Surgery has become more and more popular dramatically. Fellowships have been set up for teaching Mohs Micrographic Surgery, and recently these techniques under the auspices of American College of Graduate Medical Education (ACGME) has been renamed Procedural Dermatology. The main components of Procedural Dermatology aim at developing proficiency and skill in Mohs Surgery.

Mohs Micrographic Surgery by Keyvan Nouri is the most up to date, comprehensive and easy to comprehend textbook in the area of Mohs surgery. It includes sections on Fundamentals of Mohs Micrographic Surgery, Laboratory Processing, Mohs Micrographic Surgery by tumor and site, Pitfalls of Mohs Micrographic Surgery, Reconstructive and Adjuvant Techniques, Training and Certification in Mohs Micrographic Surgery and Patient Safety and Medicolegal Issues. The authors of the book are some of the most reputable surgeons in the field. The book also includes a section on International Perspective of Mohs Micrographic Surgery which highlights the Mohs surgical practices in various parts of the world.

To sum, I strongly recommend the textbook *Mohs Micrographic Surgery* by Dr. Keyvan Nouri and published by Springer as one of the best textbooks in this area. I congratulate Dr. Nouri and all the authors and publishers for putting together such a comprehensive and illustrious textbook.

Perry Robins
Professor Emeritus of Mohs Micrographic Surgery of NYU medical center
President of Skin Cancer Foundation

I dedicate this book to my patients, for whom it is written for.
I dedicate this book to my family and friends who have been there for me in every instance of my life.
I dedicate this book to my wife Dr. Firouzeh Miremadi and my son Kian Nouri.
I dedicate this book to my mother Mrs. Zohreh Khajavi-Noori, my father Dr. Ali Nouri, my sister Dr. Mahnaz Nouri, my uncle Dr. Farrokh Khajavi, my grandparents, and the rest of my dear family.

I love you all.
Keyvan Nouri, M.D.

Preface

Mohs micrographic surgery has revolutionized the practice of cutaneous oncology with its method of accurate, staged intraoperative histological analysis. The indications for the procedure and technique have been drastically expanded, yet the underlying principles put forth by Dr. Frederic Mohs approximately prior to 70 years remain largely unchanged. The technique evolved from the fixed tissue method utilizing zinc chloride for chemosurgery to the present day fresh frozen tissue technique. With the advent of the fresh frozen tissue technique, the ability to conduct extensive reconstructive surgery became available to dermatologic surgeons. As a result, dermatologists began performing extensive procedures that had previously been carried out by other specialties. The dermatologic surgeons then began forming organizations that were dedicated to advances in the field of dermatologic surgery and cutaneous oncology. Now immunostains are beginning to be implemented, which have expanded the utility of Mohs surgery to treat certain forms of melanomas and other rare or unusual tumors. Nearly 3.5 million new cases of skin cancer are diagnosed per annum, of which a large percentage will be treated by Mohs micrographic surgery. The indications for Mohs micrographic surgery are moving beyond the traditional basal cell and squamous cell carcinoma to include: dermatofibrosarcoma protuberans, microcystic adnexal carcinoma, atypical fibroxanthoma, sebaceous carcinoma, extramammary Paget's disease, and Merkel cell carcinoma.

This textbook attempts to explore Mohs micrographic surgery in all of its realms and presents a thorough representation of the surgical practice. Each chapter is easy to read with summary boxes to emphasize the major points. The chapters are written by well-known experts in their respective fields. We have included an international section to highlight the progression of Mohs surgery throughout the world. As we have transgressed into the modern era of the practice of Mohs surgery, the medicolegal issues along with the relevant ethical and patient safety considerations are also explored.

Overall, the reader should enjoy an up-to-date, reliable source of information discussing the important aspects of Mohs surgery. The reader will obtain a detailed understanding of this surgical practice, which will undoubtedly improve patient care.

Miami, FL, USA — Keyvan Nouri, M.D.

Acknowledgements

I sincerely thank all the authors of this textbook. These individuals are world-renowned in their respective specialties and without their time and energy, writing this book would have not been possible. These individuals have made this a comprehensive, up-to-date, and reliable source on Mohs micrographic surgery. I truly appreciate their hard work and thank them for their contributions.

Throughout my career, my family has always supported my many endeavors. I cannot thank them enough for their kind encouragement and love.

I would like to give a special thanks to Dr. Lawrence A. Schachner, Chairman of the Department of Dermatology and Cutaneous Surgery at the University of Miami Miller School of Medicine. He has been my mentor throughout my professional career. His guidance and role as an advisor over the years have influenced my efforts.

I am grateful to Dr. William H. Eaglestein, former Chairman of Dermatology at the University of Miami School of Medicine for helping and guiding me since my start in dermatology. I appreciate all of his guidance and support.

Thank you to Dr. Perry Robins, Dr. Robin Ashinoff, Dr. Vicki Levine, Dr. Seth Orlow, the late Dr. Irvin Freedberg, Dr. Hideko Kamino, and the entire faculty and staff at New York University School of Medicine Department of Dermatology. You have all created a wonderful learning and friendship experience during my surgery fellowship.

I would like to thank the faculty, dermatology residents, and staff of the Department of Dermatology and Cutaneous Surgery at the University of Miami Miller school of Medicine for their teaching, expertise, and friendship. I give special acknowledgements to the Mohs and Laser Center staff at the Sylvester Cancer Center for their hard work and support on a daily basis. I would also like to thank Maria D. Garcia, my administrative assistant, for her diligence and hard work and the rest of the Mohs staff, including Cathy Mamas, Juana Alonso, Tania Garcia, Veronica Sanchez, Liseth Velasquez, Tatania Carmouze and Lisbeth Napoles. Thank you for making my job a pleasure.

Thank you to Dr. Sonal Choudhary and Michael Patrick McLeod, my research fellows, as well as Dr. Yasser Al-qubaisy, my clinical fellow, for all their hard work and dedication to composing the book. Also, I would like to thank the medical student, Marilyn Zabielinski, and international fellow Dr. Katlein Franca, for their contributions.

I would also like to acknowledge the publishing staff Mr. Grant Weston, Ms. Linda Jacobs, Ms. Cate Rogers, and the entire Springer Publishing team for having done a superb job with the publication. It has been a pleasure working with them and this excellent project to compile the textbook.

Keyvan Nouri, M.D.

Contents

Contributors

Sumaira Z. Aasi, M.D. Department of Dermatology, Yale University, New Haven, CT, USA

Murad Alam, M.D., M.Sci. Department of Dermatology, Northwestern University, Chicago, IL, USA

Yasser A. Alqubaisy, M.D. Department of Dermatology and Cutaneous Surgery, University of Miami Hospital, Miami, FL, USA

Satoru Aoyagi, M.D., Ph.D. Department of Dermatology, Hokkaido University Graduate School of Medicine, Sapporo, Japan

Sarah G. Baker, M.D. Department of Dermatology, Northwestern University, Chicago, IL, USA

Richard J. Barlow, M.B., B.C.H., M.D., FRCP St. John's Institute of Dermatology, St. Thomas' Hospital, London, UK

Jamie L. Benenhaley Trident Dermatology, Charleston, SC, USA

Richard G. Bennett, M.D. Department of Dermatology, UCLA and USC, Santa Monica, CA, USA

Tina Bhutani, M.D. Department of Dermatology, UCSF Psoriasis and Skin Treatment Center, San Francisco, CA, USA

Diana Bolotin, M.D., Ph.D. Department of Dermatology, Northwestern University, Chicago, IL, USA

Martin Braun III, M.D. Braun Dermatology, George Washington University, Washington, DC, USA

David G. Brodland, M.D. Departments of Dermatology and Otolaryngology, Shadyside Medical Center, University of Pittsburgh Medical Center, Pittsburgh, PA, USA

Michael Campoli, M.D., Ph.D. Fellows, Zitelli & Brodland, P.C., Pittsburgh, PA, USA

Basil S. Cherpelis, M.D. Dermatology and Cutaneous Surgery, University of South Florida, Tampa, FL, USA

Sonal Choudhary, M.D. Department of Dermatology and Cutaneous Surgery, University of Miami Leonard M. Miller School of Medicine, Miami, FL, USA

Steven Chow, M.D., M.S. Department of Dermatology, University of Southern California, Santa Monica, CA, USA

Sean R. Christensen, M.D., Ph.D. Department of Dermatology, Yale University School of Medicine, New Haven, CT, USA

Daniel L. Christiansen, M.D. Department of Medicine, Division of Dermatology, Vanderbilt Medical Center, Nashville, TN, USA

Robert H. Cook-Norris, M.D. Department of Dermatology, Mayo Clinic, Rochester, MN, USA

Stephanie A. Diamantis, M.D. Department of Dermatology, Geisinger Medical Center, Danville, PA, USA

Tobechi L. Ebede, M.D. Dermatology Service, Memorial Sloan Kettering Cancer Center, New York, NY, USA

Katlein França, M.D. Department of Dermatology and Cutaneous Surgery, University of Miami Leonard M. Miller School of Medicine, Miami, FL, USA

Scott Freeman, M.D. Fellows, Zitelli & Brodland, P.C., Pittsburgh, PA, USA

Gaston Nestor Galimberti, M.D. Department of Dermatology, School of Medicine Italian Hospital, Buenos Aires, Argentina

Carlette M. Geddis, B.S., H.T.L. Trident Dermatology, Charleston, SC, USA

L. Frank Glass, M.D. Dermatology and Cutaneous Surgery, University of South Florida, Tampa, FL, USA

Hugh M. Gloster Jr., M.D. Department of Dermatology, University of Cincinnati, Cincinnati, OH, USA

David J. Goldberg, M.D., J.D. Department of Dermatology, Mount Sinai School of Medicine, New York, NY, USA

Greg Julian Goodman, M.B.B.S. (Hons), M.D., FACD, Grad. Dip. Clin. Epi. Dermatology Institute of Victoria, South Yarra, VIC, Australia

Sarah E. Grummer, M.D. Department of Mohs Surgery, Dermatology and Plastic Surgery, Key Biscayne, Dade, FL, USA

Ashraf M. Hassanein, M.D., Ph.D. Medical Director, Florida Pathology and Dermatologic Surgery & Aesthetics Institute, The Villages, FL, USA

Hatem A. Hassanein, B.Sc. Department of Microbiology and Biomedical Sciences, University of South Florida College of Medicine, Tampa, FL, USA

Misha M. Heller, B.A. Department of Dermatology, UCSF Psoriasis and Skin Treatment Center, San Francisco, CA, USA

Jennifer I. Hui, M.D. Department of Ophthalmic Plastic, Orbital Surgery and Oncology service, Bascom Palmer Eye Institute, Miami, FL, USA

Tatyana R. Humphreys, M.D. Department of Dermatology, Thomas Jefferson University, Philadelphia, PA, USA

Adam A. Ingraffea, M.D. Department of Dermatology, University of Cincinnati, Cincinnati, OH, USA

Brooke A. Jackson, M.D. Department of Dermatology, Skin Wellness Center of Chicago, SC, Chicago, IL, USA

Northwestern Medical School, Chicago, IL, USA

Lorraine M. Jennings, M.B., B.Ch., B.A.O. (Hons) Department of Mohs Micrographic Surgery, Department of Dermatology, Dana Farber Cancer Institute/Brigham and Women's Hospital, Boston, MA, USA

Hooman Khorasani, M.D. Department of Dermatology, The Mount Sinai Medical Center, New York, NY, USA

Arash Kimyai-Asadi, M.D. DermSurgery Associates, Houston, TX, USA

Richelle M. Knudson, M.D. Department of Dermatology, Mayo Clinic, Rochester, MN, USA

John Koo, M.D. Department of Dermatology, UCSF Psoriasis and Skin Treatment Center, San Francisco, CA, USA

Luis Fernando F. Kopke, M.D. Coordinator of the Department of Micrographic Surgery of the Brazilian Society of Dermatology, President of the Brazilian Society of Dermatologic Surgery, Florianopolis, Santa Catarina, Brazil

Pearon G. Lang, M.D., B.A., M.D. Trident Dermatology, Charleston, SC, USA

James A.A. Langtry, M.B.B.S., FRCP Department of Dermatology, Royal Victoria Infirmary, Newcastle Upon Tyne, Tyne and Wear, UK

Susana M. Leal-Khouri, M.D., FAAD Department of Dermatology and Cutaneous Surgery, University of Miami, Key Biscayne, Dade, FL, USA

Florida International University School of Medicine, Key Biscayne, Dade, FL, USA

Nicole R. LeBoeuf, M.D. Department of Dermatology, Dana Farber Cancer Institute/Brigham and Women's Hospital, Boston, MA, USA

Eric S. Lee, B.S. Department of Dermatology, UCSF Psoriasis and Skin Treatment Center, San Francisco, CA, USA

Boonyapat Limthongkul, M.D. Department of Dermatology, Thomas Jefferson University, Philadelphia, PA, USA

Victor J. Marks, M.D. Department of Dermatologic Surgery, Geisinger Health System, Danville, PA, USA

Ellen S. Marmur, M.D. Division of Dermatologic & Cosmetic Surgery, Department of Dermatology, The Mount Sinai Medical Center, New York, NY, USA

Michael P. McLeod, B.S., M.S. Department of Dermatology and Cutaneous Surgery, University of Miami Leonard M. Miller School of Medicine, Miami, FL, USA

Neda Mehr, M.D. Department of Dermatology,
Loma Linda University School of Medicine, Loma Linda, CA, USA

Bradley G. Merritt, M.D. Department of Dermatology,
UNC – Chapel Hill, Chapel Hill, NC, USA

Vanessa A. Morgan, M.B.B.S., FRCP
Skin and Cancer Foundation, Carlton, VIC, Australia

Kishwer S. Nehal, M.D. Dermatology Service,
Memorial Sloan Kettering Cancer Center, New York, NY, USA

Tanya Nino, M.D. Department of Dermatology,
Loma Linda University School of Medicine, Loma Linda, CA, USA

Keyvan Nouri, M.D. Department of Dermatology
and Cutaneous Surgery, University of Miami Leonard
M. Miller School of Medicine, Miami, FL, USA

Sylvester Comprehensive Cancer Center,
University of Miami Hospital and Clinics, Miami, FL, USA

Suzanne M. Olbricht, M.D. Department of Dermatology,
Lahey Clinic, Burlington, MA, USA

Howard A. Oriba, M.D. Department of Mohs Surgery,
The Skin Cancer Center, Sun City Center, FL, USA

Kapila V. Paghdal, M.D., Pharm.D. Dermatology and Cutaneous Surgery,
University of South Florida, Tampa, FL, USA

Ioulios Palamaras, M.D., Ph.D. St. John's Institute of Dermatology,
St. Thomas' Hospital, London, UK

Ilya Reyter, M.D. Department of Dermatology,
Loma Linda University School of Medicine, Loma Linda, CA, USA

Randall K. Roenigk, M.D. Division of Dermatologic Surgery,
Department of Dermatology, Mayo Clinic, Rochester, MN, USA

Thomas E. Rohrer, M.D.
SkinCare Physicians, Chestnut Hill, MA, USA

Jeffrey E. Rubenstein, D.M.D., M.S. Department of Restorative Dentistry,
University of Washington, Seattle, WA, USA

Marc Rubenzik, M.D., Ph.D. Department of Dermatology,
Thomas Jefferson University, Philadelphia, PA, USA

Tim J. Rutherford, M.B.B.S. (Hons), FACD
Victorian Dermatology & Surgery, Malnern, VIC, Australia

Paul J.M. Salmon, MBChB, FRACP, FAAD, FACMS
Dermatologic Surgery, Skin Cancer Institute,
Tauranga Bay of Plenty, New Zealand

Chrysalyne D. Schmults, M.D., M.S.C.E.
Department of Dermatologic Surgery,
MOHS Micrographic Surgery Center,
Brigham and Women's Hospital, Boston, MA, USA

Jessica M. Sheehan, M.D.
Northshore Center for Medical Aesthetics, Northbrook, IL, USA

Douglas M. Sidle, M.D., FACS Department of Otolaryngology – Head & Neck Surgery, Northwestern Feinberg School of Medicine, Chicago, IL, USA

Indira Singh, B.A. Dermatology Service,
Memorial Sloan Kettering Cancer Center, New York, NY, USA

Stephen N. Snow, M.D. Department of Dermatology,
University of Wisconsin School of Medicine & Public Health,
Madison, WI, USA

Novie Sroa, M.D. Department of Dermatology,
Roswell Park Cancer Institute, Buffalo, NY, USA

Thomas Stasko, M.D. Department of Medicine, Division of Dermatology,
Vanderbilt University, Nashville, TN, USA

Abel Torres, M.D. Department of Dermatology,
Loma Linda University School of Medicine, Loma Linda, CA, USA

David T. Tse, M.D., FACS Department of Ophthalmic Plastic, Orbital Surgery and Oncology service, Bascom Palmer Eye Institute, Miami, FL, USA

Glenn E. Turner, D.M.D., M.S.D. Department of Prosthodontics, University of Florida College of Dentistry, Gainesville, FL, USA

Edward J. Upjohn, M.B.B.S., M.Med., FACD
Skin and Cancer Foundation, Carlton, VIC, Australia

Irene Vergilis-Kalner, M.D. Assistant Professor of Dermatology, Department of Dermatology, UMDNJ, New Jersey

Andrew E. Werchniak, M.D. Department of Dermatology, Dana Farber Cancer Institute/Brigham and Women's Hospital, Boston, MA, USA

Yaohui Gloria Xu, M.D., Ph.D. Department of Dermatology,
University of Wisconsin, Madison, WI, USA

Simon Yoo, M.D. Department of Dermatology, Otolaryngology, Surgery,
Northwestern University, Chicago, IL, USA

Jeremy S. Youse, M.D. Department of Dermatology,
Mayo Clinic, Rochester, MN, USA

Marilyn Zabielinski, B.S. University of Miami, Miami, Miami, FL, USA

Nathalie C. Zeitouni, MDCM, FRCPC
Department of Dermatology,
Roswell Park Cancer Institute, Buffalo, NY, USA

John Zitelli, M.D. Fellows, Zitelli & Brodland, P.C., Pittsburgh, PA, USA

1 An Introduction to Mohs Micrographic Surgery

Michael P. McLeod, Sonal Choudhary, and Keyvan Nouri

Abstract

The founding father of Mohs micrographic surgery is Frederic E. Mohs. He was only a medical student when he began to develop his new surgical technique during the 1930s. Mohs noticed that zinc chloride could be used to "fix" a tumor so that the histologic architecture could be viewed under a microscope. In 1936, Mohs translated his research method into use for cutaneous tumors in humans. It was at this time that chemosurgery (the precursor to modern day Mohs micrographic surgery) was born. In 1941, Mohs reported his findings using fixed tissue chemosurgery in the Archives of Surgery with 440 patients. Later in 1946, he reported more results at the American Academy of Dermatology in Chicago. In 1947, he described his technique and work in the Archives of Dermatology. In 1953, Mohs was creating a video illustrating the chemosurgery technique for the eyelid. In order to speed the surgery for the video, he did not use the zinc chloride fixative. Instead, he used fresh frozen tissue to generate the horizontal sections. Hence, the birth of the present day form of Mohs Micrographic Surgery began taking shape. In 1983, the first 1-year fellowship program was formally approved by the American College of Mohs Micrographic Surgery and Cutaneous Oncology (ACMMSCO). Fourteen years after the approval of the first fellowship program, there were more than 60, 1–2-year training programs approved by the ACMMSCO. In addition, there are approved fellowships in Australia, New Zealand, and Canada. Mohs surgery is spreading across the world, and we have dedicated an entire section of this book to document its travel.

Keywords

Frederic E. Mohs • Chemosurgery • Zinc chloride • Mohs micrographic surgery

M.P. McLeod • S. Choudhary
Department of Dermatology and Cutaneous Surgery, University of Miami Leonard M. Miller School of Medicine, Miami, FL, USA

K. Nouri (✉)
Department of Dermatology and Cutaneous Surgery, University of Miami Leonard M. Miller School of Medicine, Miami, FL, USA

Sylvester Comprehensive Cancer Center, University of Miami Hospital and Clinics, Miami, FL, USA
e-mail: knouri@med.miami.edu

K. Nouri (ed.), *Mohs Micrographic Surgery*,
DOI 10.1007/978-1-4471-2152-7_1, © Springer-Verlag London Limited 2012

Summary: An Introduction to Mohs Micrographic Surgery

- Mohs was only a medical student when he began to develop his new surgical technique during the 1930s.
- In 1941, Mohs reported his findings using fixed tissue chemosurgery in the Archives of Surgery.
- In 1953, Mohs was creating a video illustrating the chemosurgery technique for the eyelid. In order to speed the surgery for the video, he did not use the zinc chloride fixative. Instead, he used fresh frozen tissue to generate the horizontal sections.
- During 1956, Mohs published his first book entitled *Chemosurgery in Cancer, Gangrene and Infections*.
- In 1967, the first meeting of the American College of Chemosurgery occurred at the Palmer House in Chicago with 23 members.
- During the 1970s, the fresh tissue technique became the main form of Mohs surgery practiced, reducing the time required for the technique, the pain experienced by the patient, and improving the cosmetic results.
- In 1983, the first 1-year fellowship program formally approved by the American College of Mohs Micrographic Surgery and Cutaneous Oncology (ACMMSCO).
- In 1985, the American College of Chemosurgery changed its name to the American College of Mohs Micrographic Surgery and Cutaneous Oncology.
- Mohs micrographic surgery is spreading across the world, and we have dedicated a section of this book to document its travel.

1.1 Introduction

The founding father of Mohs micrographic surgery, Frederic E. Mohs, was born in Wisconsin in 1910. While he was a young child, his father died, and his family moved to Madison, Wisconsin. Mohs was only a medical student when he began to develop his new surgical technique during the 1930s [1, 2]. At that time he was working under the supervision of Dr. Michael Guyer, Professor of Zoology at the University of Wisconsin. Initially, Mohs injected platinum into implanted tumors of rats and subsequently made horizontal sections to be viewed under the microscope.

At the turn of the twentieth century, Cancquin in Paris and Bougard in Brussels began investigating zinc chloride as a treatment for all types of cancer. Zinc chloride had been known to exist for at least 100 years prior when Sir Humphry Davy from Bristol took note of its "antitumor" effect. Mohs noticed that zinc chloride could be used to "fix" a tumor so that the histologic architecture could be viewed under a microscope.

In 1936, Mohs translated his research method into use for cutaneous tumors in humans. He began injecting zinc chloride into human skin cancers and taking horizontal frozen sections in thin layers to observe whether any tumors had cells extending beyond the margins of the section. It was at this time that chemosurgery, the precursor to modern day Mohs micrographic surgery, was born.

In 1941, Mohs reported his findings using fixed tissue chemosurgery in the Archives of Surgery in 440 consecutive patients involving primary cutaneous malignancies [3]. Out of those 440 patients, 409 or 93% did not experience any recurrences [3]. Dr. Mohs reported that a number of the cases that did recur were advanced in their initial presentation. Later in 1946, he reported more results at the American Academy of Dermatology in Chicago. In 1947, he described his technique and work using chemosurgery for the face [4].

After these initial reports, Dr. Mohs' clinic at the University of Wisconsin became flooded with patients who had skin cancer. In addition to skin cancer, he treated gangrene as well as cutaneous infections.

Despite the early success of Mohs' technique, there were some drawbacks to fixed tissue chemosurgery. It was labor intensive, time-consuming, and painful for the patient. The zinc chloride paste had to be left overnight in order to fix the tissue. Patients complained of great pain during the process as zinc chloride is known to be a chemical irritant. In addition, the zinc chloride paste required several weeks to be removed from the tissue so that reconstruction could be undertaken.

In 1953, Mohs was creating a video illustrating the chemosurgery technique for the eyelid. In order to speed the surgery for the video, he did not use the zinc chloride fixative. Instead, he used fresh frozen tissue to generate the horizontal sections. Hence, the birth of the present day form of Mohs micrographic surgery was beginning to take shape.

During 1956, Mohs published his first book entitled *Chemosurgery in Cancer, Gangrene and Infections*. The book was very popular and prompted many physicians to train with Mohs in Madison. Dr. Mohs' training program was noted to be very rigorous, starting at 7:00 a.m. and often going to 8:00 p.m. daily.

In 1966, Dr. Perry Robins formed the first Mohs surgery training program outside of Madison, Wisconsin, at New York University. Shortly thereafter, in 1967, the first meeting of the American College of Chemosurgery occurred at the Palmer House in Chicago with 23 members.

In 1970, Dr. Tromovitch from San Francisco demonstrated high cure rates with the fresh tissue technique at the annual meeting of the American College of Chemosurgery. Four years later in 1974, he reported the results in the Archives of Dermatology [5]. During the 1970s, the fresh tissue technique became the main form of Mohs surgery practiced, reducing the time needed for the technique, reducing the pain experienced by the patient, and improving the cosmetic results. The reconstruction could now begin on the same day of the surgery now that the zinc chloride paste was not required.

In 1983, the first one-year fellowship program formally approved by the American College of Mohs Micrographic Surgery and Cutaneous Oncology (ACMMSCO) with Dr. C. William Hanke at Indiana University. Two years later, Hanke et al. created the term Mohs micrographic surgery [6]. In 1985, the American College of Chemosurgery changed its name to the American College of Mohs Micrographic Surgery and Cutaneous Oncology as suggested by Robins and Hanke. In 1990, Picoto created the European Society for Micrographic Surgery. In 1991, Cottel created the American Board of Mohs Micrographic Surgery and Cutaneous Oncology (ACMMSO).

Fourteen years after the approval of the first fellowship program, there were more than 60, 1–2-year training programs approved by the ACMMSCO. In addition, there are approved fellowships in Australia, New Zealand, and Canada. At least 25 fellowship programs are undergoing the ACGME accreditation process.

Frederic E. Mohs died on July 1, 2002. His contributions to Dermatologic Surgery continue to live on. Mohs surgery is becoming more and more advanced, now using immunohistochemistry in combination with fresh frozen tissue to more closely delineate tumor margins. Additionally, Mohs' surgery is spreading across the world, and we have dedicated a section of this book to document its travel.

Summary: Conclusion

- The Mohs micrographic surgery was developed by Frederic Edward Mohs in the 1930s. During the 1970s, the fresh tissue technique became the main form of Mohs surgery practiced, reducing the time needed for the technique, the pain experienced by the patient, and improving the cosmetic results. It is considered the most effective procedure for certain types of skin cancer today.

1.2 Conclusion

Mohs micrographic surgery was developed by Frederic Edward Mohs in the 1930s. This technique is considered the best method for treating certain types of skin cancer with very high cure rates. His findings began after his studies in rats, noticing that zinc chloride could be used to "fix" tumors so that their histologic architecture could be viewed under a microscope.

In 1936, Mohs translated his research method into use for cutaneous tumors in humans, developing into the beginning of chemosurgery; the precursor to modern day Mohs micrographic surgery. Despite the early success of this new technique, he realized that some improvements needed to be made. The zinc chloride paste had to be left overnight in order to appropriately fix the tissue and also required several weeks to be removed from the tissue so that reconstruction could be undertaken. As a chemical irritant, it was also painful for the patient. So in 1953, he started using fresh frozen tissue to generate horizontal sections instead of zinc chloride assisted tissue fixation.

During the 1970s, the fresh tissue technique became the main form of Mohs surgery practiced, reducing the time needed for the technique, the pain experienced by the patient, and improving the cosmetic results, since the reconstruction could begin on the same day of the surgery.

Today, Mohs micrographic surgery is becoming more advanced; now using immunohistochemistry in combination with fresh frozen tissue to more closely delineate tumor margins. It is considered the most effective procedure for certain types of skin cancer today.

References

1. Swanson NA, Taylor WB. Plantar verrucous carcinoma. Literature review and treatment by the Mohs' chemosurgery technique. Arch Dermatol. 1980;116(7):794–7.
2. Shriner DL, McCoy DK, Goldberg DJ, Wagner RF. Mohs micrographic surgery. J Am Acad Dermatol. 1998;39(1): 79–97.
3. Mohs FE, Chemosurgery A. Microscopically controlled method of cancer excision. Arch Surg. 1941;42(2):279–95.
4. Mohs FE. Chemosurgical treatment of cancer of the face; a microscopically controlled method of excision. Arch Derm Syphilol. 1947;56(2):143–56.
5. Tromovitch TA, Stegman SJ. Microscopically controlled excision of skin tumors. Arch Dermatol. 1974;110:231–2.
6. Hanke CW, Temofeew RK, Miyamoto RT, Lingeman RE. Basal cell carcinoma involving the external auditory canal: treatment with Mohs micrographic surgery. J Dermatol Surg Oncol. 1985;11:1189–94.

Indications for Mohs Micrographic Surgery

2

Michael P. McLeod, Sonal Choudhary, Yasser A. Alqubaisy, and Keyvan Nouri

Abstract

Mohs micrographic surgery (MMS) can be used to treat a wide variety of tumors. General indications for Mohs micrographic surgery require that the cutaneous tumor be continuously growing. Additionally, MMS is considered particularly well suited for tumors that exhibit perineural invasion, tumors in high-risk anatomical areas, tumors that have been incompletely excised, and those with poorly defined clinical margins.

The indications for MMS for each tumor type can be divided into common and uncommon entities. The most common indications for MMS include Basal Cell Carcinoma (BCC) and Squamous Cell Carcinoma (SCC). Less common indications for MMS are not supported by as much evidence, but include: Dermatofibrosarcoma Protuberans (DFSP), Microcystic Adnexal Carcinoma (MAC), Atypical Fibroxanthoma (AFX), Superficial Leiomyosarcoma, Malignant Fibrous Histiocytoma (MFH), Sebaceous Carcinoma (SC), Melanoma, Merkel Cell Carcinoma (MCC), and Extramammary Paget's Disease (EMPD). The evidence behind using Mohs micrographic surgery will be discussed for each entity as well as the relevant results from studies used to measure recurrence rates when using Mohs micrographic surgery for these tumors.

Keywords

Mohs micrographic surgery • Mohs micrographic surgery indications • Recurrence rates • Clearance rates

M.P. McLeod • S. Choudhary
Department of Dermatology and Cutaneous Surgery, University of Miami Leonard M. Miller School of Medicine, Miami, FL, USA

Y.A. Alqubaisy
Department of Dermatology and Cutaneous Surgery, University of Miami Hospital, Miami, FL, USA

K. Nouri (✉)
Department of Dermatology and Cutaneous Surgery, University of Miami Leonard M. Miller School of Medicine, Miami, FL, USA

Sylvester Comprehensive Cancer Center, University of Miami Hospital and Clinics, Miami, FL, USA
e-mail: knouri@med.miami.edu

Summary: Introduction

- General indications for Mohs micrographic surgery require that the cutaneous tumor be continuously growing.
- MMS is considered well suited for tumors:
  - That exhibit perineural invasion
  - Tumors in high-risk anatomical areas
  - Tumors that have been incompletely excised
  - Tumors with poorly defined clinical margins

K. Nouri (ed.), *Mohs Micrographic Surgery*,
DOI 10.1007/978-1-4471-2152-7_2, © Springer-Verlag London Limited 2012

Table 2.1 Mohs versus standard excision BCC and SCC

	BCC	SCC
Mohs (MMS)	99% 5-year cure rate of primary BCC	96.9% cure rate for primary SCC
	96% cure rate with recurrent BCC	10% recurrence rate of recurrent SCC
Standard excision	10% recurrence rate of long-term primary BCC	91.9% cure rate of primary SCC
	19.9% recurrent rate for recurrent BCC with non-Mohs therapy	23% recurrence rate of recurrent SCC

2.1 Introduction

Mohs micrographic surgery can be used to treat a wide variety of tumors. It is well suited for recurrent tumors, those that have been incompletely excised, tumors in high risk anatomical areas, tumors with poorly defined clinical margins, instances of perineural invasion, tumors in immunosuppressed patients, or previously irradiated skin. The tumor should also be continuously growing in both the horizontal and vertical directions; otherwise, falsely clear margins may be observed on horizontal sections [1–3]. In addition, larger tumors greater than 2 cm on the trunk or 1 cm on the face are considered strong indications for Mohs [4–6].

The indications for Mohs micrographic surgery can be divided into common and uncommon varieties. A wealth of data exists for the most common indications, while uncommon indications are mainly supported by case series and reports.

Summary: Common Indications

- Basal Cell Carcinoma (BCC) is the most common indication for Mohs micrographic surgery (MMS).
- MMS has a 99% 5-year cure rate for primary BCC, and a 96% cure rate for recurrent BCC.
- Aggressive subtypes of BCC include micronodular, morpheaform, metatypical, and infiltrative. They are considered strong indications for MMS.
- Squamous Cell Carcinoma (SCC) is the second most common indication for MMS.
- MMS has a 96.9% cure rate for primary SCC, while it is 23.3% when treated with standard surgical excision.
- The recurrence rate for recurrent SCC treated by MMS is 10%, while it is 23.3% when treated with standard surgical excision.

2.2 Common Indications

2.2.1 Basal Cell Carcinoma (BCC)

BCC is not only the most common neoplastic condition but also the most common indication for MMS [4]. MMS has a 99% 5-year cure rate for primary BCC and a 96% cure rate with recurrent tumors [1, 3, 7]. When using standard surgical excision, the long-term recurrence rate for primary BCC is 10.1% [8] and 19.9% for recurrent BCCs treated with non-MMS therapies including radiation, excision, cryosurgery, and curettage [9] (see Table 2.1). The subtypes that are considered especially suitable for MMS are micronodular, morpheaform, metatypical, and infiltrative due to their aggressive nature.

2.2.2 Squamous Cell Carcinoma (SCC)

SCC is the second most common indication for MMS [4]. It has a 96.9% cure rate for primary tumors, while standard surgical excision yields a 91.9% cure rate [4]. The recurrence rate for recurrent SCC treated by MMS is 10%, while it is 23.3% when treated with standard surgical excision [10] (see Table 2.1).

The cure rate for SCC is largely dependent upon size and type of differentiation. Primary tumors less than 2 cm treated by MMS have a 98.1% cure rate, while those above 2 cm in size have a cure rate of 74.8% [10]. Well-differentiated SCC has a 97% clearance rate using MMS, while poorly differentiated SCC has a 67.4% clearance rate [10]. When using non-MMS treatment, well-differentiated SCC has a cure rate of only 81%, and for poorly differentiated SCC, a cure rate of 46.4% has been reported [10].

SCC in situ is also considered an indication for MMS when located on the face and genitals or when it is greater than 2 cm [4]. The in situ form of SCC, Bowen's disease, or, if located on the glans penis, erythroplasia of Queyrat is also considered an indication for MMS when located in high-risk anatomical areas such as the face or genitalia or in cases where the lesion diameter is greater than 2 cm [4]. Most recently, Hansen et al. reported a 6.3% 5-year recurrence rate for 83 SCC in situ tumors [11]. A similar recurrence rate for 95 patients with SCC in situ who completed 5 years of follow-up also had a 6.3% recurrence rate [12].

Summary: Uncommon Indications

- The uncommon indications include Dermatofibrosarcoma Protuberans (DFSP), Microcystic Adnexal Carcinoma (MAC), Atypical Fibroxanthoma (AFX), Malignant Fibrous Histiocytoma (MFH), Sebaceous Carcinoma (SC), Merkel Cell Carcinoma (MCC), Melanoma, and Superficial Leiomyosarcoma.
- The evidence underlying the indication for these tumors is limited by smaller numbers of subjects when comparing standard surgical excision and Mohs micrographic surgery.

2.3 Uncommon Indications

2.3.1 Dermatofibrosarcoma Protuberans (DFSP)

DFSP begins as a slow-growing plaque that is often skin colored. It continues to grow forming firm nodules that are red or brown in color and is comprised of spindle cells that are thought to be of fibroblastic origin. A number of small case reports and series have demonstrated recurrence rates when using MMS for DFSP to be 0–10% [13–21].

Only 3 studies in the literature have specifically compared MMS versus WLE for the treatment of DFSP. Gloster and colleagues reported 84 patients with DFSP comparing Wide Local Excision (WLE) versus MMS, with only 15 being treated by MMS [22]. They found a 6.6% recurrence rate for DFSP treated by WLE and a 10% recurrence rate for DFSP treated by MMS after 36 months of follow-up for the WLE group and 40 months of follow-up for the MMS group. It should also be noted that 56% of the tumors in this study were recurrent.

DuBay and colleagues reported results from 63 cases of DFSP comparing WLE versus MMS with only 11 patients being treated with MMS [23]. A follow-up of more than 4 years revealed that none of the tumors in either group had recurred.

Meguerditchian et al. compared MMS to WLE in 48 patients. 28 underwent WLE, while 20 were treated with MMS. At a median follow-up time of 49.9 months for the WLE group, 1/28 (3.6%) recurred, while 0/20 (0%) recurred in the MMS group at a median follow-up time of 40.4 months [24].

2.3.2 Microcystic Adnexal Carcinoma (MAC)

MAC usually develops as a flesh-colored plaque. It is most commonly observed on the head and neck (90% of cases) and more specifically on the cheek (27.3%). Perineural invasion is common and is more prevalent in recurrent tumors [25–27]. MAC is regarded as a locally aggressive tumor with little metastatic potential [28, 29]. The tumor is comprised of epithelial cords within a fibrotic stroma that can invade deeply into the dermis, subcutaneous tissue, and even to skeletal muscle. It is commonly misdiagnosed as BCC and SCC [27].

Standard surgical excision of MAC results in up to a 60% recurrence rate, although considerable variation has been noted [25, 27, 30–32]. MMS has been associated with much lower recurrence rates from 0% to 12% [26, 33–36].

2.3.3 Atypical Fibroxanthoma (AFX)

AFX presents as a rapidly growing solitary nodule on the head and neck of elderly males that may be up to 2 cm in diameter [37]. The tumor is composed of pleomorphic spindle, epithelioid, and histiocyte-like cells found in the dermis. There are also rare variants of clear cell, granular, and sclerotic atypical fibroxanthomas. In a review of 91 patients with 93 tumors, Ang and colleagues reported an overall recurrence rate of 0% for MMS (59 tumors) and 8.7% for WLE (23 tumors) with a median follow up of 8.7 years [37]. Hunter et al. found a recurrence rate of 6.9%

for MMS and 16% for other surgical methods [38]. Davis et al. reported 0/25 recurrences using MMS with a mean follow-up of 29.6 months and 3/25 recurrences using WLE with a mean follow-up of 73.6 months [39].

2.3.4 Superficial Leiomyosarcoma

Superficial Leiomyosarcoma is a rare cutaneous sarcoma that hardly ever metastasizes [40] but has a predisposition towards recurrence. The prognosis is much better compared to soft-tissue and deep leiomyosarcomas [40]. It presents as a red nodule often located on a nipple or extremity that can sometimes be painful [40]. The tumor is comprised of densely packed smooth muscle cells thought to be derived from the arrectores pilorum muscle [41]. The known recurrence rate following MMS is 14%, and for WLE, it is also 14% [38]. The tumor may act more aggressively in patients who are immunosuppressed, and clearly, more investigation needs to occur to determine the optimum treatment in those circumstances [42].

2.3.5 Malignant Fibrous Histiocytoma (MFH)

MFH most commonly presents as a nodule on the lower extremities [43]. When using traditional WLE for MFH, recurrences rates range from 30% to 40% [44, 45]. The sparse amount of literature regarding MMS demonstrated a 43% (3/7) recurrence rate over a mean of 3.8 years [38].

2.3.6 Sebaceous Carcinoma (SC)

SC is thought to arise from the Meibomian glands or glands of Zeiss [40, 46]. It most commonly presents as a slow-growing, yellow nodule on the upper eyelid of elderly women [40]. Blepharoconjunctivitis or chalazion are common misdiagnoses [40]. An extraocular form also exists and tends to present as a pink to red nodule that sometimes bleeds [47]. It was once believed that the metastatic potential of extraocular SC was lower than ocular SC; however that concept is currently under debate [48–52]. The tumor is histologically composed of irregular lobules of sebaceous cells with a foamy cytoplasm. It can histologically be confused with Basal Cell Carcinoma, especially BCC with sebaceous differentiation, and can be differentiated using an oil red O stain or Thomsen-Friedenreich (T) antigen [53, 54]. The current standard surgical excision is 5–6 mm margins with recurrence rates of 9–36% at 5 years with a mortality rate of 18–30% [55–57]. Most of the cases treated by MMS have been reported as case reports and case series. One group found an 11.1% recurrence rate when using MMS with a 3-year follow-up from 18 patients [58]. In rare cases, SC may grow in a noncontinuous fashion [47], and so MMS may not be the best surgical option in that circumstance. Although MMS appears to be promising for SC, more studies are needed to determine the exact feasibility in the treatment of SC.

2.3.7 Melanoma

A number of variations on staged surgical excision and MMS have been investigated. Dr. Zitelli and colleagues reported a 5-year recurrence rate of 0.5% using MMS for 553 tumors. This rate is equivalent to and, in some cases, better than the standard surgical excision [59]. Recently, a new 20-min MART-1 immunostaining protocol has been developed which greatly assists in evaluating frozen sections. In addition, a nuclear stain known as MITF may be helpful when used in combination of MART-1 to more closely delineate the surgical borders. There is currently a large amount of debate as to the feasibility of MMS for melanoma given the artifactual changes that occur to atypical melanocytes in frozen sections. MMS with immunohistochemistry is a very promising technique, but its evidence base is mainly limited to case reports and series.

2.3.8 Merkel Cell Carcinoma (MCC)

MCC presents as a solitary, purple, dome-like, firm nodule on the head, neck, or extremities up to 4 cm in diameter. Histologically, the tumor is comprised of small round blue cells in a nested or trabecular pattern. These tumors have a high rate of recurrence and metastasis [60]. The prognosis of MCC is considered worse than malignant melanoma [61]. A 62% survival rate over 3 years has been reported [62]. The persistence rates using WLE versus MMS are 31.7% (13/41) and 8.3% (1/12), respectively [63]. The group undergoing

MMS had a 33.3% (4/12) regional metastasis rate, while the group undergoing WLE had a 48.8% (20/41) regional metastasis rate. The group undergoing WLE had a mean 60-month follow-up, whereas the group treated with MMS had a mean 36-month follow-up.

2.3.9 Extramammary Paget's Disease (EMPD)

EMPD is manifested as a slowly growing erythematous plaque that may have associated pruritus or burning. It is usually located in the anogenital or axillary regions, making tissue conservation in those areas highly desirable [64]. The histology is typified by Paget cells, which are large, pale-staining round cells [65]. There is usually epidermal acanthosis and hyperkeratosis [65]. Debate is currently ongoing whether EMPD is a continuously growing tumor. At least one review of 48 cases demonstrated that 15 anogenital lesions were multicentric [66]. Another report of 4 lesions requiring vulvectomy demonstrated that all 4 cases demonstrated multicentric features [67]. In addition, subclinical spread can be remarkable [68]. If MMS is used for EMPD, scouting biopsies and immunostaining with cytokeratin 7 may greatly facilitate extirpating the whole tumor [68]. Recurrence rates using WLE may be up to 44% [69], whereas when MMS is used, recurrence rates up to 18.2% have been reported [65].

Summary: Conclusion

- The indications for Mohs surgery can be divided into common and uncommon entities.
- Mohs micrographic surgery is associated with the lowest long-term recurrence rates amongst currently known therapeutic options for BCC and SCC.

2.4 Conclusion

The indications for Mohs micrographic surgery can be divided into common and uncommon entities. The common entities, BCC and SCC, are backed by strong evidence that Mohs micrographic surgery is associated with the lowest long-term recurrence rates amongst currently known therapeutic options. The uncommon indications include DFSP, MAC, AFX, MFH, SC, MCC, melanoma, superficial leiomyosarcoma, and EMPD and are limited by smaller numbers of subjects in studies comparing standard surgical excision and Mohs Micrographic Surgery.

References

1. Shriner DL, McCoy DK, Goldberg DJ, Wagner Jr RF. Mohs micrographic surgery. J Am Acad Dermatol. 1998;39(1):79–97.
2. Steinman HK. Indications for Mohs surgery. In: Gross KG, Steinman HK, Rapini RP, editors. Mohs surgery fundamentals and techniques. St. Louis: Mosby Inc.; 1999. p. 9–14.
3. Martinez JC, Otley CC. The management of melanoma and nonmelanoma skin cancer: a review for the primary care physician. Mayo Clin Proc. 2001;76:1253–65.
4. Nouri K, Rivas MP. A primer of Mohs micrographic surgery: common indications. Skinmed. 2004;3(4):191–6.
5. Nouri K. What you need to know about Mohs micrographic surgery. Skin Aging. 2000;8:68–70.
6. Drake LA, Dinehart SM, Goltz RW, et al. Guidelines of care for Mohs micrographic surgery. J Am Acad Dermatol. 1995;33(2):271–8.
7. Tulli A. Mohs micrographic surgery. In: Chu T, Chu AC, Edelson RL, editors. Malignant tumors of the skin. London: Arnold; 1999. p. 381–95.
8. Rowe DE, Carroll RJ, Day CL. Long-term recurrence rates in previously untreated (primary) basal cell carcinoma: implications for patient follow-up. J Dermatol Surg Oncol. 1989;15:315–28.
9. Rowe DE, Carroll RJ, Day CL. Mohs surgery is the treatment of choice for recurrent (previously treated) basal cell carcinoma. J Dermatol Surg Oncol. 1989;15:424–31.
10. Rowe DE, Carroll RJ, Day CL. Prognostic factors for local recurrence, metastasis, and survival rates in squamous cell carcinoma of the skin, ear, and lip. J Am Acad Dermatol. 1992;26:976–90.
11. Hansen JP, Drake AL, Walling HW. Bowen's disease: a four-year retrospective review of epidemiology and treatment at a university center. Dermatol Surg. 2008;34(7):878–83.
12. Leibovitch I, Huilgol SC, Selva D, Richards S, Paver R. Cutaneous squamous carcinoma in situ (Bowen's disease): treatment with Mohs micrographic surgery. J Am Acad Dermatol. 2005;52(6):997–1002.
13. Ratner D, Thomas CO, Johnson TM, et al. Mohs micrographic surgery for the treatment of dermatofibrosarcoma protuberans. Results of a multiinstitutional series with an analysis of the extent of microscopic spread. J Am Acad Dermatol. 1997;37(4):600–13.
14. Parker TL, Zitelli JA. Surgical margins for excision of dermatofibrosarcoma protuberans. J Am Acad Dermatol. 1995;32(2 Pt 1):233–6.
15. Snow SN, Gordon EM, Larson PO, Bagheri MM, Bentz ML, Sable DB. Dermatofibrosarcoma protuberans: a report on

29 patients treated by Mohs micrographic surgery with long-term follow-up and review of the litertaure. Cancer. 2004; 101(1):28–38.
16. Tom WD, Hybarger CP, Rasgon BM. Dermatofibrosarcoma protuberans of the head and neck: treatment with Mohs surgery using inverted horizontal paraffin sections. Laryngoscope. 2003;113:1289–93.
17. Dawes KW, Hanke CW. Dermatofibrosarcoma protuberans treated with Mohs micrographic surgery: cure rates and surgical marings. Dermatol Surg. 1996;22:530–43.
18. Huether MJ, Zitelli JA, Brodland DG. Mohs micrographic surgery for the treatment of spindle cell tumors of the skin. J Am Acad Dermatol. 2001;44:656–9.
19. Ah-Weng A, Marsden JR, Sanders DS, Waters R. Dermatofibrosarcoma protuberans treated by micrographic surgery. Br J Cancer. 2002;87(12):1386–9.
20. Wacker J, Khan-Durani B, Hartschuh W. Modified Mohs micrographic surgery in the therapy of dermatofibrosarcoma protuberans: analysis of 22 patients. Ann Surg Oncol. 2004;11:438–44.
21. Jimenez FJ, Grichnik JM, Buchanan MD, Clark RE. Immunohistochemical margin control applied to Mohs micrographic surgical excision of dermatofibrosarcoma protuberans. J Dermatol Surg Oncol. 1994;20(10):687–9.
22. Gloster Jr HM, Harris KR, Roenigk RK. A comparison between Mohs micrographic surgery and wide surgical excision for the treatment of dermatofibrosarcoma protuberans. J Am Acad Dermatol. 1996;35:82–7.
23. DuBay D, Cimmino V, Lowe L, Johnson TM, Sondak VK. Low recurrence rate after surgery for dermatofibrosarcoma protuberans: a multidisciplinary approach from a single institution. Cancer. 2004;100(5):1008–16.
24. Meguerditchian A, Wang J, Lema B, Kraybill WG, Zeitouni NC, Kane JM. Wide excision or Mohs micrographic surgery for the treatment of primary dermatofibrosarcoma protuberans. Am J Clin Oncol. 2010;33(2):300–3.
25. Salerno S, Terril P. Will MAC be back? ANZ J Surg. 2003;73:830–2.
26. Snow S, Madjar Jr DD, Hardy S, et al. Microcystic adnexal carcinoma: report of 13 cases and review of the literature. Dermatol Surg. 2001;27(4):401–8.
27. Leibovitch I, Huilgol SC, Selva D, Lun K, Richards S, Paver R. Microcystic adnexal carcinoma: treatment with Mohs micrographic surgery. J Am Acad Dermatol. 2005;52(2): 295–300.
28. Bier-Lanning CM, Hom DB, Gapany M, Manivel JC, Duvall 3rd AJ. Microcystic adnexal carcinoma: management options based on long-term follow-up. Laryngoscope. 1995;105(11):1197–201.
29. Carroll P, Goldstein GD, Brown CW. Metastatic microcystic adnexal carcinoma in an immunocompromised patient. Dermatol Surg. 2000;26(6):531–4.
30. Cooper PH, MIlls SE, Leonard DD, SantaCruz DJ, Headington JT, Barr RJ. Sclerosing sweat duct (syringomatous) carcinoma. Am J Surg Pathol. 1985;9(6):422–33.
31. Cooper PH. Sclerosing carcinomas of sweat ducts (microcystic adnexal carcinoma). Arch Dermatol. 1986;122:261–4.
32. Sebastien TS, Nelson BR, Lowe L, Baker S, Johnson TM. Microcystic adnexal carcinoma. J Am Acad Dermatol. 1993;29:840–5.
33. Burns MK, Chen SP, Goldberg LH. Microcystic adnexal carcinoma. Ten cases treated by Mohs micrographic surgery. J Dermatol Surg Oncol. 1994;20:429–34.
34. Friedman PM, Friedman RH, Jiang SB, Nouri K, Amonette R, Robins P. Microcystic adnexal carcinoma: collaborative series review and update. J Am Acad Dermatol. 1999; 41(2 Pt 1):225–31.
35. Chiller K, Passaro D, Scheuller M, Singer M, McCalmont T, Grekin RC. Microcystic adnexal carcinoma: forty-eight cases, their treatment and their outcome. Arch Dermatol. 2000;136:1355–9.
36. Abbate M, Zeitouni N, Seyler M, Hicks W, Loree T, Cheney RT. Clinical course, risk factors and treatment of microcystic adnexal carcinoma: a short series report. Dermatol Surg. 2003;29:1035–8.
37. Ang GC, Roenigk RK, Otley CC, Phillips PK, Weaver AL. More than 2 decades of treating atypical fibroxanthoma at Mayo Clinic: what have we learned from 91 patients? Dermatol Surg. 2009;35(5):765–72.
38. Huether MJ, Zitelli JA, Broadland DG. Mohs micrographic surgery for the treatment of spindle cell tumors of the skin. J Am Acad Dermatol. 2001;44:656–9.
39. Davis JL, Randle HW, Zalla MJ, Roenigk RK, Brodland DG. A comparison of Mohs micrographic surgery and wide excision for the treatment of atypical fibroxanthoma. Dermatol Surg. 1997;23(2):105–10.
40. Nouri K, Rivas MP. A primer of Mohs micrographic surgery: uncommon indications. Skinmed. 2004;3(5):259–65.
41. Fields JP, Helwig EB. Leiomyosarcoma of the skin and subcutanous tissue. Cancer. 1981;47:156–69.
42. Humphreys TR, Finkelstein DH, Lee JB. Superficial leiomyosarcoma treated with Mohs micrographic surgery. Dermatol Surg. 2004;30:108–12.
43. Marcet S. Atypical fibroxanthoma/malignant fibrous histiocytoma. Dermatol Ther. 2008;21(6):424–7.
44. Weiss SW, Goldblum JR. Enzinger and Weiss's soft tissue tumors. Philadelphia: Mosby/Elsevier; 2008.
45. Helwig EB, May D. Atypical fibroxanthoma of the skin with metastasis. Cancer. 1986;57:368–76.
46. Rao NA, Hidayat AA, McLean IW, Zimmerman LE. Sebaceous carcinomas of the ocular adnexa: a clinicopathologic study of 104 cases, with five-year follow-up data. Hum Pathol. 1982;13(2):113–22.
47. Berlin AL, Amin SP, Goldberg DJ. Extraocular sebaceous carcinoma treated with Mohs micrographic surgery: report of a case and review of literature. Dermatol Surg. 2008;34: 254–7.
48. Wick MR, Goellner JR, WolfeIII JT, Su WP. Adnexal carcinomas of the skin. II. Extraocular sebaceous carcinomas. Cancer. 1985;56(5):1163–72.
49. Moreno C, Jacyk WK, Judd MJ, Requena L. Highly aggressive extraocular sebaceous carcinoma. Am J Dermatopathol. 2001;23(5):450–5.
50. Duman DG, Ceyhan BB, Celikel T, Duman RAD. Extraorbital sebaceous carcinoma with rapidly developing visceral metastases. Dermatol Surg. 2003;29(9): 987–9.
51. Bassetto F, Baraziol R, Sottosanti MV, Scarpa C, Montesco M. Biological behavior of the sebaceous carcinoma of the head. Dermatol Surg. 2004;30(3):472–6.

52. Bouraoui S, Kaddar RK, Mokni M, Badri T, Azaiez MY, Dhahri AB. Extrapalpebral sebaceous carcinoma. Ann Dermatol Venereol. 2006;133(2):165–7.
53. Ni C, Searl S, Kuo PK, Chu FR, Chong CS, Albert DM. Sebaceous cell carcinomas of the ocular adnexa. Int Ophthalmol Clin. 1982;22(1):23–61.
54. Hassanein AM. Sebaceous carcinoma and the T-antigen. Semin Cutan Med Surg. 2004;23(1):62–72.
55. Doxanas MT, Green WR. Sebaceous gland carcinoma. Arch Ophthalmol. 1984;102:245–9.
56. Botek AA, Goldberg SH. Sebaceous gland carcinoma. In: Miller SJ, Maloney ME, editors. Cutaneous oncology. Malden: Blackwell Science Inc; 1998. p. 800–10.
57. Boniuk M, Zimmerman LE. Sebaceous carcinoma of the eyelid, eyebrow, caruncle, and orbit. Trans Am Acad Ophthalmol Otolaryngol. 1968;27:619–42.
58. Spencer JM, Nossa R, Tse DT, Sequeira M. Sebaceous carcinoma of the eyelid treated with Mohs micrographic surgery. J Am Acad Dermatol. 2001;44:1004–9.
59. Zitelli JA, Brown C, Hanusa BH. Mohs micrographic surgery for the treatment of primary cutaneous melanoma. J Am Acad Dermatol. 1997;37:236–45.
60. Skelton HG, Smith KJ, Hitchcock CL, McCarthy WF, Lupton GP, Graham JH. Merkel cell carcinoma: analysis of clinical, histologic, and immunologic features of 132 cases with relation to survival. J Am Acad Dermatol. 1997;37(5 Pt 1): 734–9.
61. O'Connor WJ, Broadland DG. Merkel cell carcinoma. Dermatol Surg. 1996;22(3):262–7.
62. Mercer D, Brander P, Liddell K. Merkel cell carcinoma: the clinical course. Ann Plast Surg. 1990;25:136–41.
63. O'Connor WJ, Roenigk RK, Broadland DG. Comparison of Mohs micrographic surgery and wide excision in eighty-six patients. Dermatol Surg. 1997;23(10):929–33.
64. Lee KY, Roh MR, Chung WG, Chung KY. Comparison of Mohs micrographis surgery and wide excision for extramammary Paget's disease: Korean experience. Dermatol Surg. 2008;35:34–40.
65. O'Conner WJ, Lim KK, Zalla MJ, et al. Comparison of Mohs micrographic surgery and wide excision for extramammary Paget's disease. Dermatol Surg. 2003;29: 723–7.
66. Murata Y, Kumano K. Multicentricity of extramamary Paget's disease. Eur J Dermatol. 2007;17(2):164–5.
67. Gunn RA, Gallager HS. Vulvar Paget's disease: a topographic study. Cancer. 1980;46:590–4.
68. Hendi A, Perdikis G, Snow JL. Unifocality of extramammary Paget disease. J Am Acad Dermatol. 2008;59: 811–3.
69. Coldiron BM, Goldsmith BA, Robinson JK. Surgical treatment of extramammary Paget's disease: a report of six cases and a reexamination of Mohs micrographic surgery compared with conventional surgical excision. Cancer. 1991;67: 933–8.

Preoperative Evaluation

3

Sean R. Christensen and Sumaira Z. Aasi

Abstract

The preoperative evaluation is a critical aspect of dermatologic surgery that lays the foundation for safe and high quality surgical outcomes. In addition to establishing rapport with the patient, the preoperative evaluation allows the surgeon to anticipate the complexity of the case and make any necessary adjustments to the operative plan based on the patient's presenting lesion, past medical history, current medications, and allergies. A standard medical history form can facilitate the preoperative evaluation, although each patient's unique history should be discussed in detail. Particular attention should be paid to cardiac conditions and implantable cardiac defibrillators, which require special precautions when using electrosurgical techniques. Although anticoagulants such as warfarin may increase the incidence of local bleeding complications, there is a documented risk of serious or fatal thrombotic complications when these medications are interrupted in the perioperative period. As such, therapeutic anticoagulants and cardiac medications such as beta-blockers are continued throughout the perioperative period in most cases. While the use of preoperative antibiotics in dermatologic surgery is controversial, recent American Heart Association guidelines limit prophylactic antibiotics only to those patients with cardiac conditions at highest risk for endocarditis undergoing surgery with breach of the oral mucosa or on infected cutaneous sites.

Keywords

Dermatologic surgery • Preoperative care • Informed consent • Photography • Cardiovascular disease • Defibrillators • Immunocompromise • Anticoagulants • Antibiotic prophylaxis

S.R. Christensen (✉)
Department of Dermatology,
Yale University School of Medicine, New Haven, CT, USA
e-mail: sean.christensen@yale.edu

S.Z. Aasi
Department of Dermatology, Yale University,
New Haven, CT, USA

K. Nouri (ed.), *Mohs Micrographic Surgery*,
DOI 10.1007/978-1-4471-2152-7_3, © Springer-Verlag London Limited 2012

Summary: Introduction

- The preoperative evaluation is a critical aspect of dermatologic surgery that helps establish rapport, maximize efficiency, minimize complications, and facilitate optimal surgical outcomes.

3.1 Introduction

The preoperative evaluation is a critical but potentially overlooked aspect of dermatologic surgery. Because of the lack of general anesthesia and minimal morbidity associated with most dermatologic procedures, some practitioners may regard a systematic preoperative evaluation as superfluous or unnecessary. The skilled surgeon, however, will recognize that an appropriate preoperative evaluation lays the foundation for procedures that have safe and high quality outcomes. It helps establish rapport, creates realistic patient expectations, and allows for more efficient workflow at the time of surgery. In addition, it allows the dermatologic surgeon to anticipate and prevent intraoperative and postoperative complications, and optimize postoperative care with patient education.

Summary: Initial Consultation and Informed Consent

- The initial consultation forms the basis for all subsequent interactions between the surgeon and the patient.
- Establishing rapport, setting appropriate expectations, determining the complexity and urgency of the surgical case, and discussing the indications for and alternatives to surgery are essential aspects of the initial evaluation.
- Discussion of the risks and benefits of any procedure and documentation of patient informed consent are mandatory prerequisites to dermatologic surgery.

3.2 Initial Consultation and Informed Consent

While it is possible to have the preoperative evaluation on the same day as the surgical procedure, there are several advantages to scheduling the initial consultation as a separate visit. First, it allows for a discussion between the patient and physician regarding the diagnosis, prognosis, and indications for surgery before a commitment has been made to proceed with a given surgical treatment. Specifically, for Mohs micrographic surgery, the consult visit provides the opportunity to explain in detail the Mohs technique as well as other surgical or nonsurgical options for treatment. In addition to answering the patient's questions and preparing him or her for the logistical details of the procedure, this brief discussion builds confidence in the physician and establishes rapport. As such, it may be useful to have a family member or caregiver present at the time of initial consultation. In some circumstances, it may be a spouse or adult son or daughter who has more anxiety regarding surgery than the patient himself or herself.

Scheduling the consultative visit prior to the day of surgery also allows for a more efficient workflow on the day of the procedure. The experienced surgeon can assess the complexity of the case in consultation, including the probability of multiple stages and complicated surgical repairs. This allows for more appropriate scheduling of cases, with a more even distribution of complex and straightforward cases on any given day. In addition, scheduling the surgical procedure according to the medical urgency of the case (e.g., rapidly growing squamous cell carcinoma versus superficial basal cell carcinoma) is accomplished more effectively after an initial consultation. The need for antibiotic prophylaxis can also be assessed at the preoperative consultation, allowing appropriate treatment prior to surgery (discussed below, Sect. 3.6). Finally, holding the initial consultation in the surgical suite where the surgery will be performed allows patients to become familiar with transportation to the office and navigation within the building. It may also help to alleviate anxiety on the day of surgery if the patient is arriving at a familiar location.

Another critical aspect of the initial consultation is setting appropriate patient expectations. Although "scarless" surgery may be an ideal to strive for, any surgical intervention on visible skin will have aesthetic and possibly functional consequences. Discussion of this fact with the patient prior to surgery will improve patient satisfaction and may decrease the incidence of postprocedural misapprehension, confusion, or complaints. Similarly, patients may focus newfound attention on their facial features after surgery and may incidentally identify preexisting congenital or acquired asymmetry or anatomic variation postoperatively that is completely unrelated to the surgery. These subtle findings should be identified by the surgeon and pointed out to the patient at the preoperative evaluation. Finally, asking the patient about prior surgical procedures or trauma and examining the resulting scars can be informative in anticipating poor wound healing, spread scars, or tendency for keloid formation. This not only provides an opportunity to gain insight into the patient's understanding of wound healing but also an occasion to properly educate the patient on this process.

Informed consent is a prerequisite to any medical procedure, and Mohs micrographic surgery is no exception. As noted above, the indications and alternatives to Mohs, including standard surgical excision or no treatment, must be adequately explained to the patient so that he or she may make an informed decision to proceed. The potential risks of surgery must also be clearly explained in language that is understood by the layperson. This includes the standard procedural risks such as pain, bleeding, infection, scarring and cosmetic distortion, as well as Mohs-specific risks such as recurrence of the primary tumor and anatomically specific functional consequences such as facial nerve palsy or ectropion. Proper informed consent also includes offering a clear opportunity for the patient to ask any questions about the procedure. Ideally, the surgeon performing the procedure will be the one obtaining informed consent. A standard consent form can be a useful adjunct to this discussion and provides a clear documentation of patient consent (via signature) in the medical record. Because every surgical case has unique features, however, the preprinted consent form is no substitute for a thorough discussion between patient and physician.

Summary: History of Present Illness and Physical Examination

- Historical information can be useful to anticipate the complexity of a surgical case, and verification of the pathologic diagnosis is essential to direct appropriate therapy.
- The location of the lesion should be documented prior to surgery and confirmed with photographic records if available.
- The physical exam is focused on signs suggestive of aggressive tumor behavior and underlying medical conditions that may complicate dermatologic surgery.

3.3 History of Present Illness and Physical Examination

As with any medical evaluation, the history of the patient's chief complaint is of paramount importance. The most basic piece of historical information for the dermatologic surgeon is the duration of the lesion in question. Because most cutaneous malignancies tend to have a steady growth rate (the doubling time for basal cell carcinoma has been estimated at 6–12 months) [1], the duration of the lesion provides an estimate of the expected size and depth. Conversely, if a patient reports that a large lesion with extensive tissue destruction has been present for only a few weeks, this may imply aggressive biologic behavior or may indicate an element of neglect or psychiatric disease in the patient.

A critical historical point is whether the lesion has been treated in the past. Is the lesion a recurrence of a previously excised tumor? Was the lesion treated ineffectively with electrodessication and curettage? Was the lesion initially assumed to be benign and treated with cryotherapy or laser destruction? All these scenarios will change the interaction of the tumor with the surrounding tissue. It has been shown that recurrent basal cell carcinomas are more likely to have positive margins on the initial stage than equivalent primary lesions [2]. In addition, the presence of reactive fibrosis in the dermis may alter the microscopic appearance of the tumor, or even create "skip areas" where the tumor is not entirely contiguous, but has separate foci of invasion. Awareness of these factors will help the surgeon more effectively plan for the procedure, and potentially decrease the possibility of post-Mohs recurrence.

The remainder of the history of present illness is focused on the assessment of symptoms that are suggestive of aggressive tumor behavior. While a small amount of discomfort may be associated with reactive inflammation around a lesion, the presence of significant pain or paresthesia should alert the physician to the possibility of perineural invasion [3]. Similarly, complaints of eyebrow ptosis, slurred speech, or drooling from the angle of the mouth are signs of motor neuropathy, and suggest a poor prognosis (Fig. 3.1). Other symptoms commonly reported for skin tumors include pruritus or bleeding, although these do not necessarily provide any prognostic information.

The surgeon must also review the pathology report. It is important to note whether aggressive histologic features, such as infiltrative, acantholytic, or poorly differentiated subtypes, or evidence of vascular or

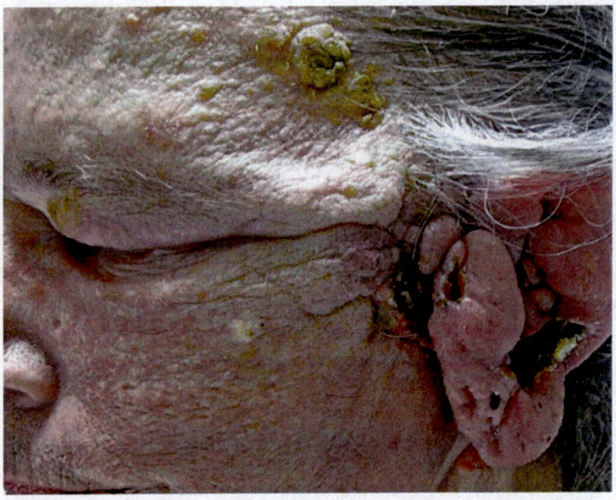

Fig. 3.1 Temporal nerve palsy caused by advanced basal cell carcinoma of the ear and pre-auricular cheek. The patient is unable to open the left eye and there is marked ptosis of the left forehead and brow. The tumor was found to invade the zygomatic and temporal bones on computed tomography

perineural invasion are documented on the pathology report. These features, in conjunction with the primary diagnosis, can be used to appropriately triage the scheduling of the case as well as prepare the surgeon for potentially larger defects and more complicated repairs. In cases of atypical variants (e.g., basosquamous carcinoma) or unusual skin tumors, it is often useful for the Mohs surgeon to request the pathologic slides for personal review, as this will provide the surgeon with the most accurate information about the specific tumor.

The preoperative evaluation should also include a brief but detailed physical examination. An obvious prerequisite to surgery is the ability to identify the lesion to be treated, but this is not always easily accomplished. Particularly in patients with extensive actinic damage, dermatitis, or multiple prior procedures, it may be difficult to define a particular healed biopsy site within a background of multiple scars and keratoses. The most reliable way to ensure that the correct site is chosen for surgery is to incorporate information from multiple sources. The consultation request and the pathology report from the initial biopsy will identify a general anatomic area but will often not be specific. The patient is a valuable source of information as well; in our practice, the patient is asked to clearly identify the site with a mirror and marking pen prior to any surgery. This practice also helps to create a shared responsibility for the treatment between patient and physician. Even so, a recent study found that patients and physicians in a Mohs surgery practice incorrectly identified surgical sites 4.4% of the time when preoperative biopsy-site photography was used to verify the correct site [4]. Quality photographs from the time of biopsy, therefore, should be used whenever possible to ensure that surgery is performed on the intended lesion (Fig. 3.2). Finally, when doubt persists about the exact location of a biopsied lesion, the referring physician should be consulted for further documentation and clarification.

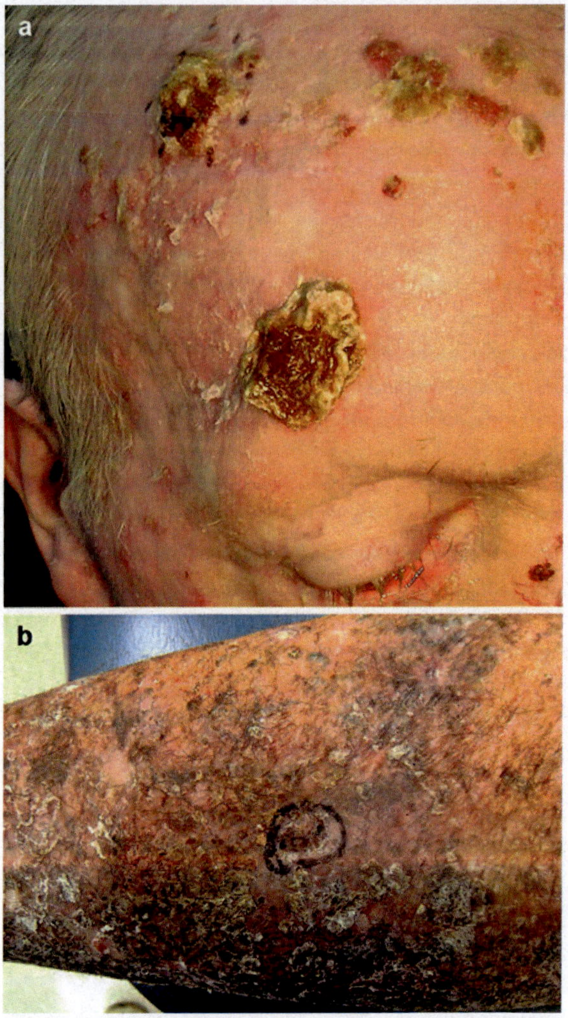

Fig. 3.2 (a-b) Preoperative biopsy site verification with photography. The dotted lesion on the scalp in panel A and the circled lesion on the lower leg in panel B were both invasive squamous cell carcinoma on biopsy. On a background of extensive actinic damage, dermatitis, dyspigmentation, and scars from previous procedures, these biopsy sites would be difficult to identify without preoperative photography

In addition to verification of the site of the lesion, several additional features of the physical exam are relevant to the preoperative evaluation. The patient's temperature, pulse, blood pressure, and respiration rate should be noted and recorded in the medical chart before any procedure is initiated. Any evidence of fever or markedly elevated pulse (greater than 120) or blood pressure (greater than 200/110) should prompt the consideration of postponing surgery. Although anxiety regarding surgery may cause mild elevations in pulse or blood pressure, uncontrolled tachycardia or hypertension are relative contraindications to cutaneous surgery. Particularly for lesions on the face or dorsal forearms, the background of actinic damage should be noted, as this can confound the assessment of keratinocyte atypia on histopathologic examination. The size of the lesion should be assessed both by visual inspection and palpation with careful assessment for fixation to or distortion of underlying muscle or bone. Similarly, facial asymmetry or ptosis can be a sign of deeper invasion causing motor neuropathy, as noted above. For all cutaneous malignancies, a brief manual examination of the draining lymph node basin must be performed at the preoperative evaluation. If there is concern for extensive involvement of deep structures or metastatic disease, it may be necessary to defer surgery until diagnostic imaging and further staging has been performed. Taking into account the gross appearance of the lesion, the presence or absence of these signs of deeper invasion, and the laxity and rhytides of the surrounding skin, the surgeon can often formulate a plan for possible reconstructive options even before the patient is scheduled for surgery.

Summary: Past Medical History

- A standard medical history form can facilitate the preoperative evaluation, although each patient's unique history should be discussed in detail.
- Dermatologic surgery can be performed in patients with cardiac conditions and implanted cardiac defibrillators with the use of proper precautions.
- Other medical conditions which may affect dermatologic surgery include diabetes, hepatic or renal disease, pregnancy, and immunosuppression.
- Overall functional status may be more important than chronologic age or specific medical conditions in predicting the response to surgery.

3.4 Past Medical History

Review of the patient's past medical history is an essential component of the preoperative evaluation. This process is made more efficient with the use of a standardized medical history form that can be completed by the patient prior to their visit or in the waiting area (Fig. 3.3). This allows the surgeon to rapidly identify the diagnoses and conditions most pertinent to the procedure at hand from a potentially complicated medical history. Any relevant details of the medical history, as well as how these will affect the planned surgical procedure, must then be discussed directly with the patient or their caregiver.

A fundamental question to be answered is whether the patient is a candidate for Mohs surgery. In general, there are no absolute contraindications to dermatologic surgery, and low risk procedures such as Mohs surgery can be safely performed in elderly patients and in those with stable comorbid conditions [5]. The individual risk-to-benefit ratio must be determined for each patient, taking into account their medical history and global functional status. An informed decision can then be made with the patient regarding the utility of the procedure and the optimal operative plan. Several factors to consider in this decision are discussed below.

For the patient with cardiac disease, it is important to determine whether the planned surgical procedure represents a significant risk for cardiac complications. Updated guidelines for preoperative cardiovascular evaluation in noncardiac surgery were published by the American College of Cardiology and American Heart Association in 2007 [6]. Dermatologic surgery is classified as a low cardiac risk procedure. As such, in cardiac patients without active cardiac conditions, the recommendation is to proceed with dermatologic surgery without further diagnostic workup. Active cardiac conditions to be excluded are unstable angina, myocardial infarction within 30 days, decompensated heart failure, symptomatic arrhythmia, and symptomatic aortic or mitral stenosis. A related historical issue is the concern for exacerbating hypertension with the administration of subcutaneous epinephrine in local anesthetics. In practice, this concern is unwarranted, as there is no significant increase in blood pressure after local epinephrine administration in dermatologic surgery, even in patients with preoperative hypertension [7]. Thus, once it has been established that a patient has stable cardiac disease and is asymptomatic, consultation with a

a

If this is your first visit to our office, please complete this section:

What is the reason for your visit today? ________________

If you are here for an evaluation of skin cancer, please answer the following questions:

Where is your skin lesion (skin cancer) located? ________________

When did you first notice this condition? ________________

Has your skin cancer been treated by a physician in the past? □ YES □ NO

If yes, type of treatment and date: ________________

Do you currently have any of the following symptoms? [REVIEW OF SYSTEMS]

□ Weight loss	□ Chest pain	□ Diarrhea	□ Changes in vision
□ Fever	□ Shortness of breath	□ Nausea/vomiting	□ Swollen lymph nodes
□ Chills	□ Abdominal pain	□ Lumps/bumps/rash	□ Bleeding tendencies
□ Night Sweats	□ Urinary problems (difficulty urinating or blood in your urine)	□ Headache	□ Depression/anxiety
□ Cough		□ Arthritis	□ Other: ______
		□ Weakness	□ NONE APPLY

Have you had any artificial joints placed within the last 6 months? □ YES □ NO

If yes, please explain: ________________

Do you have a pacemaker? □ YES □ NO

If yes, when was your pacemaker placed/serviced? ________________

Do you have an artificial heart valve? □ YES □ NO

Have you ever been diagnosed with skin cancer? □ YES □ NO

If yes, what type:

□ Basal Cell Carcinoma	□ Malignant Melanoma in situ
□ Squamous Cell Carcinoma	□ Other: ________
□ Malignant Melanoma	

Do you have a family history of skin cancer? □ YES □ NO

If yes, please explain:

Relative	Type of Cancer
________	________
________	________
________	________

Have you been diagnosed with any of the following illnesses or medical conditions? [PMH]

□ Heart Disease	□ Diabetes	□ Urinary Problems
□ Lung Problems	□ Thyroid Disease	□ Mental Illness
□ High Blood Pressure	□ GI Problems	□ Stroke

□ Other ________________

Fig. 3.3 Standard medical history form (Reprinted with permission from Yale Dermatologic Surgery and Yale Medical Group)

b

List any illness requiring hospitalization or surgeries within the past 5 years:

Operation/Illness	Hospital	City/State	Year

List and describe any ALLERGIES to medications or other substances:

____

____

List any current MEDICATIONS. Please include all prescription and non-prescription drugs.

Medication	How often taken

*****List any additional medications on the back of this form*** **□ List of medications attached**

Are you currently taking aspirin ? **□ YES □ NO**

How much alcohol do you consume each week? ______

Do you smoke? **□ YES □ NO**

If yes, how much? ______

Have you ever had a blood transfusion? **□ YES □ NO**

If yes, when?

Patient Signature ______ **Date** ______

*****FOR OFFICE USE ONLY***

Physician Signature ______ **Date** ______

Fig. 3.3 (continued)

cardiologist is generally not required. It should be noted, however, that hypertension does increase the risk of local complications, including hematoma formation [7]. The surgeon may therefore wish to postpone surgery in cases of significant hypertension until after the blood pressure has been addressed by an internist.

The presence of a cardiac pacemaker or implantable cardioverter-defibrillator (ICD) represents another potential concern for the dermatologic surgeon, particularly in regard to the use of electrosurgery. There are several reported cases of electrical interference causing pacemaker or ICD malfunction in both the dermatologic and nondermatologic literature. Although modern ICDs are equipped with better shielding and advanced software to filter out exogenous electrical interference, they are also designed for more sensitive monitoring of endogenous cardiac rhythm, respirations, and physical activity. As such, there remains a significant risk of electrical interference compromising pacemaker or ICD function when using certain electrosurgical techniques [8]. While this risk is essentially absent when using electrocautery (i.e., heat cautery) since there is no transfer of electrical current to the patient, it is greatest with electrosection and electrocoagulation, in which high amperage current passes though the patient to the grounding plate. Bipolar electrosurgery, or electrocoagulation with biterminal forceps, minimizes risk to the patient by limiting current flow to a focal area between the two prongs of the treatment forceps.

After a case presentation and review of the mechanisms of electromagnetic interference, LeVasseur et al. published guidelines for the safe use of electrosurgery in patients with cardiac devices [9]. The first of these is the recommendation to use electrocautery alone. A second option is the use of biterminal forceps for electrocoagulation. Since neither of these techniques disperses electrical current away from the operative site, the remainder of the guidelines is of secondary importance if these techniques are used. If other forms of electrosurgery must be used, it is recommended that the indifferent electrode (grounding plate) is placed to minimize current transfer near the region of the heart, that a cardiologist is consulted to determine the patient's dependence on the device, that pacemakers are placed in fixed rather than demand mode prior to surgery, that ICDs are deactivated prior to surgery if possible, that the patient is monitored preoperatively and intraoperatively with a 12-lead ECG, that electrosurgery is limited to short bursts of less than 5 s at a time, that the electrical current is minimized, and that a contingency plan is specified in the event of life-threatening arrhythmia. A survey of dermatologic surgeons in 2000 found that these guidelines are not universally followed, however [10]. While the majority of surgeons reported using short bursts of current (71%) and minimizing electrical power when possible (61%), only about half used electrocautery or biterminal forceps (34% and 19%, respectively) and a small minority pursued ICD deactivation and cardiology consultation (15% and 11%, respectively). Despite the lack of universal adherence to these measures, there were only 31 reported cases of interference in a total of 1,959 years of surgical experience, representing an incidence of 1.6 cases of electrical interference per 100 years of surgical practice. The cardiac complications due to this interference ranged from skipped beats to inappropriate ICD firing and tachyarrhythmia; there was one patient with reported hemodynamic instability, but there were no cases of cardiac resuscitation or hospital admission, and there were no deaths reported in the survey. Importantly, there were no reported cases of interference with biterminal forceps, and only one case of suspected interference with electrocautery (because of the nature of the survey, it is unclear whether this represented true interference). Overall, therefore, it appears that the risk of cardiac complications from electrosurgery in patients with pacemakers or ICDs is low in the setting of dermatologic surgery, and that this risk can be essentially eliminated with the use of electrocautery or biterminal forceps.

Several other medical conditions are relevant to the preoperative evaluation and should be explicitly discussed with the patient. Patients with diabetes have impaired wound healing and a potentially increased risk of postoperative infection, owing to inhibition of chemotaxis and phagocytosis by hyperglycemia. The slower rate of wound healing in these patients is particularly pronounced on the distal lower extremities, where coincident vascular disease impairs wound perfusion. Similarly, patients with poor nutritional status, either from dietary insufficiency, gastrointestinal malabsorption, or cachexia from systemic malignancy will have impaired healing of surgical wounds. These factors should be considered when planning the closure of large surgical defects, as complicated repairs are less likely to succeed in patients with compromised healing ability. The presence of chronic renal or hepatic disease may also inhibit wound repair and can alter the

Table 3.1 FDA pregnancy drug risk categories

A	Adequate and well-controlled studies in humans have failed to demonstrate fetal risk
B	Animal reproduction studies have failed to demonstrate a risk to the fetus, and there are no adequate and well-controlled studies in pregnant women
C	Animal reproductive studies have shown an adverse effect on the fetus, and there are no adequate and well-controlled studies in humans **Potential benefits** may warrant use of the drug in pregnant women despite potential risks
D	There is positive evidence of human fetal risk based on adverse reaction data from investigational or marketing experience or studies in humans **Potential benefits** may warrant use of the drug in pregnant women despite potential risks
X	Studies in animals or humans have demonstrated fetal abnormalities **The risks involved in use of the drug in pregnant women clearly outweigh potential benefits**

clearance of local anesthetics. Amide anesthetics such as lidocaine are metabolized by the liver then excreted by the kidneys. Patients with severe liver disease may be at particularly increased risk of lidocaine toxicity when used at doses approaching 4.5 mg/kg (the recommended maximum dose for plain lidocaine).

The presence of a bleeding diathesis, either inherited or acquired, should also be determined prior to surgery. An otherwise occult bleeding tendency may be elicited by inquiring about easy bruising, bleeding gums, or problems with prior surgical procedures. Suspicion for a hematologic disorder can be followed up with laboratory testing, including complete blood count, prothrombin time, and partial thromboplastin time. Patients with advanced liver or kidney disease are also at increased risk of postoperative bleeding, due to decreased platelet number and function. The surgeon should exercise extra precautions to ensure both intraoperative and postoperative hemostasis in these patients.

The pregnant patient presents a unique challenge to the dermatologic surgeon. While pregnancy is not a contraindication to surgery, several of the common medications used in dermatologic procedures can have adverse effects on the developing fetus. The United States Food and Drug Administration has published a rating system to define the safety of medications in pregnant patients (Table 3.1). Lidocaine is a category B medication and is thus the local anesthetic of choice in pregnant patients. Even so, lidocaine has been documented to cross the placenta, and it should be used with caution in the first trimester when fetal organogenesis occurs. The longer-acting bupivacaine, which is often mixed with lidocaine in Mohs surgery practices, is rated as category C and is not recommended due to animal studies showing increased risk of fetal death and skeletal abnormalities. The use of subcutaneous epinephrine in pregnancy remains controversial, and it is classified as pregnancy category C. Although there is a theoretical risk of uterine artery contraction with high doses of epinephrine, no clear teratogenic effects have been documented in humans despite a long history of use [11]. Adjunctive sedative or analgesic medications should generally be avoided in pregnancy. Benzodiazepine anxiolytics such as diazepam are rated as class D due to increased risk of birth defects, and narcotic analgesics such as morphine and hydrocodone are class C. Acetaminophen, however, is class B and is generally regarded as safe for postoperative analgesia. In addition to selecting appropriate anesthesia for surgery, the surgeon must also be aware of the physiologic changes of pregnancy that may impact the procedure. Perhaps the most important of these is the tendency for the gravid uterus to compress the vena cava in the second and third trimester causing hypotension, tachycardia, and dyspnea in the supine patient. This can be prevented by positioning the patient in the left lateral tilt position [11].

In addition to the general medical conditions discussed above, there are several specific conditions that have a direct impact on the treatment of cutaneous malignancy. The increased incidence and metastatic potential of squamous cell carcinoma in transplant patients on chronic immunosuppression have been well documented. In kidney or heart transplant patients, there is a 65-fold increased risk of cutaneous squamous cell carcinoma, and up to 45% of transplant patients will develop skin cancer within 10 years of their transplant, depending on climate and UV exposure [12]. In addition, the behavior of these neoplasms is more aggressive in transplant patients. The early progression and metastasis of these tumors are evidenced by the fact that in some reports cutaneous malignancy accounts for up to 27% of all deaths in transplant patients after the first 4 years [12]. The surgeon must be aware of this increased risk of progression, local recurrence, and subsequent second malignancy. In addition to expediting early surgery and adjusting the operative plan for invasive and aggressive tumors, it is also critical to ensure appropriate follow up and screening skin exams for these patients. In some practices, the dermatologic surgeon assumes primary dermatologic care for transplant patients at high risk for multiple cutaneous carcinomas. With regard to prophylactic antibiotics for prevention of surgical site infection in immunosuppressed patients, there is not sufficient clinical data to recommend this practice, and each case must be considered on an individual basis, incorporating other risk factors and the location of the surgical site (see Sect. 3.6 below).

In addition to iatrogenic immunosuppression for organ transplant, other forms of immunocompromise must be addressed prior to surgery. In particular, chronic lymphocytic leukemia (CLL) is usually an indolent hematologic malignancy associated with modest immunosuppression, but it appears to have a disproportionate effect on the behavior of cutaneous malignancy. Like patients with solid organ transplants, patients with CLL exhibit an increased incidence of BCC and SCC as well as more rapid progression and metastasis of these tumors. A retrospective study of head and neck basal cell carcinoma in patients with CLL found that these patients also had a 14-fold increased risk of BCC recurrence. Despite the use of Mohs surgery on banal-appearing tumors with typical histologic features, the recurrence of BCC at 3 and 5 years was 12% and 22%, respectively, compared to 0% and 2% in controls [13]. The use of micrographic margin control is particularly problematic in patients with CLL due to the presence of obscuring leukemic infiltrates in many patients [14]. The surgeon must be meticulous in examining histologic margins in these patients and may wish to consider taking more generous margins in certain cases. Similar to patients with immunocompromise, certain patients with inherited or acquired neoplasia syndromes appear to be at higher risk of recurrence and subsequent cutaneous malignancies. This includes genetic syndromes such as the basal cell nevus syndrome (Gorlin syndrome) and acquired conditions such as extensive actinic damage in what has been termed the actinic neoplasia syndrome [15]. Because these patients may also require a more involved surgical approach and closer postoperative monitoring, the surgeon should determine the number, type, and location of prior skin cancers in all patients during the preoperative evaluation.

Finally, psychiatric disease and social habits can also affect surgical outcomes. Patients with depression, dementia, or other psychiatric disorders are often less able to perform appropriate postoperative care and may be at higher risk for wound infection, scarring, or other complications. A caregiver or home nursing visits may be useful in these cases to ensure proper dressing care. If a patient exhibits excessive anxiety about the planned procedure during the preoperative evaluation, it may be beneficial to prescribe an anxiolytic such as diazepam. We have found that 2–5 mg of diazepam taken orally 1 h prior to surgery can be an effective adjunct in patients with moderate anxiety. As discussed above, the preoperative evaluation itself can also minimize patient anxiety by establishing an effective relationship with the patient. More intensive sedation, if required, should be performed in consultation with an anesthesiologist. The use of ethanol and tobacco can also adversely impact surgical outcomes, and patients must be questioned about these habits prior to surgery. Ethanol functions as a mild anticoagulant, and patients should be counseled to avoid alcohol consumption for 24–48 h after surgery. Nicotine, in contrast, has a vasoconstrictive and prothrombotic effect and may be more problematic for surgical patients. This is particularly true when repairs are performed with flaps or full-thickness skin grafts that require optimal vascular function to survive. A retrospective study in the plastic surgery literature found that tobacco use was strongly correlated with skin flap necrosis after face lift surgery, with an odds ratio of 12.46 [16]. Patients should be counseled to abstain from smoking for 1 week before and after surgery. Involvement of the patient's primary care physician in this process can help with compliance and may facilitate permanent abstention from tobacco use and significant overall health benefits.

Due to the disproportionate incidence of skin cancer in elderly patients, dermatologic surgeons are increasingly required to perform surgery on geriatric patients with multiple comorbid conditions as described above. In addition to the contribution of each individual condition, however, the patient's overall functional status appears to be a more important predictor of outcome after invasive procedures. One recent study found that after major surgery in patients over 65 years of age, the most important predictor of survival to 6 months was the preoperative functional status [17]. Functional status, or disability level, was defined in this case by the patient's ability to perform six activities of daily living (ADLs) without assistance, including bathing, dressing, toileting, transferring, continence, and feeding. Other commonly used and validated metrics of global function are defined by energy expenditure, such as the ability to perform light housework or walk up a flight of stairs. Although there is no published data directly addressing the role of functional status in dermatologic surgery, extrapolation of these studies suggests that global functional status could be an important prognostic indicator in dermatology as well. Thus, the surgeon should perform at least a cursory assessment of functional independence at the preoperative evaluation. This can often be inferred from observation of the patient walking down the hall, and clarified with the question, "Does anyone help you at home?" Any sign of functional disability can then be further explored, as this is likely to have an impact on the incidence of postoperative complications including dehiscence, bleeding, infection, and scar formation.

Summary: Medications and Allergies

- A detailed review of medications and allergies is an essential aspect of the preoperative evaluation.
- Although anticoagulants such as warfarin may increase the incidence of local bleeding complications, there is a documented risk of serious or fatal thrombotic complications when these medications are interrupted in the perioperative period.
- Therapeutic anticoagulants and cardiac medications such as beta-blockers are continued throughout the perioperative period in most cases.
- Over-the-counter preparations and herbal supplements may also increase hemorrhagic complications and should be suspended prior to surgery.
- Allergies or adverse reactions to systemic medications or local anesthetics must be documented in detail and may require modification of the surgical plan.

3.5 Medications and Allergies

In addition to past and current medical conditions, a patient's medications may also have significant impact on the outcome of dermatologic surgery. A detailed review of medications is particularly relevant for Mohs surgery as the majority of patients treated for skin cancer are older patients with multiple chronic conditions on multiple concurrent medications. As such, a description of medications and allergies to medications should be included in the medical history form for each patient (Fig. 3.3).

Due to the primary importance of maintaining hemostasis in surgery, anticoagulants are often the most important medications identified in the preoperative evaluation. Although anticoagulants such as warfarin, aspirin, and other nonsteroidal anti-inflammatory agents (NSAIDs) such as ibuprofen have long been associated with an increased bleeding risk, the precise contribution of these medications to bleeding complications in dermatologic surgery is not well defined. A prospective study of patients undergoing Mohs surgery found no significant difference in postoperative bleeding complications in patients taking anticoagulants, though there was a nonsignificant trend toward increased bleeding in patients taking warfarin [18]. Similarly, a larger, retrospective study of 653 patients abstracted from over 7,000 patients treated with Mohs or excisional surgery at one center did not identify a significant difference in hemorrhagic complications in patients taking warfarin, aspirin, or NSAIDs [19]. Again, however, there was a trend toward a higher rate of moderate to severe complications in patients taking warfarin (4 out of 26 cases, 15%) compared to controls (3 out of 277 cases, 1.1%). Severe complications included bleeding not stopped with pressure, hematoma, necrosis of flap or graft, or dehiscence greater than 2 mm, while moderate complications included serous oozing after 24 h, dehiscence less than 2 mm, or superficial slough of flap or graft. There were no cases of death or hemodynamically significant hemorrhage.

It appears that the use of anticoagulant medications, and warfarin in particular, results in an increased risk of postoperative bleeding, but the overall low rate of these complications in dermatologic surgery makes it difficult to quantify this risk in any given study. More definitive data was recently presented in a meta-analysis of six studies involving 122 patients taking warfarin, 472 patients on aspirin, and 779 controls undergoing dermatologic surgery for benign and malignant lesions [20]. This study found a sixfold increased risk of moderate to severe bleeding complications in patients taking warfarin compared to controls (12.3% versus 2.1%, respectively). Patients taking aspirin had a nonsignificantly increased risk of bleeding with a 4.0% rate of moderate to severe complications. Clopidogrel is a newer anticoagulant with extensive use in cardiology after intracoronary stent placement for myocardial infarction, and has synergistic antiplatelet effects when combined with aspirin. The effect of clopidogrel on bleeding complications in dermatologic surgery has not been well studied, but our own experience and published data from the general medical literature suggest that the combination of aspirin and clopidogrel is similar to warfarin in terms of bleeding risk [21]. The surgeon can therefore expect an increased incidence of postoperative bleeding in patients treated with anticoagulant medications and should take the necessary precautions to ensure adequate hemostasis in these patients. These include rigorous control of any bleeding or oozing with ligation or cautery intraoperatively and the use of pressure dressings for at least 24 h postoperatively.

Given the small but demonstrable increased risk of postoperative bleeding in patients treated with anticoagulants, it is reasonable to question whether stopping anticoagulant therapy prior to the planned procedure would mitigate this risk. Although stopping these medications was an accepted practice among dermatologic and plastic surgeons 10–20 years ago, several pharmacologic and physiologic aspects of these medications must be recognized when considering a temporary cessation of anticoagulation. First, aspirin and clopidogrel cause an irreversible inhibition of platelet function that can only be recovered by the synthesis of new platelets; the lifespan of circulating platelets is 7–10 days. Warfarin inhibits synthesis of serum coagulation proteins such as factor II, VII, IX, and X; the half-life of these factors in serum ranges from 1 to 3 days. Thus, recovery of platelet and clotting factor function requires at least 4–7 days of therapy cessation prior to any scheduled procedure. Second, resumption of the therapeutic antithrombotic effect requires another 4–7 days after the anticoagulant is initiated due to the gradual decay of serum clotting factors or inhibition of platelet function. Third, compensatory factors induced by chronic anticoagulant treatment, such as decreased levels of protein C and S or increased activity of other clotting factors, may lead to a transient hypercoagulable state when these medications are interrupted. It is therefore likely that interruption of anticoagulant therapy for a 1–2-h superficial procedure could result in up to 2 weeks of significantly increased risk of systemic thrombosis.

Several case reports in the literature have described catastrophic thrombotic events when therapeutic anticoagulation was held for cutaneous surgery. Schanbacher and Bennett reported two patients who suffered acute thrombotic stroke when warfarin was held for Mohs surgery of facial basal cell carcinoma [22]. In both cases, warfarin was held for 1 week prior to surgery, restarted the day following the procedure, and the thrombotic complications occurred 3–4 days after the procedure. Of note, anticoagulation in both cases was interrupted under consultation with the patient's internist or cardiologist. Holding therapy with antiplatelet agents can also have deleterious effects, as reported in one case of major pulmonary embolus and one case of prosthetic aortic valve thrombosis when dual anticoagulant therapy (aspirin and ticlopidine in one case and clopidogrel and ardeparin, a low-molecular weight heparin in the other, respectively) was stopped 7 days prior to surgery [23]. In both cases, the thrombotic event occurred 2–3 days after surgery. To estimate the incidence of these rare adverse events, Kovich and Otley performed a survey of Mohs surgeons to discover 46 cases of adverse thrombotic events attributed to cessation of anticoagulation therapy. These included 24 strokes, 3 cerebral emboli, 5 myocardial infarctions, and 3 deaths [24]. Based on the average rate of warfarin and aspirin use in dermatologic surgery patients and the extrapolated number of cases performed by each surgeon, the authors estimated an incidence rate of 1 in 6,219 operations for warfarin cessation and 1 in 21,448 for aspirin cessation. A more systematic review of published cases from the dental literature found 542 cases in which warfarin therapy was suspended, and 5 cases of thrombotic complications, 4 of which were fatal [25]. This nearly 1% incidence of complications is almost certainly an overestimate, however, as the previously common practice of warfarin cessation prior to oral surgery was not routinely reported in the literature.

Using data from these studies, one can determine the relative risk-to-benefit ratio of holding or continuing therapeutic anticoagulation prior to cutaneous surgery. For warfarin therapy, there does appear to be a modest increase in local bleeding complications when warfarin is continued perioperatively. As noted above, however, no cases of death or hemodynamically significant hemorrhage have been reported in cutaneous surgery from continuation of anticoagulant use. In contrast, nearly all the reported cases of thromboembolic complications associated with cessation of warfarin therapy, though rare, have resulted in death or permanent disability. The recommendation, therefore, is that warfarin treatment should not be suspended for any length of time for dermatologic surgery. Aspirin appears to have a lower risk of hemorrhagic complications when continued throughout cutaneous surgery, and it should likewise be continued in patients taking aspirin for coronary artery disease or other thrombotic tendency. While the risk-to-benefit ratio of clopidogrel has not been defined in these studies, the American College of Cardiology recommends that patients taking clopidogrel after myocardial infarction should remain on their anticoagulant therapy during minor surgical procedures such as local skin surgery [6]. One situation where anticoagulant medications should be interrupted in dermatologic surgery is when a patient is taking aspirin or other NSAIDs for pain relief, rather than for the anticoagulant effect. In this case, we advise the patient to suspend NSAIDs for 1 week before and 2 days after the surgical procedure. Pain relief in the perioperative period can then be managed with acetaminophen.

In addition to therapeutic anticoagulants, several herbal or over-the-counter (OTC) medications can have intended or unintended effects on the coagulation pathway. It is important for the surgeon to be cognizant of these medications. Because patients may not be aware of the anticoagulant effects, the surgeon must specifically question patients about use of these traditional and nontraditional medications. Several common OTC medications contain aspirin or ibuprofen as the active ingredients, such as Alka-Seltzer and Advil Cold and Sinus, respectively. Herbal medications and supplements have also been implicated in several cases of spontaneous or postoperative bleeding, including one report of serious hemorrhage requiring transfusion after uncomplicated laparoscopic cholecystectomy in an otherwise healthy 36-year-old man taking *Ginkgo biloba* supplements [26]. These reports of hemorrhagic complications are supported by mechanistic studies showing that Ginkgo extracts reduce blood viscosity and inhibit platelet activating factor. Isolated case reports and in vitro studies of platelet activation and coagulation factors have also implicated garlic, ginseng, ginger, feverfew, vitamin E, and saw palmetto in exacerbated operative and postoperative bleeding [27, 28]. For all these agents, however, definitive studies of bleeding risk have not been performed, and it remains difficult to assess whether the published case reports represent causality or coincidence. Nevertheless, because these supplements are used primarily for prevention rather than treatment and because there is no known risk of stopping these products, it is recommended that patients discontinue the use of *Ginkgo biloba*, garlic, ginseng, ginger, feverfew, vitamin E, and saw palmetto 1 week prior to surgery. Another herbal product that should also be stopped is ephedra, or ma huang, a Chinese herbal remedy with sympathomimetic properties that has been reported to cause insomnia, hypertension, arrhythmia, and stroke; these effects may be magnified when combined with epinephrine used in cutaneous surgery [27].

The use of nonselective beta-blockers such as propranolol has prompted concern for interactions with subcutaneous epinephrine since the initial report of six cases of profound intraoperative hypertension, including one case of nonfatal cardiac arrest [29]. A subsequent prospective study of ten patients on propranolol undergoing Mohs surgery, however, found no change in blood pressure after administration of typical doses of subcutaneous epinephrine [30]. All six cases of epinephrine-induced hypertension in the original report were undergoing facial and eyelid plasty, and were treated with initially large volumes of subcutaneous lidocaine with epinephrine (8–40 cc at 1:100,000 or 1:200,000 dilution); this quantity of epinephrine is not typically used in Mohs surgery in a single injection. Moreover, the majority of beta-blockers in use today (such as metoprolol and atenolol) are selective for the myocardial beta 1 receptor without pharmacologic binding to beta 2 receptors on the peripheral vasculature. Thus, these selective beta-blockers are not expected to lead to unopposed alpha receptor activity in the presence of epinephrine to the same extent as propranolol (a nonselective beta 1 and 2 blocker). In light of the clear cardioprotective effects of beta-blockers and other antihypertensive medications, particularly in the perioperative period, these medications should be continued at their usual dose in patients undergoing dermatologic surgery.

Several other medications commonly used by patients may also be relevant to dermatologic surgery and should be noted in the preoperative evaluation. Patients with diabetes mellitus should be counseled to take all of their usual medications on the day of surgery, including insulin. At the same time, they must be instructed to follow their normal eating habits on the day of surgery to prevent hypoglycemia. Similarly, diabetic patients must be monitored for symptoms of hypoglycemia during prolonged Mohs cases and provided with food or carbohydrate-rich beverages as appropriate. The increasing use of biologic agents for tumor necrosis factor alpha (TNFα) inhibition in patients with psoriasis, rheumatoid arthritis, and inflammatory bowel disease necessitates a working knowledge of the interactions of these medications with wound healing after surgery. TNFα is a cytokine with a central role in both the inflammatory phase of appropriate wound healing and in innate immune activation to limit infection. One retrospective study of rheumatoid arthritis patients found that continuing treatment with TNFα antagonists during elective orthopedic surgery resulted in a fourfold increased risk of postoperative infection compared to matched controls. Other disease-modifying antirheumatic agents such as methotrexate did not demonstrate this increased risk [31]. Although it is unclear whether similar complications can be expected from TNFα antagonists in dermatologic surgery, it may be prudent to hold these medications for 1–2 weeks perioperatively when performing larger procedures or more complex repairs. Finally, patients under the care of a dermatologist are likely to be using topical medications such as retinoids, corticosteroids, chemotherapeutics such as 5-fluorouracil, and immune modulators such as imiquimod. To prevent interference with appropriate wound healing, patients should be advised not to apply these medications to the area around the surgical site for at least 1 week before and 2 weeks after surgery, unless they are prescribed as specific adjunctive therapy for the malignancy to be treated.

Apart from documenting the patient's current medications at the preoperative evaluation, any suspected allergies to medications or skin contactants must be clearly recorded in the patient's medical record. Relevant allergies in dermatologic surgery are most often limited to antibiotics, anesthetics, preservatives in anesthetics, and adhesives in tape and dressings. Antibiotic allergies are the most common, and equivalent antibiotics from a different class are often easily substituted. Allergies to local anesthetics are unusual. When present, they often present as local contact allergies to anesthetics of the ester class such as procaine. Amide anesthetics such as lidocaine are almost universally tolerated, but there have been systemic allergic reactions reported in the literature. In one case, systemic urticaria without anaphylaxis occurred within minutes after amide anesthetic administration, and subsequent challenge confirmed amide anesthetic reactivity without any reaction to ester anesthetics or preservatives [32]. Allergies to preservatives such as methylparaben or sodium metabisulfite contained in multidose vials have also been described. When a patient reports a previous reaction to a local anesthetic, it is imperative to determine the nature of the reaction, whether the reaction was local or systemic and what anesthetic and additives were used when the reaction occurred. This can allow determination of whether there is true allergy, and whether the allergy is likely to be to anesthetics of the ester class, amide class, or preservatives. When in doubt, patients may be challenged with preservative-free (sold in single-dose ampoules) anesthetics of either class, or may be referred to an allergist for skin prick testing. This testing may be cumbersome and delay surgery, but it is clearly indicated to spare the patient from potentially unnecessary exposure to general anesthesia for the remainder of their lifetime. Although "allergic reactions" to epinephrine may be self-reported by patients, true allergy to epinephrine is physiologically implausible as this is an endogenous hormone and neurotransmitter. More often, these self-reported reactions are the expected physiologic side effect of small amounts of epinephrine reaching the systemic circulation: transient flushing, anxiety, tachycardia, or palpitations. These reactions are not a contraindication to subsequent use of subcutaneous epinephrine in cutaneous surgery. Reactions to adhesives in medical tape and wound dressings are common and should also be noted at the preoperative evaluation. Because these local reactions are often partly due to irritant dermatitis, substitution with a weaker adhesive (such as use of paper tape instead of silk or synthetic tape) is often helpful in reducing local skin irritation. Asking patients which types or brands of adhesive dressings they have tolerated in the past will also help to minimize postoperative dermatitis and patient complaints.

Summary: Assessing the Need for Infection Prophylaxis

- The incidence of transient bacteremia with dermatologic surgery on noninfected skin appears to be no greater than the incidence with routine daily activities.
- Updated guidelines from the American Heart Association and the American College of Cardiology in 2007 limit prophylactic antibiotics only to those patients with cardiac conditions at highest risk for endocarditis undergoing surgery with breach of the oral mucosa or on infected cutaneous sites.
- Prophylactic antibiotics should also be considered in patients with recent total joint replacement, or in surgical sites at high risk for postoperative wound infection.
- There is no evidence to support the use of prophylactic topical antibiotic preparations in dermatologic surgery.

3.6 Assessing the Need for Infection Prophylaxis

Dermatologic surgery is remarkably safe, but the surgical disruption of the epidermal barrier creates an inevitable risk of infection. Of particular concern is the potential for bacterial endocarditis and prosthetic joint infection in predisposed individuals. Both of these life-threatening infections involve seeding of susceptible anatomic sites (either exogenous hardware or previously damaged valves) in the setting of bacteremia. At least transient bacteremia is thought to be a prerequisite to bacterial endocarditis or septic arthritis. Reliable data suggests that the rate of bacteremia immediately following cutaneous surgery is negligible: 2.7% of 149 patients had positive blood cultures after surgery, compared with 3.3% of these patients prior to surgery and 2.1% of 240 healthy control patients without skin lesions [33, 34]. The surgeries performed in this study included basic excisional and Mohs surgery with linear, flap, and graft repair, and 31% of the skin lesions were eroded at the time of surgery. In addition, the bacteria isolated in all cases were nonpathogenic skin flora and were thought to represent contamination

Table 3.2 Cardiac conditions at high risk for infective endocarditis

Prior history of infective endocarditis
Prosthetic cardiac valve or prosthetic valvular material
Cardiac transplantation recipients who develop cardiac valvulopathy
Congenital heart disease (CHD)
Unrepaired cyanotic CHD including palliative shunts and conduits
Completely repaired CHD with prosthetic material or device during first 6 months after procedure
Repaired CHD with residual defects at site or adjacent to site of prosthesis

Data obtained from Wilson et al. [36]

rather than true infection. These studies suggest that the risk of bacterial bloodstream infections after surgery on eroded, noninfected skin is exceedingly low, and that the risk of bacteremia is not higher in Mohs surgery compared to standard excisional surgery. Although there have been published reports of bacterial endocarditis occurring after surgical procedures on noninfected skin [35], it is not clear that these procedures represent a greater risk of endocarditis than the baseline risk of normal activities.

In light of these findings and the increasing recognition of the risks associated with widespread antibiotic use, including allergic reactions, antibiotic-associated colitis, and bacterial resistance, updated guidelines from the American Heart Association (AHA) in 2007 now recommend prophylactic antibiotics only in certain patient populations under specified conditions [36]. The guidelines acknowledge that there is insufficient data to support the use of routine antibiotic prophylaxis in most surgical patients, that antibiotic prophylaxis may only prevent an exceedingly small number of cases of infective endocarditis, if any, and that the potential adverse effects associated with antibiotic use outweigh the benefit of prophylaxis for most patients. These guidelines were summarized in the dermatology literature with particular attention to dermatologic procedures in 2008 [37], and are presented in Table 3.2 and Fig. 3.4.

The first step in the algorithm (Fig. 3.4) is determining whether a patient has an underlying cardiac condition conferring significantly increased risk and exacerbated complications of infective endocarditis. These conditions are limited to prior infective endocarditis, prosthetic heart valves, valvulopathy following cardiac transplantation, and congenital heart disease as described

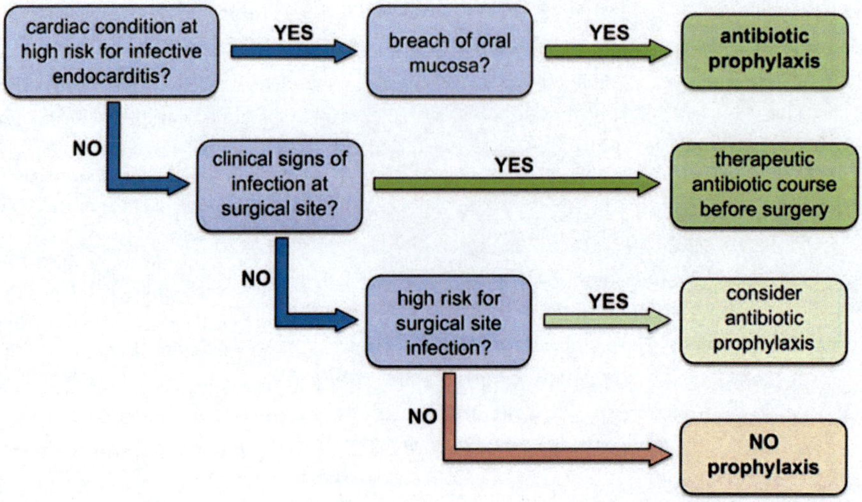

Fig. 3.4 Indications for preoperative antibiotic prophylaxis in dermatologic surgery. In the absence of breach of the oral mucosa in patients with high-risk cardiac conditions or clinical signs of infection at the operative site, there is not a definite indication for preoperative antibiotic prophylaxis. High-risk cardiac conditions are defined in Table 3.2

in Table 3.2. Other cardiac conditions such as mitral valve prolapse, mitral or aortic regurgitation, indwelling pacemakers, and intracoronary stents are not indications for antibiotic prophylaxis. The next consideration in the decision to prescribe antibiotic prophylaxis is the surgical site. Because of the increased microbial burden on mucosal sites and the difficulty in sterilizing the oral cavity preoperatively, procedures that disrupt the epithelial barrier of the oral mucosa incur a greater risk of bacteremia and subsequent endocarditis. As such, prophylaxis is recommended for surgery that penetrates the oral mucosa in patients with high-risk cardiac conditions. Surgical procedures involving the nasal mucosa are not specifically addressed in the AHA guidelines, and the decision to provide antibiotic prophylaxis for these cases must therefore be considered on a case-by-case basis. The next step is the assessment of clinical signs of infection at the operative site. The current AHA guidelines draw a distinction between surgical procedures on normal skin and infected skin, citing the evidence that procedures on normal skin have an essentially negligible risk of bacteremia, even in the presence of superficial erosions. If there is clinical evidence of local skin infection such as erythema, edema, and purulent discharge, the lesion should be cultured and the patient treated with a full course of systemic antibiotics, with delay of surgery to coincide with completion of the antibiotic regimen. In this case, antibiotic treatment is both therapeutic for local infection and prophylactic for prevention of endocarditis.

The final step in the algorithm is to determine whether the surgical site is at significantly increased risk of postoperative wound infection. The rationale for this comes from the fact that local skin infections (even in the absence of surgery) may lead to transient bacteremia, and skin infection has been associated with an increased risk of bacterial endocarditis [38]. As such, prophylactic antibiotic use to prevent postoperative wound infection is expected, but not proven, to decrease the risk of infective endocarditis. While the use of antibiotic prophylaxis for skin sites at increased risk of local infection is not specified in the AHA guidelines, this practice has been advocated in the dermatology literature [37]. Several studies have been performed to quantify the incidence of surgical site infections after dermatologic procedures. A prospective study of 5,091 Mohs and excisional surgical cases without antibiotics confirmed the overall low incidence (1.47%) of postoperative surgical site infections in dermatology and identified the following sites or repairs at greater than 5% risk of infection: any site on the lower leg below the knee (6.92%), sites in the groin (10%), wedge resection of the lip or ear (8.57%), and skin grafts at any site (8.7%) [39]. Sites on the fingers and flap repair at all sites had an intermediate risk of infection at 4.88% and 2.94%, respectively. A subsequent prospective study of 1,115 Mohs cases found an overall surgical site infection incidence of 0.7%, with only a modest increase in risk with flap repair (2.4%) and no evidence of infection in cases on the lip, ears, groin, or lower leg, although the number of cases in these sites was not reported [40]. In light of these studies, antibiotic prophylaxis may be considered in patients undergoing cutaneous surgery with elevated risk for local

Table 3.3 Selection of antibiotic dose and timing for infection prophylaxis

Surgical site	Medication restrictions	Antibiotic, route, and dose[a]
Oral	None	Amoxicillin 2 g PO
Oral	Penicillin allergy	Clindamycin 600 mg PO or Azithromycin/clindamycin 500 mg PO
Oral	Unable to take PO	Ampicillin 2 g IM/IV or Cefazolin/ceftriaxone 1 g IM/IV
Oral	Penicillin allergy, unable to take PO	Clindamycin 600 mg IM/IV
Cutaneous	None	Cephalexin 2 g PO or Dicloxacillin 2 g PO
Cutaneous	Penicillin allergy	Clindamycin 600 mg PO Azithromycin/clindamycin 500 mg PO
Cutaneous	Unable to take PO	Cefazolin/ceftriaxone 1 g IM/IV
Cutaneous	Penicillin allergy, unable to take PO	Clindamycin 600 mg IM/IV
Infected cutaneous site with known pathogen		7–14-day systemic treatment with antibiotic tailored to specific pathogen

[a]Antibiotic to be administered as single dose, 60 min prior to procedure

infection such as cases on the lower leg and groin, wedge resection of lip or ear, or cases repaired with full-thickness skin grafts. Prophylaxis may also be considered for flap repairs and repairs on the fingers, although the data is less clear in this case. It must be emphasized, however, that without data to demonstrate a clear benefit of prophylaxis for patients with these higher risk sites, definitive recommendations cannot be made.

Once the decision has been made to provide prophylactic antibiotic therapy, the AHA guidelines are clear regarding the selection, dose, and timing of antibiotic administration. For surgical procedures involving oral mucosa, the most frequent cause of subsequent bacteremia is viridans group streptococci, and antibiotic therapy should therefore be targeted against this organism. Oral amoxicillin has been shown to be the most effective with minimal side effects; a single 2-g dose given 1 h prior to surgery is therefore recommended for oral procedures. For cutaneous procedures requiring prophylaxis, either due to clinically infected skin or surgery at high risk for local infection, the most frequent pathogens are *Staphylococcus aureus* and beta-hemolytic *Streptococci*. Standard prophylaxis is therefore a single dose of oral cephalexin, 2 g given 1 h prior to surgery. Patients with penicillin allergy should be treated with either clindamycin or a macrolide antibiotic. Patients unable to take oral medication can be treated with either parenteral cephalosporins such as cefazolin or ceftriaxone, or parenteral clindamycin in the case of penicillin allergy. These recommendations, adapted from the AHA guidelines [36] and the dermatology literature, [37] are summarized in Table 3.3. It should also be noted that the most recent guidelines do not recommend an additional postoperative antibiotic dose for typical surgical procedures. For prolonged Mohs surgery lasting more than 4 h, a second dose at half strength (e.g., 1 g of cephalexin) can be given 6 h after the initial dose. The prevalence of methicillin-resistant *Staphylococcus aureus* (MRSA) of both community-acquired and healthcare-associated strains is increasing throughout the world, and postoperative local infections with MRSA have been reported after dermatologic surgery [40]. While the dermatologic surgeon must consider the possibility of MRSA and other resistant bacteria in all skin and subcutaneous surgical site infections, the lack of data regarding the true incidence of MRSA infection and the potential side effects of broad-spectrum antibiotics active against MRSA preclude the use of routine prophylaxis for this agent at this time.

Analogous to patients with prosthetic cardiac valve replacement, patients with prosthetic joint replacement exhibit an increased risk of seeding the joint space from transient bacteremia and are more likely to have significant morbidity from joint space infection than patients with native joints. The American Dental Association and the American Academy of Orthopedic Surgeons have specified guidelines to specify which patients with prosthetic joint replacement will benefit most from antibiotic prophylaxis before surgical procedures [41]. The most critical period for prosthetic joint infection is the first 2 years postoperatively, and prophylaxis is therefore only required for procedures within 2 years of joint replacement for most patients. Other patient factors are thought to increase the risk or consequences of prosthetic joint infection such that prophylaxis is recommended for oral surgical procedures occurring beyond 2 years after joint replacement. These include history of previous prosthetic joint infection, immunocompromised patients with autoimmune disease or on immunosuppressive medication, patients with insulin-dependent diabetes, HIV infection, malignancy, malnutrition, or hemophilia. Patients with orthopedic pins, plates, or screws do not require routine prophylaxis. As in the algorithm for prevention of infective endocarditis (Fig. 3.2), prophylaxis for these patients should only be given if the planned procedure will breach oral mucosa, if the surgical site shows clinical signs of local infection, or if the procedure is at high risk for surgical site infection. The choice and timing of antibiotic prophylaxis is also analogous to the prevention of endocarditis and depends upon whether the surgical site is likely to introduce mucosal or cutaneous flora (Table 3.3).

In addition to preoperative prophylaxis for endocarditis and prosthetic joint infection, many dermatologic surgeons may prescribe antibiotics either pre- or postoperatively to decrease the risk of local surgical site infection. This is a controversial subject without clear data to support clinical practice decisions and is beyond the scope of this discussion. It should be noted, however, that postoperative antibiotics are expected to have limited preventive effect since bacteria become embedded within fibrin clots intraoperatively and may be relatively sequestered from circulating antibiotics [42]. Thus, if prophylaxis is desired, it should ideally be given as a single dose 1 h prior to surgery as outlined in Table 3.3. This prophylactic regimen is also likely to minimize adverse reactions such as antibiotic-associated colitis and interaction with other medications, as well as decrease the emergence of bacterial resistance and limit medical expenditures, as total use of antibiotics is reduced. Prophylaxis for surgical site infections should also take into account patient factors that may increase the risk of postoperative infection, such as immunocompromise, diabetes, or extensive inflammatory skin disease. These factors, coupled with the site-specific and procedure-specific risk of local infection as discussed above, can help select patients most likely to benefit from antibiotic prophylaxis.

In an attempt to provide infection prophylaxis without the potential side effects of systemic antibiotics, some surgeons may prescribe topical antibiotic ointments postoperatively. This practice is not supported by the literature. A prospective, blinded trial comparing bacitracin and petrolatum ointment for postprocedure skin wounds from skin biopsies, excisions, and Mohs surgery found that while bacitracin decreased the incidence of local infection with *Staphylococcus aureus*, there was a corresponding increase in infections with gram-negative bacteria. The total rate of wound infection was no different between the groups, and 4 of 444 patients in the bacitracin group developed allergic contact dermatitis to the antibiotic [43]. A more potent topical anti-*Staphylococcal* antibiotic, mupirocin ointment, was also evaluated in a trial of postoperative surgical wounds [44]. Mupirocin was similarly found to confer no benefit for prevention of surgical site infection, although there was a higher incidence of skin edge necrosis in the mupirocin group than paraffin ointment control (1.1% versus 0.1%). The significance of the latter finding is unknown, but due to the lack of evidence for efficacy of topical antibiotic preparations in local infection prevention, routine use of these agents for prophylaxis is not recommended.

Dermatologic procedures on the cutaneous or mucosal lip induce epidermal injury and can lead to reactivation of latent herpes virus infection. Questioning patients about cold sores or fever blisters is an important part of the preoperative evaluation. Any patient with a potential history of herpes labialis under going dermatologic surgery on the lip should receive prophylaxis with oral antiviral medications. Several regimens are available, including acyclovir 400 mg three times daily, valacyclovir 500 mg twice daily, and famciclovir 250 mg twice daily. Prophylaxis should be started on the day of surgery or 1 day prior and should be continued for an additional 3–5 days. Resurfacing procedures such as dermabrasion, medium or deep chemical peels, and ablative or non-ablative laser resurfacing cause such extensive epidermal injury that a history of cold sores is not a reliable indicator of reactivation risk, and all patients undergoing these procedures should receive antiviral prophylaxis regardless of history. For resurfacing procedures, this prophylaxis should continue until reepithelialization is complete, usually within 7–10 days.

Summary: Discussion of Postoperative Care

- The preoperative evaluation can be used to initiate the discussion of postoperative care and help frame patient expectations for the postoperative course.

3.7 Discussion of Postoperative Care

A final point to be addressed in the preoperative consultation is initiating the discussion of postoperative healing and wound care. Patients should be informed of the expected wound healing process, including expected bruising and swelling, particularly on periorbital and perioral sites. Explanation of the expected time frame for discomfort, erythema, edema, ecchymosis, and bandage use at the initial consultation will prevent unwanted surprises postoperatively. Similarly, reminding patients that epidermal sutures, if placed, will require removal can help prepare for a second office visit. If it appears that a patient will have difficulty with dressing changes and wound care due to either physical disability or a difficult-to-reach operative site, the preoperative consultation is the time to begin arrangements for assistance, either from family members or a visiting nurse service. Finally, an important aspect of the treatment for skin cancer is ensuring adequate follow up screening for second malignancy, which occurs at high frequency in these patients. While the dermatologic surgeon may not be the physician performing this screening, it is important to remind patients of the need for follow up exams even before surgery has been performed. Because it is likely that patients will retain and absorb only a fraction of the counseling advice dispensed by physicians, repetition of these points at the preoperative, operative, and postoperative visits will help maximize compliance and ensure optimal surgical outcomes.

Summary: Conclusion

- Medical care of the dermatologic surgery patient begins with a simple yet complete preoperative evaluation.
- After documentation of informed consent, confirmation of the presenting lesion and diagnosis, review of the patient's past medical history and medications (with particular emphasis on anticoagulant medications), and assessment of the need for infection prophylaxis, a therapeutic plan can be tailored to the individual patient for optimal medical and surgical care.

3.8 Conclusion

When performed properly, the preoperative evaluation is a straightforward exercise that minimizes operative and postoperative complications. With adequate verification of the presenting location and diagnosis, and examination for signs of aggressive tumor behavior, an appropriate therapeutic plan can be developed with the informed consent of the patient. Modifications can then be made based on the patient's medical history and medication use. These may include electing not to use electrodessication or electrocoagulation in patients with implantable cardiac defibrillators, choosing a less invasive reconstruction method for patients with impaired wound healing and poor functional status, or advising patients to avoid over-the-counter pain relievers and herbal supplements that impair hemostasis. Awareness of the risks of interrupting therapeutic anticoagulation, coupled with continuation of these anticoagulants preoperatively, may also decrease the incidence of serious thrombotic complications in the perioperative period. Similarly, appropriate use of antibiotic prophylaxis according to recently published guidelines can minimize infectious complications of dermatologic surgery while reducing the number of patients exposed to unnecessary antibiotic therapy. Medical care of the dermatologic surgery patient begins well before the surgical procedure, and optimal delivery of this care requires a directed and precise preoperative evaluation.

References

1. Carucci JA, Leffell DJ. Basal cell carcinoma. In: Wolff K et al., editors. Fitzpatrick's dermatology in: general medicine. New York: McGraw Hill Medical; 2008. p. 1036–42.
2. Cataldo PA, Stoddard PB, Reed WP. Use of frozen section analysis in the treatment of basal cell carcinoma. Am J Surg. 1990;159(6):561–3.
3. Feasel AM et al. Perineural invasion of cutaneous malignancies. Dermatol Surg. 2001;27(6):531–42.
4. McGinness JL, Goldstein G. The value of preoperative biopsy-site photography for identifying cutaneous lesions. Dermatol Surg. 2010;36(2):194–7.
5. Rhodes LM et al. Cutaneous surgery in the elderly: ensuring comfort and safety. Dermatol Ther. 2003;16(3):243–53.
6. Fleisher LA et al. ACC/AHA 2007 Guidelines on perioperative cardiovascular evaluation and care for noncardiac surgery: executive summary: a report of the American College of Cardiology/American Heart Association Task Force on Practice Guidelines (Writing Committee to Revise the 2002 Guidelines on Perioperative Cardiovascular Evaluation for Noncardiac Surgery): Developed in Collaboration With the American Society of Echocardiography, American Society of Nuclear Cardiology, Heart Rhythm Society, Society of Cardiovascular Anesthesiologists, Society for Cardiovascular Angiography and Interventions, Society for Vascular Medicine and Biology, and Society for Vascular Surgery. Circulation. 2007;116(17):1971–96.
7. Dzubow LM. Blood pressure as a parameter in dermatologic surgery. Arch Dermatol. 1986;122(12):1406–7.
8. Rozner MA, Nishman RJ. Electrocautery-induced pacemaker tachycardia: why does this error continue? Anesthesiology. 2002;96(3):773–4.
9. LeVasseur JG et al. Dermatologic electrosurgery in patients with implantable cardioverter-defibrillators and pacemakers. Dermatol Surg. 1998;24(2):233–40.
10. El-Gamal HM, Dufresne RG, Saddler K. Electrosurgery, pacemakers and ICDs: a survey of precautions and complications experienced by cutaneous surgeons. Dermatol Surg. 2001;27(4):385–90.
11. Richards KA, Stasko T. Dermatologic surgery and the pregnant patient. Dermatol Surg. 2002;28(3):248–56.
12. Berg D, Otley CC. Skin cancer in organ transplant recipients: epidemiology, pathogenesis, and management. J Am Acad Dermatol. 2002;47(1):1–17.
13. Mehrany K et al. High recurrence rates of Basal cell carcinoma after Mohs surgery in patients with chronic lymphocytic leukemia. Arch Dermatol. 2004;140(8):985–8.
14. Albregts T et al. Squamous cell carcinoma in a patient with chronic lymphocytic leukemia. An intraoperative diagnostic challenge for the Mohs surgeon. Dermatol Surg. 1998;24(2):269–72.
15. Weinstock MA et al. Quality of life in the actinic neoplasia syndrome: the VA Topical Tretinoin Chemoprevention (VATTC) Trial. J Am Acad Dermatol. 2009;61(2):207–15.
16. Rees TD, Liverett DM, Guy CL. The effect of cigarette smoking on skin-flap survival in the face lift patient. Plast Reconstr Surg. 1984;73(6):911–5.
17. Robinson TN et al. Redefining geriatric preoperative assessment using frailty, disability and co-morbidity. Ann Surg. 2009;250(3):449–55.
18. Billingsley EM, Maloney ME. Intraoperative and postoperative bleeding problems in patients taking warfarin, aspirin, and nonsteroidal antiinflammatory agents. A prospective study. Dermatol Surg. 1997;23(5):381–3.
19. Otley CC et al. Complications of cutaneous surgery in patients who are taking warfarin, aspirin, or nonsteroidal anti-inflammatory drugs. Arch Dermatol. 1996;132(2):161–6.
20. Lewis KG, Dufresne Jr RG. A meta-analysis of complications attributed to anticoagulation among patients following cutaneous surgery. Dermatol Surg. 2008;34(2):160–4.
21. Holmes Jr DR et al. Combining antiplatelet and anticoagulant therapies. J Am Coll Cardiol. 2009;54(2):95–109.
22. Schanbacher CF, Bennett RG. Postoperative stroke after stopping warfarin for cutaneous surgery. Dermatol Surg. 2000;26(8):785–9.
23. Alam M, Goldberg LH. Serious adverse vascular events associated with perioperative interruption of antiplatelet and anticoagulant therapy. Dermatol Surg. 2002;28(11):992–8.
24. Kovich O, Otley CC. Thrombotic complications related to discontinuation of warfarin and aspirin therapy perioperatively for cutaneous operation. J Am Acad Dermatol. 2003;48(2):233–7.
25. Wahl MJ. Dental surgery in anticoagulated patients. Arch Intern Med. 1998;158(15):1610–6.
26. Fessenden JM, Wittenborn W, Clarke L. Gingko biloba: a case report of herbal medicine and bleeding postoperatively from a laparoscopic cholecystectomy. Am Surg. 2001;67(1):33–5.
27. Chang LK, Whitaker DC. The impact of herbal medicines on dermatologic surgery. Dermatol Surg. 2001;27(8):759–63.
28. Beckert BW et al. The effect of herbal medicines on platelet function: an in vivo experiment and review of the literature. Plast Reconstr Surg. 2007;120(7):2044–50.
29. Foster CA, Aston SJ. Propranolol-epinephrine interaction: a potential disaster. Plast Reconstr Surg. 1983;72(1):74–8.
30. Dzubow LM. The interaction between propranolol and epinephrine as observed in patients undergoing Mohs' surgery. J Am Acad Dermatol. 1986;15(1):71–5.
31. Giles JT et al. Tumor necrosis factor inhibitor therapy and risk of serious postoperative orthopedic infection in rheumatoid arthritis. Arthritis Rheum. 2006;55(2):333–7.
32. Cuesta-Herranz J et al. Allergic reaction caused by local anesthetic agents belonging to the amide group. J Allergy Clin Immunol. 1997;99(3):427–8.
33. Carmichael AJ et al. The occurrence of bacteraemia with skin surgery. Br J Dermatol. 1996;134(1):120–2.
34. Wilson WR, Van Scoy RE, Washington JA. Incidence of bacteremia in adults without infection. J Clin Microbiol. 1975;2(2):94–5.
35. Spelman DW, Weinmann A, Spicer WJ. Endocarditis following skin procedures. J Infect. 1993;26(2):185–9.
36. Wilson W et al. Prevention of infective endocarditis: guidelines from the American Heart Association: a guideline from the American Heart Association Rheumatic Fever, Endocarditis, and Kawasaki Disease Committee, Council on

Cardiovascular Disease in the Young, and the Council on Clinical Cardiology, Council on Cardiovascular Surgery and Anesthesia, and the Quality of Care and Outcomes Research Interdisciplinary Working Group. Circulation. 2007;116(15): 1736–54.
37. Wright TI et al. Antibiotic prophylaxis in dermatologic surgery: advisory statement 2008. J Am Acad Dermatol. 2008;59(3):464–73.
38. Strom BL et al. Risk factors for infective endocarditis: oral hygiene and nondental exposures. Circulation. 2000;102(23): 2842–8.
39. Dixon AJ et al. Prospective study of wound infections in dermatologic surgery in the absence of prophylactic antibiotics. Dermatol Surg. 2006;32(6):819–27.
40. Maragh SL, Brown MD. Prospective evaluation of surgical site infection rate among patients with Mohs micrographic surgery without the use of prophylactic antibiotics. J Am Acad Dermatol. 2008;59(2):275–8.
41. Association, A.D. and A.A.o.O. Surgeons. Antibiotic prophylaxis for dental patients with total joint replacements. J Am Dent Assoc. 2003;134(7):895–9.
42. Mangram AJ et al. Guideline for prevention of surgical site infection, 1999. Centers for Disease Control and Prevention (CDC) Hospital Infection Control Practices Advisory Committee. Am J Infect Control. 1999;27(2):96–132.
43. Smack DP et al. Infection and allergy incidence in ambulatory surgery patients using white petrolatum vs bacitracin ointment. A randomized controlled trial. JAMA. 1996; 276(12):972–7.
44. Dixon AJ, Dixon MP, Dixon JB. Randomized clinical trial of the effect of applying ointment to surgical wounds before occlusive dressing. Br J Surg. 2006;93(8):937–43.

Mohs Micrographic Surgery Operative Room Setup

4

Tobechi L. Ebede, Indira Singh, and Kishwer S. Nehal

Abstract

Office-based surgery is the standard for Mohs micrographic surgery. The design and building of a Mohs micrographic surgery suite should provide an environment for comfortable and efficient care of the patient, while meeting regulatory safety standards and the ergonomic needs of the staff. This chapter will discuss physical components of a Mohs surgery suite and operative room. Key operative room equipment will be detailed and lists of essential instruments used during Mohs surgery and reconstruction are outlined in this chapter. Finally, practice details such as photography, equipment sterilization and emergency equipment are summarized.

Keywords

Mohs surgery • Outpatient surgical suite design • Surgical equipment • Surgical instruments

Summary: Introduction

- Office-based surgery is the standard for Mohs micrographic surgery. The minimum space requirements include: a comfortable waiting room, well-equipped operative rooms, a laboratory for frozen tissue processing/histopathology slide reading, and space for cleaning and sterilizing equipment. A contractor, architect, interior designer, and occupational health specialist, knowledgeable about surgical facilities, are critical members of the development team.

T.L. Ebede (✉)
Dermatology Service, Memorial Sloan Kettering Cancer Center, New York, NY, USA
e-mail: tebede@hotmail.com

I. Singh • K.S. Nehal
Dermatology Service, Memorial Sloan Kettering Cancer Center, New York, NY, USA

K. Nouri (ed.), *Mohs Micrographic Surgery*,
DOI 10.1007/978-1-4471-2152-7_4, © Springer-Verlag London Limited 2012

4.1 Introduction

Office-based surgery is a continually growing segment of medical practice and is the standard for Mohs micrographic surgery. The American Academy of Dermatology Committee on Guidelines of Care has developed guidelines for practicing dermatologists who work in office-based surgical facilities [1, 2]. The guidelines define three classes of facilities: Class I facilities use only local, regional, or topical anesthesia; Class II facilities utilize intravenous sedative or analgesic drugs; Class III facilities use general anesthetics. This chapter will focus on operative room set-up for Mohs surgery performed in Class I office-based surgical facilities. Histopathology laboratory setup and certification will be covered in other chapters of this book.

The design and layout of an office-based Mohs surgical suite are extremely important. The minimum space requirements include: a comfortable waiting room, well-equipped operative rooms, a laboratory for frozen tissue processing/histopathology slide reading, and space for cleaning and sterilizing equipment. The space must provide an environment for comfortable and efficient care of the patient, while meeting regulatory safety standards and the ergonomic needs of the staff.

A contractor, architect, and interior designer, knowledgeable about surgical facilities, are critical in the planning process. These individuals will ensure that the facility meets local building and fire codes. Basic start-up costs will vary, but a good consultant can help save unnecessary costs through an organized and critical approach. Visiting established Mohs surgery practices can also provide useful tips regarding successful office space layout. In addition, consultation with an occupational health specialist is highly recommended for a thorough ergonomic assessment of the office space to reduce the risk of musculoskeletal disorders that can result from the repetitive nature of Mohs surgery. A potential layout of an office-based Mohs surgery suite is detailed in Fig. 4.1.

Summary: Mohs Surgery Waiting Room

- Mohs surgery patients spend several hours between Mohs stages in the waiting area. A dedicated, fully equipped waiting room can be designed to cater to their needs.

4.2 Mohs Surgery Waiting Room

Mohs surgery patients will spend several hours between Mohs stages in the waiting area. Ideally, a dedicated waiting room for Mohs surgery patients is important as patients are wearing gowns and have surgical dressings. The waiting area should accommodate a family member or friend who may accompany the patient to the procedure. This waiting room is best located near the nursing station, so that staff can remain alert to potential emergencies. Easy access to a wheelchair-accessible bathroom is also desirable. In addition, Health Insurance Portability and Accountability Act (HIPAA) regulations must be followed when discussing patient issues near this waiting room. Playing soft music, offering television viewing, or a laptop workstation in the waiting room can reduce procedure-related anxiety. Using the checklist below, the basic needs of the patients can be accommodated in the waiting room:

Mohs surgery waiting room checklist:

[] Food (bagels, crackers, or pretzels)
[] Drinks (water, juice, coffee, or tea)
[] Magazines
[] Patient education materials
[] Blankets
[] Closet/Locker (patient clothing and valuables)
[] Reclining chairs

Summary: Mohs Surgery Operative Room Planning

- Important considerations when planning a Mohs surgery operative room include: room size, storage space, and the use of durable materials on walls and floors. Digital photography needs and laser safety regulations should be addressed during the planning process

4.3 Mohs Surgery Operative Room Planning

There are multiple considerations when planning a Mohs surgery operative room. The rooms should be clustered together to increase efficiency. A flag system outside of each room can help physicians and staff prioritize patient needs. An intercom and/or phone system in the room is useful for improving communication

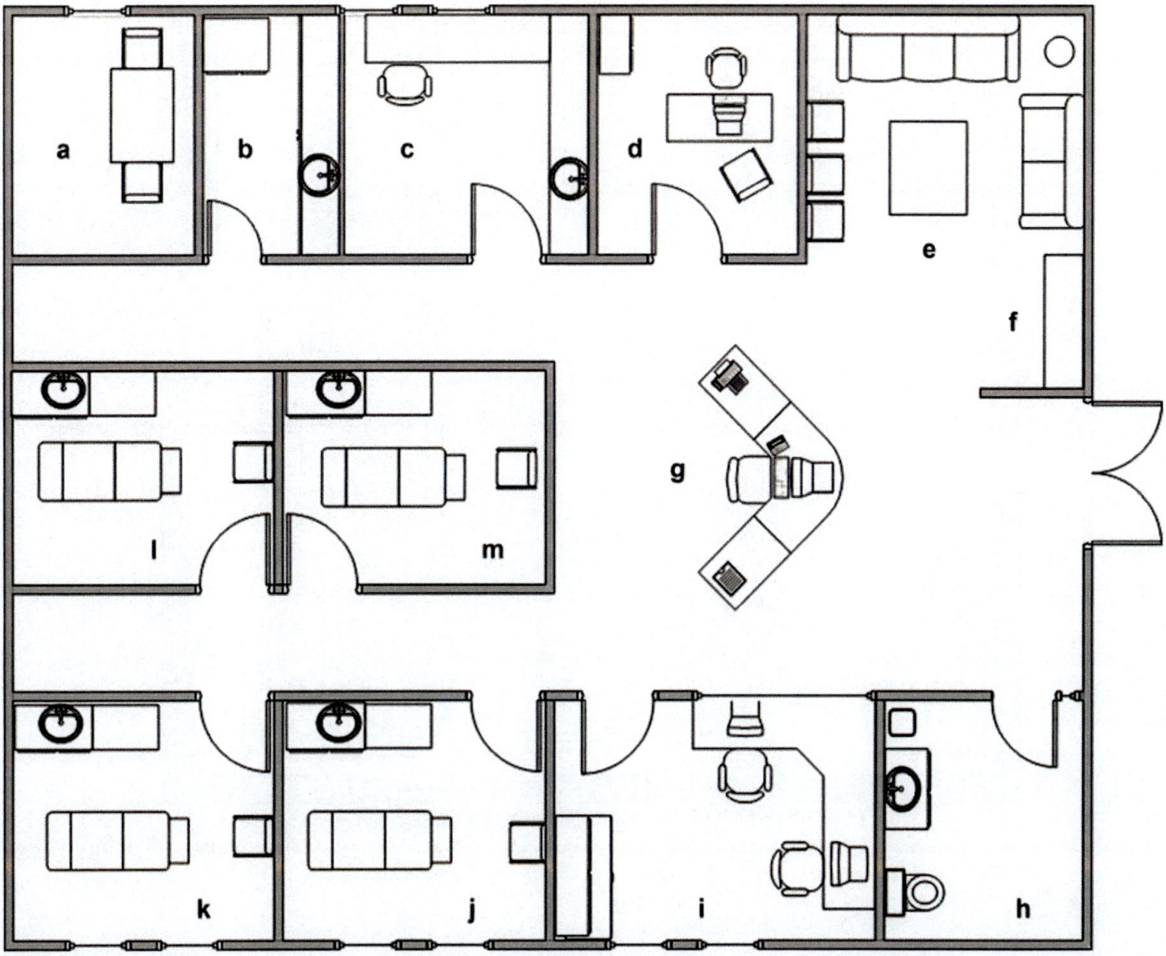

Fig. 4.1 Mohs surgery suite layout: Staff meeting area (**a**), Utility/Storage room (**b**), Histopathology lab (**c**), Physician's office (**d**), Waiting room (**e**), Snack counter (**f**), Reception area (**g**), Restroom (**h**), Nurses' station (**i**), Procedure rooms (**j**, **k**, **l**, **m**)

between staff. Important nonsurgical equipment in each room includes a desk area with chair and a computer for accessing electronic medical records and digital photographs. A sample layout of a Mohs surgery operative room is detailed in Fig. 4.2.

The recommended size of an operative room is 12×12 ft, although it can range from 10×14 to 14×20 ft [3–5]. An adequately sized room allows for free movement around the operating table, houses surgical equipment, and in the event of an emergency, can accommodate emergency equipment and personnel. The doorway should be at least 36 [3] to 44 in. [6] wide to allow stretcher or wheelchair access comfortably. It is important to consider future growth when planning an operative room. Extra space in the room can later accommodate additional equipment and supplies.

Mohs surgery operative rooms require a large amount of storage space for all the necessary equipment and supplies. Ideally, stocking all surgical supplies in the operative room avoids lost time when staff exit the room to search for items. Organizing all room layouts and cabinet arrangements in an identical manner allows the staff to efficiently locate supplies and instruments. The cabinets can be labeled with their contents and supplies should be restocked daily.

When designing an operative room, consider using durable materials for the walls and floor. Light colored latex paint or washable vinyl walls and ceilings are preferable. Linoleum or vinyl flooring is resistant to stains and easy to clean. Though carpeting creates a cozy atmosphere and reduces noise, it is not recommended in operative rooms. There is evidence that

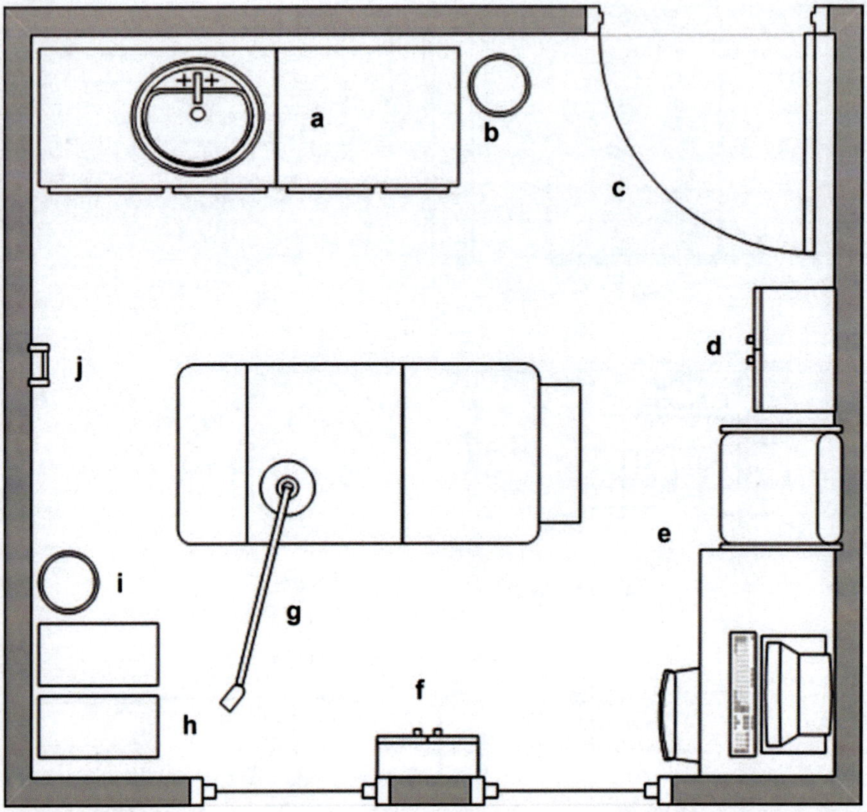

Fig. 4.2 Mohs surgery operative room layout: Overhead cabinets, counter and sink with foot pedals (**a**), Trash can (b), Curtain (**c**), Closet (**d**), Computer desk and chair (**e**), Electrosurgery unit, smoke evacuator and suction (**f**), Exam light (**g**), Mayo stands (**h**), Kick bucket (**i**), Sharps container (**j**)

carpeting does not increase the risk of bacterial contamination and may decrease dust particles in the air [4]. However, carpeting can easily become stained and soiled and is difficult to clean. This can lead to a "dirty" appearance of the room. In addition, it may be difficult to roll equipment (Mayo stand, portable devices) over carpeting. Similar to walls and floor, the ceiling covering should be light colored and washable.

4.3.1 Photography

Digital photography is essential to clinical dermatology for tracking changes in the skin, medical record keeping, and teaching purposes. Currently, digital photography is cheaper and more precise than purchasing and developing film. Costs can vary depending on the type of camera selected and accompanying equipment.

Table 4.1 Comparison of digital cameras

Camera	Pros	Cons
Point and shoot digital camera	Easy to use	Poorer image quality
	Inexpensive	No manual control
	Portable	Reliance on LCD screen to frame shot
	Quiet	
Digital single lens reflex camera (digital SLR)	High image quality	Bulky
	Manual controls	Can be complex
	Adaptability of lenses and filters	No live LCD screen
		Expensive

The Mohs surgery suite's needs, budget, layout, and staff experience with photography will determine what is suitable for the office. Comparison of digital camera options is outlined in Table 4.1.

Digital photography relies on databases that allow archiving, retrieving, and organization of digital images.

If the practice uses an electronic medical record (EMR) system, consider speaking to information technology personnel about attaching digital photographs to the EMR. Investing in photography software is another way to organize and edit images. One may use the image software enclosed with the camera or purchase an appropriate program. Another option is to purchase dermatology specific photography software. Other items to account for include equipment malfunction and the need for a backup system, such as a Polaroid camera. It is important to backup the digital photography system daily.

4.3.2 Laser Safety

For many Mohs surgeons, laser surgery is an integral part of their practice. Since lasers are often stored in the Mohs operative rooms, laser use must adhere to laser safety regulatory standards. In the US, guidance for laser safety is outlined in the ANSI (American National Standards Institute) Z136 series of standards [7]. These standards are produced by the Laser Institute of America and accepted by the US Food and Drug Administration (FDA). Overall, laser-specific goggles should be available for the patient and personnel during treatment sessions. The appropriate sign indicating the laser type must be placed on the door during laser operation. Laser shades are required on windows and must be drawn during laser use. Finally, a fire extinguisher should be easily accessible in the event of a fire.

Summary: Mohs Surgery Operative Room Equipment

- Surgical equipment for Mohs surgery operative rooms is a significant cost investment. Key items include: surgical table and surrounding ergonomic aids, lights, sink, electrosurgical equipment, suction, mayo stand/kick bucket, and waste disposal containers.

4.4 Mohs Surgery Operative Room Equipment

Surgical equipment for Mohs surgery operative rooms is a significant cost investment and should be chosen carefully for high quality and longevity. Ergonomics is an applied science that evaluates the characteristics of humans that need to be considered, when designing things people use, to make the interaction most effective and safe. In short, it is important to "buy good quality equipment and save your back" [3]. All key equipment, from the operating table to the laboratory microscope, must be designed to promote proper ergonomics. If possible, it is advisable to test large surgical equipment prior to purchase. For example, it is recommended to lie on the operating table for 10–20 min to determine its comfort since patients will lie on it for longer periods of time. When large equipment is delivered, thoroughly test it to assure proper working condition. Regular maintenance and cleaning will prolong the life of the equipment.

4.4.1 Surgical Table

The surgical table is the centerpiece of the operating room and one of the most important equipment-purchasing decisions. There are two basic types of tables, hydraulic or electric-powered. Hydraulic tables work via a pump that forces hydraulic fluid through hydraulic pistons [6]. The benefit of hydraulic tables over electric tables is that they allow faster table adjustment and last longer. Electric tables can be hand-operated, foot-operated or both. Foot operation is usually preferred, especially for intraoperative adjustments.

Variables to consider when purchasing a surgical table include table width and entry height. While a wider table may be more comfortable for a large patient, a narrower table allows the Mohs surgeon to access the surgical site more easily and maintain good ergonomic posture. Similarly, while armrests may be more comfortable for the patient and safer for senile patients that might roll, it creates a bulky operating table for the surgeon. Surgical tables with a low entry height are very important for the elderly or handicapped patients and facilitate easier transfer from wheelchairs. Other surgical table accessories to consider include headrests, armboards, footboards, and stirrups. Since Mohs surgery is often performed around the head and neck areas, small headrests are preferable for easier access.

Adjustability is another consideration when buying a surgical table. The number of "mobile" joints or break points determines the adjustability of the operating table. The options include: back elevation, foot elevation, table elevation, and tilt elevation [4]. The combination of the four positions allows flexibility in patient positioning and

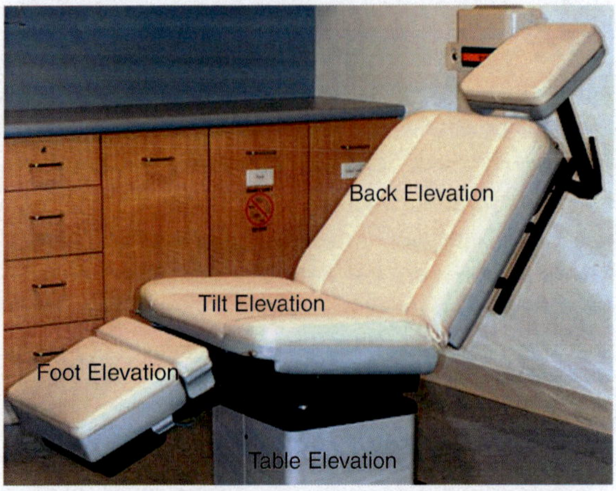

Fig. 4.3 Surgical table demonstrating four mobile joints/break points

comfort (Fig. 4.3). Some tables with programmable controls allow, with the push of a single button, configuration to a set position. All tables must allow tilt adjustment to the Trendelenburg position (head below the heart) for managing vasovagal reactions. It is the tilt adjustment that can place the patient into the Trendelenburg position.

4.4.2 Ergonomic Aids Around the Surgical Operating Table

In a recent survey of American College of Mohs Surgery members, 90% of respondents reported some type of musculoskeletal pain including neck, lower back, shoulders, and upper back (Personal communication, pending publication, Christine Liang, M.D.). Leg edema is a common complaint among Mohs surgeons due to the amount of time spent standing in static positions. In addition to compression stockings and gel insoles in shoes, other aids include: foot rails, which encourage an active stance; and antifatigue mats that reduce static stress in legs by forcing the feet to move to maintain stability [8]. Sit–stand stools and pelvic tilt chairs are other ergonomic aids around the operating table that can reduce leg edema by taking pressure off the legs. In addition, they can reduce neck, shoulder, and back pain, especially when sternal support is included.

4.4.3 Surgical Lights

Proper lighting is extremely important in all surgical procedures. Surgical lights can be mounted on the ceiling, wall, or floor. Ceiling-mounted track lights are the gold standard due to easy adjustability and not requiring floor space. Ceiling composition and height play a role when choosing surgical lights. Nine-foot ceilings are compatible with many commercial lighting fixtures [6]. Ceiling-mounted track lighting offers the greatest range of motion (360°), but it requires special structural steel beams to accommodate the weight and provide stability (Fig. 4.4). While a ceiling-mounted mini O.R. light can be used, the range of motion is limited to 300° and can be difficult to maneuver (Fig. 4.5). To avoid arm and back strain when turning ceiling-mounted lights on and off, a light switch can be placed on the wall.

There are several variables to consider when purchasing surgical lights. The intensity of light output is usually expressed in footcandles, which is related to the type of bulb and filter. Surgical lights range from 3,000 to 8,000 footcandles. Reflective dish diameter and shape (concavity) of the light determines the field size and focus depth. As the dish diameter decreases, the field size also decreases. Depth of field and focal point are related to the degree of the dish's concavity with some models having a focusing knob that sharpens the intensity of light within the depth of field. Some lights have a reflective area around the bulb that disperses the light and provides a greater field size. The reflective light also minimizes shadow and produces less heat on the surgical field. Filters can be added for color correction, giving tissue a more natural appearance [3, 9].

Eye fatigue and headaches are partially caused by bright lights and glare. Objects in the surgical field contributing to glare include skin, surgical antiseptic preparations, bloody tissue, and instruments. Reducing glare from the operative field can lessen eye fatigue and suggestions include: drying the surgical site, using goggles and glasses coated with antiglare film, and using brushed steel instead of polished steel surgical instruments [8].

4.4.4 Surgical Sink

A surgical sink with foot pedals is preferable for Mohs surgery operative rooms. While more expensive than conventional sinks, they prevent contamination of the hands when turning off sink water controls. They are often paired with foot-operated soap dispensers. A sink with a depth of 18–24 in. is recommended to decrease splash and encourage a good water stream when hand washing [4].

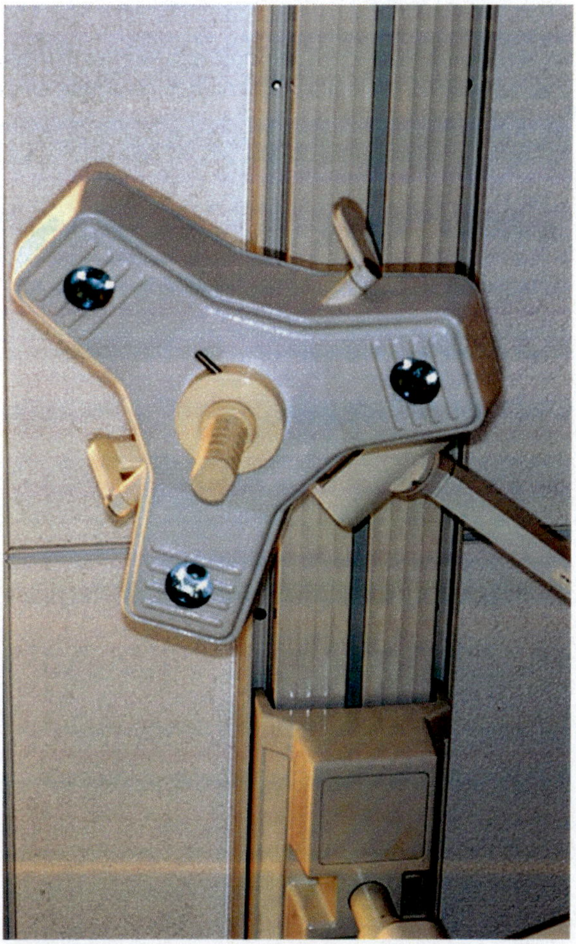

Fig. 4.4 Surgical light: ceiling-mounted track light

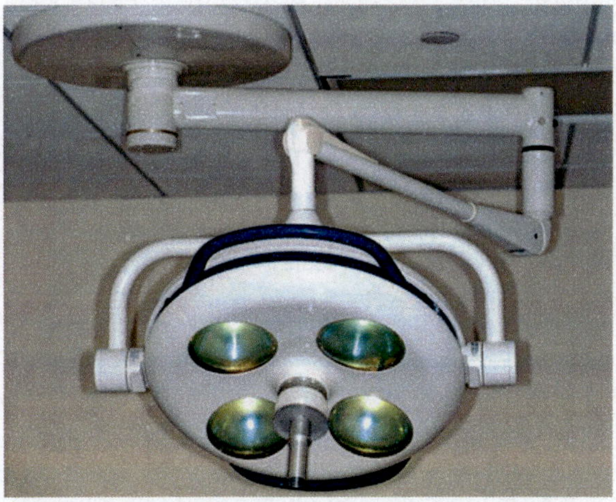

Fig. 4.5 Surgical light: ceiling-mounted mini OR light

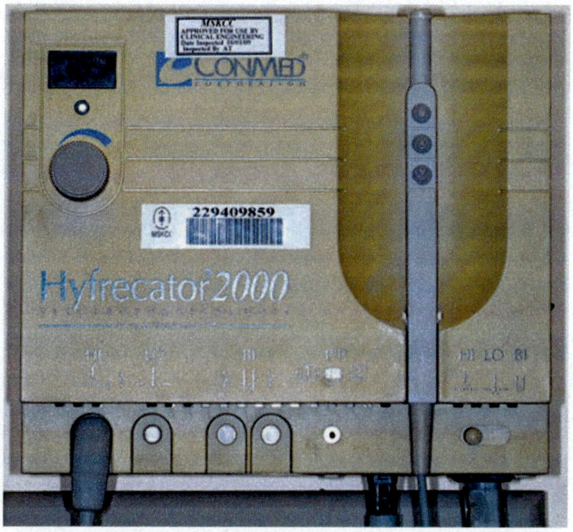

Fig. 4.6 Monoterminal electrosurgical device (Hyfrecator)

4.4.5 Electrosurgical Equipment

Electrosurgery refers to the use of electricity to cause thermal tissue damage in the form of coagulation and tissue dehydration. The two main types are high-frequency electrosurgery and electrocautery. In brief, high-frequency electrosurgery involves the passage of high-frequency alternating current through the skin where it is converted to heat and results in thermal tissue damage. Electrosurgery devices are either monoterminal or biterminal.

In monoterminal machines, commonly referred to as hyfrecators, one electrode delivers current to the patient (Fig. 4.6). The patient briefly stores the energy and then it is shed into the surrounding environment. Since current accumulates within the patient, high voltage is required to sustain current flow. These high voltage machines have low amperage (current) in order to minimize tissue damage. They cause superficial thermal tissue damage with decreased risk of scarring with lower power settings. Higher power settings can be used for electrocoagulation, but also increase the risk for superficial scarring and hypopigmentation.

Conversely, biterminal machines have a second, dispersive electrode which completes the electrical circuit from the patient back to the machine (Fig. 4.7). Thus, a lower voltage can be used to achieve increased amperage. The higher amperage causes a deeper and more thorough destruction. In addition, electrocoagulation can be achieved with less carbonization.

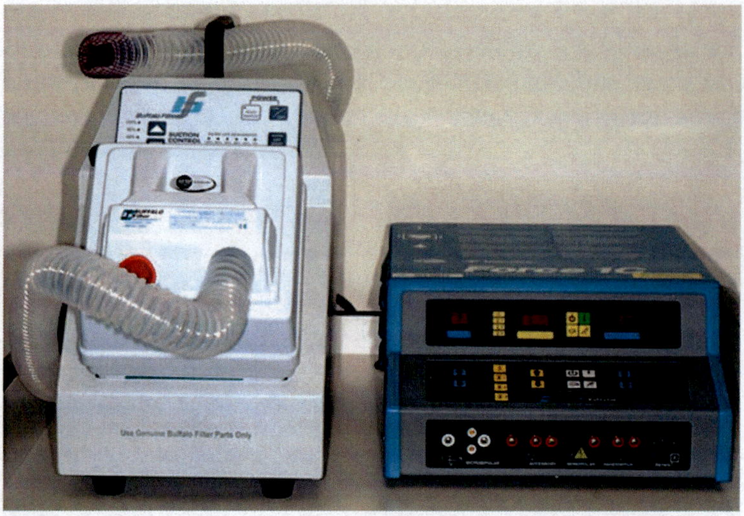

Fig. 4.7 (*left* to *right*) Smoke evacuator, biterminal electrosurgical device

Compared to electrosurgery, electrocautery differs in that direct current is used to heat an electrode that causes thermal damage by direct heat transference to tissue. Whereas the electrode remains cold in high-frequency electrosurgery, in electrocautery, it is hot. Electrocautery uses a low voltage and high amperage and is good for pinpoint hemostasis. It is the preferred electrosurgical device for patients with pacemakers and defibrillators as no current flows through the patient.

Understanding the pros and cons of each electrosurgery system can help one choose the best device for the Mohs surgery operative suite. The monoterminal hyfrecator does not provide cutting current and therefore is primarily a coagulating instrument. In addition, it requires a dry field to work effectively. The biterminal devices provide cutting and coagulating currents. These devices however can be bulky and require use of a grounding pad. Furthermore, the high amperage provided by these machines can lead to scarring when treating benign superficial lesions. A portable, battery-powered electrocautery device works well in a bloody field and can be used in patients with pacemakers and defibrillators since there is no current directly involved. However, they may not be sufficient for extensive surgical procedures and require frequent battery changes [4]. Irrespective of device choice, one must use sterile tips and have a method to sterilize the handle between patients. Disposable tips and handle covers are readily available.

Currently, there are no specific Occupational Safety and Health Administration (OSHA) standards for laser/electrosurgery smoke hazards [10]. Nonetheless, use of a smoke evacuator is recommended for several reasons (Fig. 4.7). The smell of burning skin can be disconcerting to many patients and surgical plume can lead to respiratory irritation in patients and staff. In addition, while there is no documented transmission of infectious disease through surgical smoke, there is a potential to generate infectious viral particles.

4.4.6 Suction

Electrical suction devices remove blood from the operative field during surgery. Suction units are available as mobile or wall-mounted devices. Mobile units on an equipment cart are often preferred due to ease of positioning around the patient. Wall-mounted suction outlets connected to a central suction unit save space and eliminate noise but can be very costly to install and maintain. Overall, the suction should be capable of producing a negative suction of 40–60 mmHg [3]. Disposable supplies for suction units include presterilized suction tubing and tips (Fig. 4.8).

4.4.7 Mayo Stand/Kick Bucket

Mayo stands are an essential part of a Mohs surgery operative room allowing easy access to surgical instruments during procedures. Different features on Mayo stands include: platform size and movement, mechanism for raising and lowering the platform, and number of wheels ranging from 2 to 6. Four- to six-wheeled mayo stands are preferred for ease of movement.

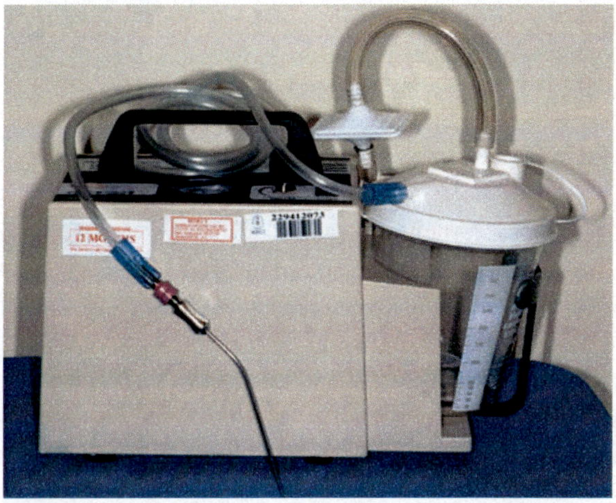

Fig. 4.8 Suction device

A stand with a modified base, either circular or tapered, accommodates a kick bucket within the base (Fig. 4.9). Two mayo stands in each operative room allow surgical instruments to be organized on one and wound dressing materials on the other. Kick buckets with wheels are convenient as they can be easily moved by foot during a procedure. They are made of stainless steel often with a protective hard rubber steel rim.

4.4.8 Waste Disposal

State and federal laws govern medical waste disposal. It is important to review relevant information from regulatory agencies to ensure that the Mohs surgery suite meets local, state and federal standards. The regulations will outline how medical waste should be handled, divided, and disposed. The Mohs surgery suite needs to be equipped with proper waste disposal devices for all sharps and biohazardous materials.

A sharps disposal container must be present in each Mohs surgery operative room. The type and volume of the sharps container chosen is based on the sharps being disposed. The sharps container should be durable, closable, and puncture and leak resistant on the bottom and sides [11]. The sharps container location is immediately accessible to the surgeon and assistant without obstacles to reduce risk of injury. Its optimal height for a standing work area is between 52" to 56"above the floor and 38" to 42" above the floor for a seated work area [11]. This configuration allows a person disposing sharps to reach the sharps container horizontally.

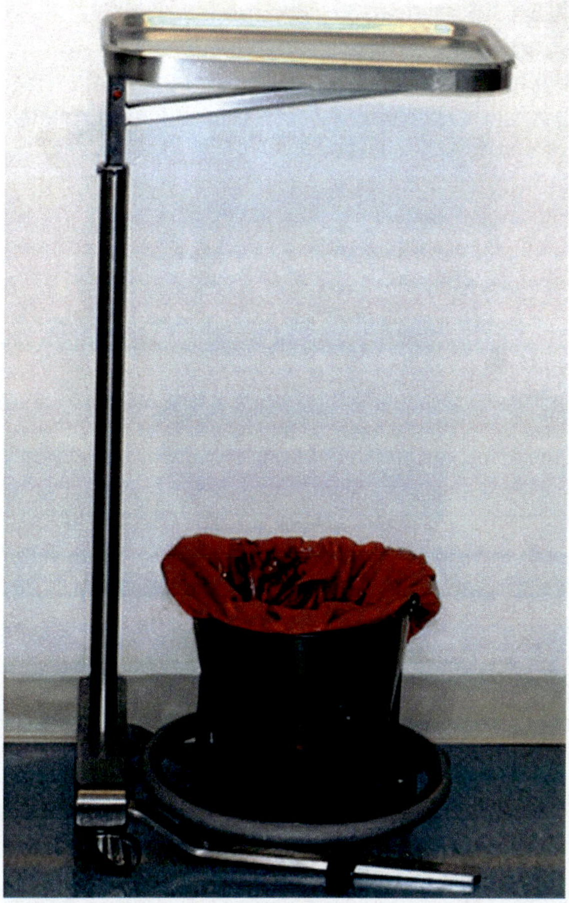

Fig. 4.9 Mayo stand with kick bucket

Containers used to transport or store regulated medical waste must have a warning label affixed to it. In lieu of biohazard signs, a red bag or red container may be used [12]. Red bags should be used in the kick bucket during surgery to discard any bloody items: gauze, suction canisters, or bandages. All other trash can be discarded as regular waste, including drapes and gowns.

Summary: Personal Protective Equipment

- Mohs surgery exposes surgeons and assistants to blood-borne pathogens. All operative rooms should be equipped with personal protective equipment (PPE) such as masks, eye protection, gowns, and gloves.

4.5 Personal Protective Equipment

OSHA defines personal protective equipment (PPE) as "specialized clothing or equipment, worn by an employee for protection against infectious materials" [12]. Since Mohs surgery exposes surgeons and assistants to blood-borne pathogens, all operative rooms should be equipped with PPE such as masks, eye protection, gowns, and gloves.

4.5.1 Masks and Eye Protection

Due to the potential for exposure to blood droplets into the eye, nose, or mouth, the surgeon and assistants must wear a face mask and safety goggles. Masks may tie at the nape of the neck and around the back of the head or fit over the ears. To provide a secure fit and prevent fogging of goggles during surgery, masks should be equipped with an adjustable aluminum nosepiece. Safety goggles that cover the eyes up to the brow bone and have anti-fog and anti-scratch coatings are ideal.

4.5.2 Gowns

Gowns offer coverage of the torso, arms, and thigh area. There are a variety of gowns available for medical wear with varying degrees of fluid resistance. Isolation gowns are made of breathable fabric, feature neck and waist ties, and protect the wearer from light splashes. For more fluid resistance, sterile operating room gowns which attach at the nape of the neck and tie around the waist are an option. These offer the highest level of protection against fluid penetration. However, single-use gowns may not be cost efficient.

4.5.3 Scrubs

Scrubs are an alternative option to surgical gowns. Because they are short sleeved, scrubs prevent the contamination of the surgical site from long sleeves dragging into the field. Scrubs also protect the wearers' body, but they are not impermeable to fluid. They are a great option for office-based surgery as they are loose and comfortable. Scrubs are also easily laundered and look professional.

4.5.4 Gloves

There are a variety of medical gloves available including latex, vinyl, nitrile, or neoprene exam gloves and sterile gloves with varying characteristics (Table 4.2). Although Mohs surgery is performed under a clean technique, using sterile gloves during defect reconstruction offers superior protection and durability. Ultimately, patients' allergies and the wearers' comfort determine the choice of gloves. For patients with true latex allergies, it is important to stock vinyl exam and sterile neoprene gloves in several sizes.

Summary: Instrumentation and Setup

- High-quality stainless steel instruments are essential in Mohs surgery. The key instruments needed during Mohs surgery, defect closures, excisions and special site surgeries are listed.

4.6 Instrumentation and Setup

Given the demands of Mohs surgery, high-quality stainless steel instruments are essential. Ideally, instruments should be stored in the Mohs surgery operative room for easy access. If there is a lack of storage space, the operative room can be stocked with a few basic instrument packages for backup and emergency situations. As the surgical instruments are delicate, they should be handled with care, and cleaned and stored properly after each use.

4.6.1 Scalpels

The two main scalpels used in Mohs surgery are the Bard Parker #3 and the Siegel handle. The Bard Parker #3 can be flat or rounded with an optional etched ruler on one side. The Siegel handle is smaller, with a hexagonal or round contour and is good for delicate work. It is also easier to use for Mohs surgeons with smaller

Table 4.2 Summary of surgical gloves

Material	Pros	Cons
Latex	Superior protection Elasticity Comfortable fit High tactile sensitivity	Latex allergy Dry irritated skin
Vinyl	Economical Latex free	Less durable synthetic Degradation with chemical exposure Poor tactile sensitivity Poor fit Lower barrier protection
Nitrile	Excellent barrier protection Highest chemical and puncture resistance Latex free	High cost
Neoprene	High tactile sensitivity Puncture resistant Excellent barrier protection Latex free	High cost Less elastic than latex

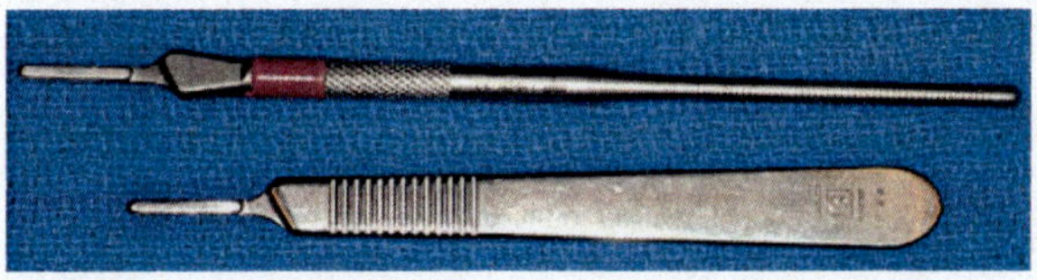

Fig. 4.10 Scalpels: (*top* to *bottom*) Siegel handle, Bard Parker #3

hands. The Siegel handle can accommodate standard blades (Fig. 4.10).

4.6.2 Blades

The #15 blade is the most commonly used blade. It has a convex shape with the sharpest point at the tip. The #15c is a smaller blade which is useful for delicate areas on the face. The #11 blade is triangular in shape with a sharp point good for precision cutting. The #10 blade is a bigger version of the #15 blade and is better for thicker skin like the back (Fig. 4.11).

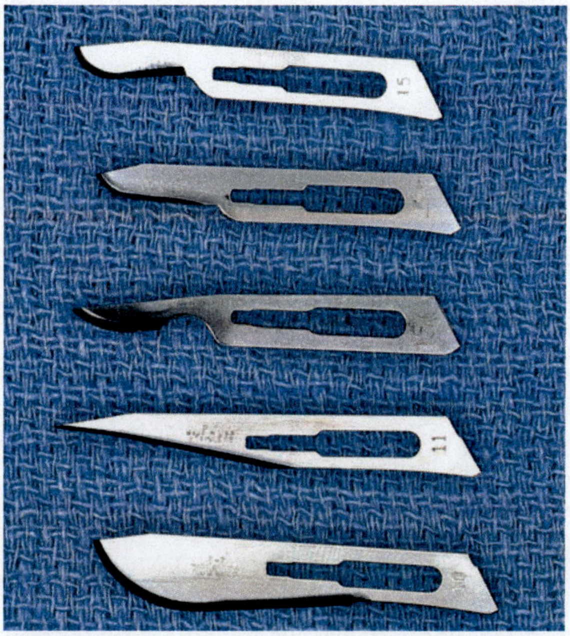

Fig. 4.11 Blades: (*top* to *bottom*) #15, #15 Personna, #15C, #11, #10

4.6.3 Standard Mohs Surgery Setup

The Mohs surgery tray for the initial stage usually consists of (Fig. 4.12):

1. 4×4 gauze and/or cotton-tipped applicator sticks
2. Fenestrated surgical drape
3. Mohs tray to transport tissue into Mohs lab
4. Hemostasis (aluminum chloride, electrosurgery, pressure)
5. Gentian violet pen or ink for tissue orientation markings
6. Fox curette – used to debulk tumors prior to removing the first layer, curette sizes range from 1 to 9.

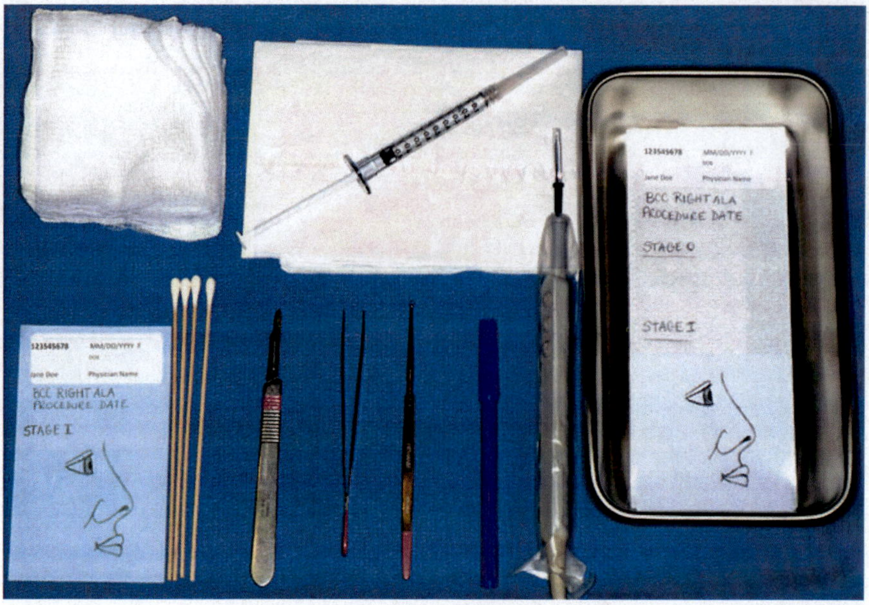

Fig. 4.12 Standard Mohs surgery stage tray: (clockwise from *top left* corner) Gauze pads, fenestrated drape with anesthesia, labeled Mohs tray, electrosurgery device, marking pen, curette, forcep, scalpel with 15 blade, cotton tip applicators, Mohs map

The number refers to the width of the opening in millimeters
7. Adson forceps – fine teeth minimize tissue damage
8. Scalpel with blade
9. Mohs map with diagram of anatomic site

4.6.4 Mohs Surgery Eye Tray

In addition to the items used in a standard Mohs surgery stage tray, the following are useful when working around the eyes (Fig. 4.13):

1. Eye shield remover
2. Plastic corneal eye shield – available in small, medium, or large sizes
3. Scalpel with blade
4. Gradle scissor
5. Adson or Bishop-Harmon forcep – useful in delicate areas to grasp small tissue pieces
6. Suction – Frazier 6 French–size tip is effective
7. Chalazion clamps – to immobilize tissue (not pictured)

4.6.5 Excision/Closure Tray for Face

The following items can be used for excisions or closures on the face (Fig. 4.14):

1. Suture cutting scissor
2. Hartman hemostat – to clamp vessels during ligation
3. Needle driver – size may vary depending on surgeon preference and comfort; size should be proportional to size of suture needle
4. Gradle scissors – optional for more delicate closures; shorter with blade slightly curved giving better control [4]
5. Skin hook – a small two-pronged skin hook is recommended to retract skin since it minimizes tissue damage compared to retractors
6. Adson forceps with suture platform – aides in stabilizing the needle while suturing
7. Scalpel handle with blade of choice
8. Miscellaneous items – gauze, cotton-tipped applicator sticks, fenestrated drapes or towels, electrosurgery pencil with a sterile plastic sheath, local anesthesia, sterile light handle cover

4.6.6 Excision/Closure Tray for Trunk

For excisions/closures on the trunk, the following modifications are made to the tray (Fig. 4.15):

1. Hemostat – medium or larger size
2. Suture-cutting scissor
3. Medium/Large Needle driver
4. Supercut Par Undermining Scissors

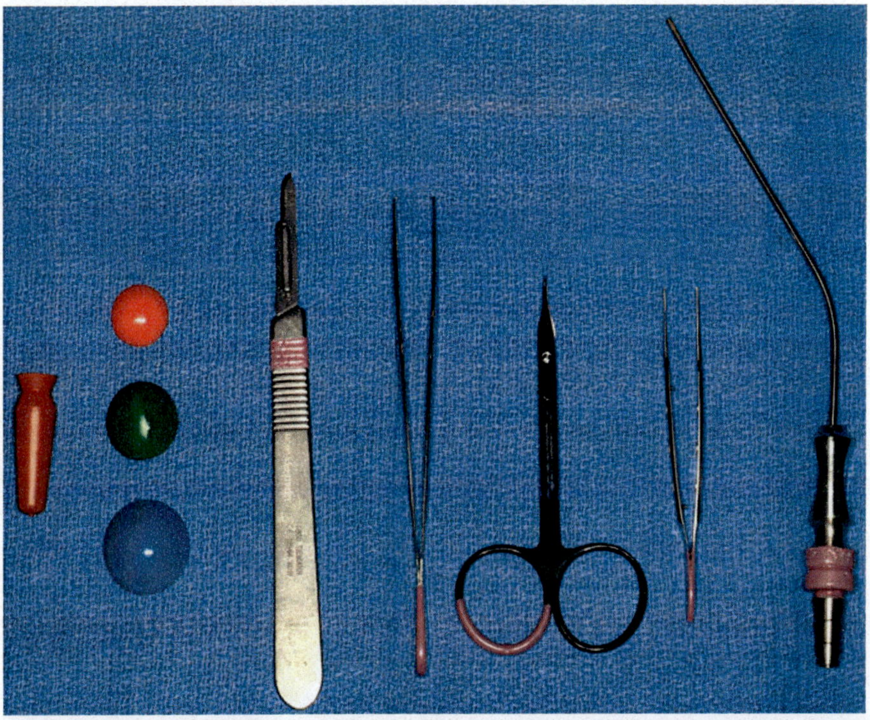

Fig. 4.13 Mohs surgery eye tray: (*left* to *right*) eye shield remover, plastic corneal eye shields in small, medium and large, scalpel with blade, Adson forcep, gradle scissors, Bishop-Harmon forcep, suction

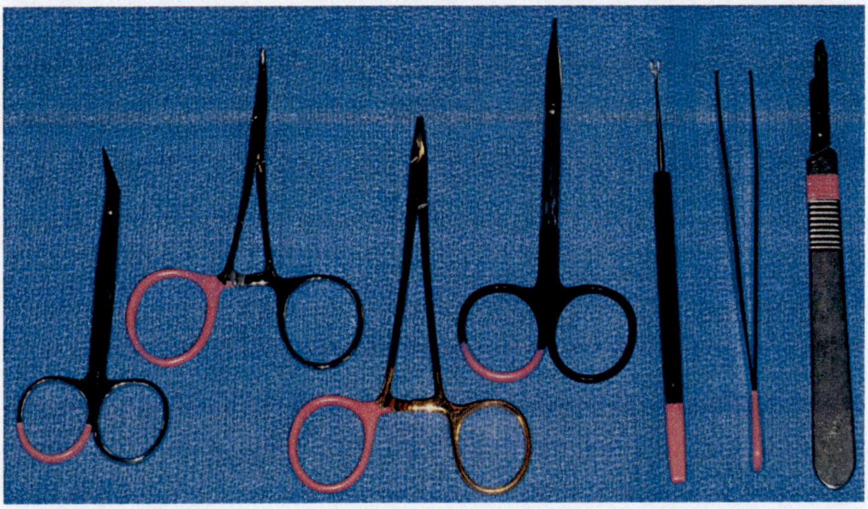

Fig. 4.14 Excision/closure tray for face: (*left* to *right*) suture scissors, hemostat, needle driver, gradle scissors, skin hook, Adson forceps, scalpel with blade

5. Skin hook – 2–4 pronged hook useful in thicker tissue
6. Adson forcep
7. Scalpel handle with blade

4.6.7 Nail Surgery Instruments

In cases where nail removal is necessary, the following instruments are recommended (Fig. 4.16):

1. Double-action nail splitter – causes minimal damage to the nailbed
2. Nail elevator
3. Nail-pulling forcep
4. Penrose tubing

4.6.8 Miscellaneous Instruments (Fig. 4.17)

1. Blade remover – to safely remove blades; forceps and needle holders should never be used as it can damage delicate instruments and risk injury

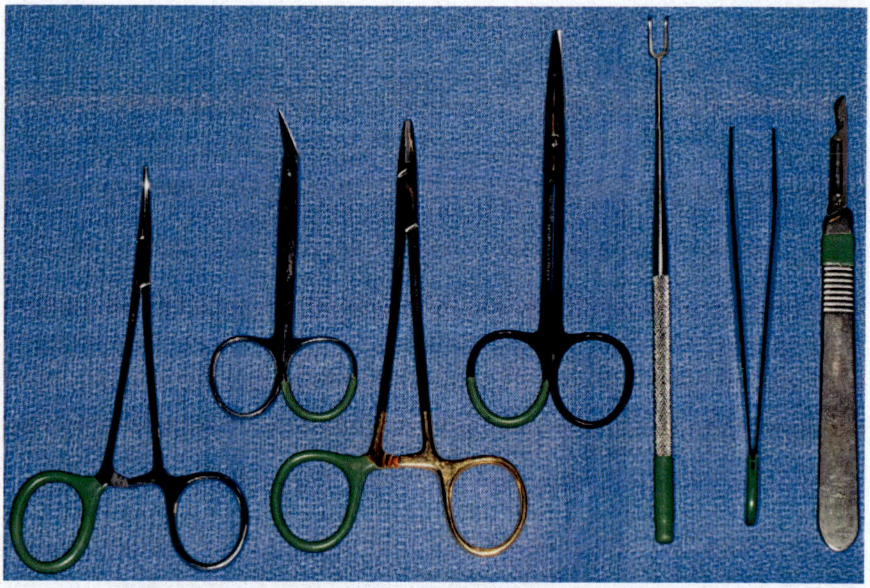

Fig. 4.15 Excision/closure tray for trunk: (*left* to *right*) hemostat, suture scissors, needle driver, Supercut Par scissors, skin hook, Adson forceps, scalpel with blade

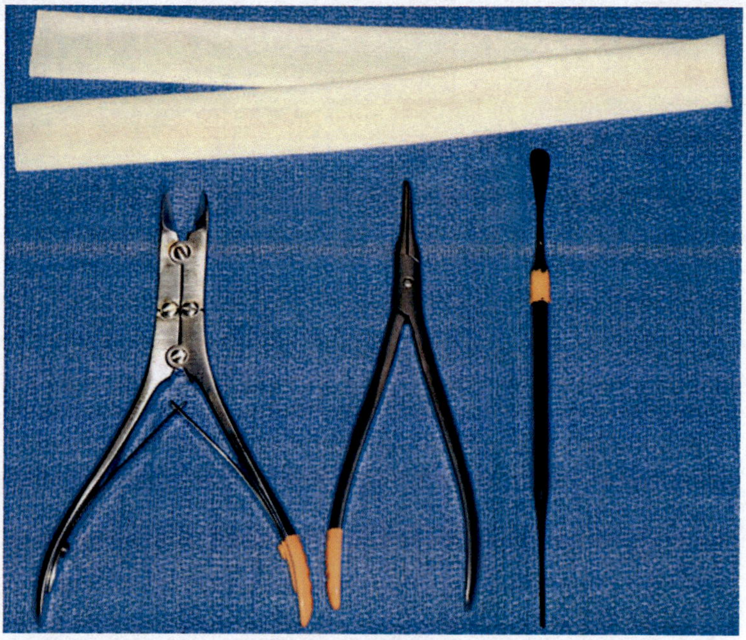

Fig. 4.16 Nail surgery instruments: (*left* to *right*) double-action nail splitter, nail pulling forcep, nail elevator, penrose tubing

2. Lister bandage scissors
3. Allis clamp – to grasp tissue such as a lipoma
4. Small metal bowl
5. Towel clamps – to secure surgical towels
6. Comedone extractor

Summary: Wound Care Dressing Materials

- The wound care materials necessary for intra and postoperative dressings are discussed.

4.7 Wound Care Dressing Materials

Mohs surgery operative rooms should be stocked with wound care dressing materials necessary for intra and postoperative dressings. If space allows, a separate area can be designated for storage of dressing supplies (i.e., on a second mayo stand). A variety of dressing materials is often necessary to accommodate the wide range of surgical procedures and anatomic sites encountered (Table 4.3).

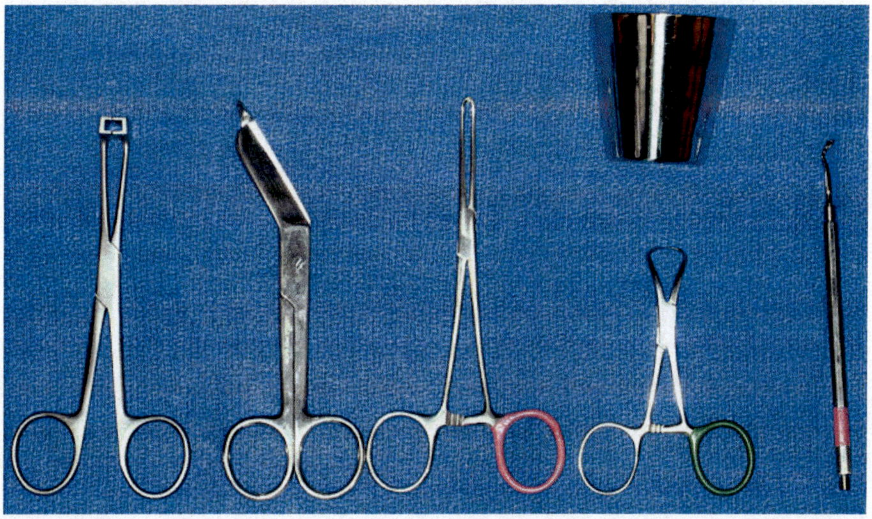

Fig. 4.17 Miscellaneous instruments: (*left* to *right*) blade remover, lister bandage scissors, Allis clamp, small metal bowl, towel clamp, comedone extractor

Table 4.3 Useful wound dressing materials

Adhesive dressings	Nonadhesive dressings	Ointments	Other
Paper tape (white and flesh colored)	Petrolatum infused gauze	Bacitracin – regular and ophthalmic	Adhesive remover
Hypafix®	Telfa	Mupirocin ointment	Mineral oil
Primapore®	Gauze	Petrolatum ointment	Cotton balls
Steri strips™	Dental rolls		Foams
Mastisol®	Surgilast tubular dressing®		
Hydrogel dressing	Coban™		
Hydrocolloid dressing			

Summary: Equipment Sterilization

- Proper cleaning and sterilization of surgical equipment is important in maintaining infection control standards. Steam autoclaving is the most practical method in an office setting.

4.8 Equipment Sterilization

Equipment sterilization depends on the composition of surgical instruments and usage. Proper cleaning and sterilization is important for maintaining infection control standards. Mohs surgery instruments are categorized as critical on the Spaulding scale, because they enter sterile tissue and could transmit microbial disease [11]. Instruments should be cleaned prior to sterilization to remove visible blood and debris and prepare instruments for safe handling. An ultrasonic cleaner is ideal because instruments are placed in a wire basket and submerged in a neutral pH detergent. The ultrasound agitation dislodges organic material in the hard to clean spaces of delicate instruments [13]. Remember that this process only renders the instruments clean not sterile.

In accordance with Center for Disease Control (CDC) guidelines, surgical instruments should be sterilized with steam if possible, or if heat sensitive, treated with Ethylene Oxide (ETO), hydrogen peroxide plasma, or liquid chemical sterilants if other methods are unsuitable [11]. Steam autoclaving is the most practical method in an office setting because it requires minimal training and has a quick treatment time. Steam autoclaves come in different sizes and the selection is based on volume of anticipated instrument usage and the size of the packaged instrument sets. Instruments that were used earlier in the day can be packaged and sterilized for usage in the afternoon. With steam sterilization, instruments are wrapped prior to sterilization, thereby maintaining sterility after processing and storage. It is a good idea to include a sterilization process indicator strip or heat sensitive tape when wrapping or packing instruments. These strips change color or darken when exposed to heat.

However, keep in mind that heat-sensitive strips confirm that packages were exposed to the sterilization process, but they do not confirm sterility. The strips are highly sensitive and can change color with heat exposure. Packages that are not yet autoclaved should not be left on top of or along the sides of the machine.

Due to federally mandated monitoring guidelines necessary for chemical or gas sterilization, particularly ETO, they are rarely used outside of hospitals. Instruments that require these methods, such as plastic corneal eyeshields can be sent to local facilities for sterilization, or the surgeon may consider purchasing eyeshields than can be autoclaved safely between 50 and 100 times before being discarded.

Summary: Monitoring and Emergency Equipment

- Office-based Mohs surgery is performed under local anesthesia without monitoring. Nonetheless, Mohs surgery offices should be equipped with an emergency kit and the office staff trained in basic life support.

4.9 Monitoring and Emergency Equipment

Although the majority of Mohs surgery cases are performed under local anesthesia without monitoring, routine vital signs such as blood pressure, heart rate and respiratory rate are often recorded. At a minimum, offices should have a thermometer, stethoscope, and manual blood pressure cuff. One can consider purchasing a pulse oximeter with an automatic blood pressure cuff that can also detect oxygen saturation [14].

Mohs surgery offices should be equipped with an emergency cart ("crash cart") or kit in case of a cardiopulmonary arrest or life-threatening drug reaction. Key office staff should be trained in basic cardiopulmonary resuscitation (CPR) and advanced cardiac life support (ACLS). In addition, an emergency plan for transporting the patient to the hospital if needed is important.

The following is a list of essential items in an emergency cart.

Essential Emergency Cart Items

- Automatic external defibrillator (AED) – these units are universally available and are part of basic CPR training
- Oropharyngeal airways
- Laryngoscope with endotracheal tubes of various sizes
- Ventilation (Ambu) bag with airways of various types and sizes
- Oxygen tank
- IV catheters of various sizes
- Bags of intravenous fluids
- Prefilled syringes/ampoules of emergency drugs including but not limited to: epinephrine, atropine, dextrose, lidocaine, sodium bicarbonate, diphenhydramine, and furosemide

Summary: Conclusion

- The careful design and building of a Mohs micrographic surgery suite will provide an environment for comfortable and efficient care of the patient, while meeting regulatory safety standards and the ergonomic needs of the staff.

4.10 Conclusion

When designing and building a Mohs surgery suite, consultation with a contractor, architect, interior designer and an occupational health specialist will ensure that the facility will meet the needs of patients and staff. Larger operative rooms will allow for future growth and longevity as will the use of durable materials on ceiling, walls and floor. All key equipment, from the operating table to the surgical instruments, should be sturdy and promote proper ergonomics. Finally, it is important to follow local, state and federal regulations regarding waste disposal, personal protection equipment, and equipment sterilization.

References

1. Drake LA, Ceilley RI, Cornelison RL, et al. Guidelines for care for office surgical facilities – Part I. J Am Acad Dermatol. 1992;26:763–5.
2. Drake LA, Ceilley RI, Cornelison RL, et al. Guidelines for care for office surgical facilities. Part II – Self-assessment checklist. J Am Acad Dermatol. 1995;33:265–70.
3. Bennett RG. Office surgical facility. In: Bennett RG, editor. Fundamentals of cutaneous surgery. 1st ed. St. Louis: Mosby; 1998.

4. Maloney M. The surgical suite. In: Grekin RC, editor. The dermatologic surgical suite, design and materials. 1st ed. New York: Churchill Livingstone; 1991.
5. Phillips P. Outpatient surgical suite. 2009. Emedicine from WebMD. http://emedicine.medscape.com/article/1128609-overview. Accessed August 3, 2010.
6. Levy R, Hanke CW. Design of the surgical suite, including large equipment and monitoring devices. In: Robinson JK, editor. Surgery of the skin: procedural dermatology. 2nd ed. New York: Mosby/Elsevier; 2010.
7. ANSI Z136 Standards. Laser Institute of America. 2010. http://www.laserinstitute.org/store/ANSI%20Z136%20Standards. Accessed September 26, 2010.
8. Esser AC, Koshy JG, Randle HW. Ergonomics in office-based surgery: a survey-guided observational study. Dermatol Surg. 2007;33:1304–14.
9. Hayes CM. Preparation of the surgical suite. In: Ratz J, editor. Textbook of dermatologic surgery. 1st ed. Philadelphia: Lippincott-Raven; 1998.
10. Laser/Electrosurgery Plume. OSHA-United States Department of Labor. 2010. http://www.osha.gov/SLTC/laserelectrosurgeryplume/index.html. Accessed September 26, 2010.
11. Rutala WA, Weber DJ, et al. Guidelines for disinfection and sterilization in healthcare facilities. Center for Disease Control. 2008. http://www.cdc.gov/ncidod/dhqp/pdf/guidelines/Disinfection_Nov_2008.pdf. Accessed August 12, 2010.
12. Bloodborne Pathogens and Needlestick Prevention. OSHA-United States Department of Labor. 2010. http://www.osha.gov/SLTC/bloodbornepathogens. Accessed August 12, 2010.
13. Bernstein G. Instrumentation for Mohs surgery. In: Mikhail GR, editor. Mohs micrographic surgery. 1st ed. Philadelphia: Saunders; 1991.
14. Gross K. Office and laboratory set-up and instrumentation in Mohs surgery. In: Gross K, editor. Mohs surgery: fundamentals and techniques. 1st ed. St. Louis: Mosby; 1999.

Anesthetic Considerations: Local Versus Regional

5

Michael P. McLeod, Sonal Choudhary, Yasser A. Alqubaisy, and Keyvan Nouri

Abstract

Local anesthesia is defined as a loss in the perception of pain over a small area of the body. Regional anesthesia is also a loss in the perception of pain, but in a larger anatomical area or region. Both local and regional anesthesia are usually achieved by pharmacological use of local anesthetic agents. There are two types of local anesthetic agents, amino-amides and amino-esters, defined by their chemical structures. Both classes achieve their effects by deactivating the sodium channels responsible for the inward flux of sodium during the depolarization phase of the action potential. The net result is an increase in the amount of stimulus required to generate an action potential as well as decreased propagation of any action potentials across the anesthetized neuron. This chapter will discuss the history, pharmacology, pharmacokinetics, metabolism, toxicities, chemical structures, as well as the clinical utility of using local anesthetics in localized and regional fashions.

Keywords

Local anesthesia • Regional anesthesia • Lidocaine • Amino-amide • Amino-ester

M.P. McLeod • S. Choudhary
Department of Dermatology and Cutaneous Surgery, University of Miami Leonard M. Miller School of Medicine, Miami, FL, USA

Y.A. Alqubaisy
Department of Dermatology and Cutaneous Surgery, University of Miami Hospital, Miami, FL, USA

K. Nouri (✉)
Department of Dermatology and Cutaneous Surgery, University of Miami Leonard M. Miller School of Medicine, Miami, FL, USA

Sylvester Comprehensive Cancer Center, University of Miami Hospital and Clinics, Miami, FL, USA
e-mail: knouri@med.miami.edu

Summary: Introduction

- Local anesthesia is a loss in the perception of pain in a small or localized area of the body.
- Regional anesthesia is also defined as a loss in sensation, but encompasses a larger area, or region, of tissue, and is usually achieved in a pharmacological and temporary fashion.

K. Nouri (ed.), *Mohs Micrographic Surgery*,
DOI 10.1007/978-1-4471-2152-7_5, © Springer-Verlag London Limited 2012

5.1 Introduction

Local anesthesia is a loss in the perception of pain over a small or localized area of the body. It is usually achieved by pharmacologically manipulating the electrochemical activity of peripheral nerves in a temporary fashion with the end result being to decrease impulse propagation or generation. Regional anesthesia is also defined as a loss in sensation, but encompasses a larger area, or region, of tissue, and is also usually achieved in a pharmacological and temporary fashion [1].

Summary: History

- The first known anesthetic was derived from the leaves of the coca plant in South America.
- The first prototype of injectable local anesthetic was procaine; a derivative of para-aminobenzoic acid (PABA).
- Lidocaine was developed in 1948 as the first amino-amide local anesthetic and is associated with less allergic reactions than its ester predecessors.

5.2 History

The first known anesthetic was derived from the leaves of the coca plant in South America and was extracted in 1860. However, the purified product of the coca plant was not used for medicinal purposes until 1884 when Freud and Koller used it as a topical agent [2]. Shortly thereafter, Halsted and Hall used cocaine for regional anesthesia by intravenously infusing it into the brachial vein [2]. The first prototype of injectable local anesthetic was procaine [3], which consists of an aromatic head, a hydrocarbon chain, and a terminal amine tail [3]. It is a derivative of para-aminobenzoic acid (PABA) and is a type of amino-ester.

Lidocaine was developed in 1948 [3], as the first amino-amide local anesthetic [3]. Its aromatic head and hydrocarbon chain are attached by an amide bond [3]. Lidocaine is associated with considerably less allergic reactions than its ester predecessors [3], because the amide bond is much more stable than the ester bond. Therefore, the highly allergenic aromatic acid does not get cleaved as in esters and stimulate an allergic response [3]. Numerous other amino-amide local anesthetics were later developed as a result of this advantageous property [3]. The chemical structure of amino-amide local anesthetics consists of an aromatic portion, and a tertiary amine which are connected by a hydrocarbon chain [4].

Summary: Pharmacology

- Local anesthetics are thought to bind to the sodium channels during their inactivated and activated states with more affinity than the resting state.
- Repeated depolarizations result in more effective anesthetic binding to the sodium channels.
- When the neuron becomes excited to a certain threshold, the membrane becomes depolarized with an inward rush of sodium ions.
- Local anesthetics target the cytoplasmic side of the receptor.
- The lower the pKa, the greater the proportion of unionized molecules for a given pH.
- Approximately, 25% of the epinephrine is degraded per week in neutral solution.
- Most local anesthetics are vasodilators.
- One way to increase the time duration by which local anesthetics exert their effect is to mix a vasoconstrictor with the local anesthetic.

5.3 Pharmacology

The resting membrane potential (RMP) of neurons is −90 mV. When the neuron becomes excited to a threshold, the membrane becomes depolarized with an inward rush of sodium ions, followed by an outward flow of potassium ions that brings the membrane potential back into equilibrium. The local anesthetics achieve their effects by inhibiting the sodium channels of neurons, thereby making it more difficult for a membrane potential to reach the threshold required for depolarization [3]. They achieve their effects on the cytoplasmic side of the receptor. In addition, it is the charged form of the local anesthetic that binds to the receptor. The charged form of the molecule cannot pass through the membrane; it can only pass through the membrane in its uncharged form. Following its

Table 5.1 Important characteristics of local anesthetics

Amino-esters	Approximate time to take effect	pK_a at 25°C	Duration of anesthetic effect (+/– epinephrine)	Max dose (with epinephrine/without)
Cocaine	5 min		2–3 h	
Procaine	Slow	9.0	30 min/90 min	1,000 mg/–
Tetracaine	Slow	8.4	4 h/8 h	Only topical and spinal
Amino-amides				
Prilocaine	Rapid	7.9	2 h	
Bupivacaine	5 min	8.1	4 h/8 h	
Lidocaine	Rapid	7.9	2 h/6 h	300 mg/500 mg
Mepivacaine	10 min	7.7	2 h/6 h	400 mg/500 mg

passage though the membrane, the molecule must become protonated to its active form so that it can interact with the sodium channels.

Local anesthetics are thought to bind to the sodium channels during their inactivated and activated states with more affinity then the resting state [3]. They dissociate from the inactivated state of the sodium channels at a much lower rate compared to the activated state. Therefore, repeated depolarizations result in more effective anesthetic binding to the sodium channels [3]. This concept is termed the "use-dependent" or "frequency-dependent" effect of local anesthesia [3]. Nerves that are more active are more likely to become anesthetized compared to inactive nerves.

A basic understanding of how pH affects local anesthetics is important to their clinical use. The Henderson-Hasselbalch equation:

$$pH = PKa + long \left[base\right] / \left[acid\right]$$

is useful to determine if a local anesthetic exists as a charged or uncharged molecule [3]. The lower the pKa, the greater the proportion of unionized molecules for a given pH [3]. Any acidic conditions such as an infective process may lead to a delay in the onset of anesthesia (see Table 5.1). Most local anesthetics have an alkaline to neutral pH. Epinephrine is rapidly degraded in an alkaline solution. Approximately, 25% of the epinephrine is degraded per week in neutral solution. Therefore, most commercial preparations of local anesthetics, such as lidocaine, are kept in an acidic solution [2]. Unfortunately, the acidic local anesthetic solution causes more pain than when a basic or neutral local anesthetic solution is injected [2]. This can be countered by adding sodium bicarbonate in a 1:10 ratio or 1 mL of 8.4% bicarbonate for every 9 mL of lidocaine [5].

Most local anesthetics are vasodilators; however, there are some exceptions. Notably, the S (–) enantiomer of ropivacaine has some vasoconstrictive activity in comparison to its R (+) enantiomer, and cocaine is a vasoconstrictor. One way to increase the time duration by which local anesthetics exert their effect is to mix a vasoconstrictor with the local anesthetic. Epinephrine is commonly used for this purpose at doses of 5 μg/mL. Care should be taken in patients who have hypertension or any predisposition to cardiac arrhythmias. It is also recommended that epinephrine not be used in areas with poor collateral flow, such as the digits.

Summary: Pharmacokinetics

- The circulatory system "washes away" the anesthetic from its local site.
- Local anesthetics that are highly lipophilic and have a high affinity for protein binding tend to stay localized to one area longer than local anesthetics that are highly hydrophilic and do not have a high affinity for protein binding.

5.4 Pharmacokinetics

Local anesthetics are unique drugs in that the circulatory system does not distribute the drug to its intended target. Instead, the circulatory system actually "washes away" the anesthetic from its local site, thereby curtailing its effect on the local tissue. The uptake of the local anesthetic via the blood can also lead to its toxicity. Local anesthetics that are highly lipophilic and have a high affinity for protein binding tend to stay localized to one area longer than local anesthetics that are highly hydrophilic and do not have a high affinity for protein binding.

Summary: Regional Anesthesia

- Regional anesthesia most often takes the form of nerve blocks.
- The advantages of regional anesthesia include: no tissue distortion at the operative site, and a much larger area can be anesthetized with less anesthetic agent.
- The anesthetic should be injected in the vicinity of the nerve, not the nerve itself, and not into a nearby blood vessel.

5.5 Regional Anesthesia

Regional anesthesia most often takes the form of nerve blocks. The most common nerve blocks performed in dermatologic surgery take place at the digital and trigeminal nerves [6]. There are some important advantages associated with regional anesthesia: there is no tissue distortion at the operative site, and a much larger area can be anesthetized with less anesthetic. Despite the advantages, there are also a number of serious complications that can occur with a nerve block, namely, physical nerve damage, hematoma, and intravascular injection. The anesthetic should be injected in the vicinity of the nerve, not the nerve itself, and should also not be injected in a nearby blood vessel. The technique may be assisted by the use of an ultrasound and muscle stimulator to help visualize proximity of the needle to vital structures and localize the correct location for injecting anesthetic.

5.6 Peripheral Nerve Fibers

Peripheral nerve fibers are classified by their diameter and the presence or absence of myelin [3]. The larger the diameter of a nerve, the faster the conduction velocity. The presence of myelin also leads to a faster conduction velocity among nerves. The spaces between each myelin sheath, i.e., unmyelinated areas, are known as nodes of Ranvier. The electrical flow of current "jumps" between the nodes of Ranvier due to the insulating property of the nodes.

When a local anesthetic is injected near a nerve, it infiltrates the nervous tissue from the outside toward the inside of the nerve; therefore, nerve fibers near the outside or mantle of a nerve are anesthetized first. Generally, the nervous fibers running along the outside of a nerve innervate more proximal anatomical structures, while those running deep innervate more distal structures [3]. The smaller nerve fibers become anesthetized before the larger nerve fibers. The nocioceptive C fibers are usually blocked before the nerves carrying pressure information, so a patient usually does not feel pain but may still perceive pressure [5].

Summary: Peripheral Nerve Fibers

- Peripheral nerve fibers are classified by their diameter and the presence or absence of myelin.
- The larger the diameter of a nerve, the faster the conduction velocity.
- When local anesthetics are injected near a nerve, they infiltrate the nervous tissue from the outside toward the inside; therefore, nerve fibers near the outside or mantle of a nerve are anesthetized first.
- The nervous fibers running along the outside of a nerve innervate more proximal anatomical structures, while those running deeply innervate more distal structures.

Summary: Metabolism

- The amino-ester molecules are metabolized via hydrolysis, while the amino-amides are metabolized via hepatic microsomal enzymes.
- Lidocaine, prilocaine, and bupivacaine are extracted from the circulatory system by the lungs.
- People who are deficient in cholinesterases are at an increased risk of developing toxic levels of amino-ester anesthetics, especially chloroprocaine.
- Lidocaine is extensively metabolized by the liver and is highly dependent upon hepatic blood flow.

5.7 Metabolism

The amino-amide and amino-ester local anesthetics are metabolized in very different ways. The amino-ester molecules are metabolized via hydrolysis by plasma cholinesterase and excreted in the kidneys, while the amino-amides are metabolized via de-alkylation and hydrolysis by hepatic microsomal enzymes [5]. In addition, lidocaine, prilocaine, and bupivacaine are extracted from the circulatory system by the lungs. The local anesthetics are lipophilic molecules, and therefore less than 5% of the injected dose is cleared by the kidneys [3].

People who are deficient in cholinesterases are at an increased risk of developing toxic levels of amino-ester anesthetics, especially chloroprocaine.

Lidocaine is extensively metabolized by the liver and is highly dependent upon hepatic blood flow. Any liver disease or medical conditions which limit blood flow to the liver such as congestive heart failure can impair the clearance of lidocaine from the plasma.

Local anesthetics cross the placenta; however, there is no data to suggest that lidocaine or tetracaine is teratogenic [6]. Local anesthetics are also secreted into breast milk.

Summary: Toxicity

- Local anesthetic toxicity generally occurs from high plasma concentrations of the drugs, or intravascular injection.
- The central nervous and cardiovascular systems are the most vulnerable to excessive plasma levels of local anesthetic.
- Allergic reactions to anesthetics are actually quite rare, and less than 1% of adverse reactions attributed to local anesthetics are considered to be allergic in nature.
- A common preservative in both amino-ester and amino-amide local anesthetics is methylparaben, which, incidentally, is similar in chemical structure to PABA and is known to be associated with type 1 hypersensitivity reactions.
- Local anesthetics can interact with MAO inhibitors, tricyclic antidepressants, phenothiazines, and non-selective beta blockers.

5.8 Toxicity

Local anesthetic toxicity generally occurs from high plasma concentrations of the drugs, or intravascular injection [3]. The central nervous and cardiovascular systems are the most vulnerable to excessive plasma levels of local anesthetic [3]. Central nervous system symptoms of local anesthetic toxicity include facial tingling, circumoral numbness, tinnitus, vertigo, and incoherent speech. At the end of this symptomatic spectrum is tonic-clonic seizures [3]. It is believed that the seizures are a result of local anesthetics depressing cortical inhibitory pathways, thereby disinhibiting excitatory pathways [3]. The seizures can lead to metabolic acidosis which can further potentiate the local anesthetic effects upon the CNS.

The cardiovascular system can be affected with high plasma concentrations of local anesthetic because it acts as a vasodilator and can result in profound hypotension [3]. Since the local anesthetics block sodium channels, they can also lead to decreased conduction of electrical impulses in the heart's conduction system [3]. This can be viewed as an increased P-R interval and widening of the QRS complex on the electrocardiogram [3].

Allergic reactions to anesthetics are actually quite rare, and less than 1% of adverse reactions attributed to local anesthetics are considered to be allergic in nature [3]. Most adverse reactions of local anesthetics are actually a result of instances in which excessive plasma concentrations were reached [3]. Despite this, the amino-ester local anesthetics are known to produce more allergic responses than the amino-amide molecules [3]. This is thought to be due to the hydrolysis of the ester bond resulting in the formation of para-aminobenzoic acid (PABA). Procaine is known to cause both type 1 and type 4 delayed hypersensitivity reactions. A common preservative in both amino-ester and amino-amide local anesthetics is methylparaben, which is similar in chemical structure to PABA and is known to be associated with type 1 hypersensitivity reactions. Typical symptoms of type 1 hypersensitivity reactions are IgE-mediated, and symptoms include angioedema, hives, bronchospasm, and rhinorrhea [2]. Therefore, if a patient is allergic to a local anesthetic, it must be determined if it is the anesthetic or the preservative in the formulation [3].

Local anesthetics may interact with MAO inhibitors, tricyclic antidepressants, phenothiazine, and non-selective β-blockers. A careful history should ascertain if the patient is taking any of the medications and appropriate medical actions taken to avoid these interactions should be discussed with the patient's healthcare team.

Summary: Method of Injection

- Infiltration of local anesthetic is the most commonly used technique of administering local anesthetic.
- Both subcutaneous and intradermal injections lead to distortion of the skin surface. This can be avoided by preoperative marking and gentle massaging of the skin.

5.9 Method of Injection

Infiltration of local anesthetic is the most commonly used technique of administering local anesthetic [4]. The smallest possible needle and syringes should be used in order to minimize pain and injection pressure [4]. Generally, 5–10-mL syringes are useful for local infiltration along with needles that are 25–30 gauge [4]. Subcutaneous injections are associated with a longer time to onset and shorter duration, while dermal injections are more painful but tend to have a shorter time to onset and longer duration of action [4]. Both subcutaneous and intradermal injections lead to distortion of the skin surface. This can be avoided by preoperative marking and gentle massaging of the skin.

Summary: Amino-Esters

- Procaine was the first injectable local anesthetic, and is associated with a significant risk of allergic reactions.

5.10 Amino-Esters

Procaine was the first injectable local anesthetic; however, it has not been used as widely since the introduction of lidocaine. Procaine is associated with a significant risk of allergic responses. Chloroprocaine has been primarily used as an epidural anesthetic in obstetrics. Its use in dermatologic surgery has not been wide spread. Tetracaine is also not commonly used in dermatologic surgery. It is used more frequently for spinal anesthesia.

Summary: Amino-Amides

- Lidocaine is the most commonly used local anesthetic in dermatologic surgery. It can be used for topical, regional, or intravenous administration.
- Mepivacaine has a slightly longer duration of action and is associated with less vasodilation than lidocaine.
- Bupivacaine is commonly used for peripheral nerve blocks, but it also is known to disrupt AV nodal conduction and depress myocardial contractility [7].
- Ropivacaine is less cardiotoxic than bupivacaine and may be more beneficial in cases where a large dose of anesthetic is required for a peripheral nerve block.
- Levobupivacaine is associated with less cardiotoxicity than bupivacaine and also may be more beneficial when large doses of anesthetic are required for a peripheral nerve block.

5.11 Amino-Amides

Lidocaine is the most commonly used local anesthetic in dermatologic surgery. It can be used for topical, regional, or intravenous situations. Mepivacaine has very similar clinical properties to lidocaine. In comparison to lidocaine, it has a marginally longer duration of action and is associated with less vasodilation [3]. It is not very effective as a topical local anesthetic and is currently not approved for use in the United States. When found in the plasma in high concentrations, its metabolism can lead to the production of ortho-toluidine which converts hemoglobin to methemoglobin leading to methemoglobinemia. Bupivacaine is commonly used for peripheral nerve blocks. It has been associated with refractory cardiac arrest when injected intravascularly at the 0.75% concentration. Bupivacaine is considered to be a "fast-in, slow-out" anesthetic because it tends to slowly dissociate from the sodium channel once it is attached [3]. It is also known to disrupt AV nodal conduction and depress myocardial contractility [7]. Ropivacaine is less cardiotoxic than bupivacaine and may be more beneficial in cases where a large dose of anesthetic is required for a peripheral nerve block [7]. It is the S (−) enantiomer homolog of mepivacaine and bupivacaine. It also has a piperidine ring with a propyl tail. Similar to ropivacaine, levobupivacaine is associated with less cardiotoxicity than bupivacaine and also may be more beneficial when large doses of anesthetic are required for a peripheral nerve block [7]. It is the S (−) enantiomer of bupivacaine.

5.11.1 Topical Anesthesia

There are different formulas for topical anesthesia, which generally exist as an oily substance at room temperature. The oily nature of the compound allows it to be easily spread over the desired area, as well as the ability to penetrate the stratum corneum. Topical anesthesia is generally not utilized during Mohs micrographic surgery.

Summary: Conclusion

- Local anesthesia is a loss in the perception of pain over a small area of the body.
- Regional anesthesia is a loss in the perception of pain in larger anatomical area.
- Two types of local anesthesia exist: amino-amides and amino-esters.

5.12 Conclusion

Local anesthesia is a loss in the perception of pain over a small area of the body. Regional anesthesia is also a loss in the perception of pain, but in a larger anatomical area or region. There are two types of local anesthetic agents, amino-amides and amino-esters, defined by their chemical structures. Both classes achieve their effects by deactivating the sodium channels responsible for the inward flux of sodium during the depolarization phase of the action potential. The net result is an increase in the amount of stimulus required to generate an action potential as well as decreased propagation of any action potentials across the anesthetized neuron. This chapter discussed the history, pharmacology, pharmacokinetics, metabolism, toxicities, chemical structures, as well as the clinical utility of using local anesthetics in localized and regional fashions.

References

1. Drake LA, Dinehart SM, Goltz RW, et al. Guidelines of care for local and regional anesthesia in cutaneous surgery. J Am Acad Dermatol. 1995;33:504–9.
2. Clark DP. Anesthesia. In: Ratz JL, Geronemus RG, Goldman MP, Maloney ME, Padilla RS, editors. Textbook of dermatologic surgery. Philadelphia: Lippincott-Raven Publishers; 1998. p. 31–40.
3. Drasner K. Local anesthetics. In: Stoelting RK, Miller RD, editors. Basics of anesthesia. Philadelphia: Churchill Livingstone/Elsevier; 2007. p. 123–34.
4. Leal-Khouri S, Lodha R, Nouri K. Local and topical anesthesia. In: Nouri K, Leal-Khouri S, editors. Techniques in dermatologic surgery. New York: Mosby; 2003. p. 47–50.
5. Leal-Khouri S, Lodha R, Nouri K. Local and topical anesthesia. In: Nouri K, editor. Techniques in dermatologic surgery. Edinburgh: Mosby; 2003. p. 47–50.
6. Bono R, Rossi G. Local anesthetic techniques. In: Rusciani L, Robins P, editors. Textbook of dermatologic surgery, vol. 1. Padova: Piccin; 2008. p. 61–72.
7. Bernards CM, Artu AA. Hexamethonium and midazolam terminate dysrhythmias and hypertension cause by intracerebroventricular bupivacine in rabbits. Anesthesiology. 1991; 74:89–96.

6 Cutaneous Anatomy in Mohs Micrographic Surgery

Diana Bolotin and Murad Alam

Abstract

Performing Mohs micrographic surgery requires an exquisite understanding of surface anatomy of the head and neck, which includes recognition both of the surface landmarks and essential subcutaneous structures. In skin surgery, an understanding of cutaneous anatomy of the head and neck is important to predicting acceptable cosmetic outcomes as well as to providing appropriate anesthesia and reducing postoperative bleeding complications. This chapter will describe the essential anatomic structures of the head and neck regions.

Keywords

Surgical anatomy • Cosmetic subunit • Cranial nerves • Motor innervation • Sensory innervations • Muscles of facial expression

Summary: Introduction

- Knowledge of cutaneous anatomy is paramount to every Mohs micrographic surgeon.
- Anatomic considerations underlie successful anesthesia as well as surgical approach.
- Appropriate and cosmetically acceptable reconstruction of defects created by Mohs micrographic surgery is rooted in knowledge of anatomic structures and boundaries.

6.1 Introduction

Every Mohs micrographic surgeon should possess a solid knowledge of anatomy. Understanding the cutaneous anatomy of the head and neck is essential in directing appropriate anesthesia, reducing postoperative complications and providing for an acceptable cosmetic outcome. Anatomy of the face will be discussed in terms of cosmetic subunits in this chapter.

Summary: Scalp and Forehead

- The soft tissue anatomy of the scalp is made up of skin, connective tissue, aponeurotic galea, loose connective tissue, and periosteum.

D. Bolotin • M. Alam (✉)
Department of Dermatology, Northwestern University, Chicago, IL, USA
e-mail: m-alam@northwestern.edu

K. Nouri (ed.), *Mohs Micrographic Surgery*,
DOI 10.1007/978-1-4471-2152-7_6, © Springer-Verlag London Limited 2012

- Undermining within the subgaleal avascular loose connective tissue space is recommended.
- Branches of both the external and internal carotid systems supply vasculature to the scalp and forehead.
- The temporal branch of the facial nerve supplies most of the motor innervations to the forehead and scalp.

6.2 Scalp and Forehead

The frontal hairline separates the forehead from the scalp superiorly and laterally, and the temporal region is separated from the scalp by the temporal hairline [1]. The forehead ends at the zygomatic arch inferiorly, while the inferior scalp is separated from the neck by the nuchal line inferiorly. The anatomy of the layers of the scalp can be recalled by the mnemonic S-C-A-L-P which refers to the skin, connective tissue, aponeurotic galeal layer, loose connective tissue, and periosteum. In its most anterior segment, the skin of the scalp measures about 3–4 mm in thickness and reaches up to 8 mm in the more posterior segments. Blood vessels, lymphatics, and cutaneous adnexa reside within the connective tissue layers, while the underlying musculature connects to the galea aponeurotica. Muscles of the forehead and scalp include frontalis, temporalis, procerus, corrugator supercilii, and superior fibers of the orbicularis oculi (Fig. 6.1). Deep to the aponeurotic layer is the loose connective tissue that is largely avascular but does contain perforating emissary veins. Lastly, the periosteum envelops the bony skull and contains another layer of vasculature.

6.2.1 Vasculature

Both the internal and external carotid arteries provide the blood supply to the forehead and scalp. The central forehead and anterior scalp are supplied by the supratrochlear and supraorbital arteries, which originate off of the ophthalmic artery branch of the internal carotid (Fig. 6.2a). The lateral forehead and scalp are supplied by the superficial temporal and posterior auricular branches of the external carotid artery (Fig. 6.2b). The posterior scalp is supplied by the occipital artery, another branch of the external carotid (Fig. 6.2b).

6.2.2 Nerves

The motor and sensory anatomy of the forehead and scalp is the key part of surgery on these subunits.

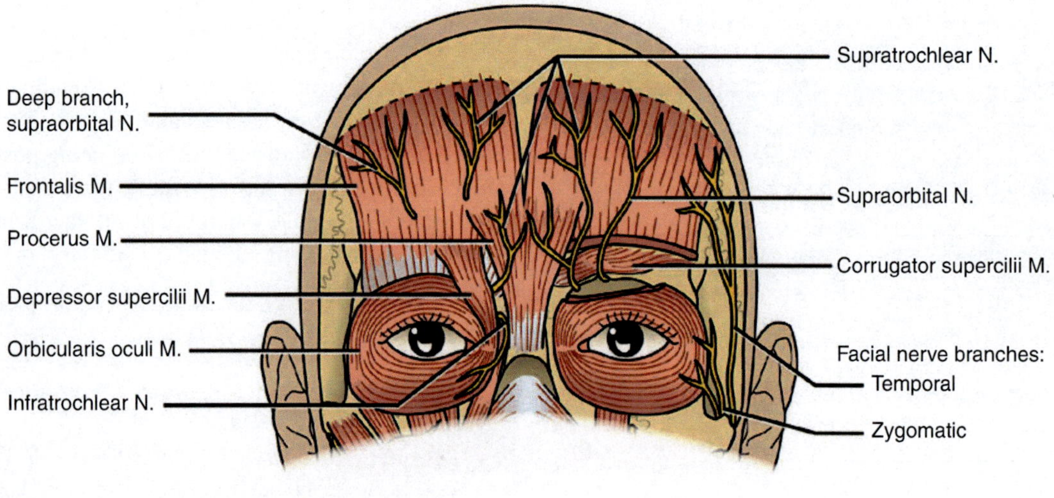

Fig. 6.1 Periorbital and forehead musculature and nerves

Motor innervation of the forehead is provided by the temporal branch of the facial nerve (CN VII). This branch is found along the zygoma but becomes more superficial superiorly to innervate the frontalis muscle at its deep surface. It is most susceptible to injury at its superficial course which may result in ipsilateral brow ptosis and pronounced asymmetry of the face (Fig. 6.1).

The sensory nerve supply to the forehead and scalp is provided by branches of all three divisions of the trigeminal nerve (CN V). The supraorbital and supratrochlear nerves branch off of the ophthalmic nerve (CN V1) to supply the scalp up to the vertex (Fig. 6.1). The zygomaticotemporal branch, arising from the maxillary division of the trigeminal nerve (CN V2), supplies sensory innervations to the anterior temple. The auriculotemporal nerve, a branch of the mandibular division (CN V3), supplies the rest of the temporal area. Branches of the cervical spinal nerves (C2, C3) innervate the posterior scalp.

6.2.3 Lymphatic Drainage

The lymphatic drainage of the scalp is collected by the occipital and posterior auricular lymph nodes (Fig. 6.3). The lymphatic basin responsible for drainage of the forehead subunit is located in the parotid glands bilaterally.

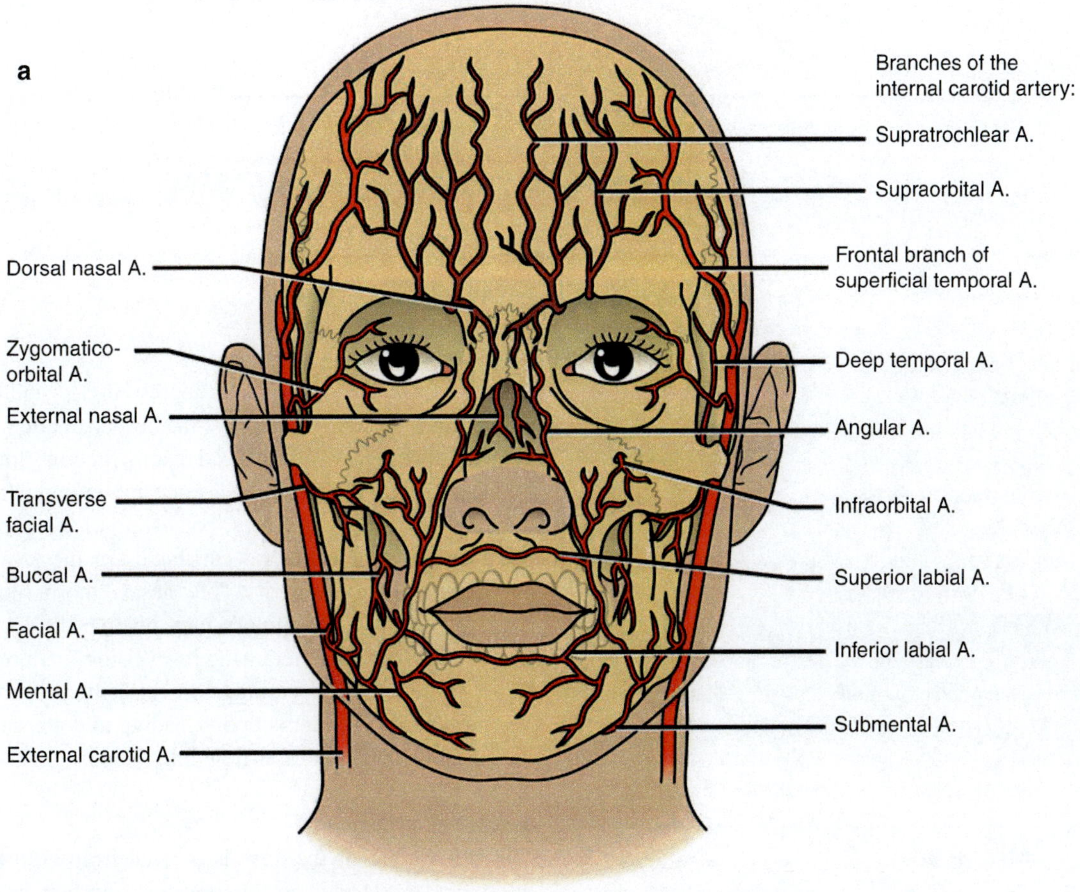

Fig. 6.2 (**a**) Facial vasculature. (**b**) Scalp vasculature

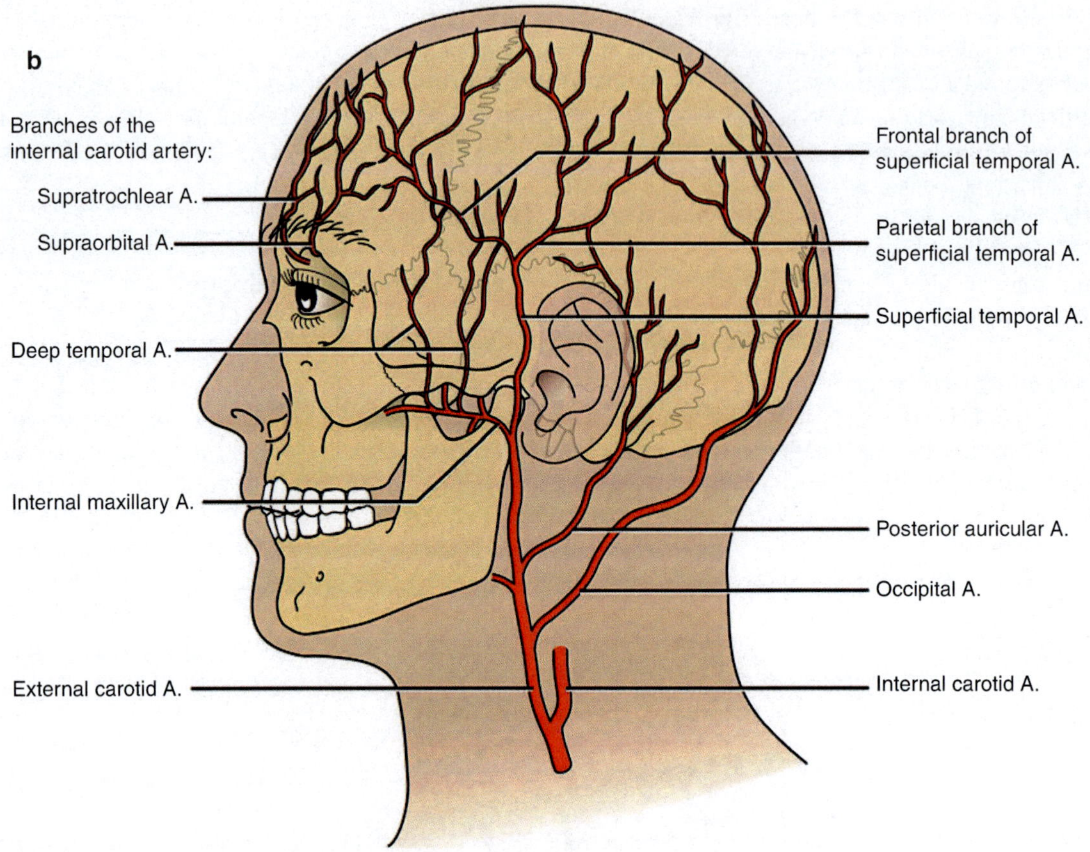

Fig. 6.2 (continued)

Summary: Midface

- Knowledge of the boundaries of the cosmetic subunits is especially important in planning reconstruction on the midface.
- Vasculature of the nose contains an essential anastomotic site between the external and internal carotid systems.
- Branches of the facial nerve (CN VII) provide motor innervations to the midface, while the maxillary and mandibular divisions of the trigeminal nerve (CN V) provide sensory input.

6.3 Midface

6.3.1 Nasal Subunit

The nasal subunit is generally subdivided into a number of cosmetic subunits [2]. These are the nasal sidewall, nasal dorsum, tip, alae, soft triangles, and the columella (Fig. 6.4). To achieve the best cosmetic outcome, incision lines during nasal reconstruction should be placed at the borders of these cosmetic units. The nasal cartilaginous structures, consisting of the lateral nasal and the lower lateral cartilage, are the key to maintaining the integrity of nasal morphology (Fig. 6.5). Infiltrative tumors may involve the lower lateral nasal cartilage, requiring its excision. Failure to repair or replace the cartilage in this situation may result in the loss of alar support, leading to collapse of the nasal ala and lack of airflow into the nose.

6.3.1.1 Vasculature

The vasculature of the nose is derived from both the internal and external carotid arteries [3]. In fact, arteries supplying the nasal area make up one of the key anastomosing sites between the internal and external carotid arteries. The dorsal nasal and external nasal branches of the ophthalmic artery, which branches off

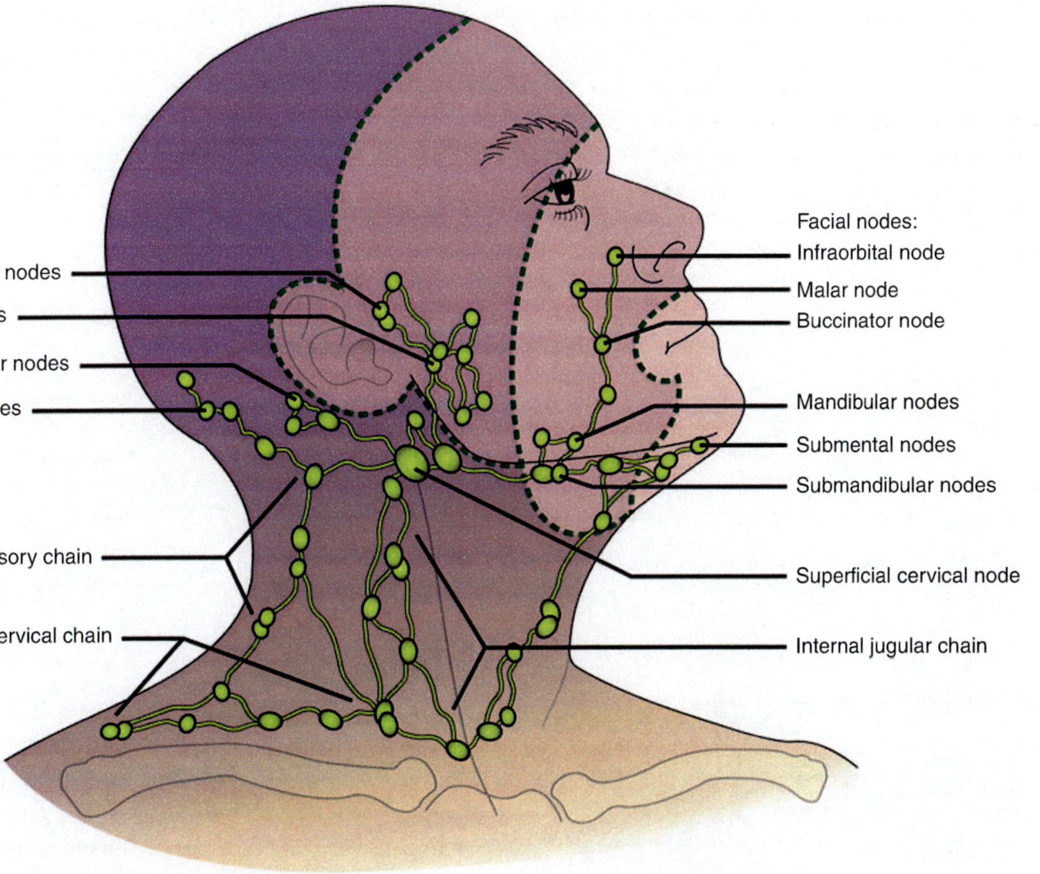

Fig. 6.3 Lymphatic drainage of the head and neck

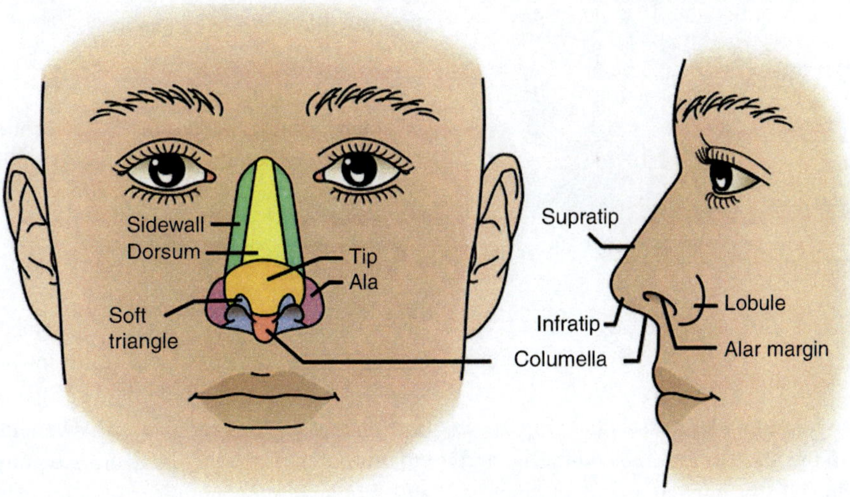

Fig. 6.4 Landmarks in nasal anatomy

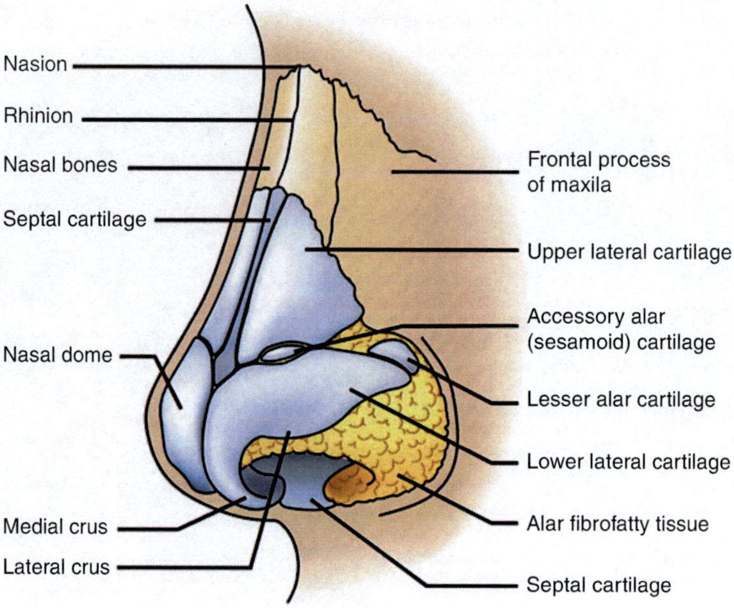

Fig. 6.5 Cartilaginous structures of the nose

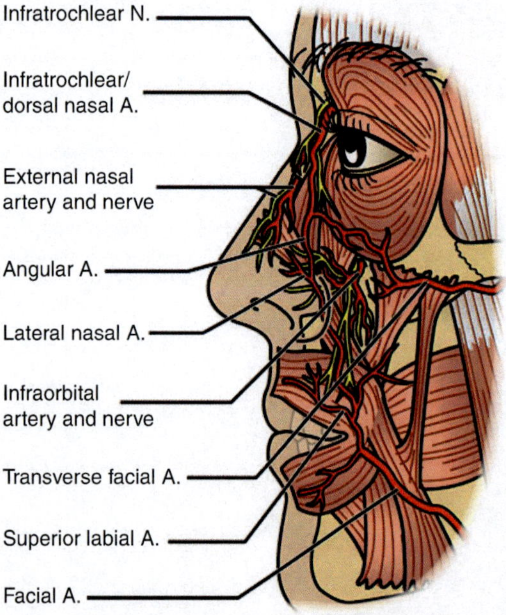

Fig. 6.6 Nasal vasculature and sensory nerves

of the internal carotid, supply the dorsal nose (Fig. 6.6). Vascular supply to the nasal sidewalls, columella, and nasal alae is provided by the angular artery, a branch of the facial artery that originates off of the external carotid (Fig. 6.6).

6.3.1.2 Nerves

The zygomatic and buccal branches of the facial nerve (CN VII) provide motor innervation to the procerus muscle at the nasal root, depressor septi nasi, and nasalis muscles (Fig. 6.6). The ophthalmic and maxillary divisions of the trigeminal nerve provide sensory innervations to the nose. The infratrochlear and external nasal branches of the ophthalmic division (CN V1) and the infraorbital branch of the maxillary division (CN V2) are the primary sources of sensory innervations for this subunit.

6.3.1.3 Lymphatic Drainage

Lymphatic drainage from the nose is collected primarily by the submandibular lymph nodes (Fig. 6.3).

6.3.2 Perioral

The surface anatomy of the lip is divided into the lateral cutaneous upper lip, philtrum, lower lip, and the vermillion border which demarcates the red and white portion of the lips (Fig. 6.7a) [4]. The underlying musculature includes orbicularis oris, zygomaticus major and minor, levator anguli oris, depressor anguli oris, levator labii superioris, depressor labii inferioris, risorius, mentalis, and the buccinator muscles (Fig. 6.7b).

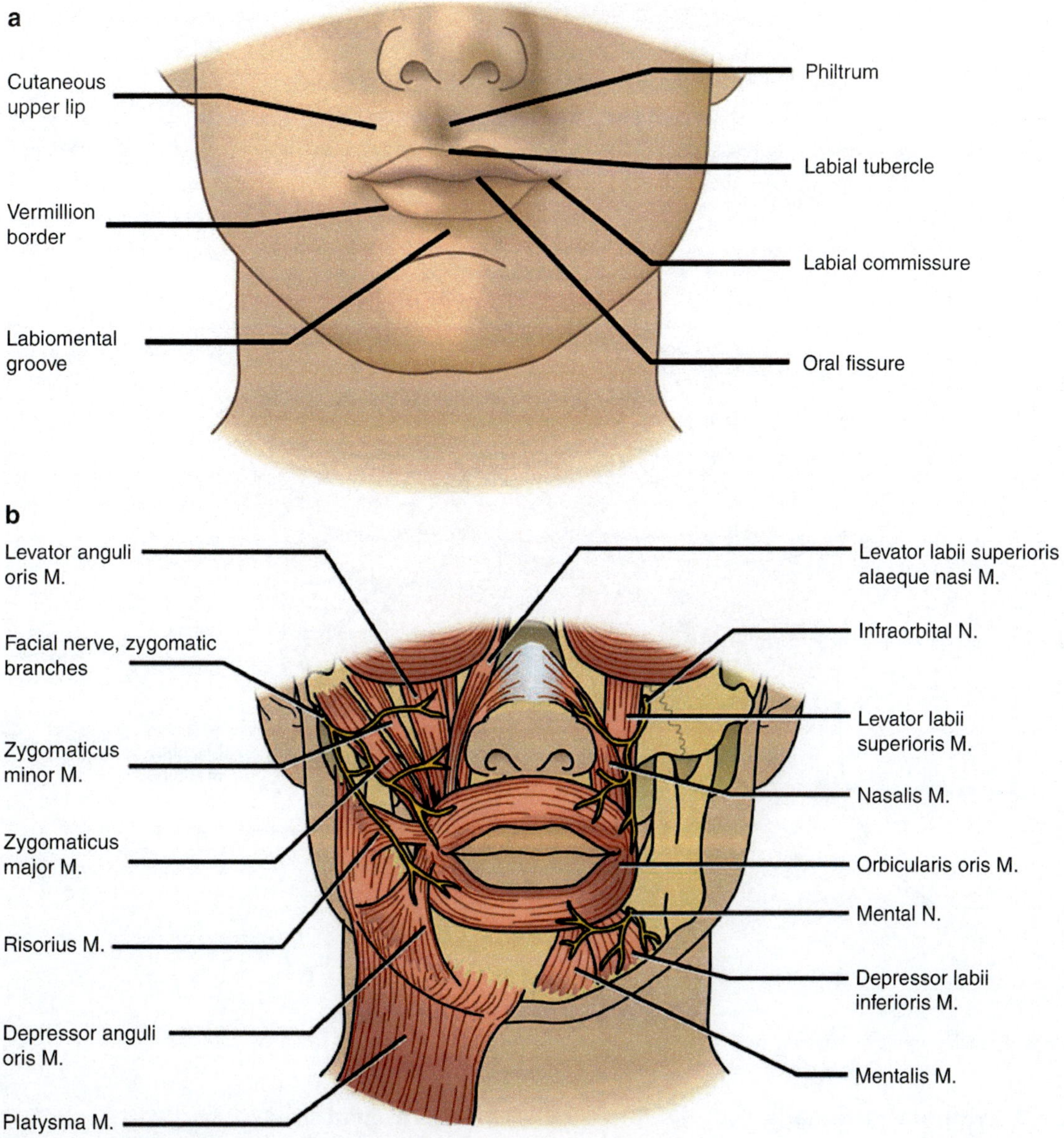

Fig. 6.7 (**a**) Perioral anatomic landmarks. (**b**) Perioral musculature

The cutaneous insertion of lip elevator musculature forms the nasolabial crease.

6.3.2.1 Vasculature

Vascular supply to the lips is provided by labial branches of the facial artery. The labial arteries are frequently resected during Mohs micrographic surgery of the perioral region. Ligation or electrosurgery of these vessels is usually sufficient to prevent excessive bleeding.

6.3.2.2 Nerves

Motor innervation to the perioral musculature is carried by the zygomatic, buccal, marginal mandibular, and cervical branches of the facial nerve (CN VII) (Fig. 6.8). The maxillary division (CN V2) provides sensory innervations to the upper perioral region via the infraorbital nerve. The mandibular division (CN V3) contributes to the sensory nerve supply of the lower lip via the mental nerve.

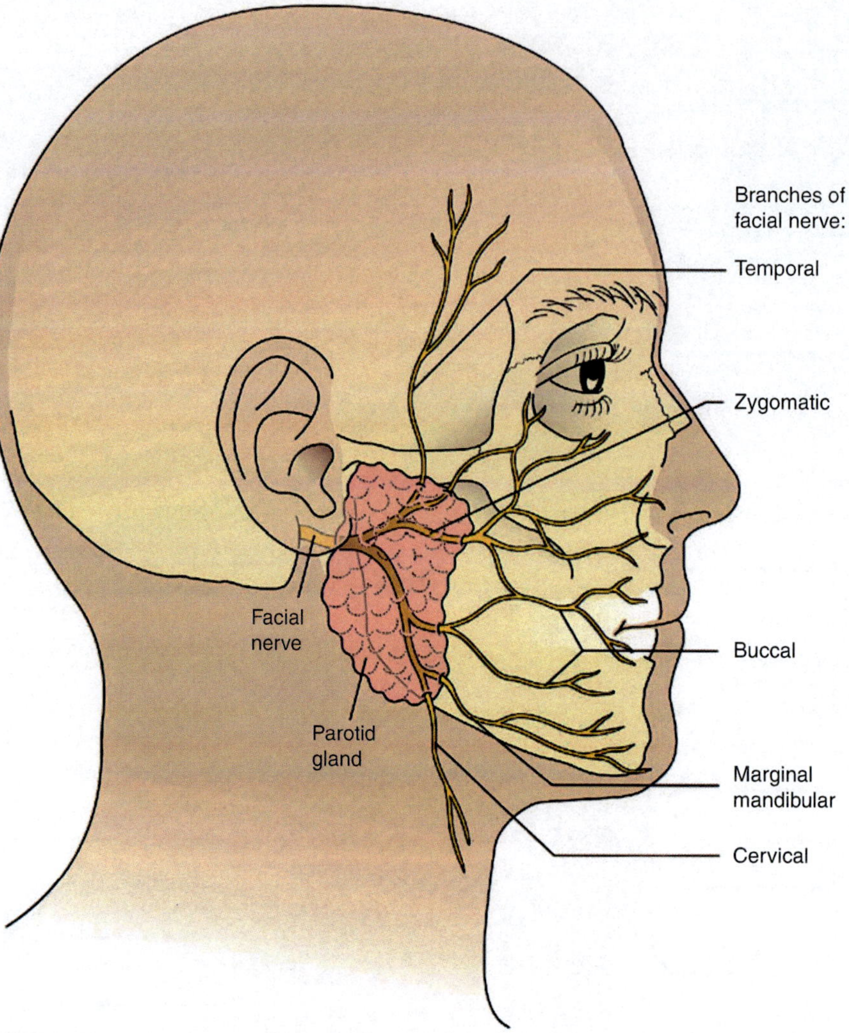

Fig. 6.8 Branches of the facial nerve (CN VII)

6.3.2.3 Lymphatic Drainage

The lymphatic drainage from the perioral region is collected by the submental lymph nodes.

6.3.3 Chin

The cosmetic subunit of the chin is separated from the cheek and lip subunits by the mentolabial crease. Surgeons must be aware of the location of the mental foramen that carries the mental nerve and vessels to the chin and is located below the second mandibular premolar tooth in the majority of the population. Musculature of the chin consists of the mentalis, depressor anguli oris, and depressor labii inferioris (Fig. 6.7b).

6.3.3.1 Vasculature

The vascular supply of the chin is provided by the mental and submental arteries which branch off the external carotid artery.

6.3.3.2 Nerves

Motor innervation to the chin is provided by the marginal mandibular branch of the facial nerve (CN VII). Injury to the marginal mandibular nerve may occur as it crosses the mandible at the masseter muscle within the superficial soft tissue (Fig. 6.8). Marginal mandibular injury is manifested as ipsilateral asymmetry of the lip and chin during smiling. The mental nerve, entering via the mental foramen, provides the sensory innervation to the chin.

6.3.3.3 Lymphatic Drainage

The submental lymph node basin receives lymphatic drainage from the chin subunit (Fig. 6.3).

Summary: Periorbital

- The canaliculi are essential for passage of tears to the lacrimal sac.
- Reconstruction of the eyelid region should avoid placing vertical tension on the eyelid free margin.
- Proper anesthesia to the eyelid region relies upon knowledge of the neural anatomy in the area.

6.4 Periorbital

Understanding of periorbital anatomy is the key to avoidance of ectropion and entropion complications of cutaneous surgery in this region. The eyelids are made up of the skin, orbicularis oculi muscle, the tarsus, and the conjunctiva [5]. The medial and lateral canthal tendons provide overall structural support to the eyelids. The superior and inferior lacrimal canaliculi are enveloped by the medial canthal tendon and are the means of passage of tears to the lacrimal sac. Transection of the canaliculi will lead to a defect in tear drainage, and therefore, a recanalization procedure may be required in these cases. Glands of Zeis and Meibomian glands are large sebaceous glands that reside in the eyelids (Fig. 6.9a). Glands of Moll are apocrine glands of the eyelids (Fig. 6.9a). Since the eyelid is a free margin, it is susceptible to distortion due to downward or upward tension. Placing the tension vector perpendicular to these free margins will lower the likelihood of postoperative distortion.

6.4.1 Vasculature

The internal and external carotid arteries provide vascular supply to the periorbital area. The dorsal nasal branch of the internal carotid system anastomoses with the angular branch of the facial artery in the vicinity of the medial canthus (Fig. 6.9b). Supraorbital and supratrochlear artery branches of the internal carotid system also supply the upper eyelid area (Fig. 6.9b). The external carotid artery supplies vasculature to the lower eyelid through the infraorbital branch of the maxillary artery and to the lateral periorbital area via the superficial temporal artery.

6.4.2 Nerves

Knowledge of neural anatomy of the periocular region is crucial to provide proper anesthesia to the eyelid region. Sensory innervation to the periocular region is provided by the ophthalmic division (CN V1). The glabella is innervated by the supratrochlear branch of the ophthalmic division. Sensation to the lower eyelid is mediated by the infraorbital nerve. The zygomatic branch of the facial nerve (CN VII) provides motor innervations to the orbicularis oculi, levator palpebrae superioris, and parts of the procerus muscles (Fig. 6.8). The temporal branch of CN VII carries motor nerves to the corrugators and procerus.

6.4.3 Lymphatic Drainage

The lymphatic drainage basin of the lateral eyelid lies primarily within the parotid lymph nodes, while the Medial canthus drains to the submandibular lymph node basin.

Summary: Cheeks

- The cheek is the largest subunit of the face and is composed of regions with various sebaceous composition and vascularity.
- The external carotid system provides vascular supply to the cheek.
- Both the parotid and submandibular lymph nodes receive drainage from the cheek.

6.5 Cheeks

The largest cosmetic subunit of the face is the cheek. Its superior border is made of the infraorbital rim and zygomatic arch. The nasolabial and melolabial folds mark the medial border, and the preauricular crease makes up the lateral border of the cheek. The cheek subunit can be further subdivided into the medial, zygomatic, buccal, and lateral cheek units. Each of these has unique surface characteristics and sebaceous component that must be taken into account during reconstruction [6].

6.5.1 Vasculature

Branches of the external carotid artery provide the vascular supply to the cheek subunit. The transverse facial artery supplies the lateral cheek. The angular branch of the facial artery and the infraorbital artery supply the medial aspects of the cheeks (Fig. 6.2a). Multiple anastomotic connections within the cheek make this subunit a highly vascularized skin surface.

6.5.2 Nerves

The muscles of the cheek are innervated by the zygomatic and buccal branches of the facial nerve (CN VII) (Fig. 6.8). The infraorbital, zygomaticofacial, and zygomaticotemporal branches of the maxillary division of the trigeminal nerve supply sensation to the medial and zygomatic aspects of the cheek. Nerves emanating from the mandibular division of the trigeminal nerve provide sensation to the rest of the cheek subunit. The auriculotemporal nerve innervates parts of the lateral cheek, with the buccal nerve providing sensation to the lateral and buccal portions. The mental nerve innervates the inferior medial aspects.

6.5.3 Lymphatic Drainage

The parotid and submandibular nodes collect the lymphatic drainage from the cheek subunit.

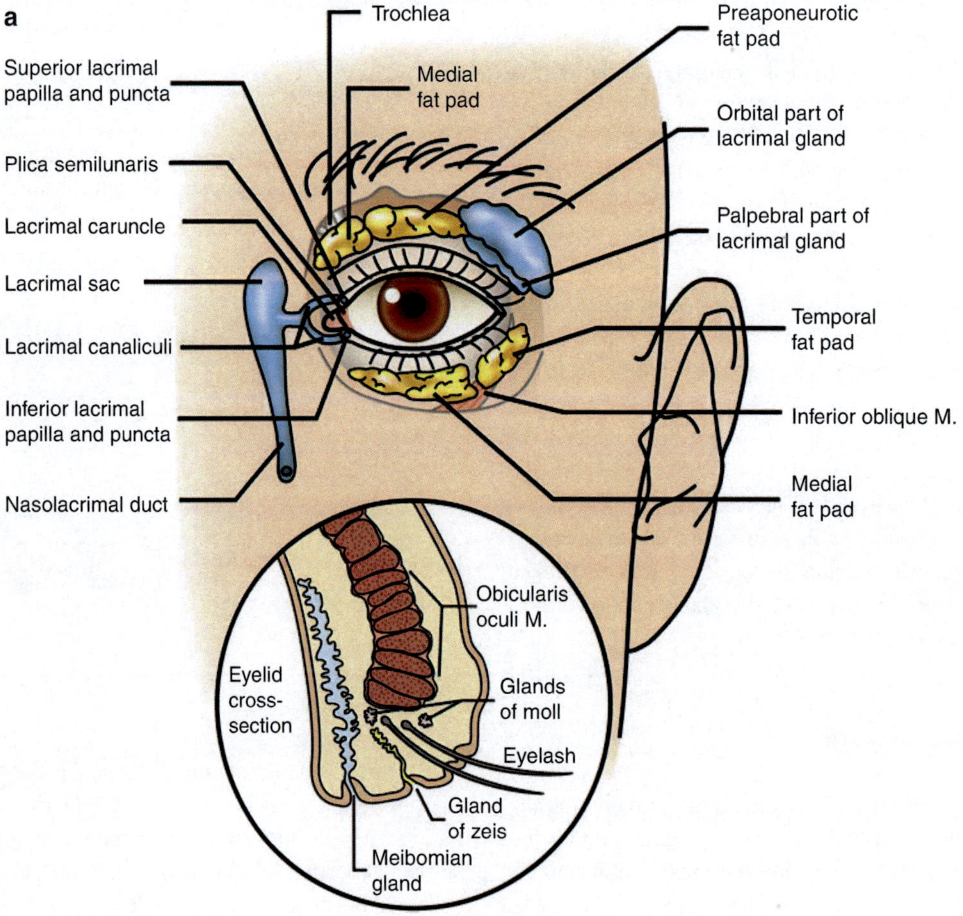

Fig. 6.9 (**a**) Lacrimal glands and periorbital fat pads. (**b**) Periorbital vascular supply

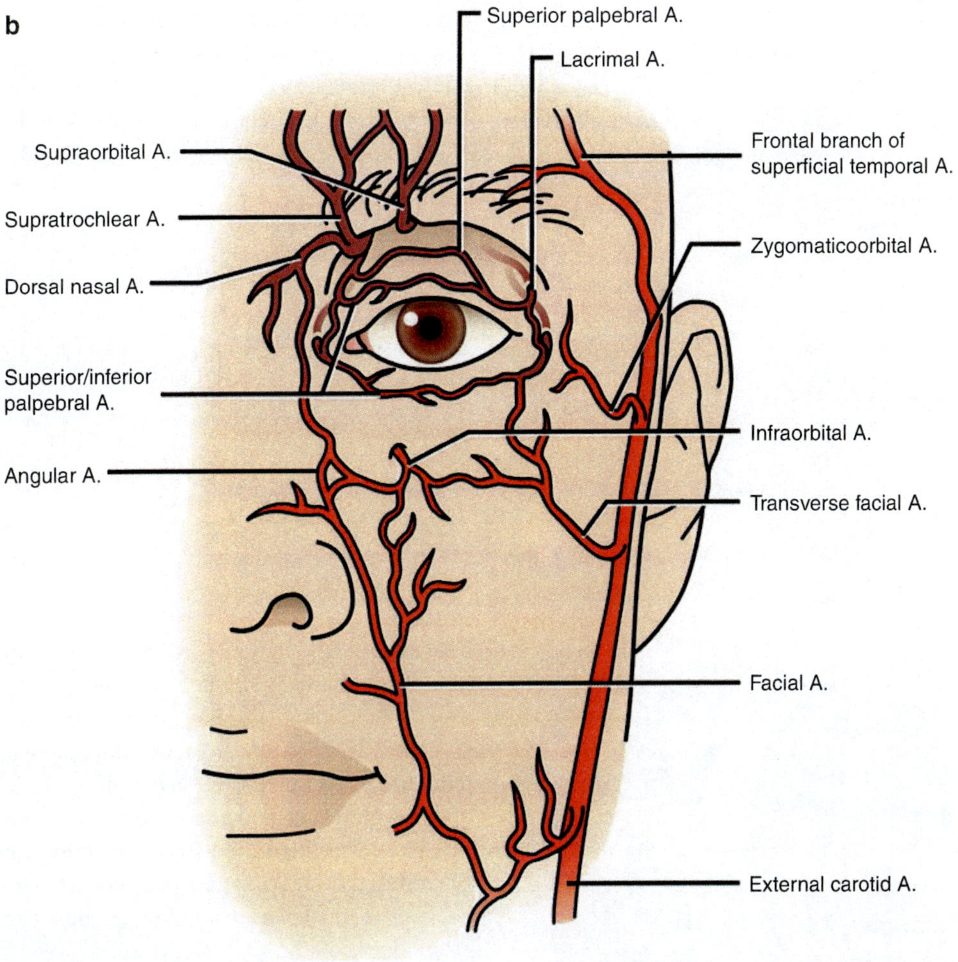

Fig. 6.9 (continued)

Summary: Auricular

- The surface topography of the ear is highly complex.
- The ear receives vascular supply exclusively from the external carotid artery system.
- Sensory innervation of the auricle is supplied by four cranial nerves and the greater auricular nerve.

6.6 Auricular

The surface anatomy of the ear is complex, with intermixing of multiple convex and concave surfaces [7]. Notable anatomic landmarks of the ear include the helix, crura, scaphoid fossa, triangular fossa, conchal bowl, antihelix, tragus, antitragus, and lobule (Fig. 6.10). The auricular cartilage is found in the upper two-thirds of the ear.

6.6.1 Vasculature

Blood supply to the auricle is derived entirely from the external carotid artery system [8]. The lobule and posterior ear are supplied by the occipital and posterior auricular arteries. The conchal bowl is supplied by branches of the posterior auricular artery. The anterior auricular artery, which branches off of the superficial temporal artery, supplies the anterior ear.

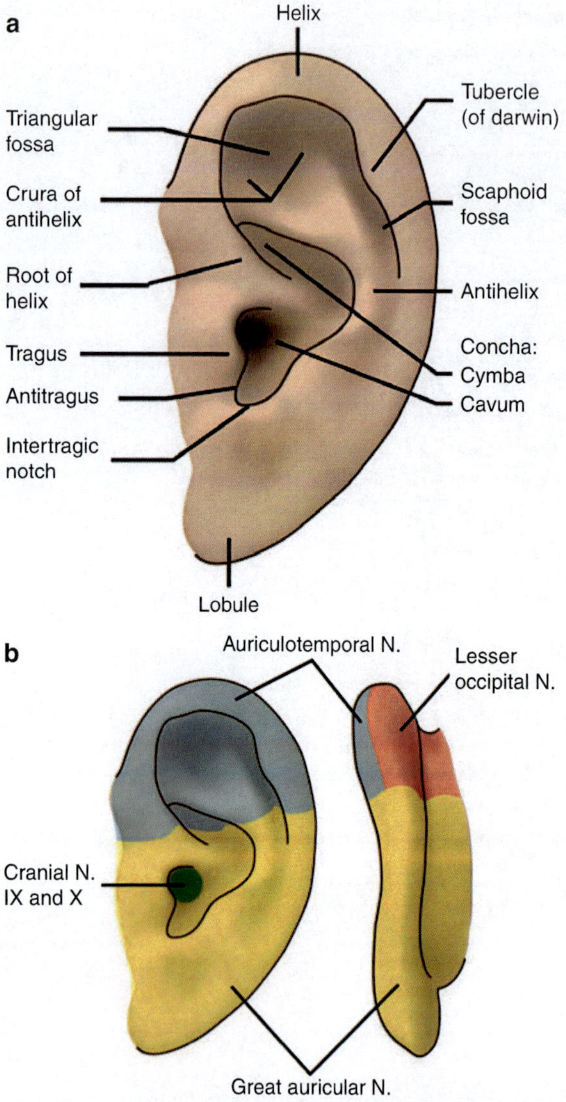

Fig. 6.10 Auricular anatomic landmarks. (**a**) Auricular anatomic landmark. (**b**) Sensory innervation of the ear

6.6.2 Nerves

Sensory innervation of the ear is complex, with the great auricular nerve (C2, C3) innervating the lower part of the lateral and posterior ear. The auriculotemporal branch (CN V3) innervates the superior lateral ear, and the lesser occipital nerve provides sensation to the superior posterior ear. The external auditory meatus and conchal bowl are supplied by fibers of the glossopharyngeal (CN IX), auricular branch of the vagus (CN X or Arnold nerve), and facial (CN VII) nerves.

6.6.3 Lymphatic Drainage

The posterior aspect of the ear drains to the occipital and posterior auricular lymph nodes. Anterior ear lymphatic drainage proceeds to the parotid nodes.

Summary: Neck

- The triangles of the neck denote important anatomic landmarks in cutaneous surgery.
- Erb's point denotes the location of the exit of the spinal accessory (CN XI) nerve, which provides motor innervation to the scapula region.

6.7 Neck

The superficial anatomy of the neck requires anatomic landmarks indicated by the triangles of the neck to help identify important underlying structures (Fig. 6.11a). The superficial musculoaponeurotic system (SMAS) is a fibrous layer of fascia that envelops the platysma and the superficial facial muscles [9]. The easily identified sternocleidomastoid muscle separates the anterior and posterior triangles of the neck. The posterior triangle contains Erb's point, a landmark of the exit of the spinal accessory (CN XI), the lesser occipital, and great auricular nerves, as well as the transverse cervical rami (Fig. 6.11b). Damage to the spinal accessory nerve may result in the inability to raise the ipsilateral shoulder. The jugular and carotid vessels run through the carotid triangle (Fig. 6.11a). The mental lymph node basin and lingual arteries occupy the submental triangle. The submaxillary triangle includes the lingual nerve, artery and vein, and hypoglossal nerve.

6.7.1 Nerves

The cervical branch of the facial nerve (CN VII) provides the motor innervations to the platysma. Sensory innervation to this area is provided by the transverse cervical, supraclavicular, and great auricular nerves.

6.7.2 Lymphatic Drainage

Lymph nodes of the neck region secondarily receive drainage from most nodes of the face. These eventually empty into the venous circulation via the thoracic duct.

- Reconstruction of the haired areas of the head and neck must proceed with caution to avoid patches of alopecia.
- Donor site selection in full-thickness skin graft reconstruction should be tailored to the hair and sebaceous gland content of the recipient site.

Summary: Special Anatomic Considerations in Mohs Micrographic Surgery

- Anatomic considerations specifically applicable to tumor extirpation by Mohs micrographic surgery include knowledge of danger zones for motor nerve injury on the face as well as awareness of free margins of the face during reconstruction.

6.8 Special Anatomic Considerations in Mohs Micrographic Surgery

6.8.1 Danger Zones

The relevant danger zones that a Mohs micrographic surgeon must be aware of revolve around several key

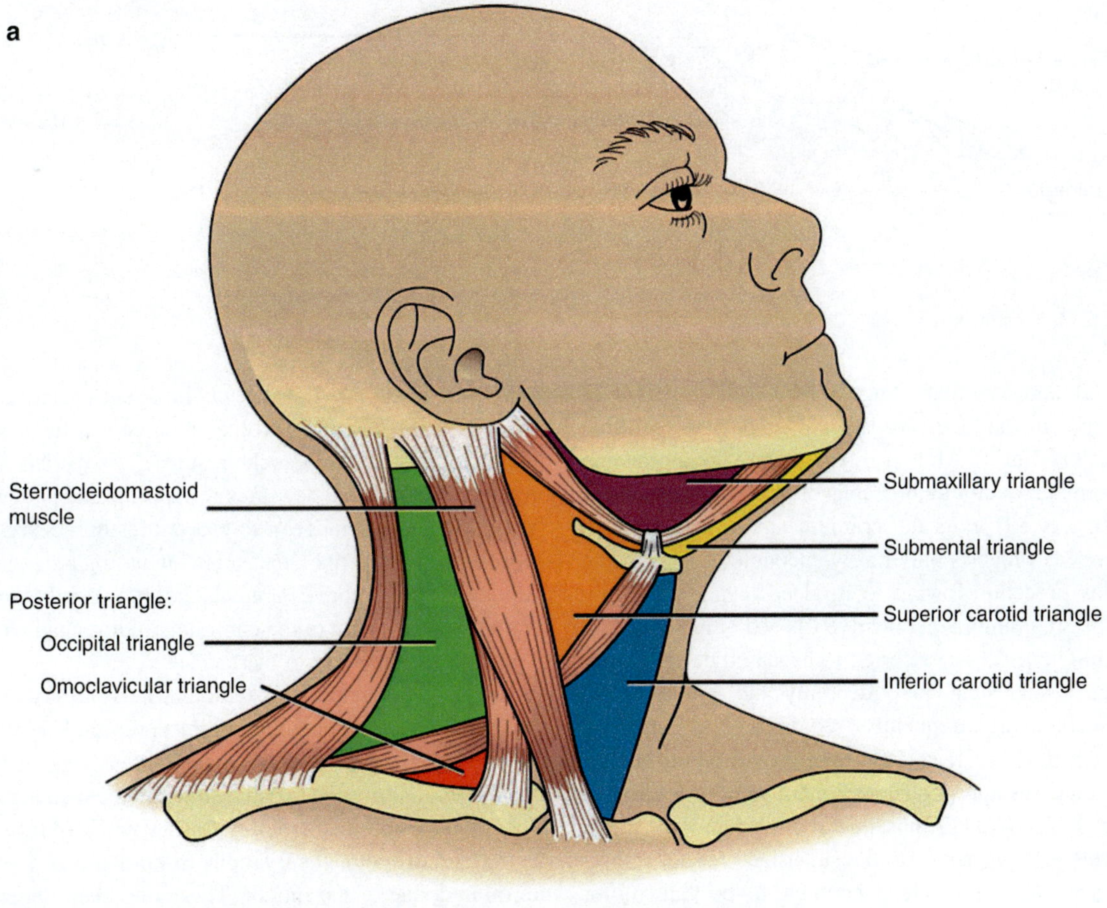

Fig. 6.11 (**a**) Anatomic triangles of the neck. (**b**) Erb's point in posterior triangle of the neck

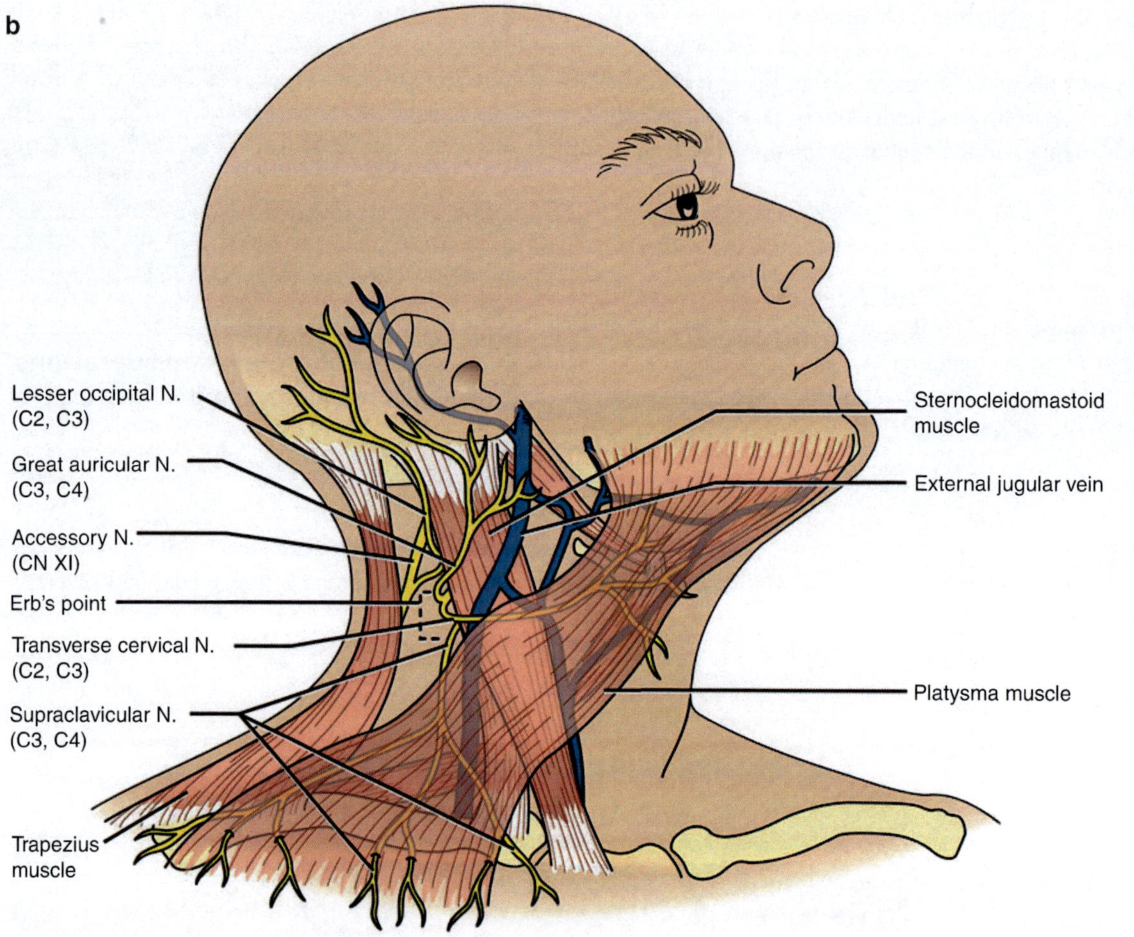

Fig. 6.11 (continued)

neural and vascular structures as well as the free margins of the face. The two nerves most susceptible to injury during Mohs surgery are the temporal and marginal mandibular branches of the facial nerve (CN VII). CN VII exits the cranium at the stylomastoid foramen, which is only rarely encountered during the Mohs procedure owing to its deep location. Deeply infiltrating tumors that involve CN VII at its exit point should generally be referred to head and neck surgery since a superficial parotidectomy and cranial nerve dissection are frequently required. The temporal branch of CN VII courses through the parotid gland and emerges approximately 2.5 cm anterior to the tragus (Fig. 6.8) [1]. Subsequently, the temporal nerve travels just superficial to the superficial fascia, a short distance from the lateral canthus, to provide motor innervations to the frontalis muscle. Avoidance of deep undermining during reconstruction is the key to preventing injury to this nerve. In some instances, however, tumor extension forces a surgeon's hand in damaging this nerve branch, resulting in ipsilateral brow ptosis and facial asymmetry. Appropriate patient discussion is essential prior to procedures in this area. Subsequent corrective measures may include an elliptical excision above the ipsilateral brow, and botulinum toxin treatment of the contralateral forehead will often restore symmetry to the face.

Similarly, the marginal mandibular nerve is susceptible to injury with deep undermining at the angle of the mandible (Fig. 6.8). Injury to this nerve branch results in an inability to purse the lips and smile on the ipsilateral side of the mouth. Cosmetic asymmetry will also result due to lack of motor innervations to lip depressors on the injured side of the mouth. Therefore, deep undermining and V to Y flap closures should be avoided in this area in order to preserve the integrity of this motor nerve. Appropriate discussion with the patient preceding surgery in this area is again essential.

The most important vascular structure encountered during Mohs surgery of the face is the angular artery, which courses superiorly along the nasal sidewall. Transection of this structure requires effective and aggressive hemostatic maneuvers. Nasolabial transposition and advancement flaps in this area are especially prone to damaging this vascular structure.

Free margins of the face include the eyelids and lips. Reconstruction of Mohs micrographic surgery defects above or below the eyelid or lip can result in ectropion or eclabion, respectively, if the tension vector is oriented parallel to the free margin. It is, therefore, imperative to orient the tension vector perpendicular to the free margin to avoid these complications.

6.8.2 Other Considerations

Several consequences of head and neck procedures may have disturbing, though not dangerous, consequences, of which Mohs surgeons should be aware. Excisions of scalp tumors carry the risk of hair loss which can be due to either superficial undermining or scar spreading. It is therefore recommended to undermine within the deep subgaleal plane on the scalp to avoid transaction of the follicular units. Closure should be oriented to reduce wound tension and scar spreading, which can result in an alopecic patch.

Not infrequently, reconstruction of Mohs surgery defects requires a full-thickness skin graft. Tissue matching between the donor and recipient sites is essential to long-term cosmesis of the graft. The general appearance, thickness, as well as hair and sebaceous density are all considerations in this process. Common donor sites include posterior auricular skin, the conchal bowl, and the supraclavicular sulcus. However, in cases where a better match is needed, the nasolabial fold, upper eyelid, and upper forehead skin may be considered as donor sites for a full-thickness skin graft.

References

1. Angelos PC, Downs BW. Options for the management of forehead and scalp defects. Facial Plast Surg Clin North Am. 2009;17(3):379–93.
2. Burget GC, Menick FJ. The subunit principle in nasal reconstruction. Plast Reconstr Surg. 1985;76(2):239–47.
3. Oneal RM, Beil RJ. Surgical anatomy of the nose. Clin Plast Surg. 2010;37(2):191–211.
4. Gassner HG, Rafii A, Young A, Murakami C, Moe KS, Larrabee Jr WF. Surgical anatomy of the face: implications for modern face-lift techniques. Arch Facial Plast Surg. 2008;10(1):9–19.
5. Most SP, Mobley SR, Larrabee Jr WF. Anatomy of the eyelids. Facial Plast Surg Clin North Am. 2005;13(4):487–92, v.
6. Dobratz EJ, Hilger PA. Cheek defects. Facial Plast Surg Clin North Am. 2009;17(3):455–67.
7. Shonka Jr DC, Park SS. Ear defects. Facial Plast Surg Clin North Am. 2009;17(3):429–43.
8. Park C, Lineaweaver WC, Rumly TO, Buncke HJ. Arterial supply of the anterior ear. Plast Reconstr Surg. 1992;90(1):38–44.
9. Mitz V, Peyronie M. The superficial musculo-aponeurotic system (SMAS) in the parotid and cheek area. Plast Reconstr Surg. 1976;58(1):80–8.

7 Mohs Surgery: Fixed Tissue Technique

Pearon G. Lang and Martin Braun III

Abstract

Today the fixed tissue technique is primarily of historical significance. A multidisciplinary approach to difficult skin cancers, the limited availability of the zinc chloride fixative, and the dwindling pool of Mohs surgeons with expertise in this technique have resulted in Mohs chemosurgery becoming a dying art.

Keywords

Fixed tissue technique • Zinc chloride fixative • Mohs chemosurgery • Zinc chloride paste • Frederic Mohs • Fresh tissue technique

Summary

- The fixed tissue technique is rarely used today.
- The fixed tissue technique was particularly useful for deeply invasive cancers and highly vascularized tumors.
- The fixed tissue technique did not permit immediate repairs
- The fixed tissue technique often required the surgery being extended over multiple days.
- The in vivo fixation process was quite painful.

7.1 Mohs Surgery-The Early Days

When Dr. Mohs initially began to develop his technique for removing skin cancer, he had concerns that transecting the cancer might result in the introduction of tumor into the lymphatics and blood vessels, thus leading to metastases. There was also concern that viable tumor cells could be implanted into the adjacent tissues resulting in a recurrence (Figs. 7.1 and 7.2). Working with the Department of Pharmacology at the University of Wisconsin, he developed a black paste, which contained zinc chloride, sanguinaria canadensis, and stibnite (Figs. 7.3 and 7.4). The application of this paste allowed the tissue to become "fixed" in vivo. This fixed tissue had the consistency of cardboard. Because of the fixation process, this tissue did not bleed when cut, and there was no sensation of pain; thus, there was no need for local anesthesia as long as one stayed within the confines of the fixed tissue. Using 20% merbromin, lines could be drawn on the floor of the wound as tissue was removed, resulting in

P.G. Lang (✉)
Trident Dermatology, Charleston, SC, USA
e-mail: pearonlang@bellsouth.net

M. Braun III
Braun Dermatology, George Washington University, Washington, DC, USA

K. Nouri (ed.), *Mohs Micrographic Surgery*,
DOI 10.1007/978-1-4471-2152-7_7,

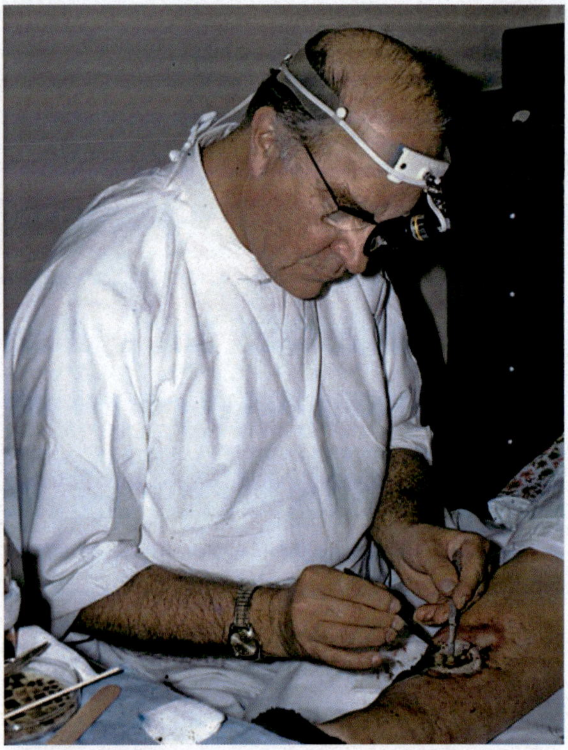

Fig. 7.1 Dr. Frederic Mohs operating on a fibrosarcoma in 1974

a grid pattern. This resulted in very accurate mapping and probably allowed for the taking of less tissue since one did not have to take into account the retraction of the wound edges as tissue was removed, as is the case with the fresh tissue technique. Also, because one could mark on the floor of the wound and create a grid pattern, the tumor could be much more precisely localized. Because removing the fixed tissue was bloodless and painless, very extensive and invasive surgery could be performed.

Although the fixed tissue technique offered a number of advantages from a surgical standpoint, it also had a number of disadvantages. The fixation of the tissue was a very painful process, often requiring narcotics for pain relief. It was also not uncommon for the patient to have fever, and swelling was common, especially around the eyes. The zinc chloride fixative was a chemoattractant for polymorphonuclear leukocytes. This rendered the microscopic interpretation of the removed tissue more difficult (Fig. 7.5). At the completion of Mohs surgery, there was usually residual fixed tissue, which might or might not be clinically obvious. This tissue would usually be sloughed within a week following the completion of the surgery.

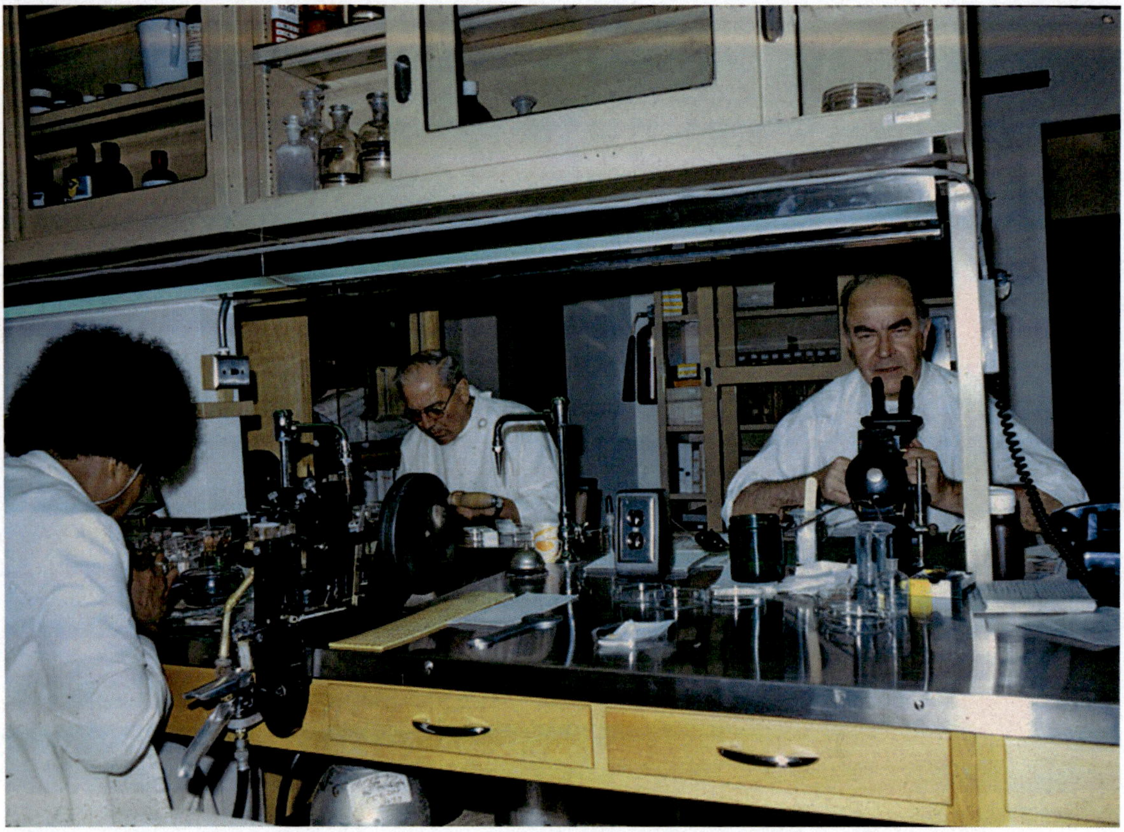

Fig. 7.2 Dr. Mohs at his single-headed microscope in his lab in 1974

Stibnite (80 mesh sieve)	40.0 gm.
Sanguinaria canadensis	10.0 gm.
Zinc chloride, saturated sol.	34.5 gm.

Fig. 7.3 Formula for the fixative

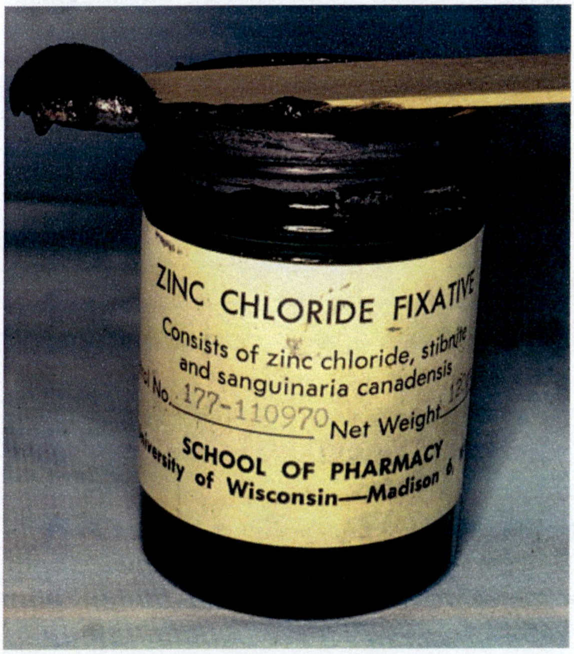

Fig. 7.4 Bottle of "the paste"

Therefore, immediate repairs were not possible. The sloughing of residual fixed tissue could also result in a full-thickness defect of a nose or ear. Also, if a large vessel had only been partially fixed, hemorrhage could occur when the slough occurred. Although the process of fixation could occur within several hours, it normally required at least 12 h. Thus, usually only one stage of Mohs surgery was done in a day. Thus, for tumors with extensive subclinical spread, the surgery could extend over many days. Because the zinc chloride fixative was routinely used in the early days of Mohs surgery, the procedure became known as chemosurgery. There were several disadvantages to this name. First of all, patients often confused the procedure with chemotherapy, with all of its side effects, and they often were afraid of undergoing surgery. Secondly, the term conjured up the idea that the procedure might be a form of quackery or witchcraft.

Typically, on the first day of surgery, the zinc chloride fixative was applied to the obvious tumor under occlusion (Fig. 7.6). Dichloroacetic acid was often applied prior to the fixative to increase its penetration. On the second day, the tumor was debulked, and the fixative was applied to the wound bed and adjacent skin. Dichloroacetic acid was applied to the adjacent epidermis prior to applying the fixative to increase its penetration. On the third and subsequent days, tissue was removed and microscopically examined for the presence of tumor. Zinc chloride was applied to any areas containing tumor, along with an occlusive dressing. The process was continued until there was no longer any residual tumor. If a repair was anticipated, this had to be delayed until the residual fixed tissue had separated; however, the majority of wounds were allowed to heal by second intent.

How deep the fixation process extended depended on a number of factors, including: (1) the thickness of the layer of paste applied, (2) the length of time the dressing was left in place (the paste was usually "used up," i.e., inactive after 18 h), (3) the vascularity of the tissue, and (4) the amount of edema that occurred. For most cases, a 1–3-mm-thick layer of paste was applied. Avascular tissue was very susceptible to fixation, and one needed to be careful if, for example, one was working in an area of prior irradiation. Over fixation could result in a full-thickness defect of an ear or nose or even the skull. Achieving a "good" fix around the eye was sometimes difficult because of the accumulation of fluid, which diluted out the paste and interfered with fixation. Intact skin was somewhat impervious to the penetration of the fixative; thus, it was necessary to pretreat with dichloroacetic acid prior to applying the fixative.

An occlusive dressing was necessary to prevent the unwanted spread of the paste and to promote its penetration. The sequence of application of the various constituents was as follows: (1) first, the dichloroacetic acid was applied to the intact epidermis surrounding the wound bed; (2) next, the fixative was applied to the wound bed and adjacent epidermis; (3) then, the area was ringed with Orabase, which helped prevent the spread of the paste (Fig. 7.6); (4) then, several layers of Vaseline-coated orthopedic cotton were applied. The piece of cotton applied first had petroleum on its outer surface, but not on its inner surface. Over this was placed gauze and tape. The next day, the patient presented for surgery. The dressing and paste were

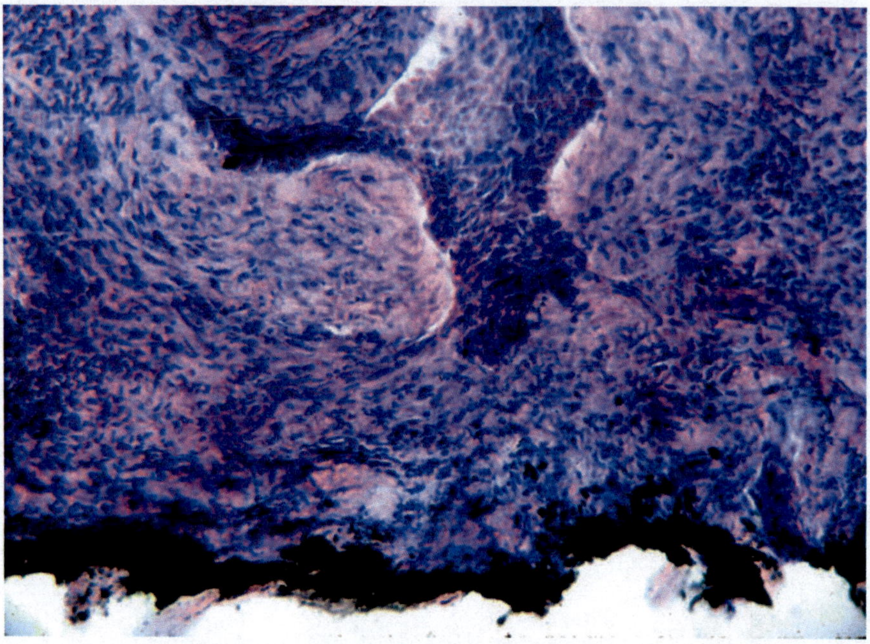

Fig. 7.5 Frozen section of fixed tissue cut with a cryotome demonstrating how thick the section is and the inflammation, which makes interpretation more difficult

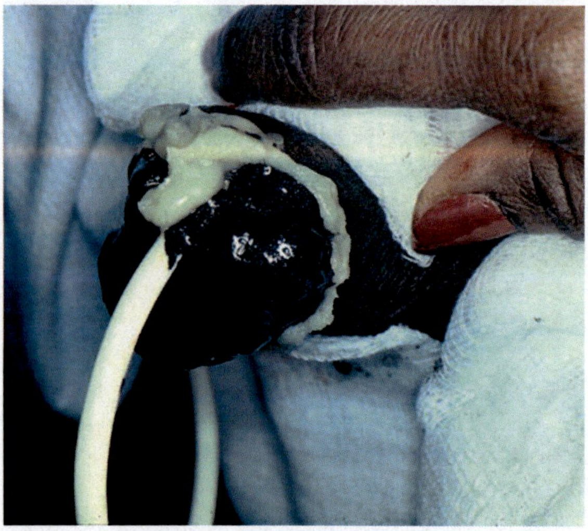

Fig. 7.6 Orabase and fixative have been applied to the lesion

removed, and surgery was initiated. The fixed tissue was very white in appearance and had the consistency of cardboard. As long as the excision was confined to the fixed tissue, there was no bleeding or pain. As the tissue was removed, 20% merbromin was used to mark on the floor of the wound, thus denoting the source of the specimens. A corresponding map was drawn. After removal, the tissue was submitted for microscopic examination utilizing frozen sections. Any areas positive for residual tumor were noted on the map of the wound. Zinc chloride fixative was applied to those areas positive for residual tumor, along with an occlusive dressing. The patient was instructed to return the following day for additional surgery, if so indicated. This sequence of events continued until the patient was tumor-free.

In the early days of Mohs surgery, most histotechnicians used a cryotome in conjunction with carbon dioxide gas and a water bath. Unfortunately, the sections generated were quite thick, which made the microscopic interpretation of these sections more difficult (Fig. 7.5). The advent of the cryostat revolutionized Mohs surgery in that ultra-thin sections could be generated quickly. These sections were, microscopically, much easier to interpret.

Although the "fixed tissue" technique had many disadvantages and thus was eventually replaced by the "fresh tissue" technique, there were situations in which it was quite helpful. For example, if one had exposed calvarium, the paste could be applied to the exposed bone. Up to 12 weeks later, if this had been done expertly, a few taps with a hammer and osteotome would result in the separation of a thin layer of bone, revealing healthy granulation tissue, which could serve as the foundation for healing by second intent or the bed for a split-thickness graft. Unfortunately, this technique was not effective if the bone had previously been irradiated. The use of the fixative also facilitated the removal of very vascular tumors and deeply invasive tumors. Deeply invasive tumors could probably be removed more safely and accurately and with less pain than with the fresh tissue technique.

In the early 1970s, Dr. Mohs [1], and Stegman and Tromovitch [2], in selected cases, would omit the zinc chloride fixative and use a local anesthetic to remove the tissue. This became known as the "fresh tissue" technique. Once it was realized that the cure rate with the "fresh tissue" technique was as good as it was with the "fixed tissue" technique and that the transection of tumor did not lead to metastases, Mohs surgery became a much less painful and much more accepted procedure for treating skin cancer. Moreover, the "fresh tissue" technique permitted immediate repairs, which eventually resulted in Mohs surgeons becoming very accomplished reconstructive surgeons. This also allowed most patients to have their surgery completed in a single day by one surgeon. The advent of the "fresh tissue" technique also resulted in a series of changes in the name of the procedure and the Mohs College. Because the "fixed tissue" technique was rarely used and the term "chemosurgery" carried with it inappropriate connotations, the term was replaced by the term "microscopically controlled surgery." However, because the use of routine frozen sections could be considered microscopically controlled surgery, it was decided that a more descriptive term be used. This resulted in the name "Mohs micrographic surgery." In tandem with these changes in the name of the procedure came changes in the name of the organization. Initially it was known as the American College of Mohs Chemosurgery. Once the use of the "fresh tissue" technique became prevalent, the College changed its name to the American College of Mohs Micrographic Surgery and Cutaneous Oncology. Although very descriptive and appropriate, it was later felt by the Public Relations Committee that it was not a name easily remembered by the public and that in order to promote the procedure and organization, it would be preferable to shorten the name to the American College of Mohs Surgery.

For many years, the pharmacy at the University of Wisconsin served as a source for the zinc chloride fixative. However, it is no longer available. One of the authors (PGL) has used other sources for this paste and did not like the preparation as well.

In addition to being used to treat skin cancer, Mohs chemosurgery proved to be useful in the management of other cancers and noncancerous conditions including gangrene, infected unresectable carcinomas, unusual cutaneous infections, and chest wall recurrences of breast cancer.

Summary: Conclusion

- The fixed tissue technique is rarely used today.
- A multidisciplinary approach to difficult skin cancers has largely supplanted the fixed tissue technique.

7.2 Conclusion

Today, the fixed tissue technique is rarely used and is mainly of historical significance. A multidisciplinary approach to difficult skin cancers has largely supplanted the need for the fixed tissue technique. This, in combination with the fact that the fixative is in short supply and that only the more senior Mohs surgeons have the expertise to use the fixative, has meant that the "fixed tissue" technique has become a dying art.

References

1. Mohs FE. Chemosurgery. Microscopically controlled surgery for skin cancer. Springfield: Charles C. Thomas; 1978. p. 106.
2. Tromivitch TA, Stegman SJ. Microscopically controlled excision of skin tumors: chemosurgery (Mohs) fixed tissue technique. Arch Dermatol. 1974;110:231–2.

Fresh Tissue Technique

8

Michael P. McLeod, Katlein França, and Keyvan Nouri

Abstract

The fresh frozen tissue technique was initially used for eyelid tumors; and since its introduction, has revolutionized the way Mohs surgery is performed. It has rapidly expanded beyond eyelid tumors and is now used for all anatomic locations. Now, reconstruction can occur immediately following complete histologic removal of the tumor; which in most instances is the same day. Additionally, the fresh frozen tissue technique is less painful, quicker, and conserves more tissue compared to the fixed tissue technique. This chapter details the introduction as well as how to perform the fresh frozen tissue technique.

Keywords

Fresh frozen tissue • Eyelid tumors • Modern mohs micrographic surgery

Summary: Introduction

- The fresh tissue technique was initially used for eyelid cancers.
- The modern approach to Mohs micrographic surgery predominantly involves the fresh tissue technique.
- Histologic preparation for microscopic examination in Mohs surgery requires skill and practice.
- Several other techniques have been described for rapidly freezing tissue and enhancing histology, including isopentane histopath, liquid nitrogen, and dry ice.

M.P. McLeod • K. França
Department of Dermatology and Cutaneous Surgery, University of Miami Leonard M. Miller School of Medicine, Miami, FL, USA

K. Nouri (✉)
Department of Dermatology and Cutaneous Surgery, University of Miami Leonard M. Miller School of Medicine, Miami, FL, USA

Sylvester Comprehensive Cancer Center, University of Miami Hospital and Clinics, Miami, FL, USA
e-mail: knouri@med.miami.edu

K. Nouri (ed.), *Mohs Micrographic Surgery*,
DOI 10.1007/978-1-4471-2152-7_8, © Springer-Verlag London Limited 2012

8.1 Introduction

Mohs Micrographic Surgery originally used fixed tissue sections. It was not until 1953, during the filming of Dr. Mohs removing a pigmented BCC from the patient's lower eyelid that the fresh tissue technique became known. In order to prevent a delay in filming the procedure, Dr. Mohs sped along the process by carrying out the last two stages using fresh frozen tissue. From that time forward Dr. Mohs used the fresh tissue technique for nearly all eyelid cancers. That way the zinc chloride paste did not risk coming into contact with the patient's eyes. However, at the time, serious doubts were raised as to whether the fresh tissue technique would be as effective as the fixed tissue technique.

In 1956, the first written material documented the fresh tissue technique in Dr. Epstein's text book, Skin Surgery. The turning point came in 1969, at the annual meeting of the American College of Chemosurgery. It was at this time that Dr. Mohs reported 100%, 5 year cure rates using the fresh tissue technique for 66 basal and squamous cell carcinomas. The following year in 1970, Dr. Tromovitch presented an additional 75 patients with the fresh tissue technique with excellent results. In 1974, Tromovitch and Stegman presented a 99% cure rate from 102 patients. The fresh tissue technique finally became accepted when Dr. Mohs reported his 5 year cure rate of 99.8% cure rate with 3,466 patients [1]. The fresh tissue technique is now well accepted and has become the predominant technique for Mohs Micrographic Surgery [2].

Summary: The Technique

- It is important to confirm the exact site of the previous biopsy and outline the tumor with a marking pen.
- After the anesthetic process, a curette should be used to debulk the tumor
- It is important to maintain specimen orientation
- The tissue should be excised with the scalpel angle 45° to the skin to facilitate the histological process and the deep margin should be excised horizontally

8.2 The Technique

Before starting the surgery, it is important to confirm the exact site of the previous biopsy and outline the tumor with a marking pen. This should be done prior to injecting the local anesthesia, because it can distort the original anatomic landmarks of the tumor.

After waiting some minutes for optimal local anesthetic effects, a curette should be used to debulk the tumor, to better delineate its extension.

The precise orientation of the specimen is important to maintain and can be carried out by making superficial scalpel incisions at the periphery of the specimen or using a substance such as methylene blue, sutures, staples, or hatch marks.

The tissue should be excised with the scalpel angle 45° to the skin to facilitate histological processing and the deep margin should be excised horizontally. The hemostasis process is achieved by using pressure, electrocautery or suture ligatures if necessary.

It is important to draw a 2-dimensional map of the tumor with markers used to orient the specimen. This map is used in orienting the specimen as well as guiding the surgeon to remove any residual neoplasm.

Summary: Histologic Preparation of the Tissue

- After excision, the tissue is carefully processed in a special lab by the technician.
- The technician must mount the tissue as it is presented, flattening it's surface in an even horizontal plane. Then, it must be cut as frozen sections, using a cryostat.
- The slides are usually stained with hematoxylin-eosin and are ready for interpretation by the Mohs surgeon.

8.3 Histologic Preparation of the Tissue

Histologic preparation for microscopic examination in Mohs surgery requires skill and practice.

After the excision, the tissue is carefully processed in a special lab by the technician.

The specimen is usually divided along the marked lines and inverted, so the dermis faces upwards. The edges of the tissue are then color-coded with tissue dyes.

The technician must mount the tissue as it is presented, flattening it's surface in an even horizontal plane. Then, it must be cut as frozen sections, using a cryostat. The horizontal sections are taken at 5–7 mm. Several other techniques have been described for rapidly freezing tissue and enhancing histology, including isopentane histopath, liquid nitrogen, and dry ice [3–5].

The epidermal margin and the entire surface of the excised specimen is thoroughly processed. Each saucerized piece of tissue is compressed and it is horizontally sectioned from the deep margin upward. The slides are usually stained with hematoxylin-eosin, and are ready for interpretation by the Mohs surgeon.

Summary: Conclusion

- The Fresh tissue technique is less painful, faster and conserves more tissue when compared with the fixed technique.
- This technique allows for immediate reconstruction.

8.4 Conclusion

The modern approach to Mohs micrographic surgery predominantly involves the fresh tissue technique. The original fixed tissue technique did not allow for immediate reconstruction. Sometimes 6-8 weeks were required for complete granulations to heal the defect when the fixed tissue technique was used. The use of the fresh tissue technique allows immediate reconstruction. It is also less painful, quicker and conserves more tissue when compared with the fixed tissue technique [2].

References

1. Mohs FE. The chemosurgical method for the microscopically controlled excision of cutaneous cancer. In: Epstein E, editor. Skin surgery. Philadelphia: Lea & Febiger; 1956.
2. Lang PG et al. Mohs micrographic surgery. Fresh-tissue technique. Dermatol Clin. 1989;7(4):613–26.
3. Erickson QL et al. Flash freezing of Mohs micrographic surgery tissue can minimize freeze artifact and speed slide preparation. Dermatol Surg. 2011;37:503–9.
4. Cecchi R et al. Micrographic surgery (fresh-tissue Tübingen technique) for treatment of basal cell carcinoma of the head: a single-centre report. J Dermatol. 2008;35:678–9.
5. Bakhtar O et al. Tissue preparation for MOHS frozen sections: a comparison of three techniques. Virchows Arch. 2007;450:513–8.

Special Considerations for Mohs Micrographic Surgery in Organ Transplant Recipients

9

Thomas Stasko and Daniel L. Christiansen

Abstract
Immunosuppressed patients have an increased risk of skin cancer, particularly virally mediated types. Squamous cell carcinomas in this population tend to behave more aggressively than in the general population. Mohs micrographic surgery is considered standard of care for treating high-risk squamous cell carcinomas.

Keywords
Immunosuppression • Merkel cell carcinoma • Organ transplant • Squamous cell carcinoma

Summary: Introduction

- Immune system compromise is theorized to play a critical role in accelerating the development of skin cancer in both organ transplant and HIV/AIDS patients. Chemotherapeutic agents may also promote carcinogenicity, and an understanding of these risk factors is essential for optimizing skin cancer management in this population.

9.1 Introduction

Immunosuppressed patients present both diagnostic and therapeutic challenges for the Mohs surgeon. In the United States alone, there are over 183,000 living organ transplant recipients [1] and 1.1 million patients with HIV [2]. New drugs and therapies have provided patients with increased survival and enabled a growing epidemic of cutaneous disease. This subset of patients not only exhibit a much higher incidence of nonmelanoma skin cancer (NMSC) when compared to the general population but also tend to develop tumors that follow a more aggressive course, portending a poorer prognosis. While the exact contributions are unknown, the likely cause of this disparity is a combination of decreased immunosurveillance and a direct carcinogenic effect of certain immunosuppressant medications. With increased transplant organ survival and the need for ongoing immunosuppression, this incidence is likely to increase.

T. Stasko (✉)
Department of Medicine, Division of Dermatology, Vanderbilt University, Nashville, TN, USA
e-mail: tom.stasko@vanderbilt.edu

D.L. Christiansen
Department of Medicine, Division of Dermatology, Vanderbilt Medical Center, Nashville, TN, USA

K. Nouri (ed.), *Mohs Micrographic Surgery*,
DOI 10.1007/978-1-4471-2152-7_9, © Springer-Verlag London Limited 2012

The importance of an intact immune system in preventing the formation of de novo malignancies was discussed by Burnett in 1970 [3]. He theorized that immune cells played a crucial role in recognizing "self" and eliminating those cells that escaped homeostatic controls. Histologic correlation of this phenomenon is evident in tumors with infiltrating cytotoxic lymphocytes [4]. This view is further supported by studies of patients with impaired immunity, namely, HIV/AIDS and solid organ transplant recipients (SOTR) on chronic immunosuppression, who have an increased risk of NMSC, – up to 250-fold higher than the general population [5–7]. Understanding the role of a compromised immune system on the development of neoplasms is critical when designing therapeutic strategies aimed at prevention and treatment in this patient population.

Summary: Solid Organ Transplant Recipients

- Solid organ transplant patients are at a higher risk of developing NMSC than the general population. Heart transplant patients are at the highest risk, followed by renal and liver transplant recipients. Some immunosuppressant medications appear to play both an indirect and direct role in promoting carcinogenesis.

9.2 Solid Organ Transplant Recipients

The first successful solid organ transplant took place in 1954 between identical twins, but frequent graft rejection and high mortality rates, outside such settings, limited its use [8]. The subsequent introduction of immunosuppressant medications, such as azathioprine and cyclosporine, substantially improved graft survival and ushered in the era of modern transplantation. New combinations of immunosuppressants and the use of targeted therapies have resulted in ever improving survival and a paradigm shift from traditional causes of mortality in this patient population (surgical complications, rejection, and acute infection) to long-term causes (diabetes, cardiovascular disease, chronic infection, and malignancies including NMSC.)

Occurring in excess of 1–2 million cases annually in the United States alone, NMSC is by far the most common human malignancy worldwide [9]. While generally considered somewhat indolent neoplasms in most immunocompetent individuals, NMSC in the solid organ transplant patient may have devastating effects [10–12]. Consequences range from frequent painful procedures, such as extensive cryotherapy, to severe disfigurement and disease-associated mortality.

Risk Factors for NMSC in SOTR

- Duration and type of immunosuppression
- History of chronic sun exposure
- Fitzpatrick skin type I–III
- Male sex
- Age at transplantation
- Number of actinic keratoses
- Exposure to human papillomavirus
- CD4 lymphopenia

In addition to the risk factors outlined above, risk of NMSC appears to vary by transplant type. Renal transplantation, the first to be performed successfully and the most common type of solid organ transplantation occurring today, with greater than 16,000 transplants annually [1], is second only to heart transplant patients in terms of increased NMSC incidence [13]. While it varies by country, the reported incidence of SCC and BCC 20 years post-renal transplant is extraordinarily high: 41% in the Netherlands [14], 48% in the United States [15], 54.4% in New Zealand [16], and 82% in Australia [17]. The majority of these skin cancers are squamous cell carcinomas, occurring at a rate of 3:1 to basal cell carcinoma [16], opposite of the observed frequency of 1:4 typically seen in immunocompetent individuals.

Heart transplantation, which first took place in 1967 [7], has the highest risk of NMSC. Historically cardiac transplantation has been associated with an increased risk of graft rejection compared with other organs which is theorized to result from an inherent increased immunogenicity of the myocardium. As a result, patients are usually placed on higher immunosuppression doses than other SOTR which has led to the inference that the higher cumulative immunosuppressive dose may play a role in promoting NMSC [13]. This is further supported by studies of liver transplant patients, typically the least immunosuppressed of all SOTR due

Table 9.1 Immunosuppressant medications [24–26, 70]

Class	Drug name	Mechanism of action	Risk of NMSC
Corticosteroids	Prednisolone, prednisone	Alters cytokine production and impairs granulocyte chemotaxis	+
Antimetabolite	Azathioprine (AZA)	Antagonizes purine metabolism and synthesis	+ + + +
Antimetabolite	Mycophenolate mofetil (MMF)	Impairs T- and B-cell proliferation by interfering with de novo guanine nucleotide synthesis	+ + + (probably an improvement over AZA)
Calcineurin inhibitor	Cyclosporine A (CSA)	Decreases T-cell activation and IL-2 production	+ + +
Calcineurin inhibitor	Tacrolimus (TAC)	Decreases T-cell activation and IL-2 production	+ + + (probably an improvement over CSA)
Polyclonal antilymphocyte antibody	Thymoglobulin	Depletes T lymphocytes through complement mediated cytolysis and apoptosis	Unknown
Monoclonal antilymphocyte antibody	OKT3	Anti-CD3 humanized monoclonal antibody to deplete T lymphocytes	+
Monoclonal anticytokine receptor antibodies	Daclizumab, basiliximab	Chimeric/humanized anti-CD25 monoclonal antibody	Unknown
Monoclonal anticytokine receptor antibody	Alemtuzumab	Humanized anti-CD52 antibody	Unknown
Monoclonal anticytokine receptor antibody	Belatacept (LEA29Y)	Fusion protein consisting of partial immunoglobulin molecule and mutated high affinity receptor for B7–1 and B7–2 that results in T-cell anergy and apoptosis	Unknown
Target of rapamycin inhibitor	Sirolimus (rapamycin)	Inhibits mammalian target of rapamycin disrupting IL-2 signaling, resultant antiangiogenic and antiproliferative effect	+, but anti-carcinogenic effect reported
Target of rapamycin inhibitor	Everolimus	Structural analogue of sirolimus	No long-term data, may be similar to sirolimus

to a lower risk of graft rejection, who have the lowest rate of NMSC. Several studies appear to support the notion that total amount of immunosuppression, rather than the type, is the most important determinant of future NMSC development [7, 18, 19].

Lung transplantation is much less commonly performed, with only 1,660 performed in 2009 [1], and the overall risk of NMSC is less well characterized in this subset of patients. Incidence appears to be most similar to renal transplant patients with approximately 0.7–6.4% of all patients studied developing SCC within 1 year of lung transplant and a similar ratio of SCC to BCC as in other SOTR of 4:1 [20–22]. The use of voriconazole in this patient population is a unique exposure not generally seen in other transplant recipients. Utilized as a prophylactic antifungal medication to prevent respiratory fungal infections, voriconazole is known to increase risk of photosensitivity [23]. Its use has been identified as an independent risk factor for SCC development in lung transplant patients [20] and may be related to the enhanced UV sensitivity which has previously been identified as a risk factor for SCC development.

In addition to voriconazole, multiple immunosuppressant medications have been proposed as playing a role in promoting NMSC. Cyclosporine A has been shown to directly increase the invasive potential of murine model cells by promoting increased TGF-B levels and inducing phenotypic alterations, independent of direct immunosuppression [24]. Whether this effect holds true in SOTR is less clear. A study comparing types of immunosuppression demonstrated that azathioprine had the highest risk of cutaneous carcinogenesis in a mouse model, followed by cyclophosphamide, cyclosporine, and lastly prednisolone [25]. Due to confounding variables it is difficult to quantify the exact role varying immunosuppressive regimens play in promoting NMSC but a general estimation of effect based on the available literature is shown in Table 9.1. A notable exception to immunosuppressant agent promotion of NMSC is sirolimus which has been shown, in limited studies, to reduce risk when added to current regimens in renal transplant patients [26].

> **Summary: HIV/AIDS**
> - HIV increases the risk of developing NMSC, particularly virally mediated types. HAART therapy may play a role in treating HIV patients with malignancy.

9.3 HIV/AIDS

Human immunodeficiency affects approximately 1 million people in the United States and is caused by a DNA retrovirus that primarily replicates in CD4+ T helper cells leading to substantial immunocompromise as lymphopenia develops [27]. Patients may ultimately develop Acquired Immunodeficiency Syndrome (AIDS) and have a three- to fivefold increased risk of NMSC [28]. Virally associated neoplasms, including Kaposi Sarcoma (KS) and human papillomavirus (HPV) associated cancers, are particularly prevalent in this population [29]. HPV dysplasia and subsequent development of SCC has been established in cervical, anal, genital, and oropharyngeal lesions. These NMSC tend to present at more advanced stages, be higher grade, and lead to shortened overall survival compared to immunocompetent hosts [29, 30]. Unlike SOTR, the ratio of SCC to BCC in HIV/AIDS patients parallels that seen in the general population at 1:7 with similar risk factors including: fair skin, age, and chronic sun exposure [31]. HIV/AIDS patients also have an increased risk of melanoma (SIR = 1.3), MCC (SIR = 11) and sebaceous carcinoma (SIR = 8.1) [32].

In recent years enormous progress has been made in the treatment of this disease, and like organ transplant recipients, patients are experiencing substantial improvement in overall survival. The advent of highly active antiretroviral therapy (HAART) has resulted in a decreased incidence of KS and melanoma in this population [28]. Treatment recommendations for NMSC and melanoma in the HIV/AIDS population parallel the general population with an emphasis on increased prevention of virally mediated cancers. HAART should be considered for all eligible patients and routine surveillance for HPV associated verrucae performed. Imiquimod has been successfully used to treat HPV and anal intraepithelial neoplasia in these patients and may be used prior to excision of SCC for cosmetically sensitive areas. Excision with or without MMS, depending on histologic subtype, site, and size, are the mainstays of treatment for SCC/BCC. Melanoma tends to follow a more aggressive course in HIV infected patients and immune reconstitution should be considered as adjuvant therapy [33]. Surgical margins will vary based on Breslow depth and the use of sentinel lymph node biopsy should be considered in tumors >1 mm.

> **Summary: Cutaneous Neoplasms**
> - The most common malignancies in transplant patients are squamous cell carcinomas, followed by basal cell carcinomas. Merkel cell carcinoma, Kaposi sarcoma, and melanoma occur more commonly in the immunosuppressed population.

9.4 Cutaneous Neoplasms

9.4.1 Actinic Keratoses and Squamous Cell Carcinoma

Actinic keratoses are widespread in the general population with a prevalence of 11–26% and are present in roughly half of all heart/renal transplant patients [34, 35]. They occur on chronically sun exposed skin and share many of the histological features of SCC in situ. Risks for developing AKs parallel those for SCC with skin type, long term UVB exposure, advanced age, and immunosuppression all conferring added risk. While the exact relationship between actinic keratoses and development of squamous cell skin cancer remains controversial, studies have shown a rate of transformation in immunocompetent individuals of approximately 0.1–0.6% per year [36, 37]. Actinic keratoses are a marker of excessive sun damage and the risk of developing SCC in SOTRs increases with higher numbers of keratotic lesions.

Due to the high risk SCC poses in this patient population prevention is increasingly being recommended

[35, 38]. Limited numbers of AKs may be treated by cryotherapy or curettage but extensive actinic damage should receive field treatments. The options available include topical fluorouracil, photodynamic therapy (PDT), imiquimod, and topical diclofenac. Topical fluorouracil and PDT are the most commonly described modalities and appear to confer a benefit in clearing actinic keratoses. Imiquimod is less well characterized in this population due to the theoretical risk of enhanced immunogenicity from activation of toll like receptor 7 but has been safely used for treating actinic keratosis in OTRs and at least one study looked closely at safety parameters [39]. Guidelines support the role of proactive field treatments in patients with extensive AKs to reduce the risk of SCC [35]. Oral retinoids have also been used in select OTR with promising results [40].

Squamous cell carcinomas (SCC) are the second most common neoplasm in the United States, with an annual incidence of at least 200,000, but are the most common malignancy in SOTR [41]. They occur most commonly on sun exposed areas, including the head and neck. SCC is 65 times more common in organ transplant patients than the general population, with increased risk conferred by cardiac transplantation and increasing number of immunosuppressant medications [7]. High risk SCC accounts for the vast majority of the 8,000 nodal metastases and 3,000 annual deaths attributed to SCC [42, 43].

SCCs in SOTR tend to behave more aggressively, with increased rates of growth, local recurrence, and metastases. Immunosuppressed patients have a 13% risk of metastatic disease compared to 6% for the general population [42]. In one case series of SOTR, 15% of patients who developed SCCs died from metastatic disease within 10 years of diagnosis [16]. The 3-year survival rate is only 48% once regional metastases occur, and distant metastases confer a 1-year survival of only 39% [45].

Other high risk clinical features include tumors greater than 2 cm in diameter and invasion of subcutaneous fat, fascia, muscle, or bone [46]. Histologically, poorly differentiated disease has a 33% risk of metastasis [42]. Tumors in SOTR are more likely to demonstrate increased proliferation rates and perineural invasion. In patients who have involvement of nerves greater than 0.1 mm in size there is a 32% risk of disease specific death [47]. Lip and ear involvement also occurs more frequently in this population and has a higher frequency of metastasis [42].

All patients with SCC should receive regional lymph node exam, and any enlarged nodes evaluated histologically [41]. Lymphadenectomy is preferred for lymph node positive disease with radiotherapy appearing to confer an additional survival benefit when appropriate [48]. Controlled studies regarding the role of radiological imaging and sentinel lymph node examination have not been performed to date for cutaneous SCC.

Low-risk SCC can be managed with standard surgical excision with 4-mm margins in tumors less than 2 cm in size producing cure in 95% of cases. Shave excision plus electrodessication and curettage has also been shown to be effective for low-risk SCC. Features of low-risk SCC are outlined in Fig. 9.1. If patients have clinically or histologically high-risk SCC based on criteria in Fig. 9.1, they should be treated with excision of at least 6-mm margins with histopathological clear margins or, preferably, Mohs micrographic surgery. If perineural invasion remains, deep structures such as bone are involved, or if clearance cannot be obtained, then adjuvant therapy should be considered. Imaging studies to assess for extension and localized radiation should be considered. Reducing immunosuppression levels should also be discussed with the patient's transplant team and, if feasible, has been shown to decrease new SCC formation and improve outcomes [49].

9.4.2 Basal Cell Carcinoma

Basal cell carcinomas are the second most common neoplasm in SOTR and occur at a rate up to ten times higher than the general population. Histologically, they are indistinguishable from those found in immunocompetent patients and tend to follow a similarly indolent course [50]. Risk factors for their development include pretransplant NMSC, duration of immunosuppression, and increasing age of recipient.

There are no standardized recommendations regarding treatment of BCC in the SOTR. While increased surveillance is suggested due to elevated risk in this population, the type of treatment modality chosen will parallel that seen in the general population. Histologic subtype, tumor size, and tumor location are the primary considerations when choosing a therapy. Superficial BCCs may be treated with a wide variety of methods based on patient/physician preference

AK/SCC treatment algorithms

Clinical presentation	Treatment	Disposition
Diffuse actinic field damage →	5-Fluorouracil, PDT, imiquimod →	3–6 month skin checks

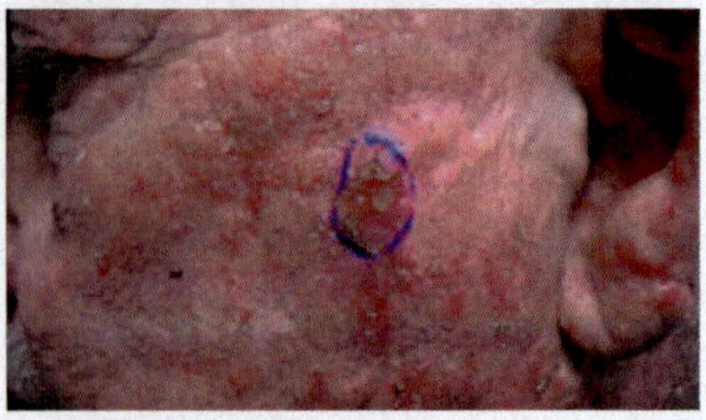

Clinical presentation	Treatment		Disposition
HAK/VV →	Cryotherapy +/– curettage → *Persists* →	Biopsy →	AK or SCC algorithm per histology

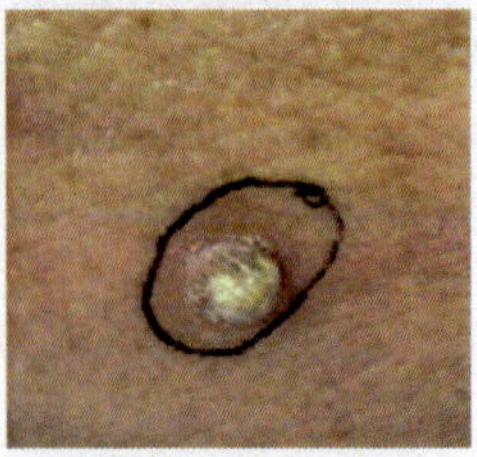

Clinical presentation	Histology	Treatment	Disposition
Low risk SCC → *Size low risk Slow growth Nonulcerated Well defined margins	In situ Keratoacanthoma Well differentiated →	ED&C, Cryosurgery, Excision, Mohs	*Resolves* → 3–6 month skin checks with regional lymph node examination *Persists* → High risk SCC algorithm

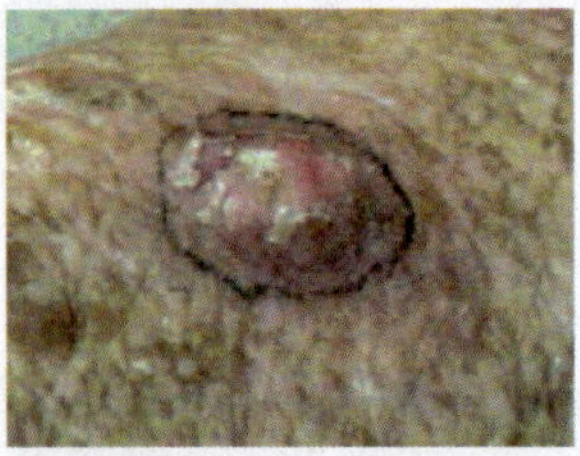

Clinical presentation	Histology	Treatment	Disposition
High risk SCC → **Size high risk Rapid growth Ulcerated Poorly defined margins	Poorly differentiated Invading subcutaneous fat Perineural invasion →	Mohs	*Resolves* → 3–6 month skin checks with regional lymph node examination *Unable to clear* *Persistent perineural invasion* *Involvement of bone or parotid* → Consider: Imaging for extension Additional tumor resection Retinoid therapy Alteration of immunosuppression

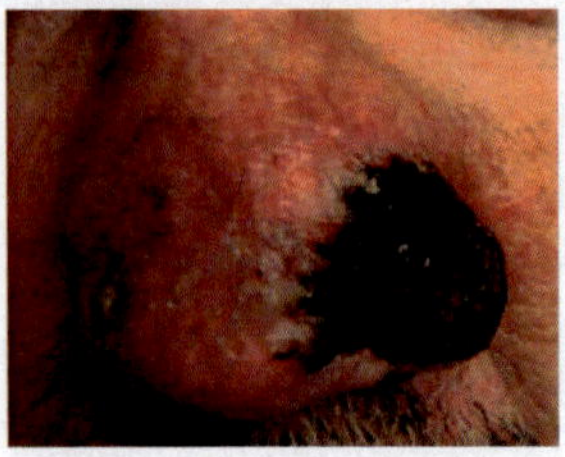

Size:

*Low risk
<0.6 cm - face (excluding cheeks, forehead, neck and scalp), ears, genitals, hands and feet
<1.0 cm - cheeks, forehead, neck and scalp
<2.0 cm - trunk and extremities

**High risk
>0.6 cm - face (excluding cheeks, forehead, neck and scalp), ears, genitals, hands and feet
>1.0 cm - cheeks, forehead, neck and scalp

Fig. 9.1 AK/SCC treatment algorithms

including: electrodessication and curettage, cryotherapy, topical chemotherapeutic agents (5-fluorouracil), topical immunomodulators (imiquimod), and photodynamic therapy [51–53]. Infiltrative and nodular basal cell carcinomas are more likely to require surgical excision, with or without micrographic margin control, for complete and sustained clearance. Cosmetically sensitive locations, such as the face, and embryonic fusion planes should generally be managed with Mohs micrographic surgery for best cosmetic outcome and lowest recurrence risk.

9.4.3 Melanoma

The incidence of melanoma is increasing at a faster rate than any other cancer in the United States with over 44,200 cases documented annually [8, 54]. Lifetime risk of developing a melanoma is now estimated at 1 in 63 [54]. Studies comparing risk of melanoma in immunocompetent patients to SOTR have yielded conflicting results, with some studies demonstrating a greater than 3.5–8-fold increased risk in renal transplant patients and others showing no appreciable increase [4, 55]. Further studies are needed to clarify risks and prognostic factors for SOTR.

Risk of melanoma recurrence after transplantation is also not well characterized. One study showed 6 of 31 patients who were in remission for an average of 2 years prior to transplant developed a recurrence, and all 6 died from metastatic melanoma [56]. Melanoma may also rarely be transmitted through transplantation itself and is associated with exceedingly poor outcomes [57].

There are no formal guidelines dictating management of melanoma in the SOTR, but similar outcomes to immunocompetent controls have been reported for thin melanoma (<1 mm) when utilizing standard therapeutic practices, with excision as the mainstay of treatment. Wide local excision should be performed with surgical margins dependent on Breslow depth. A sentinel lymph node biopsy should be considered in patients with tumors >1 mm in Breslow depth, but data regarding impact on outcome and overall survival are lacking in the SOTR. The International Transplant Skin Cancer Collaborative (ITSCC) and the Skin Care in Organ Transplant Patients Europe (SCOPE) have recently published guidelines advising decreasing immunosuppressive regimen as an adjuvant management strategy. Data is limited on the impact of this approach, but it should be considered in all patients with stage IV melanoma.

9.4.4 Merkel Cell Carcinoma

Merkel cell carcinoma (MCC) is a rare and aggressive neuroendocrine skin cancer primarily occurring in the elderly and immunosuppressed. HIV/AIDS patients and SOTR have a greater than 13-fold increased risk of developing MCC compared to the general population. The mean age of those affected is 70 years old with a male predominance. In one study, MCC developed an average of 91 months after transplantation, with over 70% of patients developing metastases and 50% dying from their disease [58]. The recent discovery of a novel polyomavirus, Merkel cell polyomavirus, in 70–80% of MCC cases has begun to shed light on the possible etiology of this rare tumor [59].

There is no formal consensus on the treatment of MCC in the immunosuppressed patients, but given the aggressive nature of this tumor, wide local excision is the preferred initial treatment modality. If this is not feasible, due to anatomic location, the use of Mohs micrographic surgery may be considered. In the immunocompetent patient, MMS has been used successfully with high cure rates [60]. Sentinel lymph node biopsy has been proposed as a useful staging tool and prognostic indicator [61]. Adjuvant radiation with 3–5-cm margins should be considered after tumor removal and some centers consider radiation to the draining lymph node basin. Clinically apparent lymph node involvement and disseminated disease may require further surgical intervention, radiation therapy, or chemotherapy. All patients should have routine follow-up and close monitoring.

9.4.5 Kaposi Sarcoma

Kaposi sarcoma is a rare endothelial tumor caused by human herpesvirus 8 (HHV-8) that is primarily seen in immunosuppressed patients. Homosexual men with acquired immunodeficiency syndrome are disproportionately affected, and increased rates of lymphopenia directly correlate with disease severity. Incidence of the disease in SOTR directly correlates with the prevalence of the disease and HHV-8 infection. In patients with AIDS and SOTR, immune reconstitution alone may be curative [28]. A switch from cyclosporine to sirolimus in a SOTR resulted in clinical regression in one case report. Additional approaches for localized disease include: cryotherapy, laser surgery, radiation, intralesional chemotherapy, imiquimod, topical retinoids, and excision. Patients with systemic disease may require chemotherapy if immune reconstitution is ineffective or not feasible.

Summary: Special Surgical Considerations in the Organ Transplant Patient

- Solid organ transplant recipients are more likely to develop high-risk and recurrent neoplasms. Mohs is considered the standard of care for treating these tumors, and frequent follow-up is necessary. The following list summarizes the key elements to managing these patients:

Preoperative Evaluation

- Type of transplantation
- History of skin cancer including size, location, and histology
- Relevant medications (may impact wound healing)

Surgical Management

- SCC (low- and high-risk subtypes) – Treatment recommendations by clinical and histologic criteria (Fig. 9.1)
- Merkel cell, Melanoma, and BCC management similar to immunocompetent patients.

Postoperative

- Notify primary transplant team for consideration of immunosuppressant regimen alteration
- 3–6-month follow-up with regional lymph node evaluations

9.5 Special Surgical Considerations in the Organ Transplant Patient

9.5.1 Preoperative Evaluation

The preoperative evaluation is an important screening tool for the dermatologic surgeon when evaluating prospective surgical candidates and is especially important when assessing the immunosuppressed patients. Special emphasis should be placed on the size, location, and histology of each skin cancer to determine the appropriate treatment modality. Patient medications should be closely evaluated, as several immunosuppressant agents (corticosteroids, sirolimus, and everolimus) have been associated with delayed or poor wound healing [62]. SOTR do not appear to be at an increased risk for scar formation, but history of keloid formation or hypertrophic scarring after transplantation should be noted. The current status of the patient's transplant should be determined, and any special precautions, such as need for antibiotic prophylaxis, be discussed.

9.5.2 Antibiotic Prophylaxis

Large scale, randomized studies examining the role of antibiotic prophylaxis in organ transplant patients undergoing dermatologic surgery do not currently exist, so consensus statements have been developed to help guide the Mohs surgeon in choosing when prophylaxis is required. The statements are to be used as guidelines but may not apply to all situations.

Although immunocompromised patients have an increased incidence of many skin and systemic infections, they are not considered at extremely high risk for surgical site infections, and prophylaxis is not routinely indicated when performing cryotherapy or electrodessication and curettage. For larger procedures, such as excision or Mohs surgery, surgical site prophylaxis should be considered utilizing the same criteria as in nonimmunosuppressed population.

Organ transplantation does not routinely require preoperative antibiotics to prevent graft infection with cutaneous procedures. The American Heart Association does recommend prophylaxis when dermatologic surgery is performed on cardiac transplant patients with valvulopathy, if performed on infected skin or the oral mucosa is breached to decrease risk of infective endocarditis [63]. Similarly, the recommendations for prophylactic antibiotics parallel use in the immunocompetent population and SOTR and HIV patients are also advised to have prophylactic antibiotics if they have had joint replacement in the past 2 years in order to minimize the risk of hematogenous joint infection [64].

9.5.3 Wound Healing

Wound healing is a particular concern in transplant patients due to the variable effects of immunosuppressant medications on the healing process. Many patients are on long-term systemic corticosteroids which have been shown to interfere with all stages of wound healing [65]. Surgeries longer than 200 min, lack of subcutaneous sutures, and use of sirolimus in kidney transplant patients have all been associated with poor wound healing, but this has not been demonstrated following Mohs surgery [66]. The immunosuppressants, azathioprine and cyclosporine, were not shown to inhibit wound healing in organ transplant patients [65]. Likewise, acitretin does not appear to significantly impede wound healing in this population, but large randomized controlled trials are lacking [67]. Additional risk factors implicated in poor wound healing for SOTR include BMI >26 and age >40 [68]. All surgical wounds should be evaluated closely at surgical follow-up to assure proper healing and perform timely interventions if needed.

9.5.4 Selection of Therapeutic Modality

As in the general population, Mohs micrographic surgery (MMS) is recommended for SOTRs with an SCC >0.6 cm in the "mask" facial area; >1 cm for cheek, forehead, and scalp; and >2 cm on the trunk or extremities. Tumors occurring on the ears, genitalia, nail units, and along anatomic fusion planes should also be managed with MMS [35]. Histologic features including depth greater than 0.4 cm, poorly differentiated tumors, and perineural invasion may also merit MMS, in addition to recurrent tumors. Wide local excision with 0.6–1.0-cm margins and intraoperative or postoperative margin evaluation may be used as an alternative if MMS is unavailable. In patients with in situ or well differentiated tumors in non-cosmetically sensitive areas, treatment approaches will vary based on patient and physician preference. Additional options include use of electrodessication and curettage, topical chemotherapeutic agents (5-fluorouracil), immunomodulators (imiquimod), photodynamic therapy, and standard excision. Because of the large number of tumors, some SOTR develop; it may be necessary to treat multiple lesions with destructive modalities such as electrodesiccation and curettage or cryosurgery with MMS applied to higher risk, more aggressive lesions and recurrent lesions. The efficacy of electrodessication and curettage in SOTR for selected lesions has been demonstrated [69].

Merkel cell carcinomas and melanomas should both be managed in the same manner as in the immunocompetent population; however, the transplant team should be notified of the diagnosis and the possibility of decreasing or altering medications discussed.

BCCs are more common in the setting of organ transplantation but behave similarly to their immunocompetent counterparts. The indications for Mohs micrographic surgery parallel those for the general population.

9.5.5 Follow-Up

Immunocompromised patients with a history of skin cancer or multiple clinical risk factors for the development of skin cancer should be seen every 3–6 months with evaluation of all sun-exposed areas and palpation of associated regional lymph nodes. A full-body skin exam with assessment of regional lymph nodes at least annually is recommended for all highly at risk SOTR. Education regarding sun avoidance should be reinforced at these visits and treatment of any actinic keratoses performed. The Mohs surgeon should have a low threshold for performing biopsies in this population given their increased risk of skin cancer [35].

Summary: Conclusion

- Mohs surgeons play a critical role in both the prevention and treatment of high-risk cutaneous neoplasms in the solid organ transplant population.

9.6 Conclusion

SOTR have benefited greatly from advances in modern day immunosuppression, with decreased graft rejection and increased survival. These medications have also had the unfortunate side effect of significantly increasing patients' chances of developing disfiguring and potentially deadly skin cancers. The Mohs surgeon has a unique opportunity to both manage high-grade neoplasms in this population and aid in prevention of further skin cancers through routine surveillance and patient education.

References

1. The U.S. Organ Procurement and Transplantation Network and the Scientific Registry of Transplant Recipients. OPTN/SRTR Annual Report: Transplant Data 1999–2008. http://optn.transplant.hrsa.gov/ar2009/. Accessed September 18, 2011.
2. Centers for Disease Control and Prevention (CDC). HIV prevalence estimates – United States, 2006. MMWR Morb Mortal Wkly Rep. 2008;57(39):1073–6.
3. Burnet FM. The concept of immunological surveillance. Prog Exp Tumor Res. 1970;13:1–27.
4. Loose D, Van De Wiele C. The immune system and cancer. Cancer Biother Radiopharm. 2009;24(3):369–76.
5. Moloney FJ, Comber H, O'Lorcain P, O'Kelly P, Conlon PJ, Murphy GM. A population-based study of skin cancer incidence and prevalence in renal transplant recipients. Br J Dermatol. 2006;154:498–504.
6. Vajdic C, van Leeuwen M. Cancer incidence and risk factors after solid organ transplantation. Int J Cancer. 2009;125:1747–54.
7. Jensen P, Hansen S, Moller B, et al. Skin cancer in kidney and heart transplant recipients and different long-term immunosuppressive therapy regimens. J Am Acad Dermatol. 1999;40(2 Pt 1):177–86.
8. Linden PK. History of solid organ transplantation and organ donation. Crit Care Clin. 2009;25(1):165–84, ix.
9. Landis SH, Murray T, Bolden S, Wingo PA. Cancer statistics, 1999. CA Cancer J Clin. 1999;49(1):8–31, 31.
10. London NJ, Farmery SM, Will EJ, Davison AM, Lodge JP. Risk of neoplasia in renal transplant patients. Lancet. 1995;346(8972):403–6.
11. Euvrard S, Kanitakis J, Claudy A. Skin cancers after organ transplantation. N Engl J Med. 2003;348(17):1681–91.
12. Penn I. Tumors after renal and cardiac transplantation. Hematol Oncol Clin North Am. 1993;7(2):431–45.
13. Collett D, Mumford L, Banner NR, Neuberger J, Watson C. Comparison of the incidence of malignancy in recipients of different types of organ: a UK Registry audit. Am J Transplant. 2010;10(8):1889–96.
14. Hartevelt MM, Bavinck JN, Kootte AM, Vermeer BJ, Vandenbroucke JP. Incidence of skin cancer after renal transplantation in the Netherlands. Transplantation. 1990;49(3):506–9.
15. Gallagher MP, Kelly PJ, Jardine M, et al. Long-term cancer risk of immunosuppressive regimens after kidney transplantation. J Am Soc Nephrol. 2010;21(5):852–8.
16. Mackenzie KA, Wells JE, Lynn KL, et al. First and subsequent nonmelanoma skin cancers: incidence and predictors in a population of New Zealand renal transplant recipients. Nephrol Dial Transplant. 2010;25(1):300–6.
17. Ramsay HM, Fryer AA, Hawley CM, Smith AG, Harden PN. Non-melanoma skin cancer risk in the Queensland renal transplant population. Br J Dermatol. 2002;147(5):950–6.
18. Caforio AL, Fortina AB, Piaserico S, et al. Skin cancer in heart transplant recipients: risk factor analysis and relevance of immunosuppressive therapy. Circulation. 2000;102(19 Suppl 3):III222–7.
19. Dantal J, Hourmant M, Cantarovich D, et al. Effect of long-term immunosuppression in kidney-graft recipients on cancer incidence: randomised comparison of two cyclosporin regimens. Lancet. 1998;351(9103):623–8.
20. Vadnerkar A, Nguyen MH, Mitsani D, et al. Voriconazole exposure and geographic location are independent risk factors for squamous cell carcinoma of the skin among lung transplant recipients. J Heart Lung Transplant. 2010;29(11):1240–4. Epub June 28, 2010.
21. Webb MC, Compton F, Andrews PA, Koffman CG. Skin tumours posttransplantation: a retrospective analysis of 28 years' experience at a single centre. Transplant Proc. 1997;29(1–2):828–30.
22. Amital A, Shitrit D, Raviv Y, et al. Development of malignancy following lung transplantation. Transplantation. 2006;81(4):547–51.
23. Denning DW, Griffiths CE. Muco-cutaneous retinoid-effects and facial erythema related to the novel triazole antifungal agent voriconazole. Clin Exp Dermatol. 2001;26(8):648–53.
24. Hojo M, Morimoto T, Maluccio M, et al. Cyclosporine induces cancer progression by a cell-autonomous mechanism. Nature. 1999;397(6719):530–4.
25. Kelly GE, Meikle W, Sheil AG. Effects of immunosuppressive therapy on the induction of skin tumors by ultraviolet irradiation in hairless mice. Transplantation. 1987;44(3):429–34.
26. Schena FP, Pascoe MD, Alberu J, et al. Conversion from calcineurin inhibitors to sirolimus: maintenance therapy in renal allograft recipients: 24-month efficacy and safety results from the CONVERT trial. Transplantation. 2009;87(2):233–42.
27. http://www.cdc.gov/hiv/resources/factsheets/us.htm. Accessed September 15, 2011.
28. Van Leeuwen MT, Vajdic CM, Middleton MG, et al. Continuing declines in some but not all HIV-associated cancers in Australia after widespread use of antiretroviral therapy. AIDS. 2009;23(16):2183–90.
29. Remick SC. Non-AIDS defining cancers. Hematol Oncol Clin North Am. 1996;10:10.
30. Nguyen P, Vin-Christian K, Ming ME, Berger T. Aggressive squamous cell carcinomas in persons infected with the human immunodeficiency virus. Arch Dermatol. 2002;138:758–63.
31. Wilkins K, Turner R, Dolev J, LeBoit P, Berger T, Maurer T. Cutaneous malignancy and human immunodeficiency virus disease. J Am Acad Dermatol. 2004;54(2):189–206.
32. Lanoy E, Dores GM, Madeleine MM, Toro JR, Fraumeni Jr JF, Engels EA. Epidemiology of nonkeratinocytic skin cancers among persons with AIDS in the United States. AIDS. 2009;23(3):385–93.
33. Coit DG, Andtbacka R, Bichakjian CK, et al. Melanoma clinical practice guidelines in oncology. JNCCN. 2009;7:250–75.
34. Salasche SJ. Epidemiology of actinic keratoses and squamous cell carcinoma. J Am Acad Dermatol. 2000;42(1 Pt 2):4–7.
35. Stasko T, Brown MD, Carucci JA, et al. Guidelines for the management of squamous cell carcinoma in organ transplant recipients. Dermatol Surg. 2004;30(4 Pt 2):642–50.

36. Fuchs A, Marmur E. The kinetics of skin cancer: progression of actinic keratosis to squamous cell carcinoma. Dermatol Surg. 2007;33(9):1099–101.
37. Marks R, Rennie G, Selwood TS. Malignant transformation of solar keratoses to squamous cell carcinoma. Lancet. 1988;1(8589):795–7.
38. Bouwes-Bavinck JN, Euvrard S, Naldi L, et al. Keratotic skin lesions and other risk factors are associated with skin cancer in organ-transplant recipients: a case-control study in The Netherlands, United Kingdom, Germany, France, and Italy. J Invest Dermatol. 2007;127(7):1647–56.
39. Ulrich C, Bichel J, Euvard S, et al. Topical immunomodulation under systemic immunosuppression: results of a multicentre, randomized, placebo controlled safety and efficacy study of imiquimod 5% cream for the treatment of actinic keratoses in kidney, heart and liver transplant patients. Br J Dermatol. 2007;157:25–31.
40. Marquez C, Bair SM, Smithberger E, Cherpelis BS, Glass LF. Systemic retinoids for chemoprevention of non-melanoma skin cancer in high-risk patients. J Drugs Dermatol. 2010;9(7):753–8.
41. Jennings L, Schmults CD. Management of high-risk cutaneous squamous cell carcinoma. J Clin Aesthet Dermatol. 2010;3(4):39–48.
42. Rowe DE, Carroll RJ, Day Jr CL. Prognostic factors for local recurrence, metastasis, and survival rates in squamous cell carcinoma of the skin, ear, and lip. Implications for treatment modality selection. J Am Acad Dermatol. 1992;26(6):976–90.
43. Brantsch KD, Meisner C, Schonfisch B, et al. Analysis of risk factors determining prognosis of cutaneous squamous-cell carcinoma: a prospective study. Lancet Oncol. 2008; 9(8):713–20.
44. Breuninger H, Schaumburg-Lever G, Holzschuh J, Horny HP. Desmoplastic squamous cell carcinoma of skin and vermilion surface: a highly malignant subtype of skin cancer. Cancer. 1997;79(5):915–9.
45. Martinez JC, Otley CC, Stasko T, et al. Defining the clinical course of metastatic skin cancer in organ transplant recipients: a multicenter collaborative study. Arch Dermatol. 2003;139:301–6.
46. Clayman GL, Lee JJ, Holsinger FC, et al. Mortality risk from squamous cell skin cancer. J Clin Oncol. 2005;23(4): 759–65.
47. Ross AS, Whalen FM, Elenitsas R, Xu X, Troxel AB, Schmults CD. Diameter of involved nerves predicts outcomes in cutaneous squamous cell carcinoma with perineural invasion: an investigator-blinded retrospective cohort study. Dermatol Surg. 2009;35(12):1859–66.
48. Veness MJ, Morgan GJ, Palme CE, Gebski V. Surgery and adjuvant radiotherapy in patients with cutaneous head and neck squamous cell carcinoma metastatic to lymph nodes: combined treatment should be considered best practice. Laryngoscope. 2005;115(5):870–5.
49. Otley CC, Maragh SL. Reduction of immunosuppression for transplant-associated skin cancer: rationale and evidence of efficacy. Dermatol Surg. 2005;31(2):163–8.
50. Harwood CA, Proby CM, McGregor JM, Sheaff MT, Leigh IM, Cerio R. Clinicopathologic features of skin cancer in organ transplant recipients: a retrospective case-control series. J Am Acad Dermatol. 2006;54:290–300.
51. Karve SJ, Feldman SR, Yentzer BA, Pearce DJ, Balkrishnan R. Imiquimod: a review of basal cell carcinoma treatments. J Drugs Dermatol. 2008;7(11):1044–51.
52. Fai D, Arpaia N, Romano I, Vestita M, Cassano N, Vena GA. Methyl-aminolevulinate photodynamic therapy for the treatment of actinic keratosis and non-melanoma skin cancer: a retrospective analysis of response in 462 patients. G Ital Dermatol Venereol. 2009;144(3):281–5.
53. Shokrollahi K, Marsden NJ, Whitaker IS, James W, Murison MS. Basal cell carcinoma treated successfully with combined CO_2 laser and photodynamic therapy in a renal transplant patient: a case report. Cases J. 2009;11:7920.
54. Zwald FO, Christenson LJ, Billingsley EM, et al. Melanoma in solid organ transplant recipients. Am J Transplant. 2010;10(5):1297–304.
55. Le Mire L, Hollowood K, Gray D, Bordea C, Wonjnarowska F. Melanomas in renal transplant recipients. Br J Dermatol. 2006;154(3):472–7.
56. Penn I. Malignant melanoma in organ allograft recipients. Transplantation. 1996;61(2):274–8.
57. Penn I. Transmission of cancer from organ donors. Ann Transplant. 1997;2(4):7–12.
58. Penn I, First MR. Merkel's cell carcinoma in organ recipients: report of 41 cases. Transplantation. 1999;68:1717–21.
59. Feng H, Shuda M, Chang Y, Moore PS. Clonal integration of a polyomavirus in human Merkel cell carcinoma. Science. 2008;319:1096–100.
60. Gollard R, Weber R, Kosty MP, Greenway HT, Massullo V, Humberson C. Merkel cell carcinoma: review of 22 cases with surgical, pathologic and therapeutic considerations. Cancer. 2000;88:1842–51.
61. Lemos BD, Storer BE, Iyer JG, et al. Pathologic nodal evaluation improves prognostic accuracy in Merkel cell carcinoma: analysis of 5823 cases as the basis of the first consensus staging system. J Am Acad Dermatol. 2010; 63(5):751–61.
62. Dandel M, Lehmkuhl HB, Knosalla C, Hetzer R. Impact of different long-term maintenance immunosuppressive therapy strategies on patients' outcome after heart transplantation. Transpl Immunol. 2010;23(3):93–103.
63. Wilson W, Taubert KA, Gewitz M, et al. Prevention of infective endocarditis: guidelines from the American Heart Association. Circulation. 2007;116(15):1736–54.
64. Wright TI, Baddour LM, Berbari EF, et al. Antibiotic prophylaxis in dermatologic surgery: advisory statement 2008. J Am Acad Dermatol. 2008;59(3):464–73.
65. Karukonda SR, Flynn TC, Boh EE, McBurney EI, Russo GG, Millikan LE. The effects of drugs on wound healing – part II. Specific classes of drugs and their effect on healing wounds. Int J Dermatol. 2000;39(5):321–33.
66. Roine E, Bjork IT, Oyen O. Targeting risk factors for impaired wound healing and wound complications after kidney transplantation. Transplant Proc. 2010;42(7):2542–6.
67. Tan SR, Tope WD. Effect of acitretin on wound healing in organ transplant recipients. Dermatol Surg. 2004;30(4 Pt 2):667–73.
68. Knight RJ, Villa M, Laskey R, et al. Risk factors for impaired wound healing in sirolimus-treated renal transplant recipients. Clin Transplant. 2007;21(4):460–5.
69. de Graaf YG, Basdew VR, van Zwan-Kralt N, Willemze R, Bavinck JN. The occurrence of residual or recurrent

squamous cell carcinomas in organ transplant recipients after curettage and electrodesiccation. Br J Dermatol. 2006;154(3):493–7.

70. Euvrard S, Ulrich C, Lefrancois N. Immunosuppressants and skin cancer in transplant patients: focus on rapamycin. Dermatol Surg. 2004;30:628–33.

Mohs Micrographic Surgery in Ethnic Skin

10

Brooke A. Jackson

Abstract

Skin cancer is the most common malignancy in the United States. While skin cancer occurs less commonly in ethnic skin, it is associated with increased morbidity and mortality as compared with Caucasian counterparts. As the demographics of the United States continue to trend toward a society with an anticipated 50% of the population with skin of color by 2050, it is imperative that physicians become familiar with the diagnosis, treatment, and prevention of skin cancer in ethnic skin. This chapter reviews special considerations when treating patients with skin of color with Mohs surgery.

Keywords

Ethnic skin • Skin of color • Skin cancer • Mohs surgery • Sun protection

10.1 Introduction

Skin cancer is the most common malignancy in the United States [1]. While skin cancer is less common in ethnic skin, it is associated with increased incidence of morbidity and mortality as compared with Caucasian counterparts [2, 3]. This imbalance raises public health concerns. While current skin cancer campaigns focus on Caucasians in high-risk groups, little is known about sun protective behaviors in patients with ethnic skin. Additionally, many physicians do not immediately associate skin cancer with ethnic skin. Published literature on skin cancer in ethnic skin is scarce, and collection of statistics for skin cancer in ethnic groups has proven difficult as non-melanoma skin cancers (NMSC) are not consistently reported to tumor registries and many NMSCs in ethnic skin are reported as melanomas. According to the 2000 census [4], 50% of the US population will be non-white by the year 2050. This changing demographics, combined with disparate morbidity and mortality in patients of color, underscores the importance for increased physician familiarity with skin cancer in ethnic skin so that we may better educate our patients on the risk factors, prevention, early detection, and treatment options of this highly treatable disease. Mohs micrographic surgery (MMS) is a highly effective treatment option for the treatment of some skin cancers [5]. While there is no difference in the MOHS surgical technique in ethnic skin, caution must be taken to minimize tension on surgical wound closures because of increased risk of keloid formation in ethnic skin [6, 7].

B.A. Jackson
Department of Dermatology, Skin Wellness Center of Chicago, SC, Chicago, IL, USA

Northwestern Medical School, Chicago, IL, USA
e-mail: bjacksonmd@mindspring.com

K. Nouri (ed.), *Mohs Micrographic Surgery*,
DOI 10.1007/978-1-4471-2152-7_10, © Springer-Verlag London Limited 2012

Summary: Histologic Differences in Skin of Color

- Ethnic skin has unique histologic features which allow some intrinsic photoprotection; however, the incidence of NMSC continues to increase in ethnic skin, suggesting there are other contributing factors.

10.2 Histologic Differences in Skin of Color

While all skin, regardless of its color, contains the same number of pigment-producing melanocytes, melanosomes in darkly complected individuals are larger and more evenly dispersed throughout the entire epidermis as compared to the less active and clumped melanocytes in white skin [8]. These larger melanocytes allow dark skin to filter almost twice as much ultraviolet B (UVB) radiation than white skin [9], resulting in an estimated sun protection factor of 13.1 in black skin [10]. These unique histologic features of dark skin serve to protect it against actinic damage, making sun-induced skin cancers less prevalent. Despite this intrinsic photoprotection, the incidence of NMSC is increasing in skin of color [10], suggesting that UV exposure may play less of a role in the development of certain skin cancers in skin of color. Known risk factors for NMSC are listed below [11].

Known Risk Factors for NMSC

- Fitzpatrick skin types I–III
- UV exposure including UV light treatment
- Male gender
- Organ transplant immunosuppression
- Genetic disorders (XP)
- Chemical exposure(arsenic, heavy metal)
- HPV

Summary: Basal Cell Carcinoma (BCC)

- Classic presentation of BCC may be difficult to appreciate in skin of color and often occurs in non-sun-exposed areas of the body. Physicians should consider biopsy of any non-healing or suspicious lesion in skin of color and educate patients with skin of color about risk factors and risk factor reduction.

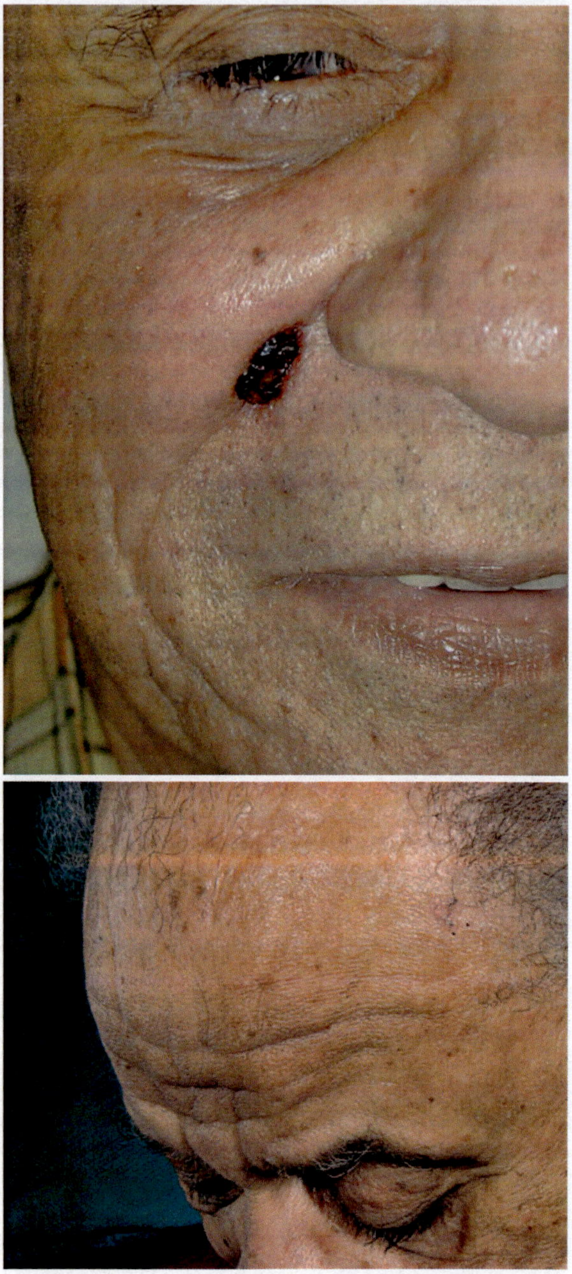

Figs. 10.1–10.2 Eighty-year-old AA golfer with nodular BCC of L frontal scalp and R NLF

10.3 Basal Cell Carcinoma (BCC)

Studies have documented the correlation of BCC in African Americans to UV light exposure [12]; however, persons of color often have a false sense of security with regard to awareness of skin cancer risk and

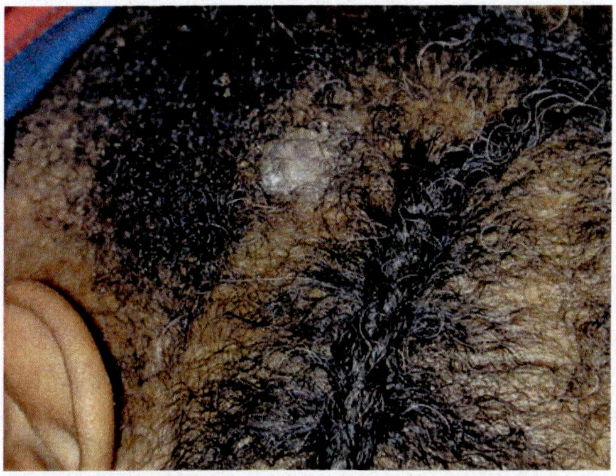

Fig. 10.3 AA woman with nodular BCC postscalp

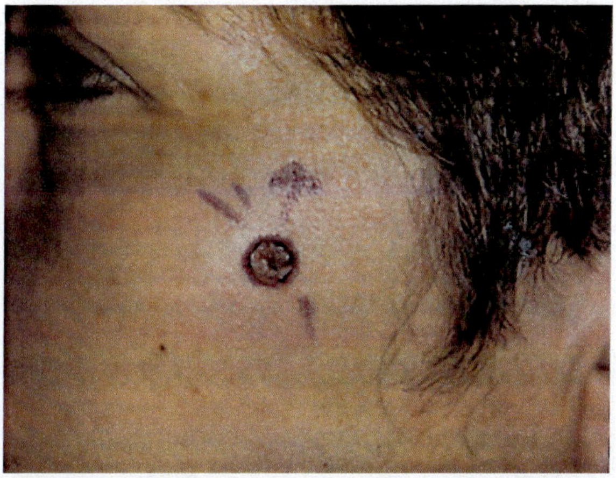

Fig. 10.4 BCC cheek of Hispanic woman

tend not to follow sun protection guidelines [13] proposed in skin cancer campaigns aimed at high-risk patients. Persons of color also have an increased incidence of medical conditions [14] such as diabetes, hypertension, and lupus necessitating the use of photosensitizing medications. These combined factors support the need for better counseling, patient education, and perhaps a distinct skin cancer awareness campaign directed toward ethnic skin.

While the classic presentation of a solitary pearly papule with rolled borders and central ulceration may occur in skin of color, pearly borders and surrounding telangiectasia may be difficult to appreciate in darker skin tones (see Figs. 10.1 and 10.2). Although BCC does occur in sun-exposed areas, in skin of color, it is seen with increasing frequency in non-sun-exposed sites [15] and often presents in an atypical manner [16], making diagnosis challenging (see Fig. 10.3). Physicians should therefore consider biopsy of any suspicious or non-healing lesion in persons of color (see Fig. 10.4). Histologically, pigmented BCC occurs more frequently in persons of color [15]. The differential diagnosis of BCC in ethnic skin is listed below.

DDX: BCC in Skin of Color
- Seborrheic keratosis
- Nevus sebaceous
- Lupus erythematosus
- Trauma (curling iron burn)
- Blue nevus
- Sarcoid
- Melanoma

Summary: Squamous Cell Carcinoma (SCC)
- Unlike Caucasian counterparts, SCC in skin of color occurs more commonly in non-sun-exposed skin and has a higher mortality rate.

10.4 Squamous Cell Carcinoma (SCC)

SCC is the most common skin cancer in African Americans [17] and the second most common skin cancer in Asians [18]. The precursor lesions to SCC, actinic keratoses, are common in Asians [19] yet tend not to occur in African Americans [20]. While SCC occurs with equal frequency on sun-exposed and non-sun-exposed skin in Caucasians, it is 8.5 times more likely to occur in non-sun-exposed areas (lower extremity, anogenital region) in African Americans, suggesting that UV radiation plays a less significant role in the development of SCC in African Americans [21, 22]. Although Bowen's disease (SCC in situ) is less common in African Americans, it often occurs on the lower extremity presenting as a hyperkeratotic plaque. Mortality rates for African Americans with SCC are as high as 29% [23, 24] and are particularly high with anogenital lesions. These alarmingly high rates may be related to delayed diagnosis of tumors in non-sun-exposed areas combined with potentially more biologically aggressive tumors [23]. Risk factors for SCC are listed in Table 10.1 [17]. Because of the increased mortality rate with African Americans, physicians should counsel their patients regarding their risks of

Table 10.1 Risk factors for SCC in skin of color

Risk factors for SCC in skin of color	
Scars from burn or trauma	Hidradenitis suppurativa
DLE/LE	Granuloma annulare
Radiation sites	HPV
Immunosuppression	Albinism
Chemical exposure (tar, arsenic)	Cutaneous ulcers

Reprinted from Jackson [25]

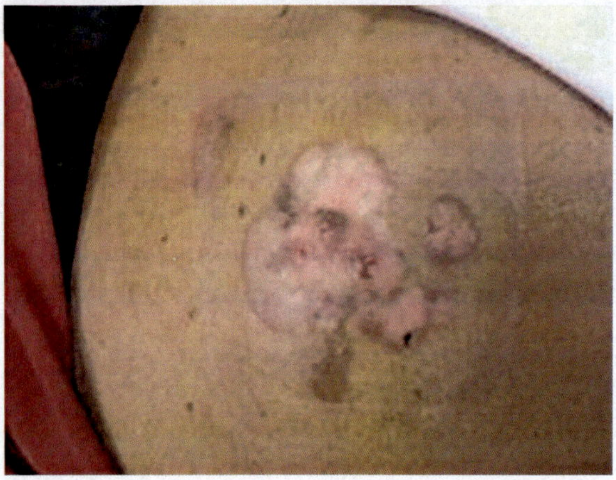

Fig. 10.5 Bowen's labelled as l cheek, it is actually l hip (close to the other cheek , lol)

SCC, evaluate new growths, and consider biopsy of any non-healing, ulcerated, or chronically inflamed lesion regardless of sun exposure (see Fig. 10.5).

> **Summary: Malignant Melanoma (MM)**
> - Patients with skin of color are more likely to present with more advanced disease with lesions occurring more commonly in non-sun-exposed areas.

10.5 Malignant Melanoma (MM)

The incidence of malignant melanoma is increasing at a rate of 2.4% per year [26], suggesting that by the year 2010, 1 in 50 Americans will be diagnosed with melanoma. Malignant melanoma is the third most commonly diagnosed cutaneous malignancy in Caucasians, African Americans, Hispanics, and Asians [27] and is

Table 10.2 DDX for MM in skin of color

Pigmented BCC	Tinea ungium
Seborrheic keratosis	Trauma (subungual hematoma)
Nev us	
Verruca	

Reprinted from Jackson [25]

the leading cause of cancer death amongst young adults [27]. While family history and UV radiation exposure are risk factors for the development of malignant melanoma in Caucasians, they do not appear to play as significant a role in the development of MM in ethnic skin. Patients with skin of color are more likely to present with more advanced disease with lesions occurring more commonly in non-sun-exposed acral and mucosal areas [28]. In a recent study [29], the most common location of MM in African Americans was the foot (38.9%) compared with 2.4% of Caucasians where the most common primary location was the trunk (35%) compared with 7.1% of tumors in African Americans. Because survival rates are directly correlated with Clark's level staging at diagnosis, early detection is critical for increased survival. Krementz et al. [30] documented that those African American patients diagnosed with early-stage MM and who received aggressive surgical treatment had the same favorable outcome as Caucasian patients. Differential diagnosis for MM in skin of color is listed in Table 10.2.

> **Summary: Treatment Techniques and Operative Considerations**
> - Increased risk of keloid formation in skin of color warrants special care with closures under minimal tension. Standard treatments for hypertrophic scars and keloids are applicable for postsurgical wounds.

10.6 Treatment Techniques and Operative Considerations

Treatment techniques for skin cancer in ethnic skin of color do not differ from those used in Caucasian patients and are addressed more fully in other chapters of this text. Keloidal scar formation can occur in any race; however, the rate of keloid formation in African

Americans has been reported to be from 5 to 15 times higher than that of the white population [6]. In Hawaii, keloids are found three times more commonly in the Japanese population and five times more commonly in the Chinese population than in white populations [7]. Because of this increased risk, care must be taken to minimize tension with wound closures. Patients should be counseled on the potential for hypertrophic scar and keloid formation, both of which may be treated with standard therapies of intralesional kenalog injection and pressure. Postoperative erythematous hypertrophic scars in Caucasians and lightly complected patients of color (skin types I–IV) may be treated with the pulsed dye laser. This author uses 595-nm at 10 mm spot, 0.5-ms pulse duration, and fluences of 3–6 J with appreciable fading in 1–3 treatments. Depressed scars may be treated with non- ablative or ablative fraxel Laser.

When treating precancerous lesions, this author avoids use of liquid nitrogen in skin of color in favor of imiquimod in an effort to avoid posttreatment loss of pigment. One may also use light electrodessication (0.9–1.2 W) and curettage but must warn the patient of potential postinflammatory hyperpigmentation.

Summary: Conclusion

- Given increased aggressiveness of certain tumors (SCC, MM) in skin of color and disparities in survival when compared to Caucasian counterparts, increased physician efforts in screening and counseling patients of color with regard to their risks of skin cancer and sun protective behavior is crucial.

10.7 Conclusion

Although less common than in Caucasians, skin cancer does occur in ethnic skin, and these patients are more likely to die from their disease. This disparate morbidity and mortality is due to both delayed diagnosis and more aggressive biologic nature of these tumors in ethnic skin. While pigmented BCC is found more commonly in skin of color than in Caucasians, SCC is the most prevalent form of NMSC in skin of color. Although malignant melanoma occurs less frequently in skin of color, the aggressive acrolentiginous form accounts for poor prognosis in these patients. While sun exposure appears to play a role in the development of BCC in ethnic skin, there is less of a correlation with SCC and MM due to the propensity of these skin cancers to occur in non-sun-exposed locations.

Little is known about the skin cancer awareness of patients with ethnic skin. Current skin cancer campaigns have focused on Caucasians in high-risk groups. Patients with ethnic skin who do not perceive themselves as being high risk are likely to ignore early warning signs of skin cancer, and physicians who do not associate skin cancer with ethnic skin may be less likely to consider it in a differential diagnosis or to counsel patients appropriately on risk prevention, surveillance, and follow-up. Better effort for public awareness must be instituted in ethnic communities. The combined efforts of physicians and improved public education will result in earlier diagnosis and better prognosis for patients with skin of color.

References

1. Centers for Disease Control and Prevention. http://www.cdc.gov/cancer/skin/statistics10/1/10.
2. Gloster Jr HM, Brodland DG. The epidemiology of skin cancer. Dermatol Surg. 1996;22:217–26.
3. Jemal A, Siegel R, Ward E, et al. Cancer statistics, 2006. CA Cancer J Clin. 2006;56:106–30.
4. US Census Bureau Population Division. Projections of the resident population by race, Hispanic origin, and dativity: middle series, 1999–2100. Washington: US Census Bureau; 2000.
5. Broadland D, Amonette R, Hanke W, et al. The history and evolution of Mohs micrographic surgery. Dermatol Surg. 2000;26:303–7.
6. LeFlore IC. Misconceptions regarding elective plastic surgery in the black patient. J Natl Med Assoc. 1980; 72:947–8.
7. Arnold HL, Franer FH. Keloids: etiology and management by excision and intensive prophylactic radiation. Arch Dermatol. 1959;80:772.
8. Montagna W. The architecture of black and white skin. J Am Acad Dermatol. 1991;24:29–37.
9. Halder RM, Bridgeman-Shah S. Skin cancer in African Americans. Cancer. 1995;75:667–73.
10. Halder RM, Ara CJ. Skin cancer and photoaging in ethnic skin. Dermatol Clin. 2003;21:725–32.
11. American Cancer Society: Non melanoma skin cancer detailed guide. http://documents.cancer.org/118.00.
12. Matsuoka LY, Schauer PK, Sordillo PP. Basal cell carcinoma in black patients. J Am Acad Dermatol. 1981;4(6):670–2.
13. Briley JJ, Chaveda K, Lynfield YL. Sunscreen use and usefulness in African Americans. J Drugs Dermatol. 2007;6(1): 19–22.

14. Ferdinand KC, Armani AM. The management of hypertension in African Americans. Crit Pathw Cardiol. 2007; 6(2):67–71.
15. Nadiminti U, Rakkhit T, Washington C. Morpheaform basal cell carcinoma in African Americans. Dermatol Surg. 2004;30:1550–2.
16. Chorun L, Norris JE, Gupta M. Basal cell carcinoma in Blacks: a report of 15 cases. Ann Plast Surg. 1994;33:90–5.
17. Mora RG, Perniciaro C. Cancer of the skin in blacks: a review of 163 black patients with cutaneous squamous cell carcinoma. J Am Acad Dermatol. 1981;5:535–43.
18. Koh D, Wang H, et al. Basal cell carcinoma, squamous cell carcinoma and melanoma of the skin: analysis of the Singapore cancer registry data 1968–1997. Br J Dermatol. 2003;148:1161–6.
19. Suzuki T, Ueda M, Naruse K, et al. Incidence of actinic keratosis of Japanese in Kasai City, Hyogo. J Dermatol Sci. 1997;16:74–8.
20. Hale EK, Jorizzo J, Nehal KS, et al. Current concepts in the management of actinic keratosis. J Drugs Dermatol. 2004; 3(2 suppl):S3–16.
21. Mora RG, Perniciaro C, Lee B. Cancer of the skin in blacks III: a review of nineteen black patients with Bowen's disease. J Am Acad Dermatol. 1984;11:557–62.
22. Sing B, Bhaya M, Shaha A, Har-El G, Lucente FE. Presentation, course and outcome of head and neck cancer in African Americans: a case controlled study. Laryngoscope. 1998;108:1159–63.
23. Fleming ID, Barnawell JR, Burlison PE, et al. Skin cancer in black patients. Cancer. 1975;35:600–5.
24. Mora RG. Surgical and aesthetic considerations of cancer of the skin in the black American. J Dermatol Surg Oncol. 1986;12:24–31.
25. Jackson BA. Skin cancer in skin of color. In: MacFarlane DF, editor. Skin cancer management: a practical approach. New York: Springer; 2010. p. 217–24.
26. Reis LAG, Eisner MP, Kosary CL, et al. SEER Cancer statistics review, 1975–2001. Bethesda: National Cancer Institute. http://www.seer.cancer.gov/csr/1975_2001.
27. Cress RD, Holly EA. Incidence of cutaneous melanoma among non-Hispanic whites, Hispanics, Asians and Blacks: an analysis of California Cancer Registry data, 1988–1993. Cancer Causes Control. 1997; 8:246–52.
28. Greenlee RT, Murray T, Bolden S, Wingo PA. Cancer statistics, 2000. CA Cancer J Clin. 2000;50(1):7–33.
29. Byrd KM, Wilson DC, Hoyler SS, Peck GL. Advanced presentation of melanoma in African Americans. J Am Acad Dermatol. 2004;50:21–4.
30. Krementz ET, Sutherland CM, Carter D, Ryan RF. Malignant melanoma in the American Black. Ann Surg. 1976;183: 533–41.

Histopathology Laboratory Setup and Necessary Instrumentation

11

Marilyn Zabielinski, Michael P. McLeod, Sonal Choudhary, and Keyvan Nouri

Abstract

A well-prepared and smoothly running office and lab are very important to performing successful Mohs micrographic surgery. The medical office of a Mohs surgeon is unique compared to most other medical offices in the sense that throughout the day, patients move frequently between the operating room and the surgical waiting room. While this is occurring, tissue specimens are being carried between the operating room, histopathology laboratory, and the microscope. It is necessary to have a well- equipped operating room, a comfortable waiting area, a laboratory to process the tissue specimens, an area for histopathology slide reading, and a space to clean and sterilize instruments properly. As each area of the office is discussed, equipment pertinent to that area will be addressed.

Keywords

Mohs micrographic surgery office • Operating room • Surgical waiting room • Histopathology laboratory

M. Zabielinski
Department of Dermatology and Cutaneous Surgery,
University of Miami Leonard M. Miller School of Medicine,
Miami, FL, USA

M.P. McLeod • S. Choudhary
Department of Dermatology and Cutaneous Surgery,
University of Miami Leonard M. Miller School of Medicine,
Miami, FL, USA

K. Nouri (✉)
Department of Dermatology and Cutaneous Surgery,
University of Miami Leonard M. Miller School of Medicine,
Miami, FL, USA

Sylvester Comprehensive Cancer Center,
University of Miami Hospital and Clinics, Miami, FL, USA
e-mail: knouri@med.miami.edu

Summary: The General Office Setup

- A well-prepared and smoothly running office and lab are very important in performing successful Mohs micrographic surgery.
- Investing in equipment and organization allows for an organized, efficient, and safe practice.

11.1 The General Office Setup

A well-prepared and smoothly running office and lab are very important in performing successful Mohs surgery. Throughout the day, patients move from the operating room to the surgical reception area. While this is occurring, tissue specimens are being transported

K. Nouri (ed.), *Mohs Micrographic Surgery*,
DOI 10.1007/978-1-4471-2152-7_11,

between the operating room, histopathology laboratory, and the microscope. Therefore, investing in quality equipment and organization allows for an organized, efficient, and safe practice.

In order to attain such a practice, it is necessary to have a properly equipped operating room, a laboratory to process the tissue specimens, an area for histopathology slide reading, and a space to clean and sterilize instruments. As each of these areas of the office is discussed, pertinent equipment and supplies will be addressed.

The general setup of the office is as important as the administration and patient scheduling in order to have an efficient practice. It is important to have an experienced and responsible office manager who can attend to the details of payment, paperwork, staff, and patient scheduling. In addition, it is also useful to have one or two medical assistants and one or two experienced nurses or physician assistants to assist with procedures.

Summary: The Operating Room (OR)

- The operating room should be well lit, ventilated, spacious, and organized.
- Medicare certification, as well as local and state regulations, may mandate certain operating room configurations, and it is important to abide by these regulations.
- Essential monitoring and emergency equipment should be readily available.
- The entire office staff should be CPR trained and certified.
- At least two digital cameras are necessary for documentation.
- Proper waste containers include one for noncontaminated, non-sharps waste, one for sharps, and one for contaminated waste.

11.2 The Operating Room (OR)

The operating room should be appropriately lit, ventilated, spacious, and organized. There needs to be adequate space for the operating table, patient monitoring equipment, multiple large Mayo stands, cabinets and storage for instruments, a sink, and electrosurgical equipment. The surgeon should be able to move 360° around the patient table and have enough space to comfortably operate standing or sitting. Medicare certification, as well as local and state regulations, may mandate certain operating room configurations, and it is important to abide by these regulations [1]. The American Academy of Dermatology has also written guidelines for office surgical facilities in the *Journal of the American Academy of Dermatology*.

The patient room should be clean and aesthetically appealing. An additional sitting chair should be available for holding the patient's belongings or can be used for seating the family member or friend. Excellent general room lighting should be supplemented with large, cool, and focusable overhead OR lights. Locking cabinets allow for storage of sutures and instruments in an organized and highly accessible fashion [1].

The surgical table should be foot operable to position and should be well padded and comfortable for the patient. For Mohs surgeons who prefer to sit while operating, a comfortable, sturdy, foot adjustable rolling surgical chair may be located on each side of the surgical table. The Mohs surgeon frequently moves from one side of the table to the other, and therefore, time will not be lost when switching sides [1].

Soothing music can be played in the operating room at an appropriate volume. It can be provided with an iPhone or iPod (or any other MP3) connected to speakers, or with a small compact disc player, although a compact disc player does not allow for selection and storage of a large variety and quantity of music. If the surgeon or the patient has a specific preference, then an iPhone or iPod can allow access to many genres of music. Meditation and classical music can also be relaxing for both the patient and the Mohs surgeon, although any soft music that is not distracting will suffice.

Although expensive, providing a high-definition screen television is a method to distract and entertain patients while they are waiting between layers (and for general dermatology patients that are waiting too). The television can be programmed to be educational or can be used to advertise other office procedures available. Another option is to have an appropriate movie playing at a low volume.

If possible, the OR temperature control should be accessible directly inside the room to allow for adjustment as needed. The Mohs surgeon may require a cooler temperature than the rest of the office that may be uncomfortable for the staff and other patients. If the Mohs surgeon usually prefers a cooler temperature, instruct patients to bring a blanket to the office for use while in the OR or have them available [1].

Essential monitoring and emergency equipment includes oxygen with a delivery system, blood pressure and pulse monitors, a manual suctioning device, fire extinguishers, an emergency eyewash station, and hands-off phone intercom capability. A convenient way to monitor all vital signs in one location is with a vital signs diagnostic station with a rolling floor stand. Additional equipment includes the following: blood pressure, pulse, and time data printer; pulse oximeter with plethsymograph display, cardiac monitor–defibrillator; battery-operated backup lighting; and full advanced cardiac life support capability. The cardiac monitor defibrillator should be light, compact, portable, and easy to use [1].

Moreover, the entire office staff should be CPR certified; this is best accomplished by having a CPR training group providing annual classes in the office. The Mohs surgeon and OR assistants should have ACLS certification in case of an emergency [1].

A device that should be available in the operating room is a high-grade manual suction device which is fast and easy to use in case the patient is at risk for aspirating vomitus or other substances and liquids. In general, electric suction devices are useful because they remove blood from the operative field during surgery. In Mohs surgery, these devices are seldom required; however, they are essential in certain situations. For example, blood can pool and accumulate in certain areas, such as the medial canthus or the ear canal, completely obscuring the surgical field. These devices are relatively inexpensive and have disposable tubing [1].

At least two digital cameras need to be available for use. There should be a designated area where they are placed in between uses. The physician assistants and medical assistants should be taught how and when to use them. The cameras are useful for several reasons. First, it is important to document all lesions, biopsies, and repairs. A suspicious lesion should be circled with a marking pen before it is biopsied so that it can be easily noted on pictures. Before a biopsy, one or two very close-up, focused pictures should be taken of the lesion and one or two should be taken farther away to orient the doctor to the anatomic location. This technique will allow the physician to better locate the biopsy site when patient returns to have the surgery performed. Pictures are also used to document intraoperative mapping and to record progress of the surgery after each Mohs stage if the repair will be performed by a reconstructive surgeon other than the Mohs surgeon. Each room should have a hand-held mirror, which is used to show patients their repair or bandages; or more importantly, it is also used to confirm tumor location before Mohs surgery if the biopsy site persists to be in question.

The operating room should contain multiple large Mayo stands to hold separate sterile surgical trays for each Mohs patient. These stands are easily height adjustable and have a flat sturdy base [1]. Each tray should be labeled with the patient's name, preventing its use for the wrong patient.

Large numbers of surgical gloves are used during Mohs surgery. Every surgeon will develop their preference for gloves, including size, brand, packaging, and whether or not they are powdered. The surgeon and physician assistant should have a large number of sterile gloves available in storage at all times.

An electrosurgical device for hemostasis is essential for Mohs surgery and other dermatological procedures. A sterile-dedicated electrode should be used for each patient; these are re-sterilizable and can be left in a sterilization envelope labeled with the patient's name between uses. The tip of the electrode stays sterile during use, but the shank does not. Use electrosurgery with caution if the patient has a pacemaker. In addition, the electrosurgical unit's "ground" may interfere with EKG monitoring and recording [1].

It is important that electrocoagulation is limited to what is necessary in order to prevent electrosurgical artifacts on successive stages, which may mimic carcinoma. The use of pressure dressings between stages minimizes the need for extensive electrocoagulation that may contribute to these artifacts. Using a jeweler's or splinter forcep for pinpoint hemostasis is another way to minimize artifact. Additionally, excessive electrocoagulation can result in a poor cosmetic outcome because it increases thermal tissue damage beyond the immediate wound. White and brown ½″, 1″, and 2″ micropore paper tapes are used to apply the pressure dressing. White Micropore paper tape, which is less expensive than brown, is used to secure the dressings between stages of Mohs surgery. Brown tape is more aesthetically pleasing as it camouflages better with skin, but it is more expensive than white tape; therefore, the brown tape is usually used at the completion of Mohs surgery. Micropore tape is also hypoallergenic and, for that reason, can also be used to substitute adhesive bandages.

Lastly, Mohs surgery generates large amounts of waste. Regulated waste has to be disposed of in containers that are closeable and constructed to contain all contents and prevent leakage of fluids during handling, storage, transport, or shipping. If outside contamination of the waste container occurs, then it needs to be placed in a second container. There are three types of waste containers necessary in the OR: a large wide-mouthed container for noncontaminated, non-sharps waste (table paper, paper towels, etc.), a sharps container, and a contaminated waste container. The sharps container has to be leak proof and puncture resistant and replaced regularly so that it does not overfill. Only dispose of appropriate materials in the sharps and contaminated waste disposal because it is expensive to manage them.

Additional miscellaneous operating room equipment useful to the Mohs surgeon is listed below [1]:

1. Magnifying glasses: Provide magnification with good working distances, allowing the Mohs surgeon better visibility of the surgical field.
2. Tool chest on wheels: For emergency resuscitation equipment and medication.
3. Surgical instrument sharpener: Used to maintain sharp equipment, including curettes, punches, and scissors. It is easy to use and highly functional. There are also services that can be purchased to sharpen instruments.
4. Gentian violet pens and pen holders: These are ethylene oxide re-sterilizable. The pen holder allows the pens to be stored point down, preventing premature loss of function.
5. Liquid gentian violet for marking deep tissue: Gentian violet can be painted on tissue with a sterile cotton tip applicator as a grid to help orient tissues that may distort or shrink after they are removed from the patient. Alternatively, an entire deep tissue plane can be painted with gentian violet. If the tissue was not completely removed, the gentian violet remains visible after the removal of the specimen. In this manner, the Mohs surgeon can be alerted to the fact that an incomplete layer was taken.
6. Alligator hair clips: Useful in keeping the patient's hair out of the surgical field and can be ethylene oxide sterilized.

Summary: Surgical Waiting Room

- The patient has to wait for the tissue specimen to be prepared and read, which usually takes about half an hour or longer.
- It is optimal to have a surgical waiting area separate from other patients.
- The surgical waiting room should be large enough to accommodate at least five patients, each with their accompanying family member or friend.
- Patient satisfaction and comfort can be enhanced with quiet music, a variety of current magazines, or even with a television.
- Bathrooms should be easily accessible, and emergency alarms should be placed in the bathrooms within easy reach.

11.3 Surgical Waiting Room

After a layer of skin is removed, the patient has to wait for the tissue specimen to be prepared and read, which usually takes about half an hour or longer. Patients can be sent back to general patient reception area, but this is not ideal. Patients may feel awkward with large dressings and other patients may feel apprehensive about sitting near surgical patients with these dressings. Therefore, it is optimal to have a discrete surgical waiting area for the Mohs patients.

The surgical waiting room should be large enough to accommodate at least five patients, each with their accompanying family member or friend. All seats should be in full view of a staff receptionist trained in CPR. The seats need to be wide enough for obese patients and have arms to support and assist older patients in standing up and sitting down. They should be arranged so that the patients can sit somewhat apart from one another but next to an accompanying family member or friend [1].

In addition to comfortable seating, patient satisfaction and comfort can be enhanced with quiet music, a variety of current magazines, or with a television. According to a systematic review in 2008, music intervention had positive effects on reducing pain and anxiety in the perioperative setting in approximately half of the reviewed studies. Music has also been shown to reduce heart rate, blood pressure, respiratory rate, and cortisol levels.

Recommendations include slow and flowing music approximately 60–80 beats per minute, nonlyrical, and maximum volume at 60 dB [2]. A television can be set to show a movie with appropriate language, content, and minimal violence or can be used to educate patients on Mohs surgery and other services the dermatology office provides. The volume level should not be distracting.

Moreover, bathrooms should be nearby. It is required that they be accessible to individuals with disabilities. Emergency alarms should be placed in the bathrooms within easy reach. Snacks and drinks should be provided as needed. The staff needs to remain alert for potential problems, for example, a patient may be bleeding through the bandage or may feel dizzy. In the occasional instant that a patient needs to lie down, take the patient to a room and notify the surgeon, who may place the patient in Trendelenburg position. Surgical patients should be supervised at all times. Overall, the surgical waiting room should be private, clean and comfortable, and regularly monitored by the staff.

Summary: The Histopathology Laboratory

- The lab should be located out of sight and hearing of patients and have a microscope slide reading area.
- The modern Mohs laboratory configuration consists of an air-conditioned room with a recirculating fume hood housing an automated slide stainer.
- The fume hood's flow rate should be approximately 380 L/s and an average face velocity of 0.5 m/s.
- The total flow rate should be 480 L/s; with 40 L/s of fresh air brought into the lab from the external environment. This system should provide at least 4.3 complete air changes per hour, taking into account the dimensions of the room.
- The lab needs to have running water, good overhead lighting, shelf space for supplies, and room for slide staining equipment.
- It is important to look up and abide by local and state regulations regarding OSHA and laboratory setup requirements, which may be variable in regards to ventilation over the staining equipment.

11.4 The Histopathology Laboratory

Each Mohs surgeon should strive to build and equip the best Mohs lab within space and budgetary limitations. Investing in a well-trained histotechnician and equipment to create the ideal laboratory is worthwhile, as this is the foundation of the surgery. A well-trained Mohs histotechnician that has access to a well-equipped lab will result in an efficient production of high-quality frozen section slides.

The lab should be located out of sight and hearing of patients and have a microscope slide reading area. It requires a cool, dry environment. It is best that the lab air-conditioning is separated from the general office air-conditioning because cryostats generate heat in the process of producing and maintaining an internally cold microtome temperature [1]. Heat inlet ducts should be fully closeable.

The Mohs laboratory has evolved significantly over the years. Older laboratories had an early-model automated slide stainer in which the technicians were required to replenish fluid levels throughout the processing. An extractor fan adjacent to the slide stainer, with a flow rate of approximately 50 L/s, allowed for ventilation. The new Mohs laboratory configuration consists of an air-conditioned room with a recirculating fume hood housing a modern automated slide stainer. Hazardous chemicals should always be handled within the fume hood. The fume hood's flow rate should be approximately 380 L/s and have an average face velocity of 0.5 m/s. Air is filtered through particulate and activated carbon filters and is then returned to the room. The lab should have its own air-conditioning system separate from the general office. The total flow rate should be 480 L/s, with 40 L/s of fresh air brought into the lab from the external environment. This system should provide at least 4.3 complete air changes per hour, taking into account the dimensions of the room [3].

The lab needs to have running water, good overhead lighting, shelf space for supplies, and room for slide staining equipment. Floor space is required for one cryostat (preferably two), and for an area where specimens can be processed (grossed, inked, and labeled) and paperwork can be completed.

Safety equipment for laboratory technicians includes safety glasses, an emergency eyewash station, nitrile gloves, and gowns. A stool should be provided even though most technicians prefer to stand while cutting tissue. The floor covering should be relatively stain resistant

[1]. It is important to look up and abide by local and state regulations regarding OSHA and laboratory setup requirements, which may be variable in regard to ventilation over the staining equipment.

Summary: Grossing and Inking

- The grossing and inking area should have a separate light task.
- A cutting board is necessary to divide specimens and to make relaxing incisions.

11.5 Grossing and Inking

The grossing and inking area should have a separate light task. A cutting board is necessary to divide specimens and to make relaxing incisions, which are also useful to line up the leading edge of the epidermis for better sectioning. Metal salt dyes can be used and are grossly colorful, but with transillumination appear indistinguishably black. The dye can be applied with pipe cleaners, cotton swabs, and wooden applicators, all which are inexpensive when bought in bulk. For a finer point, however, a paint brush is more ideal, such as an artist's No. 2 or 3 round synthetic brush with a metal ferrule [4]. Indelible marking pens for histology are used to label the glass slides because the ink they contain will not wash off during processing. Space is required for the Mohs map to be close at hand to verify the congruence between specimen inking and mapping [1].

A telephone intercom system between the lab and the OR is useful because it allows the surgeon to call the histopathology technician from the OR when a new specimen is ready to be picked up for processing. It can also be used to call the technician when there are quality assurance problems with the slide being read or if recuts are necessary [1].

Summary: Embedding and Mounting Tissue and the Cryostat

- The most important and expensive piece of equipment in the lab is the cryostat.
- Cryostats vary in cost, features, and size and dimension of the cryochamber working space.
- The microtome is the heart of the cryostat. It is a tool that can cut fresh, frozen material into very thin slices.
- Properly mounting the tissue onto the chuck is important because failing to do so may result in an uneven Mohs cut leading to skip areas on the slides.
- Flattening the tissue specimen is an important method in order to examine 100% of the surgical margin.
- All cryostats can be adjusted to produce frozen sections of varying thickness.
- Cryochamber temperature settings can also be varied although most technicians cut tissue at −20°C to −30°C.
- A backup cryostat is essential in case of unit failure.
- Preventive maintenance of cryostats is extremely important.

11.6 Embedding and Mounting Tissue and the Cryostat

The most important and expensive piece of equipment in the lab is the cryostat. The cost to purchase one varies from $2,000 to $65,000, depending on whether it is purchased used or as a top-of-the-line new cryostat. Not only is cost a factor in deciding which cryostat to purchase, but so is the desired range of features. Some of these features include the following: an ultraviolet option to disinfect the cryochamber from bacteria, spores, and viruses; memory function; self-cleaning systems; double compressors that markedly increase reliability; and programmable digital controls. In fact, portable cryostats are also now available for purchase and can also be used as a backup.

Cryostats vary in cost, features, and size and dimension of the cryochamber working space. The height of some cryostats can be widely adjusted, while others are set at a permanent height. The advantage in the ability to adjust the height is that it can allow the technician to cut tissue sitting in a standard chair [1].

The microtome is the most important part of the cryostat. It is an instrument that can cut fresh, frozen material into very thin slices. This instrument moves over a fixed knife blade and has a gear that advances the object holder a set distance with each turn of the rotating handle. The distance that the object holder advances can be adjusted and determines the thickness of the tissue sections being cut [1]. As previously mentioned, there are now cryostats available in which a memory function allows for predefined advancement of the tissue specimen to the knife blade. Another feature to consider when selecting a cryostat is the ease of removal of the microtome for cleaning. If this is difficult, there can be delay in processing tissue.

The microtome holds the chuck holder (object holder). There are two general types of chuck holders. The rectangular holder is fixed in an either upright or turned 180° in position. This fixed position is an advantage when using cryomolds to prepare tissue specimens for cutting. A cryomold is a plastic mold that holds the specimen while freezing and aids in making the surgical margin of the specimen completely even [1].

The yoke system object holder can permit 360° rotation of the tissue block and can adjust most of the cutting angle in reference to the cryostat blade [1]. There are round cryomolds that can be used with the yoke system, but they must frequently be adjusted to give a perfectly flat cutting plane.

Properly mounting the tissue onto the chuck is important because failing to do so may result in an uneven Mohs cut, leading to skip areas on the slides. An important step in tissue preparation is sufficiently flattening the specimen and placing it centrally on the chuck in a proper amount of medium [5].

Flattening the tissue specimen is critical in order to examine 100% of the surgical margin. Flattening devices may be useful when using a yoke system chuck holder. There are several devices and methods that can be used to flatten the tissue. One such way is the conventional method. A frozen tissue embedding medium, called OCT (optimal cutting temperature), is placed onto a cold chuck. A heat sink is then applied to freeze and flatten the OCT base, and afterward, the tissue specimen is placed on the center of the OCT. Fresh OCT is placed on top of that specimen, followed by placing the heat sink on the tissue again. The frozen tissue is now embedded in OCT and transferred to the cryostat [6].

The Miami Special device is also used to prepare and flatten tissue specimens (Figure 11.1). In a busy practice, frozen section preparation is the limiting step. A study has demonstrated that the CryoHist™ embedding machine allows tissue to be processed faster than Cryocup™ and the Miami Special [7]. Liquid nitrogen is required for the use of the Miami Special instrument. For fatty specimens that do not freeze well, liquid nitrogen and cooled isopentane minimize ice crystals [4].

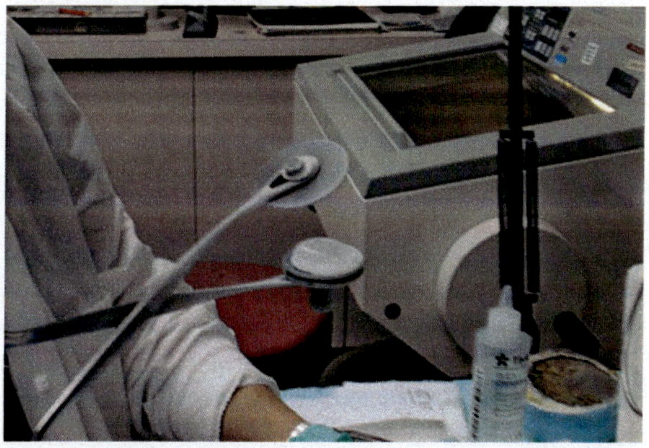

Fig. 11.1 Preparing the microtome stage for placement of the Mohs specimen

All cryostats can be adjusted to produce frozen sections of varying thickness. Most Mohs surgeons prefer sections 5–7 μm in thickness with a range of 4–10 μm. All cryostats are adjustable well beyond the range of thickness needed for Mohs surgery.

Cryochamber temperature settings can also be varied within a wide range; however, most technicians cut tissue at −20°C to −30°C. Warmer temperatures may be required to cut cartilage and colder temperatures to cut adipose tissue [1].

Cryostat knife holders can hold disposable or reusable blades. Disposable blades are available in thin and thicker, more durable varieties. Disposable blades may require an adapter for use with certain blade holders. Reusable blades are available in lengths ranging from 10 to 25 cm. An advantage of a longer blade is that if one portion dulls while cutting, another portion of the blade can be situated into position to continue cutting. A disadvantage is that a longer blade can allow for a greater chance of injury to the technician. The most common injury to a Mohs technician is cuts from the blade. For safety, a blade guard can be placed on the exposed end of a blade [1].

Blades that can be resharpened are available and are honed with an automatic blade sharpener after each use. Cryostat blades should be sharpened after each use. If the office has two cryostats, three or four blades may be purchased so that one blade is always in the sharpener. Locking blade boxes are used to store these extremely sharp blades and prevent accidental injury [1].

Once the tissue has been cut, it needs to be placed on a slide. Unfortunately, there is a tendency for frozen cuts to curl before they are placed on a glass slide. The curling can be prevented by using an anti-roll bar, or plate, and/or camel hair brushes. Camel hair brushes are also used to help orient the cut tissue sections onto the slide so that they are in perfect alignment [1]. Certain practices have found that using modern anti-roll plates uniformly provides superior sections [4]. Therefore, the anti-roll plate can be used to prevent curling, and the brushes can help orient the cut tissue onto the slides. The camel hair brushes are kept in the cryochamber on a brush shelf.

In a busy Mohs practice, a backup cryostat is essential in case of unit failure. Very large specimens can be processed on one machine, while smaller specimens from several other patients can be simultaneously processed on the backup cryostat by another technician. If the office has a backup cryostat, it is important to use it regularly so that it remains operable. If two cryostats are operated adjacent to each other in the lab, the refrigeration unit exhaust from the first unit must not be directly vented to the air intake of the second unit, or the second unit's motor could fail. If cryostat configuration and room space cannot prevent this problem, a custom plexiglass air diverter can change the direction of the hot exhaust airflow [1].

Preventative maintenance of cryostats is crucial to their continued functioning. The cryostat's moving parts should be taken apart, greased, and oiled at least quarterly. Also, before and after each cryostat use, the machine should be oiled. Maintenance logs and daily temperature logs for the cryostat should be filled out and kept up-to-date.

It may be less expensive in the long run to purchase a new, high-quality cryostat. An older machine can be less reliable and require more maintenance. The best strategy for selecting a cryostat is to attend a Mohs surgery or national dermatology or pathology meeting where the major cryostat manufacturers and suppliers exhibit their machines. Cost, features, and other specifications of the cryostats can be easily compared to each other at these events [1].

Summary: Staining Frozen Sections

- Manual slide staining is almost never used; automated slide staining results in better quality and is much more efficient.
- Most slides are 1-mm thick, have a refractive index of 1.5, and are made of glass.
- Fixation of tissue prevents cellular degradation throughout the staining process. Acid formalin is the most common fixative used in most labs.
- Hematoxylin and eosin are considered the standard for staining sections.
- After staining, it is necessary to clear excess stain. Xylene has been the classic agent, but it is neurotoxic and flammable.

11.7 Staining Frozen Sections

Slide staining can be carried out manually or using an automatic tissue stainer. Manual staining is almost never used because it can result in an uneven quality and takes a considerable amount of time. With automated staining, there is no time penalty for the technician to prepare extra slides, which can result in fewer occurrences of incomplete margins. If slides contain large amounts of cartilage, then they should be manually run though the auto stainer; if not, the cartilage may float off the slides as they advance and drop from one stain chamber to the next. Auto stainers require a water source and drain; a constant flow of fresh water results in cleaner slides [1].

Mounting and staining supplies should be located near the staining area. Different slides are available, each with their advantages. Most slides are 1-mm thick, have a refractive index of 1.5, and are made of glass. Superfrost slides adhere tissue with a small electrostatic charge and are moderately priced. The clear and frosted slides are less expensive. Frosted slides also allow the technician to quickly determine which side is "up," assisting in preventing the technician from wiping off the wrong side of the slide and ruining a specimen that was difficult to cut. The frosted end may be purchased in multiple colors, and each of these colors can represent separate patients, separate Mohs stages of each case, or may be used for other reasons [1]. It is important to note that cartilage may require adhesives for adequate attachment to the slide, such as silane and L-Lysine adhesive. Other adhesives include bovine albumin and casein glue.

Fixation of tissue is used to prevent cellular degradation throughout the staining process. Acid formalin is the most common fixative used. Acetone is a superior fixative to acid formalin for adipose tissue. Other tissue fixatives include alcohol, formaldehyde, formalin, and omnifix. Alcohol is a poor fixative for adipose tissue, and omnifix is used to preserve antigens for immunoperoxidase stains [4].

Hematoxylin and eosin are considered the standard for staining micrographic sections because not only do they provide superior cellular detail, they are also reasonably fast and cheap, and most histotechnologists are familiar with them. Toluidine blue O and safranin O are also dye stains that are occasionally used. Toluidine blue O stains keratinocytes and mucin, and can be 25% faster than hematoxylin and eosin, but there is still controversy concerning its use for squamous cell carcinoma [4].

After staining, it is necessary to clear excess stain. Xylene was once the classic agent, but it is neurotoxic and flammable. Numerous xylene substitutes are available and cost more, but should be used because they are much safer. The two main classes of substitutes are D-limonene and alkanes. An aliphatic xylene is less oily and dries more quickly [4].

Cover slips are made of glass, plastic, or quartz. The plastic cover slips are cheaper, but over several years can peel from the slide. At the end of the Mohs session, they can be placed overnight in a drying oven to prevent them from sticking together when they are filed [4].

11.8 Slide Reading

The microscope slide reading area can be located in the lab itself if there is enough space, or can be adjacent to it. There should be little distraction while the Mohs surgeon is reading slides, and the technicians and staff should be aware of the necessity of this, especially if the reading is carried out in the lab. Special sturdy microscope tables at standard height are available for purchase. The table on which slides are read must be large enough for the Mohs maps, slide trays, pencils and pens, and the microscope. A comfortable rolling stool should be available too.

A high-quality double head microscope should be used, which allows for more than one person to analyze the slide at the same time. A lighted movable pointer is useful with the double head microscope to discuss section quality with the technician, as well as when consulting with another doctor. It should be equipped with at least a 2× objective and wide-field eyepieces. The 2×, 4×, and 10× objectives will be used more than any other objectives, and therefore, an objective higher than 40× is unnecessary. Eyepieces with tilt heads are especially useful for short or tall surgeons. For those who wear glasses, the microscope can be adjusted so that the focal points of the eye pieces are a few millimeters above the surface of the eye pieces. It may also be useful to also have a dedicated pair of glasses solely for the purpose of reading slides because glasses are expensive and may become scratched, regardless [1]. Marking pens that write on glass are used for inking or dotting findings on the completely processed Mohs slides during reading and are available in multiple colors.

Summary: Slide Reading

- The microscope slide reading area can be located in the lab itself.
- There should be little distraction when the Mohs surgeon is reading slides.
- The table on which slides are read must be large enough for the Mohs maps, slide trays, pencils and pens, and the microscope.

Summary: Cleaning, Sterilization, and Maintenance of Surgical Instruments

- Sterilizing consists of several steps which include cleaning and decontamination, packaging, loading, and storage.
- Immediately after use, the instruments should be placed in the cleaner and soaked for at least 10 min, but for not more than a few hours because there are greater chances of corrosion.

- The staff that handles the decontamination should wear household cleaning rubber gloves or plastic gloves for protection.
- When packaging instruments, it is important to open all hinged instruments and disassemble all items with removable parts.
- Steam, hot air, and chemical vapor are sterilization agents that must be able to contact the instruments for an appropriate length of time.
- Alcohol- based autoclaves do not dull sharp instruments in the same way that steam autoclaves do, but they have a strong odor and need to be operated in well-ventilated areas.
- Steam autoclaves are more user and environmentally friendly, but they dull sharp instruments. Also, corrosion of instruments is possible.
- Ethylene oxide sterilization is a valuable adjunct to steam sterilization. The unit is very safe, although it may need to be exhausted to the outside to meet local and/or state regulations.
- Sterilization is monitored with chemical and biological indicators.
- Each sterilized package should have an expiration date written on it.
- Instruments need to be sharpened on a regular basis.

11.9 Cleaning, Sterilization, and Maintenance of Surgical Instruments

Maintenance of the equipment begins during the surgery. During surgery, blood should be wiped from scissors and needle holders because dried blood may result in decreased capability of them to open smoothly. Also, the knife blade should be wiped frequently on a 4×4 pad to prevent seeding of carcinoma from the scalpel blade to uninvolved tissues being excised [1].

Sterilizing consists of several steps which include cleaning and decontamination, packaging, loading, and storage. Cleaning is important to remove residues that can interfere with the sterilization process. Generally, the instruments should be presoaked in a solution of water mixed with detergent or an enzymatic cleaner immediately after use. One way to accomplish this is by conveniently placing a small metal bin in the sink filled with an enzymatic cleaner. Immediately after use, the instruments should be placed in the cleaner and allowed to soak for at least 10 min. The instruments should not be presoaked for more than a few hours because there are greater chances of corrosion. A small nylon brush is used to scrub the instruments to further clean the organic and nonorganic residue [7].

The staff that handles the decontamination should wear household cleaning rubber gloves or plastic gloves for protection against the harsh cleaners and the contaminated bodily fluids. The eyes need to be protected with face masks, and appropriate gowns need to be worn. The staff should also use forceps to retrieve the instruments from the solution.

After the instruments have been cleaned and properly dried (reduces chances of corrosion and rupture of the package), all instruments that have movement, such as needle holders, scissors, and hemostats, are lubricated with a rust inhibitor. This solution helps to prevent compromise of the working mechanisms of these instruments. Any excess solution is wiped away using a soft cloth or surgical gauze [1]. Afterward, the instruments are ready to be packaged.

When packaging instruments, it is important to open all hinged instruments and disassemble all items with removable parts. Complex instruments should be prepared and sterilized according to the manufacturer's instructions. Heavy instruments should be positioned not to damage delicate ones, and those with concave surfaces should be positioned to facilitate drainage. Having the same configuration in each pack increases efficacy and saves time. "Peel open" packages are the most convenient way to package instruments, but other more rigid containers can be purchased for heavier instruments. Sterilization wraps are sometimes necessary for certain items as well. Whatever packaging is chosen, it must allow penetration of the sterilant as well as maintain sterility.

Steam, hot air, and chemical vapor are sterilization agents that must be able to contact the instruments for an appropriate length of time. In addition to allowing proper sterilant circulation, perforated trays should be placed so that the tray is parallel to the shelf, non-perforated containers should be placed on their edge, and small items should be loosely placed in wire baskets. Peel packs should be placed on perforated or mesh bottom racks.

There are several machines used to sterilize instruments. Alcohol- based autoclaves do not dull sharp instruments in the same way that steam autoclaves do, but they have a strong odor and need to be operated in well-ventilated areas. Also, during operation, no staff members should be in the room. Steam autoclaves are more user and environmentally friendly, but they dull sharp instruments. Also, corrosion of instruments is possible.

Ethylene oxide sterilization is a valuable adjunct to steam sterilization. Nearly anything can be ethylene oxide sterilized. It is affordable and relatively easy to install. The unit is very safe, although it may need to be exhausted to the outside to meet local and/or state regulations.

Sterilization is monitored with chemical and biological indicators. Chemical indicators are markings on pouches that change color after exposure to the sterilizing agent. They indicate that the item has been exposed to the agent, but they do not analyze for microbial kill. Therefore, routine spore testing should be done to assure that sterilization is occurring properly. Spore testing is a biological indicator used to test that sterilization is indeed effective. Spore testing should be done at least weekly. It can be assumed that if the spores are destroyed, then destruction of viruses and bacteria occurred since they are more easily inactivated.

Each sterilized package should have an expiration date written on it. Peel packages and wrapped packs sealed in 3/1,000 in. polyethylene overwrap are reported to be sterile for as long as 9 months after sterilization. If the package is wet, punctured, or torn, the instruments are no longer sterile, and they need to be repackaged and processed. Packages should be stored in a safe place, free of moisture, or possibility of contamination. Once a package becomes wet, it is not sterile anymore. Closed or covered cabinets can be a way to store the packages to prevent moisture damage. If the package falls on the floor, it must be examined for tears.

In addition to lubrication, instruments also need to be sharpened on a regular basis, such as scissors, curettes, and other sharp instruments. There are services which can come to the office on a regular basis to sharpen instruments.

Summary: Conclusion

- Proper setup is important for an efficient, profitable, and safe Mohs practice.
- The basis of a well-run office is an experienced, reliable office manager and a well-trained staff consisting of histotechnicians, medical assistants, and physician assistants and/or nurses.

11.10 Conclusion

Proper setup is important for an efficient, profitable, and safe Mohs practice. The basis of a well-run office is an experienced, reliable office manager and a well-trained staff consisting of histotechnicians, medical assistants, and physician assistants and/or nurses. All staff taking direct care of patients need to be CPR certified and ACLS certified and trained. The operating room needs to be organized and spacious and have all the essential instruments and equipment prepared and readily available. The surgical waiting area needs to be discrete, comfortable, and in view of staff in case of an emergency. The laboratory needs to be configured to allow for proper ventilation. The cryostat is an important investment and should have features that allow the histotechnicians to produce high-quality frozen sections. It should be easy to clean and needs to be maintained daily. The microscope reading area should be free of distraction. All instruments should be cleaned and sterilized appropriately. The proper setup is the basis of a successful Mohs practice.

References

1. Gross K. Office and laboratory set-up and instrumentation for Mohs surgery. In: Baxter S, Gunter A, Achenbach F, editors. Mohs surgery: fundamentals and techniques. Saint Louis: Mosby; 1999. p. 15–55.
2. Nilsson U. The anxiety- and pain-reducing effects of music interventions: a systematic review. AORN J. 2008;87(4): 780–807.
3. Gunson TH, Smith HR, Vinciullo C. Assessment and management of chemical exposure in the Mohs laboratory. Dermatol Surg. 2011;37:1–9. Epub November 11, 2010.
4. Davis DA, Pellowski DM, Hanke CW. Preparation of frozen sections. Dermatol Surg. 2004;30(12 Pt 1):1479–85.
5. Bakhtar O, Close A, Davidson TM, Baird SM. Tissue preparation for MOHS' frozen sections: a comparison of three techniques. Virchows Arch. 2007;450(5):513–8.
6. Desciak EB, Maloney ME. Artifacts in frozen section preparation. Dermatol Surg. 2000;26(5):500–4.
7. Hanke CW, Leonard AL, Reed AJ. Rapid preparation of high-quality frozen sections using a membrane and vacuum system embedding machine. Dermatol Surg. 2008;34(1):20–5.

Tissue Transport and Initial Processing Cryostat Preparation of Slides

12

Michael P. McLeod, Sonal Choudhary, Katlein França, and Keyvan Nouri

Abstract

The major goal during tissue transport and initial processing is to maintain specimen orientation. Once the specimen is removed from the surgical site and hemostasis is achieved, the Mohs map can be drawn. Then the specimen is transported to the histopathology laboratory. The specimen should be cut into as few sections as possible in order to avoid orientation error, while still producing high-quality slides. Colored ink is used to assist in maintaining orientation. Optimum cutting temperature (OCT) is used to facilitate specimen adhesion to the microtome chuck. Following microtome sectioning, the specimen is stained, most commonly with hematoxylin and eosin. After application of the coverslip, the slides are ready to be analyzed by the Mohs surgeon.

Keywords

Mohs map • Tissue transport • Hematoxylin and eosin • Mohs micrographic surgery initial processing

Summary: Tissue Transport

- The major goal of transporting tissue from the surgical site to the histology processing center is to maintain specimen orientation.
- The 12 o'clock position of the specimen should be oriented to line up with the 12 o'clock position of the transferring device.
- The specimen should be transferred with toothed forceps, and care must be taken to avoid damaging or dropping the specimen.
- After transferring the specimen and sufficient hemostasis is achieved, the Mohs' map should be drawn.
- A standard system should be devised and strictly followed for designating specific details of a map.

M.P. McLeod • S. Choudhary • K. França
Department of Dermatology and Cutaneous Surgery,
University of Miami Leonard M. Miller School of Medicine,
Miami, FL, USA

K. Nouri (✉)
Department of Dermatology and Cutaneous Surgery,
University of Miami Leonard M. Miller School of Medicine,
Miami, FL, USA

Sylvester Comprehensive Cancer Center,
University of Miami Hospital and Clinics, Miami, FL, USA
e-mail: knouri@med.miami.edu

K. Nouri (ed.), *Mohs Micrographic Surgery*,
DOI 10.1007/978-1-4471-2152-7_12, © Springer-Verlag London Limited 2012

12.1 Tissue Transport

The major goal of transporting tissue from the surgical site to the histology processing center is to maintain specimen orientation [1]. There is ample opportunity for orientation error, and every precaution should be made to safeguard against it. A transferring device such as an index card or gauze on a plate with the 12 o'clock position marked is very useful for maintaining orientation and preventing specimen dropping [1]. Guards around the plate can prevent unexpected movement of air from changing the specimen's orientation. The device should be held closely to the wound when transferring the specimen from the surgical site to the plate in order to avoid dropping the specimen or placing it in the incorrect orientation. The 12 o'clock position of the specimen should be oriented to line up with the 12 o'clock position of the transferring device. The specimen should be transferred with toothed forceps, and care must be taken to avoid damaging or dropping the specimen.

After transferring the specimen and sufficient hemostasis is achieved, the Mohs' map should be drawn. Care should be taken to draw the precise shape of the specimen. It should be at least the same size of the specimen if not larger so that it can demonstrate important details of subsequent stages. A standard system should be devised and strictly followed for designating specific details of a map. For example, short radiating lines are commonly used to denote borders with epithelial margins. Wavy lines can be used to denote nonepithelized margins. Subsequent stages should also be drawn with reference to the previous stage so that a "pictorial story" can be followed until the end of the procedure [1].

Summary: Initial Processing

- The specimen should be divided into as few sections as possible because more sections can lead to orientation confusion.
- Tissue scores or relaxing incisions can also be implemented that allow the specimen to flatten for placement onto the microscope slide.
- Inks can also be very useful in keeping proper specimen orientation throughout histologic processing.
- The cryostat uses a refrigerated microtome to cut histological sections of tissue that are placed onto slides.
- The specimen is placed upon a microtome chuck, and optimum cutting temperature (OCT) is used to fix the tissue to the chuck.
- The slides should be labeled with the patient's medical record number, stage of surgery, and procedure date prior to sectioning the specimen with the microtome to avoid confusion and ease the work flow.
- Staining of the slides must occur so that colorless cellular material can be visualized underneath the microscope.
- The most commonly used stain for Mohs micrographic surgery is hematoxylin and eosin (H&E).
- Following transport and initial processing of the slides, the specimen is now ready to be analyzed by the Mohs micrographic surgeon

12.2 Initial Processing

The Mohs map and transferring device with specimen are then carefully transported to the histological processing center. If the specimen is too large to fit on the slides, it must be divided. The specimen should be divided into as few sections as possible because more sections can lead to orientation confusion [1]. There are a few different ways to divide the specimen. Depending on the specimen shape, it can be divided in half so that there is a top and bottom or left and right. If the specimen is very large, it can be divided into numerous sections. Tissue scores or relaxing incisions can also be implemented that allow for the specimen to flatten for placement onto the microscope slide. These incisions should be superficial enough to allow the tissue to flatten but should not extend deep enough to distort the histology [1].

Inks can also be very useful in keeping proper specimen orientation throughout histologic processing. The color coding scheme should be decided upon and strictly followed as any deviation could lead to orientation error. Colors that are clearly distinct from one another should be used in order to avoid confusion. Sections should be inked one at a time and placed back into the transfer device to avoid orientation error. In addition, the ink should be placed approximately 1–2 mm underneath the surface of each section [1].

The cryostat uses a refrigerated microtome to cut histological sections of tissue that are placed onto slides. The specimen is placed upon a microtome chuck, and optimum cutting temperature (OCT), a type of tissue glue, is used to fix the tissue specimen to the chuck. There are a number of methods used to freeze the specimen. Each cryostat is equipped with a small workstation (the freeze bar) that is approximately 20–30°C below the temperature of the rest of the cryostat [1]. This lower temperature results in an area where tissue can be quickly frozen.

The basic method of tissue freezing and fixing to the chuck involves placing the chuck directly on the freeze bar and placing OCT on its surface. As soon as the OCT begins to turn opaque, the specimen is placed with the deep margin facing upwards and the superior margin directly touching the OCT. A heat extractor can be used to flatten the tissue as it lies upon the OCT so that the peripheral margins come into the same plane as the deep margins. Additional OCT is then placed over top of the specimen after it is frozen [1].

When processing very small specimens, a technique that uses a glass slide may be helpful. The specimen is placed with the superior margin touching the glass slide surface. The lateral edges are then gently pushed down on the slide so that they are in plane with the deep margin. OCT is then placed on top of the specimen with the slide on the freeze bar. The microtome chuck is also placed on the freeze bar, and OCT is placed on it as well. While the OCT on the microtome is in a solid state, the glass slide is inverted and placed on top of the chuck containing the OCT. The glass slide containing the specimen is kept on top of the OCT on the microtome until it freezes. After the OCT freezes, a small amount of heat is placed on top of the glass slide with a finger, and the glass slide is gently removed from the frozen OCT. Additional OCT is then placed over the specimen. Upon freezing of the OCT, the specimen is now ready to be positioned for cutting with the microtome [1].

Another technique is to directly place the specimen with its deep margin touching the freeze bar. Again, the lateral margins should be gently pushed downward to maintain the same plane. Next, OCT is poured directly over the specimen. The OCT covering the specimen should be allowed to freeze. The chuck is again placed on the freeze board, and OCT is poured onto it until it reaches a semisolid state at which time the specimen, frozen in OCT, should be inverted and placed in the semisolid OCT on the microtome chuck. Additional OCT is then added to the specimen on the chuck as required [1].

The specimen can also be prepared using a cryomold in combination with the microtome chuck. The specimen is placed with its superior margin against the surface of the chuck. OCT is poured into the mold on top of the specimen. After that, the mold along with the chuck is placed on the freeze bar and allowed to freeze making sure that the specimen does not change orientation. Once the specimen is frozen in place, additional OCT is poured into the cryomold so that the specimen is covered. When the entire specimen is frozen in OCT, the cryomold can be peeled away leaving the specimen for sectioning [1].

The slides should be labeled with the patient's medical record number, stage of surgery, and procedure date prior to sectioning the specimen with the microtome to avoid confusion and ease the work flow. Electrostatically charged slides are highly recommended as they encourage the specimen to adhere to the slide when being cut with the microtome. In addition, different slide colors can be used to demarcate particular Mohs stages.

Once the specimen is prepared on the chuck and properly placed on the microtome, sectioning the tissue may commence. Whenever possible, the epidermis should be placed perpendicular to the microtome blade in order to prevent tissue folding. The cryostat temperature should be set at –20°C to –29°C [1]. A temperature that is too low can lead to specimen shattering when the microtome blade cuts a section. On the other hand, when the temperature is too high, the tissue can "aggregate" together instead of creating a thin line of OCT and specimen on the microtome stage. Sometimes, the digital temperature reported on the cryostat is not accurate. In order to ensure that the microtome blade and stage are at the desired temperature, a thermometer can be placed in close approximation to these structures and compared to the digital display. In addition to the temperature, the microtome blade should be monitored for dullness and buildup of OCT and/or specimen [1].

When first beginning to rotate the microtome blade, the outer layers of OCT have to be cut away until reaching the actual specimen. Upon reaching the specimen, it may require realignment to achieve as flat a specimen as possible to create uniform slides. The sections should be approximately 5–10 μm thick. At this point, the anti-roll plate should be engaged, and the slides should be appropriately labeled and ready for "picking up" the specimen from the microtome stage. The slides should be kept at room temperature, so that when the slide is gently placed upon the microtome stage, the cold freshly cut specimen quickly adheres to the slide. The specimen should be consistently placed on the slides in the same manner so that orientation confusion is not introduced [1].

Staining of the slides must occur so that colorless cellular material can be visualized underneath the microscope. The most commonly used stain for Mohs micrographic surgery is hematoxylin and eosin (H&E) [1]. Newer stains including immunohistochemical stains are discussed in Chapter 15. Hematoxylin is derived from the logwood tree. When combined with a metal salt, hematoxylin becomes a cation known as hematein. Since hematein has a positive charge, it can bind to negatively charged molecules. In the case of molecular structures, this is most commonly RNA and DNA, which are negatively charged. On the other hand, eosin is a negatively charged molecule and stains other molecules such as proteins that have a positive charge. Hematoxylin stains structures blue, while eosin stains the structures that it binds pink. Slide staining can occur manually or using an automated device. The automated slide staining technique has developed widespread use because it uses fewer reagents and does not demand as much time from the histotechnician (Figure 12.1). For example, in the manual method, the histotechnician must continually change the water-rinse areas; however, the automated staining device continually fills these areas with fresh water [1].

There are many different protocols available for staining slides with H&E. It is important for a Mohs histology processing center to use a protocol that yields the highest quality slides. Protocols can be modified based upon experience and preferences.

First, the tissue can be fixed. If using frozen sections, fixation is not necessary, but 10% neutral buffered formalin can be used. Next, water can be used to hydrate the slides. It is recommended to use distilled water as regular tap water can exhibit different alkalinities. Next, the dye is added. Hematoxylin is most commonly used first as a regressive stain. Following the regressive stain, the "bluing" step uses ammonia or alkaline salts to enhance the nuclear structures stained by the hematoxylin. Eosin is used to counterstain the specimen and dye the cytoplasmic proteins different shades of pink. The last step is dehydration and clearing. This step uses 95% alcohol and is important for determining how much pink to red color remains on the slide. The alcohol removes the excess water from the slide. All the water must be removed before the clearing step is used to improve the transparency of slides. Traditionally, xylene has been used as the predominant clearing agent; however, it has been found to be toxic. Less toxic substitutes have been developed and now include aliphatic hydrocarbons and essential oils [1].

The last step in the preparation of standard H&E slides is applying the coverslip. When removing the

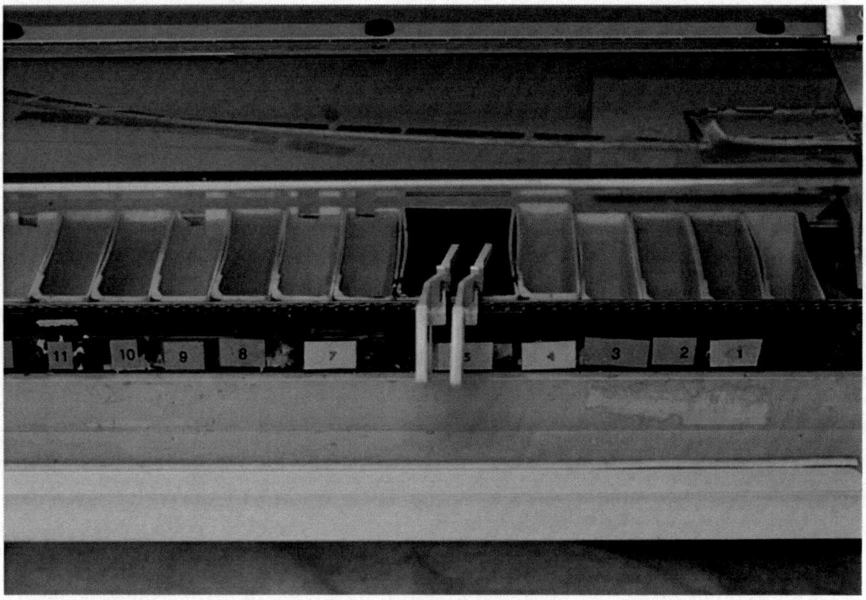

Fig. 12.1 Automated H&E staining device with two slides actively being stained

slide from the staining solution, the side with the specimen should be carefully noted. One must be absolutely sure that the clearing reagent and the mounting media are compatible. The mounting media should be nonaqueous as it lasts longer and does not desiccate as quickly as aqueous media. The correct size of coverslip must also be chosen and applied to the slide. The mounting media can be applied to the cover slip or to the slide. The end result is to not have any air bubbles on the slide, while preserving the integrity of the specimen [1]. Following transport and initial processing of the slides, the specimen is now ready to be analyzed by the Mohs micrographic surgeon.

Summary: Conclusion

- The major goal during tissue transport and initial processing is to maintain the proper specimen orientation. The sample should be cut into as few sections as possible to minimize error orientation. After being sectioned in the microtome, it is stained, most commonly with hematoxylin and eosin. After the coverslip is placed on the slide, the analysis can be made by the Mohs surgeon.

12.3 Conclusion

The major goal during tissue transport and initial processing is to maintain the proper specimen orientation. After the specimen is removed from the surgical site and hemostasis is complete, the Mohs map can be drawn. The specimen can then be transported to the histopathology laboratory. It should be cut into as few sections as possible, that way orientation error is minimized. Colored ink is generally used to maintain orientation. Optimum cutting temperature (OCT) is used to attach the specimen to the microtome chuck. After being sectioned in the microtome, the specimen is stained, most commonly with hematoxylin and eosin. After the coverslip is placed on the slide, the slides are ready to be analyzed by the Mohs surgeon.

Reference

1. Steinman HK. Specimen Transport and Preliminary Tissue Processing. In: Mohs Surgery: Fundamentals and Techniques. Gross KG, Steinman HK, Rapini RP, editors. Saint Louis: Mosby; 1999. p. 91–96.

Histopathologic Interpretation of Mohs Slides

13

Ashraf M. Hassanein and Hatem A. Hassanein

Abstract

Interpretation of Mohs slides is the most critical step in MMS. Mohs surgeons should be adept in identifying different cutaneous structures and in detecting different skin neoplasms. Missing a focus of tumor will result in tumor recurrence. Likewise, interpreting slides with missing pieces of tissue may result in tumor recurrence. Technical errors represent the most common cause of local recurrence after MMS. Consequently, Mohs surgeons should verify that 100% of the margin is evaluated including the entire deep margin and all epidermal peripheries. Tumor prognosis could be dependent on the identification of certain changes in the Mohs slides such as angiovascular invasion or perineural invasion. On the other hand, lack of experience in identifying cutaneous structures such as a bulge, a mantle, a folliculocentric basaloid proliferation (funny follicle), or an atypical reactive endothelial cell may result in unnecessary extra stages which would lead to unnecessarily larger defects. This would negate the purpose of MMS in producing the smallest possible defect with clear margins.

Keywords

Interpretation • Mohs slides • Histopathology • Mohs surgery • Skin neoplasms

A.M. Hassanein (✉)
Medical Director, Florida Pathology, Dermatologic Sugery & Aesthetics Institute,
The Villages, FL, USA
e-mail: floripathol@aol.com

H.A. Hassanein
Department of Microbiology and Biomedical Sciences,
University of South Florida College of Medicine
Tampa, FL, USA
e-mail: hatem.h@gmail.com

Summary: Introduction

- The Mohs surgeon should communicate with the laboratory personnel to ensure the production of high-quality Mohs slides.
- The Mohs surgeon should be aware of all the technical issues related to the Mohs laboratory, since technical errors represent the most common cause of local recurrence after MMS.

K. Nouri (ed.), *Mohs Micrographic Surgery*,
DOI 10.1007/978-1-4471-2152-7_13,

13.1 Introduction

The success of MMS is contingent upon high-quality frozen tissue sections for histopathologic interpretation. The Mohs slide is the product of the Mohs surgeon's performance and the laboratory personnel's experience. Strong communication between the Mohs surgeon and the laboratory personnel is a key for production of high-quality Mohs slides. For example, some Mohs surgeons do not bevel the Mohs layers. This will require special tissue processing such as compression with Miami spatula to produce slides showing a complete tissue with epidermis. The low recurrence rate and the tissue-sparing benefit associated with MMS require accurate interpretation of the frozen sections by the Mohs surgeon [1]. Mohs surgeons should be aware of all the technical issues related to the Mohs laboratory. Frozen tissue section processing results in approximately 10–20% tissue shrinkage. The Mohs surgeon should pay attention to any discrepancy in the size of the tissue on the slide compared to the tissue excised. Discrepancy in the tissue size or large holes could be due to missing tissue and is definitely associated with incomplete margin. Technical errors represent the most common cause of local recurrence after MMS [2].

Summary: Histopathologic Scanning of Mohs Slides

- Histopathologic scanning of Mohs slides should include all tissue sections on the slide.
- Mohs surgeons should evaluate all the tissue on the slides in a systematic way by examining all of the peripheral margin (i.e., the epidermis) and the deep margin. This should entail evaluation of 100% of the margin.
- Overlooking a piece of tissue or evaluating a suboptimal slide with missing tissue or containing a hole may result in tumor recurrence.
- Routine scanning should be performed under the low power (20× and 40×) magnification. Positive areas of a residual tumor can be easily seen upon scanning. Any suspicious areas should be examined under high-power (100× and 200×) magnification.

13.2 Histopathologic Scanning of Mohs Slides

The MMS layer is typically a thin slice of skin that is removed by curvilinear excision. Sections are usually divided into subunits to facilitate flattening of the tissue so that the epidermis (the peripheral margin) and the deep margins lie on the same plane. Consequently, Mohs slides contain only margins and interpretation of Mohs slides entails literally 100% evaluation of specimen margins [3, 4]. This is in contrary to routine dermatopathology slides that are meant mostly for diagnostic reasons. Routine surgical pathology, grossing and processing of excisional specimens show only less than 1% of the actual margin. When you examine a Mohs slide, you are actually evaluating the entire bottom and the whole periphery of the specimen.

Mohs slides should be examined in numerical order corresponding to the map. Any residual tumor identified can be located with its exact site on the map based upon the colors of the margins (Chap. 12). Mohs slides should be routinely scanned under the low power (20× and 40×) magnification. If microscopic evaluation reveals malignancy at one point in the slides, it should be assumed that the corresponding point in the patient is positive. Scanning of Mohs slides should be done the same way dermatopathologists examine their slides. A routine and systematic way of evaluation of cutaneous structures should be followed. We always teach our new dermatopathology fellows to scan slides at low power in the same fashion a photocopier machine or scanner does. One should scan slides starting at one side of the specimen and sweep, up and down until reaching the other side. Practically speaking, it is advisable to go up and down, perpendicular to the epidermis, after evaluating the epidermis itself and consequently the dermo-epidermal junction. The latter is of utmost importance in scanning Mohs slides for melanoma.

The time needed to scan Mohs slides depends upon the experience of the Mohs surgeon; it is usually a few seconds. Positive areas of residual tumor can be easily seen on scanning. If any suspicious areas are found, high-power (100× and 200×) examination is needed. The Mohs surgeon should scan and examine all the sections on the slide. The histotechnician usually puts multiple tissue sections on one slide. This helps

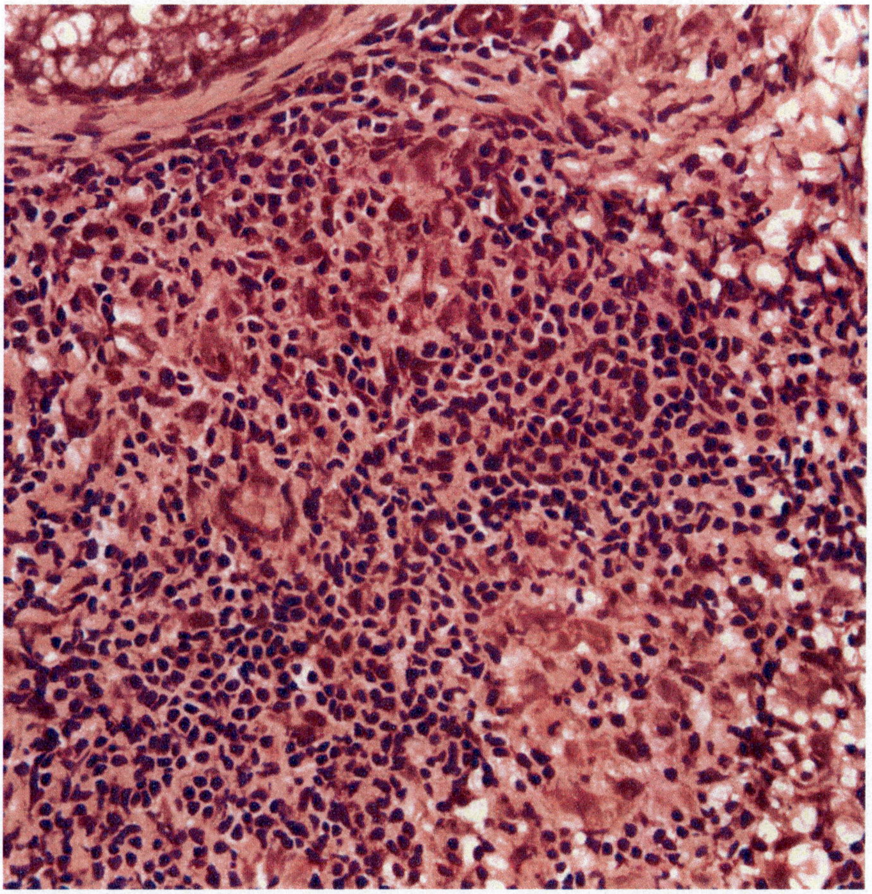

Fig. 13.1 High-power view of a rosacea granuloma showing multinucleated giant cells and lymphohistiocytic cellular infiltrate

specifically if a part of one section is missing or folded and also helps track a particular suspicious structure that is mimicking cancer.

Higher magnification facilitates evaluation of certain structures and small groups of malignant cells. For instance, perineural invasion definitely needs high-power examination. Dense inflammatory infiltrate is said to be the pathologist's enemy. Higher-power examination of dense inflammatory infiltrate is important to rule out any hidden individual cells, groups of tumor cells or perineural invasion. Patients with chronic lymphocytic leukemia and solid-organ transplant recipients have a 36% and 13% incidence, respectively, of dense inflammatory infiltrates seen in Mohs slides; as opposed to 1% seen in controls [5]. Dense inflammatory infiltrate does not normally obscure residual tumors of BCC [6] or SCC [7]. In the author's experience, high-power evaluation and/or recuts usually resolve any problem interpreting dense inflammatory infiltrate. Permanent sections should always be obtained in these cases as a frozen section control. It is important to note that these permanent sections (frozen section control) are routinely obtained for all frozen sections performed in the surgical pathology department. It is advisable to do them only in controversial Mohs cases and in cases of aggressive cancers such as melanoma, sebaceous carcinoma, and merkel cell carcinoma. On the other hand, dense inflammatory infiltrate can be reactive or represent a chronic skin disease. This is not uncommon in Mohs slides of facial tumors that may show a variable degree of rosacea. The presence of multinucleated giant cells and/or granulomas within the lymphohistiocytic infiltrate is helpful in identifying rosacea (Fig. 13.1).

Summary: Histopathologic Recognition of Cutaneous Structures

- The Mohs surgeon should be able to recognize different cutaneous structures and tumors with special reference to the histopathologic differential diagnosis.
- Actinic keratosis should be differentiated from Bowenoid (full thickness) atypia and squameous cell carcinoma in situ.
- Squamous eddies of irritated seborrheic keratosis or inverted follicular keratosis should be differentiated from the epithelial pearls of SCC. The former are numerous, small, monotonous rounded or oval collections of reactive keratinocytes, whereas the latter are less in number, variable in size, and larger with focal or diffuse keratinocytic atypia and mitoses.
- Incidental acantholytic dyskeratosis or epidermolytic hyperkeratosis (granular degeneration) should be differentiated from acantholytic SCC.
- Pseudoepitheliomatous hyperplasia should be differentiated from SCC by the lack of cytologic atypia and atypical mitoses.
- The Mohs surgeon should be aware of the presence of large, atypical melanocytes in sun-damaged skin when interpreting Mohs slides for melanoma.
- The Mohs surgeon should be able to recognize different cross-sections of hair follicles at different levels. The presence of perifollicular fibrous tissue sheeth helps differentiate them from BCC tumor formations that are usually surrounded by immature mucinous stroma.
- The bulge is the follicular protrusion at the site of attachment of the arrector pili muscle. Horizontal sections of the bulge may create a rounded or oval basaloid cell structure with a blend of suprabulbar and isthmic cellular features which should be differentiated from BCC tumor formations.
- The mantle is a ribbon of basaloid cells extending from the upper portion of the hair follicles and they represent the origin of, or "the resting stage," of mature sebaceous gland lobules. The mantle should be differentiated from BCC tumor formations.
- Folliculocentric basaloid proliferations (funny looking follicles) are reactive irregular strands of basaloid cells emanating from the upper portion of some hair follicles and should be differentiated from BCC tumor formations. They are believed to be hyperplasia of the mantle epithelium.
- Dense desmoplastic reaction can sometimes create a picture that mimics perineural invasion and is referred to as peritumoral fibrosis.
- Dense perineural inflammation has been associated with a higher incidence of perineural invasion. Examination of other tissue sections on the slide or deeper levels may be warranted to rule out perineural invasion.
- Reactive endothelial cells may show prominent cytologic atypia and should be differentiated from different cutaneous neoplasms such as SCC.

13.3 Histopathologic Recognition of Cutaneous Structures

13.3.1 Recognition of Epidermal and Epithelial Components and Their Neoplasia

13.3.1.1 The Epidermis

The Mohs surgeon should be adept in understating the normal histology of the skin to recognize cutaneous pathology. The epidermal thickness varies depending on the site on the body, the age of the patient, and the degree of sun damage in sun-exposed areas. Mucosal epithelium is usually glycogenated and appears vacuolated, which could be interpreted as a freezing artifact by an inexperienced Mohs surgeon (Fig. 13.2). Tangential cutting of rete ridges and/or epidermis may sometimes resemble basal or squamous cell carcinoma tumor formations (Fig. 13.3).

A variable degree of keratinocytic atypia and rare normal mitotic figures at the basal cell layer can be seen in sun-damaged skin. The incidental presence of a common benign epidermal tumor should be evaluated cautiously with comparison to the original cancer. For instance, a focus of irritated seborrheic keratosis

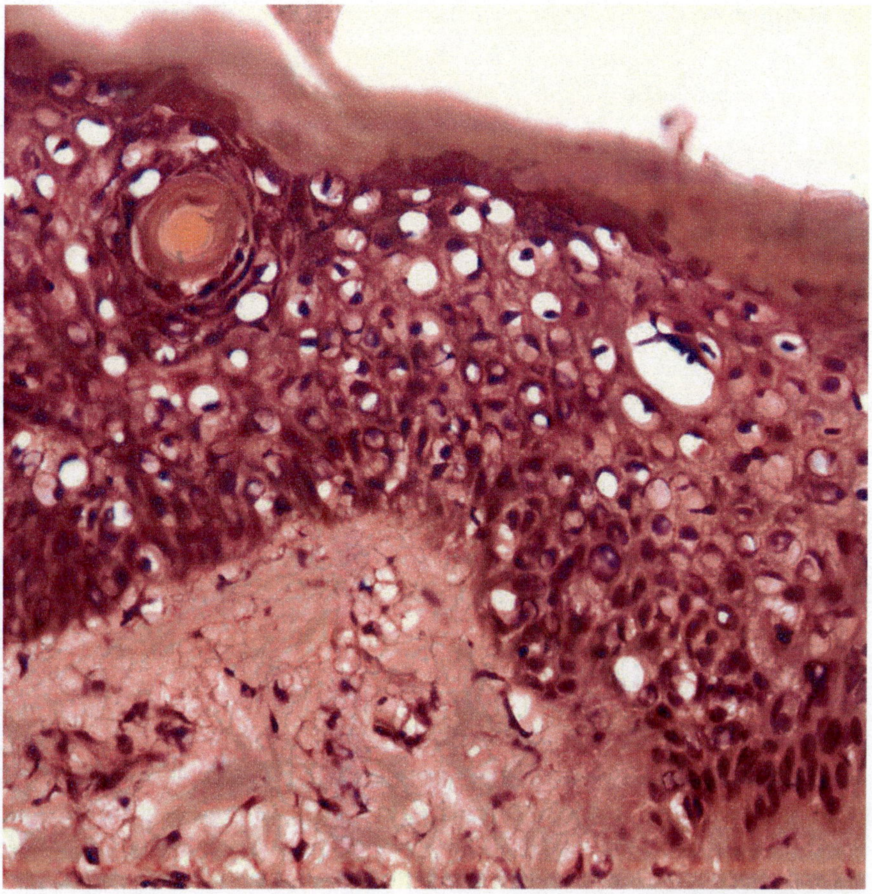

Fig. 13.2 High-power view of a Mohs section showing prominent freezing artifacts

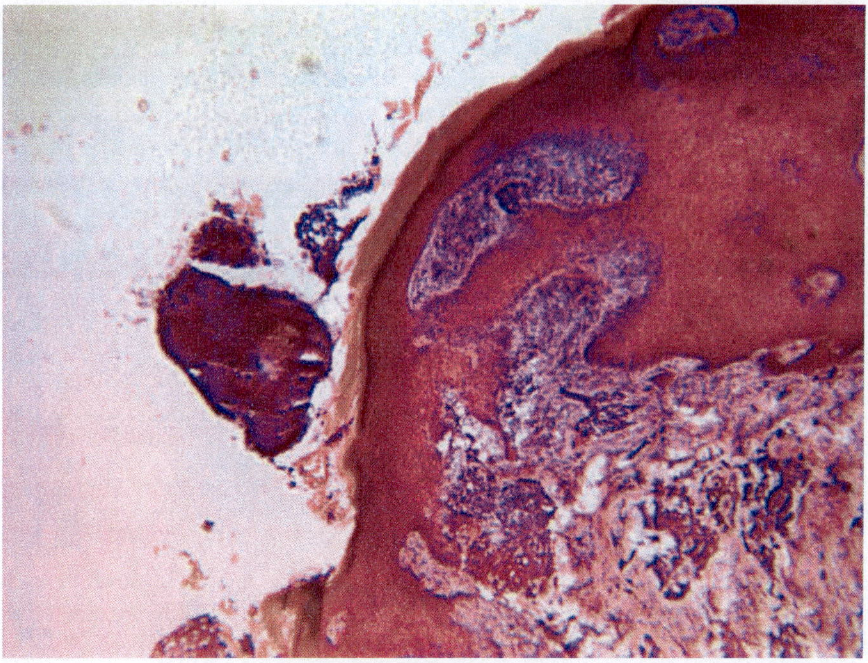

Fig. 13.3 Intermediate-power view of a Mohs section showing tangential cutting of the epidermis (on the *right*) which could mimic SCC. This particular case shows positive residual infiltrating BCC in the center. Note the presence of a BCC floater on the surface of the epidermis

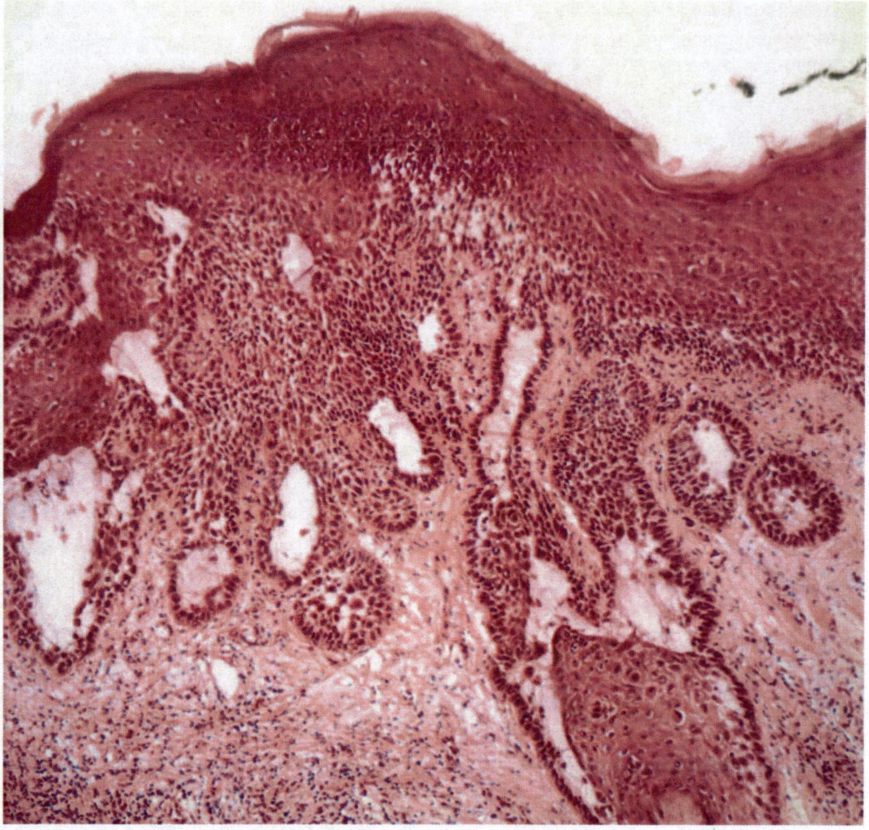

Fig. 13.4 Intermediate-power view of a Mohs slide showing a superficially infiltrating acantholytic SCC

with squamous eddies or clonal seborrheic keratosis poses a challenge in a case of SCC, but not BCC.

Furthermore, acantholysis (that could be mechanical due to a biopsy bandage) or the incidental focal acantholytic dyskeratosis or epidermolytic hyperkeratosis (granular degeneration) may mimic a focus of acantholytic SCC (Fig. 13.4). Inverted follicular keratosis and irritated seborrheic keratosis can mimic SCC. The former usually shows many small, uniform squamous eddies compared to the large, irregular squamous and keratin pearls seen in SCC (Fig. 13.5a, b). Adenoid and reticulated seborrheic keratosis (Fig. 13.6) show thin epithelial strands which interlace with each other, creating an adenoid feature that could be mistaken for adenoid BCC. The presence of horn cysts and the identification of keratinocytic desmosomes under high-power magnification, together with the surrounding mature fibrous stroma differentiate them from BCC (Fig. 13.7). The latter shows immature mucinous stroma around the basaloid tumor formations. Large cell acanthoma shows large keratinocytes with large nuclei and disordered arrangement, but without mitotic activity (Fig. 13.8) or overt dysplasia that differentiates it from Bowen disease (Fig. 13.9). Actinic keratosis is usually easy to identify and differentiate from Bowen disease (Fig. 13.10). However, tangential cutting of the epidermis at the basal epidermal third may create a picture that mimics the full thickness atypia seen in Bowen disease. In this case, the differentiation can be tough, however, the oblique arrangement of cells and rete ridges, if present, would greatly help in such differentiation.

When interpreting Mohs slides for MMS of Paget disease, the Mohs surgeon should be careful in identifying freezing artifacts, and glycogenated clear mucosal cells that could mimic Paget cells or Pagetoid Bowen disease (Fig. 13.11). The latter are larger-showing paler vacuolated cytoplasm and lack intercellular bridges. When in doubt, and if immunohistochemistry laboratory is available, CEA immunostaining should decorate Paget cells, but not keratinocytes.

Finally, pseudoepitheliomatous (pseudocarcinomatous) hyperplasia [8] may create an indistinguishable picture from SCC for some Mohs surgeons. The most important and probably the only criteria for differentiation are the lack of cytologic atypia and lack of atypical/bizarre

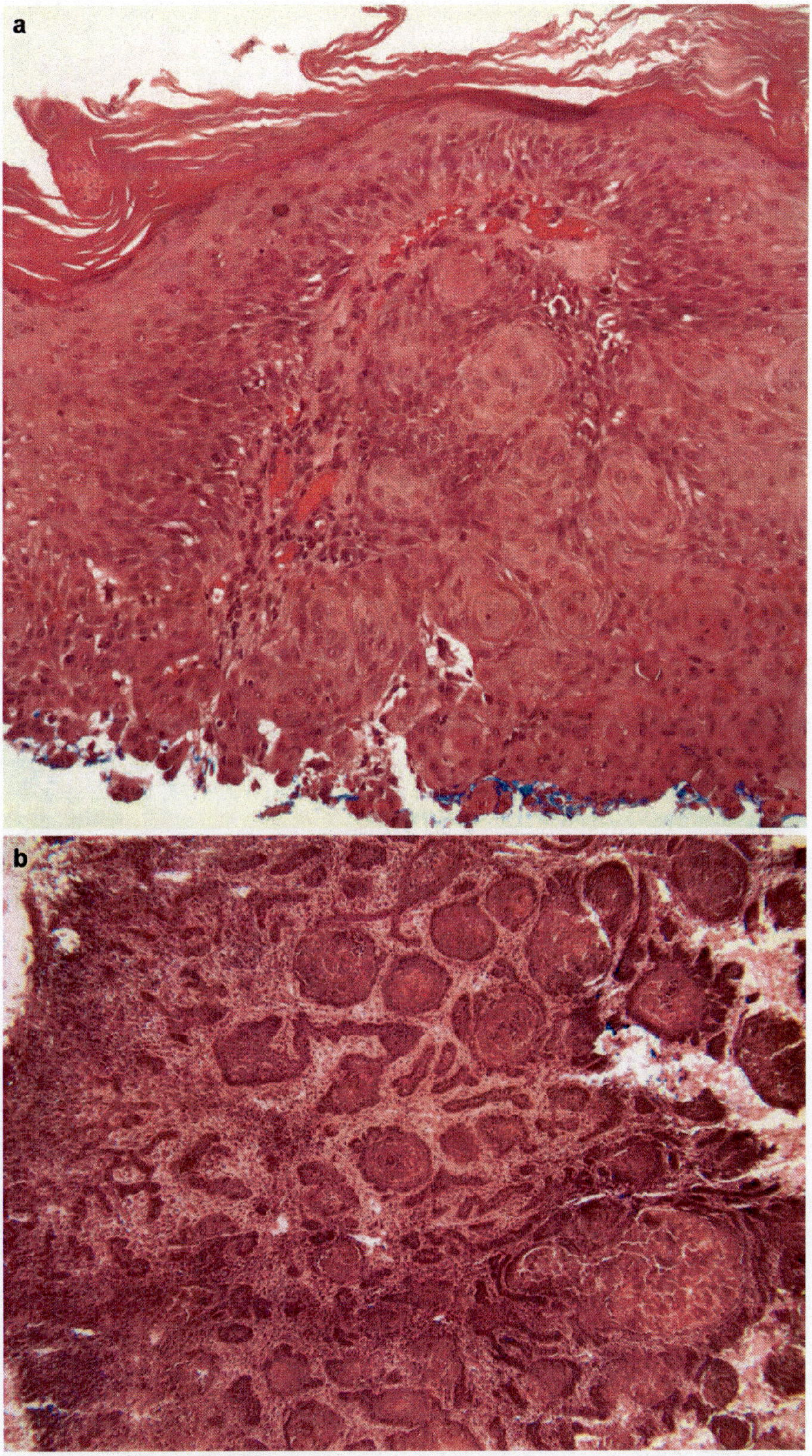

Fig. 13.5 (**a**) High-power view of an irritated seborrheic keratosis showing multiple, monotonous small squamous eddies. Note there is no overt cytologic atypia or atypical mitoses. (**b**) Intermediate-power view of a Mohs section showing prominent residual SCC with multiple, variably sized, larger epithelial pearls

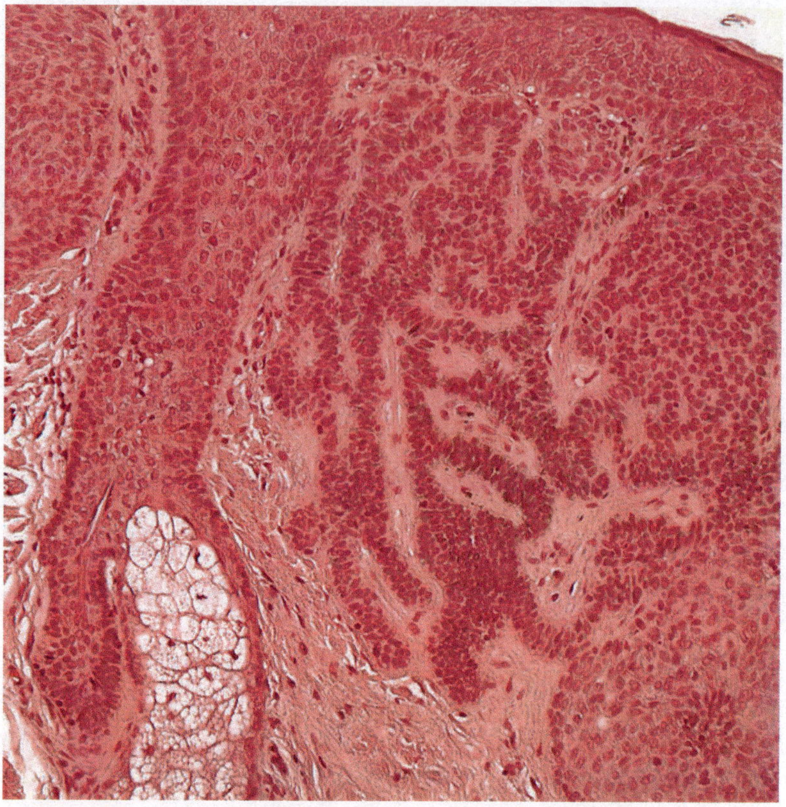

Fig. 13.6 Intermediate-power view of a permanent section showing pigmented, reticulated seborrheic keratosis

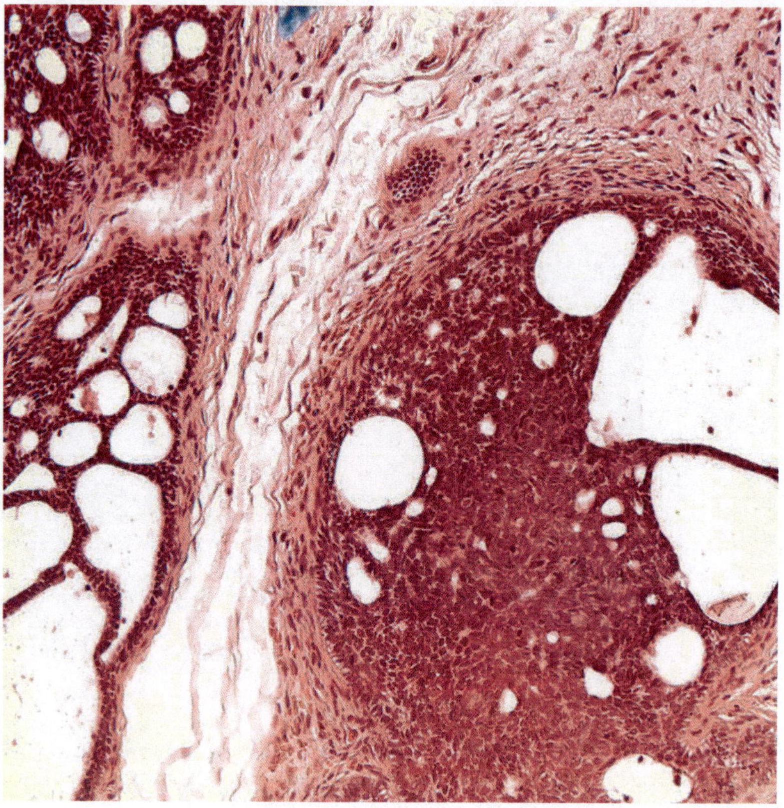

Fig. 13.7 Intermediate-power view of a permanent section showing adenoid BCC. Note the large basaloid tumor formations with peripheral palisading and prominent spaces creating an adenoid (*gland-like*) picture

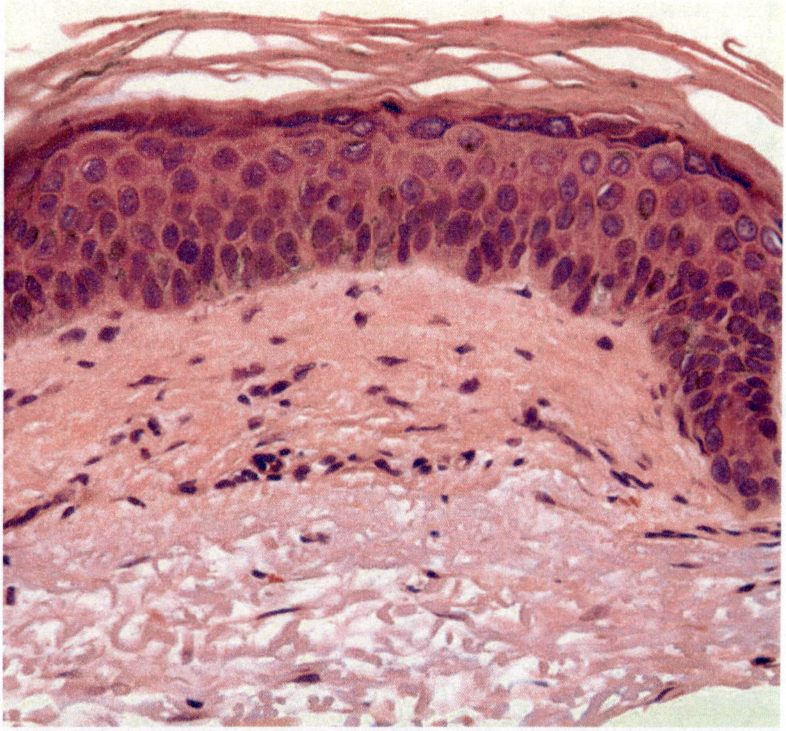

Fig. 13.8 High-power view of a permanent section showing large cell acanthoma with large, somewhat atypical keratinocytes with large nuclei and disordered arrangement. No overt mitotic activity or dysplasia is seen

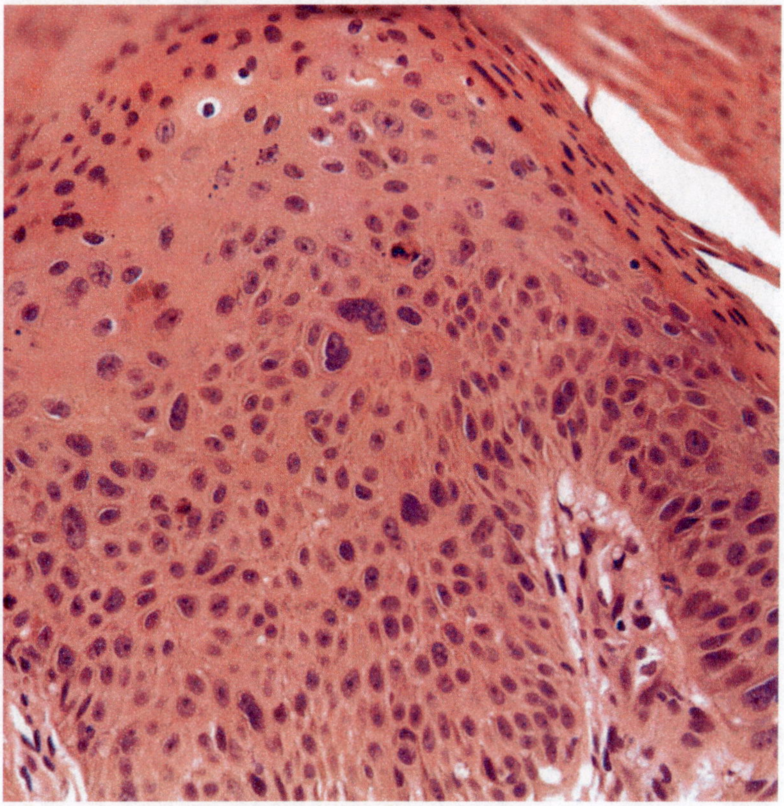

Fig. 13.9 High-power view of a permanent section showing Bowen disease with full thickness keratinoctyic atypia, lack of surface maturation and overlying parakeratosis

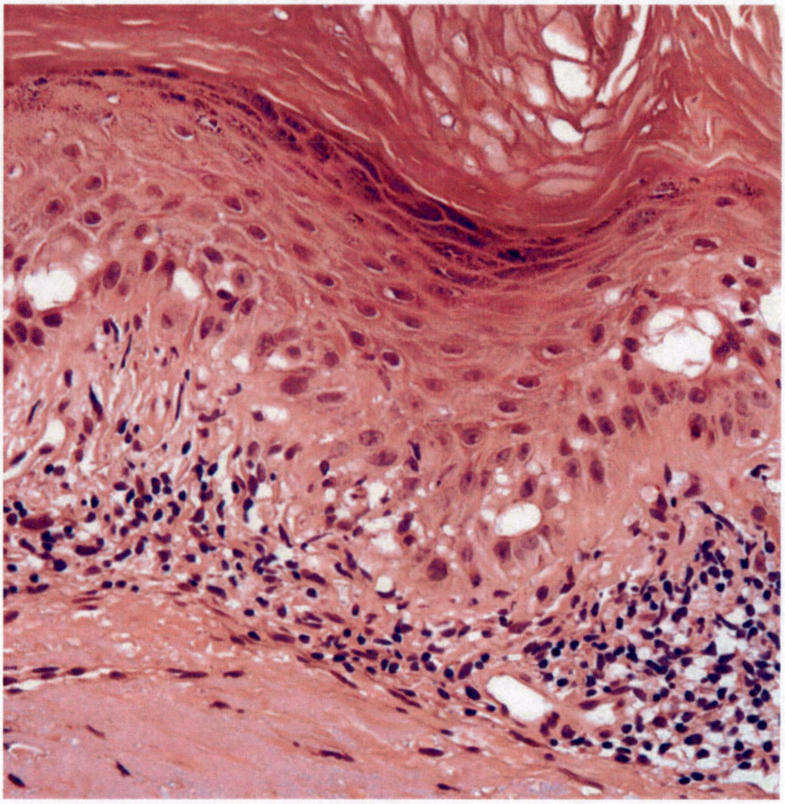

Fig. 13.10 High-power view of a permanent section showing acantholytic actinic keratosis with keratinocytic atypia that is limited only to the lower third of the epidermis. Note the lichenoid lymphocytic infiltrate

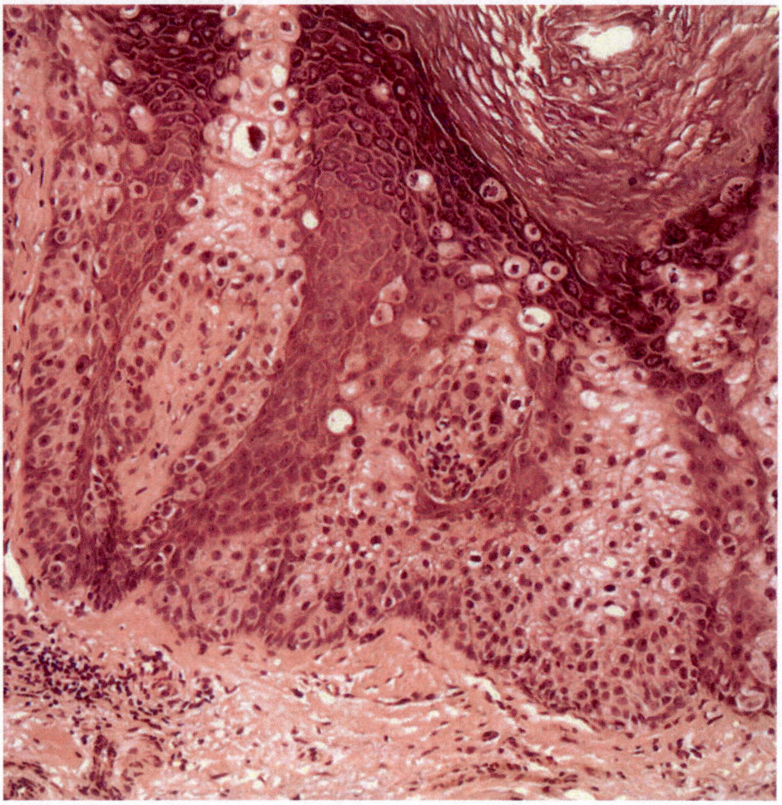

Fig. 13.11 High-power view of a permanent section showing pagetoid Bowen disease with full thickness keratinocytic atypia and lack of surface maturation. Note the vacuolated, large atypical keratinocytes (Pagetoid cells)

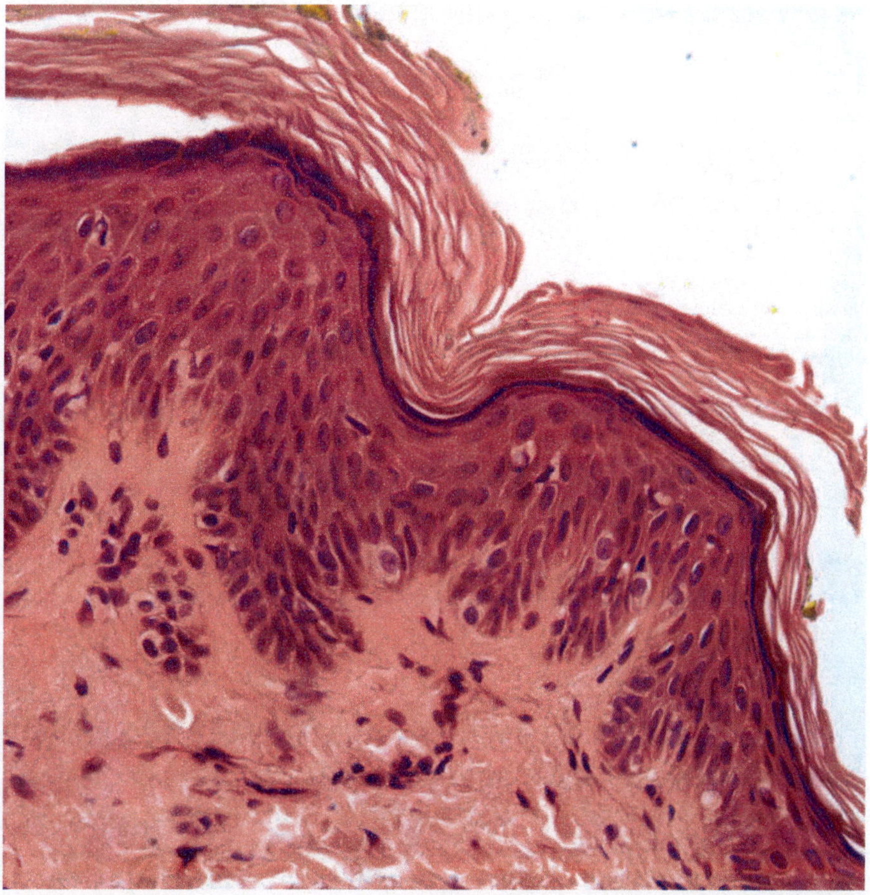

Fig. 13.12 High-power view of a permanent section taken from sun damaged skin showing increased number of large mildly atypical melanocytes. Note the absence of confluence and overt atypia

mitoses seen in SCC. All other criteria of SCC can, unfortunately, be seen in pseudoepitheliomatous hyperpasia including irregular infiltration by variably sized groups of keratinocytes with mitoses and surrounding host's inflammatory reaction. Subepidermal clefting could be due to artifacts or due to dense lichenoid/interface lymphocytic infiltrate or due to falling of a superficial component of BCC. A request for a recut from the Mohs surgeon is warranted in this situation.

13.3.1.2 Melanocytes and the Melanocytic Lesions

Evaluation of melanocytic lesions in frozen sections can be challenging. Mohs sections for melanoma should be thin (2–4 μm) and properly stained. The two main challenging questions are, (1) is this a melanocyte and, if so, (2) is it a malignant melanocyte or not. Normally, melanocytes are seen within the basal cell layer of the epidermis, hair bulbs and outer root sheath of hair follicles [9]. In hematoxylin–eosin-stained sections, the dendrites of epidermal melanocytes are not seen and the cells are usually surrounded by small spaces or a clear halo, due to the lack of attachment by desmosones and shrinkage during processing. When interpreting Mohs slides for melanoma, the Mohs surgeon should be aware of the normal variation of the number of melanocytes within the body regions. The number of melanocytes increases with exposure to ultraviolet light, but the average number of melanocytes to keratinocytes in the basal epidermal cell layer is approximately 1:10 in normal skin [9, 10]. The highest numbers of melanocytes are seen on the face and the male genitals, and the lowest is on the trunk [11]. There is no significant variation in the density of distribution of melanocytes for a given region of the skin between Caucasoid and African American skin. Melanocytes tend to be larger and more dendritic in African American skin than in Caucasoid skin [12]. It is expected to see more melanocytes in sections taken from the face and the dorsal hand, as opposed to the back. In long standing sun-exposed skin, there is a moderate increase in the number of melanocytes to approximately 3–6 adjacent melanocytes without exhibiting overt confluence, Pagetoid spread, or nesting [13] (Fig. 13.12). It is also important to know

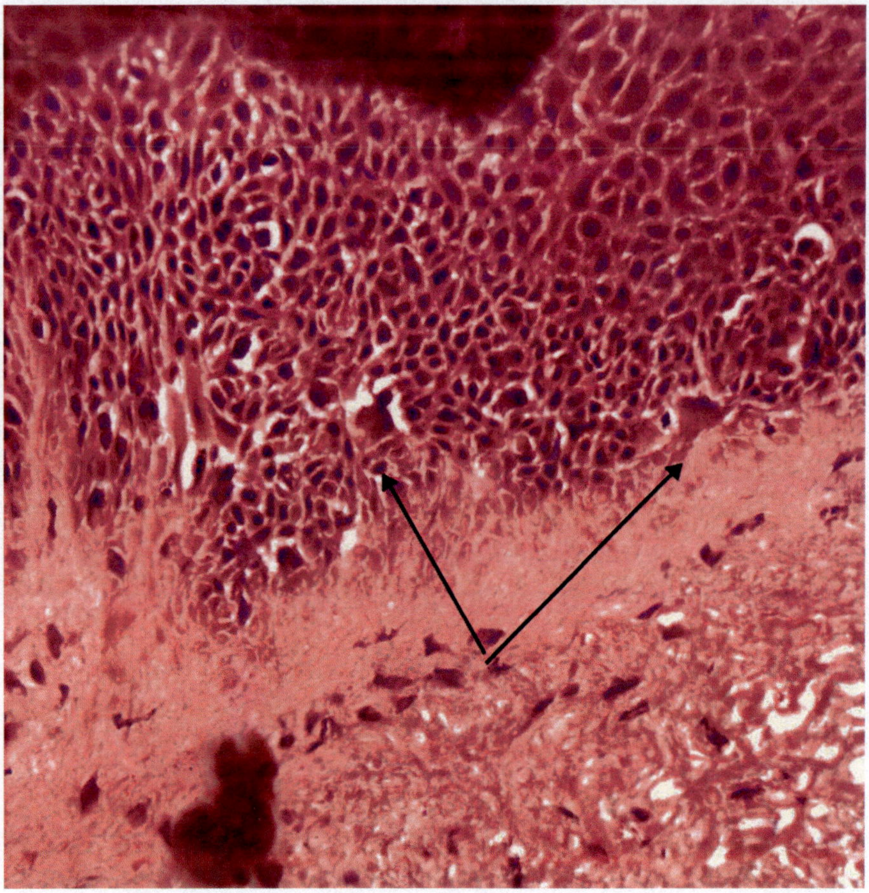

Fig. 13.13 High-power view of a Mohs section showing prominent residual melanoma in situ. Note the confluence of large, atypical melanocytes with large, irregular nuclei. There are larger, atypical melanocytes (in the *middle* and to the *right* of the dermo-epidermal junction) which are referred to as starburst cells (*arrows*)

that the process of melanin transfer from melanocytes to keratinocytes is normal and increases with ultraviolet light exposure. Hence, in sun-damaged skin, melanocytes increase in number and in size. The mere presence of melanin pigmentation in melanoma margins does not indicate a positive margin. The Mohs surgeon should be careful in interpreting sections of melanoma from patients with dark skin color. We found that Mohs sections of acral lentiginous melanoma and melanoma of the genital skin can be challenging. In these circumstances, we found that some Mohs surgeons rely on pigmentation alone to assess the margin if there is no melanocyte. If the next stage does not show any overt melanocytic proliferation and shows only pigmentation, this should be interpreted as a negative margin and sent for permanent section control, provided that an adequate margin was excised depending on the Breslow's thickness of the tumor [14]. Some Mohs surgeons take an extra stage, if pigmentation alone is present, to assure complete excision. Again, this last stage should be sent for permanent section control.

Margins of melanoma pose a challenging point not only to the Mohs surgeon but also to some dermatopathologists. Most dermatopathologists comment on the presence of large, somewhat, atypical melanocytes in the margin. The most important point in differentiating positive from negative melanoma margins is the presence of confluence, Pagetoid spread, or nesting. Sometimes, solitary, large hyperchromatic, and atypical melanocytes can be seen, signifying a positive margin. Unfortunately, there is no immunohistochemical marker that helps in such differentiation. HMB-45 stains both normal and neoplastic epidermal melanocytes. Immunohistochemical staining for Melan-A or Mart-1 is sensitive and specific for melanocytes, but we found that a thin cut and properly stained Mohs section minimizes the need for immunohistochemical staining. The latter should only be used in equivocal cases.

13.3.1.3 Interpretation of Melanoma in Frozen Sections

Generally speaking, the histologic criteria for melanoma in situ include (Fig. 13.13): (1) confluence of

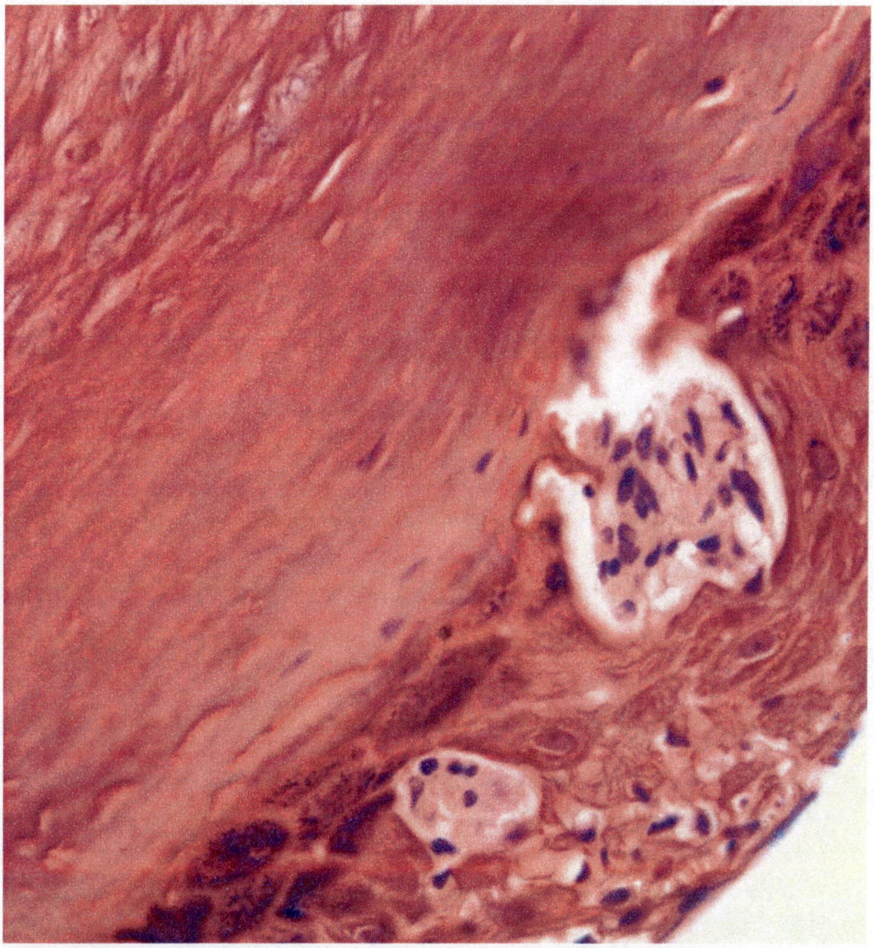

Fig. 13.14 High-power view showing collections of Langerhans cells. This should be differentiated from a melanoma nest by the absence of associated confluence and pagetoid spread of large atypical melanocytes. Note the horn to the left

atypical melanocytes along the dermo-epidermal junction with extension along adnexal structures with or without nesting. (2) Extension of atypical melanocytes at the upper reaches of the epidermis (Pagetoid spread) and (3) presence of large starburst/giant cells. The latter should be differentiated from large Bowen cells in cases of Pagetoid Bowen disease. Immunohistochemical staining is greatly helpful where Melan-A or Mart-1 stains melanoma cells, but not Bowen cells [15].

Invasive melanoma shows infiltration of the dermis by individual cells or atypical, variably sized groups or sheats of melanocytes. These invasive melanocytes can exhibit different cytologic features: epithelioid, nevoid, or even spindle shape. They do not express the normal maturation with descent seen in banal nevi. Melanoma cells show large/open-face nuclei with prominent nucleoli. A variable degree of mitotic activity can be seen. Destruction or effacement of adnexal structures can be seen and sometimes angiovascular invasion can be noted.

MMS for melanoma should only be performed by an experienced Mohs surgeon who is well adept and is very familiar with the histologic changes of different melanocytic lesions. The most common histologic challenges in MMS for melanoma are (1) the melanocytic hyperplasia seen in sun-damaged skin, actinic keratosis, and lentigines. These can mimic melanoma in situ, especially when they are tangentially cut. They should be differentiated from melanoma in situ by the absence of melanocytic atypia and the absence of confluence or nesting of melanocytes. (2) The presence of an associated benign melanocytic nevus. The latter is identified by its benign cytology, maturation with descent, and the symmetry of the lesion. (3) Pagetoid Bowen disease, which can be differentiated from Pagetiod melanoma, as discussed earlier. (4) Collections of Langerhans cells at the upper reaches of the epidermis can be seen as an incidental finding and can mimic melanoma in situ (Fig. 13.14). S-100 is not helpful since it stains both melanocytes and Langerhans cells. CD-la is helpful

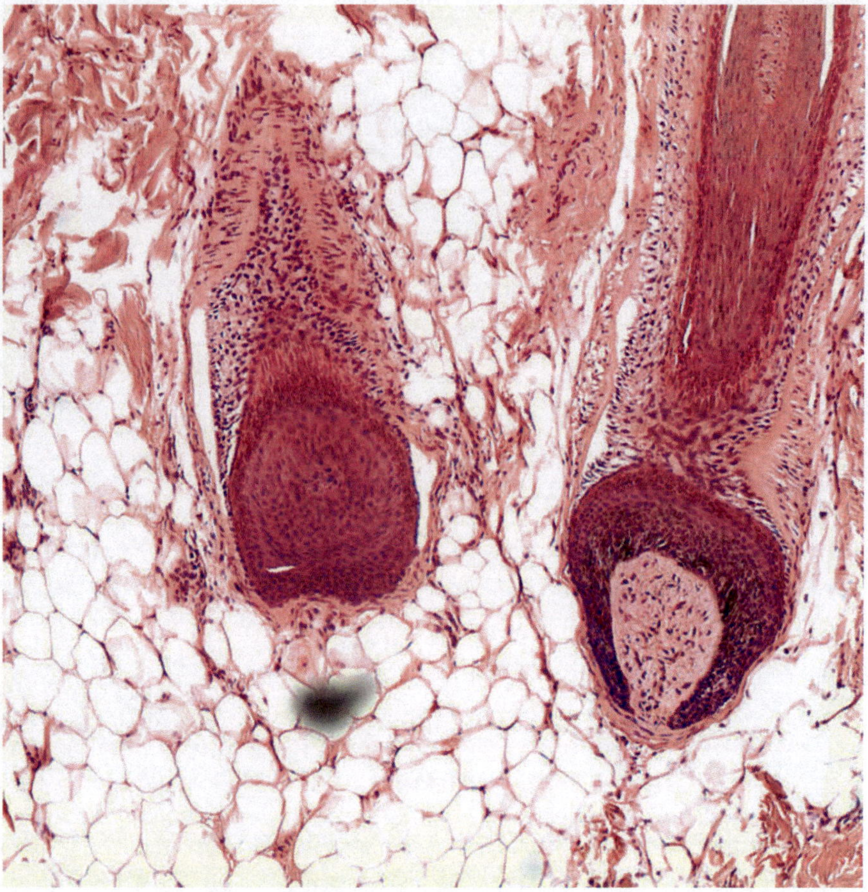

Fig. 13.15 Intermediate-power view of a Mohs section showing two hair follicles. To the left, the follicle shows a section through the bulbar epithelium without dermal papilla. The follicle on the right shows a dermal papilla with surrounding, focally pigmented bulbar epithelium. At the level of the suprabulbar zone, you can identify the presence of inner and outer root sheeths and the decrease and absence of matrix cells

because it decorates Langerhans cells specifically. Immunohistochemical staining for Melan-A and Mart-1 is very helpful in this situation [16]. (5) Dermal reactive fibrohistiocytic infiltrates can mimic invasive melanoma. The latter shows large atypical melanocytes arranged in groups, sheets, or fascicles and show the classic melanocytic cytology. In cases of desmoplastic melanoma, the differentiation can sometimes be difficult and immunohistochemical staining for Melan-A is usually helpful. (6) Tangentially cut reactive endothelial cells can mimic epithelioid melanocyte. Deeper levels would help in identifying the anatomic location of these cells in relation to a vessel, and again Melan-A is a helpful tool in such differentiation, CD31 and Factor VIII–related antigen stain endothelial cells but not melanocytes. (7) A tangentially cut intraepidermal sweat gland duct can sometimes mimic a melanocytic nest. Deeper section showing the duct or a cuticular material can be helpful in such differentiation. Immunohistochemical staining for cytokeratin (positive duct and negative melanoma) can be helpful.

13.3.1.4 The Pilosebaceous Unit

The hair follicle is divided into four zones from bottom to top: the hair bulb, the suprabulbar zone (where different layers of the hair follicle starts to appear), the isthmus (between the insertion of the arrector pili muscle and the entrance of the sebaceous duct), and the infundibulum (uppermost part of the hair follicle and greatly resembles the epidermis histologically). The bulb of terminal hairs lies deep in the dermis at the junction with or within the upper subcutaneous adipose tissue. If one sees a bulbar structure at the upper dermis, it is either a vellus hair or a telgen hair (the resting stage of the hair follicle). A cross section of the latter shows irregular island of basaloid cells with a variable degree of peripheral palisading. This can be easily differentiated from basal cell carcinoma by the irregular outline, the surrounding mature perifollicular fibrous sheath, and sometimes, if the fibrous follicular stella or part of it is seen in the section. The follicular stella is an angiofibrotic streamer extending from the telogen hair follicle down to the subcutaneous fat (to the former position of the bulb) [17].

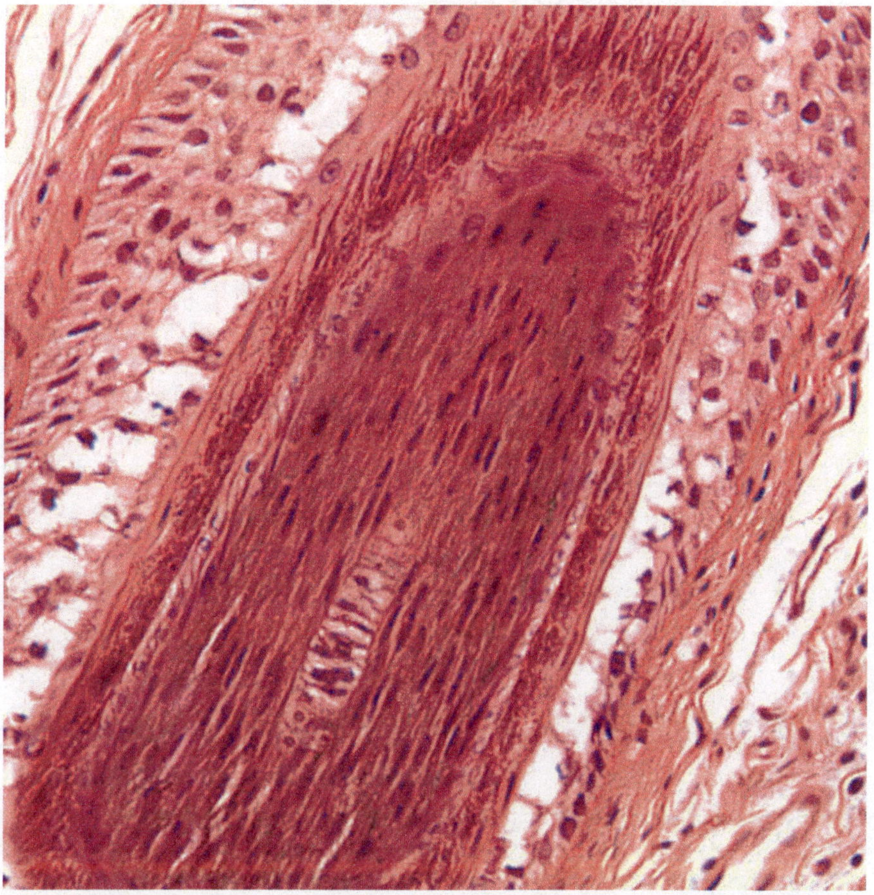

Fig. 13.16 High-power view showing an oblique cut of a hair follicle at the level of the suprabulbar zone and the isthmus. Note the presence of keratohyaline granules, inner and outer root sheeths and the perifollicular fibrous tissue sheeth

Cross sections at the level of the bulb would show a central island of fibrous tissue corresponding to the dermal papilla, which makes it very easy to identify. If the dermal papilla is not seen due to tangential sectioning, one can identify it by the presence of the hair matrix cells, and of course the surrounding perifollicular fibrous sheath. At the level of the suprabulbar zone, one can identify the presence of inner and outer root sheaths and decreased or absent matrix cells and the surrounding perifollicular fibrous tissue sheath (Fig. 13.15). At the isthmus level, one can see the hair shaft surrounded by the trichilemmal, abruptly keratinized cuticle and the inner root sheath, the outer root sheath, and the perifollicular fibrous tissue sheath (Fig. 13.16). At the infundibulum level, the epidermal keratinization with granular layer can be seen. Finally, follicular germs and papillae seen in embryonic development and the very early anagen stage can be recapitualized by BCC and some other follicular adnexal neoplasms such as trichoblastomas.

13.3.1.5 The Bulge

The bulge is the follicular protrusion at the attachment of the arrector pili muscle (Fig. 13.17). Horizontal sectioning of the bulge shows rounded or oval basaloid structure with a blend of suprabulbar and isthmic cellular features with surrounding perifollicular fibrous tissue sheath (Fig. 13.18). Again, the latter differentiates the bulge from BCC, which is usually surrounded by immature mucinous stroma. The latter is not usually seen in infiltrating and morpheaform BCC, which are identified by the unique strands/ribbons of basaloid cells with characteristic stroma, rather than groups of basaloid cells with peripheral palisading (Fig. 13.19a, b).

The "bleb" of the isthmus [18] is probably a misshapen cystic bulge lined by isthmic epithelium with corneocytes arrayed in concentric, lamellar fashion. They are surrounded by a prominent basement membrane. Bulges and blebs can be encountered in frozen sections and should be differentiated from BCC.

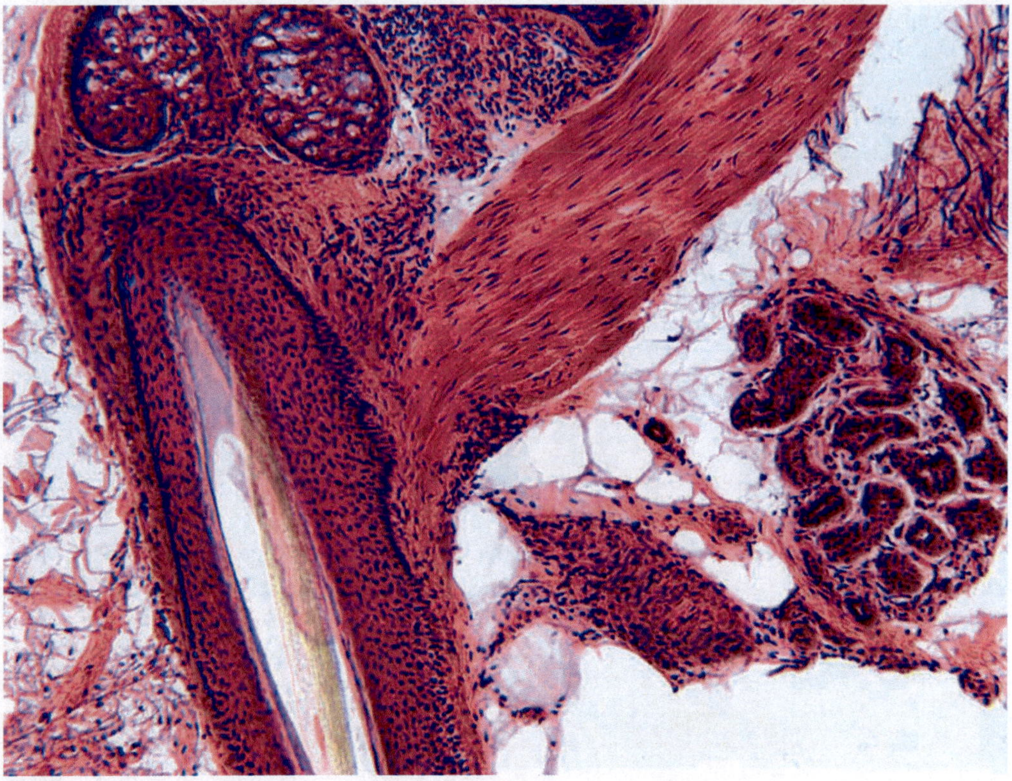

Fig. 13.17 Intermediate-power view of a Mohs section showing the bulge area at the level of the insertion of the arrector pili muscle

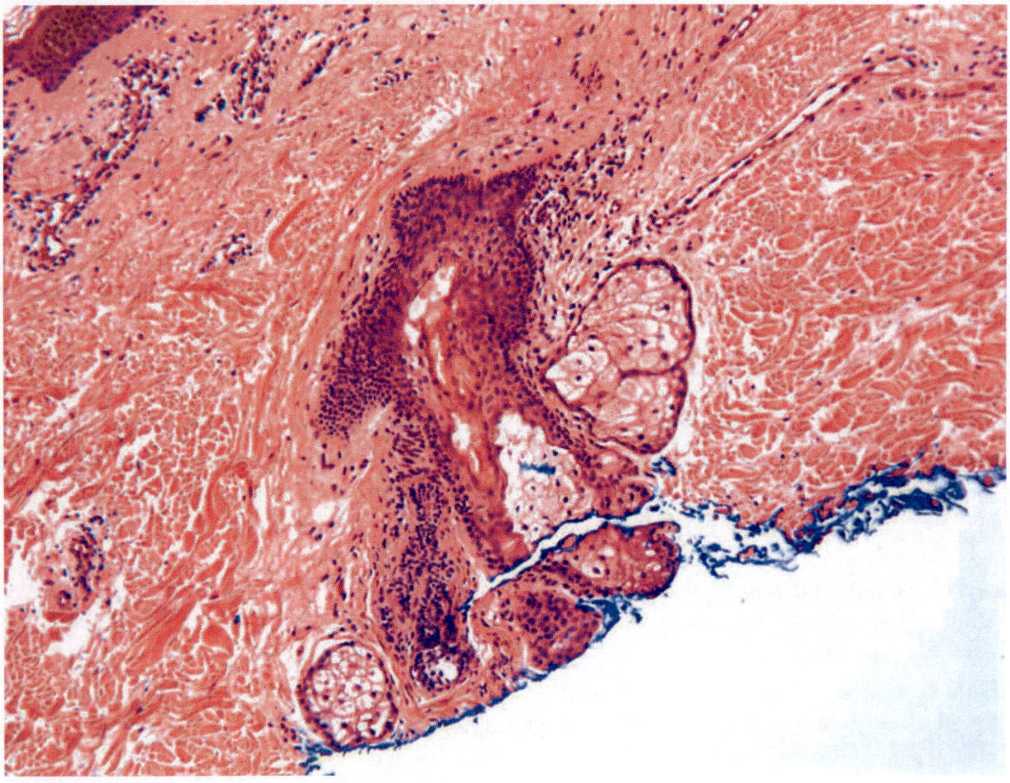

Fig. 13.18 Intermediate-power view of a permanent section showing the bulge area with somewhat immature basaloid cell aggregates

13.3.1.6 The Mantle and Sebaceous Glands

Mantles are symmetrically distributed cords of basaloid cells extending from the upper portion of the hair follicles, (lower infundibulum) and they represent the origin of, or "the resting stage" of mature sebaceous gland lobules (Fig. 13.20). They should be differentiated from BCC by the variable degree of early sebaceous differentiation and their characteristic "skirt-like" appearance with elongated ribbons of basaloid cells (Fig. 13.21).

Sebaceous gland lobules pour their holocrine secretions in the infundibulum via the sebaceous ducts. The sebaceous duct is a crenulated channel connecting the sebaceous gland lobules with the infundibulum and consequently is lined by thin, stratified keratinocytic epithelium. Its lumen contains fine particles representing the holocrine sebaceous secretions. Horizontal sectioning of sebaceous ducts should be differentiated from epithelial pearls of SCC by lacking: cytologic atypia and atypical mitoses and by the presence of a granular layer and crenulated lining. Sebaceous gland lobules are surrounded by a layer or two of immature basaloid germinative cells. When the latter is cut tangentially, they may produce a group of basaloid cells that mimic BCC. The presence of foam cells can help resolve that mimicry. BCC with sebaceous differentiation is a debatable entity, however, in the author's experience, it does exist [19, 20]. Looking at the original biopsy is priceless in this situation, so that the Mohs surgeon would be familiar with the histologic and cytologic nature of the original neoplasm. There is an increasing number of MMS performed on sebaceous carcinoma (SC). The presence of doubtful basaloid cells with mantle-like

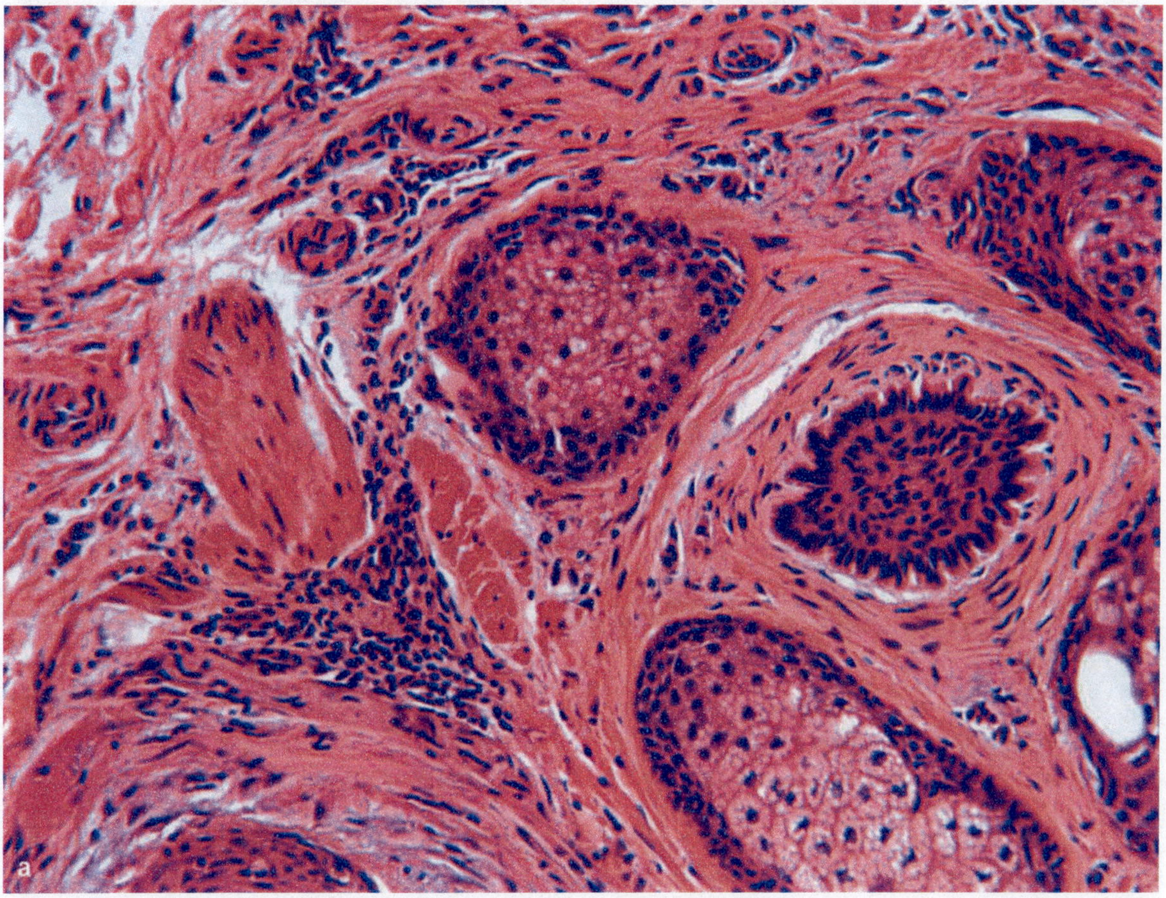

Fig. 13.19 (**a**) Intermediate-power view of a permanent section showing a hair follicle at the isthmic level above the bulge with some telogen features showing crenulated, irregular border with surrounding prominent perifollicular fibrous tissue sheeth. Note the arrector pili muscle at the left. (**b**) Intermediate power view of a Mohs section showing residual BCC. Note the basaloid tumor formation is surrounded by immature mucinous stroma

Fig. 13.19 (continued)

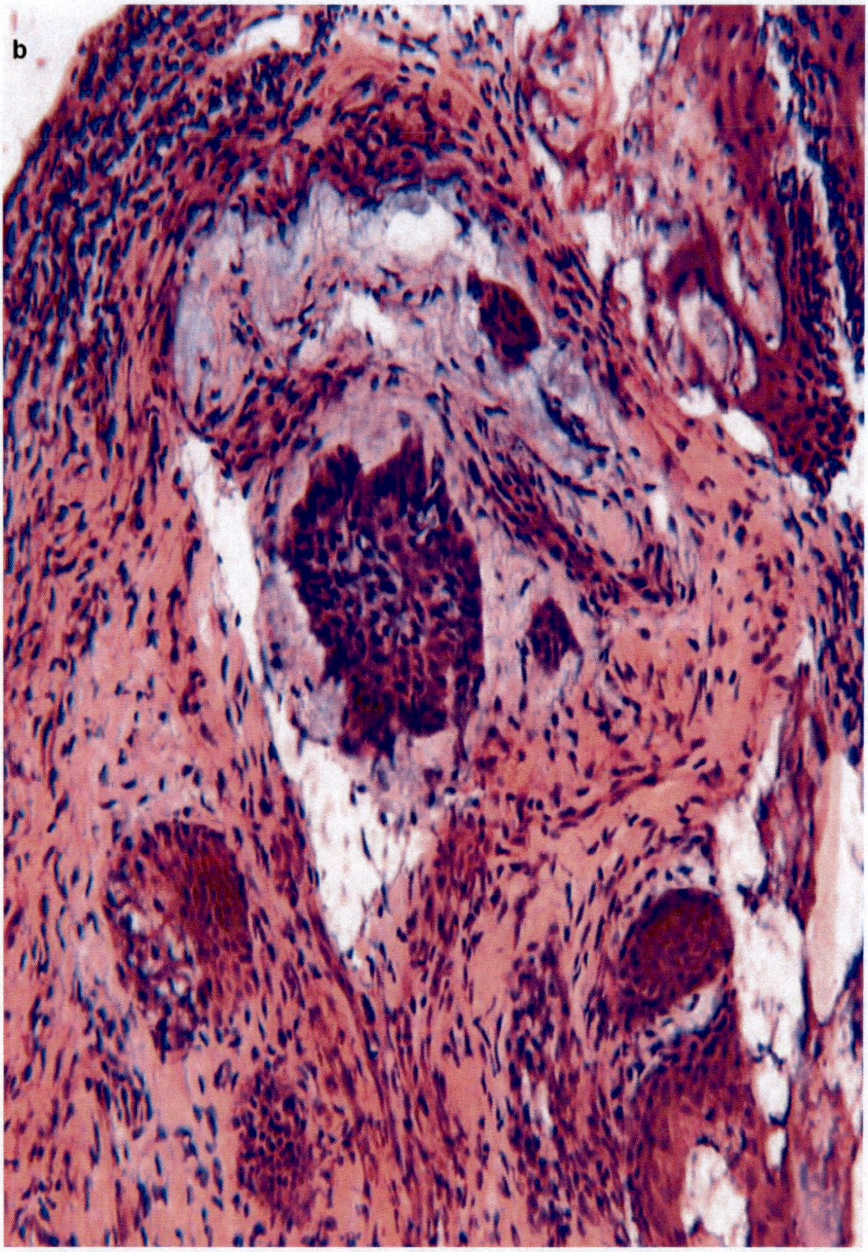

changes can pose a problem in interpreting Mohs slides for sebaceous carcinoma. In this case, the Mohs surgeon should consider these groups as a positive part of sebaceous carcinoma and perform an extra stage. These authors classified SC into: (1) SC in situ, (2) SC, infiltrating, low-grade with or without Pagetoid spread, (3) SC, infiltrating, high-grade, with or without Pagetoid spread, and (4) SC with extra ocular and extra cutaneous involvement, including metastases. The dermatopathology report should mention the grade and the presence or absence of Pagetoid spread [20]. The lipid stain oil red O is not routinely used in the Mohs laboratory. It can be very helpful though, especially in cases of sebaceous carcinoma of the eyelid. Goblet cells, normally present at the eyelid, are oil red O-negative [21].

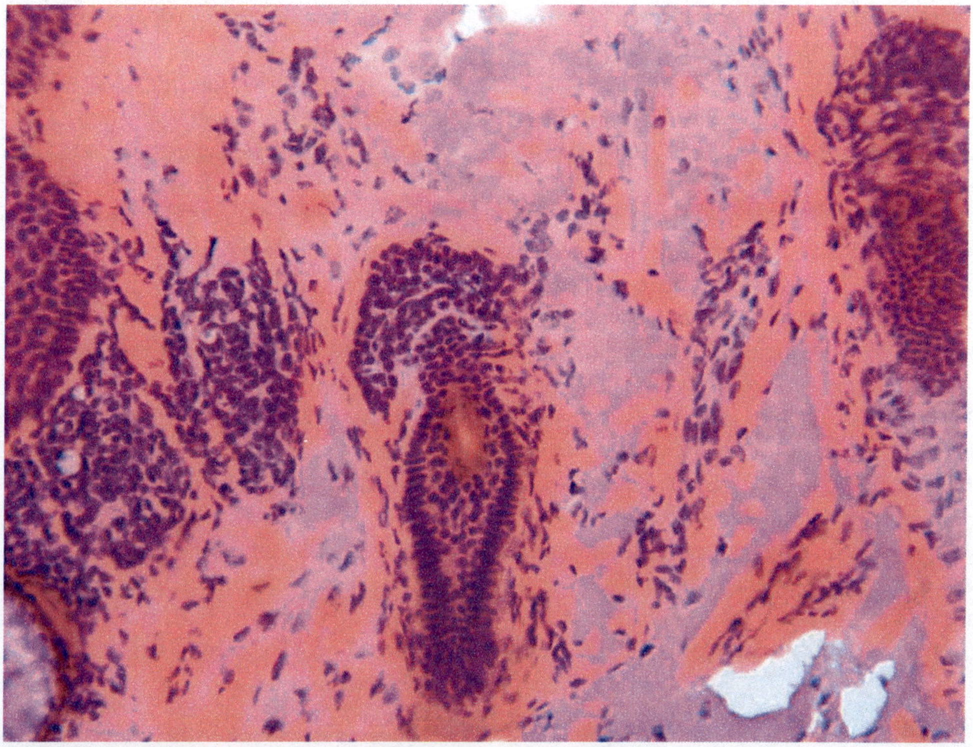

Fig. 13.20 Intermediate-power view of a Mohs section showing a mantle that is composed of two layers of immature basaloid cells creating a "skirt-like" appearance

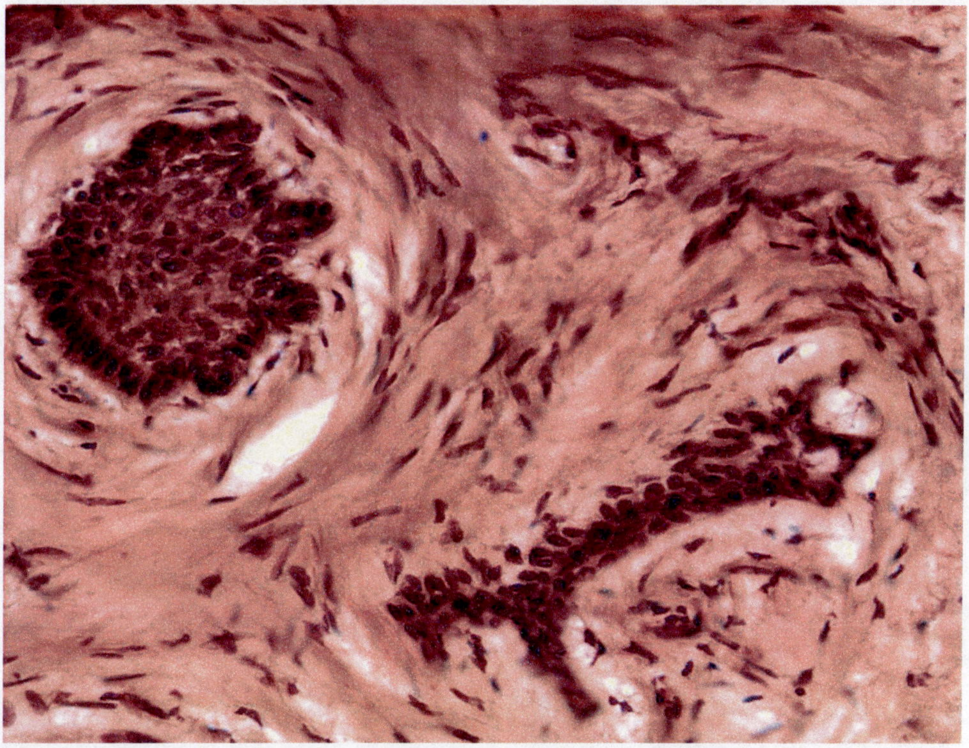

Fig. 13.21 High-power view of a Mohs slide showing a mantle to the right and a follicle to the left. Note that the mantle is composed of a ribbon of 2–3 layers of immature basaloid cells. Focal, early sebaceous differentiation can be appreciated

13.3.1.7 The Folliculocentric Basaloid Proliferations (FBP)

FBP or "funny looking follicles" are irregular strands of basaloid cells emanating from the upper portion of the hair follicles (Fig. 13.22a, b). They are most likely a reactive phenomenon to irritation and can be seen in normal skin, margins of BCC, or in a myriad of neoplastic and non-neoplastic skin conditions [22]. Moreover, they are most commonly associated with tumors of skin with abundant hair follicles, such as nasal and perinasal skin. They were originally thought to be hyperplasia of the bulge epithelium, but are believed now to be hyperplasia of the mantle epithelium [18]. FBPs can sometimes be difficult to distinguish from BCCs. Factors that help differentiate FBPs from BCCs are: (1) vertical orientation in relation to a hair follicle, (2) radial pin wheel or lattice-like orientation along an axis, (3) superficial location with or without epidermal attachment, (4) presence of basement membrane material around them, and (5) absent retraction artifacts, stromal mucinous material, cytologic, and nuclear atypia, or atypical mitoses.

Moreover, some BCCs show overt follicle-like structures. These types are BCC with follicular differentiation, infundibulocystic BCC, and BCC with matrical differentiation. In this situation, and when in doubt, whether a particular basaloid cell formation is actually a part of BCC with follicular differentiation or a benign follicular structure, the Mohs surgeon should take an extra stage to be confident that all of the tumor is removed. Factors that help identify benign follicular differentiation include: (1) follicular papillae and papillary mesenchymal bodies, (2) follicular bulbs, (3) presence of outer root sheath cells (pale cells), (4) trichohyaline granules, (5) shadow cells, and (6) hair shafts. Finally, follicular induction or basaloid cellular hyperplasia can be seen overlying some skin lesions, such as dermatofibroma or nevus sebaceus. This usually represents a reactive process and is not a true BCC. Some rare cases of true neoplasms, however, were reported in this setting [23]. The original clinical diagnosis should be very helpful when evaluating frozen sections in these cases.

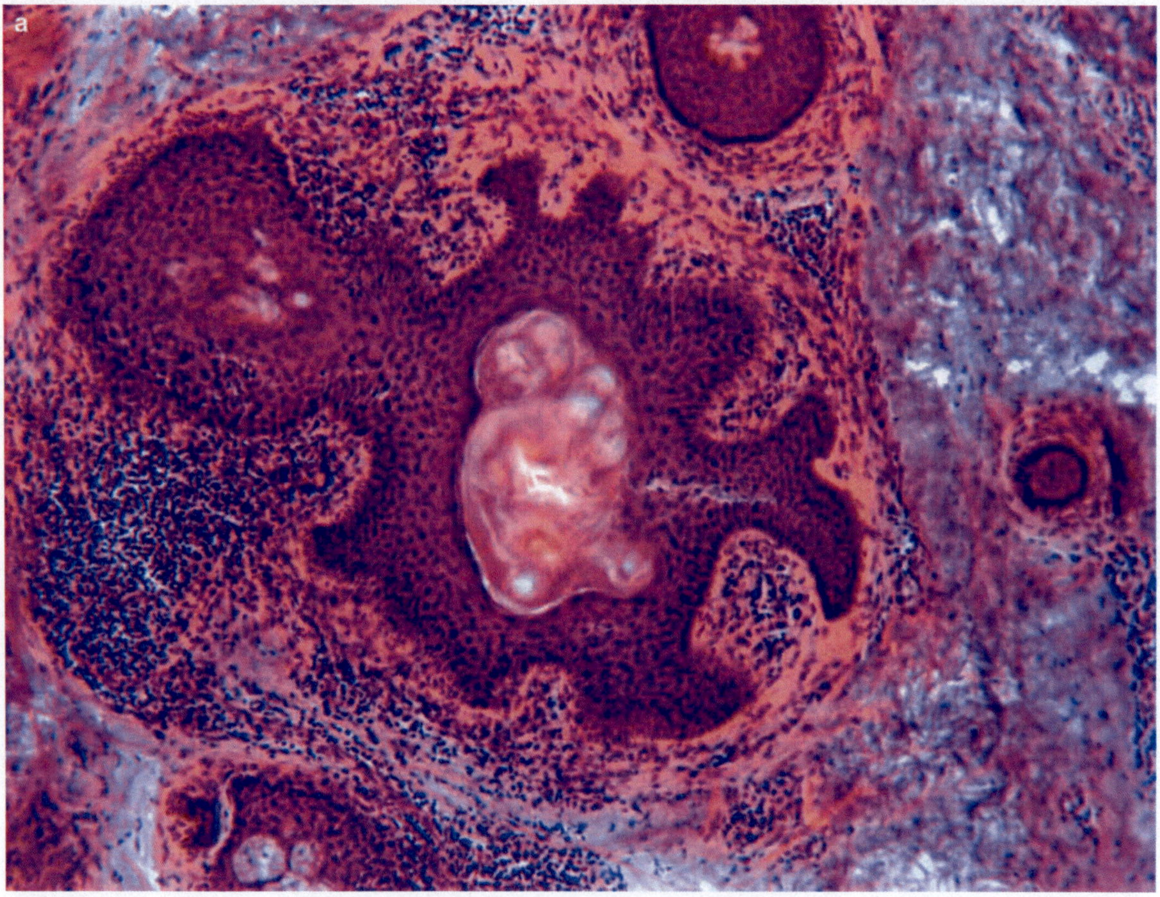

Fig. 13.22 (**a**) Intermediate-power view of a Mohs section showing FBP with irregular strands of basaloid cells emanating from a hair follicle. (**b**) Low power view of a Mohs section showing a FBP with characteristic pin wheel appearance

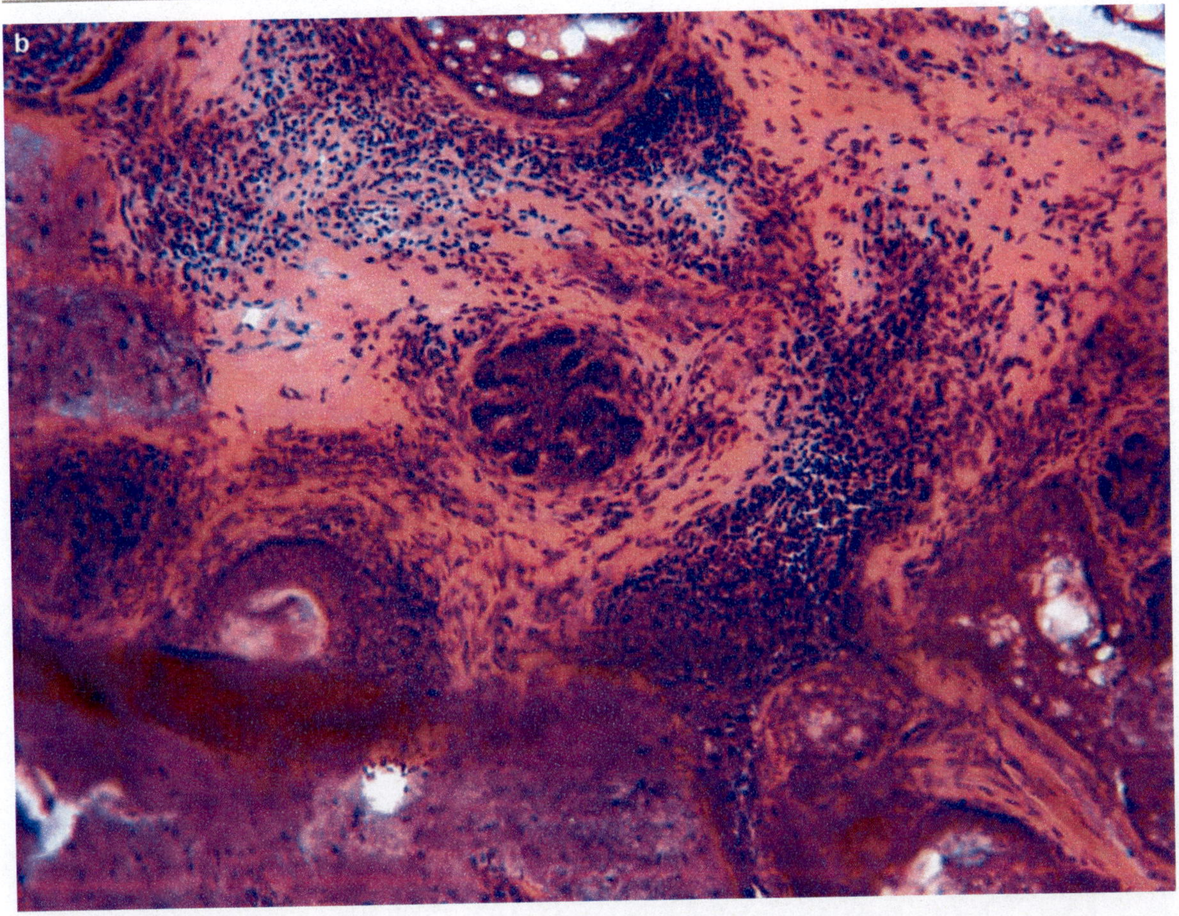

Fig. 13.22 (continued)

13.3.2 Histopathologic Recognition of Dermal Components

The Mohs surgeon should be able to easily recognize different dermal structures. In this section, we will briefly discuss the histologic criteria for some pathologic changes associated with some dermal structures.

13.3.2.1 Fibrous Tissue, Desmoplasia, and Nerves

The dermal fibrous tissue is composed of wavy collagen bundles and spindled fibroblasts. Desmoplasia is a dense reactive fibrous tissue surrounding tumors. It is claimed that some tumors release fibroblast growth factor and are associated with this surrounding florid desmoplasia. We described this specific pattern of fibrosis noted in BCC and SCC which we called peritumoral fibrosis [24]. It shows concentric layers of fibrous tissue surrounding and/or surrounded by tumor formations and resembles carcinomatous perineural and/or intraneural invasion (Fig. 13.23). Mohs micrographic surgeons should be aware of this phenomenon to avoid triggering unnecessary steps in managing these cases, such as irradiation. Dense perineural inflammation has been associated with a higher incidence of perineural invasion [25]. Immunohistochemical staining for S-100 protein decorates nerve fibrils, but not fibrous tissue bundles (Fig. 13.24a, b). One should be careful interpreting S-100 stained sections for the presence of positive dermal dendrocytes in peritumoral fibrosis. This is easily differentiated from the uniformly positive nerve fibrils.

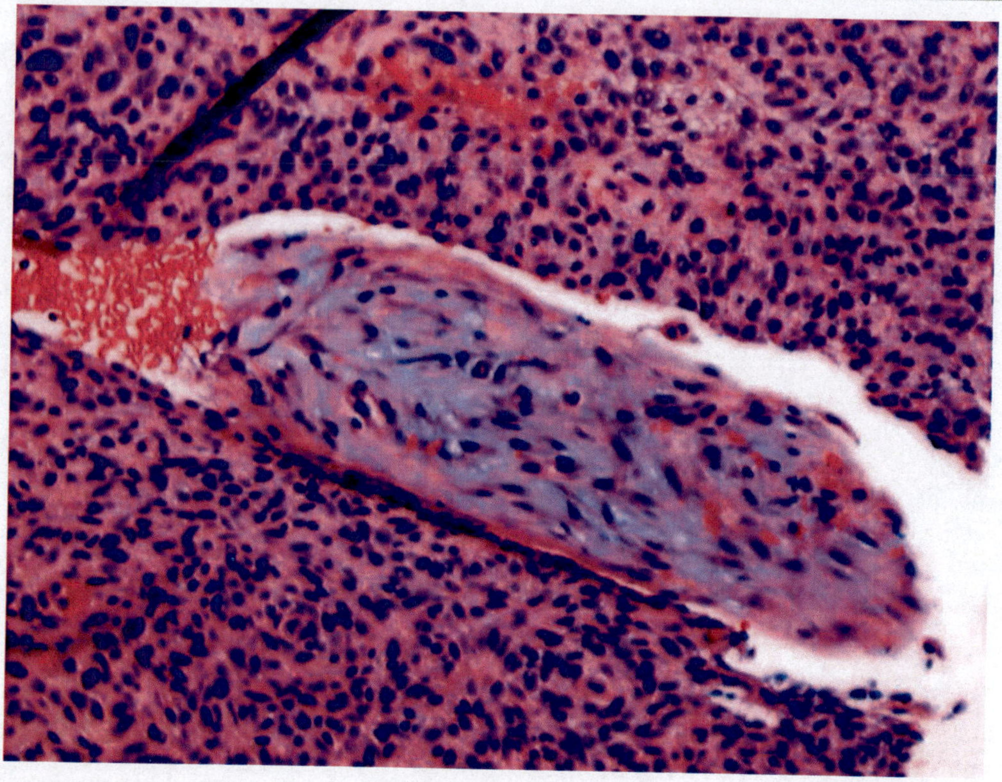

Fig. 13.23 High-power view of a Mohs section of a SCC showing a dense strand of desmoplastic fibrous tissue mimicking a nerve fibril. This phenomenon is described as peritumoral fibrosis

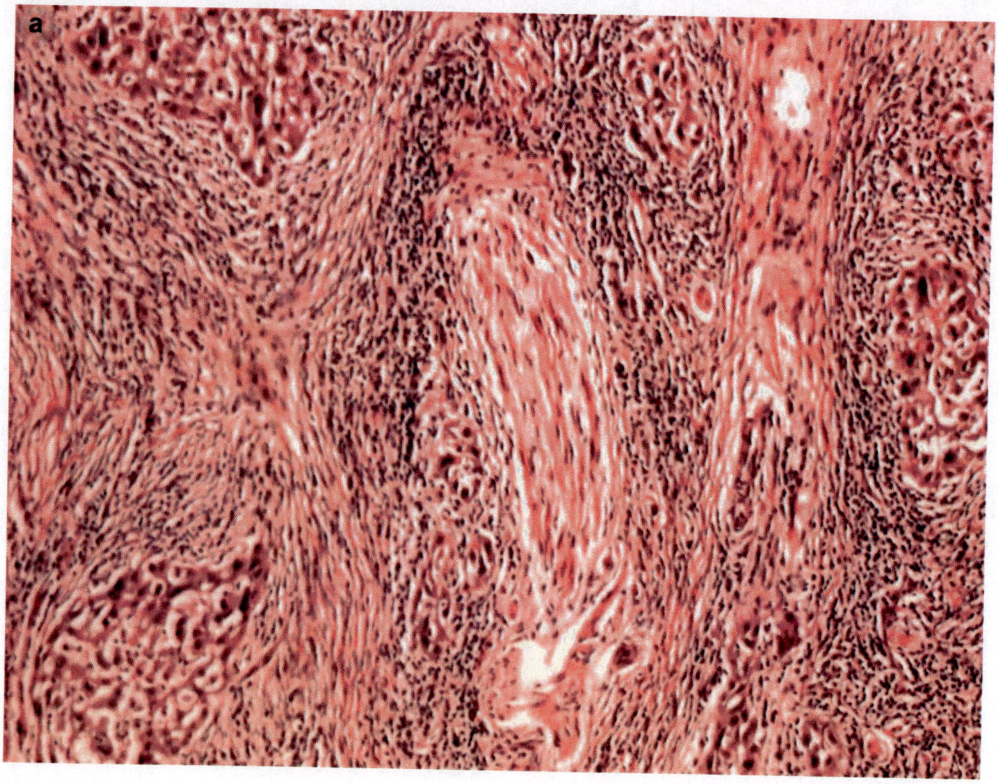

Fig. 13.24 (**a**) Intermediate-power view of a Mohs section showing prominent perineural inflammation and invasion by SCC. (**b**) Immunohistochemical staining with S-100 protein decorating the nerve fibril ([24] Copyright Wiley & Sons. Used by permission)

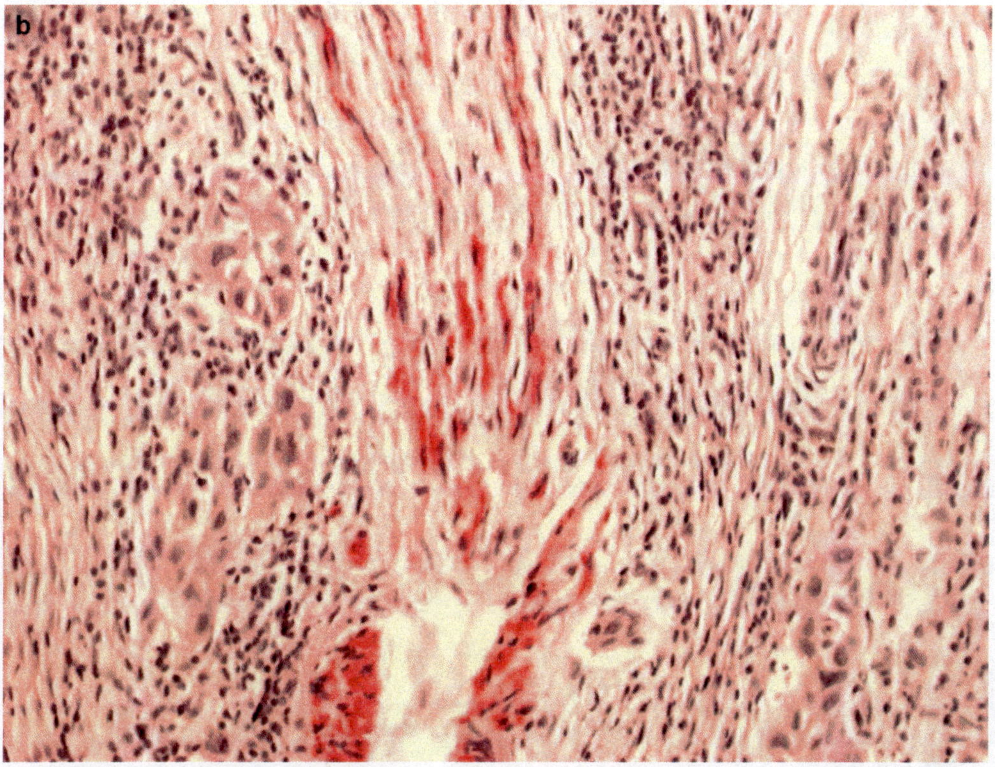

Fig. 13.24 (continued)

13.3.2.2 The Dermal Microvascular Unit

The Mohs surgeon should be familiar with the histologic changes seen within the dermal vessels. Different inflammatory diseases of the skin are usually associated with reactive endothelial cellular changes. When these vessels are cut tangentially, they could produce cytologic changes that may closely mimic carcinoma cells mainly SCC or sometimes epithelioid melanoma cells. A common example of this is the reactive endothelial cells associated with the dense lymphohistiocytic infiltrate seen in some cases of rosacea. Deeper sections would help identify the relationship of these cells to a blood vessel. One should note also that dermal blood vessels usually run in parallel with/or associated with nerve fibrils, the so-called neurovascular bundles. Tissue compression may create abnormal pictures depicting vessels and nerves in different positions which could mimic perineural invasion (Fig. 13.25). Dense dermal lymphocytic infiltrate can be seen in cutaneous deposits of leukemia, Jessner's lymphocytic infiltrate, and prior treatment with 5-FU or Imiquimod 5% [26].

13.3.2.3 Dermal Muscles, Cartilage, and Subcutaneous Adipose Tissue

In addition to arrector pili muscle, cutaneous smooth muscles can be seen with cross-section/tangential cutting of blood vessels. Mohs surgeons should be able to identify these normal smooth muscles and differentiate them from malignant spindle cells seen in cutaneous leiomyosarcoma. Cytologic features of malignancy in the form of cytomegally, hyperchromasia, pleomorphism, and atypical mitoses would help differentiate benign from malignant smooth muscles. Skeletal muscles can be encountered in most sections of the lips, neck (platysma), face, and deeply infiltrating cancers such as DFSP.

Cartilage is frequently seen in Mohs sections of the nose and ears. It is usually easy to interpret Mohs sections with cartilage. The latter is normally basophilic with routine H&E staining showing small, rounded, or oval chondrocytes with surrounding halos and homogeneous, structureless stroma. Cartilage tends to wash off the slides, so special slides should be used routinely for better results. These slides electrostatically attract frozen and formalin-fixed tissue sections and bind them, while improving tissue adherence. Superfrost®

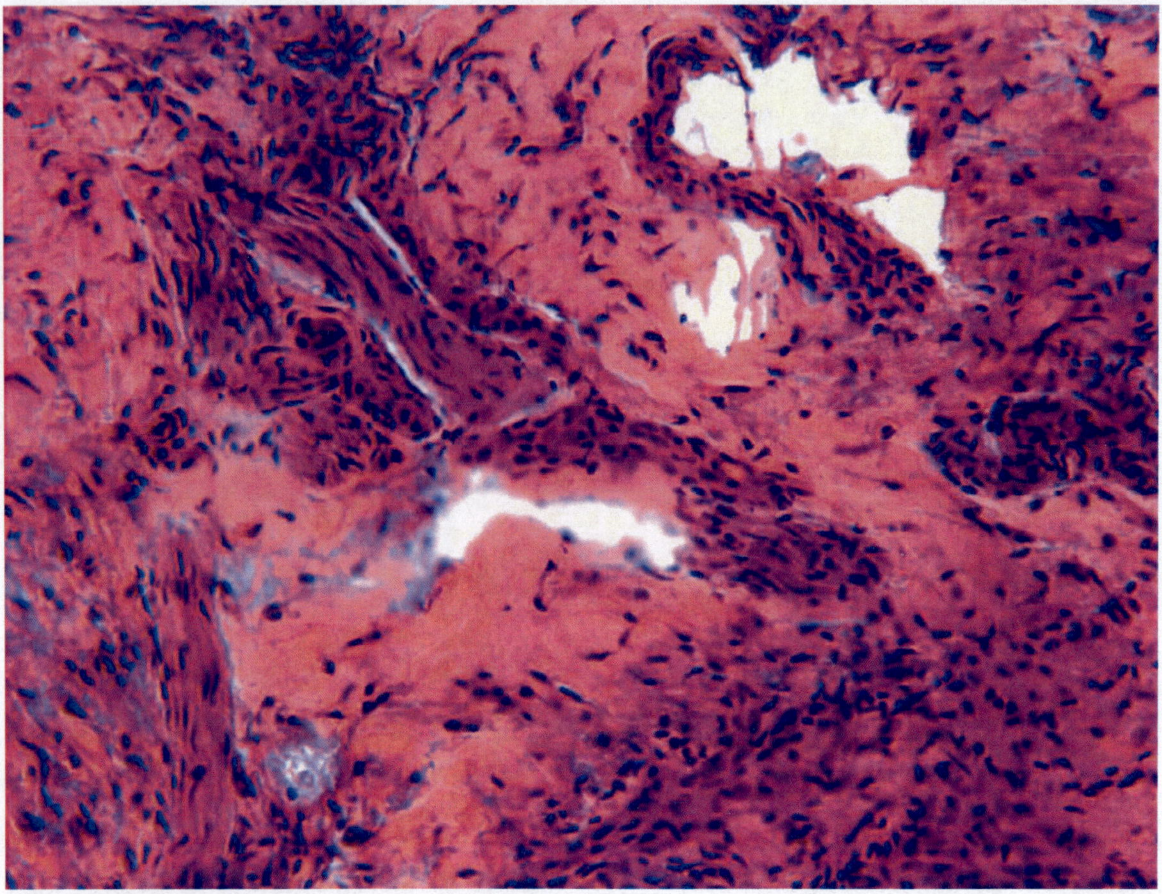

Fig. 13.25 Intermediate-power view of a Mohs section showing a compressed neurovascular bundle. Note the nerve fibril is surrounded by vascular endothelial cells mimicking perineural invasion

Plus Slides are made by a process that places a permanent positive charge on the slide. Tissue sections adhere better to Plus glass slides without the need for labor intensive special adhesives or protein coatings. Plus slides virtually eliminate background staining in standard H&E stains.

Subcutaneous adipose tissue is difficult to cut. Infiltration by tumors makes it easier to cut the sections due to the surrounding tumor stroma. Mohs technicians usually freeze the tissue to a colder degree and cut thicker sections in order to obtain a good Mohs slide with adipose tissue.

Summary: Conclusion

- The success of MMS depends on the correct interpretation of Mohs slides.
- Tumor recurrence may result from missing a focus of tumor or evaluating a suboptimal slide with missing pieces of tissue. However, over reading can result in unnecessary extra stages that will produce a larger Mohs defect.
- Technical errors are the most common cause of local recurrence after MMS.

13.4 Conclusion

The high rate of cure associated with MMS is contingent upon different surgical and laboratory steps. Thorough and correct interpretation of Mohs slides is probably the most important step in the Mohs technique. Missing a focus of tumor or evaluating a suboptimal slide with missing pieces of tissue may result in tumor recurrence. Over reading due to lack of experience identifying different cutaneous structures such as a bulge or a mantle will result in unnecessary extra stages which will produce a larger Mohs defect. Proper training of Mohs fellows, dermatology residents, and young dermatologists in dermatopathology and particularly in skin frozen section interpretation is very important for the practice of MMS. Finally, it is important to note that technical errors represent the most common cause of local recurrence after MMS.

References

1. Mariwalla K, Aasi SZ, Glusac EJ, Leffell DJ. Mohs micrographic surgery histopathology concordance. J Am Acad Dermatol. 2009;60(1):94–8.
2. Hruza GJ. Mohs micrographic surgery local recurrences. J Dermatol Surg Oncol. 1994;20:573–7.
3. Yu Y, Finn DT. Crescent versus rectangle: is it a true negative margin in second and subsequent stages of Mohs surgery? Dermatol Surg. 2010;36(2):171–6.
4. Whalen J, Leone D. Mohs micrographic surgery for the treatment of malignant melanoma. Clin Dermatol. 2009;27(6): 597–602.
5. Mehrany K, Byrd DR, Roenigk RK, et al. Lymphocytic infiltrates and subclinical epithelial tumor extension in patients with chronic leukemia and solid-organ transplantation. Dermatol Surg. 2003;29:129–34.
6. Katz KH, Helm KF, Billingsley EM, et al. Dense inflammation does not mask residual primary basal cell carcinoma during Mohs micrographic surgery. J Am Acad Dermatol. 2001;45:231–8.
7. Albregts T, Orengo I, Salasche S, et al. Squamous cell carcinoma in a patient with chronic lymphocytic leukemia. An intraoperative diagnostic challenge for the Mohs surgeon. Dermatol Surg. 1998;64:269–72.
8. Tuttle MS, Rosenberg AS, Winfield HL, Somach SC. Pseudocarcinomatous hyperplasia with follicular differentiation overlying basal cell carcinoma. Am J Dermatopathol. 2009;31(6):557–60.
9. Cochran AJ. The incidence of melanocytes in normal skin. J Invest Dermatol. 1970;55:65–70.
10. Dean NR, Brennan J, Haynes J, et al. Immunohistochemical labeling of normal melanocytes. Appl Immunohistochem Mol Morphol. 2002;10:199–204.
11. Gilchrest BA, Blog FB, Szabo G. Effects of aging and chronic sun exposure on melanocytes in human skin. J Invest Dermatol. 1979;73:141–3.
12. Toda K, Kathak MA, Parrish JA, et al. Alteration of racial differences in melanosome distribution in human epidermis after exposure to ultraviolet light. Nature. 1972;236:143–5.
13. Hendi A, Brodland DG, Zitelli JA. Melanocytes in long-standing sun-exposed skin: quantitative analysis using the MART-1 immunostain. Arch Dermatol. 2006;142(7): 871–6.
14. Zitelli JA, Brown CD, Hanusa BH. Surgical margins for excision of primary cutaneous melanoma. J Am Acad Dermatol. 1997;37(3 Pt 1):422–9.
15. Zalla MJ, Lim KK, Dicaudo DJ, Gagnot MM. Mohs micrographic excision of melanoma using immunostains. Dermatol Surg. 2000;26:771–84.
16. Florell SR, Zone JJ, Gerwels JW. Basal cell carcinomas are populated by melanocytes and Langerhans cells. Am J Dermatopathol. 2001;23(1):24–8.
17. Whiting DA. Histology of normal hair. In: Hordinsky MK, Sawaya ME, Scher RK, editors. Atlas of hair and nails. Philadelphia: Churchill Livingstone; 2000. p. 17.
18. Ackerman AB, Reddy VB, Soyer HP. Anatomic, histologic, and biological aspects. In: Neoplasms with follicular differentiation. New York, NY: Ardor Scribendi Publishers; 2001. p. 80.
19. Hassanein AM, Al-Quran SZ, Kantor GR, et al. Thomsen-Friedenreich (T) antigen: a possible tool for differentiating sebaceous carcinoma from its simulators. Appl Immunohistochem Mol Morphol. 2001;9(3):250–4.
20. Hassanein AM. Sebaceous carcinoma and the T-antigen. Semin Cutan Med Surg. 2004;23(1):62–72.
21. Rao NA, Hidayat AA, McLeon IW. Sebaceous carcinomas of the ocular adnexa: a clinicopathologic study of 104 cases, with five-year follow-up data. Hum Pathol. 1982;13:113–22.
22. Holecek B-U, Ackerman AB. Bulge-activation hypothesis: is it valid? Am J Dermatopathol. 1993;15:235.
23. Herman KL, Kantor GR, Katz SM. Squamous cell carcinoma in situ overlying dermatofibroma. J Cutan Pathol. 1990;17(6):385–7.
24. Hassanein AM, Proper SA, Depcik-Smith ND, Flowers FP. Peritumoral fibrosis in basal cell and squamous cell carcinoma mimicking perineural invasion: potential pitfall in Mohs micrographic surgery. Dermatol Surg. 2005;31(9 Pt 1):1101–6.
25. Abbas O, Bhawan J. Cutaneous perineural inflammation: a review. J Cutan Pathol. 2010;37(12):1200–11.
26. Moehrle M, Breuinger H, Schippert W, Häfner HM. Letter: Imiquimod 5% cream as adjunctive therapy for primary, solitary, nodular basal cell carcinomas before Mohs micrographic surgery: a randomized, double-blind, vehicle-controlled study. Dermatol Surg. 2010;36(3):428–30.

14 Tissue Specimen Documentation, Record Keeping, and Sample Storage

Jeremy S. Youse, Robert H. Cook-Norris, Richelle M. Knudson, and Randall K. Roenigk

Abstract

A busy practice specializing in Mohs micrographic surgery (MMS) will treat several dozen or more patients and generate hundreds or perhaps even thousands of frozen section pathology slides in a typical week. Over a year, this means that a practice must manage tens of thousands of glass slides in addition to the paper or electronic documentation associated with each patient. A single mislabeled, lost, or switched specimen may lead to devastating consequences for a patient. To reduce and prevent medical errors, developing a detailed plan for handling this volume of frozen section pathologic specimens is necessary. This chapter highlights the importance of proper methods for documentation, storage, and record keeping that are vital to providing high-quality care for patients undergoing MMS.

Keywords

Tissue • Specimen • Documentation • Labeling • Identification • Storage • Record keeping • Medical errors

J.S. Youse • R.H. Cook-Norris • R.M. Knudson
Department of Dermatology,
Mayo Clinic, Rochester, MN, USA
e-mail: youse.jeremy@mayo.edu;
cooknorris.robert@mayo.edu and knudson.richelle@mayo.edu

R.K. Roenigk (✉)
Consultant, Department of Dermatology,
Mayo Clinic, Rochester, Minnesota;
Professor of Dermatology, College of Medicine,
Mayo Clinic. Rochester, Minnesota, 55905, USA

Abbreviations

AAD	American Academy of Dermatology
CLIA	Clinical Laboratory Improvement Amendments
CLSI	Clinical and Laboratory Standards Institute
MMS	Mohs micrographic surgery

K. Nouri (ed.), *Mohs Micrographic Surgery*,
DOI 10.1007/978-1-4471-2152-7_14, © Springer-Verlag London Limited 2012

Summary: History

- Proper identification, labeling, and documentation of patients and tissue samples are important aspects of patient safety.
- System-based quality improvement offers a systematic approach to reducing medical errors in all medical specialties, including dermatology and MMS.
- Simple medical procedures, such as obtaining a skin biopsy, are fraught with many potential medical errors, especially errors associated with misidentification and mislabeling.

14.1 History

In the past several decades, patient safety and medical errors have become the focus of broad quality improvement initiatives. System-based quality improvement has evolved into a driving force within the field of medicine, in part as a result of the high number of medical errors uncovered by a 1999 Institute of Medicine report [1]. System-based improvements have focused on proper patient identification, specimen handling, medication errors, and result reporting, among others. These system-based improvements are pertinent to MMS practices for two reasons. First, system-based quality measures such as proper identification of patients and tissues reduce medical errors and lead to improved patient care. Proper identification of patients and tissue specimens is perhaps the most important system-based quality measurement in dermatology and MMS practices. The simple act of obtaining a skin biopsy and submitting the specimen for pathologic evaluation has the potential for dozens of medical errors, some of which may cause the patient serious harm. Recently, the dermatology literature has emphasized medical errors related to the transfer of patient care and tissue specimens between providers [2].

Continuum of Care for a Patient with a Presumed Malignant Melanoma

1. PCP (primary care provider) sees patient and places dermatology referral for suspect pigmented lesion.[1]
2. Patient keeps the appointment and is seen by the dermatologist, and a biopsy is performed.
3. The specimen is labeled and requisition form is completed.*
4. The specimen is placed in a bin for the pathology courier.*
5. The courier signs for the specimen and transports it to the laboratory.*
6. The dermatopathology laboratory receives the specimen and enters it into their computer system.*
7. A technician grosses the specimen and places it into a labeled cassette for processing.*
8. The gross dictation is sent to transcription.*
9. A histology technician places the cassette into a tissue processor.*
10. After processing, a technician embeds each piece of the tissue in a correctly labeled block.*
11. Sections are cut from the paraffin blocks and placed on correctly labeled slides.*
12. The labeled slide is stained, and a cover slip is applied.
13. The slides are reunited with the correct paperwork and delivered to the pathologist.*
14. The pathologist reviews the slides and dictates or enters a diagnosis into a computer program.*
15. If the report is dictated rather than entered directly into a computer, it must pass to transcription;* then the completed report is returned to the pathologist for review and signature.*
16. The report is generated and sent to the dermatologist on paper or electronically.*
17. The dermatologist contacts the patient and sends a message to the appointments pool to schedule an appointment for definitive treatment.*
18. The diagnosis and treatment plan are communicated to the PCP.
19. Treatment is completed.*
20. The appropriate interval of follow-up is scheduled.*
21. The patient keeps all subsequent follow-up appointments.*

Patient identity and specimen labeling are important sources of medical errors in this process. Eliminating medical errors associated with these handoff points in a patient's care is vital to improving overall patient safety. The second reason system-based improvements are important to MMS is the requirement for a well-developed written manual detailing the policies and processes for collection, labeling, processing, evaluation, reporting, and storage of tissue specimens in order to obtain laboratory certification by oversight bodies.

Summary: Regulation and Certification

- The Clinical Laboratory Improvement Amendments (CLIA) sets basic quality standards for medical laboratories.
- Under CLIA, MMS practices are considered high-complexity laboratories.
- There are multiple organizations associated with medical laboratory accreditation.
- Many resources are available to assist MMS practices with the laboratory accreditation process.

14.2 Regulation and Certification

In 1988, the federal government passed the Clinical Laboratory Improvement Amendments (CLIA). These amendments were established to set quality standards and to ensure the integrity of medical laboratories. CLIA requires that medical laboratories be certified by the Secretary of the Department of Health and Human Services. CLIA defines a laboratory as any facility used for the testing and examination of human-derived tissue for the purpose of providing information for the diagnosis, prevention, or treatment of disease. Different levels of CLIA certification are given on the basis of the complexity of testing performed. CLIA stratifies the levels of certification into the following categories: waiver of certification, provider-performed microscopy procedures, moderate complexity, and high complexity. Laboratories involved in complex testing processes, such as histopathology, immunohistochemistry, microbiology, blood chemistries, and others, are considered as "High Level of Complexity" under CLIA. MMS laboratories are included in this high-complexity classification. Application for CLIA certification may be done through state CLIA offices or via an alternative private physician-directed accreditation program, such as COLA (Commission on Office Laboratory Accreditation) or the College of American Pathologists (CAP). These organizations have been granted authority to inspect clinical laboratories and issue accreditation. In short, CLIA certification requires the laboratory to meet various quality standards for facility safety, process quality assessment, personnel training, and proficiency testing and to agree to routine inspections every 2 years [3–6].

This chapter is meant to highlight the importance of proper methods for documentation, record keeping, and storage of tissue specimens for MMS practices and to provide guidance and a starting point for obtaining accreditation. A detailed discussion of CLIA certification requirements and accreditation processes is beyond the scope of this chapter. Regulations vary from state to state; contact your state CLIA office, COLA, or the College of American Pathologists [7] for detailed information (www.cms.hhs.gov/CLIA/downloads/CLIA.SA.pdf). For an MMS surgeon in a solo practice, the accreditation process may seem arduous and complicated. However, other additional resources and organizations are available to simplify and streamline the accreditation process (see "Additional Resources").

Summary: CLSI and Path of Workflow

- The Clinical and Laboratory Standards Institute (CLSI) is an international organization dedicated to developing best practice guidelines for collection, processing, and documentation of tissue specimens.
- CLSI organizes clinical laboratory processes into three phases: preexamination, examination, and postexamination.
- The CLSI framework for clinical laboratory processes, also called the total testing process, or path of workflow, can be easily applied in MMS labs.

14.3 CLSI and Path of Workflow

The Clinical and Laboratory Standards Institute (CLSI, formerly National Committee for Clinical Laboratory Standards) is an international organization dedicated to development of consensus guidelines and standards for patient examination. Given the broad consensus obtained in their development, CLSI standards are used as a model for most laboratories to assist with development of best practices for proper collection, processing, documentation, and storage of tissue specimens [8–11]. Sample documents available from CLSI are a valuable reference in the development of a complete policy and procedure manual. CLSI regularly updates numerous

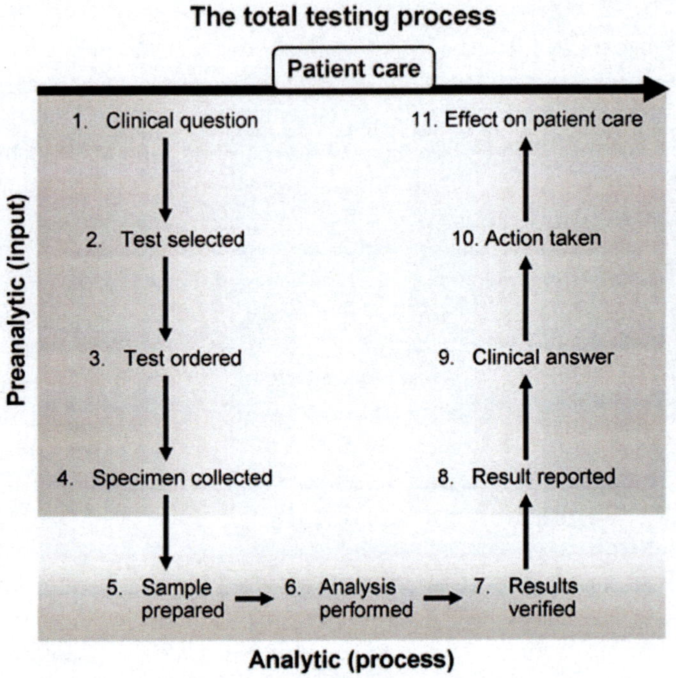

Fig. 14.1 An overview of the entire total testing process, also called the path of workflow. Any step in the process may lead to medical errors. Note that the process always begins and ends with patient care (Adapted from Barr and Schumacher [12]. Reproduced with permission of The McGraw-Hill Companies)

resources dedicated to continually improving patient care and quality from medical laboratories, including a quality management system focused on path of workflow.

A thorough understanding of the path of workflow in a clinical laboratory, also called the testing process, is essential to understanding the importance of proper tissue specimen documentation, record keeping, and storage. The path of workflow allows clinical laboratories to provide quality results and reduce medical errors. Regardless of the specimen, whether a blood sample or a Mohs layer, a defined sequential process is followed to transform a physician's order into a usable result. This process is called the path of workflow, and it is often subdivided into three separate processes: preexamination, examination, and postexamination. All of the specific policies and procedures for a given laboratory should stem from this simple path of workflow. Development of an organized, thorough, and well-understood path of workflow is the foundation of quality laboratory results. An overview of the path of workflow, also known as the total testing process, is shown in Fig. 14.1 [12]. During inspections, demonstration of appropriate documentation, understanding, training, and execution of a well-organized path of workflow is important to obtaining and maintaining accreditation.

Consider the path of workflow for an MMS practice. All the processes from the time of patient check-in through the preparation of tissue slides make up the preexamination process. The microscopic evaluation of Mohs frozen tissue sections on glass slides is the examination step. The recording, documentation, and notification of results, as well as the storage of slides and tissue, are part of the postexamination process. The American Academy of Dermatology (AAD) has prepared a sample policy and procedure manual that details the individual steps in the path of workflow for an MMS practice. This document is available for AAD members on the AAD Web site (www.aad.org/pm/compliance/clia). Pertinent features for each of these processes in the path of workflow specific to an MMS surgical practice are discussed next.

Summary: Preexamination Process

- Preexamination process involves collection, transport, receipt, and initial processing of tissue specimens.
- Rate of medical errors is higher in the preexamination process.
- Medical errors occurring in the preexamination process are often preventable.

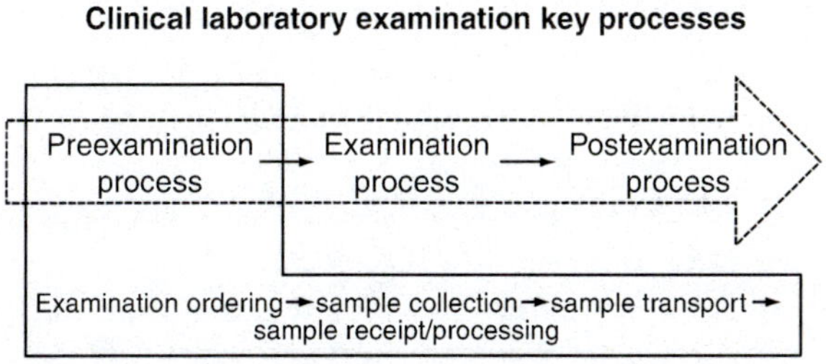

Fig. 14.2 Overview of the preexamination process with permission from NCCLS [10]

14.4 Preexamination Process

The preexamination process includes all of the processes from ordering of the examination to collection, transport, receipt, and processing of the specimen (Fig. 14.2). Each step in this process requires appropriate documentation. A example of the preexamination process for a Mohs surgery patient is shown in Fig. 14.3.

The rate of medical errors for the preexamination process is higher than that for the rest of examination process [13, 14]. Decreasing errors in the preexamination process has become the focus of system-based improvement initiatives and quality measures. The focus on the preexamination process is partly because these errors are more common and can potentially lead to serious negative outcomes and partly because many errors are preventable by modifying the system of specimen collection. Preexamination errors include those related to failure to verify patient identity and incorrect labeling of specimens. Medical errors related to mislabeling of specimens represents a common, serious, and often preventable error. Specimen labeling errors are estimated to occur at rates of 0.1–5% [13–16]. A recent prospective trial found a rate of 4.3 per 1,000 for mislabeling of surgical specimens over a 6-month period. Skin specimens were the second most common tissue involved with labeling errors. Compared with specimens obtained in an operating room, specimens obtained in the outpatient setting were more likely to be mislabeled with the incorrect patient, site, or laterality or to involve an empty container [14]. The potential for patient harm related to mislabeled specimens may result from treatment delay, repeat biopsy procedures, unnecessary treatment, or procedures to the wrong site or wrong patient.

In an effort to reduce these types of errors, the Joint Commission requires the use of two patient identifiers in specimen labels and a preoperative Universal Protocol consisting of a preprocedure verification process, marking of the procedure site, and performing a time-out before any procedure [17]. In addition to creation of standardized processes for specimen collection and labeling, procedures such as use of radiofrequency identification of specimens, introduction of a paperless pathology requisition process, and confirmation of correct site and correct patient by two health care providers have been shown in other studies to decrease errors [11, 18]. CLSI guidelines and standards with sample documents are available to assist with development of standardized labeling and identification systems for both patients and specimens [19–21]. These documents set standards for labels including exact specifications on the content, size, and arrangement of clinical data on the label. A sample label adhering to these recommendations is shown in Fig. 14.4.

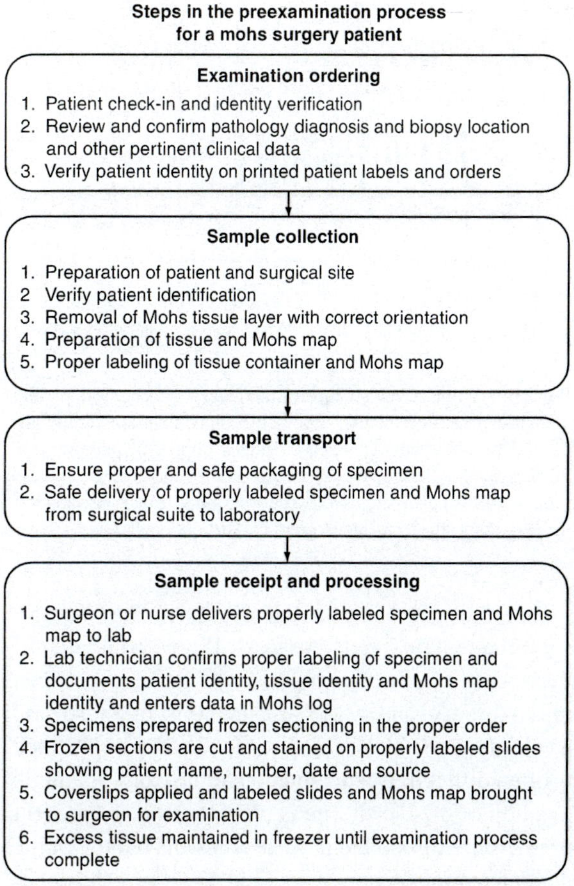

Fig. 14.3 Steps in the preexamination process for a Mohs surgery patient

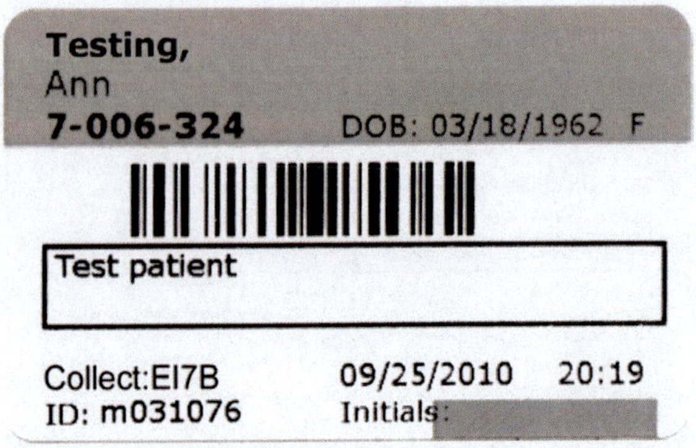

Fig. 14.4 Sample Mayo Clinic patient label. This sample patient label illustrates key features of a well-designed patient label highlighted by standardized arrangement of important patient data. Standardized labeling is a key component of the preexamination process [19–21] (Figure used by permission of Mayo Foundation for Medical Education and Research. All rights reserved)

Some aspects of the preexamination process deserve special attention in relation to MMS, including identification of a previous biopsy site. The time between initial biopsy and MMS treatment is often several weeks. Identification of biopsy sites that are well healed is often difficult. Documentation of the exact anatomic location of the biopsy site is often lacking. To prevent or minimize this problem, we recommend photographic documentation of biopsy sites and modifying the documentation of the biopsy site to include a measurement from a fixed anatomic point (e.g., "biopsy site is located 6 cm in the 9 o'clock position from the tragus"). The use of photography to document biopsy sites has been shown to decrease errors in biopsy site identification [22]. After drawing the proposed surgical plan with a surgical marker at the MMS appointment, it is recommended to verbally and visually verify the biopsy site with the patient using a handheld mirror.

Summary: Examination Process

- Examination process involves the evaluation of a tissue specimen and recording of results.
- Special emphasis on MMS examination phase given the unique importance of tissue orientation in recording results and because a single provider is obtaining, evaluating tissue, recording results, and then providing treatment based upon those results.

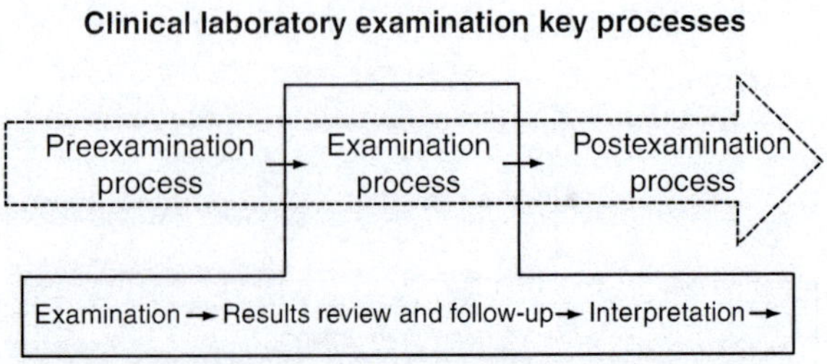

Fig. 14.5 Overview of the examination process with permission from NCCLS [10]

14.5 Examination Process

The examination process must provide accurate and reliable results in order to be successful. The examination process in MMS involves the surgeon evaluating the frozen sections and recording the results of the evaluation on the Mohs map. The process itself is straightforward and involves two steps: evaluation and recording (Fig. 14.5). As has been emphasized previously, special attention should be given to continuing to verify the identity of the specimen and ensure that it matches the identity on the Mohs map with each handoff. The most important and complex step in the examination process is the accurate evaluation of Mohs frozen section histopathologic samples for the presence or absence of tumor. This examination process is somewhat unique in MMS for several reasons. First, correct orientation of the tissue is absolutely vital to treatment. Second, the surgeon is often the only person evaluating the slides, marking results on the Mohs map, and providing treatment for a patient with skin cancer on the basis of the results. This places much responsibility on the surgeon to carefully examine each slide for the presence or absence of tumor, to determine the accurate location and orientation within the tissue block, and to properly record and orient the results on the Mohs map. A successful Mohs surgeon must recognize the importance of these steps in the examination process for MMS (Fig. 14.6).

The process of converting the histopathologic evidence of tumor on a Mohs section both to a diagnosis and to proper recording of the tumor on the Mohs map is difficult to standardize. This complex and poorly understood process is valueless if the results are recorded on the wrong Mohs map. Thus, it is important for the Mohs surgeon to constantly verify that the

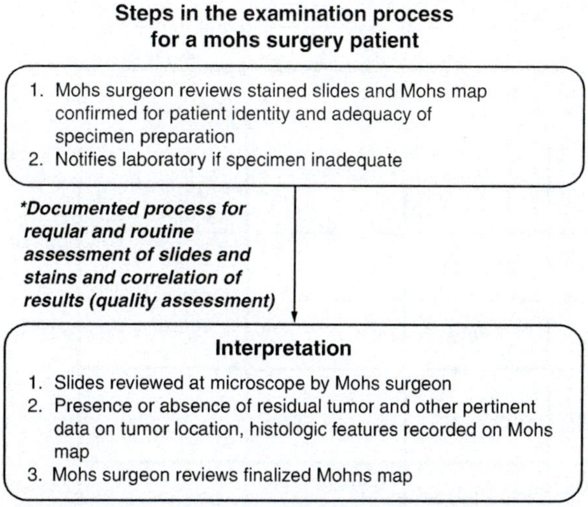

Fig. 14.6 Steps in the examination process for a Mohs surgery patient

orientation, specimen, and Mohs map are correct. Implementation of a well-documented standardized process for regular quality control to ensure that the preparation, staining, tracking, and evaluation of specimens are consistent will limit preventable errors in the examination process. This will allow the Mohs surgeon to devote his or her full attention to the often challenging task of interpreting slides rather than wondering if the examined sections belong to the correct patient.

In our practice, quality checks are regularly performed by randomly selecting both positive and negative slides for blinded peer review by fellow MMS colleagues. Results of the quality assurance measures are recorded, and discrepancies in results undergo careful root cause analysis. Ultimately, the goal of the examination process is to produce a usable result that will guide further patient care. Once all slides have been evaluated and results have been properly recorded, the postexamination process begins.

Summary: Postexamination Process

- Postexamination process involves reporting of results and archiving of records and specimens.
- Postexamination process is streamlined in a MMS practice where results are obtained and acted upon in the same day.

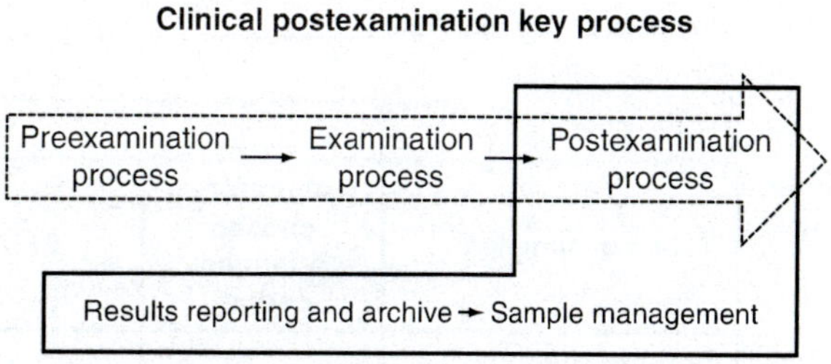

Fig. 14.7 Overview of the postexamination process with permission from NCCLS [10]

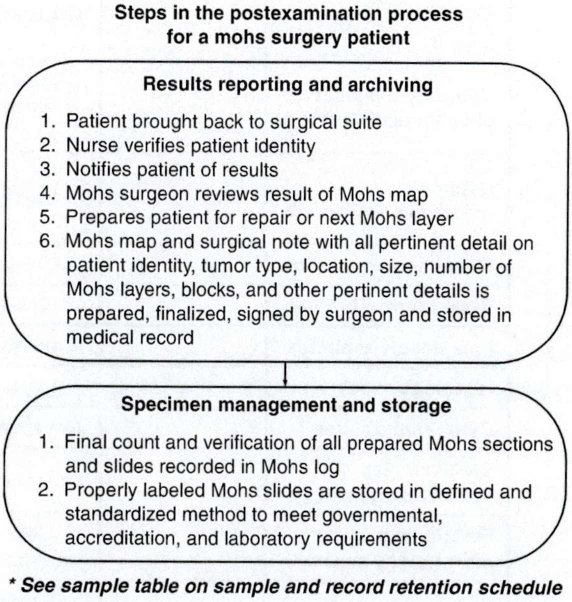

Fig. 14.8 Steps in the postexamination process for a Mohs surgery patient

14.6 Postexamination Process

The postexamination process involves reporting of results and archiving of records and specimens (Fig. 14.7). This process is simplified and streamlined by the nature of MMS practice, which usually involves same-day specimen collection, processing, and notification of results overseen by one Mohs surgeon (Fig. 14.8). This same-day processing inherently simplifies the postexamination process compared with that in a large clinical laboratory that must record and interpret clinical results for critical values and have a standardized system for relaying results to a multitude of ordering providers. Thus, the most salient feature of the postexamination process for the MMS practice is

Laboratory name: ______________________________

	Sample retention period				
Types of samples	**[Laboratory's chosen retention period]**	**CLIA**	**CAP**	**JCAHO**	**[Other organization]**
Serum/CFS/body fluids		Not specified	24 hours		
Blood films, body fluid slides (normal)		Not specified	7 days		
Blood films, body fluid slides (abnormal)		Not specified			
Cytology (negative slides/unsatisfactory)		5 years from examination date	5 years	5 years from examination date	
Cytology (positive/suspicious)		10 years	5 years	5 years from examination date	
Bone marrow smears		10 years	10 years		
Bone marrow biopsy		10 years			
Fine needle aspirates		10 years	10 years		
Histology slides		10 years		10 years	
Cytogenetic slides		Not specified			
DNA samples (molecular genetics)		Not specified			
Fertility testing lab morphology slides		Not applicable			
Wet and formalin-fixed tissue		Until final report is issued	2 weeks after final report	7 days after final report	
Paraffin blocks		2 years from examination date	5 years	2 years from examination date	

This example was modified from the table contributed by the Department of Laboratory Medicine and Pathology, Mayo Clinic, Rochester, MN, USA

Fig. 14.9 Example of sample retention schedule with permission from NCCLS [10]. A schedule for retention of various tissue specimens. The rules for retention of tissue specimens vary according to institutional, state, and local regulations

having a system for proper retention and storage of records and specimens. Regulations regarding proper storage and retention of various tissue specimens and associated records vary by state law, accrediting organization, and institution. Examples of tissue sample and document retention schedules are shown in Figs. 14.9 and 14.10.

In our practice, photographs of the treated area(s) are obtained before and after treatment and after repair. The patient photographs and the finalized Mohs map are double-checked for correct labeling and then scanned and loaded into each patient's electronic medical record for permanent storage. An MMS surgical note also is entered, which contains all pertinent

Types of records	[Laboratory's chosen retention period]	CLIA	CAP	JCAHO	[Other organization]
	Governmental/accreditation organization – Retention Period				
Calibration records		2 years	2 years	2 years	
Photographed images and work lists containing patient results for Molecular Genetics and Cytogenetics		2 years			
Instrument/equipment • Preventative maintenance (daily, monthly, quarterly, yearly) records • Service repair and record		2 years	2 years	2 years for daily, weekly or monthly performance examination and function checks Life of instrument-major repairs, parts replacement, and annual maintenance	
Records of monitoring of temperature controlled spaces, heating and cooling devices		2 years			
Quality control (QC) records Quality assurance (QA) records		2 years	2 years 5 years for immuno-hematology	5 years: immuno-hematology, histo-compatibiliy, and tissue banking 2 years: all others	
Methodology changes, normal range changes, reporting unit changes		Not specified	2 years		
Proficiency testing (records of examination handling, preparation, processing, examination, results of reporting, the signed attestation statement, and feedback reports)		2 years	2 years	2 years	

Fig. 14.10 Example of record retention schedule with permission from NCCLS [10]. Similar to rules regarding retentions of specimens, the rules for retention of records vary according to institutional, state, and local regulations

Employee continuing education **Employee training including safety training** **Employee competence**		2 years			
Employee medical record (contains the record of vaccinations against Hepatitis B or the signed statement declining vaccination)		Not specified			

This example was modified from the table contributed by the Department of Laboratory Medicine and Pathology, Mayo Clinic, Rochester, MN, USA
NOTE: Regional or local requirements may apply to access to patient medical records

Fig. 14.10 (continued)

patient identification data, tumor type, precise location, preoperative and postoperative size, relevant pathologic features, number of Mohs layers, number of blocks, and details of repair. The Mohs log is prepared and maintained by the MMS laboratory technicians. The glass slides are double-checked for proper labeling and stored in temporary storage in the Mohs laboratory. Within 30 days, the slides are prepared and labeled for long-term storage. The slides are kept on-site in the Mohs laboratory for 2 years and then transferred to off-site storage for at least 10 years to comply with current CAP and CLIA guidelines. These processes are all performed in compliance with relevant federal, state, and institutional policies. Further information regarding the rules for individual states is available in the "Additional Resources."

Summary: Conclusion

- A well-organized path of workflow is the foundation for a quality clinical laboratory.
- Adherence to a well-planned path of workflow reduces medical errors and improves patient safety.
- Clinical laboratories, including MMS practices, should constantly monitor and adapt their path of workflow to maintain the highest quality standards.

14.7 Conclusion

The process of careful documentation, record keeping, and storage of tissue specimens in MMS is an important aspect of patient care and patient safety. The process of establishing a consistent, standardized procedure and process manual for tissue specimen documentation and storage may seem tedious, but it is a vital step to providing excellent Mohs surgical care. Although this chapter focuses largely on the path of workflow in relation to tissue specimens, the same principles of quality management systems can and should be applied to all aspects of a Mohs surgical practice from maintenance of equipment to inventory control processes. The investment of time and effort to develop a thorough, well-understood, well-executed, and regularly reviewed path of workflow for tissue specimen collection provides a framework for safe and effective Mohs surgical care that will have benefits for both the practice and the patient.

Additional Resources

College of American Pathologists Web site: www.cap.org

CLIA Web site: www.cms.gov/CLIA/

State CLIA office for detailed information: www.cms.hhs.gov/CLIA/downloads/CLIA.SA.pdf

COLA Web site: www.cola.org

American Academy of Dermatology Web site: www.aad.org/pm/compliance/clia/

Acknowledgment We thank Audrey Anderson, Mayo Clinic Department of Dermatology and Department of Laboratory Medicine and Pathology, for her assistance in the preparation of this manuscript.

References

1. Kohn LT, Corrigan JM, Donaldson MS, editors. To err is human: building a safer health system. Washington: National Academy Press; 2000.
2. Elston DM, Stratman E, Johnson-Jahangir H, et al. Part II. Opportunities for improvement in patient safety. J Am Acad Dermatol. 2009;61:193–205.
3. Centers for Medicare and Medicaid Services, U.S. Department of Health and Human Services. Chapter IV Part 493 – Laboratory Requirements. http://www.access.gpo.gov/nara/cfr/waisidx_04/42cfr493_04.html
4. Chaudhari R. Answers to frequently asked questions about CLIA standards for lab testing. Dermatol World. 2009;19 (11):8–9.
5. COLA. www.cola.org. Accessed September 1, 2010.
6. Centers for Medicare and Medicaid Services, U.S. Department of Health and Human Services. Clinical laboratory improvement amendments. http://www.cms.gov/CLIA/. Accessed September 1, 2010.
7. Lawson NS, Howanitz PJ. The College of American Pathologists, 1946–1996: quality assurance service. Arch Pathol Lab Med. 1997;121:1000–8.
8. Clinical and Laboratory Standards Institute (CLSI). www.clsi.org. Accessed September 1, 2010.
9. NCCLS. A quality management system model for health care; Approved guideline. 2nd ed. NCCLS document HS1-A2 [ISBN 1–56238–554–2].
10. NCCLS. Application of a quality management system model for laboratory services; Approved guideline. 3rd ed. NCCLS document GP26-A3 [ISBN 1–56238–553–4].
11. Clinical and Laboratory Standards Institute (CLSI). Laboratory documents: development and control; Approved guideline. 5th ed. CLSI document GP2-A5 (ISBN 1–56238–600-X).
12. Barr JT, Schumacher GE. The total testing process applied to therapeutic drug monitoring. In: Schumacher GE, editor. Therapeutic drug monitoring. Norwalk: Appleton & Lange; 1995. p. 47–82.
13. Howanitz PJ. Errors in laboratory medicine: practical lessons to improve patient safety. Arch Pathol Lab Med. 2005;129:1252–61.
14. Makary MA, Epstein J, Pronovost PJ, et al. Surgical specimen identification errors: a new measure of quality in surgical care. Surgery. 2007;141:450–5.
15. Wagar EA, Stankovic AK, Raab S, et al. Specimen labeling errors: a Q-probes analysis of 147 clinical laboratories. Arch Pathol Lab Med. 2008;132:1617–22.
16. Sandbank S, Klein D, Westreich M, et al. The loss of pathological specimens: incidence and causes. Dermatol Surg. 2010;36:1084–6.
17. The Joint Commission. Accreditation program: office-based surgery. National Patient Safety Goals. 2010. http://www.jointcommission.org/assets/1/6/2011_NPSGs_OBS.pdf.
18. Francis DL, Prabhakar S, Sanderson SO. A quality initiative to decrease pathology specimen-labeling errors using radiofrequency identification in a high-volume endoscopy center. Am J Gastroenterol. 2009;104:972–5.
19. Clinical and Laboratory Standards Institute (CLSI). Accuracy in patient and sample identification; Approved guideline. CLSI document GP33-A (ISBN 1–56238–721–9).
20. Clinical and Laboratory Standards Institute (CLSI). Specimen labels: content and location, fonts, and label orientation; Proposed standard. CLSI document AUTO12-P (ISBN 1–56238–715–4).
21. NCCLS. Laboratory automation: data content for specimen identification; Approved standard. NCCLS document AUTO7-A [ISBN 1–56238–537–2].
22. McGinness JL, Goldstein G. The value of preoperative biopsy-site photography for identifying cutaneous lesions. Dermatol Surg. 2010;3:194–7.

Immunostains

15

Kapila V. Paghdal, Basil S. Cherpelis, and L. Frank Glass

Abstract

Mohs micrographic surgery (MMS) is a frozen section technique well suited for removal of some of the more difficult cutaneous malignancies. The primary emphasis of the procedure is histologic examination of the entirety of surgical margins, which is done intraoperatively prior to wound closure. There are, on occasion, instances where the microscopic interpretation during Mohs is hindered by, dense inflammation abundant scar tissue, and additional cases where subtle perineural or skeletal muscle invasion may go undetected in frozen sections. For melanoma patients, the problem is difficulty in locating melanocytes on H & E stained frozen sections, especially for tumors that arise on chronically sun-damaged skin. Immunostains can be extremely helpful for visualizing tumor in frozen sections and are being used more frequently by Mohs surgeons when H & E alone is deemed insufficient. We intend to review the full spectrum of immunostaining techniques used in Mohs, many of which are simply modifications of immunoperoxidase protocols employed in permanent sections. A perceived drawback is the delay in surgery associated with tissue processing and the technical aspects of immunostaining. The time required to process each Mohs layer varies with the antibody, but many of the newer protocols require as little as 20 min to complete. Currently, immunostains are used during MMS for melanoma, basal cell carcinoma, squamous cell carcinoma, dermatofibrosarcoma protuberans, extramammary Paget's disease, granular cell tumor, primary mucinous carcinoma, and trichilemmal carcinoma, and these immunostains are summarized in this chapter.

Keywords

Immunostain • Immunohistochemistry • Immunoperoxidase • Mohs micrographic surgery • Melanoma • Basal cell carcinoma • Squamous cell carcinoma • Dermatofibrosarcoma protuberans • Extramammary Paget's disease • Granular cell tumor Primary mucinous carcinoma • Trichilemmal carcinoma

K.V. Paghdal (✉) • B.S. Cherpelis • L.F. Glass
Dermatology and Cutaneous Surgery,
University of South Florida, Tampa, FL, USA
e-mail: kpaghdal@health.usf.edu

K. Nouri (ed.), *Mohs Micrographic Surgery*,
DOI 10.1007/978-1-4471-2152-7_15,

Summary: Introduction

- Mohs micrographic surgery (MMS) is a surgical technique utilized for skin cancers that allows for 100% visualization of the lateral and deep margins of the excision specimen.
- During excision of squamous cell or basal cell carcinoma with Mohs, frozen section slides may occasionally be difficult to interpret with H & E staining if there is fibrosis, inflammation, or perineural and muscle invasion.
- Permanent sections stained with H & E allow for better visualization of nuclear detail and cell morphology of melanocytes compared to frozen sections.
- Immunostaining is an indispensible adjunctive technique during MMS to visualize certain tumors in frozen section slides that are difficult to see on H & E.

15.1 Introduction

Mohs micrographic surgery (MMS) has proven to be an effective technique for the excision of various skin cancers as it allows visualization of the complete peripheral and deep margins of surgery [1]. It results in excellent cure rates with minimal recurrences; for example, only 1% for primary basal cell carcinoma (BCC) and 3–8% for recurrent basal BCC. In contrast, standard excisional surgery permits examination of only 1–2% of the surgical margin and is associated with higher recurrence rates of up to 10% for primary lesions and 5–40% for recurrent tumors [2, 3].

For most cases of BCC and squamous cell carcinoma (SCC) submitted for MMS, delineating margins is relatively straightforward in frozen sections (FS). However, there are occasional cases with extensive inflammation or where there is dense fibrosis masking the tumor relative to its surrounding. Occasionally, the tumor may infiltrate skeletal muscle or nerve bundles.

The problem with Mohs for melanoma is that it may be difficult to differentiate melanocytes from atypical keratinocytes in the background of sun-damaged skin, and there is risk of freeze artifact. The use of formalin-fixed paraffin-embedded sections (FFPES, or "permanent sections") permits better visualization of melanocytes than in FS and provides more detail of nuclear and cellular morphology, such as, for example, the perinuclear "halo" that pathologist rely upon to recognize melanocytes in permanent sections.

Table 15.1 Various immunostains used during Mohs micrographic surgery

Neoplasm	Immunostain
Melanoma	Melan-A or MART-1, HMB-45, Mel-5, S-100, MITF
Squamous cell carcinoma	Cytokeratins
Basal cell carcinoma	Cytokeratins, Ber-EP4
Dermatofibrosarcoma protuberans	CD34
Extramammary Paget's disease	CEA, Cytokeratin 7
Primary mucinous carcinoma	Cytokeratins
Granular cell tumor	S100
Trichilemmal carcinoma	Cytokeratin 17

To improve the accuracy and quality of frozen sections for both melanoma and nonmelanoma skin cancers, it has become common to use immunostaining or immunohistochemistry as an adjunct to routine H & E staining for the more difficult or recurrent and high-risk tumors.

Its use for cutaneous tumors was first reported in 1984 by Drs. Robinson and Gottschalk for the staining of antibodies to fibrous keratin in deeply invasive basal and squamous cell carcinomas [4]. Now, immunohistochemistry is used mostly for patients with melanoma, basal cell carcinoma, squamous cell carcinoma, extramammary Paget's disease, dermatofibrosarcoma protuberans, granular cell tumor, and trichilemmal carcinoma (Table 15.1).

Summary: Review of Immunofluorescence and Immunoperoxidase Techniques

- Immunoperoxidase and immunofluorescence staining techniques are both utilized to identify specific antigens in tissue.
- Immunofluorescence is conducted on frozen section material, but is not applicable to MMS because it requires special UV microscopy and its staining is not durable.
- Immunohistochemistry using a DAB chromophore permanently stains tissue sections and can be viewed with a light microscope; ideal of MMS.
- Methods such as heating tissue sections and the use of polymers during immunohistochemistry reduce processing time, which may range from 1 h to less than 20 min per stage.

15.2 Review of Immunofluorescence and Immunoperoxidase Techniques

Initially, immunohistochemistry for frozen sections was prohibitively time consuming; some cases taking over an hour for results. Now, newer techniques employ rapid and even ultrarapid protocols and can produce reliable results is as little as 19 min [2]. It is still, however, paramount that immunohistochemistry-trained laboratory personnel perform these protocols due to the complex and precise nature of these stains.

As a review, immunostaining techniques are generally divided into immunofluorescence (IF) and immunoperoxidase (IMP). Immunofluorescence includes both direct and indirect techniques. Direct IF utilizes frozen sections that are incubated at room temperature with fluorescein isothiocyanate (FITC) antisera. The resulting fluorescent green deposits are visualized by the use of special ultraviolet microscopy. Paraffin-embedded sections are generally not recommended, but perhaps could be attempted after pretreatment with proteolytic enzymes and 0.1% aluminum hydroxide. Indirect immunofluorescence detects serum polyclonal or monoclonal antibodies by incubating the serum with normal skin substrates obtained from volunteers. If the antibody is present and becomes attached to the substrate, then it is detected via incubation with FITC-labeled antisera [5].

Immunoperoxidase staining is reliable in both FS and FFPES. Techniques that have been developed include the peroxidase–antiperoxidase method (PAP), the avidin–biotin–peroxidase complex procedure (ABC), and the alkaline phosphatase–antialkaline phosphatase procedure (APAAP). The initial studies used a direct method that involved a single antibody conjugated with an enzyme (i.e., peroxidase), which then bound to antigen. After the substrate was introduced, the peroxidase enzyme would oxidize the chromagen and produce an insoluble colorized product (Fig. 15.1). The limitation of this method is its low sensitivity and the need for higher concentrations of the antibody to produce results [6]. Indirect methods were developed to shorten the procedure, enhance its sensitivity, and decrease the quantity of antibody required. There may be increased background staining using indirect staining and a diminishment in the specificity of this method. A negative control is recommended for comparison [6].

In the PAP method, after the tissue is exposed to the primary antibody, it is then washed and incubated with a secondary antibody labeled with horseradish peroxidase. The peroxidase oxidizes the chromagen detection system, forming an insoluble precipitate, corresponding to the localization of the entire complex (Fig. 15.2). The most commonly used chromagens include 3,3′-diaminobenzidine hydrochloride (DAB), which forms a brown product, or 3-amino-9-ethylcarbazole (AEC), which forms a red product.

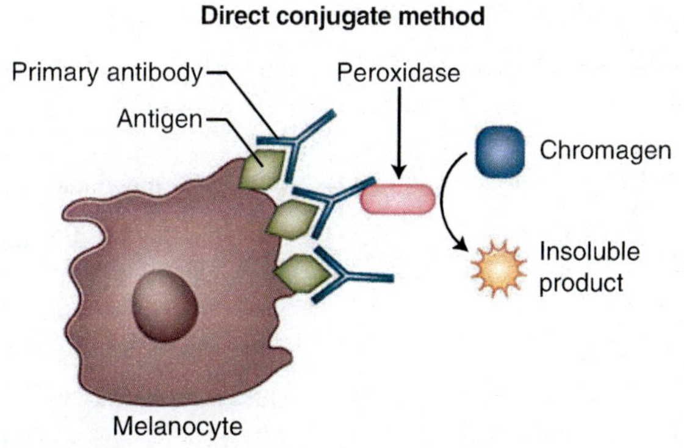

Fig. 15.1 The peroxidase is conjugated to the primary antibody

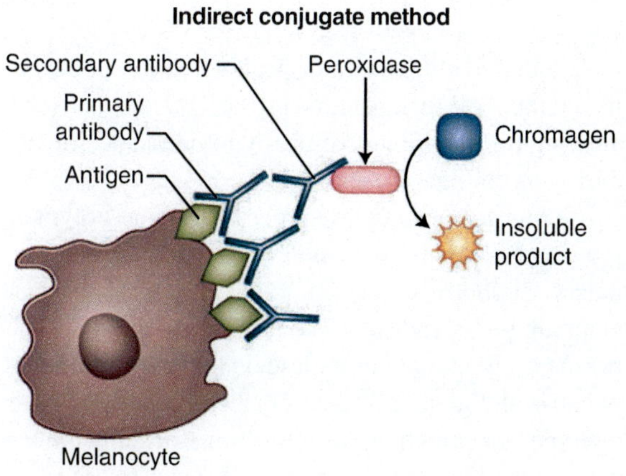

Fig. 15.2 The peroxidase is conjugated to the secondary antibody

The ABC procedure is an alternative technique that utilizes the natural attraction between biotin bound to the primary antibody, and avidin, which is conjugated to the secondary antibody, whereby creating tertiary complexes of avidin, biotin, and horseradish peroxidase. This produces a higher degree of sensitivity compared to PAP. Finally, the APAAP method utilizes intestinal-type alkaline phosphatase instead of horseradish peroxidase and uses fast red instead of DAB as the chromagen. The advantage of this technique is that endogenous tissue peroxidase does not need to be quenched unlike in the PAP and ABC methods because the alkaline phosphatase enzyme has activity specific to intestinal mucosa. A protein blocking step can also

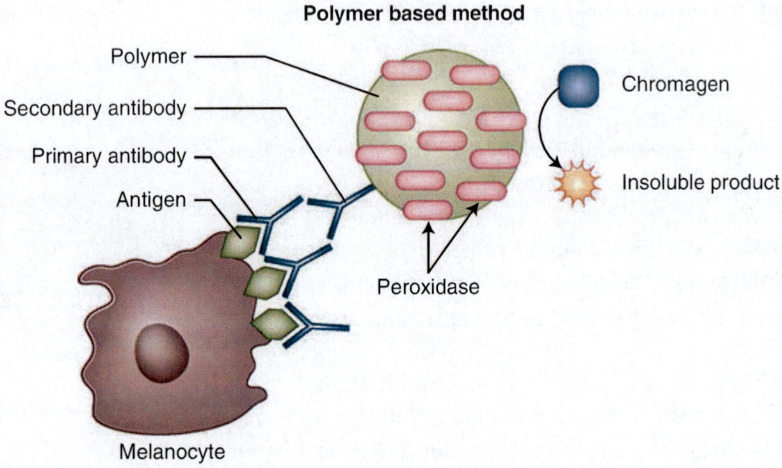

Fig. 15.3 Multiple peroxidase enzymes are conjugated to the spherical polymer

be included to eliminate nonspecific IgG antibodies in the vicinity of Ig receptors in the cutaneous tissue, allowing for the primary antibody to more specifically bind to the antigen [7].

In order to speed up the processing time, polymer-based techniques have been developed, where the secondary antibody is bound to a spherical polymer containing horseradish peroxidase (Fig. 15.3) [7]. The increased amount of peroxidase on the polymer is correlated with the increased chromagen activation [7].

Some newer methods of immunohistochemistry use enhanced techniques of antigen retrieval to improve upon the sensitivity of the stain because antigens are often obscured by the fixation process. One such example involves using microwave heating combined with citrate buffers or heavy metal–containing solutions leading to enhanced immunoperoxidase staining of antigen. Again, there may be increased background staining and a resultant decrease in specificity [5, 8].

A major advantage of immunohistochemistry, compared to immunofluorescence, is that the resultant staining is durable if not permanent within FS and FFPES sections, rather than fading with time. The staining is clearly visible with light microscopy, rather than special ultraviolet microscopy, and the sensitivity is substantially greater than immunofluorescence [4, 8].

Summary: Melanoma

- Frozen section H & E stained slides may not always permit clear visualization of melanoma cells because they are usually recognized by an artifact seen in formalin-fixed paraffin-embedded processing.
- With specific immunostains, melanocytes are readily identified in frozen sections, which facilitate determination of surgical margins for melanoma with MMS.
- MART-1 or Melan-A is the most commonly used immunostain for melanoma; however, HMB-45, Mel-5, S100, and MITF may also be useful in some cases.

15.3 Melanoma

The standard treatment of melanoma (MM) is wide local excision, and size of the margins varies with tumor depth. Application of frozen section techniques like MMS for resection of melanoma is still considered controversial, but gradually becoming mainstream for the more ill-defined and difficult to remove melanomas like lentigo maligna (LM). The most significant limitation of this technique is that melanocytes can be difficult to find and distinguish from atypical keratinocytes along the dermal epidermal junction in chronically sun-damaged skin. The microscopic feature of "retraction artifact" seen in permanent sections stained with H & E, which pathologists depend on to recognize melanocytes, is not consistently present on FS, and without precise identification of melanocytes, MMS cannot be considered a viable approach to interpreting surgical margins for MIS, that is, without the aid of immunostains (Fig. 15.4). On the contrary, investigators have reported that some architectural features in FS can be used to signal the presence of MIS. The basal layer may be disordered, and nesting of cells may be present.

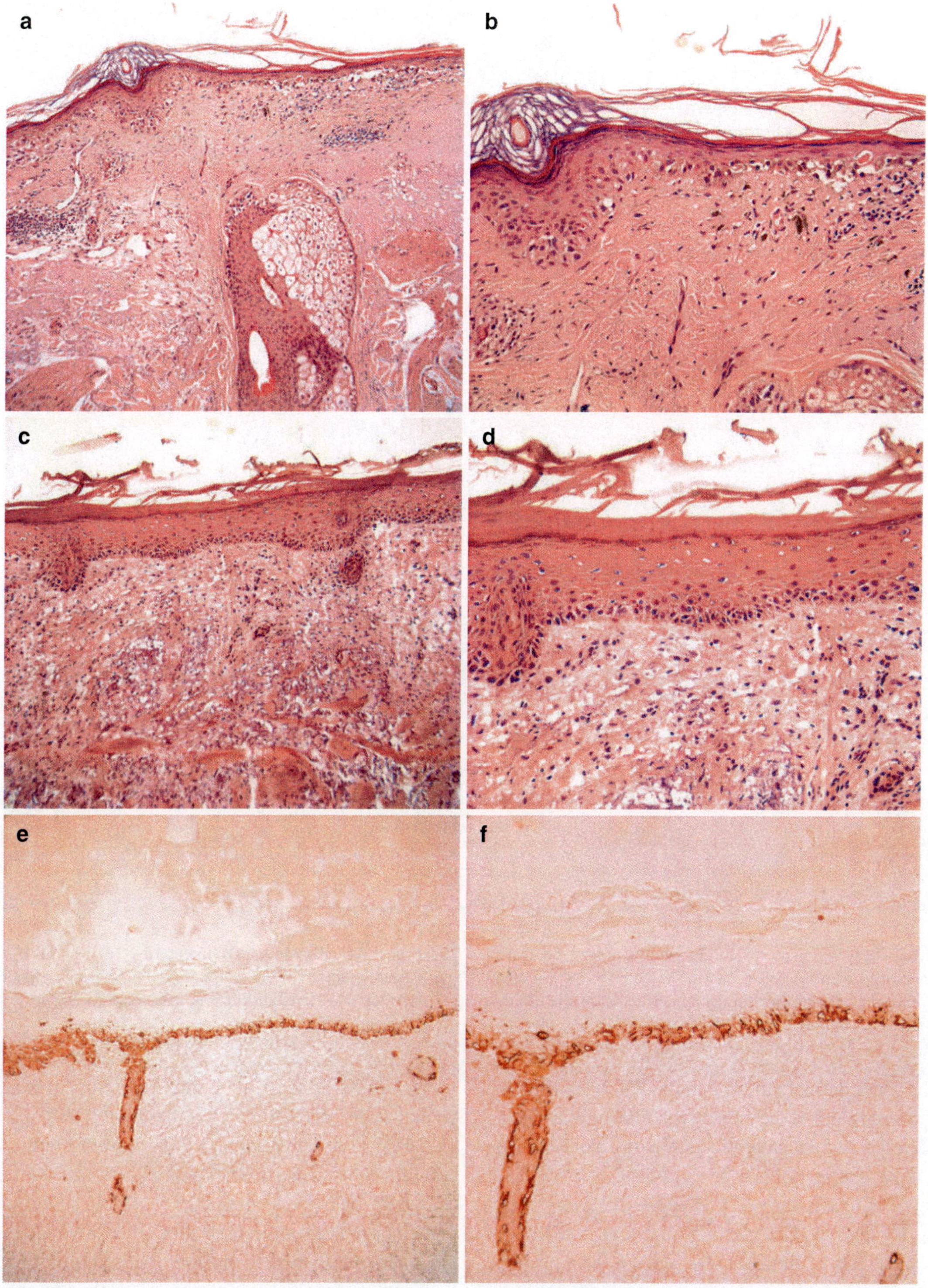

Fig. 15.4 Biopsy of melanoma in situ in a permanent section stained with H & E at (**a**) 10×, and (**b**) 20× magnification, compared to a frozen section obtained during Mohs surgery at (**c**) 20× and (**d**) 40× magnification. The features of melanoma in situ, including confluence and nesting, are far more apparent in the permanent section compared to the frozen section. MART-1 highlights (**e**) confluence of melanocytes along the interface and nesting within a follicular unit at 20× and (**f**) 40×

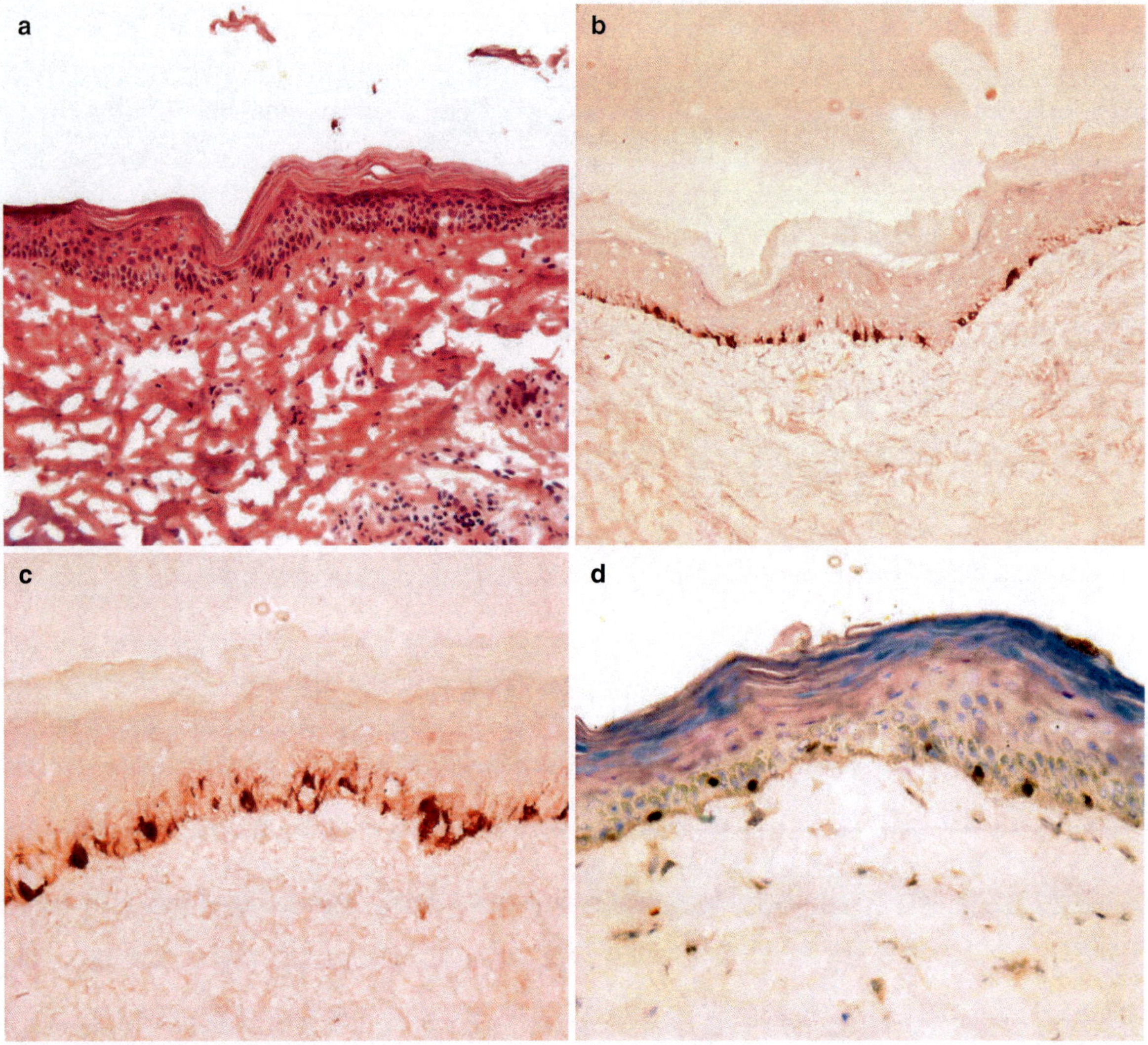

Fig. 15.5 Negative margins during Mohs surgery on frozen section stained with (**a**) H & E and (**b**) MART-1 (20×). The distribution of melanocytes within the epidermis is difficult to discern by H & E staining, but they label with MART-1. There is a "false positive" pattern of confluence by (**c**) MART-1, but a more clear depiction of the density and diameter of melanocytes by (**d**) MITF at 40× magnification, indicating a "negative" margin for melanoma

Also, a dense dermal infiltrate immediately beneath the interface may signal the presence of melanoma [9].

Regardless of the theoretical limitations of MMS for melanoma, the recurrence rate after the procedure for primary lesions is only 1%, and for recurrent melanoma, about 10% [10]. In a 5-year study, MMS for melanoma with FS analysis was found to be equivalent or better than a historic control of wide local excisions for melanoma, with a recurrence rate of 0.5%. The average margin for MMS was 6 mm which cleared 83% of the patients [9], and the sensitivity and specificity values for the identification of melanoma ranges from 73% to 100% and 68% to 90%, respectively [11, 12].

With the advent of immunostaining, enhanced visualization of melanocytes has facilitated the use of MMS for melanoma. The immunostain most commonly used currently for melanoma is Melan-A or MART-1 (Figs. 15.4 and 15.5). Using immunohistochemistry, the requirements for reliable MMS results have been described as follows: the tumor cells must be visually identifiable in the section, the tumor must be contiguous to avoid false negatives, the mapping and staining component must be technically feasible, and the total tissue processing time should be short enough to allow for a staged excision and repair on the same day [13].

Melan-A or MART-1 is a 22 kDa cytoplasmic melanosome-associated glycoprotein recognized by mouse monoclonal antibodies A-103 and M2–7 C10 [6, 14]. It is a melanocyte differentiation antigen similar to gp100, gp75, and tyrosinase [6, 14]. It is present in 80–100% of melanomas and is also found in benign melanocytes within nevi and normal skin [15].

The sensitivity of this marker for melanocytes has been reported to be 75–92%, while the specificity is 97–100% [16]. Several studies have found this marker to be more sensitive than HMB-45, or more specific compared to S100 [15, 17, 18]. However, there are reports that MART-1 may not be very helpful in regard to differentiating pigmented actinic keratoses from MIS in heavily sun-damaged skin. In one study, MART-1, HMB-45, S100, and tyrosinase were used to stain unequivocal pigmented actinic keratosis to determine the usefulness of these markers in sun-damaged skin [18]. MART-1 was found to stain numerous melanocytes in the areas of the actinic keratoses as well as adjacent sun-damaged skin, exceeding staining observed with the other markers [18]. In addition, four of ten cases stained with MART-1 revealed focal clusters suggestive of melanocytic nests [18]. This increased staining could be explained by an increased number of melanocytes, making this stain nonspecific in patients with sun-damaged skin or possibly due to the expression of MART-1 in keratinocytes or other nonmelanocytic cells damaged by inflammation [18–20]. As it applies to MMS, this can potentially lead the surgeon to excise greater margins in areas that appear to be melanoma but are in fact a false positive [21].

In one study, investigators used MART-1 immunostaining of FS material in hopes of differentiating melanoma from melanocytic hyperplasia in individuals with severely chronically sun-damaged skin. The study found that in normal sun-exposed skin, the melanocyte density is 15–20 per high-power field, confluence of up to nine melanocytes, and melanocytes were noted to extend along hair follicles [19]. They also noted the lack of pagetoid spread and nesting, but as previously mentioned, the MART-1 staining at times may stain clusters of cytoplasmic material that can simulate nests [18, 19]. The use of negative and positive controls can aid in interpreting the specimens. Some studies have used a biopsy from a similarly exposed body site, sometimes the contralateral side of the face, while others have utilized dog ears removed during reconstruction to serve as negative controls [7, 14–16, 18, 22]. The initial debulking specimen taken from the center of the tumor, and often processed for a permanent section to assess Breslow depth, can also serve as a positive control. In addition, some surgeons may use two or more immunostains if margins still appear equivocal after the primary immunostain; however, this is not always feasible or cost-effective [17].

The results with MART-1-stained FS were found to correlate 100% with FFPES, in a study of patient with LM [15]. The MART-1 stain can take up to 2–3.5 h; however, various investigators have been able to shorten this time considerably. In one study of 40 patients with melanoma (24 MIS, 16 MM), the authors utilized a polymer-based immunoperoxidase stain which considerably shortened the blocking step of the procedure and eliminated the linking step where the chromagen would be linked to the secondary antibody (Fig. 15.3). This shortened the protocol to just 1 h, while still maintaining quality MART-1-stained sections in frozen material [7]. There have been other reports of processing time shortened to 19 min without significant differences in histologic features, including the number of keratinocytes, nuclear diameter of keratinocytes or melanocytes, number of melanocytes, the presence of confluence, pagetoid spread, and melanocytic nesting or atypical melanocytes when compared to H & E [22].

Another marker is HMB-45, human melanoma black-45, which is one of the first melanoma-specific markers, and a mouse monoclonal antibody that recognizes the 30–35 kDa cytoplasmic premelanosomal glycoprotein gp100 [6, 16]. This marker is present in stages I and II of melanosomes in neoplastic melanocytes and stages II and III of melanosomes in fetuses and infants [23]. There is a complete absence of keratinocyte staining with HMB-45, and it does not stain normal adult benign melanocytes [14, 24].

The sensitivity for HMB-45 ranges from 69% to 93%, with a higher range for primary melanoma (77–100%) as compared to metastatic melanoma (56–83%) [16]. This marker has a greater specificity than S100, but a decreased sensitivity. Of particular note is that desmoplastic, spindle cell, and amelanotic melanomas may be negative for HMB-45, though with newer antigen retrieval techniques, the sensitivity increases to 75% for spindle cells melanomas [14, 25]. Due to the decreased sensitivity for MM and the weaker staining of the deeper component of the tumor, some authors recommend this stain be performed in conjunction with other stains [16]. This staining technique takes 90 min [24].

In one study of 20 patients (18 MIS, 2 MM) with melanoma, HMB-45 staining was found to be positive in 11 patients, which is equivalent to results with permanent sections. The sensitivity was 100%, and the specificity was 95% as there was one false positive [24]. In a case of a patient with recurrent acral melanoma, H & E–stained FS, FFPESs, and HMB-45-stained FSs were utilized. The authors found that the HMB-45 stain was comparable to the H & E–stained FS and FFPES, but was also strongly positive in areas where the FFPESs were equivocal or negative [10]. While it appears to be useful in some cases, HMB-45 is generally not commonly used for immunostaining during MMS.

S100 is a 21 kDa acidic calcium-binding protein, given its name because of solubility in 100% saturated ammonium sulfate solution [6, 14, 16]. S100 is present in the nucleus and cytoplasm of melanocytes. It stains benign melanocytic lesions, melanomas, glial cells, Schwann cells, skeletal and cardiac muscle, histiocytes, chondrocytes, and salivary and sweat glands. The sensitivity and specificity of this marker is 92–100% and 75–87%, respectively; consequently, it is more sensitive than HMB-45 and MART-1, but less specific than MART-1 [16]. This nonspecificity leads to increased background staining making the interpretation of the slide more difficult. It is superior to HMB-45, MART-1, and Mel-5 for the deeper component of tumors, but does not stain the epidermal component as reliably. Furthermore, it is the preferred stain for desmoplastic and spindle cell melanoma [17].

Mel-5, a mouse monoclonal antibody, recognizes the most ample glycoprotein in melanocytes, gp75. It is in the tyrosinase-related family of proteins and is found in melanosomes, particularly in stages III and IV. It stains normal fetal and adult melanocytes in the epidermis, benign nevi and melanoma, as well as areas of melanosome transfer such as the basal layer of the epidermis [14]. Therefore, this stain would appear useful for in situ melanomas. The specificity was found to be better than S100 but less than HMB-45 [14]. An increase in specificity generally correlates with a decrease in background staining. In a large study of 200 patients (158 LM, 42 LM melanoma), with both primary and recurrent tumors, Mel-5 immunostaining was utilized resulting in a 99.5% cure rate over a 38.4 follow-up period. This method added 40 additional minutes per stage, with half the time required if an autostainer was utilized [26].

In a study comparing MART-1, HMB-45, Mel-5, and S-100, 68 patients with melanoma (46 MIS, 22 MM) underwent MMS. MART-1 was found to be the most crisp with regular staining of basilar epithelial cells and easily interpretable stain with 96% of tumors staining positively. While S100 stained 100% of tumors positive, it had increased background staining making it difficult to interpret. Interestingly, in this study, only 50% of patients with MIS cleared with margins of </= 6 mm, while 96% cleared with 15 mm margins [14]. This is triple that of the wide local excision margins recommended currently for MIS, highlighting the benefits of MMS and immunostaining. Another study concluded with similar results in regard to the superiority of MART-1, with HMB-45 and S100 failing to recognize melanocytic proliferations in certain cases [27].

MITF, microphthalmia transcription factor, is a phosphorylation target in the Steel/c-kit signaling pathway. Stimulation of c-Kit results in MAP kinase–mediated phosphorylation of MITF producing transcriptional superactivation [28]. It is a transcription factor of the tyrosinase gene and is involved in development, survival, and differentiation of melanocytes [29]. MITF demonstrates nuclear staining, compared to stains such as HMB-45 or S-100 which are more cytoplasmic or diffuse. In one study of 76 patients (19 MIS, 50 MM, 7 metastatic melanoma), MITF stained 100% of melanomas on FFPES, including the amelanotic variant, while HMB-45 staining and S100 were 91% and 93% positive, respectively. The authors summarize that the nuclear staining pattern is useful as it helps reduce the background staining as well as diminish architectural changes (Fig. 15.5) [28].

Recently, a 35-min protocol for MITF on FS was made possible with the elimination of the surfactant in the buffer and use of diaminobenzidine hydrochloride and Giemsa counterstaining. The group compared FFPES to FS of sun-damaged and MIS specimens stained with MITF and MART-1. They found no difference in nuclear diameter or density between frozen and permanent sections for MITF, but did find a decrease in melanocytic density on FS compared to MART-1 from previously published data by the same group using FS material. They concluded that while it was a useful stain due to the nuclear staining pattern, allowing for easier identification of the melanocytes, they prefer to use the MITF stain concomitantly with the MART-1 stain [30].

Summary: Basal Cell and Squamous Cell Carcinoma

- Basal cell carcinoma (BCC) and squamous cell carcinoma (SCC) are easily recognized in frozen section with H & E or toluidine blue during Mohs, but in cases where there is extensive inflammation, fibrosis, or perineural and muscle invasion, immunostaining may be necessary to locate residual tumor.
- Cytokeratin stains, such as AE1/AE3, can be used to identify epidermal-derived tumor cells within the background of stromal cells and collagen.
- Cytokeratin immunostains generally stain both BCC and SCC, while Ber-EP4 staining is mostly for BCC.

15.4 Basal Cell and Squamous Cell Carcinoma

Determination of margins of resection of basal cell carcinoma (BCC) and squamous cell carcinoma (SCC) with Mohs is generally straightforward and based entirely on H & E staining on FS material. In a 2001 survey, dermatologic surgeons reported the use of H & E in 87% of BCC and 95% of SCC, and toluidine blue was used for 13% of BCC and 5% of SCC [31].

There may be, however, a role for FS immunostaining in difficult or indeterminate cases (Fig. 15.6). In a study of 400 patients with both BCCs and SCCs, 36 frozen sections were deemed difficult to interpret due to a dense inflammation, perineural invasion, or subtle morpheaform infiltration. The authors utilized the broad-spectrum antibody cytokeratin AE1/AE3 and cytokeratin 14 to assist in determination of margins. The processing time took an hour, but they found it useful in identification of morpheaform cords of tumor and perineural infiltration; furthermore, it was particularly useful in unmasking the tumor from the dense inflammation [32].

Immunostains commonly used for BCCs and SCCs include cytokeratin (CK) stains and Ber-EP4. Cytokeratins are intermediate-filament protein polymers that are present in nearly all animal cells. They are responsible for maintenance, communication between adjacent epithelial cells, and protection from trauma [29, 33]. Currently, there are 20 CKs, classified by their molecular weight or pH. Cytokeratin 9–20 are Type 1, acidic keratins that are encoded by chromosome 17q12–21, and CK 1–8 are Type 2, basic keratins regulated by genes located on chromosome 12q11–13 [33]. Cytokeratin antibodies are useful in differentiating between epidermal and mesodermal tumor cells [29]. BCCs express CK 5, 14, 15, and 17, and SCCs express 5, 6, 8, 14, 17, and 18 [6]. The CKs that immunostain AE1 detects are high molecular weight (HMW) CK 10, 14, 15, 16 and low molecular weight (LMW) CK 19; while AE3 detects HMW CK 1, 2, 3, 4, 5, 6 and LMW CK 7 and 8 [2, 6]. Combining AE1 and AE3 will help stain most SCCs and BCCs regardless of depth and differentiation, as the keratin expression is still present [2].

The initial studies with cytokeratin immunostaining for Mohs conducted in the mid 1980s were promising, but the processing, took several hours [4]. A 1-h protocol was developed years later utilizing AE1. Twenty patients with extensive, recurrent, or aggressive SCC underwent MMS. In the final stage, all slides were confirmed negative by H & E and underwent staining with AE1. Eight of twenty patients were found to have tumor hidden in either dense inflammation or perineural/muscle invasion. The authors noted that because adnexal structures are also cytokeratin positive, they can be a source of confusion when interpreting margins [34]. In another study, the AE1/AE3 immunostaining protocol was shortened to only 19 min. The results in FS were comparable to permanent sections stained with H & E and AE1/AE3. The authors found that cytokeratin immunostaining was particularly useful in areas of dense inflammation and perineural involvement, and avoided unnecessary additional layers and time [2]. An anticytokeratin stain, MNF116, which detects CK 5, 6, 8, 17, and 19, along with p63, may be helpful in cases of poorly differentiated SCCs that present with an atypical, infiltrative single-cell pattern. In one study, MNF116-stained slides were also compared to matched H & E "cleared" slides. Only 1 of 143 slides was mismatched, a recurrent aggressive growth BCC, which stained positive for MNF 116 while negative for H & E. They concluded that H & E is sufficient for the majority of BCC, but cytokeratin immunostaining may be a useful adjunctive for more aggressive subtypes of tumor [35]. Another possible use for cytokeratin staining may be for Mohs in patients with hematological malignancies such as chronic lymphocytic leukemia (CLL). Due to the

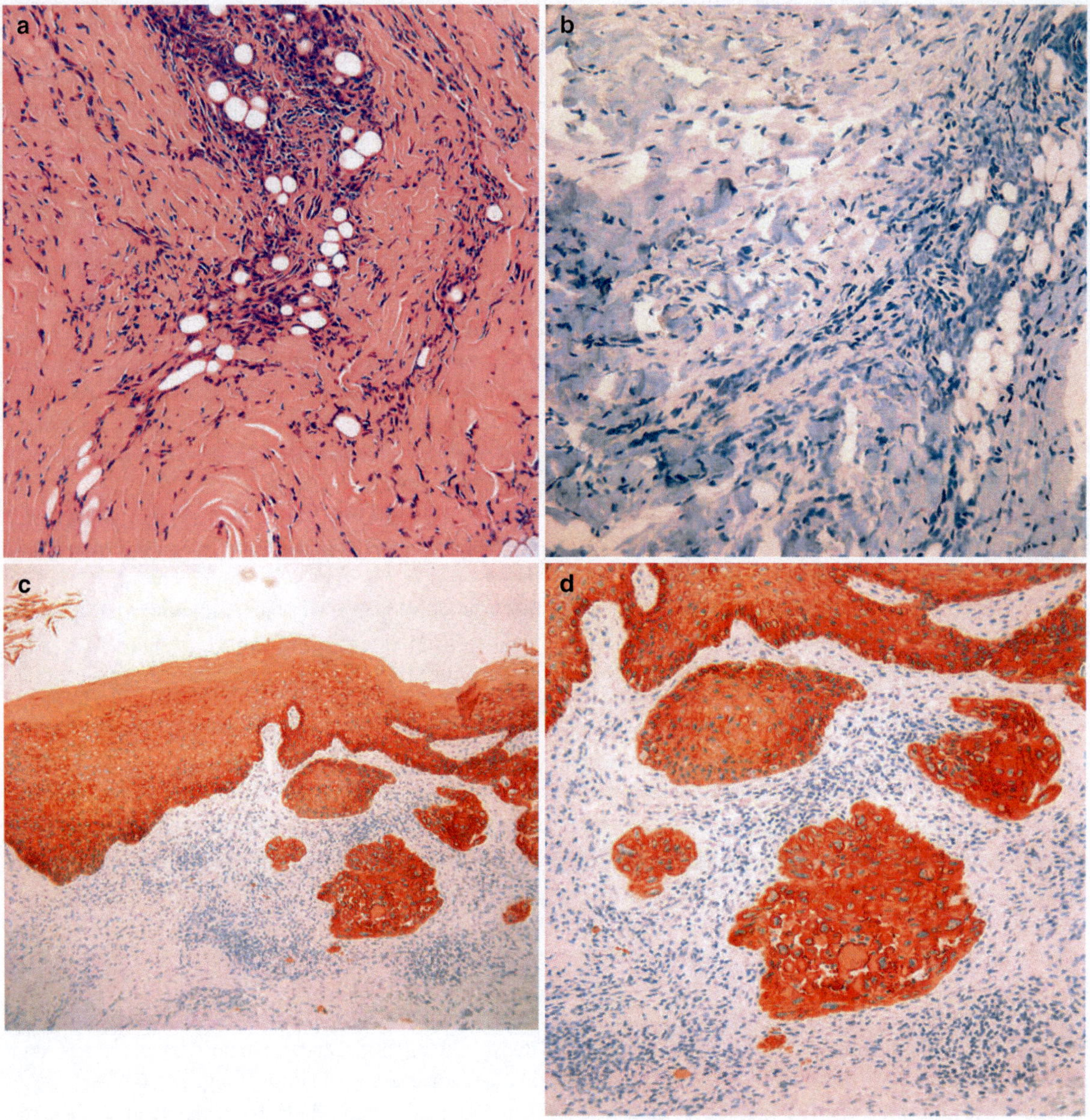

Fig. 15.6 (**a**) H & E–stained frozen section of a margin during Mohs surgery for BCC with scar tissue and dense inflammation within the panniculus that could mask tumor cells (40×). (**b**) Frozen section stained with AE1/AE3 CK immunostain confirms that no tumor is buried within the infiltrate (40×), indicating a negative margin for basal cell carcinoma. In the control specimen, AE1/AE3 CK immunostaining demonstrates lobules of tumor within the dermis in frozen section at (**c**) 10× and (**d**) 20× magnification

abundant leukemic infiltrate, it may be difficult to find the tumor [36].

Ber-EP4, a monoclonal antibody directed against two 34 kDa and 39 kDa glycopeptide chains, stains BCC but not SCC [37]. It is expressed in all normal epithelial tissues, preferentially at the basement membrane in a basolateral location, in both cutaneous and noncutaneous tumors [37]. It also stains adnexal epithelium, such as eccrine and apocrine glands and ducts, and the base of the hair bulb, but does not stain the keratinocytes of the remainder of the follicular unit [38]. In one study, 43 cases of BCCs and SCCs were stained with Ber-EP4, and Ber-EP4 was positive in all of the BCCs, regardless of differentiation, while staining none of the SCCs. In addition, the authors noted that the general lack of hair follicle staining was useful in differentiating certain hair follicles that may otherwise be confused with a BCC [38].

Some authors found Ber-EP4 useful in unmasking tumors surrounded by inflammation. In one study, 27 slides of BCCs were stained with H & E and Ber-EP4. All slides stained with Ber-EP4, and 13/27 slides provided an enhanced view of the tumor compared to H & E. In addition, 2 of 27 slides revealed a morpheaform BCC while the H & E interpretation was negative [39]. Conversely, a group found that the use of Ber-EP4 actually resulted in cases of overdiagnosis of BCC where there were dense inflammatory infiltrates. They found that in 48% of cases that were Ber-EP4 positive, no tumor could be identified when the slides were reviewed. In fact, when tumors were surrounded by dense inflammation, the tumors could be revealed by deeper sections. Infiltrative BCC were found to be most closely associated with dense infiltrates (73%), while nodular BCC were least associated (30%). Because the authors were able to detect all cases of tumor surrounded by dense inflammation with deeper H & E sections, it was concluded that Ber-EP4 was not necessary in "unmasking" the tumor [40].

While Ber-EP4 stains primarily the base of the hair bulb, many authors have detected "patchy" staining in other portions, making it difficult to distinguish BCC from folliculocentric basaloid proliferation (FBP) [39–41]. One study explored the use of monoclonal anti-desmoglein antibody, 33–3D, which recognizes the cytoplasmic domain of desmoglein, which is conducted in a 60-min protocol. In 18 biopsy-proven BCC patients where it was difficult to differentiate FBP from BCC, the 33–3D stain was utilized. In 4/18 patients, the perimembranous staining pattern typical of normal follicles was absent and instead revealed a confluent cytoplasmic staining pattern leading the authors to take another layer. A follow-up period of 6–24 months resulted in no recurrence [41].

Differentiating BCC from trichoepithelioma (TE) is also a diagnostic challenge. Both tumors are comprised of basaloid strands of epithelium embedded in fibrocellular stroma. BCC is associated with characteristic peripheral palisading, stromal retraction, and an increased mitotic rate, among other diagnostic findings, while trichoepithelioma is more lobular and associated with papillary mesenchymal bodies. Twenty cases each of BCC and TE were stained with the immunostains Bcl-2, p53, Ki67, and PCNA. Bcl-2 and p53 were not useful in differentiating both tumors, while Ki67 and PCNA demonstrated more diffuse and frequent staining in BCC and less frequent and peripheral staining of TEs [42].

Summary: Dermatofibrosarcoma Protuberans

- Dermatofibrosarcoma protuberans (DFSP) is a locally aggressive fibrohistiocytic tumor with a high recurrence rate following wide local excision.
- CD34 is commonly used to differentiate DFSP from dermatofibroma, keloids, and sarcomas such as malignant fibrous histiocytoma and atypical fibroxanthoma. It is used in Mohs to find the edge of the DFSP for margin assessment.

15.5 Dermatofibrosarcoma Protuberans

Dermatofibrosarcoma protuberans (DFSP) is a locally aggressive fibrohistiocytic sarcoma that accounts for approximately 0.1% of all malignancies [43]. This tumor can be a challenge to remove because it can have projections of tumor that can extend in all directions at the periphery, between collagen bundles, and even invading muscle and fascia. This tumor has recurrence rates as high as 43–50% after wide local excision [43, 44]. MMS may provide an opportunity for tissue sparing, while identifying areas of extension. Recurrence rates in the literature after MMS have been reported to be 0–6.6% [43, 45].

CD34 immunostaining may be helping in discerning tumor margins in difficult cases of DFSP. CD34 is a 115 kDa single chain transmembrane glycoprotein found on normal human hematopoietic progenitor cells, endothelial cells, and a characteristic population of dermal dendritic cells [46, 47]. It is a helpful stain in differentiating DFSP from dermatofibroma (DF), malignant fibrous histiocytoma (MFH), atypical fibroxanthoma (AFX), and keloids. The sensitivity of utilizing CD34 in some reports for FFPES is 84–100%, as authors have found it does not uniformly stain all DFSP, and on occasion can stain DFs leading to false positives [44].

An anti-CD34 mouse monoclonal antibody immunostain was reportedly utilized in MMS in a difficult case in order to discern the tumor from the adjacent stroma to provide reassurance that the margins were negative. The authors recommended that a positive control, such as tissue from the first stage, be used initially to determine CD34 positivity [47]. Interestingly, in another case where the FFPES was negative for CD34, the frozen section slide revealed strong positive staining. The authors caution that while it is a useful stain, there is considerable variability of staining for CD34, therefore recommending that CD34 negative slides be sent for paraffin-embedded sections as well [46].

Summary: Extramammary Paget's Disease

- Extramammary Paget's disease (EMPD) is an adenocarcinoma usually located in the skin of the anogenital and axillary region.
- Complete excision of EMPD may be difficult, and despite numerous surgical procedures and significant morbidity, the recurrence rate is still high.
- CK7 and CEA are useful markers during MMS for EMPD and differentiate Paget's cells from atypical keratinocytes and melanocytes.

15.6 Extramammary Paget's Disease

Extramammary Paget's disease (EMPD) is a rare cutaneous adenocarcinoma with potential for metastases. It is associated with the apocrine glands and is found primarily in the anogenital or axillary area [48]. Paget's cells, usually restricted to the epidermis, are large, vacuolated cells with pale staining cytoplasm and a central or laterally displaced large reticulated nucleus [48, 49]. Radical surgeries such as local excision, wide local excision, vulvectomy, or abdominoperineal resection are associated with increased morbidity. Despite these sometimes disfiguring surgeries, recurrence rates following these procedures may still be as high as 31–61% [50, 51]. In some cases, EMPD can be difficult to differentiate from a squamous cell – in situ or melanoma histologically [52].

In 1979, Frederic Mohs reported the use of his fresh tissue technique for the treatment of EMPD. He studied five cases, four of which utilized the fresh tissue technique and one utilized the fixed tissue technique. Three of the fresh tissue cases were recurrent and one was newly diagnosed. All showed no signs of recurrences with follow-ups ranging from 4 months to 4 years; consequently, he concluded that the ability to visualize 100% of the margins through his technique provided a reliable alternative to radical surgery to allow for tissue sparing. In addition, he noted that Paget's cells in the adnexal structures should not be considered invasive malignancy [49].

Subsequent studies have shown that recurrence after MMS for EMPD has been at least 23%, compared to 33% for standard surgical excision [51]. One study noted that the recurrence rate for primary and recurrent tumors is 16% and 50%, respectively. The average margin required to clear 97% of patients in this study was 5 cm [50]. The mean time to recurrence after MMS has been reported to be 2.5 years; therefore, long-term monitoring of the patient is necessary to assess efficacy [51].

Paget's cells can stain with carcinoembryonic antigen (CEA), epithelial membrane antibody (EMA), gross cystic disease fluid protein (GCDFP), and LMW cytokeratins such as CK 7, 8, 18, and 19 [48, 52]. These cytokeratins are found in the simple and glandular nonstratified squamous epithelium of eccrine and apocrine structures [52]. In a study conducted on EMPD and mammary Paget's disease patients, FFPES were stained with CK7, CK20, carcinoembryonic antigen (CEA), Ber-EP4, and CAM 5.2 (CK 8 and 18). Anti-CK 7 was found to be the most sensitive stain and produced the strongest staining in each case with the lowest amount of background staining [52].

CK7 was also studied on FS in 4/12 patients, while CEA was used in two of these four patients treated with MMS [48]. The investigators reported that CK7 is the intraoperative immunostain of choice, but cautioned that distinguishing between an ordinary eccrine coil and dermal EMPD can be difficult. It may be prudent to send tissue from the debulking layer during MMS for FFPES preparation and CK immunostaining for confirmation. It should be noted, however, that one of the four patients enrolled in the study went on to have a local recurrence in 1 year [48].

Another marker found in eccrine and apocrine glands is CEA, which also has been shown to be sensitive and specific in differentiating Paget's cell from keratinocytes or melanocytes. It may be difficult to distinguish Paget's disease from Bowen's disease. CEA immunostaining was utilized in a patient with EMPD with adjacent keratinocytic intraepidermal dysplasia. Negative staining in keratinocytes and melanocytes and variable cytoplasmic staining intensity in the

Paget's cell compared to more uniform cytoplasmic staining for the normal eccrine and apocrine glands established the diagnosis of Paget's disease [53].

Summary: Other Rare Tumors

- Granular cell tumor (GCT) is a benign neural tumor that may rarely become malignant with the possibility of metastases.
- S100 is an immunostain useful during MMS for detecting granular cell tumor, especially through the proper identification of perineural extension.
- Primary mucinous carcinoma (PMC) is a sweat gland tumor that can be identified in FS with low molecular weight cytokeratin (LMW CK).
- Trichilemmal carcinoma (TC), an adnexal tumor that in rare cases can demonstrate local invasion, can be detected by Cytokeratin 17 (CK 17) staining in difficult cases.

15.7 Other Rare Tumors

15.7.1 Granular Cell Tumor

Granular cell tumors (GCT) are rare soft tissue tumors of neural origin, likely derived from Schwann cells [54, 55]. The majority of these tumors are benign, while 1–3% can become malignant, with a possibility of metastases [54, 55]. Histologically, the cells have a granular cytoplasm with small, round, centrally located basophilic nuclei [56]. An aggressive tumor is identified by increased mitosis, necrosis, and spindling of the cells [56]. If excised with adequate margins, the recurrence rate ranges from 2% to 8% [54, 56].

MMS has been utilized for the treatment of GCT and is especially helpful in determining perineural involvement. In 2002, a group reported the use of the S-100 immunostain on FS material during MMS, as this antigen is expressed in the nucleus and cytoplasm of granular cells [57]. Later studies reported similar findings, where the use of S100 compared to H & E staining was particularly beneficial in preventing additional unnecessary layers due to the proper identification of perineural extension [56, 57].

15.7.2 Primary Mucinous Carcinoma

Primary Mucinous Carcinoma (PMC) is an extremely rare sweat gland tumor, possibly related to the eccrine secretory coils [58]. Cutaneous metastases from a visceral adenocarcinoma would have similar histology, and although it would be extremely uncommon, it would be imperative to exclude the possibility. Histologically, it is characterized by pools of pale-staining mucin surrounding islands of basaloid nests which can have duct-like differentiation with dark and pale cells [58, 59]. PMC is a locally recurrent tumor (27%); however, it can rarely present with regional and distant metastases of 11% and 3%, respectively [59]. MMS was reported for the treatment of PMC in a few cases in the literature, and patients were found to have no recurrences in the 2–5 year follow-up period [59, 60].

PMC has stained positively on FFPES with LMW CK and epithelial membrane antigen (EMA), while CEA and S100 are variable [58, 61]. One study utilized the immunostains LMW CK, pan-keratin, EMA, CEA, and a vimentin-specific monoclonal antibody during MMS for the treatment of PMC. The authors found that the LMW CK immunostain stained strongly positive, while EMA was weakly positive. CEA and vimentin immunostains were negative. They concluded that LMW CK, which labels the nonsquamous epithelium, not the neural tissue or mesenchyme, is a useful stain when residual tumor is difficult to identify on H & E. The patient was reported to be tumor free for the 3-year follow-up period [58].

15.7.3 Trichilemmal Carcinoma

Trichilemmal carcinoma (TC) is a rare adnexal cutaneous malignancy that is not generally associated with perineural spread or vascular invasion. However, one study reported the utility of MMS with immunostaining for a rare case that recurred many times and demonstrated perineural extension. They employed CK 17, CK 15, and c-erb-B2 immunostains and found strong cytoplasmic staining on FS material with CK17 and c-erb-B2. CK17 is typically expressed in the outer root sheath (ORS) of hair follicles, while CK 15 is normally expressed in the bulge area of the ORS. The authors suggested that since TC can demonstrate follicular ORS differentiation, CK 17 is a helpful immunostain in identifying TCs during MMS. They noted that since not all follicular ORS produce CK 15, it may be negative. C-erb-15 was found to be a stain that correlated with aggressive behavior [62].

Summary: Conclusions

- Immunostaining is an adjunctive technique for MOHs micrographics surgery that is helpful in determining tumor extension when it is unclear with H & E stained frozen sections due to inflammation, fibrosis, or muscle and nerve invasion.

15.8 Conclusions

MMS has been utilized for a variety of cutaneous tumors especially in cosmetically sensitive areas, and in particular, tumors with ill-defined extensions into the surrounding tissue and recurrent tumors. Immunostaining has been a helpful adjunct in many cases on FS to determine the extent of the tumor, when this assessment would be difficult, if not impossible to accomplish with routine H & E. It results in smaller margins of resection and less recurrences, which is likely to reduce health care costs associated with managing recurrences. In a study conducted in 2001, 13 of 108 (12%) laboratories were utilizing immunostains on frozen sections [31]. However, with new protocols with faster processing times reported in the literature, increased cost-effectiveness, as well as enhanced familiarity with the technique, immunostaining will likely be more widely used by dermatologic surgeons in the future.

References

1. Drake LA et al. Guidelines of care for Mohs micrographic surgery. American Academy of Dermatology. J Am Acad Dermatol. 1995;33(2 Pt 1):271–8.
2. Cherpelis BS et al. Innovative 19-minute rapid cytokeratin immunostaining of nonmelanoma skin cancer in Mohs micrographic surgery. Dermatol Surg. 2009;35(7):1050–6.
3. Lane JE, Kent DE. Surgical margins in the treatment of nonmelanoma skin cancer and Mohs micrographic surgery. Curr Surg. 2005;62(5):518–26.
4. Robinson JK, Gottschalk R. Immunofluorescent and immunoperoxidase staining of antibodies to fibrous keratin. Improved sensitivity for detecting epidermal cancer cells. Arch Dermatol. 1984;120(2):199–203.
5. Maize J, BW, Hurt M, LeBoit P, Metcalf, J, Smith T, Solomon A. Cutaneous Pathology. Philadelphia: Churchill Livingstone; 1998.
6. El Tal AK et al. Immunostaining in Mohs micrographic surgery: a review. Dermatol Surg. 2010;36(3):275–90.
7. Bricca GM, Brodland DG, Zitelli JA. Immunostaining melanoma frozen sections: the 1-hour protocol. Dermatol Surg. 2004;30(3):403–8.
8. Mondragon RM, Barrett TL. Current concepts: the use of immunoperoxidase techniques in Mohs micrographic surgery. J Am Acad Dermatol. 2000;43(1 Pt 1):66–71.
9. Zitelli JA, Brown C, Hanusa BH. Mohs micrographic surgery for the treatment of primary cutaneous melanoma. J Am Acad Dermatol. 1997;37(2 Pt 1):236–45.
10. Griego RD, Zitelli JA. Mohs micrographic surgery using HMB-45 for a recurrent acral melanoma. Dermatol Surg. 1998;24(9):1003–6.
11. Zitelli JA, Moy RL, Abell E. The reliability of frozen sections in the evaluation of surgical margins for melanoma. J Am Acad Dermatol. 1991;24(1):102–6.
12. Cohen LM et al. Successful treatment of lentigo maligna and lentigo maligna melanoma with Mohs' micrographic surgery aided by rush permanent sections. Cancer. 1994;73(12): 2964–70.
13. Gross EA, Andersen WK, Rogers GS. Mohs micrographic excision of lentigo maligna using Mel-5 for margin control. Arch Dermatol. 1999;135(1):15–7.
14. Zalla MJ et al. Mohs micrographic excision of melanoma using immunostains. Dermatol Surg. 2000;26(8):771–84.
15. Kelley LC, Starkus L. Immunohistochemical staining of lentigo maligna during Mohs micrographic surgery using MART-1. J Am Acad Dermatol. 2002;46(1):78–84.
16. Ohsie SJ et al. Immunohistochemical characteristics of melanoma. J Cutan Pathol. 2008;35(5):433–44.
17. Thosani MK, Marghoob A, Chen CS. Current progress of immunostains in Mohs micrographic surgery: a review. Dermatol Surg. 2008;34(12):1621–36.
18. El Shabrawi-Caelen L, Kerl H, Cerroni L. Melan-A: not a helpful marker in distinction between melanoma in situ on sun-damaged skin and pigmented actinic keratosis. Am J Dermatopathol. 2004;26(5):364–6.
19. Hendi A, Brodland DG, Zitelli JA. Melanocytes in long-standing sun-exposed skin: quantitative analysis using the MART-1 immunostain. Arch Dermatol. 2006;142(7): 871–6.
20. Maize Jr JC et al. Ducking stray "magic bullets": a Melan-A alert. Am J Dermatopathol. 2003;25(2):162–5.
21. Geisse JK. Re: Questionable utility of Melan-A/Mart-1 immunoperoxidase staining while doing Mohs surgery for melanoma. Dermatol Surg. 2005;31(4):495.
22. Cherpelis BS et al. Comparison of MART-1 frozen sections to permanent sections using a rapid 19-minute protocol. Dermatol Surg. 2009;35(2):207–13.
23. Kikuchi A, Shimizu H, Nishikawa T. Expression and ultrastructural localization of HMB-45 antigen. Br J Dermatol. 1996;135(3):400–5.
24. Menaker GM et al. Rapid HMB-45 staining in Mohs micrographic surgery for melanoma in situ and invasive melanoma. J Am Acad Dermatol. 2001;44(5):833–6.

25. Skelton HG et al. HMB45 negative spindle cell malignant melanoma. Am J Dermatopathol. 1997;19(6):580–4.
26. Bhardwaj SS, Tope WD, Lee PK. Mohs micrographic surgery for lentigo maligna and lentigo maligna melanoma using Mel-5 immunostaining: University of Minnesota experience. Dermatol Surg. 2006;32(5):690–6; discussion 696–7.
27. Albertini JG et al. Mohs micrographic surgery for melanoma: a case series, a comparative study of immunostains, an informative case report, and a unique mapping technique. Dermatol Surg. 2002;28(8):656–65.
28. King R et al. Microphthalmia transcription factor. A sensitive and specific melanocyte marker for melanoma diagnosis. Am J Pathol. 1999;155(3):731–8.
29. Stranahan D et al. Immunohistochemical stains in Mohs surgery: a review. Dermatol Surg. 2009;35(7):1023–34.
30. Glass LF et al. Rapid frozen section immunostaining of melanocytes by microphthalmia-associated transcription factor. Am J Dermatopathol. 2010;32(4):319–25.
31. Robinson JK. Current histologic preparation methods for Mohs micrographic surgery. Dermatol Surg. 2001;27(6):555–60.
32. Jimenez FJ et al. Immunohistochemical techniques in Mohs micrographic surgery: their potential use in the detection of neoplastic cells masked by inflammation. J Am Acad Dermatol. 1995;32(1):89–94.
33. Jacques C, de Aquino AM, Ramos-e-Silva M. Cytokeratins and dermatology. Skinmed. 2005;4(6):354–60; quiz 360–1.
34. Zachary CB et al. Rapid cytokeratin stains enhance the sensitivity of Mohs micrographic surgery for squamous cell carcinoma. J Dermatol Surg Oncol. 1994;20(8):530–5.
35. Smeets NW et al. Adjuvant cytokeratin staining in Mohs micrographic surgery for basal cell carcinoma. Dermatol Surg. 2003;29(4):375–7.
36. Albregts T et al. Squamous cell carcinoma in a patient with chronic lymphocytic leukemia. An intraoperative diagnostic challenge for the Mohs surgeon. Dermatol Surg. 1998;24(2):269–72.
37. Latza U et al. Ber-EP4: new monoclonal antibody which distinguishes epithelia from mesothelial. J Clin Pathol. 1990;43(3):213–9.
38. Tellechea O et al. Monoclonal antibody Ber EP4 distinguishes basal-cell carcinoma from squamous-cell carcinoma of the skin. Am J Dermatopathol. 1993;15(5):452–5.
39. Kist D et al. Anti-human epithelial antigen (Ber-EP4) helps define basal cell carcinoma masked by inflammation. Dermatol Surg. 1997;23(11):1067–70.
40. Katz KH et al. Dense inflammation does not mask residual primary basal cell carcinoma during Mohs micrographic surgery. J Am Acad Dermatol. 2001;45(2):231–8.
41. Krunic AL et al. The use of antidesmoglein stains in Mohs micrographic surgery. A potential aid for the differentiation of basal cell carcinoma from horizontal sections of the hair follicle and folliculocentric basaloid proliferation. Dermatol Surg. 1997;23(6):463–8.
42. Abdelsayed RA et al. Immunohistochemical evaluation of basal cell carcinoma and trichepithelioma using Bcl-2, Ki67, PCNA and P53. J Cutan Pathol. 2000;27(4):169–75.
43. Gloster HM, Harris Jr KR, Roenigk RK. A comparison between Mohs micrographic surgery and wide surgical excision for the treatment of dermatofibrosarcoma protuberans. J Am Acad Dermatol. 1996;35(1):82–7.
44. Haycox CL et al. Immunohistochemical characterization of dermatofibrosarcoma protuberans with practical applications for diagnosis and treatment. J Am Acad Dermatol. 1997;37(3 Pt 1):438–44.
45. Roh MR, Bae B, Chung KY. Mohs' micrographic surgery for dermatofibrosarcoma protuberans. Clin Exp Dermatol. 2010;35:849–52.
46. Garcia C et al. Dermatofibrosarcoma protuberans treated with Mohs surgery. A case with CD34 immunostaining variability. Dermatol Surg. 1996;22(2):177–9.
47. Jimenez FJ et al. Immunohistochemical margin control applied to Mohs micrographic surgical excision of dermatofibrosarcoma protuberans. J Dermatol Surg Oncol. 1994;20(10):687–9.
48. O'Connor WJ et al. Comparison of Mohs micrographic surgery and wide excision for extramammary Paget's disease. Dermatol Surg. 2003;29(7):723–7.
49. Mohs FE, Blanchard L. Microscopically controlled surgery for extramammary Paget's disease. Arch Dermatol. 1979;115(6):706–8.
50. Hendi A, Brodland DG, Zitelli JA. Extramammary Paget's disease: surgical treatment with Mohs micrographic surgery. J Am Acad Dermatol. 2004;51(5):767–73.
51. Coldiron BM, Goldsmith BA, Robinson JK. Surgical treatment of extramammary Paget's disease. Cancer. 1991;67(4):933–8.
52. Smith KJ et al. Cytokeratin 7 staining in mammary and extramammary Paget's disease. Mod Pathol. 1997;10(11):1069–74.
53. Harris DW et al. Rapid staining with carcinoembryonic antigen aids limited excision of extramammary Paget's disease treated by Mohs surgery. J Dermatol Surg Oncol. 1994;20(4):260–4.
54. Chilukuri S, Peterson SR, Goldberg LH. Granular cell tumor of the heel treated with Mohs technique. Dermatol Surg. 2004;30(7):1046–9.
55. Gardner ES, Goldberg LH. Granular cell tumor treated with Mohs micrographic surgery: report of a case and review of the literature. Dermatol Surg. 2001;27(8):772–4.
56. Abraham T et al. Mohs surgical treatment of a granular cell tumor on the toe of a child. Pediatr Dermatol. 2007;24(3):235–7.
57. Smith SB et al. Mohs micrographic surgery for granular cell tumor using S-100 immunostain. Dermatol Surg. 2002;28(11):1076–8.
58. Marra DE, Schanbacher CF, Torres A. Mohs micrographic surgery of primary cutaneous mucinous carcinoma using immunohistochemistry for margin control. Dermatol Surg. 2004;30(5):799–802.
59. Ortiz KJ et al. A case of primary mucinous carcinoma of the scalp treated with Mohs surgery. Dermatol Surg. 2002;28(8):751–4;discussion 754.
60. Cecchi R, Rapicano V. Primary cutaneous mucinous carcinoma: report of two cases treated with Mohs' micrographic surgery. Australas J Dermatol. 2006;47(3):192–4.
61. Bellezza G, Sidoni A, Bucciarelli E. Primary mucinous carcinoma of the skin. Am J Dermatopathol. 2000;22(2):166–70.
62. Allee JE et al. Multiply recurrent trichilemmal carcinoma with perineural invasion and cytokeratin 17 positivity. Dermatol Surg. 2003;29(8):886–9.

Basal Cell Carcinoma

16

Michael P. McLeod, Sonal Choudhary,
Yasser A. Alqubaisy, and Keyvan Nouri

Abstract

BCC is the most common neoplasm encountered in humans. It is also the most common indication for Mohs micrographic surgery (MMS). MMS has a 99% 5-year cure rate for primary BCCs. For recurrent BCCs, the 5-year cure rate is 96%. Infiltrating, micronodular, and morpheaform subtypes are considered more aggressive forms of BCC, and MMS should be the primary treatment for those subtypes. Inflammatory cells, hair follicles, and folliculocentric basaloid proliferations are benign conditions that can resemble BCC when using horizontal frozen sections. Malignant processes such as metastatic breast cancer, ameloblastoma, cloacogenic carcinoma, eccrine spiradenoma, pilomatricomas, and trichoepitheliomas can also mimic BCC. Additionally, BCC may differentiate to simulate many structures such as hair follicles, sweat glands, and sebaceous glands. The evidence behind MMS for BCC is strong with studies backed by a high number of patients along with very low recurrence rates. It is especially well suited for aggressive histological subtypes of BCC and for BCCs in anatomical regions where tissue conservation is paramount.

Keywords

Basal cell carcinoma • Mohs micrographic surgery • Nodular BCC • Superficial BCC • Morpheaform BCC • Infiltrative BCC • Folliculocentric basaloid proliferations

M.P. McLeod • S. Choudhary
Department of Dermatology and Cutaneous Surgery, University of Miami Leonard M. Miller School of Medicine, Miami, FL, USA

Y.A. Alqubaisy
Department of Dermatology and Cutaneous Surgery, University of Miami Hospital, Miami, FL, USA

K. Nouri (✉)
Department of Dermatology and Cutaneous Surgery, University of Miami Leonard M. Miller School of Medicine, Miami, FL, USA

Sylvester Comprehensive Cancer Center, University of Miami Hospital and Clinics, Miami, FL, USA
e-mail: knouri@med.miami.edu

Summary: Introduction

- Basal cell carcinoma (BCC) is the most common malignant neoplasm found in humans.
- Approximately 800,000 new cases of BCC are diagnosed in the USA per annum.
- Mohs micrographic surgery (MMS) has a 99% 5-year cure rate for primary BCCs and a 96% 5-year cure rate for recurrent BCCs.

K. Nouri (ed.), *Mohs Micrographic Surgery*,
DOI 10.1007/978-1-4471-2152-7_16,

16.1 Introduction

Basal cell carcinoma (BCC) is the most common malignant process encountered in humans as well as the most common indication for Mohs micrographic surgery (MMS) [1]. In fact, nearly 30% of all BCCs are treated with MMS in the USA [2]. Approximately 800,000 new BCC cases are diagnosed in the USA per year [3]. BCC accounts for approximately 90% of all known skin cancers [4]. Fair skin, sun exposure, immunosuppression, and a low Fitzpatrick skin type are known risk factors for BCC; additionally, the average Caucasian individual has a 30% chance of developing BCC [5]. Individuals with darker skin types are 19 times less likely to develop BCC [6]. As stated in Chap. 2 on General Indications, MMS has a 99% 5-year cure rate for primary tumors and a 96% cure rate with recurrent tumors [7–9].

Summary: Etiology

- The predominant cause of BCC is thought to be an interaction between UVB and DNA resulting in the formation of dipyrimidine dimers in the DNA.
- The dipyrimidine dimers are formed in three genes, PTCH1, SMO, and SHH, and cause the Sonic hedgehog pathway to become constitutively activated.

16.2 Etiology

BCC is thought to occur largely as a result of interactions between UVB and DNA forming DNA pyrimidines [10, 11]. These mutations cause inappropriate activation of the hedgehog signaling pathway so that it becomes constitutively active [12]. Within the hedgehog pathway, these mutations occur in primarily three genes, PTCH1, SMO, and SHH. Mutations leading to PTCH1 inactivation or deletion are believed to occur in 30–60% of sporadic BCCs [13, 14], while mutations in SMO (Smoothened) are thought to account for 10–20% of sporadic BCC. If one combines the mutations in PTCH1 and SMO, they account for 90% of sporadic BCCs [15].

Summary: Histological Findings Using Horizontal Frozen Sections

- BCC tumors are comprised of nests of small, uniform, round basaloid cells.
- BCC usually demonstrates cytologic atypia, mitotic activity, and peripheral palisading.
- Nodular BCC consists of dermal, nodular aggregates of tumor that commonly arises from the epidermis and extends into the epidermis.
- In superficial BCC, the basaloid cells usually only penetrate to the papillary dermis. The tumor tends to have buds which branch in different directions with palisading along the periphery of the tumor.
- In morpheaform BCC, a firm, dense stroma develops, and the basaloid cells are found in the "crevices" of the stroma.
- Infiltrative BCCs have elongated strands of cells only a few layers thick that can deeply invade the tissue.
- Micronodular BCC exhibits micronodules of basaloid tumor cells.
- Adenoid BCCs have tubular or gland-like structures.
- Granular BCCs contain basaloid cells with clear cytoplasm.

16.3 Histological Findings Using Horizontal Frozen Sections

BCC tumors are comprised of nests of small, uniform, and round basaloid cells. In distinction to SCC, the BCC cells are considered more immature in their differentiation and are less eosinophilic in their cytoplasm. BCC usually demonstrates cytologic atypia, mitotic activity, and peripheral palisading. BCCs usually do not demonstrate abnormal mitoses even in rare cases where metastasis occurs. Cystic spaces due to cellular dyshesion as well as necrosis of the tumor may be observed [16]. Mucin has also been noted in the stroma around the nests of BCCs leading to the stromal retraction that is often observed on sectioning (Fig. 16.1). Another characteristic feature is calcification. In rare cases, basaloid cells can be multi-nucleated, exhibit large hyperchromatic nuclei, and demonstrate "starburst" mitoses. Despite these findings, the clinical outcome remains the same as BCCs that do not exhibit these findings [17, 18].

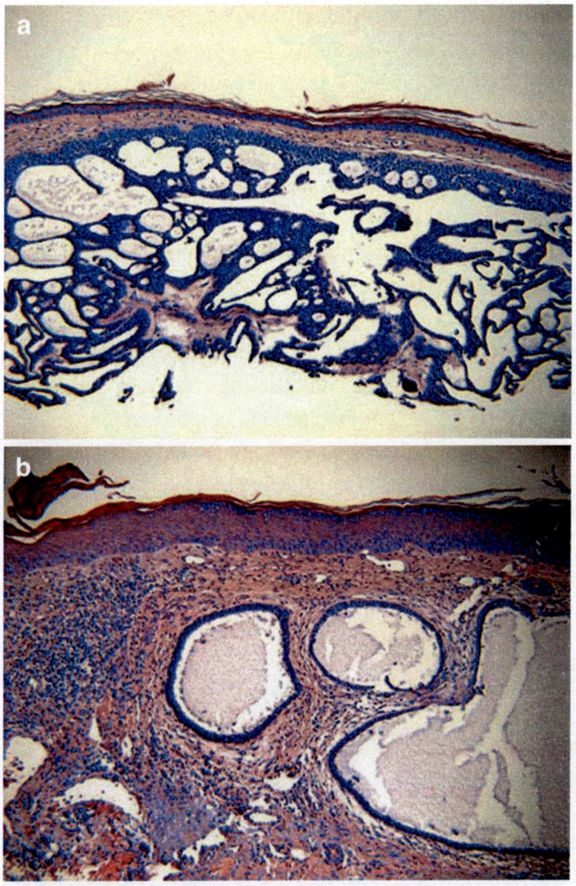

Fig. 16.1 Mucinous BCC (**a**) cystic to reticulated appearing basaloid neoplasm with large sometimes interconnecting spaces in which (**b**) large amounts of mucin can be observed. Courtesy of Dr. Evangelos Badiavas

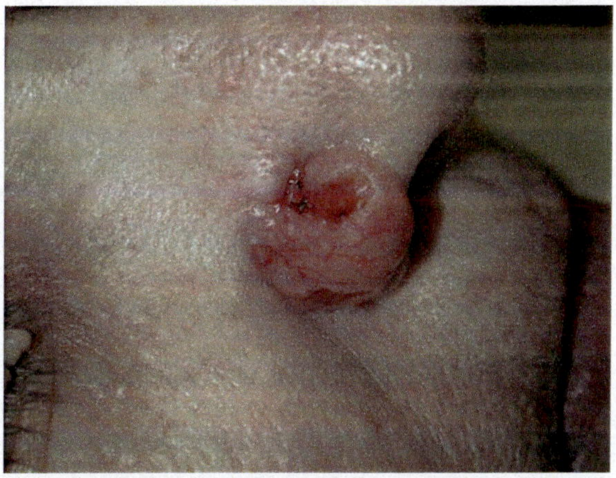

Fig. 16.2 Nodular BCC located on the right nasal ala

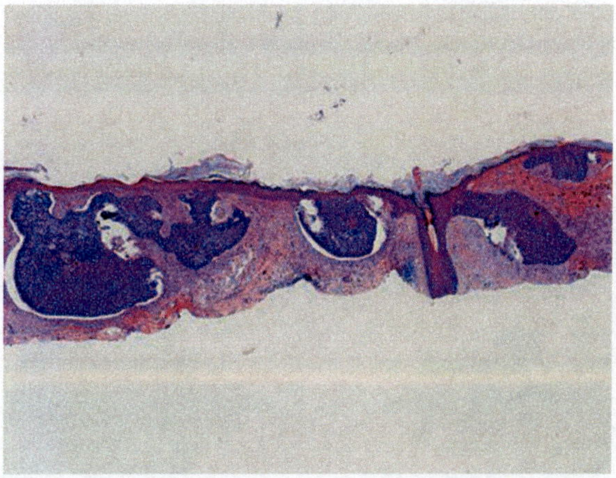

Fig. 16.3 Superficial BCC: Neoplasm extends into the superficial dermis and is multifocal. Larger surface areas can be involved with limited invasion into the mid or deep dermis. Courtesy of Dr. Evangelos Badiavas

There are several histologic subtypes that are often observed when using MMS. BCC is comprised of multiple subtypes, and a biopsy suggesting one subtype does not necessarily mean that a tumor will be entirely comprised of that one subtype.

Nodular BCC consists of nodular aggregates of tumor that commonly arises from the dermis and extends into the epidermis (Fig. 16.2). Clinically, nodular BCC resembles a pearly papule that can be ulcerated or even eroded, and often demonstrates telangiectasia.

In superficial BCC, the basaloid cells only penetrate to the papillary dermis. The tumor tends to have buds, which branch into different directions with palisading along the periphery of the tumor (Fig. 16.3). An inflammatory infiltrate is often observed in the papillary dermis. When viewed under the microscope, it may look as though the different buds are not connected, and the term multifocal has been used to describe the tumor. Indeed, the buds are actually connected and have been described as "net-like." The "net-like" histological morphology can complicate the Mohs procedure, and one has to be careful not to leave a bud outside the margin of sectioning. Clinically, superficial BCC tends to be macular to slightly papular and has an eczematous or scaly appearance.

In morpheaform BCC, a firm, dense stroma develops, and the basaloid cells tend to be found within the "crevices" of the stroma (Fig. 16.4). Morpheaform is less well demarcated than nodular BCC and tends to resemble a flat, yellow plaque. It appears similar to morphea or scleroderma, hence its name. Morpheaform BCC can be associated with significant subclinical spread as the average tumor spread is 7.2 mm outside the clinically observed tumor [19].

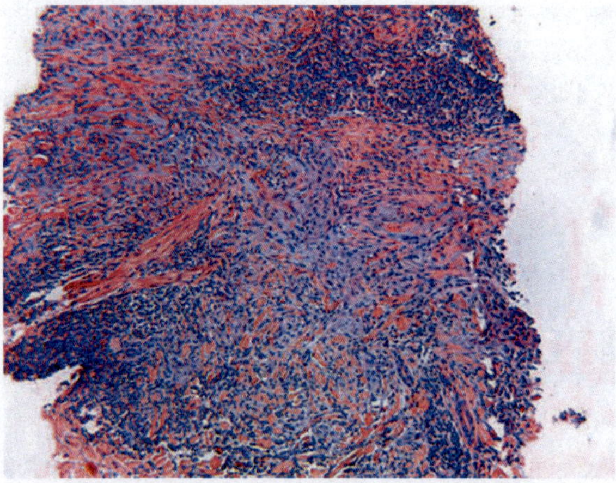

Fig. 16.4 Morpheaform BCC: Strands of basaloid cells extending into a fibrotic dermis and between thickened eosinophilic collagen bundles. The central portion of the neoplasm can often appear more scar-like. Courtesy of Dr. Evangelos Badiavas

Infiltrative BCC typically has elongated strands of cells only a few layers thick that can deeply invade the tissue. There is usually little to no peripheral palisading. This BCC subtype is also known to frequently invade nerves and can also invade bone (Fig. 16.5).

Micronodular BCC usually exhibits micronodules of basaloid tumor cells just as the name implies. Adenoid BCCs have tubular or gland-like structures. The basaloid cells form nodular-appearing structures with a "lace" type of pattern within those structures. Granular BCCs are exemplified by basaloid cells with clear cytoplasm (Fig. 16.6). Pigmented BCCs are histologically very similar to nodular BCCs except that they contain brown pigment in areas of the tumor, and may require smaller surgical margins than nodular BCC [20] (Fig. 16.7). Their biological behavior is also similar to nodular BCCs.

In general, perineural invasion is known to occur in BCC approximately 1% of the time [21]. When it does

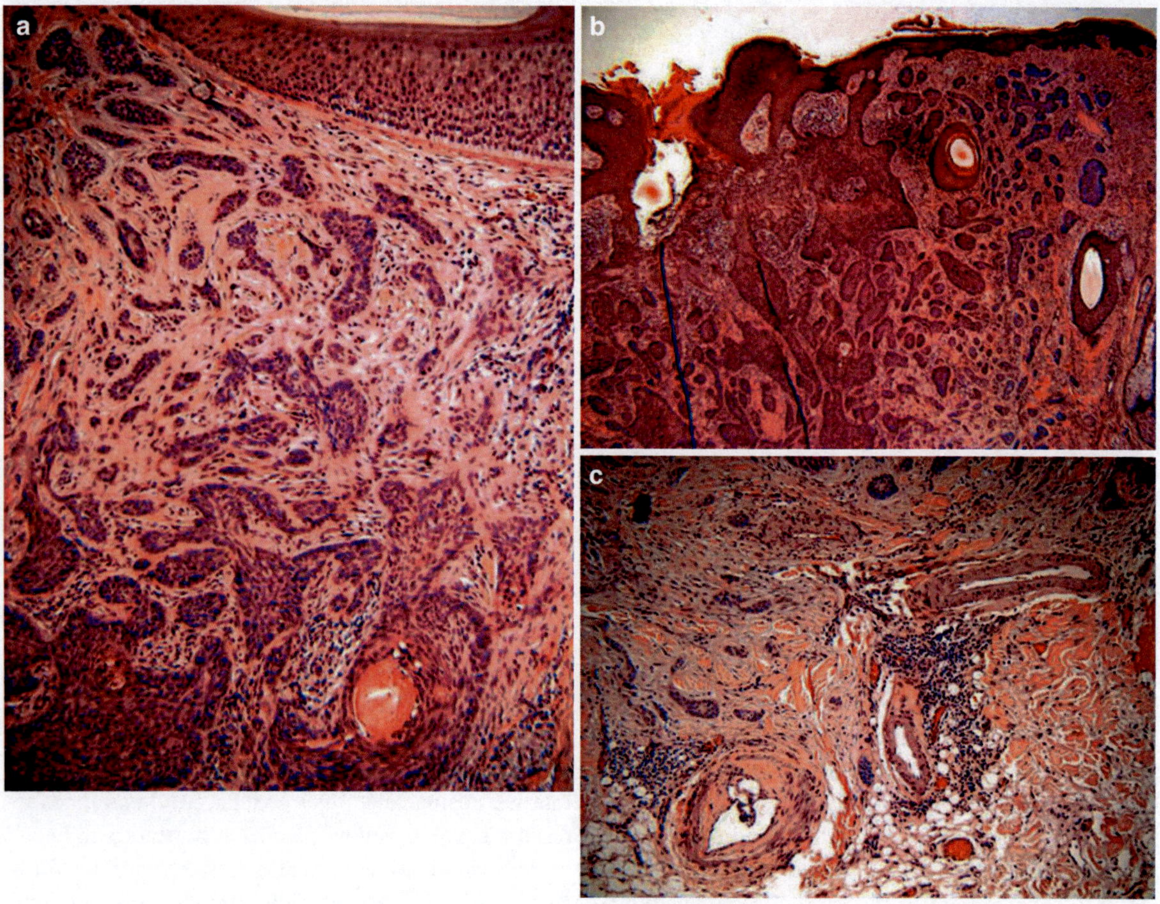

Fig. 16.5 (**a**) BCC with infiltrative features. (**b**) The basal cell carcinoma is more nodular in the central aspect of the lesion. (**c**) In the neoplasm thin strands splay collagen bundles and in places are only two cells thick. Coutesy of Dr. Evangelos Badiavas

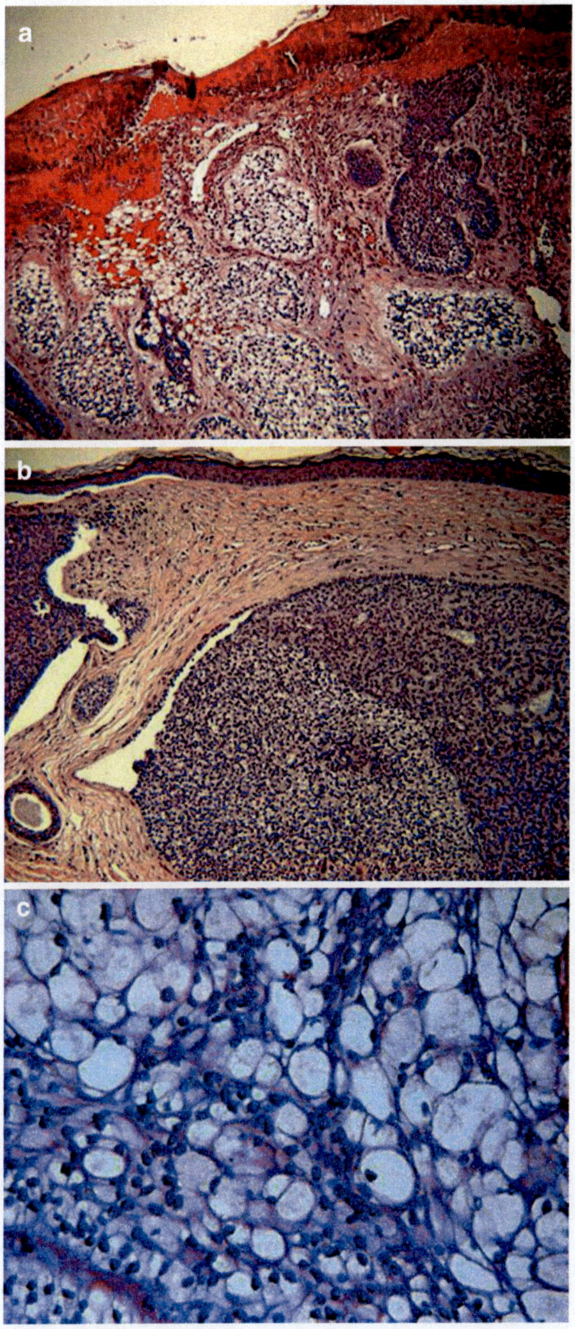

Fig. 16.6 (**a**) Clear cell basal cell carcinoma: areas of typical appearing basal cell carcinoma with several nests exhibiting marked clear cell features. (**b**) Some nests contain both typical and clear cell features that are sharply demarcated. (**c**) Clear cells with nuclei at the periphery of the cell with central clear to bluish expanded cytoplasm that is not lobulated such as in sebaceous cells. Courtesy of Dr. Evangelos Badiavas

occur, the trigeminal and facial nerve branches are the most commonly involved [21]. Prior to the Mohs procedure, the surgeon should ascertain whether the patient has experienced paresthesias, pain, numbness, or paresis in the vicinity of suspicious BCCs. These symptoms could suggest perineural invasion. On horizontal frozen sections, perineural invasion is exemplified by basophilic basaloid cells wrapping around the nerve.

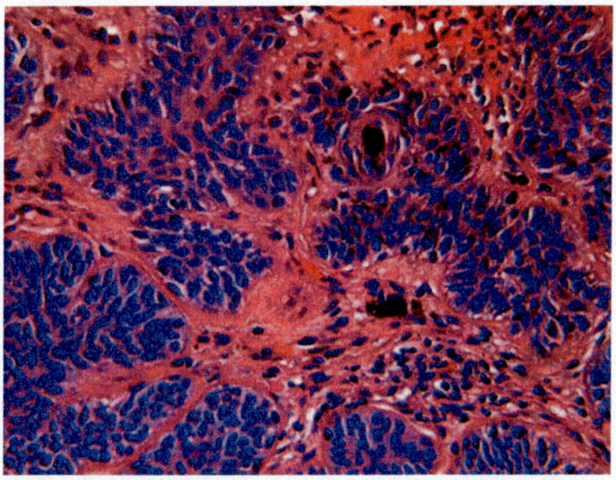

Fig. 16.7 Pigmented BCC: Basaloid neoplasm with areas of melanin pigment deposistion. Courtesy of Dr. Evangelos Badiavas

BCCs are typically stromal dependent, which is thought to be one of the reasons behind why BCCs do not usually metastasize. Incisions to the level of the adipose tissue are usually sufficient; however, occasionally, BCCs create their own stroma as they invade into underlying structures. More aggressive BCCs such as infiltrating, micronodular, and morpheaform have been known to use the already laid down stoma and invade into fascia, muscle, cartilage, and even bone. It has also been reported that BCCs without peripheral palisading tend to be more aggressive [22].

Summary: Non-cancerous Conditions That May Be Histologically Similar to BCC

- Several benign conditions can simulate BCC, notably hair follicles, inflamed adnexal structures, and endothelial cells.

16.4 Non-cancerous Conditions That May Be Histologically Similar to BCC

The frozen horizontal sections containing normal epidermis and adnexal structures can actually resemble BCC. Significant experience needs to be gained in order to adequately differentiate normal basal cells from the abnormal basaloid cells. On H & E, hair follicles tend to stain lighter than BCC. One should note that adnexal structures can sometimes develop atypia in areas that are inflamed. Often, scanning at low power helps to avoid over-analyzing for atypia and mitoses. The overall pattern should be analyzed rather than discreet areas under high magnification. Similar to BCC, certain parts of the hair follicle can display peripheral palisading, but it should not demonstrate stromal retraction. Follicles can also have mucin around them, but usually not in the proportion that is found around BCCs.

Inflammatory cells such as T cells, B cells, and plasma cells can look like BCC, especially when aggregated. These inflammatory cells are usually smaller and more round than the basaloid cells seen in BCC. Nests of inflammatory cells may be observed around BCCs as a reaction to the tumor. However, these same nests may be observed around the follicles of acne and rosacea patients and in areas where a previous biopsy occurred. Inflammatory cells can also be observed "swarming" around blood vessels, and indeed, the endothelial cells can also mimic BCC, more specifically morpheaform BCC.

Summary: Cancerous Conditions That May Be Histologically Similar to BCC

- Several other cancerous conditions can appear similar to BCC including: metastatic breast cancer, ameloblastomas, cloacogenic carcinomas, eccrine spiradenomas, pilomatricomas, trichoepitheliomas, cylindromas, and mucinous carcinomas.

16.5 Cancerous Conditions That May Be Histologically Similar to BCC

There are a number of other neoplastic conditions that appear histologically similar to BCC. Metastatic breast cancer may be observed when performing MMS on a lesion in the patient's chest. It can be distinguished from BCC by a lack of connection to the epidermis or adnexal structures. Ameloblastomas appear nearly identical to BCC but occur in the mouth. Cloacogenic carcinomas are found in the perianal area. Eccrine spiradenomas are also not connected to the epidermis and demonstrate a rosette pattern. Pilomatricomas are comprised of basaloid cells with dermal or subcutaneous nodules containing keratin and transitional cells, as well as shadow cells. Calcifications along with ossifications are commonly observed. Trichoepitheliomas have basaloid cells that closely resemble those of BCCs. Papillary mesenchymal cells can be found in close proximity to the basaloid-like nests in distinction to BCC. Trichoepitheliomas also do not exhibit the stromal retraction commonly found in BCCs. Cylindromas contain an eosinophilic "cylinder" located around basaloid cells. They are most commonly observed in the scalp. Mucinous carcinomas have basaloid cell groups, but unlike BCC, the aggregates are suspended in mucin pools along with fibrous bands of tissue.

Summary: Adnexal Differentiation Observed in BCC

- BCCs are considered immature in their differentiation and therefore can exhibit features of hair follicles, sweat glands, and sebaceous glands.
- When this occurs, it is difficult to determine if the tumor will biologically behave like a BCC or more like the entity it has differentiated toward.
- Folliculocentric basaloid proliferations appear as "pinwheels" of basaloid-appearing cells. They are benign and can be confused with BCC.

16.6 Adnexal Differentiation Observed in BCC

The basaloid cells of BCC are considered immature in their differentiation and harbor some ability to differentiate into other structures. The most commonly observed features include those of hair follicles, sweat glands, or sebaceous glands.

Basaloid differentiation toward hair follicles can be problematic in the sense that it is not known if the tumor will act more like a hair follicle tumor or more like a BCC. Trichoepithelioma, trichoblastoma, and basaloid follicular hamartoma may fall into this category. In these circumstances, it is probably better to excise the tumor in a similar fashion as BCC without these differentiation features.

When BCC with adnexal features exists, the tumor may actually be considered an eccrine epithelioma, sebaceous epithelioma, apocrine epithelioma, and BCC with sebaceous differentiation. One must take note that some of these tumors are considered more aggressive than BCC.

One variant is called microcystic adnexal carcinoma (MAC). It shows differentiation toward both sweat ductal and follicular structures and is discussed in detail in Chap. 20.

16.6.1 Folliculocentric Basaloid Proliferation (FBP) Observed in BCC

FBPs are considered benign and resemble BCCs. They are typically comprised of basaloid cells that form a "pinwheel" or "head of medusa" around a follicle [23]. They are very common and can make it difficult to distinguish from BCC. They tend to connect to the epidermis and do not have stromal retraction, necrosis, atypia, or mitoses. FBPs can be distinguished from BCC using the immunostain 33–3D antidesmoglein [24].

Summary: Basosquamous Differentiation

- Basosquamous cell carcinoma demonstrates histologic features of both BCC and squamous cell carcinoma (SCC).
- Histologically, basosquamous carcinoma is comprised of basaloid cells with peripheral palisading and stromal retraction along with the keratin pearls and the more eosinophilic cytoplasm that is associated with SCC.
- These tumors tend to metastasize more often than BCC, and several authors suggest that the metastatic potential is similar to squamous cell carcinoma.

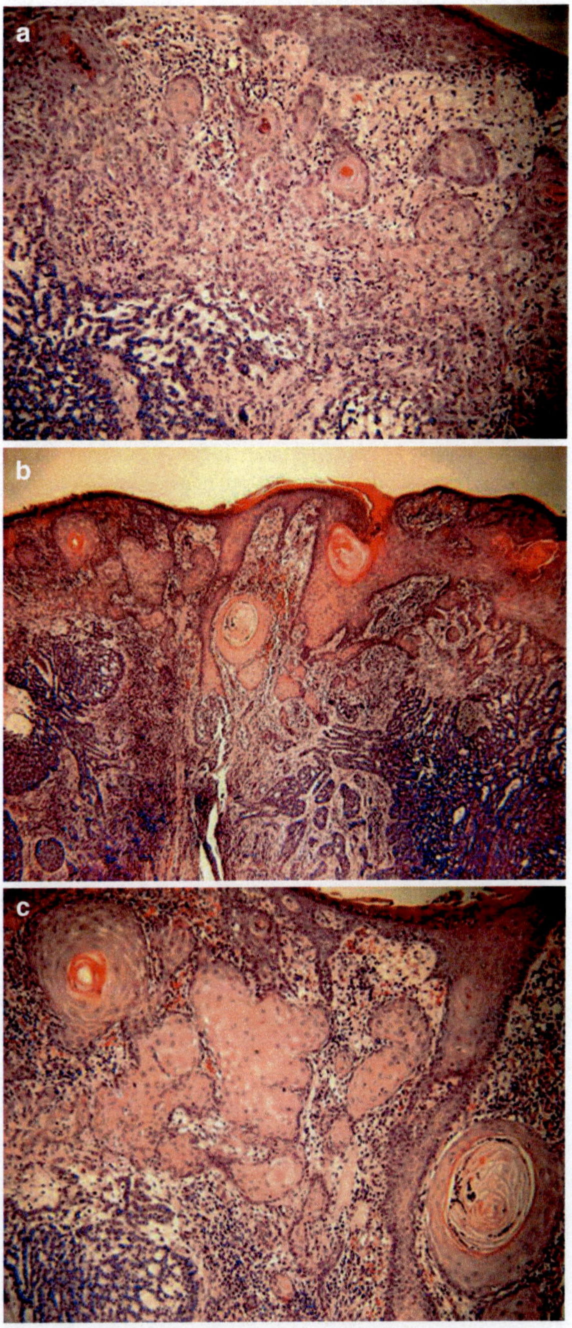

Fig. 16.8 (**a**) BCC with squamous differentiation (**b**) Basaloid neoplasm that is continuous with an eosinophilic neoplasm. (**c**) Note the keratinizing features and small cysts. Courtesy of Dr. Evangelos Badiavas

16.7 Basosquamous Differentiation

Basosquamous cell carcinoma demonstrates histologic features of both BCC and squamous cell carcinoma (SCC) (Fig. 16.8). There is some controversy regarding the exact definition of basosquamous carcinoma; however, most dermatologists now consider it a BCC subtype [25]. Approximately 1.2–2.7% of BCCs are actually considered basosquamous carcinomas. [25] Histologically, basosquamous carcinoma is comprised of basaloid cells with peripheral palisading and stromal retraction along with the keratin pearls. They generally have more eosinophilic cytoplasm that is more similar to that observed in SCC. These tumors tend to metastasize more often than BCC, and several authors suggest that the metastatic potential is similar to squamous cell carcinoma with an overall metastatic rate of approximately 9.7% [25–33]. One Australian prospective trial examined 98 cases of basosquamous carcinoma with 4 (4%) recurrences and 2 (2%) lymph node metastases over 5 years [25, 34]. A review of 17 cases of metastatic BCC, of which 10 lesions were available for analysis, demonstrated that 8 of them were either basosquamous or metatypical [35]. Another study found that from 170 metastatic BCC cases, 15% of the cases had areas resembling squamous differentiation [36]. Since basosquamous carcinoma is considered an aggressive BCC subtype, it is considered a strong indication for Mohs micrographic surgery similar to other aggressive BCC subtypes [25].

Summary: Therapeutic Options

- BCC has a very low rate of metastasis ranging from 0.003% to 0.55% of cases.
- Nonsurgical therapies include imiquimod, 5-fluorouracil, and radiotherapy.
- Surgical therapies include curettage and electrodessication, conventional surgical excision, and MMS.

16.8 Therapeutic Options

BCC has a very low metastatic rate with rates ranging from 0.003% to 0.55% of cases [12, 37, 38]. The primary goal of treatment is to prevent recurrence with full removal of the tumor while preserving function and if possible, cosmesis [12]. The treatment modality chosen relies on a number of clinical parameters, notably anatomical location, age, overall health of the patient, and biological behavior characteristics of histological subtypes [9].

Nonsurgical options include imiquimod, 5-fluorouracil, and radiotherapy. Imiquimod can be used for primary BCCs that are less than 2.0 cm in diameter and located on the neck, arms, legs, or trunk. It should not be used for nodular, infiltrative, or morpheaform BCCs. Side effects include erythema, edema, vesiculation, erosion/ulceration, flaking, headache, nausea, and vomiting [39]. It binds to Toll-like receptors 7 and 8 on macrophages and stimulates release of interferon gamma and tumor necrosis factor, likely upregulating the TH_1 response against the tumor [39].

5-Fluorouracil (5-FU) interferes with the production of thymine with the end result being to cause cell death to the tumor cells [1]. It can be used for superficial BCCs for 4–6 weeks, usually causing superficial erosions and erythema at the site of application [1]. Patients applying this medication should be closely followed during this time because substantial pruritus and irritation can develop [39–41]. 5-FU is broken down in the liver by dihydropyrimidine dehydrogenase (DHPDH). Patients who lack DHPDH constitute 1–3% of the population, and 0.1% of the population have a total deficiency of the enzyme [42]. In these patients, care should be taken not to use the topical cream over a large surface area of the body as the unmetabolized 5-FU could potentially lead to a toxic dose, albeit this is more of a concern in IV 5-FU [43] than with topical application.

Radiotherapy uses ionizing energy to destroy tumor cells usually in the form of fractionated doses of superficial X-rays, orthovoltage, or electron beam therapy [1]. The treatment is usually painless, and 63% of patients have good long-term cosmetic results [44]. This is lower than curettage and electrodessication and conventional surgical excision as 91% and 84%, respectively, of patients treated with these modalities have a good long-term cosmetic outcome [44]. Radiation therapy should also not be used in certain situations such as poorly defined BCCs, anatomical locations of the hands, feet, legs, and genitalia, and in patients with genodermatoses that generate a large number of BCCs [1]. It may be useful in cases where the patient cannot undergo surgical procedures [1].

Surgical therapy options include curettage and electrodessication (C&E), cryosurgery, conventional surgical excision, and Mohs micrographic surgery (MMS) [1]. C&E works well due to BCC's propensity to form fewer connections to the basement membrane. It can be used for small, well-defined, and superficial BCCs with nonaggressive subtypes and not in high-risk anatomical locations; however, the technique is limited by its lack of histological analysis and requirement for 4–6 weeks of wound healing [1]. It may be particularly advantageous for patients whose BCC meets the above criteria because the patient would not have to limit physical activity postoperatively; which is required when using conventional surgical excision or MMS [1].

Conventional surgical excision uses margins of 3–6 mm and can be used for BCCs less than 2 cm in low-risk anatomical areas with low-risk histological subtypes [1]. Nearly 95% of BCCs with low-risk histological subtypes are completely removed using a surgical margin of 4 mm [1]. At least one study directly compared conventional surgical excision versus cryotherapy and found a 5-year recurrence rate of 17.6% for cryotherapy versus 8.2% for conventional surgical excision, albeit the authors reported that this result was not statistically significant [45]. Similar recurrence rates were noted for other studies involving cryotherapy with recurrence rates ranging from 4.2% to 39% with 2 years of follow-up for cryotherapy [46–50]. Conventional surgical excision is associated with recurrence rates of 1.1–2.9% [51–54]. It should be noted that BCCs within the H zone of the face as well as the nose and ears are associated with a higher recurrence rate when using surgical excision at 8.4% [54, 55]. Conventional surgical excision is a good option when the patient does not have access to a Mohs surgeon or has a low-risk histological subtype of BCC.

Summary: Mohs Micrographic Surgery

- Mohs micrographic surgery (MMS) is considered the treatment of choice for micronodular, morpheaform/sclerosing, and infiltrative subtypes of BCC.
- For primary BCCs less than 3 cm in diameter, MMS cures the tumor 99% of the cases; however, primary BCCs greater than 3 cm only have a cure rate of 93%.
- There are a number of factors including size, location, and histologic subtype that can affect the tumor's cure rate.
- BCCs located on the face have higher recurrence rates.

16.9 Mohs Micrographic Surgery

Mohs micrographic surgery (MMS) is considered the treatment of choice for micronodular, morpheaform/sclerosing, and infiltrative subtypes of BCC because these subtypes are associated with unpredictable clinical spread with margins that are best observed using horizontal sections [1, 7]. In addition, these subtypes may also leave behind small strands of tumor cells when excised by conventional surgical excision and analyzed by vertical sectioning [56]. MMS offers the advantages of removing the tumor with the smallest necessary surgical margins. For primary BCCs less than 3 cm in diameter, MMS cures the tumor 99% of the cases; however, primary BCCs greater than 3 cm only have a cure rate of 93% [7, 9].

The largest series of patients for which the results of using MMS have been reported was by Dr. Frederic Mohs involving 7,575 patients with a 5-year follow-up. It was noted that 11% of the tumors were primary and had diameters greater than 2 cm, while 18.3% of the tumors were recurrent. The overall reported 5-year recurrence rate was only 0.7%! [57]. Another study, the second largest, involved 6,982 BCCs with 49% of those tumors being recurrent and 67% being greater than 1.9 cm with 2,960 tumors having 5 years of follow-up. From those 2,960 tumors, a 1.8% recurrence rate for primary BCCs and a 3.4% recurrence rate for recurrent tumors were reported [58]. Drs. Mohs and Robins later reported 5-year cure rates using MMS for periocular BCC of 98% out of 1,414 cases and 98.1% for primary and 93.6% out of 631 recurrent BCCs [59, 60].

Further evidence behind using MMS for BCC can be gained from the perspective of tissue conservation. At least two studies have examined the predicted defect size using conventional surgical excision and actual MMS. One study involved 71 auricular tumors in which 40 were BCC and 29 were SCC [61]. The predicted conventional surgical margins were determined to be 8 mm for primary BCCs less than 3 cm, 1 cm for primary SCC less than 3 cm, and 1.5 cm for recurrent tumors and those greater than 3 cm [61]. If conventional surgical excision had been used, 180% of tissue beyond the MMS defect in primary BCCs and 27% beyond the Mohs defect in recurrent BCCs would have been removed [61]. Additionally, more than one stage of conventional surgical excision would have been required in nine primary tumors as well as eight recurrent tumors [61]. Downes et al. also compared post-surgical wound defects in periorbital BCC between MMS and conventional surgical excision and demonstrated that a local repair, direct closure, or graft could be used in 15 out of 22 patients undergoing Mohs while those methods could only be used in 6 of 22 patients if conventional surgical excision was used [62]. In fact, the extent of surgery was much less complicated in 41% of the Mohs cases compared to if conventional surgical excision had been carried out [62].

MMS is the primary treatment for aggressive BCCs (those with aggressive histological subtypes) as well as those in precarious anatomical locations such as the face or the genitalia due to its tissue-conserving property [7, 63–65]. Strictly speaking, there are a number of factors including size, location, and histologic subtype that can affect the tumor's cure rate [7]. If the BCC is greater than 3 cm, then the cure rate is 93% versus 99% if the tumor is less than 3 cm [7]. Primary periocular and perioral BCCs have a 98% cure rate [7]. BCCs located on the face have higher recurrence rates following MMS as one study reported a 5-year recurrence rate of 6.5% for primary BCCs and 10% for recurrent BCCs, with the temple having the highest number of recurrences [66]. Another study demonstrated that 2.5% of primary facial BCCs and 2.4% of recurrent facial BCCs recurred over a 5-year period [67]. Smeets et al. reported that primary facial BCCs recurred 2% of the time with 5 years of follow-up, while none of the recurrent facial BCCs recurred over 5 years [68].

Remarkably, morpheaform BCC has been demonstrated to subclinically spread 7.2 mm on average from the clinically visible tumor [19]. Infiltrative BCCs are known to invade the perineural tissues at higher rates than other BCC subtypes [69, 70]. Additionally, a number of reports have demonstrated that approximately 65% of infiltrative BCCs have a micronodular or infiltrating component [22, 70–75]. Following conventional surgical excision, micronodular BCC has been found to have a positive margin in 18.6% of cases versus only 6.4% of nodular BCC cases with farther tumor extensions being noted in the micronodular BCC cases [7, 76]. This demonstrates the importance of intraoperative histological analysis in micronodular BCC cases. Although superficial BCC is considered a nonaggressive subtype (noninfiltrative) of BCC, it is actually associated with the highest rate of recurrence out of the BCC subtypes [71].

Summary: Conclusions

- BCC is the most common neoplasm diagnosed in humans.
- BCC is the most common indication for MMS with nearly 30% of all BCC cases in the USA treated by MMS.
- The evidence behind using MMS as a surgical therapy for BCC is strong, with studies backed by a high number of patients along with very low recurrence rates reported.

16.10 Conclusion

In conclusion, BCC is the most common neoplasm diagnosed in humans. Interactions between UVB and DNA lead to dipyrimidine formation, which causes constitutive activation of the Sonic hedgehog pathway. BCC is the most common indication for MMS with nearly 30% of all BCC cases in the USA treated by MMS. Infiltrating, micronodular, and morpheaform are considered more aggressive subtypes of BCC. Inflammatory cells, hair follicles, and folliculocentric basaloid proliferations are benign conditions that can resemble BCC when using horizontal frozen sections. More malignant processes such as metastatic breast cancer, ameloblastoma, cloacogenic carcinoma, eccrine spiradenoma, pilomatricomas, and trichoepitheliomas can also mimic BCC. Additionally, BCC may differentiate to simulate many structures such as hair follicles, sweat glands, and sebaceous glands. The evidence behind MMS as a surgical therapy for BCC is strong with studies backed by a high number of patients along with very low recurrence rates reported. It is especially well suited for aggressive histological subtypes of BCC and for BCCs in anatomical regions where tissue conservation is paramount due to intraoperative histological analysis that allows the Mohs surgeon to observe nearly 100% of the surgical borders.

References

1. Neville JA, Welch E, Leffell DJ. Management of nonmelanoma skin cancer in 2007. Nat Clin Pract Oncol. 2007;4(8):462–9.

2. Welch ML, Anderson LL, Grabski WJ. How many nonmelanoma skin cancers require Mohs' micrographic surgery? J Dermatol Surg. 1996;22:711–3.
3. ACS. Cancer Facts & Figures 2001. http://www.cancer.org/downloads/STT/F&F2001.pdf (2001). Accessed March 19, 2002.
4. Iwasaki JK, Srivastva D, Moy RL, Lin HJ, Kouba DJ. The molecular genetics underlying basal cell carcinoma pathogenesis and links to targeted therapeutics. J Am Acad Dermatol. Epub Aug 25, 2010.
5. Lear JT, Schmith AG. Basal cell carcinoma. Postgrad Med. 1997;73:538–42.
6. Roewer-Huber J, Lange-Asschenfeldt B, Stockfleth E, Kerl H. Epidemiology and aetiology of basal cell carcinoma. Br J Dermatol. 2007;157 Suppl 2:47–51.
7. Shriner D, McCoy DK, Goldberg DJ, WagnerJr R. Mohs micrographic surgery. J Am Acad Dermatol. 1998;39:79–97.
8. Tulli A. Mohs micrographic surgery. In: Chu T, Chu AC, Edelson RL, editors. Malignant tumors of the skin. London: England; 1999. p. 381–95.
9. Martinez JC, Otley CC. The management of melanoma and nonmelanoma skin cancer: a review for the primary care physician. Mayo Clin Proc. 2001;76:1253–65.
10. Xie J, Murone M, Luoh SM, et al. Activating smoothened mutations in sporadic basal-cell carcinoma. Nature. 1998;391:90–2.
11. Zedan W, Robinson PA, Markham AF, High AS. Expression of the Sonic Hedgehog receptor "PATCHED" in basal cell carcinomas and odontogenic keratocytes. J Pathol. 2001;194:473–7.
12. Rubin AI, Chen EH, Ratner D. Basal-cell carcinoma. N Engl J Med. 2005;353:2262–9.
13. Hahn H, Wojnowski L, Miller G, Zimmer A. The patched signalling pathway in tumorigenesis and development; lessons from animal models. J Mol Med. 1999;77:459–68.
14. Bonifas JM, Bare JW, Kerschmann RL, Maser SP, Epstein Jr EH. Paternal origin of chromosome 9q22.3-q31 lost in basal cell carcinomas from basal cell nevus Syndrome patients. Hum Mol Genet. 1994;3:447–8.
15. Donovan J. Review of the hair follicle origin hypothesis for basal cell carcinoma. Dermatol Surg. 2009;35:1311–23.
16. Kirkham N. Tumors and cysts of the epidermis. In: Elder DE, Elenitsas R, Johnson BL, Murphy GF, Xiaowei X, editors. Lever's histopathology of the skin. 10th ed. Philadelphia: Lippincott Williams & Wilkins; 2008. p. 1048.
17. Okun MR, Blumental G. Basal cell epithelioma with giant cells and nuclear atypicality. Arch Dermatol. 1964;89:598.
18. Rupec M, Vakilzadeh F, Korb G. Über das vorkommen von mehrkernigen riesenzellen in basaliomen. Arch Klin Exp Dermatol. 1969;235:198.
19. Salasche SJ, Amonette R. Morpheaform basal-cell epitheliomas: a study of subclinical extensions in a series of 51 cases. J Dermatol Surg Oncol. 1981;7:387–93.
20. Aoyagi S, Nouri K. Difference between pigmented and nonpigmented basal cell carcinoma treated with Mohs micrographic surgery. Dermatol Surg. 2006;32:1375–9.
21. Terashi H. Perineural and neural involvement in skin cancers. Dermatol Surg. 1997;22:259.
22. Lang PG, Maize JC. Histologic evolution of recurrent basal cell carcinoma and treatment implications. J Am Acad Dermatol. 1986;14:186.
23. Leshin B, White WL. Folliculocentric basaloid proliferation. The bulge (der Wulst) revisited. Arch Dermatol. 1990;126(7):900–6.
24. Krunic AL, Garrod DR, Viehman GE, Madani S, Buchanan MD, Clark RE. The use of antidesmoglein stains in Mohs micrographic surgery. Dermatol Surg. 1997;23(6):463–8.
25. Garcia C, Poletti E, Crowson AN. Basosquamous carcinoma. J Am Acad Dermatol. 2009;60:137–43.
26. Borel DM. Cutaneous basosquamous carcinoma: review of the literature and report of 35 cases. Arch Pathol. 1973;95:293–7.
27. Crowson AN. Basal cell carcinoma: biology, morphology and clinical implications. Mod Pathol. 2006;19(Suppl):S127–47.
28. de Lopes FJ, Nunes PH. Basosquamous cell carcinoma of the skin with metastases. Histopathology. 1988;12:85–94.
29. Martin RC, Edwards MJ, Cawte TG, Sewell CL, McMasters KM. Basosquamous carcinoma: analysis of prognostic factors influencing recurrence. Cancer. 2000;88:1365–9.
30. Jones MS, Helm KF, Maloney ME. The immunohistochemical characteristics of the basosquamous cell carcinoma. Dermatol Surg. 1997;23:181–4.
31. Maloney ML. What is basosquamous carcinoma? Dermatol Surg. 2000;26:505–6.
32. Barksdale SK, O'Connor N, Barnhill R. Prognostic factors for cutaneous squamous cell and basal cell carcinoma: determinants of risk of recurrence, metastasis, and development of subsequent skin cancers. Surg Oncol Clin N Am. 1997;6:625–38.
33. Randle HW. Basal cell carcinoma: identification and treatment of the high-risk patient. Dermatol Surg. 1996;22:255–61.
34. Leibovitch I, Huilgol SC, Selva D, Richards S, Paver R. Basosquamous carcinoma: treatment with Mohs micrographic surgery. Cancer. 2005;104:170–5.
35. Farmer ER, Helwig EB. Metastatic basal cell carcinoma: a clinicopathologic study of seventeen cases. Cancer. 1980;46:748–57.
36. VonDomarus H, Stevens PJ. Metastatic basal cell carcinoma: report of five cases and review of 170 cases in the literature. J Am Acad Dermatol. 1984;10:1043–60.
37. Tavin E, Persky MS, Jacobs J. Metastatic basal cell carcinoma of the head and neck. Laryngoscope. 1995;105:814–7.
38. Schuller D, Berg JW, Sherman G, Krause CJ. Cutaneous basosquamous carcinoma of the head and neck: a comparative analysis. Otolaryngol Head Neck Surg. 1979;87(4):420–7.
39. Schon MP, Schon M. Imiquimod: mode of action. Br J Dermatol. 2007;157(S2):8–13.
40. Goette DK. Topical chemotherapy with 5-fluorouracil. J Am Acad Dermatol. 1981;6:633–49.
41. Acarturk TO, Edington H. Nonmelanoma skin cancer. Clin Plast Surg. 2005;32:237–48.
42. Cancer M-AGI. Toxicity of fluorouracil in patients with advanced colorectal cancer: effect of administration schedule and prognostic factors. J Clin Oncol. 1998;16(11):3537–41.
43. Serdar AM, Sertoğlu E, Uyanik M, Tapan S, Akin O, Cihan M. Determination of 5-fluorouracil and dihydrofluorouracil levels using a liquid chromatography-tandem mass spectrometry method for evaluation of dihydropyrimidine dehydrogenase enzyme activity. Cancer Chemother Pharmacol. 2011;68:525–9. Epub 24 Nov 2010.

44. Silverman MK, Kopf AW, Gladstein AH, Bart RS, Grin CM, Levenstein MJ. Recurrence rates of treated basal cell carcinomas. Part 4: X-ray therapy. J Dermatol Surg Oncol. 1992;18(7):549–54.
45. Kuijpers DI, Thissen MR, Berretty PJ, Ideler FH, Nelemans PJ, Neumann MH. Surgical excision plus cryosurgery in the treament of basal cell carcinoma. Dermatol Surg. 2007;33:579–87.
46. Kokoszka A, Scheinfeld N. Evidence-based review of the use of cryosurgery in treatment of basal cell carcinoma. Dermatol Surg. 2003;29:566–71.
47. Mallon E, Dawber R. Cryosurgery in the treatment of basal cell carcinoma. Assessment of one and two freeze-thaw schedules. Dermatol Surg. 1996;22:854–8.
48. Thissen MR, Nieman FH, Ideler AH, Berretty PJ, Neumann HA. Cosmetic results of cryosurgery versus surgical excision for primary uncomplicated basal cell carcinomas of the head and neck. Dermatol Surg. 2000;26:759–64.
49. Wang I, Bendsoe N, Klinteberg CA, et al. Photodynamic therapy vs. cryosurgery of basal cell carcinomas: results of a phase III clinical trial. Br J Dermatol. 2001;144(4):832–40.
50. Hall VL, Leppard BJ, McGill J, Kesseler ME, White JE, Goodwin P. Treatment of basal-cell carcinoma: comparison of radiotherapy and cryotherapy. Clin Radiol. 1986;37(1):33–4.
51. Werlinger KD, Upton G, Moore AY. Recurrence rates of primary nonmelanoma skin cancers treated by surgical excision compared to electrodesiccation-currettage in a private dermatological practice. Dermatol Surg. 2002;28:1138–42.
52. Germann G, Bernstein-Sommer B, Petrovici V, Steinau HU. Differential, oncologically adequate therapy of basalioma. Handchir Mikrochir Plast Chir. 1992;24(3):151–8.
53. Bauer M, Loosli RM, Anderl J, Wilflingseder P. Surgical treatment of malignant skin epitheliomas. Principles, methods, results. Chirurg. 1977;48(3):170–9.
54. Silverman MK, Kopf AW, Bart RS, Grin CM, Levenstein MS. Recurrence rates of treated basal cell carcinomas. Part 3: surgical excision. J Dermatol Surg Oncol. 1992;18(6):471–6.
55. Bogdanov-Berezovsky A, Cohen AD, Glesinger R, Cagano E, Krieger Y, Rosenberg L. Risk factors for incomplete excision of basal cell carcinomas. Acta Derm Venereol. 2004;84(1):44–7.
56. LangJr PG, Osguthorpe JD. Indications and limitations of Mohs micrographic surgery. Dermatol Clin. 1989;7: 627–44.
57. Mohs FE. Chemosurgery. Microscopically controlled surgery for skin cancer. Springfield: Charles C Thomas; 1978. p. 153.
58. Robins P. Chemosurgery: my 15 years experience. J Dermatol Surg Oncol. 1981;7:779–89.
59. Mohs FE. Micrographic surgery for the microscopically controlled excision of eyelid cancer. Arch Ophthalmol. 1986;104:901–9.
60. Robins P, Rodriquez-Sains R, Rabinovitz H, Rigel D. Mohs surgery for periocular basal cell carcinomas. J Dermatol Surg Oncol. 1985;11:1203–7.
61. Bumsted RM, Ceilley RI, Panje WR, Curmley RL. Auricular malignant neoplasms. When is chemotherapy (Mohs' technique) necessary? Arch Otolaryngol. 1981;107:721–4.
62. Downes RN, Waker NPJ, Collin JRO. Micrographic (Mohs) surgery in the management of periocular basal cell epitheliomas. Eye. 1990;4:160–8.
63. Swanson NA. Mohs Surgery. Technique, indications, applications and the future. Arch Dermatol. 1983;119:761–73.
64. Cottell WI, Proper S. Mohs' surgery, fresh tissue technique. J Dermatol Surg Oncol. 1982;8:576–87.
65. Rappini RP. On the definition of Mohs surgery and how it determines appropriate surgical margins. Arch Dermatol. 1992;128:673–8.
66. Wennberg AM, Larko O, Stenquist B. Five-year results of Mohs' micrographic surgery for aggressive facial basal cell carcinoma in Sweden. Acta Derm Venereol. 1999;79:370–2.
67. Mosterd K, Krekels GAM, Nieman FHM, et al. Surgical excision versus Mohs' micrographic surgery for primary and recurrent basal-cell carcinoma of the face: a prospective randomised controlled trial with 5-years' follow-up. Lancet Oncol. 2008;9(12):1149–56.
68. Smeets NWJ, Krekels GAM, Ostertag JU, et al. Surgical excision vs Mohs' micrographic surgery for basal-cell carcinoma of the face: randomised controlled trial. Lancet. 2004;364:1766–72.
69. Bennett RG. Current concepts in Mohs micrographic surgery. Dermatol Clin. 1991;9:777–88.
70. Mehregan AH. Aggressive basal cell epithelioma on sunlight-protected skin: report of eight cases, one with pulmonary and bone metastases. Am J Dermatopathol. 1983;5:221–9.
71. Sloane JP. The value of typing basal cell carcinomas in predicting recurrence after surgical excision. Br J Dermatol. 1977;96:127–32.
72. Jacobs GH, Rippey JJ, Altinbi M. Prediction of aggressive behavior in basal cell carcinoma. Cancer. 1982;49:533–7.
73. Thackray AC. Histological classification of rodent ulcers and its bearing on their prognosis. Br J Cancer. 1951;5:213–24.
74. Dellon AL. Histologic study of recurrent basal cell carcinoma. Plast Reconstr Surg. 1985;75:853–9.
75. Siegle RJ, MacMillan J, Pollack SV. Infiltrative basal cell carcinoma: a nonsclerosing subtype. J Dermatol Surg Oncol. 1986;12:830–6.
76. Hendrix JD, Parlette JL. Micronodular basal cell carcinoma: a deceptive histologic subtype with frequently clinically undetected tumor extension. Arch Dermatol. 1996;132:295–8.

Squamous Cell Carcinoma

17

Nicole R. LeBoeuf, Lorraine M. Jennings,
Andrew E. Werchniak, and Chrysalyne D. Schmults

Abstract

Cutaneous squamous cell carcinoma (SCC) is the second most common cutaneous malignancy in the USA, accounting for 20% of non-melanoma skin cancers. Among Caucasians, it is the second most common cancer overall. Although the great majority of cases are cured by surgery or other treatments, deaths from SCC may be nearly as common as those from melanoma. Identification of patients at risk for untoward outcomes as well as clarity regarding appropriate staging and management, particularly of high-risk tumors, is imperative. This chapter discusses the current state of knowledge regarding the pathophysiology leading to cutaneous SCC, risk factors for its development, and the clinical spectrum of squamous dysplasia with particular attention given to high-risk and invasive disease. It provides an in-depth discussion of the available data regarding surgical and non-surgical management of cutaneous SCC, particularly of high-risk tumors.

Keywords

Squamous cell carcinoma (SCC) • Immunosuppression • Human papilloma virus (HPV) • Organ transplant recipient (OTR) • Ultraviolet (UV) light • Radiation • Mohs surgery

N.R. LeBoeuf (✉)
Department of Dermatology, Dana Farber Cancer Institute/
Brigham and Women's Hospital,
Boston, MA, USA
e-mail: nleboeuf@partners.org

L.M. Jennings
Department of Mohs Micrographic Surgery, Department of Dermatology, Dana Farber Cancer Institute/Brigham and Women's Hospital,
Boston, MA, USA

A.E. Werchniak
Department of Dermatology, Dana Farber Cancer Institute/
Brigham and Women's Hospital,
Boston, MA, USA

C.D. Schmults
Department of Dermatologic Surgery, MOHS Micrographic Surgery Center, Brigham and Women's Hospital,
Boston, MA, USA

Summary: Introduction

- Cutaneous squamous cell carcinoma is increasing in frequency, and based on incidence data, may result in as many deaths as melanoma in some regions of the US. Prognostic models predicting who is at risk of metastasis and death are lacking. Subsequently, there is little consensus regarding staging and management of high-risk patients.

K. Nouri (ed.), *Mohs Micrographic Surgery*,
DOI 10.1007/978-1-4471-2152-7_17, © Springer-Verlag London Limited 2012

17.1 Introduction

Cutaneous squamous cell carcinoma is the second most common malignancy in white persons [1]. Various studies have estimated its annual incidence to be between 87,000 and 760,000 with an increasing incidence over time and much higher incidences in the south and southwest USA [2–9]. A white male born in the USA in 1994 has an estimated lifetime risk of 9–14% of developing a cutaneous SCC, while a white woman's estimated risk is 4–9% [8]. Despite very high cure rates for most SCC, approximately 4% metastasize to lymph nodes and 1.5% result in death [10]. It can be estimated from these figures that SCC accounts for 1,300–11,000 deaths annually in the USA. As a point of reference, melanoma kills 8,600 persons annually. Nearly all deaths occur in those who have tumors with known risk factors [11]. Therefore, understanding classic and highly curable SCC and differentiating it from high-risk disease are crucial in appropriately managing SCC. However, as will be discussed, the subset of SCC which carries a high risk of metastasis and death has not been well defined, and the risks have not been well quantified. Subsequently, there is currently little consensus regarding optimal staging and treatment for high-risk patients making it difficult for clinicians to advise these patients with confidence [12].

Summary: Pathophysiology (Risk Factors for SCC Development)

- In order to prevent squamous cell carcinoma and effectively manage it once it occurs, physicians should be familiar with mechanisms of disease development, including risk factors associated with tumor formation. Genetic factors as well as external influences contribute to tumor development.

17.2 Pathophysiology (Risk Factors for SCC Development)

Cutaneous squamous cell carcinoma is a neoplasm arising from epidermal keratinocytes. Identification of the host and environmental factors associated with the development of cutaneous SCC has provided insights into the mechanisms leading to tumor development. Intrinsic host risk factors include age, skin phototype, the presence of immunodeficiency disorders, and genodermatoses resulting in defective DNA repair (xeroderma pigmentosa), defective melanin production (oculocutaneous albinism), or chronic cutaneous inflammation (epidermolysis bullosa) [13–15]. Immunosuppressive conditions such as leukemia and lymphoma result in an increased risk of SCC as well. Extrinsic or environmental factors are many and include, most commonly, exposure to medical ultraviolet (UV) light treatments or natural UV radiation. The latter accounts for higher skin cancer rates in geographic latitudes nearer the equator and in people with outdoor occupations [1, 15]. Other iatrogenic factors include exposure to ionizing radiation, organ transplantation, immunosuppressive medications, and treatment with psoralens prior to UVA radiation. Infectious contributors include high-risk strains of the human papilloma virus (in anogenital SCC), HIV/AIDS, and chronic infections such as osteomyelitis. Chronically injured skin is at increased risk, as with chronic radiation dermatitis, sinus tracts, ulcers, and burn scars. In particular, patients with dystrophic epidermolysis bullosa have a very high risk of mortality from SCC. Chemical carcinogens include arsenic and polycyclic aromatic hydrocarbons [4, 13, 14, 16–23].

17.2.1 Ultraviolet Light

The most common cause of cutaneous SCC is exposure to ultraviolet radiation, with UVB (290–320 nm) accounting for most of the carcinogenic effect. UVA (320–400 nm) plays a lesser, but additive, role. Cutaneous SCC may arise de novo, or from a precursor lesion. Most commonly, UV radiation generates pyrimidine dimers within the sequence of the p53 tumor suppressor gene. When both copies of p53 within the keratinocyte are mutated or dysfunctional, the cell undergoes clonal expansion. This results in the formation of actinic keratoses, squamous cell carcinoma in situ, and, with persistent proliferation, invasive SCC. P53 is mutated in 90% of SCC [24]. While it is difficult to determine the likelihood of an individual AK progressing into an invasive SCC, this has been estimated at 0.1–10% [25–27]. The presence of multiple AKs serves as a marker of increased risk of developing SCC. Patients with greater than 10 AKs have a 14% probability of developing an SCC within 5 years [28]. Their presence further serves as a marker of high cumulative lifetime sun exposure and therefore an increased risk of other UV-related malignancies such as basal cell carcinoma.

17.2.2 Human Papilloma Virus

Both bowenoid papulosis and the autosomally inherited disorder epidermodysplasia verruciformis (EDV) are premalignant disorders that may progress to invasive SCC. Both disorders are associated with human papilloma viruses (HPVs), small, double stranded DNA viruses which have a specific tropism for stratified squamous epithelium. While bowenoid papulosis is most commonly associated with high-risk HPV types 16 and 18 (genus *alpha-papilloma virus*), EDV subtypes (genus *beta-papilloma virus*) include 23 variants. In patients *without* EDV, beta species 1 HPV types (HPV 5, 8, 12, 14, 19, 20, 21, 24, 25, 36, 47, and 93) have been shown to be more commonly associated with benign warts, while beta species 2 HPV types (HPV 9, 15, 17, 22, 23, 37, 38, and 80) have been shown to be associated with SCC [29]. Conversely, in patients *with* the inherited disorder of EDV, HPV 5 and 8 appear most commonly and have been identified in up to 90% of SCCs in these patients [30, 31]. In solid-organ-transplant recipients, an increased prevalence of the *beta*-HPV subtypes is seen, with 90% of SCCs in renal transplant patients containing HPV-*beta* DNA. However, a pathogenic role of HPV has not been established in transplant-associated SCC.

While the role of HPV in cutaneous SCC in transplant patients remains debated, the presence of HPV (most commonly 16) in 70–90% of anogenital SCC [32–34] has lead to an accepted causal association. While the incidence of anal cancer is increasing at a rate of 2% per year [35], HIV infected men and women are at substantially increased risk of developing all types of anogenital HPV-associated in situ and invasive malignancies. For patients under 30 who are HIV positive, the relative risk of vulvovaginal and penile cancer is 37, and for anal cancer >100 [36].

The oncogenic mechanism of action of high-risk HPV types is via the ability of the E6 protein, primarily of types 16 and 18, to promote the ubiquitin-dependent degradation of the tumor suppressor, p53. Similarly, the oncoprotein E7 interacts with the tumor suppressor pRb, inducing the degradation of the Rb protein, and activating telomerase, which leads to cell cycle progression [37, 38]. While all subspecies of HPV possess the E6 and E7 proteins, their malignant potential in the HPV-*beta* subspecies is thought to be weaker than in the high-risk types. The importance of intact cytotoxic T-lymphocyte activity against HPV E6 and E7 proteins is hypothesized to play a critical role in clearance of the virus and is impaired in those infected with HIV. This may partially explain why HPV infection is so strongly linked to anogenital SCC in this patient group [39].

17.2.3 Molecular and Genetic Factors Impacting SCC Development

While knowledge regarding the importance of p53 and HPV in the development of SCC has grown over many years, recent discoveries regarding the role of the immune system in SCC and the genetic and molecular mechanisms underlying keratinocyte proliferation and migration allow for better potential understanding of invasive tumor development, particularly in immunosuppressed patients. The point at which keratinocytes develop the capacity for invasion has been linked to the loss of expression or function of p16 [40], a protein that is not expressed during the normal wound healing process. Concomitantly, laminin-332 has been shown to be co-expressed with p16 at the transition point from in situ to invasive disease. Further study has revealed that a precursor form of laminin-332 may be responsible for the induction of the coordinated production of functional laminin-332 and p16 leading to hypermobility and growth arrest during wound healing and early invasion of neoplastic keratinocytes [41]. Additional studies have shown that there is increased lymphatic vessel density within SCC as well as increased expression of VEGF-C, important in lymphangiogenesis, in the peritumoral microenvironment [42]. Differential gene expression studies in SCC as compared with non-malignant hyperproliferative disease have implicated multiple tumor suppressor genes, the WNT signaling pathway, and variable expression of matrix metalloproteinases in the pathogenesis of SCC [43]. Additionally, the areas surrounding SCC tumors contain an abundance of T-lymphocytes which fail to control tumor growth. Interestingly, approximately 50% of T-cells surrounding SCCs have been shown to be FOXP3+ T regulatory cells (Tregs) which are immunosuppressive and thus may allow tumors to evade destruction by the immune system and continue to grow. Additionally, SCCs do not express E-selectin on tumor vessels, and therefore cutaneous lymphocyte antigen (CLA) 4+ skin-homing memory T-cells cannot enter the tumor tissue [44]. The CLA4+ cells are crucial for immune surveillance. In mice, treatment of SCCs with imiquimod reverses many of these effects; this results in expression of vascular E-selectin, decreased Treg density [44], and increased CLA4+ effector T-cells with resultant interferon-γ (IFN-γ) production and resulting tumor regression [45]. Thus, the development and growth of invasive squamous cell carcinoma appears to involve complex genetic and immunologic alterations within the tumor and the surrounding microenvironment, all of which serve as potential portals for further understanding of high-risk disease and the development of novel therapies.

Summary: Clinical Disease Spectrum

- The spectrum of cutaneous neoplasms with squamous dysplasia is broad ranging from superficial focal actinic keratoses to highly aggressive, invasive SCC. The etiology of a particular tumor may correlate with a specific presentation and course, as in bowenoid papulosis and verrucous carcinoma. Understanding variations in presentation and diagnosis allows for appropriate diagnosis and management of the SCC disease spectrum.

17.3 Clinical Disease Spectrum

Evaluation of the patient with known or suspected cutaneous SCC involves obtaining a thorough history evaluating for common risk factors and those associated with high-risk disease. While most typical SCCs are brought to the physicians' attention by the patient or relative and are generally asymptomatic, a careful history can help distinguish those patients at high risk for recurrence and metastases. Rate of growth should be assessed, as well as symptoms of numbness, tingling, pain, or weakness, which may reflect the presence of perineural involvement (PNI); this has prognostic and management implications [46]. History of immunosuppression, especially exposure to immunomodulatory drugs or diagnosis of chronic lymphocytic leukemia (CLL), should be obtained as high-risk disease is more common in these patients.

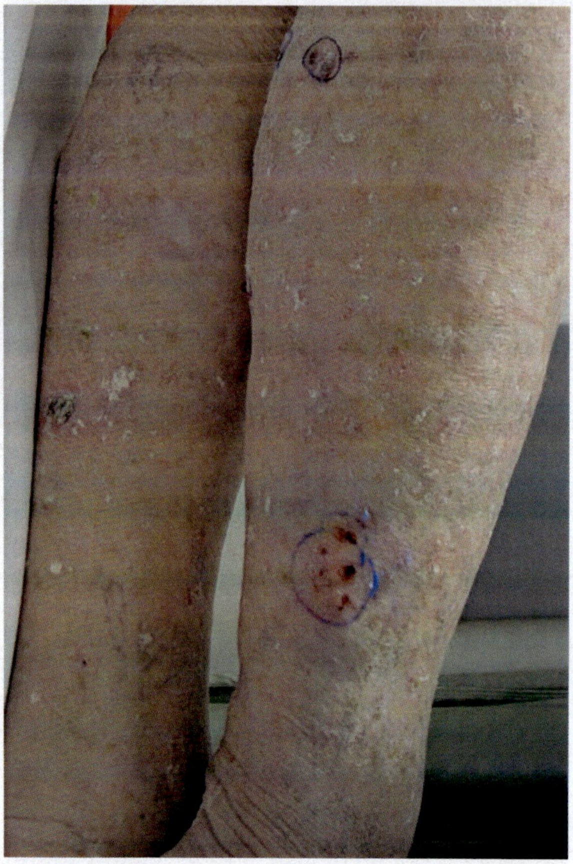

Fig. 17.1 Dermally invasive SCCs on a background of diffuse actinic damage and SCCIS on the posterior legs

17.3.1 Actinic Keratosis

Actinic keratoses (AK) are the third most common diagnosis made on dermatologic consultation [47]. Clinically, they are typically rough, keratotic skin-colored papules 2–6 mm in diameter. Patients with diffuse actinic damage are more likely to develop multiple SCCs. Such patients with multiple tumors in a background of diffuse actinic damage (Fig. 17.1) can be considered clinical entities in and of themselves, requiring special consideration with regard to evaluation and management. These patients with diffuse precancerous and cancerous lesions can present a management challenge. Referral to a high-risk or immunosuppression dermatology subspecialty clinic for close follow-up and field therapy may be considered. See the section on field cancerization below for a step-wise approach to management.

17.3.2 Squamous Cell Carcinoma In Situ

Squamous cell carcinoma in situ is a histologic diagnosis defined by full thickness keratinocyte atypia. The breadth of the lesion is often not considered pathologically. Thus, a small microscopic focus of full-thickness atypia seen in a background of actinic keratosis is still diagnosed as SCCIS. The natural history of SCCIS, including the percentage of SCCIS lesions that progress to invasive SCC, is not known. However, it is assumed they have the potential for invasion, similar to actinic keratoses, so treatment is generally advised. Clinically, SCCIS may be indistinguishable from AK. Classic Bowen's disease is a well-demarcated pink plaque of SCCIS arising in a non-sun-exposed area. An example of this is erythroplasia of Queyrat, Bowen's disease of the glans penis. Also occurring in the genital region, bowenoid papulosis presents with hyperpigmented papules of the pubic region, with histologic findings identical to Bowen's disease. It is most commonly associated with HPV 16 and 18. The significance of distinguishing the particular clinical variant of SCCIS is relevant when implementing treatment plans, as these entities have different potentials for invasion; the risk of developing invasive disease in erythroplasia of Queyrat is reported to be 30% [48, 49] while that potential for bowenoid papulosis is less than 1% [50]. Thus, clinicopathologic correlation is quite important in developing management and follow-up plans for the various subtypes of SCCIS.

17.3.3 Invasive Squamous Cell Carcinoma

Typical invasive cutaneous SCC arises most commonly on sun-exposed skin of the head and neck or distal extremities and presents as a firm pink keratotic papule or plaque (Fig. 17.2). They may also be exophytic without hyperkeratosis (Figs. 17.3 and 17.4, superior) or relatively flat and ill defined (Fig. 17.4, inferior). The presence of a nodule lacking surface change should raise suspicion of a metastatic tumor.

Cutaneous SCCs commonly associated with HPV include periungual and anogenital disease. The periungual

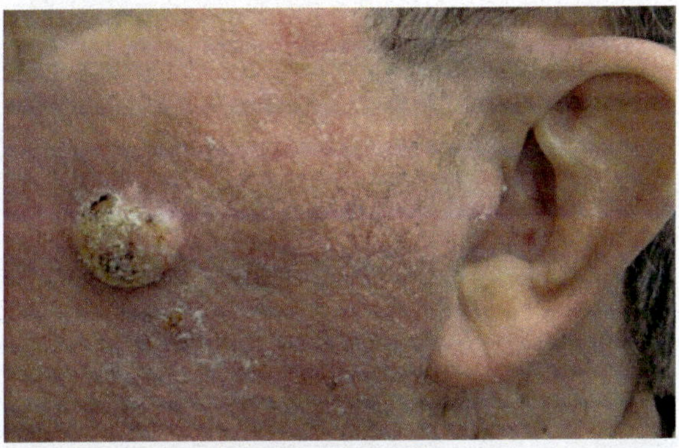

Fig. 17.2 SCC with associated hyperkeratosis

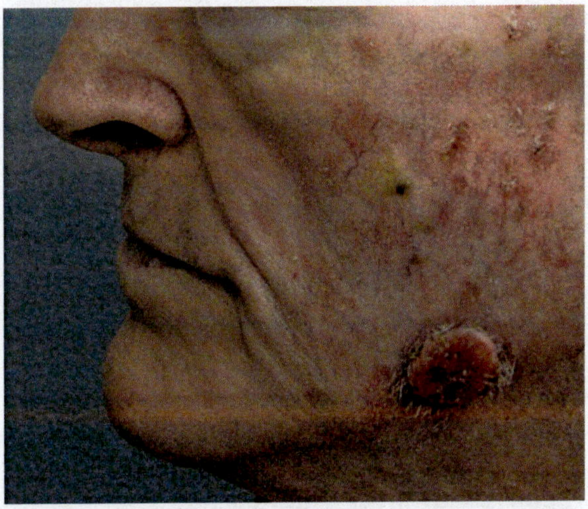

Fig. 17.3 Exophytic SCC without hyperkeratosis on a background of actinically damaged skin

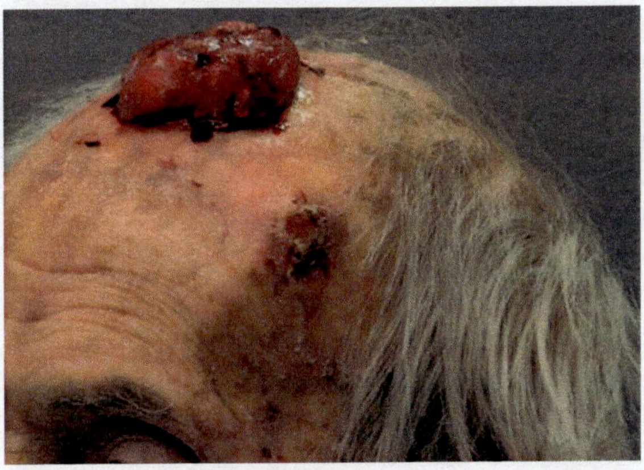

Fig. 17.4 Two clinical presentations of SCC: A large friable exophytic tumor with hemorrhagic crust removed on the anterior central scalp (*superior*) and a thinner but more ill-defined lesion just above the left temple (*inferior*)

variant is often mistaken for a recalcitrant wart frequently causing a delay in diagnosis. Clinicians should have a low threshold for biopsy, particularly when initial treatment fails [51]. Anogenital SCCs commonly present as moist red, indurated, or ulcerated plaques.

The keratoacanthoma (KA) type of squamous cell carcinoma is a well differentiated, rapidly growing crateriform nodule with a central keratin plug. It is considered a self-healing neoplasm with a particular history and histologic architecture. While the metastatic potential of a keratoacanthoma is minimal, KA can be indistinguishable histologically from invasive SCC [52]. Given the potential morbidity and mortality of an error in diagnosis or predicted biologic behavior, KA is best considered and treated as a well-differentiated SCC taking the patient, the history, and the risks and benefits of treatment into consideration.

Verrucous carcinoma is a slow-growing variant of invasive SCC that can be locally destructive but has low metastatic potential. When found in the anogenital region, these lesions are referred to as Buschke–Lowenstein tumors. When found in the mouth, they are termed oral florid papillomatosis, and on the foot, epithelioma cuniculatum. Despite their low metastatic potential, their propensity toward local destruction can be quite severe, particularly in immunosuppressed patients.

17.3.4 Differential Diagnosis

The differential diagnosis of cutaneous SCC includes its precursor lesions, actinic keratoses, and SCCIS, as well as basal cell carcinoma and verruca. Atypical fibroxanthoma and merkel cell carcinoma may present similarly to some SCCs and often occur in similar locations. Additionally, ulcerative diseases, such as pyoderma gangrenosum, may be in the clinical differential in the case of a non-healing ulcer. Biopsy is required for definitive diagnosis and, given the ease and low morbidity associated with it, should be done when there is any concern for SCC.

Summary: Management of Invasive Cutaneous SCC

- The management of cutaneous SCC is a mainstay of Mohs surgical practice. However, the treating surgeon should always consider both surgical and non-surgical treatment options.

17.4 Management of Invasive Cutaneous SCC

In approaching the patient with cutaneous SCC, it is important to rule out high-risk disease (see high-risk section below). If the tumor is not high risk, surgical excision is the mainstay of care for invasive SCC. Radiation as primary therapy will also be discussed. Non-surgical modalities such as curettage, electrocautery, cryosurgery, topical creams (5-fluorouracil and imiquimod), and photodynamic therapy are generally reserved for in situ disease since cure rates are generally inferior to surgery, and non-surgical methods do not allow for evaluation of histologic margins [53]. However, non-surgical approaches play a central role in the treatment of in situ field cancerization (see below).

17.4.1 Surgical Options

Complete surgical clearance of invasive SCC is of paramount importance since negative surgical margins are critical for achieving cure. When clear histologic margins are confirmed, results are excellent (local recurrence risk 5%, lymph node metastasis 5%, distant metastasis 1%, disease-specific death 1%) [54].

Standard excision is considered appropriate for well-defined tumors in areas where tissue sparing is not critical. For well-defined tumors <2 cm, a 4-mm margin is curative 95% of the time. However, high rates of positive margins after standard excision are reported for tumors on the ear, infiltrative SCC, and recurrent or re-excised tumors [55]. Therefore, for larger tumors (>2 cm) or infiltrative growth patterns with deeper invasion, a 6-mm margin or, preferably, Mohs micrographic surgery or another method of total margin-controlled excision is generally preferred [56, 57].

Mohs micrographic surgery is the recommended therapy for high-risk cutaneous SCC (see below) and tumors located in anatomically critical or cosmetically sensitive areas. Mohs histologic sectioning allows for visualization of nearly the entire surgical margin; <1% of the margin is examined following standard excision. 5-year cure rates support the importance of meticulous margin evaluation, as traditional surgical excision cures 92% of primary tumors, while Mohs cures 97%. For recurrent disease, standard excision has a 77% cure rate, while Mohs is able to cure 90–94% [11, 58, 59].

For very large tumors which are difficult to approach with local anesthesia, a multidisciplinary surgical approach may be employed.

Controlled comparative studies of Mohs versus standard excision have not been carried out for SCC. However, given the compelling case series data, and Mohs' ability to fully examine the marginal surface, Mohs is considered the standard of care for high-risk SCC and tumors on the head by most American dermatologists. A comparative study would be helpful in identifying a single surgical standard of care for SCC across multiple specialties, including plastic surgery, head and neck surgery, and surgical oncology specialists who routinely manage SCC with standard excision.

17.4.2 Radiation Therapy as Primary Therapy

While *radiation* can be used as a primary treatment option for cutaneous SCCs, reported outcomes are worse than surgical therapy. In addition to the long-term cutaneous risks of radiation, tumors that do respond tend to quickly recur, and radiation is far more cumbersome for patients than surgery [60]. Its appropriate use as a primary therapy is therefore limited to a subset of patients with early disease where surgery would lead to unacceptable cosmetic or functional impairment or in patients with inoperable tumors [61]. Given the high rates of recurrence, inconvenience, and the inability to confirm clear margins with radiation, surgery remains the most effective approach for treating primary SCC.

Summary: Identification and Management of High-Risk Squamous Cell Carcinoma

- The rare risks of metastasis and death should be considered by physicians managing invasive SCC. The precise risk of these poor outcomes for individual patients is unknown. This, coupled with a lack of clinical trials, makes decision-making regarding the need for nodal staging and adjuvant therapy difficult. This section summarizes the information currently available.

17.5 Identification and Management of High-Risk Squamous Cell Carcinoma

The evaluation of a patient with invasive cutaneous SCC is incomplete without considering the risk for recurrence or metastasis. Although for the vast majority of patients this risk is minute, for a subset of patients, the risk appears to be substantial. Tumors with features that have been associated with metastasis and death have been termed high-risk cutaneous SCC (HRSCC). To date, there is no consensus for defining HRSCC. The potential for aggressive disease can be attributed to both tumor and host factors. As there is no prognostic model available, it is unknown how various risk factors combine and lead to recurrence or metastasis. Therefore, estimating these risks for an individual patient remains challenging. Current recommendations are summarized in the table below and indicate that there are significant areas of ambiguity of opinion regarding management of high-risk tumors. This uncertainty has been further demonstrated in a recent survey study of Mohs surgeons which indicated that there is only agreement at the far ends of the high-risk spectrum. Opinion regarding nodal staging and adjuvant radiation varies widely for most HRSCC cases (Table 17.1) [12, 62–67].

17.5.1 Tumor Factors Associated with High-Risk SCC

Location: Cutaneous SCC arising in skin that has been previously injured, such as a scar, chronic wound, ulcer, or burn site, has a higher risk of recurrence and metastasis [11, 68–70]. Recurrence rates have been reported as high as 58% and 5-year survival only 52% [71]. Tumor location appears to impact prognosis. The largest review of available data suggests that location on the lip and ear have higher rates of metastases (14% and 9%, respectively) than other sun-exposed sites [11]. A three-fold higher risk of metastasis from lesions on the ear has been shown in a prospective study [10]. Anogenital SCC has shown high metastatic rates, ranging from 15% to 74% [72–75]. However, studies to evaluate the prognostic importance of anatomic location relative to other risk factors have been underpowered. Thus, the question of the impact of location on outcomes remains open.

Table 17.1 Expert consensus recommendations for the management of high-risk SCC

Source	Recommendations				
	Surgical	Radiotherapy	Adjuvant therapy	Staging	Comments
Miller [62]	Treat all high-risk[a] SCC with surgery (Mohs or excision with complete pathologic assessment of all circumferential and deep marginal surfaces)	Option for primary therapy in non-surgical candidates, usually reserved for patients over 60 due to long-term sequelae	Recommend adjuvant radiation for any NMSC that involves "more than just a few small sensory nerve branches or has large nerve involvement"	NR regarding SLN biopsy. Imaging studies for all patients as clinically indicated for extensive disease	MRI if large nerve involvement is suspected to rule out skull involvement
	If there is pathologic evidence of lymph node involvement, preferred treatment is regional lymph node dissection	Option for treatment of lymph node basin if surgery is not feasible. Reconsider surgery following radiation	Considered for all patients with regional disease on trunk and extremities who have undergone lymph node dissection		Consider oral retinoids
			Recommended postoperatively for all patients with lymph node involvement of the head and neck		Consider dose reduction in immunosuppression in OTRs in favor of mTOR inhibitors
Breuninger [63]	Complete surgical excision with microscopic control of margins Prophylactic lymph node dissection may be done for tumors with a high risk of metastasis (precise indications not specified)	If complete excision is not possible, salvage radiation therapy is the best option, sometimes in combination with chemotherapy and/or immunotherapy	NR for indications for adjuvant radiation	NR regarding radiologic nodal staging Sentinel lymph node biopsy can be incorporated into the staging procedure, (precise indications not specified)	
Stasko[b] [64]	For aggressive SCC[c], surgical excision should be done via Mohs micrographic surgery or excision with margin control For incomplete clearance, consider further tumor resection whenever possible	If there is PNI or invasion of deep structures, if one is unable to clear margins, If patient is unable to tolerate surgery, or if tumor is inoperable, may consider primary radiation therapy	If there is PNI or invasion of deep structures or if one is unable to clear margins, consider adjuvant radiation therapy	If there is PNI or invasion of deep structures or if one is unable to clear margins, then: • Consider radiologic imaging to assess local extension • Consider SLN biopsy and node dissection NR regarding indications for radiologic nodal staging	If there is PNI or invasion of deep structures or if one is unable to clear margins, then consider reduction of immunosuppression
Motley [65]	Surgical excision (including Mohs surgery) should be considered treatment of first choice for all cutaneous SCC		NR for when adjuvant radiotherapy should be used	NR for nodal staging	Patients with a high-risk SCC should ideally be managed by a multidisciplinary cutaneous oncology team[d]

Miller [66]	Treat all high-risk SCC with surgery (Mohs or excision with complete pathologic assessment of all circumferential and deep marginal surfaces)	Salvage radiotherapy for positive surgical margins	Recommend adjuvant radiotherapy for extensive perineural or large nerve involvement	NR regarding nodal staging	Consider sentinel lymph node mapping "in certain high-risk lesions"
Committee on Guidelines of care [67]	Mohs micrographic surgery is efficacious for treatment of recurrent lesions and tumors displaying one or more of the anatomic, clinical, or histologic factors associated with increased biologic aggressiveness[e]		NR for indications for adjuvant radiation	NR for nodal staging	No specific recommendations for high-risk SCC

NR no recommendations made, *PNI* perineural involvement, *NMSC* non-melanoma skin cancer, *OTR* organ transplant recipient, *mTOR* mammalian target of rapamycin

[a]Any high-risk feature places tumor in the high-risk category: >2.0 cm on trunk and extremities, >1.0 cm on cheeks, forehead, scalp, and neck, >0.6 cm on remaining "mask" area of face; poorly defined borders, recurrent tumor, moderately or poorly differentiated, adenoid/acantholytic adenosquamous or desmoplastic subtypes, Clark level IV,V or depth >0.4 cm, rapid growth, neurologic symptoms, occurring in a site of prior RT or chronic inflammation and occurring in the setting of immunosuppression

[b]Guidelines for treatment of cutaneous SCC, specifically in organ transplant recipients

[c]Size >0.6 cm on "mask" areas of the face, >1.0 cm on cheeks, forehead, neck, and scalp, >2.0 cm on trunk and extremities, location on scalp, ear, lip, midface, genitalia, or nail unit, rapid growth, poorly defined margins, ulceration, poorly differentiated histology, perineural involvement, and invasion to subcutaneous fat

[d]A multidisciplinary cutaneous oncology team has the following available: A dermatologist, pathologist, Mohs surgeon, surgical oncologist, medical oncologist, and a clinical nurse

[e]Size >1 cm, rapid growth, ulceration, immunocompromised host, recurrent tumors, location on mucous membranes, ear, temple, scalp, or eyelid, undifferentiated histology, depth into and beyond the subcutaneous fat, perineural invasion, lymphatic invasion

Diameter: Tumor diameter correlates with risk of metastasis with most series reporting tumors greater than 2 cm as higher risk [11, 69, 76]. Smaller tumors of the lip and ear can metastasize, and cut points of 1.0 or 1.5 cm have sometimes been used to connote higher risk in these locations [77].

History of recurrence after surgical excision: Local recurrence has been associated with distant metastatic disease; 30–50% of metastatic tumors occur in patients with a prior local recurrence [11, 78].

Histologic characteristics: Histologic features associated with increased rates of recurrence, metastasis, and death, assessed via case series and small prospective studies, include tumor depth, perineural involvement (PNI) and poorly differentiated histology [11, 79].

Tumor thickness and the tissue level of invasion (e.g., fat, fascia, muscle, or bone) may predict metastatic disease. The millimeter depth that defines a high-risk tumor and the magnitude of that risk are not well defined. Reported rates of metastasis correlating with depths of 4–6 mm are 16–46% depending on the series [10, 11, 80]. The wide range may be due to small numbers of subjects and the biases of case-series, single-center data. Patients with tumors <2 mm thick appear to have a very low risk of metastasis [10]. Tumors infiltrating through subcutaneous fat are associated with disease-specific death [79].

Histologic grade appears to be a very important prognostic factor. The estimated cure rate for poorly differentiated tumors is 37%. In contrast, it reaches 88% for well-differentiated disease and 59% in moderately differentiated cases [69]. A 33% risk of metastasis has also been reported in patients with poorly differentiated tumors [11]. Desmoplastic or infiltrative SCCs have a tendency toward local recurrence and regional metastasis; this risk increases with increasing tumor thickness. Infiltrative cutaneous SCCs have been reported to have six times the rate of lymph node metastases and ten times the rate of local recurrence compared to non-infiltrative tumors [80].

Perineural invasion (PNI) is associated with a high incidence of recurrence, metastasis, and death [11, 79, 81]. However, the spectrum of PNI is vast varying from involvement of tiny dermal nerve twigs to cranial nerve extension inside the skull. Patients may have evidence of cranial nerve involvement on physical exam, most commonly in fifth and seventh nerves [82], or they may be asymptomatic. Patients with symptomatic involvement of named nerves have a particularly poor prognosis. The risk of death from SCC in patients with involvement of nerves 0.1 mm or greater was reported to be 32% in a small cohort study. Conversely, those with involvement of smaller nerve twigs less than 0.1 mm had a good prognosis with only rare local recurrence and no metastasis or death [83].

17.5.2 Host Factors Associated with High-Risk SCC

Immunosuppressed patients are at substantially greater risk of developing SCC than the immunocompetent, and they have a higher risk of poor outcomes. The rate of metastasis is twice as high in the immunocompromised, with rates of 13% described [11]. The type of immunodeficiency correlates with varying degrees of increased risk.

Organ transplant recipients (OTRs) have a 65-fold increased incidence of cutaneous SCCs when compared to the general population [84]. The ratio of SCCs to basal cell carcinomas (BCCs) is 3:1, which is reversed compared to the general population [85, 86]. Degree of immunosuppression may impact risk. For example, there is a nearly three times greater incidence of SCCs in heart transplant recipients when compared to kidney transplants [84], presumably because heart transplant patients need to receive higher doses of immunosuppression to avoid rejection. When additional risk factors are added to a history of organ transplantation, such as fair skin and extensive sun exposure, incidence rates approach 70% [53]. Additionally, the cumulative incidence of developing skin cancer increases with longer duration of immunosuppression; in one Australian study rates were 7% after 1 year, 45% after 11 years, and 70% after 20 years [53]. A history of one cutaneous SCC in OTRs has been shown to correlate with a 66% chance of developing a second primary tumor within 5 years [87]. Unfortunately, OTRs present more commonly with high-risk cutaneous SCCs with a greater tendency toward metastasis; since tumors are more often deep and poorly differentiated [88]. Heart transplant patients have been shown to have a 4% incidence of aggressive and poorly differentiated cutaneous SCC within 10 years of transplant. The risk of death from high-risk SCC 20 years after heart transplantation has been shown to be extraordinarily high at 66% in one small study [89]. The occurrence of in-transit cutaneous metastases which carry a high (65%) associated mortality is also higher in OTRs [90].

Chronic lymphocytic leukemia (CLL) and small-cell lymphocytic lymphoma (SLL) are well known to be associated with cutaneous malignancy. SCC is reported most frequently [91] and is commonly aggressive with high rates of recurrence and metastasis [20]. The cumulative 5-year recurrence rate for cutaneous SCC in patients with CLL/SLL has been reported at 19%, seven times higher than controls [20]. While the number of patients with CLL/SLL developing SCC is less than 5%, tumors in these patients tend to be more aggressive, with more than half in patients with CLL/SLL meeting high-risk criteria [91]. One quarter of the tumors in these patients recur or metastasize despite standard therapy, and 41% of cutaneous SCC patients with CLL/SLL have been reported to die from their skin cancer [91]. The behavior of the tumors may correlate with the status of their underlying lymphoproliferative disorder; if neoplasms suddenly become more aggressive, their CLL/SLL very well may be progressing, and the treating oncologist should be notified.

While there is a well-documented increase in anogenital cutaneous SCC in association with HPV in HIV patients, a definitive association with high-risk cutaneous SCC has not been made. Small case series have described patients with HIV who developed aggressive SCC, with 50% mortality at 7 years [21]. It is reasonable to conclude that caution should be used when managing patients with poorly controlled HIV or AIDS who develop cutaneous SCC, particularly high-risk tumors.

Other host conditions have been associated with high-risk cutaneous SCC and worse outcomes. These include iatrogenic psoralen-ultraviolet-A (PUVA) or ionizing radiation exposure, environmental arsenic exposure, and chronic inflammatory states. In patients with recessive dystrophic epidermolysis bullosa (RDEB), cutaneous SCC is the leading cause of death, with an 80% mortality rate within 5 years of diagnosis of the neoplasm [92]. Other chronic autoimmune diseases, treated with immunosuppression, may also be associated with a higher risk of developing cutaneous SCC [93]; this may be related to both therapy and the disease itself.

17.5.3 Work-Up (Staging of Primary Tumor and Nodal Basins)

Examination of draining lymph node basins is important in evaluating a patient with high-risk SCC. If nodes are palpable on exam, a fine-needle aspiration (FNA) or excisional biopsy should be performed. Different from its counterpart melanoma, most patients with lymph node metastasis from cutaneous SCC are curable if the tumors are operable, and therefore evaluation of the nodal basin and early identification of disease are critical.

Radiologic imaging is the most common approach used to detect subclinical tumor extension and nodal disease. The gold standard imaging modality of choice, as well as which patients require imaging, has not been established in cutaneous SCC. However, there is data evaluating imaging for oronasopharyngeal SCC. This data suggests that CT, MRI, PET, and ultrasound all have variable specificity and sensitivity and commonly result in false positives and negatives. The addition of PET to CT improves sensitivity; however, because it has not yet shown an impact on outcomes, justifying its cost can be difficult for routine cases. For detecting nodal necrosis, extracapsular spread, and bone or cartilage involvement, CT is generally most useful. MRI is the better choice if the goal is to evaluate tissue plains, distinguish soft tissues, or gauge extent of large-nerve invasion [94, 95]. Given their different strengths, both MRI and CT may be helpful in planning a surgery. They may be of particular use in SCC thought to be involving LNs or deeper bone, glands, or major nerves. CT scanning and MRI appear to have little utility in detecting asymptomatic perineural invasion (PNI). However, when PNI is visible on imaging, outcomes are often poor; the 5-year survival with positive imaging is reported at 50% versus 86% with negative imaging [46]. PET scanning and ultrasound-guided FNA may be useful screening tools in detecting subclinical nodal metastases, but their utility and likelihood of altering management have been minimally studied [96, 97]. The use of 18F-fluorodeoxyglucose positron emission tomography (FDG-PET) to detect nodal metastasis may be a useful staging tool, but there is very limited data on its effectiveness in cutaneous SCC. Its utility lies in its ability to detect metastasis where radiotherapy has resulted in necrosis, fibrosis, and dense scarring [98].

While radiologic imaging in cutaneous SCC requires further study to determine which patients are likely to benefit from which study, imaging is safe. Given its low risk, it should be considered in those with high-risk neoplasms to evaluate the draining nodes and when deeper tissue involvement is suspected, for surgical planning.

Sentinel lymph node (SLN) biopsy is another method of evaluating clinically negative nodal basins. Again, because there have been no controlled studies in cutaneous SCC, its impact remains unknown. Review of the English literature [99] consisting of case reports and small case series in which SLN biopsy was used in high-risk SCC showed 21% of cases to have a positive SLN in non-anogenital SCC and 24% in anogenital cases. False negatives were rare and mostly from studies prior to the use of combination lymphoscintigraphy with methylene blue dye. Rates of morbidity from SLN in the literature are low and generally mild. It is not known whether early detection of LN metastasis will improve outcomes for patients with SCC. This awaits further study. Considering that only 5–10% of cases are SLN positive in most melanoma series, it may be that SLN biopsy is underutilized in high-risk SCC. Unlike melanoma, SCC with nodal involvement is highly curable (73% 5-year survival), so early detection via SLN biopsy may more readily impact outcomes than it does in melanoma. However, the right target group for SLN staging in high-risk SCC has yet to be defined.

17.5.4 Surgical Management

As described above, Mohs is an excellent choice for management of SCC and, in particular, of high-risk disease. However, in cases with advanced local extension, surgical clearance may require a multidisciplinary team, particularly if there is bone invasion or intracranial involvement of major nerve branches. A multidisciplinary team approach (Fig. 17.5) using preoperative radiologic imaging and/or SLN biopsy is ideal. Mohs surgeons may establish the peripheral margin while craniofacial or head and neck surgeons manage PNI of major nerves, parotid involvement, and bone extirpation to complete the tumor clearance. Using Mohs under local anesthesia to establish the peripheral margin minimizes general anesthesia time and allows the head and neck or craniofacial surgeon to focus on clearing the deep margin and the reconstruction.

Because high-risk tumors have features that may make it difficult to interpret margins or to track subtle PNI, the addition of cytokeratin immunohistochemical (IHC) stains [100, 101] may help to improve the sensitivity of Mohs in selected cases. IHC helps make individual tumor cells, which are otherwise difficult to identify, more visible than on hematoxylin- and eosin-stained sections. However, the costs of staining large marginal surfaces can be prohibitive.

17.5.5 Radiation as Primary Therapy

For high-risk SCC, the cure rate with radiation as monotherapy is generally inferior to surgery with local recurrence rates of 15–20% [62]. However, maintenance of oral function and cure rates similar to surgery have been reported with the use of radiation in treating cutaneous SCC of the lower lip [102]. Radiation as primary therapy is generally reserved for select cases of locally advanced SCC in which the prognosis is poor (in which case it may be delivered with palliative rather than curative intent), and/or attempting surgical clearance would introduce risk or morbidity unacceptable to the patient such as blindness or an inability to eat or speak.

17.5.6 Adjuvant Therapy

Radiation: It is accepted that adjuvant radiation therapy (ART) should be considered with certain tumors, particularly those with significant PNI (named nerves or larger-caliber nerves), although no controlled studies have evaluated outcomes; the utility of adjuvant radiation is therefore unknown [54]. There is no clear data regarding which patients should receive ART. However, it is known that patients with surgically clear margins prior to ART have better outcomes [103]. This is seen even when there is invasion of major nerves [81]. Although PNI is the most commonly cited reason for considering ART, data on its impact in this patient group is limited [54]. However, these tumors have high recurrence rates even with clear surgical margins [54, 81, 83]. Therefore, in cases of PNI involving larger nerves, ART should be considered, despite the lack of proof of its utility. Additionally, when surgical clearance of PNI is not possible, salvage radiotherapy may be helpful, but mortality rates as high as 30% have been reported in this setting [60]. In the case of nodal disease, this should be first managed by aggressive surgical resection of all local and regional disease, including LN dissection of multiple nodal basins if indicated. Addition of adjuvant radiation to lymphadenectomy can result in high cure rates, which have been reported as 73% 5-year disease-free survival (DFS) [104].

In summary, it is reasonable to consider ART in the highest-risk patients, particularly those with involvement of nerves >0.1 mm in diameter, and those in whom the surgical margin is uncertain such as in

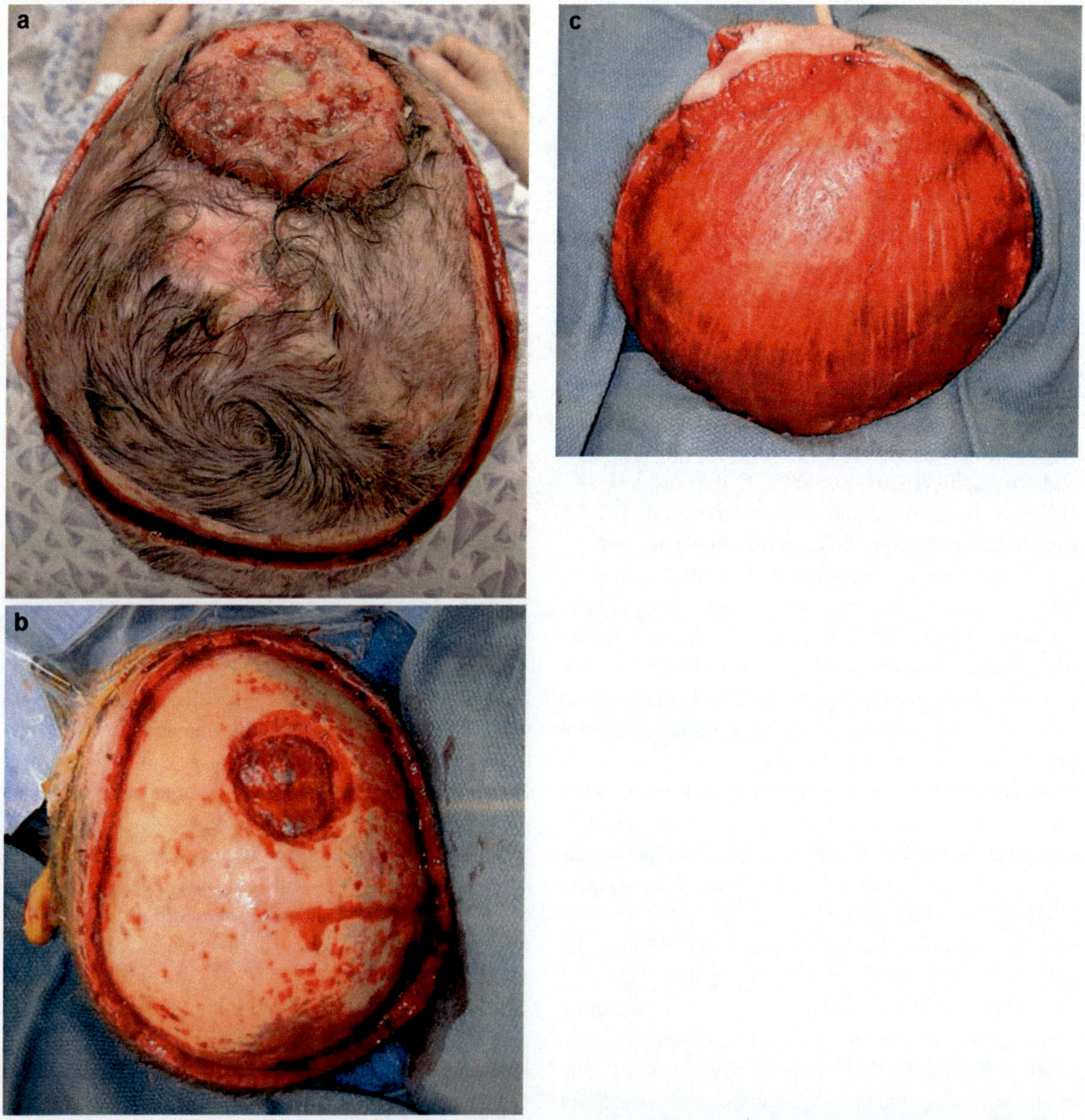

Fig. 17.5 (**a**) A very large SCC of the scalp with bone invasion confirmed on MRI. Multiple surrounding areas of shallow erosion were also SCC on biopsy. Mohs was used to establish a clear peripheral margin including periosteum. An 8-cm zone of tissue was left intact anteriorly to prevent tissue necrosis in the event of a delay of the planned complete resection. The wound was closed with a single running suture. (**b**) The next day, the entire region defined by Mohs was removed by a head and neck surgeon, including bone immediately below the tumor Photo courtesy of Dr. Don Annino, Brigham and Women's Head and Neck Surgery. (**c**) A latissimus dorsi free flap reconstruction was performed by the head and neck surgeon. The patient remained disease-free for over 2 years before death from an unrelated cause. Photo courtesy of Dr. Don Annino, Brigham and Women's Head and Neck Surgery

poorly differentiated tumors with single-cell spread, multiply recurrent tumors, or tumors with in-transit local metastasis.

Chemotherapy: The use of chemotherapy in the treatment of high-risk cutaneous SCC remains is a relatively new concept. Retinoids have been the most well studied and reported in these patients. This class of medications is known to slow the development of new tumors but do not alter the course of an existing tumor. They act to promote differentiation, downregulate proto-oncogenes, and regulate growth in the hyperproliferative epidermis [105, 106]. They are used as prophylactic agents, particularly in OTRs, when there is diffuse actinic damage [106–110]. Doses ranging from 10 to 30 mg/day have proven efficacious, and low-dose therapy is usually sufficient and must be continued indefinitely, as patients usually return to baseline on discontinuation of treatment. Dose escalation, beginning with 10 mg every other day and increasing to an effective tolerated dose, is an acceptable reported method [111]. Once efficacy is achieved, tapering to the lowest effective maintenance dose is reasonable, given the need for indefinite therapy. In the treatment of existing tumors, randomized trials of 13-cis retinoic acid (isotretinoin), either used alone for adjuvant treatment of established mucosal SCC of the head and neck [112] or in combination with interferon [113] for established cutaneous SCC, have shown no benefit. There have been no controlled trials evaluating the use of acitretin in treating existing disease, although in patients with metastatic or inoperable disease, the use of full-dose retinoids can be considered for a possible chemotherapeutic or suppressive effect [111].

In cases of advanced cutaneous SCC, cisplatin-based combination regimens have been tried. These have included combination regimens with 5-fluorouracil (5-FU), methotrexate, bleomycin, and doxorubicin. Outcomes have varied, and patients have reported the onset of 5-FU-related adverse effects. Capecitabine (Xeloda, Roche Laboratories, Inc), the oral 5-FU prodrug, is metabolized selectively to 5-FU within tumor cells, with the goal of less resulting systemic toxicity. There have been some reports of improved outcomes when capecitabine is used alone [114] or with subcutaneous interferon [115] to treat locally advanced cutaneous SCC. Capecitabine, when used with cisplatin or paclitaxel [116, 117] or in combination with radiation [118], has shown favorable outcomes in phase II trials of patients with mucosal SCC of the head and neck.

Epidermal growth factor receptor (EGRF) is expressed in normal basal layer and appendageal epidermal keratinocytes [119] and may be over-expressed in deposits of cutaneous SCC [120]. Therefore, the (EGFR) inhibitors have been used off-label in a handful of case reports in the treatment of cutaneous SCC to control proliferation, cell cycle progression, survival, angiogenesis, and metastasis. Cetuximab has had reported success in cases of inoperable tumors, in-transit metastases, in metastatic SCC with and without epidermolysis bullosa, and as combination therapy with celecoxib [121–125]. Gefitinib has been reported to result in palliative tumor shrinkage in a single case report [126]; however, phase II [127] and III [128] trials in metastatic mucosal head and neck SCC failed to show a survival benefit.

While there is a persistent lack of evidence, adjuvant chemotherapy may still be considered in cases of cutaneous SCC that is locally advanced or metastatic. Consultation with medical oncology should be considered in these cases. The available treatments are well tolerated with low risk of serious adverse effects. Further evaluation is needed to determine which patients are most likely to benefit from which adjuvant chemotherapeutics and to determine whether there is a subgroup of high-risk patients who would benefit from adjuvant chemotherapy after surgery to prevent recurrence.

17.5.7 Assessment of Immune Status

All patients with cutaneous SCC require a thorough history and exam to evaluate for the presence of any underlying process that might impair their immune status, placing them at higher risk of a poor outcome. Particularly in OTRs and CLL patients, immunosuppression is the primary cause of an elevated risk of recurrent and metastatic cutaneous SCCs. Accelerated skin cancer formation with multiple invasive cutaneous SCCs may be a marker of worsening immunity. In the case of OTRs, immunosuppression can result in the rapid development of new tumors. When immunosuppression is reduced, the number of new SCCs declines, and outcomes in patients with known aggressive disease improve [111]. Therapy with a single agent is less problematic than multi-agent immunosuppression. Specific newer immunosuppressive agents, particularly sirolimus, an inhibitor of the mammalian target of rapamycin (mTOR), are associated with a lower incidence of cutaneous SCC when compared to older calcineurin inhibitors (CNIs) [129, 130]. Further, when switched from traditional CNIs to sirolimus, patients' tumors were thinner with reduced vascularization [131]; this is in line with the known anti-angiogenic properties of mTOR inhibitors. However, sirolimus has other side effects which limit its use. Changes in dose or class of immunosuppression in OTRs should be carried out with the transplant physician to avoid impairment in graft function and rejection. The risks posed by SCC must be balanced with the risks of a new immunosuppressive regimen and rejection. The transplant physician should be advised by the dermatologist or Mohs surgeon of the impact of SCC on the patient's quality of life and estimates of morbidity and mortality for high-risk tumors conveyed.

17.5.8 Follow-Up for High-Risk SCC Patients

Because patients with nodal disease can be cured up to 73% of the time [104], patients with cutaneous SCC should be closely followed for recurrence; early detection and treatment are crucial. Full skin and lymph node exam by a dermatologist every 3–6 months is advised with 95% of local recurrences and metastases occurring within 5 years [11]. A neurological exam should be performed if indicated. Aggressive management of actinic keratoses and early biopsy of suspicious or persistent lesions are recommended. For more advanced cases, such as with PNI, with multiple recurrences, or in those who are at higher risk of aggressive tumor behavior secondary to immunosuppression, re-imaging of the draining nodal basin can be considered every 6 months.

Summary: Treatment of Field Cancerization

- The treatment of the immunosuppressed patient with diffuse actinic damage and innumerable atypical squamous tumors requires field therapy, applied sequentially. The treatment of "field cancerization" is likely to improve the quality of life of such patients, ideally limiting the development of invasive disease and the time spent in health care facilities.

17.6 Treatment of Field Cancerization

Patients with diffuse actinic damage on the AK/SCCIS spectrum, termed "field cancerization," who develop multiple SCCs, particularly OTRs, must be approached differently than the typical sun-damaged patient with one or few tumors. These field-damaged patients spend a considerable amount of time in health care facilities, and their tumors may adversely affect their quality of life in addition to their long-term survival.

As stated above, the first step in an immunocompromised patient is to address and improve their immune status when possible. This should be followed by clearing all invasive SCCs. Histologic margins should be examined for all invasive SCCs, and electrodessication and curettage should be avoided. One approach that is acceptable to patients due to its efficiency is the use of disc excision without prior biopsy to clear numerous invasive SCCs on the body. Invasion can often be determined clinically by the presence of dermal induration. Patients can be seen monthly, and multiple tumors can be removed at each visit. Wound care instructions for secondary intention healing are provided. Tumors that are appropriate for Mohs (large lesions and those on the head, below the knees, and hands) may be biopsied and then treated via Mohs excision. This "clean-up" phase to remove invasive tumors may require several months of frequent visits.

Concurrently, hypertrophic actinic keratoses and suspected early SCCIS are curetted to remove hyperkeratotic overlying scale (Fig. 17.6). This is followed immediately by topical 5-fluorouracil (5-FU) twice a day for a month to a given field. Such a regimen can markedly improve field cancerization (Fig. 17.7). Application of petrolatum every 3–6 h to the treated area can reduce the burning sensation and increase tolerability. Imiquimod is less useful in this setting given the eroded skin surface and large areas of involvement which can lead to increased systemic absorption and severe flu-like side effects. Similarly, cryotherapy has a limited role in the treatment of field cancerization, as it cannot be applied to large surface areas. Curettage of hyperkeratotic AKs and SCCISs followed by 5-FU may be repeated as needed. Patients with severe dermatoheliosis may need re-treatment every 6–12 months to maintain control of their disease. Lesions that fail to clear must be biopsied or treated with disc excision [132].

Another option for the treatment of field cancerization includes cyclic photodynamic therapy (PDT). The use of 20% 5-aminolevulinic acid (ALA) under plastic wrap occlusion followed by PDT with blue light (417 nm) every 2–4 months has been shown to reduce cutaneous SCC formation by 95% when compared to the year preceding the initiation of this method [133].

If patients continue to develop multiple cancers 6–12 months after instituting the above methods for field treatment, the addition of low-dose oral retinoids, dosed as discussed above, should be considered for tumor prophylaxis. Again, patients are likely to require

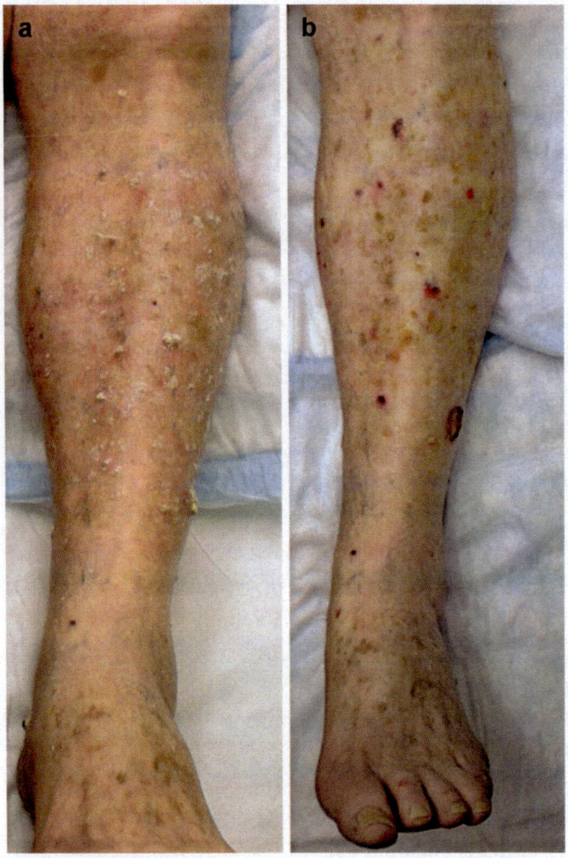

Fig. 17.6 (**a**) Diffuse hyperkeratoic actinic keratoses and SCCIS with a dermally invasive tumor on the infero-lateral aspect of left leg. (**b**) The same patient after Mohs excision of the invasive SCC and light curettage of the AKs and SCCISs. He immediately began a 4-week course of 5% 5-fluorouracil cream twice daily with good clearance of disease although re-treatment every 6 months is required to maintain the effect. Few invasive tumors are developing with this intensive approach

lifelong therapy given the probability of returning to their pretreatment baseline upon discontinuing retinoids. Dose reduction, including alternate day therapy, should be considered, rather than discontinuation, when possible.

Summary: Conclusions

- Cutaneous SCC is common and can be aggressive, with high morbidity and mortality particularly in the immunocompromised. A thorough understanding of disease development as well as all available treatment options is critical in optimizing patient care.

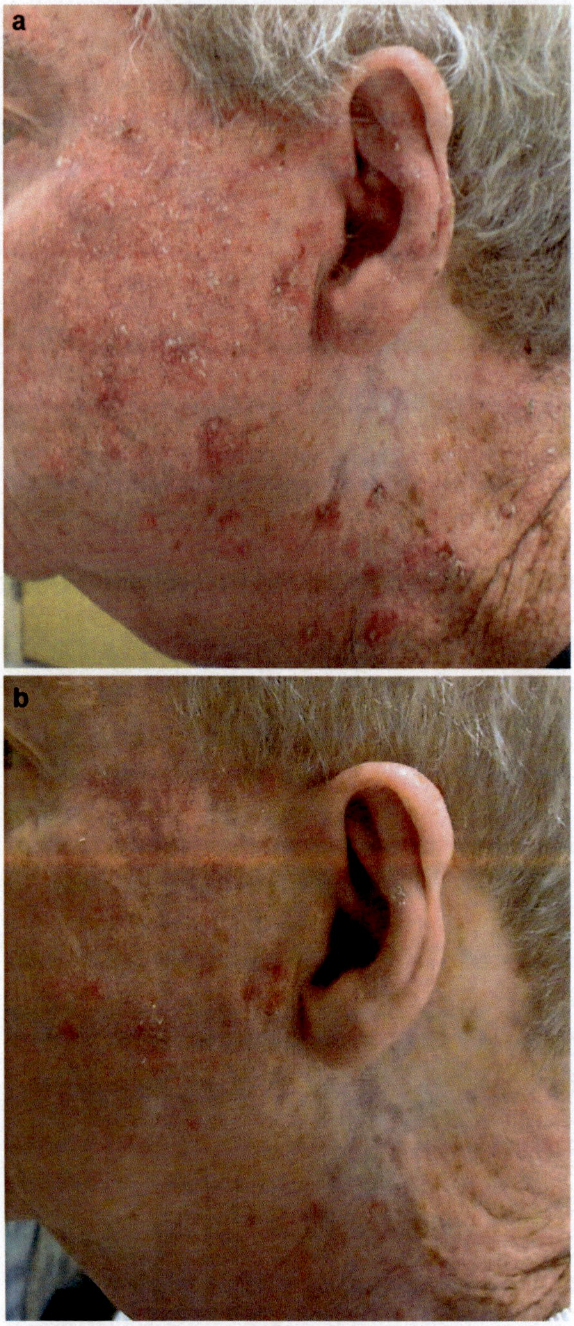

Fig. 17.7 (**a**) Diffuse actinic keratoses and SCCIS. (**b**) The same patient after a 4-week course of 5% 5-fluorouracil cream twice daily with marked improvement

17.7 Conclusions

SCC is the second most common malignancy in white persons, and despite its visibility on the skin, accounts for thousands of deaths annually in the USA. Although most tumors are easily cured with surgical excision, identification of high-risk SCC is imprecise. Without reliable prognostic models, there is ambiguity in treatment guidelines and the optimal care of high-risk patients. Current practice standards have developed from clinician experience and primarily uncontrolled case-series data. Based on the information currently available, invasive cutaneous SCC is best managed by detecting disease early, identifying high-risk tumors and patients, initiating surgical treatment with clear margins whenever possible, utilizing Mohs surgery for all high-risk tumors, and considering staging of draining nodal basins and adjuvant radio or chemotherapy when appropriate. Close follow-up is important in high-risk cases to detect any recurrences early. Prospective, multicenter studies are necessary to more accurately stratify risk and define optimal management. Development of reliable prognostic models will greatly aid treatment decisions in cutaneous SCC. Controlled clinical trials of staging and adjuvant therapy for high-risk patients and of non-surgical treatments for low-risk disease should ultimately decrease morbidity and improve overall survival for SCC patients.

References

1. Johnson TM, Rowe DE, Nelson BR, Swanson NA. Squamous cell carcinoma of the skin (excluding lip and oral mucosa). J Am Acad Dermatol. 1992;26:467–84.
2. Landis SH, Murray T, Bolden S, Wingo PA. Cancer statistics, 1999. CA Cancer J Clin. 1999;49(1):8–31.
3. Scotto J, Kopf AW, Urbach F. Non-melanoma skin cancer among Caucasians in four areas of the United States. Cancer. 1974;34(4):1333–8.
4. Fears TR, Scotto J. Estimating increases in skin cancer morbidity due to increases in ultraviolet radiation exposure. Cancer Invest. 1983;1(2):119–26.
5. Chuang TY, Reizner GT, Elpern DJ, Stone JL, Farmer ER. Nonmelanoma skin cancer in Japanese ethnic Hawaiians in Kauai, Hawaii: an incidence report. J Am Acad Dermatol. 1995;33(3):422–6.
6. Harris RB, Griffith K, Moon TE. Trends in the incidence of nonmelanoma skin cancers in southeastern Arizona, 1985–1996. J Am Acad Dermatol. 2001;45(4):528–36.
7. Athas WF, Hunt WC, Key CR. Changes in nonmelanoma skin cancer incidence between 1977–1978 and 1998–1999 in Northcentral New Mexico. Cancer Epidemiol Biomarkers Prev. 2003;12(10):1105–8.
8. Miller DL, Weinstock MA. Non-melanoma skin cancer in the United States: incidence. J Am Acad Dermatol. 1994; 30: 774–8.
9. Karagas MR, Greenberg ER, Spencer SK, Stukel TA, Mott LA. Increase in incidence rates of basal cell and squamous cell skin cancer in New Hampshire, USA. New Hampshire Skin Cancer Study Group. Int J Cancer. 1999;81(4):555–9.
10. Brantsch KD, Meisner C, Schonfisch B, et al. Analysis of risk factors determining prognosis of cutaneous squamous-cell carcinoma: a prospective study. Lancet Oncol. 2008;9(8):713–20.
11. Rowe DE, Carroll RJ, Day CL. Prognostic factors for local recurrence, metastasis, and survival rates in squamous cell carcinoma of the skin, ear, and lip. Implications for treatment modality selection. J Am Acad Dermatol. 1992;26(6):976–90.
12. Jambusaria-Pahlajani A, Hess SD, Katz KA, Berg D, Schmults CD. Uncertainty in the perioperative management of high-risk cutaneous squamous cell carcinoma among Mohs surgeons. Arch Dermatol. 2010;146(11):1225–31.
13. Alam M, Ratner D. Cutaneous squamous-cell carcinoma. N Engl J Med. 2001;344(13):975–83.
14. Kwa RE, Campana K, Moy RL. Biology of cutaneous squamous cell carcinoma. J Am Acad Dermatol. 1992; 26(1):1–26.
15. English DR, Armstrong BK, Kricker A, Winter MG, Heenan PJ, Randell PL. Demographic characteristics, pigmentary and cutaneous risk factors for squamous cell carcinoma of the skin: a case-control study. Int J Cancer. 1998;76(5):628–34.
16. Leiter U, Garbe C. Epidemiology of melanoma and non-melanoma skin cancer – the role of sunlight. Adv Exp Med Biol. 2008;624:89–103.
17. Masini C, Fuchs PG, Gabrielli F, et al. Evidence for the association of human papillomavirus infection and cutaneous squamous cell carcinoma in immunocompetent individuals. Arch Dermatol. 2003;139(7):890–4.
18. Wong SS, Tan KC, Goh CL. Cutaneous manifestations of chronic arsenicism: review of seventeen cases. J Am Acad Dermatol. 1998;38(2 Pt 1):179–85.
19. Herman S, Rogers HD, Ratner D. Immunosuppression and squamous cell carcinoma: a focus on solid organ transplant recipients. Skinmed. 2007;6(5):234–8.
20. Mehrany K, Weenig RH, Lee KK, Pittelkow MR, Otley CC. Increased metastasis and mortality from cutaneous squamous cell carcinoma in patients with chronic lymphocytic leukemia. J Am Acad Dermatol. 2005;53(6):1067–71.
21. Nguyen P, Vin-Christian K, Ming ME, Berger T. Aggressive squamous cell carcinomas in persons infected with the human immunodeficiency virus. Arch Dermatol. 2002;138(6):758–63.
22. Mallipeddi R. Epidermolysis bullosa and cancer. Clin Exp Dermatol. 2002;27(8):616–23.
23. Preston DS, Stern RS. Nonmelanoma cancers of the skin. N Engl J Med. 1992;327:1649–62.
24. Leffell DJ. The scientific basis of skin cancer. J Am Acad Dermatol. 2000;42(1 Pt 2):18–22.
25. Marks R, Jolley D, Dorevitch AP, Selwood TS. The incidence of non-melanocytic skin cancers in an Australian population: results of a five-year prospective study. Med J Aust. 1989;150(9):475–8.
26. Marks R, Rennie G, Selwood T. The relationship of basal cell carcinomas and squamous cell carcinomas to solar keratoses. Arch Dermatol. 1988;124(7):1039–42.
27. Dobson JM, DeSpain J, Hewett JE, Clark DP. Malignant potential of actinic keratoses and the controversy over treatment: a patient-oriented perspective. Arch Dermatol. 1991;127:1029–31.
28. Moon TE, Levine N, Cartmel B, et al. Effect of retinol to prevent squamous cell skin cancer in moderate-risk subjects. Cancer Epidemiol Biomarkers Prev. 1997;6:949–56.

29. Forslund O, Iftner T, Andersson K, et al. Cutaneous human papillomaviruses found in sun-exposed skin: beta-papillomavirus species 2 predominates in squamous cell carcinoma. J Infect Dis. 2007;196(6):876–83. Epub August 6, 2007.
30. Orth G, Jablonska S, Jarzabek-Chorzelska M, et al. Characteristics of the lesions and risk of malignant conversion associated with the type of human papillomavirus involved in epidermodysplasia verruciformis. Cancer Res. 1979;39:1074–82.
31. Karagas MR, Nelson HH, Zens MS, et al. Squamous cell and basal cell carcinoma of the skin in relation to radiation therapy and potential modification of risk by sun exposure. Epidemiology. 2007;18(6):776–84.
32. Daling J, Madeleine M, Johnson LG, et al. Human papillomavirus, smoking, and sexual practices in the etiology of anal cancer. Cancer. 2004;101:270–80.
33. Frisch M, Fenger C, van den Brule ACJ, et al. Variants of squamous cell carcinoma of the anal canal and perianal skin and their relation to human papillomaviruses. Cancer Res. 1999;59:753–7.
34. Bjorge T, Engeland A, Luostarinen T, et al. Human papillomavirus infection as a risk factor for anal and perianal skin cancer in a prospective study. Br J Cancer. 2002;87:61–4.
35. Johnson LG, Madeleine MM, Newcomer LM, Schwartz SM, Daling JR. Anal cancer incidence and survival: the surveillance, epidemiology and end results experience, 1973–2000. Cancer. 2004;101:281–8.
36. Frisch M, Biggar R, Goedert JJ. Human papillomavirus-associated cancers in patients with human immunodeficiency virus infection and acquired immunodeficiency syndrome. J Natl Cancer Inst. 2000;92:1500–10.
37. Liu X, Dakic A, Zhang Y, Dai Y, Chen R, Schlegel R. HPV E6 protein interacts physically and functionally with the cellular telomerase complex. Proc Natl Acad Sci U S A. 2009;106(44):18780–5.
38. Muench P, Probst S, Schuetz J, et al. Cutaneous papillomavirus E6 proteins must interact with p300 and block p53-mediated apoptosis for cellular immortalization and tumorigenesis. Cancer Res. 2010;70(17):6913–24.
39. Farhat S, Nakagawa M, Moscicki A. Cell-mediated immune responses to human papillomavirus 16 E6 and E7 antigens as measured by IFN gamma ELISpot in women with cleared or persistent HPV infection. Int J Gynecol Cancer. 2009;19(4):508–12.
40. Natarajan E, Saeb M, Crum CP, et al. Co-expression of p16^{INK4A} and laminin 5γ2 by microinvasive and superficial squamous cell carcinomas in vivo and by migrating wound and senescent keratinocytes in culture. Am J Pathol. 2003;163:477–91.
41. Natarajan E, Omobono JD, Guo Z, et al. A keratinocyte hypermobility/growth arrest response involving laminin 5 and p16^{INK4A} activated in wound healing and senescence. Am J Pathol. 2006;168:1821–37.
42. Moussai D, Mitsui H, Pettersen JS, et al. The human cutaneous squamous cell carcinoma microenvironment is characterized by increased lymphatic density and enhanced expression of macrophage-derived VEGF-C. J Invest Dermatol. 2011;131(1):229–36. Epub September 9, 2010.
43. Haider AS, Peters SB, Kaporis H, et al. Genomic analysis defines a cancer-specific gene expression signature for human squamous cell carcinoma and distinguishes malignant hyperproliferation from benign hyperplasia. J Invest Dermatol. 2006;126:869–81.
44. Clark RA, Huang SJ, Murphy GF, et al. Human squamous cell carcinomas evade the immune response by down-regulation of vascular E-selectin and recruitment of regulatory T cells. J Exp Med. 2008;205:2221–34.
45. Huang SJ, Hijnen D, Murphy GF, et al. Imiquimod enhances IFN-γ production and effector function of T cells infiltrating human squamous cell carcinomas of the skin. J Invest Dermatol. 2009;129:2276–685.
46. Williams LS, Mancuso AA, Mendenhall WM. Perineural spread of cutaneous squamous and basal cell carcinoma: CT and MR detection and its impact on patient management and prognosis. Int J Radiat Oncol Biol Phys. 2001;49(4):1061–9.
47. Feldman SR, Fleischer Jr AB, McConnell RC. Most common dermatologic problems identified by internists, 1990–1994. Arch Intern Med. 1998;158(7):726–30.
48. Wieland U, Jurk S, Weisenborn S, Krieg T, Pfister H, Ritzkowsky A. Erythroplasia of Queyrat: coinfection with cutaneous carcinogenic human papillomavirus type 8 and genital papillomaviruses in a carcinoma in situ. J Invest Dermatol. 2000;115:396–401.
49. Bleeker M, Heideman D, Snijders P, Horenblas S, Dillner H, Meijer C. Penile cancer: epidemiology, pathogenesis and prevention. World J Urol. 2009;27:141–50.
50. Patterson JW, Kao GF, Graham JH, Helwig EB. Bowenoid papulosis. A clinicopathologic study with ultrastructural observations. Cancer. 1986;57(4):823–36.
51. Sau P, McMarlin SL, Sperling LC, Katz R. Bowen's disease of the nail bed and periungual area. A clinicopathologic analysis of seven cases. Arch Dermatol. 1994;130(2):204–9.
52. Cribier B, Asch P, Grosshans E. Differentiating squamous cell carcinoma from keratoacanthoma using histopathological criteria. Is it possible? A study of 296 cases. Dermatology. 1999;199:208–12.
53. Bouwes Bavinck JN, Hardie DR, Green A, et al. The risk of skin cancer in renal transplant recipients in Queensland, Australia. A follow-up study. Transplantation. 1996;61(5):715–21.
54. Jambusaria-Pahlajani A, Miller CJ, Quon H, Smith N, Klein RQ, Schmults CD. Surgical monotherapy versus surgery plus adjuvant radiotherapy in high-risk cutaneous squamous cell carcinoma: a systematic review of outcomes. Dermatol Surg. 2009;35(4):574–85.
55. Tan PY, Ek E, Su S, Giorlando F, Dieu T. Incomplete excision of squamous cell carcinoma of the skin: a prospective observational study. Plast Reconstr Surg. 2007;120(4):910–6.
56. Brodland DG, Zitelli JA. Surgical margins for excision of primary cutaneous squamous cell carcinoma. J Am Acad Dermatol. 1992;27(2 Pt 1):241–8.
57. Sober A. Cutaneous squamous cell carcinoma and other cutaneous carcinomas, Chapter 29. In: Edge SB, Byrd DR, Compton CC, Fritz AG, Greene FL, Trotti A, editors. AJCC cancer staging manual. 7th ed. New York: Springer; 2010.
58. Lawrence N, Cottel WI. Squamous cell carcinoma of skin with perineural invasion. J Am Acad Dermatol. 1994;31(1):30–3.
59. Leibovitch I, Huilgol SC, Selva D, Hill D, Richards S, Paver R. Cutaneous squamous cell carcinoma treated with Mohs micrographic surgery in Australia I. Experience over 10 years. J Am Acad Dermatol. 2005;53(2):253–60.
60. Kwan W, Wilson D, Moravan V. Radiotherapy for locally advanced basal cell and squamous cell carcinomas of the skin. Int J Radiat Oncol Biol Phys. 2004;60(2):406–11.

61. Veness M, Richards S. Role of modern radiotherapy in treating skin cancer. Australas J Dermatol. 2003;44(3):159–66; quiz 67–8.
62. Miller S, Alam M, Andersen J, et al. Basal cell and squamous cell skin cancers. J Natl Compr Canc Netw. 2010;8: 836–64.
63. Breuninger H, Bootz F, Hauschild A, et al. Short German guidelines: squamous cell carcinoma. J Dtsch Dermatol Ges. 2008;6 Suppl 1:S5–8.
64. Stasko T, Brown MD, Carucci JA, International Transplant-Skin Cancer Collaborative; European Skin Care in Organ Transplant Patients Network, et al. Guidelines for the management of squamous cell carcinoma in organ transplant recipients. Dermatol Surg. 2004;30(4 Pt 2):642–50.
65. Motley R, Kersey P, Lawrence C. Multiprofessional guidelines for the management of the patient with primary cutaneous squamous cell carcinoma. Br J Dermatol. 2002;1 46(1):18–25.
66. Miller SJ. The National Comprehensive Cancer Network (NCCN) guidelines of care for nonmelanoma skin cancers. Dermatol Surg. 2000;26(3):289–92.
67. Committee on Guidelines of Care; Task Force on Cutaneous Squamous Cell Carcinoma. Guidelines for care for squamous cell carcinoma. J Am Acad Dermatol. 1993;28(4):628–31.
68. Cherpelis BS, Marcusen C, Lang PG. Prognostic factors for metastasis in squamous cell carcinoma of the skin. Dermatol Surg. 2002;28(3):268–73.
69. Mullen JT, Feng L, Xing Y, et al. Invasive squamous cell carcinoma of the skin: defining a high-risk group. Ann Surg Oncol. 2006;13(7):902–9.
70. Moller R, Reymann F, Hou-Jensen K. Metastases in dermatological patients with squamous cell carcinoma. Arch Dermatol. 1979;115(6):703–5.
71. Edwards MJ, Hirsch RM, Broadwater JR, Netscher DT, Ames FC. Squamous cell carcinoma arising in previously burned or irradiated skin. Arch Surg. 1989;124(1):115–7.
72. Ayyappan K, Ananthatkrishnan N, Sankaran V. Can regional lymph node involvement be predicted in patients with carcinoma of the penis? Br J Urol. 1994;73:549–53.
73. Magrina JF, Gonzalez-Bosquet J, Weaver AL, et al. Primary squamous cell cancer of the vulva: radical versus modified radical vulvar surgery. Gynecol Oncol. 1998;71:116–21.
74. Gerard JP, Chapet O, Samiei F, et al. Management of inguinal lymph node metastases in patients with carcinoma of the anal canal: experience in a series of 270 patients treated in Lyon and review of the literature. Cancer. 2001;92: 77–84.
75. Stehman FB, Bundy BN, Ball H, et al. Sites of failure and times to failure in carcinoma of the vulva treated conservatively: a Gynecologic Oncologic Group study. Am J Obstet Gynecol. 1996;174:1128–33.
76. Kraus DH, Carew JF, Harrison LB. Regional lymph node metastasis from cutaneous squamous cell carcinoma. Arch Otolaryngol Head Neck Surg. 1998;124(5):582–7.
77. Dinehart SM, Pollack SV. Metastases from squamous cell carcinoma of the skin and lip. An analysis of twenty-seven cases. J Am Acad Dermatol. 1989;21(2 Pt 1):241–8.
78. Tavin E, Persky M. Metastatic cutaneous squamous cell carcinoma of the head and neck region. Laryngoscope. 1996;106(2 Pt 1):156–8.
79. Clayman GL, Lee JJ, Holsinger FC, et al. Mortality risk from squamous cell skin cancer. J Clin Oncol. 2005;23(4):759–65.
80. Breuninger H, Schaumburg-Lever G, Holzschuh J, Horny HP. Desmoplastic squamous cell carcinoma of skin and vermilion surface: a highly malignant subtype of skin cancer. Cancer. 1997;79(5):915–9.
81. Goepfert H, Dichtel WJ, Medina JE, Lindberg RD, Luna MD. Perineural invasion in squamous cell skin carcinoma of the head and neck. Am J Surg. 1984;148(4):542–7.
82. Mendenhall WM, Amdur RJ, Hinerman RW, et al. Skin cancer of the head and neck with perineural invasion. Am J Clin Oncol. 2007;30(1):93–6.
83. Ross AS, Whalen FM, Elenitsas R, Xu X, Troxel AB, Schmults CD. Diameter of involved nerves predicts outcomes in cutaneous squamous cell carcinoma with perineural invasion: an investigator-blinded retrospective cohort study. Dermatol Surg. 2009;35(12):1859–66.
84. Jensen P, Hansen S, Moller B, et al. Skin cancer in kidney and heart transplant recipients and different long-term immunosuppressive therapy regimens. J Am Acad Dermatol. 1999;40(2 Pt 1):177–86.
85. Adamson R, Obispo E, Dychter S, et al. High incidence and clinical course of aggressive skin cancer in heart transplant patients: a single-center study. Transplant Proc. 1998; 30(4):1124–6.
86. Ong CS, Keogh AM, Kossard S, Macdonald PS, Spratt PM. Skin cancer in Australian heart transplant recipients. J Am Acad Dermatol. 1999;40(1):27–34.
87. Euvard S, Kanitakis J, Decullier E, et al. Subsequent skin cancers in kidney and heart transplant recipients after the first squamous cell carcinoma. Transplantation. 2006;81(8):1093–100.
88. Smith KJ, Hamza S, Skelton H. Histologic features in primary cutaneous squamous cell carcinomas in immunocompromised patients focusing on organ transplant patients. Dermatol Surg. 2004;30(4 Pt 2):634–41.
89. Veness MJ, Quinn DI, Ong CS, et al. Aggressive cutaneous malignancies following cardiothoracic transplantation: the Australian experience. Cancer. 1999;85(8):1758–64.
90. Carucci JA, Martinez JC, Zeitouni NC, et al. In-transit metastasis from primary cutaneous squamous cell carcinoma in organ transplant recipients and nonimmunosuppressed patients: clinical characteristics, management, and outcome in a series of 21 patients. Dermatol Surg. 2004;30(4 Pt 2):651–5.
91. Frierson Jr HF, Deutsch BD, Levine PA. Clinicopathologic features of cutaneous squamous cell carcinomas of the head and neck in patients with chronic lymphocytic leukemia/small lymphocytic lymphoma. Hum Pathol. 1988;19(12):1397–402.
92. Fine JD, Johnson LB, Weiner M, Li KP, Suchindran C. Epidermolysis bullosa and the risk of life-threatening cancers: the National EB Registry experience, 1986–2006. J Am Acad Dermatol. 2009;60(2):203–11.
93. Kinlen LJ. Incidence of cancer in rheumatoid arthritis and other disorders after immunosuppressive treatment. Am J Med. 1985;78(1A):44–9.
94. Yousem DM, Som PM, Hackney DB, Schwaibold F, Hendrix RA. Central nodal necrosis and extracapsular neoplastic spread in cervical lymph nodes: MR imaging versus CT. Radiology. 1992;182(3):753–9.
95. Ginsberg LE. MR imaging of perineural tumor spread. Magn Reson Imaging Clin N Am. 2002;10(3):511–25.
96. Land R, Herod J, Moskovic E, et al. Routine computerized tomography scanning, groin ultrasound with or without fine needle aspiration cytology in the surgical management of

primary squamous cell carcinoma of the vulva. Int J Gynecol Cancer. 2006;16(1):312–7.
97. Cho SB, Chung WG, Yun M, Lee JD, Lee MG, Chung KY. Fluorodeoxyglucose positron emission tomography in cutaneous squamous cell carcinoma: retrospective analysis of 12 patients. Dermatol Surg. 2005;31(4):442–6; discussion 6–7.
98. Bailet JW, Abemayor E, Jabour BA, Hawkins RA, Ho C, Ward PH. Positron emission tomography: a new, precise imaging modality for detection of primary head and neck tumors and assessment of cervical adenopathy. Laryngoscope. 1992;102(3):281–8.
99. Ross AS, Schmults CD. Sentinel lymph node biopsy in cutaneous squamous cell carcinoma: a systematic review of the English literature. Dermatol Surg. 2006;32(11): 1309–21.
100. Zachary CB, Rest EB, Furlong SM, Arcedo PN, McGeorge BC, Kist DA. Rapid cytokeratin stains enhance the sensitivity of Mohs micrographic surgery for squamous cell carcinoma. J Dermatol Surg Oncol. 1994;20(8):530–5.
101. Cherpelis BS, Turner L, Ladd S, Glass LF, Fenske NA. Innovative 19-minute rapid cytokeratin immunostaining of nonmelanoma skin cancer in Mohs micrographic surgery. Dermatol Surg. 2009;35(7):1050–6.
102. Veness MJ, Ong C, Cakir B, Morgan G. Squamous cell carcinoma of the lip. Patterns of relapse and outcome: reporting the Westmead Hospital experience, 1980–1997. Australas Radiol. 2001;45(2):195–9.
103. Cox J, editor. Radiation oncology: rationale, techniques, results. 8th ed. Philadelphia, PA: Mosby; 2003.
104. Veness MJ, Morgan GJ, Palme CE, Gebski V. Surgery and adjuvant radiotherapy in patients with cutaneous head and neck squamous cell carcinoma metastatic to lymph nodes: combined treatment should be considered best practice. Laryngoscope. 2005;115(5):870–5.
105. Chambon PT. The retinoid signaling pathway: molecular and genetic analysis. Semin Cell Biol. 1999;5:115–25.
106. Wright TI, Spencer JM, Flowers FP. Chemoprevention of non-melanoma skin cancer. J Am Acad Dermatol. 2006;54:933–46.
107. Harwood CA, Leedham-Green M, Leigh IM, Proby CM. Low-dose retinoids in the prevention of cutaneous squamous cell carcinomas in organ transplant recipients: a 16-year retrospective study. Arch Dermatol. 2005;141(4): 456–64.
108. Bavinck JN, Tieben LM, Van der Woude FJ, et al. Prevention of skin cancer and reduction of keratotic skin lesions during acitretin therapy in renal transplant recipients: a double-blind, placebo controlled study. J Clin Oncol. 1995;13:1933–8.
109. McKenna DB, Murphy GM. Skin cancer chemoprophylaxis in renal transplant recipients: 5 years experience using low-dose acitretin. Br J Dermatol. 1999;140:656–60.
110. Marquez C, Bair SM, Smithberger E, Cherpelis BS, Glass LF. Systemic retinoids for chemoprevention of non-melanoma skin cancer in high-risk patients. J Drugs Dermatol. 2010;9(7):753–8.
111. Otley CC, Maragh SL. Reduction of immunosuppression for transplant-associated skin cancer: rationale and evidence of efficacy. Dermatol Surg. 2005;31(2):163–8.
112. Toma S, Bonelli L, Sartoris A, et al. 13-cis retinoic acid in head and neck cancer chemoprevention: results of a randomized trial from the Italian Head and Neck Chemoprevention Study Group. Oncol Rep. 2004;11(6):1297–305.
113. Brewster AM, Lee JJ, Clayman GL, et al. Randomized trial of adjuvant 13-cis-retinoic acid and interferon alfa for patients with aggressive skin squamous cell carcinoma. J Clin Oncol. 2007;25(15):1974–8.
114. Cartei G, Cartei F, Interlandi G, et al. Oral 5-fluorouracil in squamous cell carcinoma of the skin in the aged. Am J Clin Oncol. 2000;23(2):181–4.
115. Wollina U, Hansel G, Koch A, Kostler E. Oral capecitabine plus subcutaneous interferon alpha in advanced squamous cell carcinoma of the skin. J Cancer Res Clin Oncol. 2005;131(5):300–4.
116. Hitt R, Jimeno A, Rodriguez-Pinilla M, et al. Phase II trial of cisplatin and capecitabine in patients with squamous cell carcinoma of the head and neck, and correlative study of angiogenic factors. Br J Cancer. 2004;91(12):2005–11.
117. Bentzen JD, Hansen HS. Phase II analysis of paclitaxel and capecitabine in the treatment of recurrent or disseminated squamous cell carcinoma of the head and neck region. Head Neck. 2007;29(1):47–51.
118. Kim JG, Sohn SK, Kim DH, et al. Phase II study of concurrent chemoradiotherapy with capecitabine and cisplatin in patients with locally advanced squamous cell carcinoma of the head and neck. Br J Cancer. 2005;93(10):1117–21.
119. Nanney LB, Magid M, Stoscheck CM, King LE. Comparison of epidermal growth factor binding and receptor distribution in normal human epidermis and epidermal appendages. J Invest Dermatol. 1984;83(5):385–93.
120. Shimizu T, Izumi H, Oga A, et al. Epidermal growth factor receptor overexpression and genetic aberrations in metastatic squamous-cell carcinoma of the skin. Dermatology. 2001;202(3):203–6.
121. Suen JK, Bressler L, Shord SS, Warso M, Villano JL. Cutaneous squamous cell carcinoma responding serially to single-agent cetuximab. Anticancer Drugs. 2007;18(7):827–9.
122. Bauman JE, Eaton KD, Martins RG. Treatment of recurrent squamous cell carcinoma of the skin with cetuximab. Arch Dermatol. 2007;143(7):889–92.
123. Arnold AW, Bruckner-Tuderman L, Zuger C, Itin PH. Cetuximab therapy of metastasizing cutaneous squamous cell carcinoma in a patient with severe recessive dystrophic epidermolysis bullosa. Dermatology. 2009;219(1):80–3.
124. Jalili A, Pinc A, Pieczkowski F, Karlhofer FM, Stingl G, Wagner SN. Combination of an EGFR blocker and a COX-2 inhibitor for the treatment of advanced cutaneous squamous cell carcinoma. J Dtsch Dermatol Ges. 2008;6(12):1066–9.
125. Miller K, Sherman W, Ratner D. Complete clinical response to cetuximab in a patient with metastatic cutaneous squamous cell carcinoma. Dermatol Surg. 2010;36(12): 2069–74. Epub October 11, 2010.
126. Baltaci M, Fritsch P, Weber F, et al. Treatment with gefitinib (ZD 1839) in a patient with advanced cutaneous squamous cell carcinoma. Br J Dermatol. 2005;153(1):234–6.
127. Cohen EE, Rosen F, Stadler WM, et al. Phase II trial of ZD1839 in recurrent or metastatic squamous cell carcinoma of the head and neck. J Clin Oncol. 2003;21(10):1980–7.

128. Stewart JS, Cohen EE, Licitra L, et al. Phase III study of gefitinib compared with intravenous methotrexate for recurrent squamous cell carcinoma of the head and neck [corrected]. J Clin Oncol. 2009;27(11):1864–71.
129. Abou Ayache R, Thierry A, Bridoux F, et al. Long-term maintenance of calcineurin inhibitor monotherapy reduces the risk for squamous cell carcinomas after kidney transplantation compared with bi- or tritherapy. Transplant Proc. 2007;39(8):2592–4.
130. Schena FP, Pascoe MD, Alberu J, et al. Conversion from calcineurin inhibitors to sirolimus maintenance therapy in renal allograft recipients: 24-month efficacy and safety results from the CONVERT trial. Transplantation. 2009;87(2):233–42.
131. Rival-Tringali AL, Euvrard S, Decullier E, Claudy A, Faure M, Kanitakis J. Conversion from calcineurin inhibitors to sirolimus reduces vascularization and thickness of post-transplant cutaneous squamous cell carcinomas. Anticancer Res. 2009;29(6):1927–32.
132. Jennings L, Schmults CD. Management of high-risk cutaneous squamous cell carcinoma. J Clin Aesthet Dermatol. 2010;3(4):39–48.
133. Willey A, Mehta S, Lee PK. Reduction in the incidence of squamous cell carcinoma in solid organ transplant recipients treated with cyclic photodynamic therapy. Dermatol Surg. 2010;36(5):652–8.

Mohs Micrographic Surgery for the Treatment of Cutaneous Melanoma

18

Michael Campoli*, Scott Freeman*,
David G. Brodland, and John Zitelli

Abstract

Melanoma is a clinically and biologically diverse malignancy for which complete surgical excision offers the only chance for cure. Current guidelines for surgical excision margins are based on consensus recommendations, and clear, evidence-based data to guide the surgeon in each case is limited. Mohs micrographic surgery (MMS) offers the surgeon the ability to assess 100% of the surgical margin, far better than margins evaluated with the standard bread-loaf sectioning technique. Immunohistochemical stains such as MART-1 allow for the reliable identification of melanoma in frozen sections and produce cure rates at least as good as standard excision with traditional margins.

Keywords

Mohs micrographic surgery • Melanoma • Clinical margins • Excision margins • Immunohistochemical stains

M. Campoli • S. Freeman • J. Zitelli (✉)
Fellows, Zitelli & Brodland, P.C., Pittsburgh, PA, USA
e-mail: mcampoli@gmail.com; scottrfreeman@gmail.com

D.G. Brodland
Departments of Dermatology and Otolaryngology,
Shadyside Medical Center,
University of Pittsburgh Medical Center,
Pittsburgh, PA, USA

*Both authors contributed equally to the manuscript.

K. Nouri (ed.), *Mohs Micrographic Surgery*,
DOI 10.1007/978-1-4471-2152-7_18,

Summary: Introduction

- Incidence and mortality of cutaneous melanoma continue to rise, despite improvements in diagnosis of early stage disease.
- Surgical excision of primary invasive melanoma is presently the only effective treatment and is the standard of care for melanomas of all depths.
- While early stage melanoma is highly curable with surgery, advanced stage melanoma is relatively resistant to conventional therapeutic regimens and is often fatal.

18.1 Introduction

Malignant melanoma represents the most deadly form of skin cancer [1]. Its incidence and mortality rates have risen steadily across all age groups since at least the middle of the twentieth century [1]. Current estimates indicate that its incidence is increasing at a rate of 5% per year [1]. It is anticipated that the lifetime risk of developing melanoma in the United States is now between 1 in 75 and 1 in 39, versus 1 in 1,500 in 1935 [1, 2]. In spite of significant improvements in diagnosis of early stage disease [3], the mortality rate for melanoma has been continually increasing over the past decade, and the disease represents one of the most common fatal malignancies of young adults [1]. While early stage melanoma is highly curable with surgery [4], advanced stage melanoma is relatively resistant to conventional therapeutic regimens and is often fatal [5–7]. Although promising results have been obtained with B-Raf and MEK inhibitors in recent clinical trials [8–10], the lack of effective conventional therapies for the treatment of advanced stage disease has stimulated interest in the application of novel strategies for the treatment of patients with malignant melanoma. Nonetheless, clinical trials have failed to reproduce the therapeutic benefit shown in animal models [11–16]. To date, surgical excision of primary invasive melanoma is the only effective treatment and is the standard of care for melanomas of all depths [17–20].

In this chapter, we will first review the current recommendations for the surgical treatment of melanoma as well as their associated pitfalls. Second, we will discuss the role of Mohs micrographic surgery (MMS) in the surgical treatment of melanoma including the different techniques utilized, the use of frozen versus formalin-fixed tissue as well as the advantages and disadvantages of the available immunohistochemical (IHC) stains. Third, we will discuss the long-term clinical responses in patients with melanoma treated with MMS. Lastly, we will discuss potential strategies to improve the surgical treatment of melanoma.

Summary: Surgical Treatment of Melanoma

- The goal of surgical treatment of melanoma is complete removal of the primary tumor.
- Recommended surgical margins are largely based on consensus.
- Melanomas are clinically and biologically diverse, and therefore reliable standardized margins do not exist to guide the surgeon in every case.

18.2 Surgical Treatment of Melanoma

Surgical excision of primary invasive melanoma is the standard of care of all depths [17–20]. The goal of surgical treatment for cutaneous melanoma is complete removal of the primary tumor. Complete removal of the primary tumor prior to metastasis eliminates the chance for local recurrence, nodal metastasis, distant metastasis, and death from melanoma. Although the recommended margins for standard excision are well recognized (Table 18.1), they continue to remain a source of some controversy. Until recently, margins of 5 cm or more were standard, but these were based more on personal bias and surgical dogma than scientific evidence. It was not until Clark et al. [21] and Breslow [22] established that level and thickness of the primary melanoma could be used to predict the prognosis accurately that groups of patients with a similar prognosis could be collected to compare the outcome

Table 18.1 Recommended surgical margins for excision of primary cutaneous melanoma

Tumor thickness (Breslow)	Excision margin (cm)
In situ	0.5
≤2 mm	1
≥2 mm	2

Derived from [29, 30]

of different surgical margins. To date, only five prospective randomized studies have been conducted to investigate surgical excision margins for primary cutaneous melanoma [23–28]. These studies have failed to show any difference in overall survival in patients with tumors of various thickness treated with narrow (1–2 cm) versus wide (3–5 cm) surgical margins. Although today's standards for excision of primary cutaneous melanoma are somewhat based on the results of the aforementioned trials, it must be stressed that the current guidelines continue to be largely based on consensus recommendations [29, 30]. It is key for the dermatologic surgeon to recognize that there is no evidence to demonstrate that today's standards for excision of primary cutaneous melanoma are superior to the narrowest margin that removes the tumor in its entirety. The ability to remove a tumor in its entirety utilizing the narrowest surgical margins reflects the aim of MMS.

Many surgeons continue to rely on the excision of wide margins of normal skin because of the possibility that these wider margins may contain micrometastases with the assumption that removal of micrometastases will limit recurrences and improve survival. There is no evidence to support these claims. The presence of micrometastases within surgically excised primary cutaneous melanomas is statistically associated with disease-free survival [31], and those patients have a prognosis similar to that of patients with known in transit or nodal metastatic disease [32–37]. These findings suggest that micrometastases are merely indicators of distant metastatic disease. Therefore, wider surgical margins are unable to remove all metastatic disease. Again, it must be stressed that the available evidence suggests that narrower margins are as good as wider margins in the excision of primary cutaneous melanoma with no difference in overall survival [29, 30]. Taken together the available evidence supports the notion that the distance of the margin of excision from the edge of the tumor is immaterial as long as the tumor has not metastasized and is removed in its entirety.

Melanomas are clinically and biologically diverse, and therefore reliable standardized margins do not exist to guide the surgeon in every case. There is particularly limited data to provide guidelines for the treatment of (1) melanomas more than 4 mm thick; (2) melanomas on the head, neck, hands, feet, and genitals; and (3) in situ melanomas. Moreover, while there is some evidence supporting the current guidelines for width of excision of primary cutaneous melanoma, there is a paucity of data supporting the appropriate depth of excision [38–40]. In 1992, a National Institutes of Health (NIH) Consensus Panel suggested that MIS be excised to subcutaneous tissue while invasive melanoma should be excised to fascia [41]. However, these recommendations regarding depth of excision have been based only on the personal opinions of the panel members. To the best of our knowledge, there is no clinical evidence to support or refute the current depth of excision recommendations. Current guidelines, including those of the National Comprehensive Cancer Network (NCCN) Melanoma Panel [42], the British Association of Dermatologists [43], and the American Academy of Dermatology (AAD) Guidelines/Outcomes Committee [44], do not make recommendations with regard to depth of excision. The NIH Consensus Panel has stated that the recommendation of excision of invasive melanomas to fascia is "based on the anatomic understanding that the lymphatics drain to the regional lymph nodes in the subcutaneous tissue extending to the underlying muscle fascia" [45]. Nevertheless, to the best of our knowledge, there is currently no sound scientific evidence for or against excision of melanoma to the fascia.

The only "correct" surgical margin is that which removes the entire tumor and conserves the most normal tissue. It is paramount to understand that melanomas often have indistinct clinical margins and may be amelanotic at the periphery, making proper surgical planning difficult. Furthermore, melanomas of the head and neck, which represent 17–25% of all melanomas [46], as well as those on the hands, feet, and genitals often exist near vital structures that compromise the ability to excise the standard margins without causing serious functional or cosmetic deformities. One- to two-centimeter margins in these locations are generally impractical and strongly favor the most tissue conservative approach in the excision of the tumor. Moreover, local recurrence rates on the head, neck, hands, feet, and genitals range from 9% to 20% with standard excisional margins, far higher than the 3% rate reported on the trunk [47–51]. Given these high recurrence rates, some have suggested amputation as surgical treatment of cutaneous melanoma in areas such as the hands and feet [52, 53].

The local recurrence rates on the head, neck, hands, feet, and genitals may reflect both technical as well as biologic variables. From a biologic viewpoint, this high recurrence rate may reflect the ability of melanomas to grow with invisible subclinical extensions analogous to other cutaneous malignancies. As will be discussed below, these extensions may be missed by conventional histopathologic examination of excised tissue. Although melanin pigment helps to define the margins for melanomas, pigment is not always present and is least visible in nests of tumor cells at the periphery. In areas of chronic sun damage such as the head and neck, these extensions are often camouflaged by ephelides, pigmented actinic keratoses, lentigines, nevi, seborrheic keratoses, or thick stratum corneum. Lastly, unique anatomic features of the hands and feet include the nail plate and nail fold, which often make determining the clinical margins of melanoma difficult.

From a technical viewpoint, some surgeons may be more conservative with their surgical margins and not adhere to established standards in areas such as the head, neck, hands, feet, and genitals. This is due to the problems associated with radical excision in these cosmetically and functionally sensitive areas. Further, it must be stressed that conventional histopathologic evaluation of surgically removed tissue using vertical sectioning lacks the ability to completely identify tumor margins. Specifically, when excisional specimens are sent to the pathology laboratory to check the margins for residual tumor, serial thin sections are cut from the tissue perpendicular to the epidermis. Representative vertical sections are often taken at 2–4 mm intervals throughout the tissue specimen. For a well-defined tumor, this may suffice, but the 2–4 mm between sections is not examined. A tumor determined to have clear margins by this bread loaf method may, in fact, have extensions of tumor in the unexamined intervals, as <1% of the margins are actually visualized [54]. Therefore, conventional histopathologic examination of the tumor margin is more likely to lead to false negative margin assessment and may be an explanation for a higher marginal recurrence rate after a tumors "complete excision." Whatever the reason for the high rate of local recurrence of melanomas on the head, neck, hands, feet, and genitals, it is important to realize that failure to completely remove a primary melanoma surgically has important clinical consequences. Tumors recurring after incomplete excision often are of increased Breslow's depth, one of the most important predictors of survival in patients with cutaneous melanoma [55].

Summary: MMS for Cutaneous Melanoma

- Evidence supports the notion that the distance of the margin of excision from the edge of the tumor is immaterial as long as the tumor is removed in its entirety.
- Microscopic margin control eliminates the problem of indistinct clinical margins seen in photodamaged skin and conserves normal tissue.
- Up to 8% of primary cutaneous melanomas surgically treated with the current recommended NIH guidelines are inadequately excised.

18.3 MMS for Cutaneous Melanoma

As discussed above, the available evidence suggests that wide margins do not improve survival or decrease the risk of satellite metastases when compared with more narrow margins as long as the primary melanoma is completely excised [29, 30]. MMS uses the microscope to allow for histologic examination of 100% of the peripheral tumor margin in a three-dimensional fashion. Microscopic margin control eliminates the problem of indistinct clinical margins seen in photodamaged skin and conserves normal tissue, thereby minimizing functional and cosmetic disfigurement. As will be discussed below, the use of MMS in combination with the IHC technique (Fig. 18.1) has greatly expanded our capacity to treat a wide array of malignancies using MMS, especially melanoma. The use of MMS to determine surgical margins is not unique to primary cutaneous melanoma since MMS has been used to measure the difference between the clinical diameter and the subclinical diameter of other skin cancers to establish guidelines for excisional margins for basal cell carcinoma, squamous cell carcinoma, dermatofibrosarcoma protuberans, and recurrent cutaneous melanomas [56–59]. In primary cutaneous melanoma, local recurrence as well as overall cure rates of patients with melanoma treated with MMS is at least as good as surgery with standard wide surgical excision margins [46, 60–66]. Zitelli et al. have reported statistically significant decreased local recurrence rates at 5 years in patients treated with MMS compared to historical controls treated with wide local excision [46, 66]. In these studies, the 5-year local recurrence rates for MIS and invasive melanoma were between 0% and 0.5% [46, 66]. Bricca et al. have expanded these studies demonstrating that patients with mela-

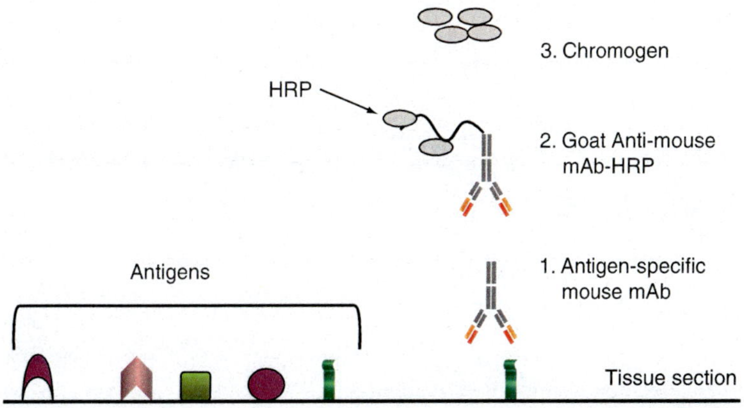

Fig. 18.1 Illustrative example of the immunohistochemical method. The antigen to be detected in the tissue section is indicated in *green*. (1) A specific antibody to that antigen is added (also called primary antibody). (2) The antigen-antibody binding reaction is detected adding a secondary antibody, which is labeled with many molecules of an enzyme (e.g., horse radish peroxidase (HRP)) depicted as *dark gray circles*. (3) The immunologic reaction is detected by adding a substrate and a chromagen that will produce a colored reaction visible under the microscope

noma of the head and neck treated with MMS have improved or equivalent 5-year disease-specific survival rates when compared to historical controls treated with wide local excision [66]. In these studies, the surgical margin for the excision of primary cutaneous melanoma was found to be dependent on tumor location, diameter, and depth (Table 18.2a, b) [46, 66]. Moreover, the surgical margins derived from these studies demonstrate that 59% of primary cutaneous melanomas surgically treated with the current recommended guidelines are excised with an excess margin greater than 5 mm, including 23% that would be in excess of 1 cm. Even more disconcerting is that ~8% of primary cutaneous melanomas are inadequately excised with the current recommended guidelines [46, 66] (Table 18.2a, b). It should be noted that these findings have also been confirmed with others [67–71]. Most of these inadequately excised melanomas are MIS located on the head and neck, suggesting that the consensus panel recommendation of narrow margins (5 mm) is inadequate. This prediction for inadequate excision is similar to the reported recurrence rates for melanomas on the head, neck, hands, and feet after standard surgery [47–51].

Table 18.2 Surgical margins for primary cutaneous melanoma derived from MMS based on (**a**) tumor depth and (**b**) tumor location and diameter

(a)

Tumor thickness (Breslow)	Excision margin (cm)
In situ	0.9
≤1.01 mm	0.9
1.01–2.0 mm	1.2
2.01–4.0 mm	1.2
>4 mm	>1.2

(b)

Tumor location	Tumor diameter (cm)	Excision margin (cm)
Trunk and extremity	<2	1.0
Trunk and extremity	>2	1.5
Head, neck, hands, or feet	<3	1.5
Head, neck, hands, or feet	>3	2.5

Derived from [46, 66]

Summary: Application of MMS for the Treatment of Cutaneous Melanoma: IHC Stains

- Several melanocytic markers have been applied to MMS for the treatment of melanoma, with MART-1 being the most common.
- MART-1-specific monoclonal antibodies have high sensitivity (75–92%) and specificity (95–100%) for melanoma.
- Atypical melanomas, like spindle cell and desmoplastic melanomas, often pose a diagnostic dilemma due to atypical morphology, and their IHC profiles are different from and not as distinctive as those of other types of melanomas.
- Other melanocytic differentiation markers are currently being investigated.

18.4 Application of MMS for the Treatment of Cutaneous Melanoma

18.4.1 IHC Stains

Most neoplasms treated with MMS can be identified in standard hematoxylin and eosin (H&E)-stained frozen sections with very high certainty. However, in certain tumors, especially melanoma, identifying the tumor in

Table 18.3 Antigens utilized in the diagnosis of melanoma

Antigen	Sensitivity	Specificity
MART-1	75–92%	95–100%
S100	97–100%	75–87%
HMB-45	69–93%	77–100% (primary); 56–83% (metastatic)
Tyrosinase	84–94%	97–100%
MITF	81–100%	88–100%
NKI/C3	86–100%	Poor

Derived from [75, 82–111, 115, 116, 120]

frozen sections can be more challenging. We, as well as others, have reported that the sensitivity and specificity of H&E-stained frozen sections for the evaluation of surgical margins of MIS and primary cutaneous melanoma are 100% and 90%, respectively [66–70, 72–74]. Although frozen sections are proven to be reliable in margin assessment of primary cutaneous melanoma, they are not recommended for diagnosis or prognostic staging. Moreover, it can be difficult to differentiate atypical melanocytic proliferations from true melanoma utilizing light microscopy.

The application of the IHC technique (Fig. 18.1) to MMS has greatly expanded our capacity to treat a wide array of malignancies using MMS, especially melanoma. In this regard, the use of IHC staining of frozen tissue sections removed during MMS overcomes the problem of interpreting atypical melanocytes in frozen sections. Furthermore, an advantage of IHC staining of the frozen sections processed during MMS rather than formalin-fixed, paraffin-embedded sections is the preservation of antigenic epitopes which can often be lost in fixation of tissues with formalin and their subsequent embedding with paraffin [75]. To date, several melanocytic markers have been applied to MMS for the treatment of melanoma (Table 18.3). Currently, the most widely utilized marker is the melanoma differentiation antigen known as melanoma antigen recognized by T cells (MART-1) or Melan-A. MART-1 is a cytoplasmic protein of melanosomal differentiation recognized by T cells [76–81]. Two clones of MART-1-specific monoclonal antibody (mAb) are available: M2-7C10, referred to as MART-1, and A103, referred to as Melan-A. The reactivity of these MART-1-specific mAb is not restricted to melanoma since both label mesenchymal tumors consisting of perivascular epithelioid cells and some clear cell sarcomas and mAb A103 also labels adrenal cortical tumors and gonadal steroid tumors [75, 82–94]. These MART-1-specific mAb show sensitivity (75–92%) and specificity (95–100%) for melanoma that is similar to HMB-45. There is a decrease in the percentage of stained cells in metastatic melanomas relative to primary melanomas. However, these mAb generally show more diffuse and intense staining than HMB-45 and do not show reduced staining in the dermal component of melanomas; this property makes them easier to interpret especially in metastatic melanomas [76–81].

Of the other melanocytic markers that have been applied to MMS for the treatment of melanoma, HMB-45, a marker of the cytoplasmic premelanosomal glycoprotein gp100, was one of the first melanoma-specific markers discovered [86, 87, 90–105]. The reported sensitivity of HMB-45 for melanoma ranges from 69% to 93%, and expression is maximal in primary melanoma specimens (77–100%) and less in metastases (58–83%). Staining may be patchy, and melanoma cells are less diffusely positive than with other markers. There may be strong staining with HMB-45 in the epidermal component of primary melanomas with gradually weaker staining in the deeper vertical growth phase. HMB-45 is very specific for melanomas; however its expression has been detected in angiomyolipomas, lymphangiomyomatosis, sweat gland tumors, meningeal melanocytomas, clear cell sarcoma of the tendons and aponeuroses, ovarian steroid cell tumors, breast cancers as well as renal cell carcinomas [86, 87, 90–105]. Decreased sensitivity of HMB-45 has also been noted in metastatic melanoma.

Other melanocytic differentiation markers are currently being investigated and are not yet in widespread clinical use including multiple myeloma oncogene-1 (MUM-1), melanocortin-1, the microphthalmia transcription factor (MITF), SM5-1, TRP-1/2, and PNL2 [75, 76, 88, 106–120]. However, none of these newer markers have yet shown significant advantages over the immunostains currently in clinical use.

It should be noted that spindle cell or desmoplastic melanomas often pose a diagnostic dilemma because their morphology is atypical and their IHC profiles are different from and not as distinctive as those of other types of melanomas [82, 84–88, 91, 95]. All the markers that are more specific for melanoma also show very poor sensitivity for spindle/desmoplastic lesions (Table 18.4). Histologically, desmoplastic melanoma is characterized as a mainly intradermal ill-defined lesion composed of elongated hyperchromatic spindle cells distributed singly or in bundles, fascicles, or nests, between variably increased collagen fibers of the papillary and the reticular dermis. Both primary and metastatic desmoplastic melanomas lesions usually show immunoreactivity with S-100 protein and NKI/C3 but not with HMB-45,

Table 18.4 Sensitivity of melanoma-associated antigen in spindle cell and desmoplastic melanoma

Antigen	Sensitivity (%)
MART-1	~20
S100	~98
HMB-45	~15
Tyrosinase	~25
MITF	~25

Derived from [75, 82, 84–88, 90, 91, 95]

MART-1, or other antibodies (Table 18.4) [82, 84–88, 90, 91, 95, 120, 121]. Nevertheless, negativity does not exclude the diagnosis when the clinical picture and/or histology are characteristic. In this regard, recent evidence suggests the human chondroitin sulfate proteoglycan-4 is more sensitive than HMB-45 and MART-1 for IHC diagnosis of primary and metastatic desmoplastic melanoma lesions [122]. Whether this marker can be applied to MMS remains to be determined.

Summary: Technical Application of MMS and Interpretation of IHC Stains

- The margins of the remaining melanoma or biopsy site should be identified prior to anesthesia using bright surgical lighting.
- Fat must be removed from the Mohs specimen prior to staining with IHC so that extremely thin (2–4 μm) sections can be cut by the histotechnician without artifact or distortion.
- Well-maintained equipment, including high-grade cryostats, liquid nitrogen to lower the temperature of fatty specimens, and very sharp cryostat blades, is essential.
- Accurately interpreting the labeling patterns of melanocytes with MART-1-specific mAb using the IHC technique requires knowledge of the melanocytic staining patterns of normal and sun-damaged skin.

18.4.2 Technical Application of MMS and Interpretation of IHC Stains

Prior to MMS, patients receive detailed information regarding prognosis and alternative treatments and are taught to perform both skin and lymph node self-exams. Patients should be encouraged to ask each and every question they may have regarding their disease. All patients are staged by complete history and physical examination including palpation of pertinent lymph node basins. Chest roentgenography and serum lactate dehydrogenase (LDH) levels may be performed in patients with melanomas greater than 1 mm thick, though the utility of these tests is questionable. The surgeon should be ready to discuss topics such as sentinel lymph node (SLN) biopsy, completion nodal dissection, and systemic therapies and be familiar with local research trials patients may qualify for. For those patients requesting SLN biopsy, it should be noted that wide local excision prior to SLN biopsy does not adversely impact the ability to identify the draining SLN [123–125]. Moreover, the SLN has been shown to accurately reflect the status of the regional lymph node basin in patients with melanoma previously treated with wide local excision [123–125].

To initiate MMS for the treatment of a melanoma, the remaining tumor or surgical scar is confirmed with the patient. Prior to anesthesia and using bright surgical lighting along with magnification, the margin of the remaining melanoma or biopsy site scar is outlined with a surgical marking pen. For melanomas with clinically indistinct margins, a Wood's lamp can be used to assist in establishing the clinical margins. MMS is initiated by excising the remaining visible tumor or biopsy site scar with a 3-mm surgical margin through the dermis into the subcutaneous tissue plane deep enough to remove all adnexal structures. This "debulking" specimen may be submitted for permanent step sectioning using conventional histopathologic techniques to determine the maximum Breslow thickness. After debulking, a second 3-mm margin is excised to the subcutis for complete examination of the margin by means of the MMS technique. Subsequently, the epidermis and dermis are trimmed from the subcutis (Fig. 18.2) since production of consistently readable melanoma slides on frozen sections is dependent on the meticulous preparation of thin 2–4 μm sections without artifact or distortion. Once the epidermis and dermis have been removed from the fat, the specimen is then precisely mapped and color-coded. Very thin, 2–4 μm sections are then stained with both H&E [126] and immunostained with MART-1-specific mAb [79]. As noted above, MART-1-specific mAb are favored for IHC staining by the authors because of its superior sensitivity and specificity. Summarized in Table 18.5, the authors utilize the 1-h protocol consisting of a polymer-based detection system as previously described [79]. It is noteworthy that

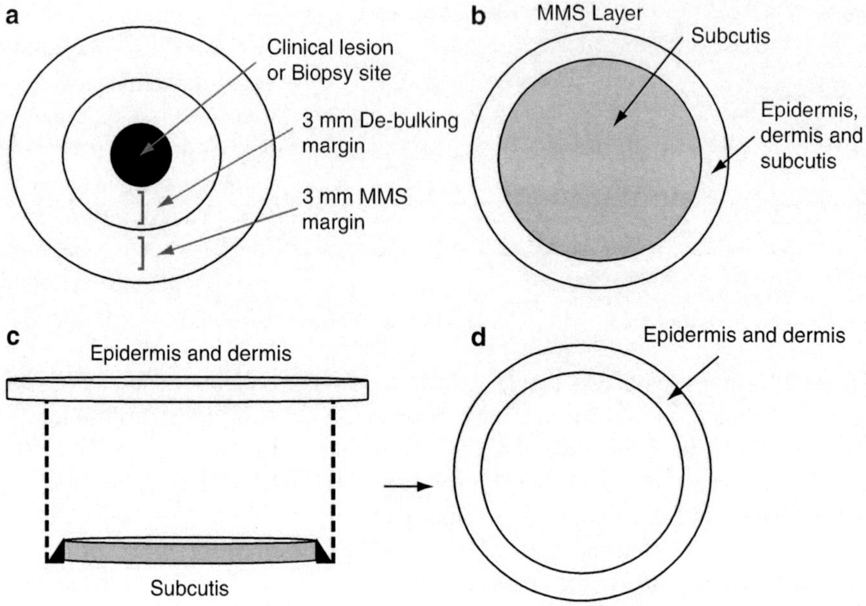

Fig. 18.2 Tissue processing during the application of MMS for the treatment of melanoma. (**a**) The remaining tumor or biopsy scar is identified, and the margin is outlined. MMS is initiated by excising the remaining visible tumor or biopsy site scar with a 3-mm surgical margin through the dermis into the subcutaneous tissue plane deep enough to remove all adnexal structures. (**b**) After debulking, a second 3-mm margin is excised vertically for complete examination of the margin. (**c, d**) Prior to tissue staining with both H&E and MART-1-specific mAb, the epidermis and dermis are trimmed from the fat

Table 18.5 Protocol for staining frozen sections with MART-1-specific mAb

Tissue preparation	Tissue staining
1. Cut thin (2–4 μm) sections	1. Apply blocking agent (5 min)
2. Mount on positively charged IHC slides	2. Shake off, do not rinse
3. Air dry at room temperature (5 min)	3. Apply MART-1-specific mAb (10 min)
4. Heat on 60°C plate (5 min)	4. Rinse in Tris buffer (3 min)
5. Fix in acetone (3 min)	5. Apply polymer HRP (10 min)
6. Air dry at room temperature (5 min)	6. Rinse in Tris buffer (3 min)
7. Rehydrate in Tris buffer (4 min)	7. Apply chromogen (2 min)
	8. Rinse in distilled water (2 min)
	9. Counterstain with hematoxylin (2 s)
	10. Dehydrate in alcohol and mount (5 min)

Derived from [79]

thick sectioning, freeze artifact and folding are common pitfalls when preparing tissue for frozen section evaluation as well as IHC staining. It must be stressed that even with proper tissue preparation, consistently readable melanoma slides processed with the IHC technique on frozen sections require well-trained technicians and proper, well-maintained equipment.

Accurately interpreting the labeling of melanocytes with MART-1-specific mAb using the IHC technique requires knowledge of the melanocytic staining patterns of normal and sun-damaged skin. Criteria for identifying positive margins have been published and include: nests of three or more atypical melanocytes, upward migration of melanocytes in the epidermis (pagetoid spread), and "nonuniform" contiguous melanocytic hyperplasia along the basement membrane [127] (Fig. 18.3). Atypical melanocytes are defined as those that contain mitoses, pleomorphic and hyperchromatic nuclei, or pleomorphic shape. Other nondiagnostic histologic findings that may occasionally be observed in association with melanoma include extension of atypical, crowded melanocytes down adnexal structures, nonuniform distribution of pigment, increased number of melanophages, and/or brisk inflammatory infiltrate. Positive margins are indicated on the map, and the corresponding tissue is then excised with additional 3-mm margins. The above steps are repeated until all margins are free of tumor, and then surgical wound management is performed. Distinguishing benign melanocytic hyperplasia from melanoma in situ can prove challenging even for the most experienced Mohs surgeon. In this regard, increased melanocytic density has been noted in up to one quarter of samples of normal sun-damaged skin with a mean number of melanocytes per high power field of 20.3 [127]. In the most severe areas of melanocyte confluence, the number of adjacent melanocytes did not exceed 9 in the study population [127].

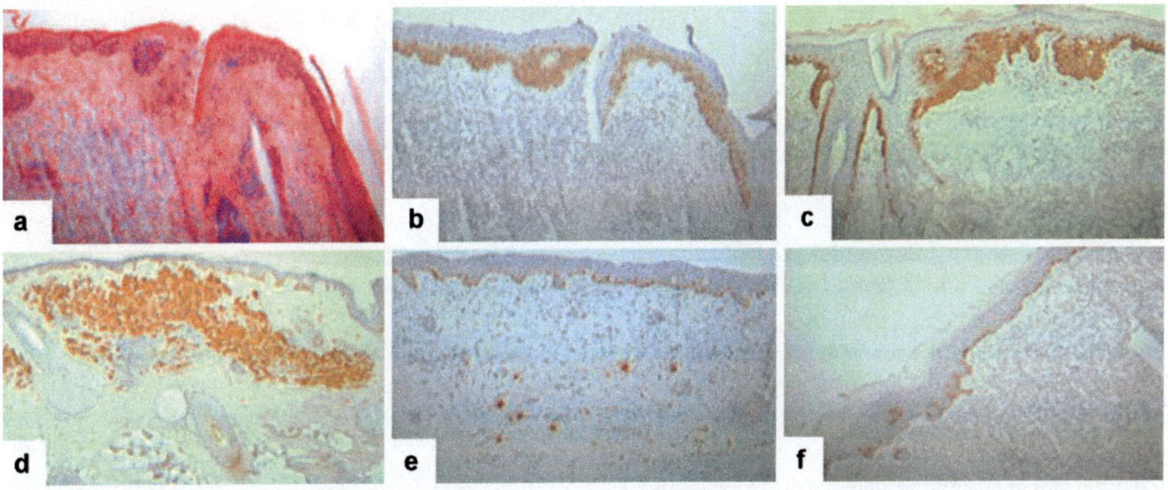

Fig. 18.3 Examples of immunohistochemical staining of frozen sections with MART-1-specific mAb. Malignant melanocytes were stained by H&E (**a** 5×). MART-1-specific staining in the immunoperoxidase reaction is performed in melanoma in situ (**b** 5×, **c** 10×) and in invasive melanoma (**d** 10×). Normal sun-exposed skin stained with MART-1-specific mAb (**e** 5×, **f** 5×) and nonspecific staining of dermal cells (**e** 5×) (**f**) demonstrates "pseudopagetoid" pattern of melanocytes along tangentially cut rete

Importantly, nonspecific staining of dermal cells was observed in about half of the specimens. These cells consistently stained after repeating the MART-1 protocol in the absence of the MART-1-specific mAb, supporting the notion that this labeling pattern may be indicative of nonspecific uptake of secondary antibody [127]. Certain histologic features of melanocytes in sun-damaged skin allow for reliable distinction from MIS. These features include focal confluence of basilar melanocytes without pagetoid spread and the absence of melanocyte nesting [127] (Fig. 18.3).

Summary: Conclusion

- The mortality rate for melanoma has been continually increasing over the past decade, and effective therapies for advanced stage melanoma are lacking.
- MMS is important in the management of cutaneous melanoma, especially for lesions with poorly defined clinical margins and those occurring in areas where tissue conservation is critical.
- MMS for the treatment of cutaneous melanoma depends critically on both surgical and pathological experience as well as the ability to produce high-quality thin frozen sections without artifact.

18.5 Conclusion

In the last 20 years, there has been significant progress in the diagnosis of melanoma, the molecular mechanisms underlying its pathogenesis, and the role the immune system plays in the clinical course of the disease. The information we have acquired has greatly contributed to our understanding of the unique features of this disease. Nevertheless, the mortality rate for melanoma has been continually increasing over the past decade, and effective therapies for advanced stage melanoma are lacking. To date, surgical excision of primary invasive melanoma is the only effective treatment for cutaneous melanoma and is the standard of care for melanomas of all depths [17–20]. Despite our advances, today's surgical standards are still largely based on consensus recommendations [29, 30].

Cutaneous oncologic surgeons caring for patients with melanoma must have a comprehensive knowledge of the disease and continually review pertinent literature in order to provide the most appropriate treatment. This is necessary in order to discuss staging as well as surgical techniques and adjuvant therapies with patients. Surgical excision of primary invasive melanoma continues to be the only effective treatment for primary cutaneous melanoma. MMS clearly has a role in the management of cutaneous melanoma, especially for lesions with poorly defined clinical margins and those occurring in areas where tissue conservation is critical. Moreover, recent advances in IHC staining have made it practical to incorporate the use of immunostains, such as MART-1, during MMS in order to identify melanocytes on frozen sections. These improvements have greatly expanded our capacity to treat cutaneous melanoma by overcoming the problem of identifying atypical melanocytes as well as atypical melanocytic pattern or proliferations on frozen sections. The major advantages of MMS for melanoma are (1) low local recurrence rates, (2) smaller wounds, and (3) evaluation of 100% of the surgical margin. These advantages lead to optimal local recurrence, metastasis, and 5-year disease-specific survival rates and simplify reconstruction of surgical wounds especially in areas where functional and cosmetic outcomes are paramount. A secondary benefit of MMS is that it occurs in the outpatient setting under local anesthesia, and patients often wait with their family and/or friends in a comfortable environment for pathology results. Perhaps the most important benefit is that evaluation of 100% of the surgical margin in every case alleviates the need to depend on broad consensus recommendations for surgical margins, thereby enhancing the certainty of ensuring complete tumor removal on the day of surgery and prior to reconstruction. Clearly, future prospective studies comparing MMS to WLE, specifically comparing tumors occurring in different anatomic locations, would be beneficial in order to more appropriately define surgical margins. Moreover, as new classes of melanocyte and/or melanoma-specific antigens become available, it will be important to determine if these antigens can enhance the identification of atypical melanocytes in MMS.

References

1. MacKie RM, Hauschild A, Eggermont AM. Epidemiology of invasive cutaneous melanoma. Ann Oncol. 2009;20 Suppl 6:1–7.
2. Rigel DS, Russak J, Friedman R. The evolution of melanoma diagnosis: 25 years beyond the ABCDs. CA Cancer J Clin. 2010;60:301–16.
3. Terando A, Sabel MS, Sondak VK. Melanoma: adjuvant therapy and other treatment options. Curr Treat Options Oncol. 2003;4:187–99.
4. Crosby T, Mason M, Savage P. Malignant melanoma (non-metastatic). Clin Evid. 2005;14:2058–72.
5. Cooper JS. Radiation therapy of malignant melanoma. Dermatol Clin. 2002;20:713–6.
6. Cascinelli N, Santinami M, Maurichi A, Patuzzo R, Pennacchioli E. World Health Organization experience in the treatment of melanoma. Surg Clin North Am. 2003;83:405–16.
7. Soengas MS, Lowe SW. Apoptosis and melanoma chemoresistance. Oncogene. 2003;22:3138–51.
8. Bollag G, Hirth P, Tsai J, et al. Clinical efficacy of a RAF inhibitor needs broad target blockade in BRAF-mutant melanoma. Nature. 2010;467:596–9.
9. Flaherty KT, Hodi FS, Bastian BC. Mutation-driven drug development in melanoma. Curr Opin Oncol. 2010;22:178–83.
10. Flaherty KT, Puzanov I, Kim KB, et al. Inhibition of mutated, activated BRAF in metastatic melanoma. N Engl J Med. 2010;363:809–19.
11. Campoli M, Ferrone S. T-cell-based immunotherapy of melanoma: what have we learned and how can we improve? Expert Rev Vaccines. 2004;3:171–87.
12. Basu B, Biswas S, Wrigley J, Sirohi B, Corrie P. Angiogenesis in cutaneous malignant melanoma and potential therapeutic strategies. Expert Rev Anticancer Ther. 2009;9:1583–98.
13. Jandus C, Speiser D, Romero P. Recent advances and hurdles in melanoma immunotherapy. Pigment Cell Melanoma Res. 2009;22:711–23.
14. Campoli M, Ferris R, Ferrone S, Wang X. Immunotherapy of malignant disease with tumor antigen-specific monoclonal antibodies. Clin Cancer Res. 2010;16:11–20.
15. Hashmi MH, Van Veldhuizen PJ. Interleukin-21: updated review of phase I and II clinical trials in metastatic renal cell carcinoma, metastatic melanoma and relapsed/refractory indolent non-Hodgkin's lymphoma. Expert Opin Biol Ther. 2010;10:807–17.
16. Mouawad R, Sebert M, Michels J, Bloch J, Spano JP, Khayat D. Treatment for metastatic malignant melanoma: old drugs and new strategies. Crit Rev Oncol Hematol. 2010;74:27–39.
17. Morton DL. Current management of malignant melanoma. Ann Surg. 1990;212:123–4.
18. Balch CM, Urist MM, Karakousis CP, et al. Efficacy of 2 cm surgical margins for intermediate-thickness melanomas 1–4 mm. Ann Surg. 1993;218:262–9.
19. Breslow A, Macht SD. Optimal size of resection margin for thin cutaneous melanoma. Surg Gynecol Obstet. 1997;145:691–2.
20. Heaton KM, Sussman JJ, Gershenwald JE, et al. Surgical margins and prognostic factors in patients with thick (>4 cm) primary melanoma. Ann Surg Oncol. 1998;5:322–8.
21. Clark Jr WH, From L, Bernardino EA, Mihm MC. The histogenesis and biologic behavior of primary human malignant melanomas of the skin. Cancer Res. 1969;29:705–27.
22. Breslow A. Thickness, cross-sectional areas and depth of invasion in the prognosis of cutaneous melanoma. Ann Surg. 1970;172:902–8.
23. Veronesi U, Cascinelli N, Adamus J, et al. Thin stage I primary cutaneous malignant melanoma: comparison of excision with margins of 1 or 3 cm. N Engl J Med. 1988;318:1159–62.

24. Cascinelli N. Margin of resection in the management of primary melanoma. Semin Surg Oncol. 1998;14:272–5.
25. Cohn-Cedermark G, Rutqvist LE, Andersson R, et al. Long term results of a randomized study by the Swedish Melanoma Study Group on 2-cm versus 5-cm resection margins for patients with cutaneous melanoma with a tumor thickness of 0.8–2.0 mm. Cancer. 2000;89:1495–501.
26. Balch CM, Soong SJ, Smith T, et al. Long-term results of a prospective surgical trial comparing 2 cm vs. 4 cm excision margins for 740 patients with 1–4 mm melanomas. Ann Surg Oncol. 2001;8:101–8.
27. Khayat D, Rixe O, Martin G, et al. Surgical margins in cutaneous melanoma (2 cm versus 5 cm for lesions measuring less than 2.1-mm thick). Cancer. 2003;97:1941–6.
28. Thomas JM, Newton-Bishop J, A'Hern R, et al. Excision margins in high-risk malignant melanoma. N Engl J Med. 2004;350:757–66.
29. Sladden MJ, Balch C, Barzilai DA, et al. Surgical excision margins for primary cutaneous melanoma. Cochrane Database Syst Rev. 2009;4:CD004835.
30. Leiter U, Eigentler TK, Forschner A, et al. Excision guidelines and follow-up strategies in cutaneous melanoma: facts and controversies. Clin Dermatol. 2010;28:311–5.
31. Nagore E, Oliver V, Botella-Estrada R, Moreno-Picot S, Insa A, Fortea JM. Prognostic factors in localized invasive cutaneous melanoma: high value of mitotic rate, vascular invasion and microscopic satellitosis. Melanoma Res. 2005;15:169–77.
32. Day Jr CL, Harrist TJ, Gorstein F, et al. Malignant melanoma. Prognostic significance of "microscopic satellites" in the reticular dermis and subcutaneous fat. Ann Surg. 1981;194:108–12.
33. Day Jr CL, Mihm Jr MC, Lew RA, et al. Prognostic factors for patients with clinical stage I melanoma of intermediate thickness (1.51 - 3.39 mm). A conceptual model for tumor growth and metastasis. Ann Surg. 1982;195:35–43.
34. Harrist TJ, Rigel DS, Day Jr CL, et al. Microscopic satellites" are more highly associated with regional lymph node metastases than is primary melanoma thickness. Cancer. 1984;53:2183–7.
35. León P, Daly JM, Synnestvedt M, Schultz DJ, Elder DE, Clark Jr WH. The prognostic implications of microscopic satellites in patients with clinical stage I melanoma. Arch Surg. 1991;126:1461–8.
36. Mraz-Gernhard S, Sagebiel RW, Kashani-Sabet M, Miller 3rd JR, Leong SP. Prediction of sentinel lymph node micrometastasis by histological features in primary cutaneous malignant melanoma. Arch Dermatol. 1998;134:983–7.
37. Balch CM, Gershenwald JE, Soong SJ, et al. Final version of 2009 AJCC melanoma staging and classification. J Clin Oncol. 2009;27:6199–206.
38. Macht SD. Depth of excision of melanomas. JAMA. 2001;286:167–8.
39. Wolf Y, Balicer RD, Amir A, Feinmesser M, Hauben DJ. The vertical dimension in the surgical treatment of cutaneous malignant melanoma – how deep is deep? Eur J Plast Surg. 2001;24:74–7.
40. Charles CA, Yee VS, Dusza SW, et al. Variation in the diagnosis, treatment, and management of melanoma in situ: a survey of US dermatologists. Arch Dermatol. 2005; 141:723–9.
41. NIH consensus conference: diagnosis and treatment of early melanoma. JAMA. 1992;268:1314–9.
42. Coit DG, Andtbacka R, Bichakjian CK, NCCN Melanoma Panel, et al. Melanoma. J Natl Compr Canc Netw. 2009; 7:250–75.
43. Roberts DLL, Anstey AV, Barlow RJ, et al. U.K. guidelines for the management of cutaneous melanoma. Br J Dermatol. 2002;146:7–17.
44. Sober AJ, Chuang TY, Duvic M, Guidelines/Outcomes Committee, et al. Guidelines of care for primary cutaneous melanoma. J Am Acad Dermatol. 2001;45:579–86.
45. Johnson TM, Sondak VK. A centimeter here, a centimeter there: does it matter? J Am Acad Dermatol. 1995;33: 532–4.
46. Bricca GM, Brodland DG, Ren D, Zitelli JA. Cutaneous head and neck melanoma treated with Mohs micrographic surgery. J Am Acad Dermatol. 2005;52:92–100.
47. Urist MM, Balch CM, Soong SJ, Shaw HM, Milton GW, Maddox WA. The influence of surgical margins and prognostic factors predicting the risk of local recurrence in 3445 patients with primary cutaneous melanoma. Cancer. 1985;55:1398–402.
48. O'Brien CJ, Coates AS, Peterson-Schaefer K, et al. Experience with 998 cutaneous melanomas of the head and neck over 30 years. Am J Surg. 1991;162:310–4.
49. Anderson AP, Gottlieb J, Drzewlecki KT, Hou-Jensen K, Sondergaard K. Skin melanoma of the head and neck. Prognostic factors and recurrence-free survival in 512 patients. Cancer. 1992;69:1153–6.
50. Brown CD, Zitelli JA. The prognosis and treatment of true local cutaneous recurrent malignant melanoma. Dermatol Surg. 1995;21:285–90.
51. Karakousis CP, Balch CM, Urist MM, Ross MM, Smith TJ, Bartolucci AA. Local recurrence in malignant melanoma: long-term results of the multiinstitutional randomized surgical trial. Ann Surg Oncol. 1996;3:446–52.
52. Furukawa H, Tsutsumida A, Yamamoto Y, et al. Melanoma of thumb: retrospective study for amputation levels, surgical margin and reconstruction. J Plast Reconstr Aesthet Surg. 2007;60:24–31.
53. Cohen T, Busam KJ, Patel A, Brady MS. Subungual melanoma: management considerations. Am J Surg. 2008;195: 244–8.
54. Kimyai-Asadi A, Katz T, Goldberg LH, et al. Margin involvement after the excision of melanoma in situ: the need for complete en face examination of the surgical margins. Dermatol Surg. 2007;33:1434–9.
55. Debloom JR, Zitelli JA, Brodland DG. The invasive growth potential of residual melanoma and melanoma in situ. Dermatol Surg. 2010;36:1251–7.
56. Wolf DJ, Zitelli JA. Surgical margins for basal cell carcinoma. Arch Dermatol. 1987;123:340–4.
57. Brodland DG, Zitelli JA. Surgical margins for excision of primary cutaneous squamous cell carcinoma. J Am Acad Dermatol. 1992;27(2 Pt 1):241–8.
58. Parker TL, Zitelli JA. Surgical margins for excision of dermatofibrosarcoma protuberans. J Am Acad Dermatol. 1995;32:233–6.
59. Paradisi A, Abeni D, Rusciani A, et al. Dermatofibrosarcoma protuberans: wide local excision vs. Mohs micrographic surgery. Cancer Treat Rev. 2008;34:728–36.

60. Mohs FE. Chemosurgery for melanoma. Arch Dermatol. 1977;113:285–91.
61. Mohs FE. Chemosurgery: microscopically controlled surgery for skin cancer. Springfield: Charles C Thomas; 1978. p. 225–48.
62. Mohs FE. Microscopically controlled surgery for periorbital melanoma: fixed-tissue and fresh-tissue techniques. J Dermatol Surg Oncol. 1985;11:284–91.
63. Fewkes J, Mohs FE. Microscopically controlled surgical excision (the Mohs technique). In: Fitzpatrick TB, Eisen AZ, Wolff K, et al., editors. Dermatology in general medicine. New York: McGraw-Hill; 1987. p. 2557–63.
64. Mohs FE. Fixed tissue micrographic surgery for melanoma of the ear. Arch Otolaryngol Head Neck Surg. 1988;114: 625–31.
65. Zitelli JA, Mohs FE, Larson P, Snow S. Mohs micrographic surgery for melanoma. Dermatol Clin. 1989;7:833–43.
66. Zitelli JA, Brown C, Hanusa BH. Mohs micrographic surgery for the treatment of primary cutaneous melanoma. J Am Acad Dermatol. 1997;37:236–45.
67. Cohen LM, McCall MW, Hodge SJ, Freedman JD, Callen JP, Zax RH. Successful treatment of lentigo maligna and lentigo maligna melanoma with Mohs micrographic surgery aided by rush permanent sections. Cancer. 1994;73: 2964–70.
68. Robinson JK. Margin control for lentigo maligna. J Am Acad Dermatol. 1994;31:79–85.
69. Cohen LM, McCall MW, Zax RH. Mohs micrographic surgery for lentigo maligna and lentigo maligna melanoma. A follow-up study. Dermatol Surg. 1998;24:673–7.
70. Bienert TN, Trotter MJ, Arlette JP. Treatment of cutaneous melanoma of the face by Mohs micrographic surgery. J Cutan Med Surg. 2003;7:25–30.
71. Temple CL, Arlette JP. Mohs micrographic surgery in the treatment of lentigo maligna and melanoma. J Surg Oncol. 2006;94:287–92.
72. Zitelli JA, Moy RL, Abell E. The reliability of frozen sections in the evaluation of surgical margins for melanoma. J Am Acad Dermatol. 1991;24:102–6.
73. Ferrciro JA, Meyers JL, Bostwick DG. Accuracy of frozen section diagnosis in surgical pathology: review of a 1-year experience with 24,880 cases at Mayo Clinic Rochester. Mayo Clin Proc. 1995;70:1137–41.
74. Snow SN, Mohs FE, Oriba HA, Dudley CM, Leverson G, Hetzer M. Cutaneous malignant melanoma treated by Mohs surgery: review of the treatment results of 179 cases from the Mohs Melanoma Registry. Dermatol Surg. 1997;23: 1055–60.
75. Dabbs DJ. Diagnostic immunohistochemistry. Philadelphia: Churchill Livingstone; 2002.
76. Zalla MJ, Lim KK, Dicaudo KK, Gagnot MM. Mohs micrographic excision of melanoma using immunostains. Dermatol Surg. 2000;26:771–84.
77. Albertini JG, Elston DM, Libow LF, Smith SB, Farley MF. Mohs micrographic surgery for melanoma: a case series, a comparative study of immunostains, an informative case report, and a unique mapping technique. Dermatol Surg. 2002;28:656–65.
78. Kelley LC, Starkus L. Immunohistochemical staining of lentigo maligna during Mohs micrographic surgery using MART-1. J Am Acad Dermatol. 2002;46:78–84.
79. Bricca GM, Brodland DG, Zitelli JA. Immunostaining melanoma frozen sections: the 1-hour protocol. Dermatol Surg. 2004;30:403–8.
80. Davis DA, Kurtz KA, Robinson RA. Ultrarapid staining for cutaneous melanoma: study and protocol. Dermatol Surg. 2005;31:753–6.
81. Bhardwaj SS, Tope WD, Lee PK. Mohs micrographic surgery for lentigo maligna and lentigo maligna melanoma using Mel-5 immunostaining: University of Minnesota experience. Dermatol Surg. 2006;32:690–6.
82. Jungbluth AA, Busam KJ, Gerald WL, et al. A103: an anti-Melan-A monoclonal antibody for the detection of malignant melanoma in paraffin-embedded tissues. Am J Surg Pathol. 1998;22:595–602.
83. Kaufmann O, Koch S, Burghardt J, Audring H, Dietel M. Tyrosinase, Melan-A, and KBA62 as markers for the immunohistochemical identification of metastatic amelanotic melanomas on paraffin sections. Mod Pathol. 1998;11:740–6.
84. Busam K, Jungbluth A. The new melanoma markers: MART- 1 and Melan-A (the NIH experience): author's response. Am J Surg Pathol. 1999;23:610–3.
85. Fetsch PA, Marincola FM, Abati A. The new melanoma markers: MART-1 and Melan-A (the NIH experience). Am J Surg Pathol. 1999;23:607–10.
86. Orchard GE. Comparison of immunohistochemical labeling of melanocyte differentiation antibodies Melan-A, tyrosinase and HMB45 with NKIC3 and S100 protein in the evaluation of benign nevi and malignant melanoma. Histochem J. 2000;32:475–81.
87. Clarkson KS, Sturdgess IC, Molyneux AJ. The usefulness of tyrosinase in the immunohistochemical assessment of melanocytic lesions: a comparison of the novel T311 antibody (anti-tyrosinase) with S-100, HMB45, and A103 (anti-melan-A). J Clin Pathol. 2001;54:196–200.
88. Miettinen M, Fernandez M, Franssila K, Gatalica Z, Lasota J, Sarlomo-Rikala M. Microphthalmia transcription factor in the immunohistochemical diagnosis of metastatic melanoma: comparison with four other melanoma markers. Am J Surg Pathol. 2001;25:205–11.
89. Granter SR, Weilbaecher KN, Quigley C, Fisher DE. Role for microphthalmia transcription factor in the diagnosis of metastatic malignant melanoma. Appl Immunohistochem Mol Morphol. 2002;10:47–51.
90. Sundram U, Harvell JD, Rouse RV, Natkunam Y. Expression of the B-Cell proliferation marker MUM1 by melanocytic lesions and comparison with S100, gp100 (HMB45), and MelanA. Mod Pathol. 2003;16:802–20.
91. Zubovits J, Buzney E, Yu L, Duncan LM. HMB-45, S-100, NK1/C3, and MART-1 in metastatic melanoma. Hum Pathol. 2004;35:217–23.
92. Hornick JL, Fletcher CDM. PEComa: what do we know so far? Histopathology. 2006;48:75–82.
93. Mai KT, Belanger EC. Perivascular epithelioid cell tumour (PEComa) of the soft tissue. Pathology. 2006;38:415–20.
94. Dim DC, Cooley LD, Miranda RN. Clear cell sarcoma of tendons and aponeuroses: a review. Arch Pathol Lab Med. 2007;131:152–6.
95. Ordonez NG, Xiaolong J, Hickey RC. Comparison of HMB-45 monoclonal antibody and S-100 protein in the immunohistochemical diagnosis of melanoma. Am J Clin Pathol. 1988;90:385–90.

96. Wick MR, Swanson PE, Rocamora A. Recognition of malignant melanoma by monoclonal antibody HMB-45. An immunohistochemical study of 200 paraffin-embedded cutaneous tumors. J Cutan Pathol. 1988;15:201–7.
97. Swanson PE, Wick MR. Clear cell sarcoma: an immunohistochemical analysis of six cases and comparison with other epithelioid neoplasms of soft tissue. Arch Pathol Lab Med. 1989;113:55–60.
98. Unger PD, Hoffman K, Thung SN, Pertsemlides D, Wolfe D, Kaneko M. HMB-45 reactivity in adrenal pheochromocytomas. Arch Pathol Lab Med. 1992;116:151–3.
99. Bishop PW, Menasce LP, Yates AJ, Win NA, Banerjee SS. An immunophenotypic survey of malignant melanomas. Histopathology. 1993;23:159–66.
100. Trefzer U, Rietz N, Chen Y, et al. SM5–1: a new monoclonal antibody which is highly sensitive and specific for melanocytic lesions. Arch Dermatol Res. 2000;292:583–9.
101. Deavers MT, Malpica A, Ordonez NG, Silva EG. Ovarian steroid cell tumors: an immunohistochemical study including a comparison of calretinin with inhibin. Int J Gynecol Pathol. 2003;22:162–7.
102. Turhan T, Oner K, Yurtseven T, Akalin T, Ovul I. Spinal meningeal melanocytoma. Report of two cases and review of the literature. J Neurosurg. 2004;100:287–90.
103. Argani P, Lae M, Hutchinson B, et al. Renal carcinomas with the t(6;11)(p21;q12): clinicopathologic features and demonstration of the specific alpha-TFEB gene fusion by immunohistochemistry, RT-PCR, and DNA PCR. Am J Surg Pathol. 2005;29:230–40.
104. McKee PH, Calonje E, Granter SR. Pathology of the skin with clinical correlations. 3rd ed. Philadelphia: Elsevier Mosby; 2005.
105. O'Brien DF, Crooks D, Mallucci C, et al. Meningeal melanocytoma. Childs Nerv Syst. 2006;22:556–61.
106. Hofbauer GFL, Kamarashev J, Geertsen R, Boni R, Dummer R. Tyrosinase immunoreactivity in formalin-fixed, paraffin- embedded primary and metastatic melanoma: frequency and distribution. J Cutan Pathol. 1998;25:204–9.
107. Castelli C, Rivoltini L, Andreola G, Carrabba M, Renkvist N, Parmiani G. T-cell recognition of melanoma-associated antigens. J Cell Physiol. 2000;182:323–31.
108. Busam KJ, Iversen K, Coplan KC, Jungbluth AA. Analysis of microphthalmia transcription factor expression in normal tissues and tumors, and comparison of its expression with S-100 protein, gp100, and tyrosinase in desmoplastic malignant melanoma. Am J Surg Pathol. 2001;25:197–204.
109. King R, Weilbaecher KN, McGill G, Cooley E, Mihm M, Fisher DE. Microphthalmia transcription factor: a sensitive and specific melanocyte marker for melanoma diagnosis. Am J Pathol. 1999;155:731–8.
110. King R, Googe PB, Weilbacher KN, Mihm Jr MC, Fisher DE. Microphthalmia transcription factor expression in cutaneous benign, malignant melanocytic, and nonmelanocytic tumors. Am J Surg Pathol. 2001;25:51–7.
111. Makhlouf HR, Ishak KG, Shekar R, Sesterhenn IA, Young DY, Fanburg-Smith JC. Melanoma markers in angiomyolipoma of the liver and kidney. Arch Pathol Lab Med. 2002;126:49–55.
112. Salazar-Onfray F, López M, Lundqvist A, et al. Tissue distribution and differential expression of melanocortin 1 receptor, a malignant melanoma marker. Br J Cancer. 2002;87:414–22.
113. Trefzer U, Chen Y, Herberth G, et al. The monoclonal antibody SM5–1 recognizes a fibronectin variant which is widely expressed in melanoma. BMC Cancer. 2006;6:8.
114. Reinke S, Königer P, Herberth G, et al. Differential expression of MART-1, tyrosinase, and SM5–1 in primary and metastatic melanoma. Am J Dermatopathol. 2005;27: 401–16.
115. Busam KJ, Kucukgol D, Sato E, Frosina D, Teruya-Feldstein J, Jungbluth AA. Immunohistochemical analysis of novel mono-clonal antibody PNL2 and comparison with other melanocyte differentiation markers. Am J Surg Pathol. 2005;29:400–6.
116. Roma AA, Magi-Galluzzi C, Zhou M. Differential expression of melanocytic markers in myoid, lipomatous, and vascular components of renal angiomyolipomas. Arch Pathol Lab Med. 2007;131:122–5.
117. Morris LG, Wen YH, Nonaka D, et al. PNL2 melanocytic marker in immunohistochemical evaluation of primary mucosal melanoma of the head and neck. Head Neck. 2008;30:771–5.
118. Meije CB, Swart GW, Lepoole C, Das PK, Van den Oord JJ. Antigenic profiles of individual-matched pairs of primary and melanoma metastases. Hum Pathol. 2009; 40:1399–407.
119. Mitra D, Fisher DE. Transcriptional regulation in melanoma. Hematol Oncol Clin North Am. 2009;23:447–65.
120. Glass LF, Raziano RM, Clark GS, et al. Rapid frozen section immunostaining of melanocytes by microphthalmia-associated transcription factor. Am J Dermatopathol. 2010;32:319–25.
121. Fernando SS, Johnson S, Bate J. Immunohistochemical analysis of cutaneous malignant melanoma: comparison of S-100 protein, HMB-45 monoclonal antibody and NKI/C3 monoclonal antibody. Pathology. 1994;26:16–9.
122. Campoli M, Ferrone S, Wang X. Functional and clinical relevance of chondroitin sulfate proteoglycan 4. Adv Cancer Res. 2010;109:73–121.
123. McCready DR, Ghazarian DM, Hershkop MS, Walker JA, Ambus U, Quirt IC. Sentinel lymph-node biopsy after previous wide local excision for melanoma. Can J Surg. 2001;44:432–4.
124. Leong WL, Ghazarian DM, McCready DR. Previous wide local excision of primary melanoma is not a contraindication for sentinel lymph node biopsy of the trunk and extremity. J Surg Oncol. 2003;82:143–6.
125. Gannon CJ, Rousseau Jr DL, Ross MI, Johnson MM, Lee JE, Mansfield PF, et al. Accuracy of lymphatic mapping and sentinel lymph node biopsy after previous wide local excision in patients with primary melanoma. Cancer. 2006;107:2647–52.
126. Wheeland RG, Ratz JL, Bailin PL. Mohs micrographic surgery technique. In: Roenigk RK, Roenigk HH, editors. Dermatologic surgery: principles and practice. New York: Marcel Dekker; 1997. p. 731–44.
127. Hendi A, Brodland DG, Zitelli JA. Melanocytes in long-standing sun-exposed skin: quantitative analysis using the MART-1 immunostain. Arch Dermatol. 2006;142: 871–6.

Dermatofibrosarcoma Protuberans

19

Novie Sroa and Nathalie C. Zeitouni

Abstract

Dermatofibrosarcoma protuberans (DFSP) is a rare but locally aggressive spindle cell neoplasm accounting for less than 2% of all soft tissue sarcomas and less than 0.1% of all malignancies. Immunohistochemical and ultrastructural studies indicate that the tumor is of a fibroblastic origin. DFSP commonly occurs in the dermis and has the potential to invade through fascial planes into muscle and bone. It may occur on any part of the body with a predilection for the trunk. The tumor rarely exhibits metastasis, but it has the propensity for subclinical involvement. Complete surgical excision is the mainstay of therapy. DFSP can be resected with either wide local excision (WLE) or Mohs micrographic surgery (MMS). The exact role of neoadjuvant imatinib mesylate in the management of DFSP remains unclear. Successful treatment outcome is dependent on achieving negative surgical margins while preventing functional deficits.

Keywords

Dermatofibrosarcoma protuberans • Imatinib mesylate • Mohs micrographic surgery • Wide excision • Platelet-derived growth factor receptor

Summary: Introduction

- Dermatofibrosarcoma protuberans is a rare intermediate grade spindle cell neoplasm, which rarely metastasizes.
- It accounts for less than 0.1% of all malignancies.
- It can invade through fascial planes onto muscle and bone.
- Complete surgical excision is the mainstay of therapy.

N. Sroa • N.C. Zeitouni (✉)
Department of Dermatology,
Roswell Park Cancer Institute, Buffalo, NY 14263, USA
e-mail: nathalie.zeitouni@roswellpark.org

K. Nouri (ed.), *Mohs Micrographic Surgery*,
DOI 10.1007/978-1-4471-2152-7_19, © Springer-Verlag London Limited 2012

19.1 Introduction

Dermatofibrosarcoma protuberans (DFSP) is a rare but locally aggressive spindle cell neoplasm accounting for less than 2% of all soft tissue sarcomas and less than 0.1% of all malignancies [1]. Immunohistochemical and ultrastructural studies indicate that *the tumor* is of a fibroblastic origin [2]. This intermediate-grade cutaneous malignancy commonly occurs in the dermis and has the potential to invade through fascial *planes into muscle* and bone. It may occur on any part of the body with a predilection for the trunk. *DFSP* rarely exhibits metastases, but it has the propensity of subclinical involvement [3, 4].

Treatment generally focuses on *surgical* removal of the tumor to prevent local recurrence. Clinical exam alone cannot predict the extent of involvement. DFSP can be resected with either wide local excision (WLE) or Mohs micrographic surgery (MMS) [4–8]. Successful treatment outcome is dependent on achieving negative surgical margins while preventing functional deficits.

Summary: Epidemiology

- DFSP accounts for approximately 0.1% of all human cancers.
- Patients between the third and fifth decades have the highest age-specific annual incidence rates.
- Overall, African-Americans represent the highest annual incidence rate among all the races, followed by Caucasians.

19.2 Epidemiology

According to the descriptive epidemiology study of cancer registries of the Surveillance, Epidemiology, and End Results (SEER) program from 1973 to 2002, the overall incidence of DFSP is 4.2 per million. DFSP accounts for approximately 0.1% of all cancers in the database. Standardized for race and gender, the data indicated that patients between the third and fifth decades have the highest age-specific annual incidence rates. Overall, African-Americans represent the highest annual incidence rate among all the races, followed by Caucasians. There is no gender predilection. However, beyond the sixth decade, men were found to have higher incidence rates than women [1].

Summary: Pathogenesis

- Dermatofibrosarcoma protuberans may be related to previous trauma, vaccination, burns, or insect bites.
- The p53 pathway and microsatellite instability causing DNA mismatch repair are implicated in tumor progression.
- Up to 95% of DFSPs are characterized by genetic abnormalities of t(17;22) causing fusion of collagen type 1 alpha 1 (*COL1A1*) gene on chromosome 17 with the platelet-derived growth factor B (*PDGFB*) chain gene on chromosome 22.
- Constitutive activation of platelet-derived growth factor receptor (*PDGFR*) by *PDGFB* may lead to uninhibited growth of neoplastic cells.

19.3 Pathogenesis

The exact etiology of DFSP is unknown, and its pathogenesis remains controversial. A history of previous local trauma is often elicited. There are reports of DFSP occurring in sites of previous vaccinations including immunizations for smallpox, yellow fever, tetanus, and tuberculosis [9, 10]. DFSP has been reported to arise in burn scar in two patients and from an infected insect bite in one case report [11–13]. The development of malignancy has been attributed to the persistent inflammation and/or wound healing associated with vaccine components, constant irritation, chronic ulceration, the release of local toxins following injury, poor lymphatic regeneration, repeated trauma, or exposure to noxious environmental agents [14, 15]. In addition, accelerated growth of DFSP has been reported during pregnancy. DFSPs appear to express low levels of hormone receptors, which may be one factor that accounts for their accelerated growth during pregnancy [16, 17].

Molecular studies of pathogenesis of DFSP are limited. It is hypothesized that the *p53* pathway may be involved in DFSP tumorigenesis, and more specifically, in the fibrosarcomatous areas of DFSP. Point and missense mutations of *p53* gene were found in metastatic DFSPs but not in non-fibrosarcomatous variants of DFSPs [18, 19]. In addition, microsatellite analyses of DFSPs have revealed defective DNA mismatch repair in tumor replication via microsatellite polymorphisms. This microsatellite instability has been implicated in tumor progression of DFSP in both non-fibrosarcomatous and fibrosarcomatous variants [20].

Cytogenetic analyses have demonstrated that up to 95% of DFSPs are characterized by anomalies of chromosomes 17 and 22 consisting of a supernumerary ring chromosome deriving from t(17;22) or a reciprocal translocation t(17;22)(q22;q13) [21, 22]. The frequency of each of these cytogenetic abnormalities is unknown [22, 23]. These cytogenetic abnormalities fuse collagen type 1 alpha 1 (*COL1A1*) gene on chromosome 17 with the platelet-derived growth factor B (*PDGFB*) chain gene on chromosome 22 (Fig. 19.1).

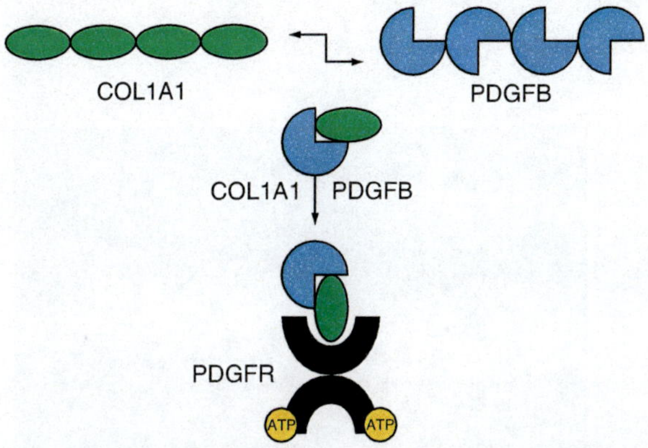

Fig. 19.1 Dermatofibrosarcoma protuberans, cytogenetics. Collagen type 1 alpha 1 (*COL1A1*) gene on chromosome 17 fuses with the platelet-derived growth factor B (*PDGFB*) chain gene on chromosome 22. The resultant *COL1A1-PFGFB* fusion protein undergoes posttranslational processing to form functional *PDGFB*, the ligand for the cell surface receptor, tyrosine kinase platelet-derived growth factor receptor (*PDGFR*). *COL1A1* collagen type 1 alpha 1 gene, *PDGFB* platelet-derived growth factor B, *PDGFR* kinase platelet-derived growth factor receptor

The reported breakpoint of PDGFB is constant at exon 2, whereas the breakpoint in *COL1A1* is variable and may occur on exons 6–49 [23]. The resultant *COL1A1-PFGFB* fusion protein undergoes posttranslational processing to form functional *PDGFB*, the ligand for the cell surface receptor, tyrosine kinase platelet-derived growth factor receptor (*PDGFR*). It is thought that deregulated expression of *PDGFB*, with concomitant autocrine stimulation of *PDGFR*, could be a critical molecular event in the pathogenesis of DFSP [24–26]. Constitutive activation of *PDGFR* may cause uninhibited growth of connective tissue cells and tumor proliferation [27].

These molecular changes in DFSP can be detected cytogenetically by polymerase chain reaction (PCR) or fluorescent in situ hybridization (FISH) techniques (Fig. 19.2) [28]. The combination of FISH and comparative genomic hybridization (CGH) techniques has been valuable in identifying the composition of the DFSP ring chromosomes [22, 29, 30]. Reverse transcription–polymerase chain reaction (RT-PCR) assays can be used to detect the COL1A1-PDGFB fusion transcripts in DFSP specimens either frozen or paraffin-embedded [31]. Takahira et al. have amplified and quantified PDGFB gene copies and PDGFB/PDGFRB mRNA levels by a real-time PCR system for DFSP samples in which the fusion transcripts had been successfully detected. The authors found no correlation between the PDGFRB expression level and histologic subtype of DFSP [32]. Quantification of PDGF-B RNA by real-time polymerase chain reaction (RT-PCR) has shown higher expression of PDGF-B gene in DFSP than standard PCR, yielding less false-negative results in distinguishing DFSP from its benign counterpart, dermatofibroma [33].

Fig. 19.2 Dermatofibrosarcoma protuberans, fluorescence in situ hybridization. Multiple signals in the spindle cells of a DFSP specimen indicating fusion between chromosomes 17 and 22 (*magnification ×1000*) (Reprinted from Najarian et al. [28], copyright 2010, with permission from John Wiley & Sons Ltd)

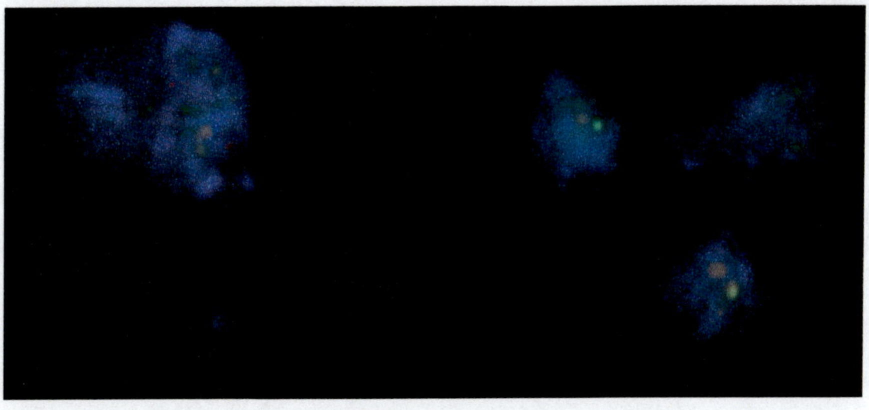

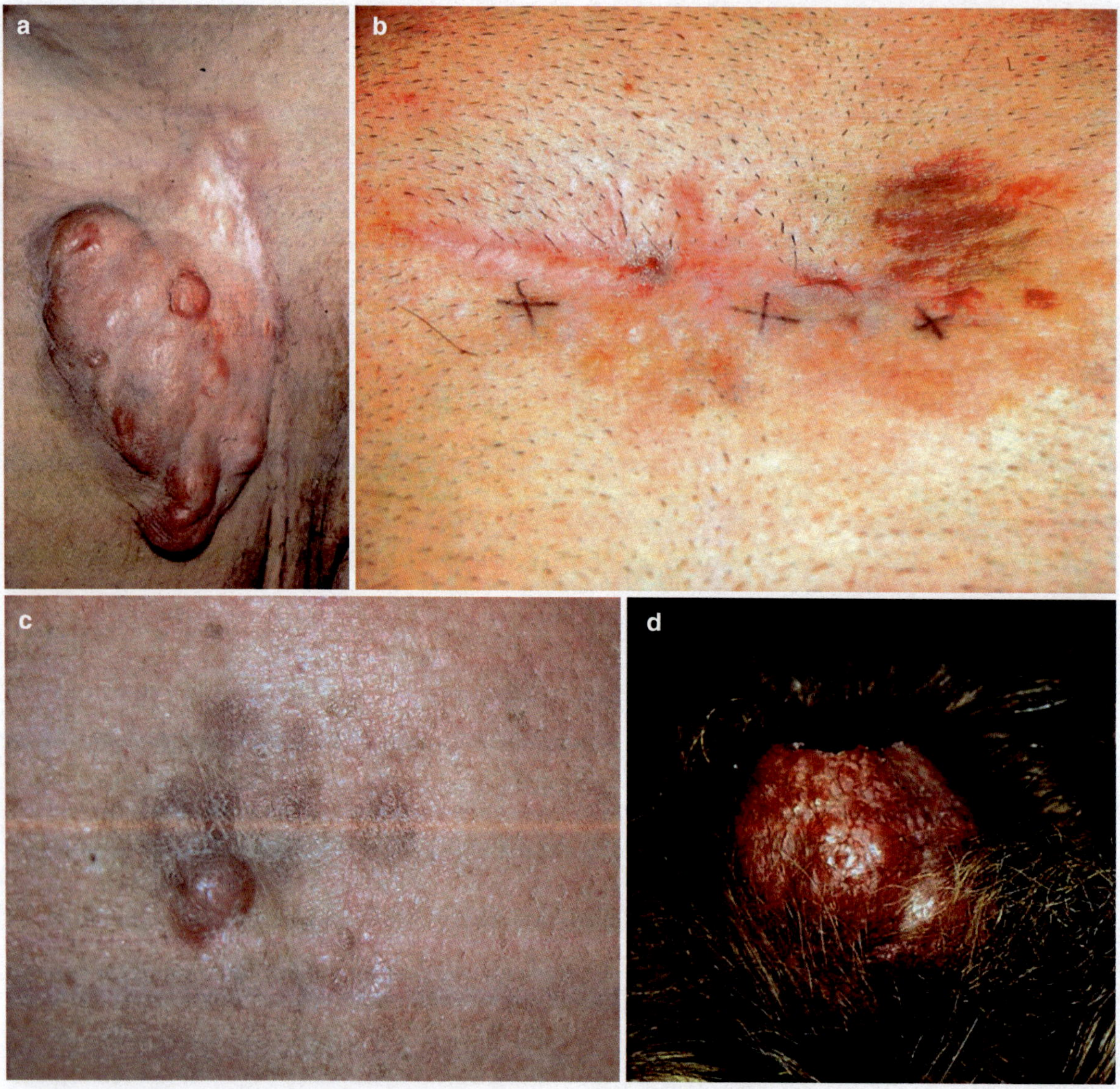

Fig. 19.3 Dermatofibrosarcoma protuberans. (**a**) A multinodular plaque on groin/medial thigh area. (**b**) Erythematous, pigmented scar-like plaque arising in area of previous DFSP excision. (**c**) Erythematous-brown atrophic plaque and nodule on back. (**d**) Telangiectatic and flesh-colored tumor mass on the scalp (Photo courtesy of Dr. Mark DeLacure)

Summary: Clinical Features

- Dermatofibrosarcoma protuberans typically presents *as a flesh-colored*, blue-red plaque, nodule, or subcutaneous mass.
- It most commonly occurs on the trunk and extremities followed by the head and neck region.
- Tumor invasion into underlying fascia, muscle, and bone can be observed.
- Pediatric DFSP accounts for 6% of all DFSP cases.

19.4 Clinical Features

DFSP initially manifests itself as an asymptomatic flesh-colored, blue-red to hyperpigmented patch, patch, plaque, nodule, or subcutaneous mass (Fig. 19.3). Although DFSP may occur anywhere on the body, the most common location is the trunk (up to 72%), followed by the extremities (up to 30%). Head and neck involvement ranges from 5% to 15% [1, 34]. DFSP may not always present as the prototypical protuberant mass. Some cases exhibit overlying telangiectasias, suggesting vascular lesions. Others have demonstrated atrophy in the form of atrophoderma or morphea [35, 36]. A less commonly described clinical variant is the multiple clustered dermatofibroma (MCDF) which should be distinguished from multiple eruptive dermatofibromas (MEDF). MCDF portends a benign course, whereas MEDF is associated with immunosuppression [37]. Exhibiting indolent behavior, DFSP may remain quiescent over an extended interval of months to years before becoming symptomatic [38]. By gradually infiltrating adjacent tissue, it can become multifocal, large, painful, and ulcerative. Tumor invasion and fixation to underlying fascia, muscle, and bone can be observed late in the course of disease [39, 40].

Pediatric DFSP, although rare, accounts for 6% of all DFSP cases in children younger than 16 years of age. Congenital DFSP is even rarer with approximately 61 cases reported in literature. Variable clinical presentations as flesh-colored, blue, or red nodules/plaques often lead to misdiagnoses as vascular malformations, nevi, or fibromatoses [35, 41]. There is a 5-year average delay between initial presentation and the final diagnosis. The frequency of pediatric DFSP cases may be underestimated due to subtle clinical findings. Some cases diagnosed during adulthood may have represented congenital or childhood DFSP [35, 42]. Giant cell fibroblastoma (GCF), a benign neoplasm rarely encountered in children, must be distinguished from DFSP [43, 44].

Summary: Pathology

- Dermatofibrosarcoma protuberans consists of cytologically bland spindle cells in a whorled or storiform pattern infiltrating into subcutaneous tissue.
- It stains positively for CD34 and nestin and negatively for factor XIIIa.
- The fibrosarcomatous variant is characterized by a herringbone pattern of hypercellular spindle cell proliferation and is associated with high a risk of metastasis.

19.5 Pathology

Histologically, DFSP appears as a well-differentiated tumor with fascicular proliferation of cytologically bland spindle cells in a whorled or storiform pattern (Fig. 19.4a). Patch lesions may demonstrate tumor-free epidermis, while nodular lesions have cells infiltrating deep into subcutaneous tissue, described as honeycomb architecture (Fig. 19.4b). Long-standing DFSP invades the neighboring dermis, subcutis and underlying fascia by pseudopod-like, irregular projections of monomorphous cells with low mitotic activity. These infiltrative and asymmetric characteristics on light microscopy make the tumor border ambiguous and partly account for the high rate of recurrences [4, 45]. The spindle cell proliferation of DFSP can be confused with other fibrohistiocytic neoplasms including, but not limited to, dermatofibroma, dermatomyofibroma, fibrosarcoma, and atypical fibroxanthoma [36].

Immunohistochemical studies can facilitate the diagnosis of DFSP, and more importantly to distinguish it from dermatofibroma (DF), the benign counterpart. DFSP typically stains positively for CD34 and negatively for factor XIIIa, whereas DF stains negatively for CD34 and positively for Factor XIIIa (Fig. 19.5). However, the diagnostic value is not absolute since 20% of DFSPs will stain negatively for CD34 and 20% will stain positively for Factor XIIIa [2, 46]. In addition, CD163, a hemoglobin scavenger receptor, is expressed by DF in 83–89% of cases and may differentiate cellular DF from DFSP [2, 47]. Nestin, a neuroepithelial stem cell marker, preferentially labels DFSP in contrast with DF, with the exception of intralesional blood vessels. Several authors have concluded that CD34, Factor XIIIa, CD163, and nestin can aid in histopathological differential diagnosis of the two disorders [48, 49].

Several histopathologic variants have been described including pigmented DFSP or Bednar tumor, myxoid DFSP, fibrosarcomatous DFSP (FS-DFSP), granular cell DFSP, DFSP/FS-DFSP with foci of myoid/myofibroblastic differentiation, DFSP with areas of giant cell fibroblastoma, palisading, and Verocay body prominent DFSP [50]. A rare variant of DFSP, Bednar tumor constitutes less than 5% of all cases of DFSP. Variable number of melanosome-containing dendritic cells are found in classic DFSP, which accounts for the black discoloration of the tumor on light microscopy [51, 52].

The fibrosarcomatous (FS) variant, a rare phenomenon, deserves special mention since it has a high rate of metastasis. FS change is characterized by a hypercellular spindle cell proliferation with a herringbone or fascicular architecture (Fig. 19.6). FS areas resembling pleomorphic sarcoma have also been identified [53, 54]. Unlike classic DFSP, FS-DFSP loses CD34

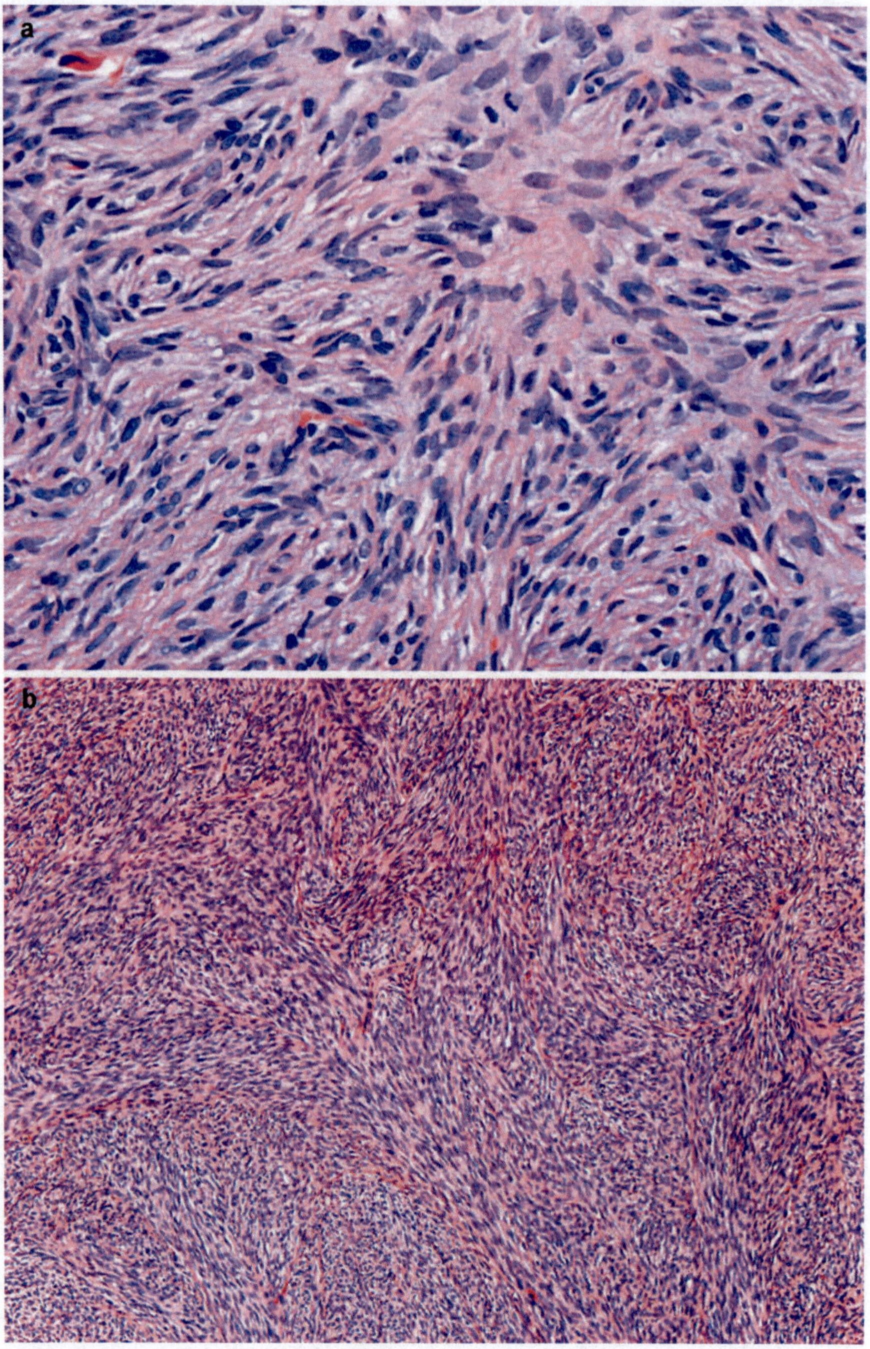

Fig. 19.4 Dermatofibrosarcoma protuberans. (**a**) The bland spindle cells are arranged in a whorled or storiform pattern (hematoxylin and eosin, original magnification ×400). (**b**) Spindle cells infiltrating deep into subcutaneous tissue with honeycomb pattern (hematoxylin and eosin, original magnification ×100)

positivity and possesses a high MIB-1 labeling index, a feature that may be used an adjunctive tool to identify fibrosarcomatous areas in DFSP [55, 56]. The true incidence of FS change in DFSP is unknown but has been estimated to be 7–27%. There is no consensus on the risk of recurrence incurred by the FS variant. However, the local metastasis rate of FS-DFSP in the literature is between 10% and 15% with lung being the most common site of metastases [54, 55, 57]. Abbott et al. report that metastases occurred in patients with less than 15% FS change in DFSP. They emphasize the importance of addressing even focal FS changes in DFSP with long-term clinical follow-up of the patient [55].

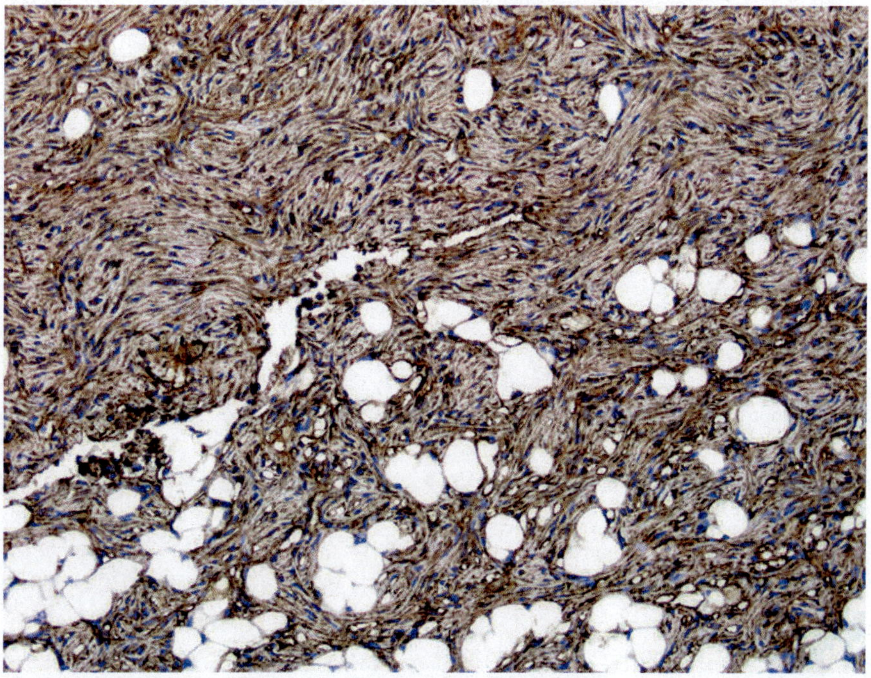

Fig. 19.5 Dermatofibrosarcoma protuberans. CD34 positive spindle cells infiltrating the subcutaneous fat (hematoxylin and eosin, original magnification ×100)

Summary: Differential Diagnose

- Dermatofibrosarcoma protuberans can clinically mimic keloid, dermatomyofibroma, morphea, verrucous pigmented nevus, infantile fibromatoses, among others.
- Other spindle cell neoplasms should be excluded: neurofibroma, schwannoma, leiomyosarcoma, spindled squamous cell carcinoma, and malignant peripheral nerve sheath tumor.
- Desmoplastic melanoma can resemble dermatofibrosarcoma protuberans and should be excluded by immunostains.

19.6 Differential Diagnoses

Clinically, DFSP can be mistaken for its benign counterpart, dermatofibroma, in its nodular stage. The plaque stage of DFSP can be confused with keloid, dermatomyofibroma, and morphea. In children, DFSP is commonly misdiagnosed as hemangioma, vascular malformations, fibrosarcoma, rhabdomyosarcoma, verrucous pigmented nevus, infantile fibromatoses, mastocytoma, and xanthomatous hamartoma [35, 36, 50]. Clinicopathologic correlation is necessary to render the correct diagnosis. Table 19.1 lists several lesions that can simulate DFSP.

The pathologic differential diagnoses DFSP includes entities characterized by spindle cell proliferations. DFSP can be misdiagnosed as dermatofibroma, with its variants of cellular and deeply penetrating dermatofibromas, which may extend to subcutaneous tissue. Dermatofibromas are negative for CD34 and positive for Factor XIIIa while vice versa is true for DFSP [45, 58]. DFSP can mimic neurofibromas histologically in areas with wavy nuclei and schwannomas in areas with palisaded nuclei in Verocay body formations. Both proliferations S-100 positive but fail to stain with CD34 [59]. Smooth muscle markers, such as muscle actin, desmin, and vimentin, can help in distinguishing leiomyoma and leiomyosarcoma from DFSP [60]. In less differentiated areas of oval nuclei arranged in fascicles alternating with hypocellular areas with increased mitotic activity, consideration should be given to the diagnosis of malignant peripheral nerve sheath tumor [61, 62]. It is of utmost importance to exclude desmoplastic melanoma as it can mimic DFSP with characteristic loosely textured mild to moderately atypical spindle cells in collagenous matrix that may infiltrate

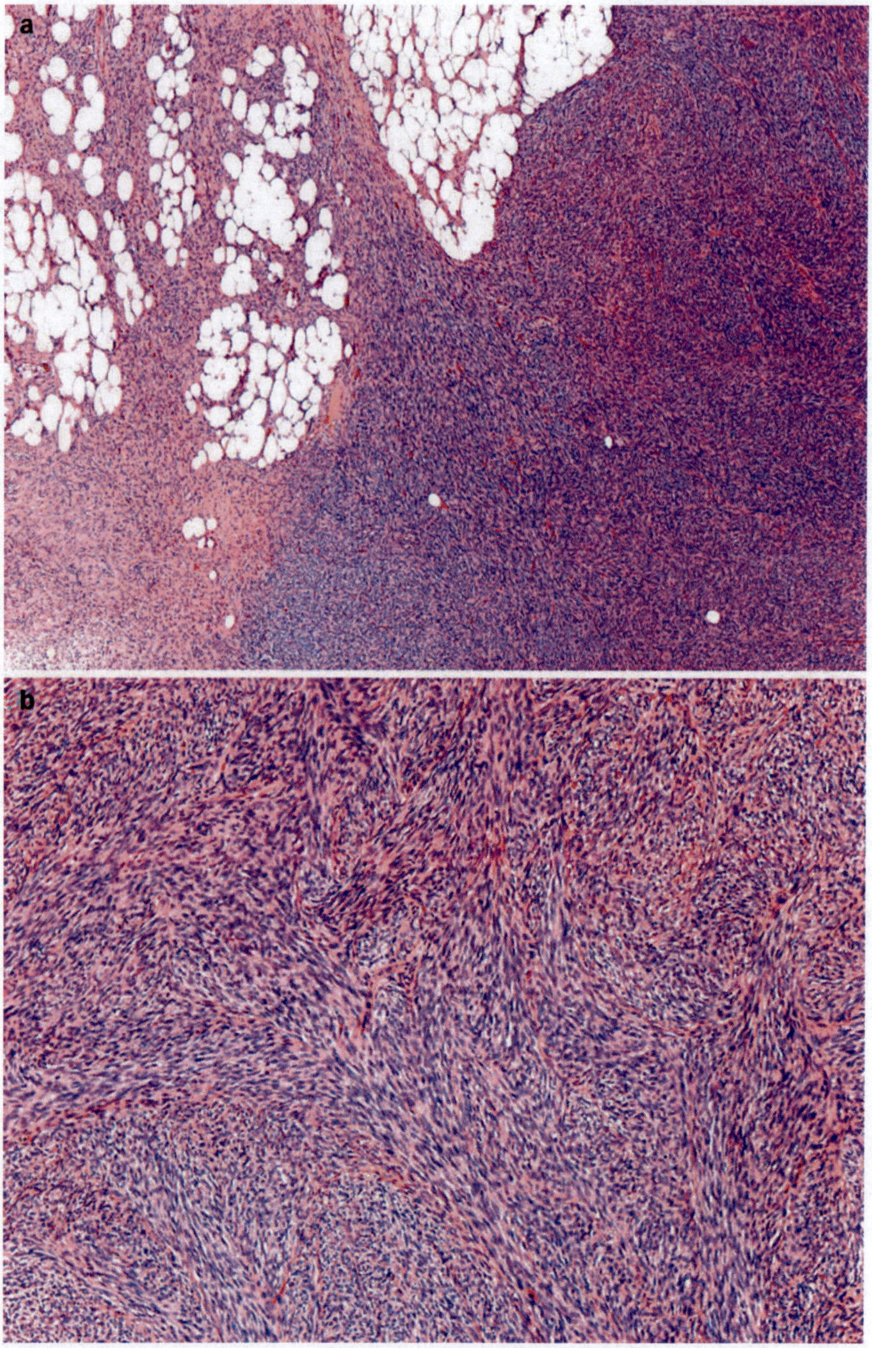

Fig. 19.6 Dermatofibrosarcoma protuberans – fibrosarcomatous variant. (**a**) The transition zone between bland, hypocellular DFSP spindle cells on the left side of field and the hypercellular FS variant of DFSP on the right side of field (hematoxylin and eosin, original magnification ×200). (**b**) FS variant with hypercellular spindle cells with herringbone architecture (hematoxylin and eosin, original magnification ×400)

subcutaneous tissue. Many cases have evident intraepidermal melanocytic proliferation and typically stain positive for S-100 [62, 63]. A panel of antibodies can be used to better delineate a spindle cell tumor for its line of differentiation and aid in diagnosis (Table 19.2).

Summary: Management

- Dermatofibrosarcoma protuberans can be treated either with Mohs micrographic surgery *or* wide local excision.

- The role of radiation therapy remains controversial since radiation-induced dermatofibrosarcoma protuberans has been reported.
- Imatinib mesylate competes for the ATP binding site of *PDGFR*, inhibiting tyrosine phosphorylation of proteins involved in *COL1A1-PDGFB* related signal transduction.
- Imatinib is approved for use in adults patients with unresectable, recurrent, and metastatic disease and may be beneficial as neoadjuvant therapy.
- Magnetic resonance imaging may play a role in evaluation of patients with large tumor size, history of recurrence, location in critical anatomic regions, or in cases of re-excision of positive surgical margins.

Table 19.1 Differential diagnoses of dermatofibrosarcoma protuberans

Clinical	Pathological
• Dermatofibroma • Dermatomyofibroma • Keloid • Fibromatoses, infantile • Fibrosarcoma • Hemangioma • Hamartoma, xanthomatous • Mastocytoma • Rhabdomyosarcoma • Nevus, verrucous and/or pigmented • Vascular malformation	• Dermatofibroma, cellular, and deeply penetrating • Fibrosarcoma • Leiomyoma • Leiomyosarcoma • Liposarcoma, myxoid • Malignant peripheral nerve sheath tumor • Melanoma, desmoplastic • Neurofibroma • Schwannoma • Squamous cell carcinoma, spindled

19.7 Management

19.7.1 Surgery

19.7.1.1 Wide Local Excision

WLE with histologically negative margins has historically been the mainstay of treatment for DFSP. There is no consensus regarding the precise adequate resection margins to achieve local control. In a literature review of studies where WLE was performed with >2 cm margins, the total rate of local recurrence was 8.8%, while the range was 0–41%. Most recurrences occurred within the first 3 years after excision [3, 40, 64, 65]. Head and neck DFSP, in particular, has higher rates of local recurrence with WLE when compared with more common trunk and extremity locations. Recurrence range of 50–75% has been reported in the literature. Marks et al. reported a local recurrence rate of 60% in their series of 15 head and neck disease patients treated with WLE [66–68]. Several case series evaluating optimal excision margins and recurrence rates have produced conflicting results.

More recently, Farma et al. have reported a recurrence rate of 1% at 5-year follow-up for 206 DFSP lesions utilizing a median excision width of 2 cm (range: 0.5–3 cm) [5]. In their series of 38 patients, Heuvel et al. reported local failure rate of 7% with 2–3 cm margins at a median follow-up of 89 months [69]. Increasing recurrence-free survival rates have been observed with increasing margins of resection [70–72]. In a series 66 patients with DFSP, a statistically significant difference rate of 47% versus 7% was observed in tumors resected with less than 3 cm margins and tumors resected with margins from 3 to 5 cm, respectively [70].

Table 19.2 Comparison of immunohistochemical stains in spindle cell tumors MPNST, malignant peripheral nerve sheath tumor

	Dermatofibrosarcoma protuberans	Dermatofibroma	Leiomyosarcoma	Melanoma	MPNST
CD34	+	–	–	–	–
Factor XIIIa	–	+	–	–	–
CD163	±	+	–	–	–
Actin	–	–	+	–	–
Desmin	–	–	+	–	–
S-100 protein	–	–	–	+	+

19.7.1.2 Mohs Micrographic Surgery

MMS has several advantages over WLE which include (1) inspection of 100% of tissue margins for residual tumor, (2) intraoperative pathologic assessment of three-dimensional view of clinical margins, (3) preservation of maximum amount of normal tissue, and (4) functional and cosmetic sensitivity in anatomically challenging areas [73–75].

The decision to treat DFSP with MMS versus WLE depends on the anatomic location, tumor size, availability of MMS, and physician preference. The efficacy of MMS in the treatment of DFSP has been well documented in the literature. Recurrence rates as low as 0–6.6% have been reported with MMS [76–79]. In the most recent study evaluating MMS as the sole treatment for DFSP, MMS yielded a local recurrence rate of 0% at an average of 39 months follow-up in 39 DFSP cases. Four cases were recurrent tumors and 31 were primary [78]. Another study by Nelson et al. reported no tumor recurrence in their series of 44 DFSP patients over a 3.3 years average follow-up [79]. Deep margin resection during MMS should go down to and include fascia or periosteum [66].

Only three studies formally examine the utility of MMS compared to WLE, and each study reported different recurrence rates between the two modalities. The Mayo Clinic case series consisting of 84 DFSP patients reported lower recurrence rates of 6.6% for MMS and 10% for WLE at 36 and 40 months follow-up, respectively. Only 15 patients (18%) underwent MMS. The study also included 56% of patients with recurrent tumors which *may not* allow for an unbiased assessment of the true efficacy of MMS in comparison to WLE [80]. Dubay et al. described 63 DFSP cases with no recurrence in any of the three groups of patients assigned to three different treatment regimens: 11 (17%) cases of MMS, 44 (70%) cases of WLE, and 9 (14%) cases of combination treatment (MMS and/or WLE and/or radiation). Two WLE cases received additional treatment with radiation after maximal excision for positive microscopic margins. This study also included least 11 recurrent DFSP tumors, 8 of which were treated with WLE, 1 with MMS, and 2 with combination treatment [3].

A third case series with 48 DFSPs reported 3.6% recurrence rate with WLE (28/48 cases, 58%) versus 0% with MMS (20/48 cases, 42%) at a median follow-up of 49.9 and 40.4 months, respectively. The authors of the study commented that although WLE resulted in more frequent positive margin resection, local control was ultimately similar for both surgical modalities. They also noted that WLE proved to be a more time-efficient procedure with significantly lower operative time at 77 min versus 257 min for MMS. However, the opportunity to perform definitive resection in the case of positive margins on the same day was lost. The authors concluded that the choice of WLE versus MMS should be based on patients and tumor characteristics as well as institutional expertise in these modalities [74].

Postoperative defect sizes can be large requiring advanced reconstruction. Nelson et al. reported defect sizes ranging from 7.2 to 168.0 cm^2 in their series of 44 DFSP patients treated with MMS. Fifty percent of the patients underwent plastic reconstruction, while the rest underwent primary closure by the Mohs surgeon [69]. Multidisciplinary approach is often needed for tumors adjacent to or involving vital structures on scalp, face, breast, and eyes, among others. Several cases in the literature have illustrated the joint efforts of specialties such as ophthalmology, plastic surgery, and head and neck surgery in optimal reconstruction of tissue defects [3, 66, 81–83].

Adjuvant immunohistochemistry can facilitate the accurate delineation of DFSP margins intraoperatively during MMS. The most common and practical immunohistochemical marker used in MMS is CD34, an antigen typically found in hematopoietic stem cells, endothelium, dermal dendritic cells, and endoneuronal dendritic cells. Staining tumor specimens with CD34 has enhanced the yield of negative margins by clearly delineating the extent of tumor involvement and unmasking areas of tumor cells surrounded by inflammation [84, 85]. The increased time for immunostaining limits its practical use during MMS. Alternatively, after complete excision of the tumor with MMS via frozen sections, a final layer can be sent for permanent sections to be stained with CD34, thereby providing more corroboratory means of assessing margin control [86, 87]. Caution must be exercised since DFSP cells may have variable CD34 expression depending on tumor characteristics of plaque or nodular components [88].

19.7.2 Radiotherapy

The role of radiation therapy for DFSP remains controversial. In combination with surgery, radiotherapy has been utilized in patients who cannot undergo invasive procedures due to medical or technical reasons. Eternal beam radiation therapy (EBRT) is usually administered in the range of 59–65 gray (Gy) [89]. Dagan et al. reported disease-free follow-up ranging from 1.8 to

15.5 years in ten DFSP patients who underwent resection before EBRT. Four patients had negative surgical margins, while the rest had either or <5 mm of microscopically positive margins. Only one patient, who had the FS variant of DFSP, experienced local recurrence 3 months after treatment [90]. In another case series of 35 DFSP patients who underwent surgery alone (24 patients) and combined surgery with radiation (11 patients), local control rates after 7-year follow-up were 28% and 80%, respectively. One of the 11 patients receiving adjuvant radiation initially had inoperable tumor and received palliative preoperative radiation. The remaining ten patients underwent radiation due to either surgeon's preference (four patients) or inadequate resection margins (six patients) [91].

Radiation-induced DFSP has also been reported in the literature. DFSP should be included in the differential diagnosis of postradiation fibrohistiocytic tumors [92–94]. The pathogenesis of postradiation DFSP is not clear. It has been speculated that fibroblasts transform into DFSP cells under long-term stimulation by various radiation-induced cytokines, especially transforming growth factor-B (*TGF-B*) [95].

19.7.3 Molecularly Targeted Therapy

Imatinib mesylate (imatinib, STI 571) is a low-molecular weight, synthetic, 2-phenylaminopyridine derivative, and a tyrosine kinase inhibitor. Initially developed to inhibit the tyrosine kinase *BCR-ABL*, imatinib also showed clinical efficacy against *ABL*-related kinase, *KIT*, *PDGFRs*. It is marketed as Gleevec® in North America and Glivec® in Europe by Novartis Pharmaceuticals and is available as 100 and 400 mg capsules [96]. Imatinib has revolutionized treatment of chronic myelogenous leukemia (CML) as well as gastrointestinal stromal tumors (GISTs). It is clinically indicated and approved by the Food and Drug Administration (FDA) for Philadelphia (Ph) chromosome positive CML, refractory Ph chromosome positive acute lymphoblastic leukemia, hypereosinophilic syndrome, systemic mastocytosis, myelodysplastic disorders, GISTs, and DFSP. Imatinib has become the model of targeted therapy in oncology and a novel treatment modality for DFSP [27, 97].

The introduction of imatinib-targeted therapy into the treatment of DFSP was possible due to the advances in the understanding of the molecular pathogenesis of DFSP. *PDGFB* is overexpressed in DFSP and constitutively stimulates its tyrosine kinase receptor, *PDGFR*. The adenosine triphosphate (ATP) binding site of

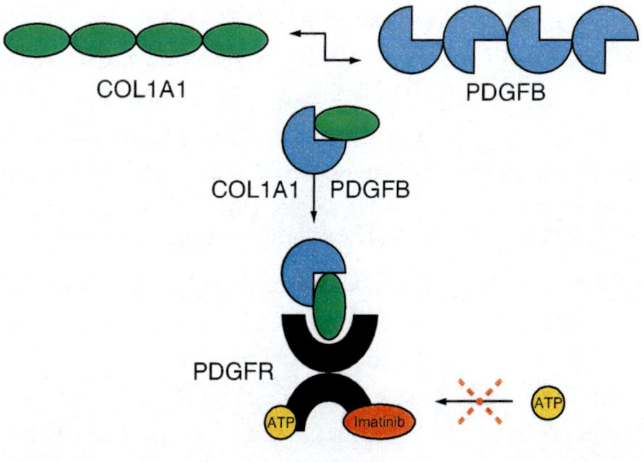

Fig. 19.7 Pathomechanism of imatinib mesylate. *Imatinib* inhibits the tyrosine phosphorylation of proteins involved in *COL1A1-PDGFB* related signal transduction by binding to the adenosine triphosphate (ATP) binding site of *PDGFR*. *ADP* adenosine diphosphate, *ATP* adenosine triphosphate, *PDGFB* platelet-derived growth factor B, *PDGFR* kinase platelet-derived growth factor receptor

PDGFR is inhibited by imatinib, a tyrosine kinase inhibitor. By competing for the ATP binding site of the kinase, imatinib inhibits the tyrosine phosphorylation of proteins involved in *COL1A1-PDGFB* related signal transduction (Fig. 19.7). It is hypothesized that imatinib reduces proliferation of DFSP cells, causing a decrease in tumor size [24–26].

Initial use of off-label imatinib involved cases of unresectable or metastatic DFSP to the lungs. Some cases showed a treatment response characterized by reduction in tumor size or tumor resolution with a dose of 400 mg daily [98–100]. These results led to a phase II open label study in 2004 using imatinib 800 mg daily (400 mg bid) in ten patients, eight patients with primary DFSP, and two patients with metastatic disease. All nine of nine cases of DFSP with t(17;22), including one case of metastatic DFSP, showed either partial or complete response. The one case lacking *PDGFB* rearrangement also had metastatic disease and showed no improvement [101]. Based on the results of this study and other case reports, the FDA approved imatinib for use in adults patients with (1) unresectable DFSP, (2) recurrent DFSP, if additional resection would lead to unacceptable functional or cosmetic outcomes, and (3) metastatic DFSP [8].

Additional clinical trials have demonstrated the effectiveness and safety of imatinib in inducing partial or complete remission. A phase II clinical study on 25 DFSPs (longest diameter: 25 cm, median diameter: 4.5 cm) using 600 mg/day imatinib daily for 2 months demonstrated clinical response rate of 36%. The primary endpoint was a decrease in tumor size by at least 30%. The *COL1A1-PDGFB* fusion gene was detected in 21 patients, 13 of which failed to respond to imatinib [102].

A nearly 50% response rate was demonstrated in pooled analysis of two phase II clinical trials on 24 DFSP patients for 14–16 weeks. No significant difference in efficacy was noted between imatinib doses of 400 or 800 mg daily. The use of neoadjuvant imatinib in facilitating complete surgical excision has also been substantiated. Four patients achieved complete remission after WLE in an EORTC (European Organisation for Research and Treatment of Cancer) study using 800 mg of imatinib for 14 weeks. Rutkowski et al. reported disease-free survival of 47% in 7 out of 15 patients undergoing WLE after 400–800 mg imatinib daily. The median time from the initiation of imatinib therapy to WLE of residual tumor was 3.3 months (range: 3–8 months) [103].

Several pediatric DFSP case reports have illustrated the use of adjuvant imatinib mesylate therapy in the management of DFSP [104–106]. The largest pediatric case series to date used 400–500 mg/m^2/day imatinib over 6–12 months as preoperative management in three children (age range: 1–14 years old). The patients had previous history of multiple recurrences or anatomically challenging tumor location. Partial response, as defined by response evaluation criteria in solid tumors (RECIST), was noted in all three patients. The patients remain free of disease at an average of 2-year follow-up [104].

Imatinib has a favorable safety profile with most patients experiencing mild-moderate and well-tolerated side effects of edema, asthenia, nausea, and maculopapular rash. These were easily managed by supportive medical management, dose reduction or interruption. Rare serious adverse event has included transaminitis, anemia, neutropenia, leukopenia thrombocytopenia, and Stevens–Johnson syndrome [8, 107].

Clinical benefit of imatinib is lacking in DFSP without t(17;22) as these tumors may not be dependent on signal transduction through *PDGFR*s. As a result, the National Comprehensive Cancer Network (NCCN) guidelines recommend that cytogenetic analysis may be useful prior to the institution of imatinib therapy. Cytogenetic confirmation for the tyrosine kinase receptor may be done via FISH or RT-PCR [8, 108]. The use of neoadjuvant imatinib therapy to reduce tumor burden prior to surgery may also have its limitations. It has been suggested that the therapeutic actions of imatinib on DFSP may be non-uniform. The resultant skip areas of tumor could potentially be missed during surgery with margin control [8, 109].

For appropriately selected patients, imatinib may minimize functional and cosmetic disfigurement while enhancing surgical outcomes. The optimal duration of preoperative imatinib therapy in DFSP patients is unknown. Further studies are needed to evaluate imatinib's clinical efficacy and long-term outcomes with respect to local control and disease-free survival in DFSP.

19.7.4 Imaging Studies

The extent of DFSP involvement cannot be ascertained based solely on clinical examination. Large tumor size does not necessarily indicate subclinical extension. Several imaging modalities are being used to characterize tumor size and extent including ultrasound and magnetic resonance imaging (MRI).

Shin et al. described the ultrasonographic features of four DFSPs as a subcutaneous mass abutting the skin with lobulated margin and hypoechogenicity or an irregular margin and mixed echogenicity. The study also correlated the pathologic findings with the corresponding sonographic aspects of DFSP [110, 111]. A hypoechoic DFSP exhibits high cellularity, with spindle cells arranged in a distinct storiform pattern, whereas the hyperechoic areas are a mixture of DFSP cells and fibrous tissue infiltrating the subcutaneous fat. The sensitivity and specificity of ultrasound for detection of DFSP is, however, unknown at the present [110, 111].

Perioperative MRI has been utilized to assess muscle and tendon involvement. MRI appears to be the superior imaging modality for DFSP because of its high soft tissue resolution and contrast. In the largest study to date evaluating the utility of MRI in DFSP assessment, three out of ten histologically confirmed DFSPs with clinically obscure extent of tumor demonstrated fascial and muscle involvement. The actual tumor size ranged from 2 to 8 cm with an average of 4 cm. Either T1 or T2-weighted MRI images may be used. DFSP is isointense or slightly hypointense compared with skeletal muscle with a lower intensity signal than subcutaneous fat on T1-weighted images. T2-weighted imaging portrays DFSP as hyperintense or isointense compared with fat. Fat suppression techniques are routinely used in T1-weighted images since the brightness of the fat signal can obscure DFSP [112, 113].

Studies suggest that preoperative MRI may play a role in evaluation of DFSP with large tumor size, history of recurrence, location in critical anatomic regions, or in cases of re-excision with positive surgical margins.

Routine MRI prior to surgery is not warranted in most cases of DFSP. In pediatric DFSP cases where delineation of tumor from critical anatomic structures is ambiguous, MRI has aided in appropriate determining extent of tumor, surgical planning, and post-therapy follow-up [114, 115]. MRI has also been utilized in intraoperative resection of DFSP. Gould et al. used MRI to confirm clearance of DFSP after excision in three cases of DFSP with subcutaneous extension. They concluded that MRI-guided resection is a valuable tool for achieving surgical clearance of soft tissue sarcomas while reducing the amount of non-involved tissue removed and the need for subsequent reconstructive surgery [116]. No studies exist in the current literature regarding the accuracy and limitations of MRI in predicting tumor extension of DFSP or its utility in postoperative surveillance.

Summary: Prognosis

- *Metastases are rare with lung being the most common site.*
- Indicators of poor prognosis are fibrosarcomatous variant, high mitotic index, and increased cellularity, history of prior recurrence, age greater than 50, and anatomic location of head and neck.
- Patients with history of recurrent tumors or probable metastatic disease should undergo physical examination with elicitation of review of systems.
- A thorough metastatic workup, including imaging of chest, abdomen, and pelvis, may be performed if signs and symptoms of malignancy are present.

19.8 Prognosis

Generally, the prognosis for DFSP is good. Metastases rarely occur with DFSP with an estimated rate of 1%. In the SEER database study, 57% cases of DFSP were classified as "localized" disease restricted to skin, while only 0.4% were reported as having distant metastases. The remaining 43% exhibited "regional" disease limited to localized lymph nodes [1]. Lung is the most common site of metastases [40]. Metastatic foci can be evaluated in suspicious cases via CT or MRI scans. In addition, tumor activity can also be detected on fluorodeoxyglucose (FDG)-positron emission tomography with increased FDG uptake signifying hypermetabolic state of tumor formation [117].

Due to its infiltrative nature, DFSP has high potential for recurrence. Most recurrences occurring within a mean of 3 years [40, 74]. Several factors are associated with increased morbidity from recurrence. Most commonly, inadequate resection margins are implicated in high rates of local recurrence. Histologically, the fibrosarcomatous variant of DFSP, high mitotic index, and increased cellularity are predictors of poor clinical outcome. History of prior recurrence, age greater than 50, and location of head and neck are also unfavorable. Interestingly, tumor size or depth and gender do not confer an increased risk for local recurrence [74].

After complete excision of DFSP, patients should be closely monitored for signs of recurrence. The NCCN recommends cutaneous examination intervals of 6–12 months for inspection of the primary DFSP site and biopsy of any suspicious areas [118]. Patients with history of recurrent tumors or probable metastatic disease should undergo physical examination with elicitation of review of systems. A thorough metastatic workup, including imaging of chest, abdomen, and pelvis, may be performed if signs and symptoms of malignancy are present. It has been suggested that the histopathological diagnosis of DFSP should be confirmed by cytogenetics for *PDGFB* overexpression, and inoperable tumors expressing *PDGFB* should receive imatinib before surgical resection [119].

Summary: Conclusion

- DFSP is a rare and locally aggressive soft tissue sarcoma with varying clinical presentation and high rate of recurrence.
- The mainstay of DFSP therapy is margin-controlled surgical resection by either MMS or WLE.
- All DFSP patients need careful monitoring of disease recurrence and regular clinical follow-up.

19.9 Conclusion

DFSP is a rare and locally aggressive soft tissue sarcoma with varying clinical presentation and high rate of recurrence. It most commonly presents in adults, and it is increasingly being reported in children. Early diagnosis and prompt pathological evaluation can aid in institution of appropriate treatment. The mainstay of DFSP therapy is margin-controlled surgical resection by either MMS or WLE. Radiotherapy provides limited benefit, and its utility is controversial. Imatinib is approved for use in adults patients with unresectable, recurrent, and metastatic DFSP. It is unclear whether imatinib is beneficial as neoadjuvant therapy. All DFSP patients need careful monitoring of disease recurrence and regular clinical follow-up to promote tumor-free survival.

References

1. Criscione VD, Weinstock MA. Descriptive epidemiology of dermatofibrosarcoma protuberans in the United States, 1973 to 2002. J Am Acad Dermatol. 2007;56:968–73.
2. Sachdev R, Sundram U. Expression of CD163 in dermatofibroma, cellular fibrous histiocytoma, and dermatofibrosarcoma protuberans: comparison with CD68, CD34, and Factor XIIIa. J Cutan Pathol. 2006;33:353–60.
3. Dubay D, Cimmino V, Lowe L, Johnson TM, Sondak VK. Low recurrence rate after surgery for dermatofibrosarcoma protuberans: a multidisciplinary approach from a single institution. Cancer. 2004;100:1008–16.
4. Bowne WB, Antonescu CR, Leung DH, Katz SC, Hawkins WG, Woodruff JM, et al. Dermatofibrosarcoma protuberans: a clinicopathologic analysis of patients treated and followed at a single institution. Cancer. 2000;88:2711–20.
5. Farma JM, Ammori JB, Zager JS, Marzban SS, Bui MM, Bichakjian CK, et al. Dermatofibrosarcoma protuberans: how wide should we resect? Ann Surg Oncol. 2010;17:2112–8.
6. Roh MR, Bae B, Chung KY. Mohs' micrographic surgery for dermatofibrosarcoma protuberans. Clin Exp Dermatol. 2010;35(8):849–52.
7. Paradisi A, Abeni D, Rusciani A, Cigna E, Wolter M, Scuderi N, et al. Dermatofibrosarcoma protuberans: wide local excision vs. Mohs micrographic surgery. Cancer Treat Rev. 2008;34:728–36.
8. Johnson-Jahangir H, Sherman W, Ratner D. Using imatinib as neoadjuvant therapy in dermatofibrosarcoma protuberans: potential pluses and minuses. J Natl Compr Canc Netw. 2010;8:881–5.
9. Morman MR, Lin RY, Petrozzi JW. Dermatofibrosarcoma protuberans arising in a site of multiple immunizations. Arch Dermatol. 1979;115:1453.
10. McLelland J, Chu T. Dermatofibrosarcoma protuberans arising in a BCG vaccination scar. Arch Dermatol. 1988;124:496–7.
11. Seo JK, Cho KJ, Kang JH, Lee D, Sung HS, Hwang SW. Dermatofibrosarcoma protuberans arising from a burn scar. Ann Dermatol. 2009;21:416–8.
12. Tanaka A, Hatoko M, Tada H, Kuwahara M, Iioka H, Niitsuma K. Dermatofibrosarcoma protuberans arising from a burn scar of the axilla. Ann Plast Surg. 2004;52:423–5.
13. Zaiden R, Latif N, Pham D, Hosenpud J. Dermatofibroma protuberans arising from an infected insect bite. Clin Adv Hematol Oncol. 2009;7:404–8.
14. Hendrick MJ. Feline vaccine-associated sarcomas: current studies on pathogenesis. J Am Vet Med Assoc. 1998;213:1425–6.
15. Turegun M, Nisanci M, Guler M. Burn scar carcinoma with longer lag period arising in previously grafted area. Burns. 1997;23:496–7.
16. Morrison AE, Lang PG. Case of rapidly enlarging dermatofibrosarcoma protuberans during pregnancy followed by metastasis in the absence of local recurrence. Dermatol Surg. 2006;32:125–7.
17. Parlette LE, Smith CK, Germain LM, Rolfe CA, Skelton H. Accelerated growth of dermatofibrosarcoma protuberans during pregnancy. J Am Acad Dermatol. 1999;41:778–83.
18. Diaz-Cascajo C, Bastida-Inarrea J, Borrego L, Carretero-Hernandez G. Comparison of p53 expression in dermatofibrosarcoma protuberans and dermatofibroma: lack of correlation with proliferation rate. J Cutan Pathol. 1995;22:304–9.
19. Hisaoka M, Okamoto S, Morimitsu Y, Tsuji S, Hashimoto H. Dermatofibrosarcoma protuberans with fibrosarcomatous areas. Molecular abnormalities of the p53 pathway in fibrosarcomatous transformation of dermatofibrosarcoma protuberans. Virchows Arch. 1998;433:323–9.
20. Takahira T, Oda Y, Tamiya S, Yamamoto H, Kawaguchi K, Kobayashi C, et al. Microsatellite instability and p53 mutation associated with tumor progression in dermatofibrosarcoma protuberans. Hum Pathol. 2004;35:240–5.
21. Patel KU, Szabo SS, Hernandez VS, Prieto VG, Abruzzo LV, Lazar AJ, et al. Dermatofibrosarcoma protuberans COL1A1-PDGFB fusion is identified in virtually all dermatofibrosarcoma protuberans cases when investigated by newly developed multiplex reverse transcription polymerase chain reaction and fluorescence in situ hybridization assays. Hum Pathol. 2008;39:184–93.
22. Pedeutour F, Simon MP, Minoletti F, Sozzi G, Pierotti MA, Hecht F, et al. Ring 22 chromosomes in dermatofibrosarcoma protuberans are low-level amplifiers of chromosome 17 and 22 sequences. Cancer Res. 1995;55:2400–3.
23. Llombart B, Sanmartin O, Lopez-Guerrero JA, Monteagudo C, Serra C, Requena C, et al. Dermatofibrosarcoma protuberans: clinical, pathological, and genetic (COL1A1-PDGFB) study with therapeutic implications. Histopathology. 2009;54:860–72.
24. Simon MP, Pedeutour F, Sirvent N, Grosgeorge J, Minoletti F, Coindre JM, et al. Deregulation of the platelet-derived growth factor B-chain gene via fusion with collagen gene COL1A1 in dermatofibrosarcoma protuberans and giant-cell fibroblastoma. Nat Genet. 1997;15:95–8.
25. O'Brien KP, Seroussi E, Dal CP, Sciot R, Mandahl N, Fletcher JA, et al. Various regions within the alpha-helical domain of the COL1A1 gene are fused to the second exon of the PDGFB gene in dermatofibrosarcomas and giant-cell fibroblastomas. Genes Chromosomes Cancer. 1998;23:187–93.
26. Shimizu A, O'Brien KP, Sjoblom T, Pietras K, Buchdunger E, Collins VP, et al. The dermatofibrosarcoma protuberans-associated collagen type Ialpha1/platelet-derived growth factor (PDGF) B-chain fusion gene generates a transforming protein that is processed to functional PDGF-BB. Cancer Res. 1999;59:3719–23.
27. Duffaud F, Le CA. Imatinib in the treatment of solid tumours. Target Oncol. 2009;4:45–56.
28. Najarian DJ, Morrison C, Sait SN, Meguerditchian AN, Kane III J, Cheney R, et al. Recurrent giant cell fibroblastoma

treated with Mohs micrographic surgery. Dermatol Surg. 2010;36:417–21.
29. Pedeutour F, Coindre JM, Nicolo G, Bouchot C, Ayraud N, Carel CT. Ring chromosomes in dermatofibrosarcoma protuberans contain chromosome 17 sequences: fluorescence in situ hybridization. Cancer Genet Cytogenet. 1993; 67:149.
30. Iwasaki H, Ohjimi Y, Ishiguro M, Isayama T, Fujita C, Kaneko Y, et al. Supernumerary ring chromosomes and nuclear blebs in some low-grade malignant soft tissue tumours: atypical lipomatous tumours and dermatofibrosarcoma protuberans. Virchows Arch. 1998;432:521–8.
31. Wang J, Hisaoka M, Shimajiri S, Morimitsu Y, Hashimoto H. Detection of COL1A1-PDGFB fusion transcripts in dermatofibrosarcoma protuberans by reverse transcription-polymerase chain reaction using archival formalin-fixed, paraffin-embedded tissues. Diagn Mol Pathol. 1999;8: 113–9.
32. Takahira T, Oda Y, Tamiya S, Higaki K, Yamamoto H, Kobayashi C, et al. Detection of COL1A1-PDGFB fusion transcripts and PDGFB/PDGFRB mRNA expression in dermatofibrosarcoma protuberans. Mod Pathol. 2007;20:668–75.
33. Muchemwa FC, Wakasugi S, Honda Y, Ihn H. PDGFB quantification is a useful tool in the diagnosis of dermatofibrosarcoma protuberans: a study of 10 cases. Clin Exp Dermatol. 2010;35:295–9.
34. Fiore M, Miceli R, Mussi C, Lo VS, Mariani L, Lozza L, et al. Dermatofibrosarcoma protuberans treated at a single institution: a surgical disease with a high cure rate. J Clin Oncol. 2005;23:7669–75.
35. Love WE, Keiler SA, Tamburro JE, Honda K, Gosain AK, Bordeaux JS. Surgical management of congenital dermatofibrosarcoma protuberans. J Am Acad Dermatol. 2009;61: 1014–23.
36. Martin L, Piette F, Blanc P, Mortier L, Avril MF, Delaunay MM, et al. Clinical variants of the preprotuberant stage of dermatofibrosarcoma protuberans. Br J Dermatol. 2005;153: 932–6.
37. Gershtenson PC, Krunic AL, Chen HM. Multiple clustered dermatofibroma: case report and review of the literature. J Cutan Pathol. 2010;37:e42–5.
38. Marcus JR, Few JW, Senger C, Reynolds M. Dermatofibrosarcoma protuberans and the Bednar tumor: treatment in the pediatric population. J Pediatr Surg. 1998;33: 1811–4.
39. Kricorian GJ, Schanbacher CF, Kelly AP, Bennett RG. Dermatofibrosarcoma protuberans growing around plantar aponeurosis: excision by Mohs micrographic surgery. Dermatol Surg. 2000;26:941–5.
40. Lemm D, Mugge LO, Mentzel T, Hoffken K. Current treatment options in dermatofibrosarcoma protuberans. J Cancer Res Clin Oncol. 2009;135:653–65.
41. Checketts SR, Hamilton TK, Baughman RD. Congenital and childhood dermatofibrosarcoma protuberans: a case report and review of the literature. J Am Acad Dermatol. 2000;42:907–13.
42. Reddy C, Hayward P, Thompson P, Kan A. Dermatofibrosarcoma protuberans in children. J Plast Reconstr Aesthet Surg. 2009;62:819–23.
43. Terrier-Lacombe MJ, Guillou L, Maire G, Terrier P, Vince DR, de Saint Aubain SN, et al. Dermatofibrosarcoma protuberans, giant cell fibroblastoma, and hybrid lesions in children: clinicopathologic comparative analysis of 28 cases with molecular data – a study from the French Federation of Cancer Centers Sarcoma Group. Am J Surg Pathol. 2003;27:27–39.
44. Shmookler BM, Enzinger FM, Weiss SW. Giant cell fibroblastoma. A juvenile form of dermatofibrosarcoma protuberans. Cancer. 1989;64:2154–61.
45. Gloster Jr HM. Dermatofibrosarcoma protuberans. J Am Acad Dermatol. 1996;35:355–74.
46. Wood L, Fountaine TJ, Rosamilia L, Helm KF, Clarke LE. Cutaneous CD34+ spindle cell neoplasms: histopathologic features distinguish spindle cell lipoma, solitary fibrous tumor, and dermatofibrosarcoma protuberans. Am J Dermatopathol. 2010;32(80):764–8.
47. Pouryazdanparast P, Yu L, Cutlan JE, Olsen SH, Fullen DR, Ma L. Diagnostic value of CD163 in cutaneous spindle cell lesions. J Cutan Pathol. 2009;36:859–64.
48. Mori T, Misago N, Yamamoto O, Toda S, Narisawa Y. Expression of nestin in dermatofibrosarcoma protuberans in comparison to dermatofibroma. J Dermatol. 2008;35: 419–25.
49. Sellheyer K, Nelson P, Krahl D. Dermatofibrosarcoma protuberans: a tumour of nestin-positive cutaneous mesenchymal stem cells? Br J Dermatol. 2009;161:1317–22.
50. Oliveira-Soares R, Viana I, Vale E, Soares-Almeida LM, Picoto A. Dermatofibrosarcoma protuberans: a clinicopathological study of 20 cases. J Eur Acad Dermatol Venereol. 2002;16:441–6.
51. Bisceglia M, Vairo M, Calonje E, Fletcher CD. [Pigmented fibrosarcomatous dermatofibrosarcoma protuberans (Bednar tumor). 3 case reports, analogy with the "conventional" type and review of the literature]. Pathologica. 1997;89:264–73.
52. Suehara Y, Yazawa Y, Hitachi K. Metastatic Bednar tumor (pigmented dermatofibrosarcoma protuberans) with fibrosarcomatous change: a case report. J Orthop Sci. 2004;9: 662–5.
53. Goldblum JR, Reith JD, Weiss SW. Sarcomas arising in dermatofibrosarcoma protuberans: a reappraisal of biologic behavior in eighteen cases treated by wide local excision with extended clinical follow up. Am J Surg Pathol. 2000; 24:1125–30.
54. Mentzel T, Beham A, Katenkamp D, Dei Tos AP, Fletcher CD. Fibrosarcomatous ("high-grade") dermatofibrosarcoma protuberans: clinicopathologic and immunohistochemical study of a series of 41 cases with emphasis on prognostic significance. Am J Surg Pathol. 1998;22:576–87.
55. Abbott JJ, Oliveira AM, Nascimento AG. The prognostic significance of fibrosarcomatous transformation in dermatofibrosarcoma protuberans. Am J Surg Pathol. 2006;30:436–43.
56. Goldblum JR. CD34 positivity in fibrosarcomas which arise in dermatofibrosarcoma protuberans. Arch Pathol Lab Med. 1995;119:238–41.
57. Minter RM, Reith JD, Hochwald SN. Metastatic potential of dermatofibrosarcoma protuberans with fibrosarcomatous change. J Surg Oncol. 2003;82:201–8.
58. Labonte S, Hanna W, Bandarchi-Chamkhaleh B. A study of CD117 expression in dermatofibrosarcoma protuberans and cellular dermatofibroma. J Cutan Pathol. 2007;34:857–60.
59. Kovarik CL, Hsu MY, Cockerell CJ. Neurofibromatous changes in dermatofibrosarcoma protuberans: a potential

pitfall in the diagnosis of a serious cutaneous soft tissue neoplasm. J Cutan Pathol. 2004;31:492–6.
60. Nielsen GP, Rosenberg AE, Koerner FC, Young RH, Scully RE. Smooth-muscle tumors of the vulva. A clinicopathological study of 25 cases and review of the literature. Am J Surg Pathol. 1996;20:779–93.
61. Bahrami A, Folpe AL. Adult-type fibrosarcoma: a reevaluation of 163 putative cases diagnosed at a single institution over a 48-year period. Am J Surg Pathol. 2010;34:1504–13.
62. Edelweiss M, Malpica A. Dermatofibrosarcoma protuberans of the vulva: a clinicopathologic and immunohistochemical study of 13 cases. Am J Surg Pathol. 2010;34:393–400.
63. Hoang MP, Selim MA, Bentley RC, Burchette JL, Shea CR. CD34 expression in desmoplastic melanoma. J Cutan Pathol. 2001;28:508–12.
64. Popov P, Bohling T, Asko-Seljavaara S, Tukiainen E. Microscopic margins and results of surgery for dermatofibrosarcoma protuberans. Plast Reconstr Surg. 2007;119:1779–84.
65. Chang CK, Jacobs IA, Salti GI. Outcomes of surgery for dermatofibrosarcoma protuberans. Eur J Surg Oncol. 2004;30:341–5.
66. Loss L, Zeitouni NC. Management of scalp dermatofibrosarcoma protuberans. Dermatol Surg. 2005;31:1428–33.
67. Kasper B, Lossignol D, Gil T, Flamen P, De Saint AN, Awada A. Imatinib mesylate in a patient with metastatic disease originating from a dermatofibrosarcoma protuberans of the scalp. Anticancer Drugs. 2006;17:1223–5.
68. Marks LB, Suit HD, Rosenberg AE, Wood WC. Dermatofibrosarcoma protuberans treated with radiation therapy. Int J Radiat Oncol Biol Phys. 1989;17:379–84.
69. Heuvel ST, Suurmeijer A, Pras E, Van Ginkel RJ, Hoekstra HJ. Dermatofibrosarcoma protuberans: recurrence is related to the adequacy of surgical margins. Eur J Surg Oncol. 2010;36:89–94.
70. Monnier D, Vidal C, Martin L, Danzon A, Pelletier F, Puzenat E, et al. Dermatofibrosarcoma protuberans: a population-based cancer registry descriptive study of 66 consecutive cases diagnosed between 1982 and 2002. J Eur Acad Dermatol Venereol. 2006;20:1237–42.
71. Stojadinovic A, Karpoff HM, Antonescu CR, Shah JP, Singh B, Spiro RH, et al. Dermatofibrosarcoma protuberans of the head and neck. Ann Surg Oncol. 2000;7:696–704.
72. Yu W, Tsoukas MM, Chapman SM, Rosen JM. Surgical treatment for dermatofibrosarcoma protuberans: the Dartmouth experience and literature review. Ann Plast Surg. 2008;60:288–93.
73. Ratner D, Thomas CO, Johnson TM, Sondak VK, Hamilton TA, Nelson BR, et al. Mohs micrographic surgery for the treatment of dermatofibrosarcoma protuberans. Results of a multiinstitutional series with an analysis of the extent of microscopic spread. J Am Acad Dermatol. 1997;37:600–13.
74. Meguerditchian AN, Wang J, Lema B, Kraybill WG, Zeitouni NC, Kane III JM. Wide excision or Mohs micrographic surgery for the treatment of primary dermatofibrosarcoma protuberans. Am J Clin Oncol. 2010;33:300–3.
75. Snow SN, Gordon EM, Larson PO, Bagheri MM, Bentz ML, Sable DB. Dermatofibrosarcoma protuberans: a report on 29 patients treated by Mohs micrographic surgery with long-term follow-up and review of the literature. Cancer. 2004;101:28–38.
76. Wacker J, Khan-Durani B, Hartschuh W. Modified Mohs micrographic surgery in the therapy of dermatofibrosarcoma protuberans: analysis of 22 patients. Ann Surg Oncol. 2004;11:438–44.
77. Rutgers EJ, Kroon BB, Albus-Lutter CE, Gortzak E. Dermatofibrosarcoma protuberans: treatment and prognosis. Eur J Surg Oncol. 1992;18:241–8.
78. Thomas CJ, Wood GC, Marks VJ. Mohs micrographic surgery in the treatment of rare aggressive cutaneous tumors: the Geisinger experience. Dermatol Surg. 2007;33:333–9.
79. Nelson RA, Arlette JP. Mohs micrographic surgery and dermatofibrosarcoma protuberans: a multidisciplinary approach in 44 patients. Ann Plast Surg. 2008;60:667–72.
80. Gloster Jr HM, Harris KR, Roenigk RK. A comparison between Mohs micrographic surgery and wide surgical excision for the treatment of dermatofibrosarcoma protuberans. J Am Acad Dermatol. 1996;35:82–7.
81. Haas AF, Sykes JM. Multispecialty approach to complex dermatofibrosarcoma protuberans of the forehead. Arch Otolaryngol Head Neck Surg. 1998;124:324–7.
82. Hobbs ER, Wheeland RG, Bailin PL, Ratz JL, Yetman RJ, Zins JE. Treatment of dermatofibrosarcoma protuberans with Mohs micrographic surgery. Ann Surg. 1988;207:102–7.
83. King M, Ocheltree I. Dermatofibrosarcoma protuberans treatment and reconstruction: a case study. Plast Surg Nurs. 1996;16:77–82.
84. Stranahan D, Cherpelis BS, Glass LF, Ladd S, Fenske NA. Immunohistochemical stains in Mohs surgery: a review. Dermatol Surg. 2009;35:1023–34.
85. Robinson JK. Dermatofibrosarcoma protuberans resected by Mohs' surgery (chemosurgery). A 5-year prospective study. J Am Acad Dermatol. 1985;12:1093–8.
86. Jimenez FJ, Grichnik JM, Buchanan MD, Clark RE. Immunohistochemical techniques in Mohs micrographic surgery: their potential use in the detection of neoplastic cells masked by inflammation. J Am Acad Dermatol. 1995;32:89–94.
87. Jimenez FJ, Grichnik JM, Buchanan MD, Clark RE. Immunohistochemical margin control applied to Mohs micrographic surgical excision of dermatofibrosarcoma protuberans. J Dermatol Surg Oncol. 1994;20:687–9.
88. Garcia C, Viehman G, Hitchcock M, Clark RE. Dermatofibrosarcoma protuberans treated with Mohs surgery. A case with CD34 immunostaining variability. Dermatol Surg. 1996;22:177–9.
89. Demiri EC, Dionyssiou DD, Kirkos JM, Panayotopoulou C, Papadimitriou DK. Multiple recurrent dermatofibrosarcoma protuberans of the hand. J Plast Reconstr Aesthet Surg. 2008;61:842–5.
90. Dagan R, Morris CG, Zlotecki RA, Scarborough MT, Mendenhall WM. Radiotherapy in the treatment of dermatofibrosarcoma protuberans. Am J Clin Oncol. 2005;28:537–9.
91. Sun LM, Wang CJ, Huang CC, Leung SW, Chen HC, Fang FM, et al. Dermatofibrosarcoma protuberans: treatment results of 35 cases. Radiother Oncol. 2000;57:175–81.
92. Huber GF, Matthews TW, Dort JC. Radiation-induced soft tissue sarcomas of the head and neck. J Otolaryngol. 2007;36:93–7.
93. McLoughlin PM, Girach M, Wood GA. Dermatofibrosarcoma protuberans of the scalp. Br J Oral Maxillofac Surg. 1992;30:401–3.

94. Argiris A, Dardoufas C, Aroni K. Radiotherapy induced soft tissue sarcoma: an unusual case of a dermatofibrosarcoma protuberans. Clin Oncol (R Coll Radiol). 1995;7:59–61.
95. Kamiya T, Saga K, Kaneko R, Ono I, Kawada M, Maeda Y. Postradiation dermatofibrosarcoma protuberans. Acta Derm Venereol. 2006;86:152–3.
96. Champagne MA, Capdeville R, Krailo M, Qu W, Peng B, Rosamilia M, et al. Imatinib mesylate (STI571) for treatment of children with Philadelphia chromosome-positive leukemia: results from a Children's Oncology Group phase 1 study. Blood. 2004;104:2655–60.
97. Barr RD. Imatinib mesylate in children and adolescents with cancer. Pediatr Blood Cancer. 2010;55:18–25.
98. Maki RG, Awan RA, Dixon RH, Jhanwar S, Antonescu CR. Differential sensitivity to imatinib of 2 patients with metastatic sarcoma arising from dermatofibrosarcoma protuberans. Int J Cancer. 2002;100:623–6.
99. Rubin BP, Schuetze SM, Eary JF, Norwood TH, Mirza S, Conrad EU, et al. Molecular targeting of platelet-derived growth factor B by imatinib mesylate in a patient with metastatic dermatofibrosarcoma protuberans. J Clin Oncol. 2002;20:3586–91.
100. Labropoulos SV, Razis ED. Imatinib in the treatment of dermatofibrosarcoma protuberans. Biologics. 2007;1:347–53.
101. McArthur GA, Demetri GD, van Oosterom A, Heinrich MC, Debiec-Rychter M, Corless CL, et al. Molecular and clinical analysis of locally advanced dermatofibrosarcoma protuberans treated with imatinib: Imatinib Target Exploration Consortium Study B2225. J Clin Oncol. 2005;23:866–73.
102. Kerob D, Porcher R, Verola O, Dalle S, Maubec E, Aubin F, et al. Imatinib mesylate as a preoperative therapy in dermatofibrosarcoma: results of a multicenter phase II study on 25 patients. Clin Cancer Res. 2010;16:3288–95.
103. Rutkowski P, Van GM, Rankin CJ, Ruka W, Rubin BP, Debiec-Rychter M, et al. Imatinib mesylate in advanced dermatofibrosarcoma protuberans: pooled analysis of two phase II clinical trials. J Clin Oncol. 2010;28:1772–9.
104. Gooskens SL, Oranje AP, van Adrichem LN, de Waard-van der Spek FB, den Hollander JC, van de Ven CP, et al. Imatinib mesylate for children with dermatofibrosarcoma protuberans (DFSP). Pediatr Blood Cancer. 2010;55:369–73.
105. Price VE, Fletcher JA, Zielenska M, Cole W, Viero S, Manson DE, et al. Imatinib mesylate: an attractive alternative in young children with large, surgically challenging dermatofibrosarcoma protuberans. Pediatr Blood Cancer. 2005;44:511–5.
106. Ahmed AA, Ostlie D, Fraser JD, Newell B, Cooley L. Dermatofibrosarcoma protuberans in the breast of a 2-year-old girl. Ann Diagn Pathol. 2010;14:279–83.
107. Wolf D, Rumpold H. A benefit-risk assessment of imatinib in chronic myeloid leukaemia and gastrointestinal stromal tumours. Drug Saf. 2009;32:1001–15.
108. Haycox CL, Odland PB, Olbricht SM, Piepkorn M. Immunohistochemical characterization of dermatofibrosarcoma protuberans with practical applications for diagnosis and treatment. J Am Acad Dermatol. 1997;37:438–44.
109. Mehrany K, Swanson NA, Heinrich MC, Weenig RH, Lee KK, White Jr CR, et al. Dermatofibrosarcoma protuberans: a partial response to imatinib therapy. Dermatol Surg. 2006;32:456–9.
110. Shin YR, Kim JY, Sung MS, Jung JH. Sonographic findings of dermatofibrosarcoma protuberans with pathologic correlation. J Ultrasound Med. 2008;27:269–74.
111. Lee SJ, Mahoney MC, Shaughnessy E. Dermatofibrosarcoma protuberans of the breast: imaging features and review of the literature. AJR Am J Roentgenol. 2009;193:W64–9.
112. Torreggiani WC, Al-Ismail K, Munk PL, Nicolaou S, O'Connell JX, Knowling MA. Dermatofibrosarcoma protuberans: MR imaging features. AJR Am J Roentgenol. 2002;178:989–93.
113. Riggs K, McGuigan KL, Morrison WB, Samie FH, Humphreys T. Role of magnetic resonance imaging in perioperative assessment of dermatofibrosarcoma protuberans. Dermatol Surg. 2009;35:2036–41.
114. Navarro OM, Laffan EE, Ngan BY. Pediatric soft-tissue tumors and pseudo-tumors: MR imaging features with pathologic correlation: part 1. Imaging approach, pseudotumors, vascular lesions, and adipocytic tumors. Radiographics. 2009;29:887–906.
115. Thornton SL, Reid J, Papay FA, Vidimos AT. Childhood dermatofibrosarcoma protuberans: role of preoperative imaging. J Am Acad Dermatol. 2005;53:76–83.
116. Gould SW, Agarwal T, Benoist S, Patel B, Gedroyc W, Darzi A. Resection of soft tissue sarcomas with intra-operative magnetic resonance guidance. J Magn Reson Imaging. 2002;15:114–9.
117. Mizutani K, Tamada Y, Hara K, Tsuzuki T, Saeki H, Tamaki K, et al. Imatinib mesylate inhibits the growth of metastatic lung lesions in a patient with dermatofibrosarcoma protuberans. Br J Dermatol. 2004;151:235–7.
118. National Comprehensive Cancer Network. Dermatofibrosarcoma protuberans. Clinical practice guidelines in oncology. J Natl Compr Canc Netw. 2004;2:74–8.
119. Mattox AK, Mehta AI, Grossi PM, Cummings TJ, Adamson DC. Response of malignant scalp dermatofibrosarcoma to presurgical targeted growth factor inhibition. J Neurosurg. 2010;112:965–77.

Microcystic Adnexal Carcinoma

20

Ioulios Palamaras and Richard J. Barlow

Abstract

Microcystic adnexal carcinoma (MAC) is a rare adnexal tumor often found on the head and neck and usually presenting as an ill-defined, yellowish, or faintly erythematous plaque. It is characterized by aggressive local infiltration and has a high propensity for perineural invasion (PNI).

Most cases have been reported in white patients aged 40–60 years, and there is no sexual predilection. The tumor also occurs in other ethnic groups and across a much wider age range.

An adequately sized biopsy is necessary for diagnosis.

Surgery is the treatment of choice. The poorly defined clinical margins and propensity for perineural spread make Mohs micrographic surgery (MMS) preferable to standard surgical excision. When nerve involvement is present, MMS with formalin-fixed, paraffin-embedded sections should be considered.

The prognosis is good, and the 10-year survival rate is higher than 85%. Metastases are rare.

Keywords

Microcystic adnexal carcinoma • Mohs micrographic surgery • Syringomatous carcinoma • Perineural invasion • Radiotherapy • Surgical excision

Summary: Introduction

- Microcystic adnexal carcinoma (MAC) is a rare skin tumor and was firstly described in 1982. Slow growth, as well as subtle clinical and histological signs, may delay the diagnosis. Similarly, tumor size may be underestimated, and a standard excision may be incomplete.

I. Palamaras (✉)• R.J. Barlow
St. John's Institute of Dermatology, St. Thomas' Hospital, London, UK
e-mail: drioulios@hotmail.com

K. Nouri (ed.), *Mohs Micrographic Surgery*,
DOI 10.1007/978-1-4471-2152-7_20,

20.1 Introduction

Microcystic adnexal carcinoma (MAC) is an uncommon, locally invasive adnexal skin tumor which usually presents on the head and neck. It was described in 1982 by Goldstein et al., who considered it to be of follicular or eccrine origin and possibly to derive from a pluripotential adnexal cell [1]. Other authors have favored at least partial sebaceous or apocrine lineage [2]. The current consensus seems to be that MAC is a separate clinicopathologic entity, probably synonymous with at least some of the low-grade sweat gland carcinomas reported variously as eccrine epithelioma, syringomatous carcinoma, malignant syringoma, syringoid eccrine carcinoma, aggressive trichofolliculoma, and also as the sclerosing sweat gland carcinomas [3, 4].

MAC is a rare tumor but is associated with high morbidity. It can infiltrate subcutaneous fat as well as along fascial planes and nerves, perichondrium, and periosteum [5–8].

Summary: Epidemiology

- Most cases seem to occur in whites, though Asians and African Americans have also been affected. There is no significant sexual predilection, and most cases present between 40 and 60 years of age.

20.2 Epidemiology

Only about 300 microcystic adnexal carcinomas have been reported in the literature [9], most in the white population. Other ethnic groups may also be affected, and at least 50 Japanese [10] and 7 African American patients have been reported in the literature [9, 11–15].

Most affected individuals are 40–60 years of age, although the reported age range is very wide (10–102 years) [16–18]. Although there is no significant sexual predilection, it is possible that among affected individuals, there is a female preponderance [8, 16, 18–20].

Summary: Pathogenesis

- The pathogenesis of MAC is unknown. Loss of a tumor suppressor gene on the long arm of chromosome 6 may play a role. Although not confirmed, other possible risk factors include UV exposure, radiotherapy, and immune compromise.

20.3 Pathogenesis

The molecular pathophysiology of MAC is unknown. Unlike other more common skin tumors, a p53 gene mutation seems not to play a role [2, 21]. Abbate et al. reported MAC in two sisters and, on this basis, suggested a genetic predisposition [22]. Cytogenetic analysis in another affected individual showed a chromosome deletion on arm 6q [23]. The same deletion has also been documented in all major types of malignant salivary gland tumors, prompting some authors to postulate the loss of a tumor suppressor gene on that locus [24, 25].

Although their relative significance has not yet been established, potential risk factors associated with MAC may include UV exposure, radiotherapy, and being immunocompromised. A role for UV exposure was raised in a review of 48 North American patients in which 24 out of 48 patients had MAC on the left side of the head and neck region, compared with nine on the right side and nine on the midline [16]. The author postulated that this may be a consequence of driving on the left side of the road [16]. The opposite would be expected to apply to patients in two Australian studies, though comparative data are not available [17, 19]. Whatever the role of UV exposure, MAC also occurs in unexposed areas, such as the tongue, axilla, vulva, buttocks, and perianal skin [26].

A history of radiation therapy was noted in five out of ten patients in one study [22] and in two out of ten patients in a second [27]. In a third study [28], there was a history of radiotherapy in 2 out of 13 patients, of whom one was also a renal transplant patient on immunosuppression. In a review [29] of 274 published cases of MAC, a history of radiation exposure is reported to have preceded development of the tumor in 14 of 84 patients in whom a history was available, an incidence of 19.5%.

Three cases of MAC have been reported in immunosuppressed patients – two in renal transplant recipients [28, 30] and one in a patient with chronic lymphocytic leukemia [31].

Summary: Clinical Features and Diagnosis

- MAC characteristically presents as a poorly defined, yellowish or slightly erythematous, and indurated plaque. Nerve involvement may cause paresthesia or dysesthesia. The tumor may extend for several centimeters beyond the clinical margins.

20.4 Clinical Features and Diagnosis

An indolent growth history is a characteristic feature and may contribute to delayed diagnosis, which is common [32]. In one patient, MAC was diagnosed as the cause of asymptomatic and gradually expanding alopecia which had been present for 31 years [13]. Also, a review of 50 Japanese patients included a patient who was considered to have had an undiagnosed MAC for 50 years [10].

MAC has a predilection for the head and neck, accounting for 74% of cases in a review of all patients with MAC reported between 1973 and 2004 in the Surveillance, Epidemiology, and End Results database of the National Cancer Institute of the USA [18]. This was followed by the trunk (9%), the arms (8.5%), and legs (5.4%). Two tumors were present on the labia majora [18].

MAC is often mistaken for morpheaform basal-cell carcinoma (BCC), which it can resemble clinically. Like this, MAC usually presents as a nontender, poorly defined, indurated plaque (Fig. 20.1) which is yellowish or faintly erythematous in color. Ulceration is uncommon, and subcutaneous extension may result in deeper, nodular swelling.

The true size of the tumor can be considerably underestimated because of subclinical extension which can sometimes extend to several centimeters. Different case series have measured a 3- to 14.4-fold discrepancy between the presumed clinical size and the wound after Mohs micrographic surgery (MMS) (Fig. 20.2) [16, 20, 28, 33, 34].

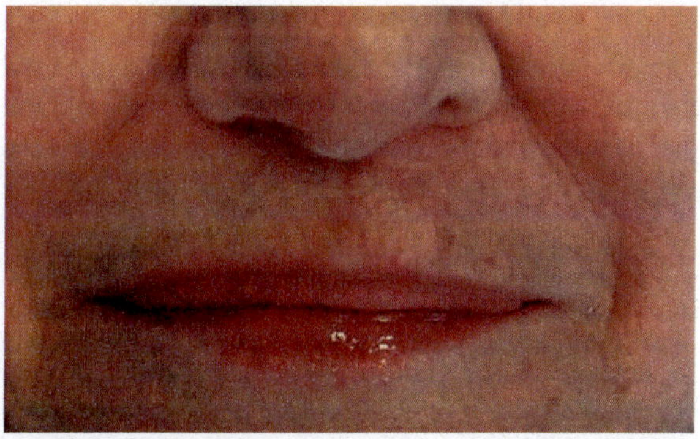

Fig. 20.1 Photograph of a patient with MAC on the philtrum, illustrating the difficulty in determining the clinical margins of the tumor

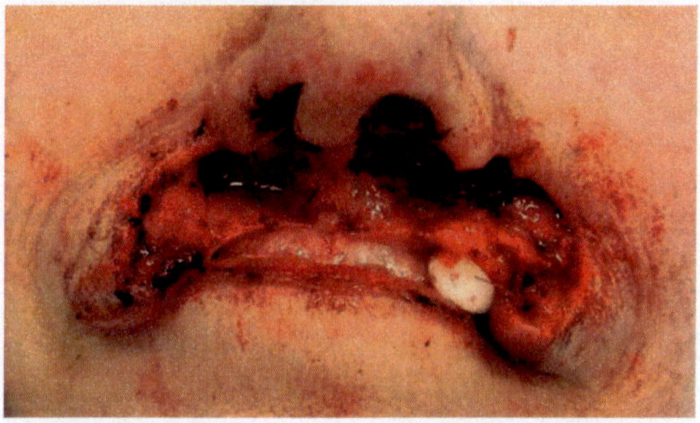

Fig. 20.2 Photograph after Mohs micrographic surgery, illustrating the extent of subclinical spread

Symptoms such as numbness, burning, stinging, or paresthesia may be present and should alert the examiner to the possibility of perineural infiltration [8].

Summary: Histopathological Features

- An adequately sized biopsy is needed to assess the architectural pattern of the tumor and its perineural involvement. MAC has a superficial component consisting of keratin cysts lined with eosinophilic squamous epithelium and a deeper component comprising nests and cords of basaloid cells. The associated inflammatory infiltrate is characteristically scanty.

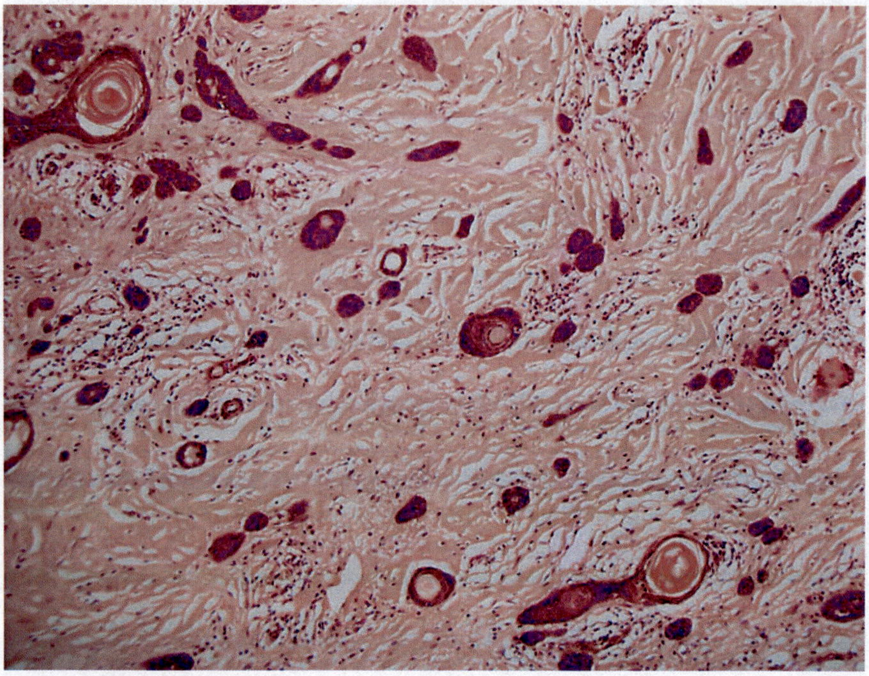

Fig. 20.3 Photomicrograph of a diagnostic paraffin section showing keratin cysts and small islands of tumor cells deep in the dermis. There is a scanty inflammatory infiltrate (hematoxylin and eosin stain; original magnification ×40) (Courtesy of Dr. Alistair Robson, Consultant Dermatopathologist at St. John's Institute of Dermatology, London, UK)

20.5 Histopathological Features

An adequately sized biopsy is critical both for diagnosis and for assessment of perineural involvement. Interpretation of the histology may be particularly difficult in a small shave or superficial punch biopsy in which it is not possible to assess the architectural pattern. In the largest published case series, the diagnosis of MAC was made in only 70% of initial biopsy specimens [10, 16, 17]. In periocular skin, this figure seems to be even lower, applying to only 19% of all 35 periocular MAC reported in the English language literature [35]. It is possible that this is because smaller biopsies are taken at this site, making a correct diagnosis more challenging.

These are aggressive tumors which can infiltrate subcutaneous tissue. The cytology is often bland, with little pleomorphism and mitotic activity (Fig. 20.3). The relative proportions of the cellular components differ, the first consisting of keratin cysts lined with eosinophilic squamous epithelium. Deeper in the tumor are nests and cords of usually basaloid epithelial cells. Some of these show central keratinization or calcification, and some show duct formation and a tadpole appearance that may cause diagnostic confusion with syringomas [1, 3]. Perineural invasion is characteristic [5]. The tumor cells frequently elicit a desmoplastic stromal response [1, 2, 5, 6]. It is possible that a variant characterized by nuclear pleomorphism, hyperchromasia, vascular invasion, and necrosis behaves more aggressively and may metastasize [36].

Toluidine blue is the preferred staining technique of many Mohs surgeons and may be useful in this context because it stains tumor strands with a distinctive pink halo. Where tumor is present around nerves, a maroon tint is seen [37].

The differential diagnosis includes syringoma and desmoplastic trichoepithelioma, though these do not extend deeply into the dermis or subcutis and do not show perineural invasion [1, 3, 38].

A morphoeic basal-cell carcinoma is likely to show epidermal contiguity and can be excluded by the presence of ductal differentiation in MAC (though this can sometimes occur in nodular BCC) and by the presence of intracytoplasmic lumen formation. Likewise, a desmoplastic squamous cell carcinoma can usually be excluded on the basis of epidermal involvement and the absence of ductal structures.

There is no specific immunohistochemical stain for MAC, but immunohistochemistry may nevertheless be helpful in making a diagnosis. Of particular use is p63, the nuclear staining pattern of which is highly expressed in morphoeic BCC and desmoplastic trichoepitheliomas [39]. In MAC, staining is scattered and peripheral, particularly in deeper parts of the tumor. Epithelial membrane antigen is positive in MAC and helps differentiate from morphoeic BCC [40]. Staining for cytokeratin 15 may be useful in excluding basal-cell and squamous cell carcinoma but not desmoplastic trichoepithelioma [41].

Summary: Treatment

- Surgery is the mainstay of treatment. Mohs micrographic surgery (MMS) is associated with fewer complications and a lower recurrence rate than standard surgical excision (SSE). When perineural infiltration is noted on the diagnostic biopsy or when MAC persists after previous treatment, it is possible that MMS using formalin-fixed, paraffin-embedded sections should be considered as an alternative to the frozen section technique. Otherwise, the fresh tissue technique can be used until tumor-free margins are achieved, followed by an additional layer for paraffin sections.
- Primary or adjuvant radiotherapy and chemotherapy have been attempted with ambivalent results.

20.6 Treatment

Surgery is the treatment of choice, though radiotherapy has been attempted as either primary or adjuvant therapy in a small number of patients. These have usually had extensive locoregional disease, and treatment has usually been unsuccessful [29]. In one patient, the tumor is even thought to have recurred in a more extensive and aggressive form 6 months after primary radiotherapy [42]. Furthermore, previous radiation exposure has been implicated as a possible risk factor for MAC.

There have been no randomized controlled studies comparing Mohs micrographic surgery (MMS) with standard surgical excision (SSE). The rationale for using the former would be the characteristic poorly defined clinical margins of this tumor and its predilection for perineural spread.

For the purposes of writing this chapter, we have assessed all of the 13 reported case series consisting of five patients or more (Table 20.1). MMS was used to treat MAC in six of these, with a total of 113 patients and an average follow-up of 4.3 years (range, 3 months–13.3 years) [17, 20, 27, 28, 33, 34]. Of these, 5.8% of tumors persisted (exact 95%; CI, 1.9–13). On the other hand, SSE was used in four studies, with a total of 95 cases and an average follow-up of 6.9 years (range, 4 months–29 years) [5, 10, 19, 43]. Among these, 32.2% persisted (exact 95%; CI, 22.75–42.9).

The remaining three studies employed either MMS or SSE in 72 patients (MMS, $n=39$ and SSE, $n=33$), with a mean follow-up of 2 years in the MMS group and 2.7 years in the SSE group [2, 16, 22]. The percentage of tumors persisting in the MMS and SSE groups was 5.4% (exact 95%; CI, 0.6–18.2) and 12.9% (exact 95%; CI, 3.6–29.8), respectively. There was no true randomization in these studies, and all three series contained patients in whom SSE had resulted in incomplete excision and as a result of which, they were referred for MMS.

A second disadvantage of SSE over MMS would seem to be higher morbidity. In the studies reviewed, incomplete SSE was reported in 17.6–58% of patients subjected to SSE [2, 16, 19, 22, 43]. In one study [43], a mean of 1.6 non-Mohs excisions was required to achieve clear surgical margins in primary tumors, and a mean of 2.5 excisions in recurrent MAC. Others reported a mean of 2.75 [16] and 1.5 [2] non-Mohs excisions to obtain clear margins in mixed primary and persistent tumors.

MMS can be undertaken with either the frozen tissue technique or using formalin-fixed, paraffin-embedded sections ("Slow Mohs"). Frozen sections seem reliable for treating primary MAC not associated with perineural and/or intraneural infiltration [20]. However, involvement of nerves is often present and may not be readily apparent on frozen sections stained with hematoxylin and eosin (H&E) (Fig. 20.4) [20, 44]. Adding to this difficulty are the characteristic absence of a marked inflammatory infiltrate and the difficulty in distinguishing between small strands of tumor and adnexal tissue (Fig. 20.5) [20, 44]. As a consequence, some authors have recommended that the fresh tissue technique is used until tumor margins appear clear on frozen sections and that an additional layer is then sent for paraffin sections [35, 45]. An alternative to this may be the use of toluidine blue, possibly together with H&E stains on the same tissue blocks [37]. As noted above, toluidine blue stains the tumor stroma with a pink halo, owing to

Table 20.1 Results of comparison of MMS and SSE for MAC

	Pretreatment MAC			Recurrent MAC (posttreatment)		
Study	Comments	No. of cases	Patients lost to follow-up	No. of recurrent patients	Recurrence rate (%)	Exact 95% CI (%) – recurrence rate
Only Mohs micrographic surgery (MMS)						
Palamaras et al. [20]		9	2	1	14.3	0.36–57.9
Thomas CJ et al. [34]		26	1	3	12	2.55–31.22
Leibovitch et al. [17]		44	24	1	5	0.13–24.9
Snow et al. [28]		13	–	0	0	0–20.5
Friedman et al. [27]		11	–	0	0	0–23.8
Burns et al. [33]		10	–	0	0	0–25.9
Recurrence rate, mean					*5.8 (5/86)*	*1.9–13*
Average follow-up: 4.3 years (range, 3 months–13.3 years)						
Only standard surgical excision (SSE)						
Gabillot-Carre et al. [43]	3 patients had adjuvant Rx	7	–	4	57.14	18.4–90.1
Salerno et al. [19]		17	–	2	11.8	1.46–36.45
Ohtsuka et al. [10]		51	–	16	31.4	19.1–45.9
Cooper et al. [5]		20	5	7	46.6	21.3–73.4
Recurrence rate, mean					*32.2 (29/90)*	*22.75–42.9*
Average follow-up: 6.9 years (range, 4 months–29 years)						
MMS or SSE						
Abbate et al. [22]	MMS	6	–	0	0	0–39.3
	SSE	4	–	1	25	0.63–80.6
Chiller et al. [16]	MMS	25	–	2	8	0.98–26
	SSE	20	–	1	5	0.13–24.8
Le Boit et al. [2]	MMS	8	2	0	0	0–39.3
	SSE	9	2	2	28.6	3.6–71
Recurrence rate, mean	*MMS*				*5.4 (2/37)*	*0.6–18.2*
Recurrence rate, mean	*SSE*				*12.9 (4/31)*	*3.6–29.8*
Average follow-up: MMS 2.07; SSE 2.7 years (range, 0 months–11.1 years)						

MMS Mohs micrographic surgery, *SSE* standard surgical excision, *MAC* microcystic adnexal carcinoma, *Recurrence rate* total number of recurrences divided by the total number of patients observed during follow-up, *Rx* radiotherapy

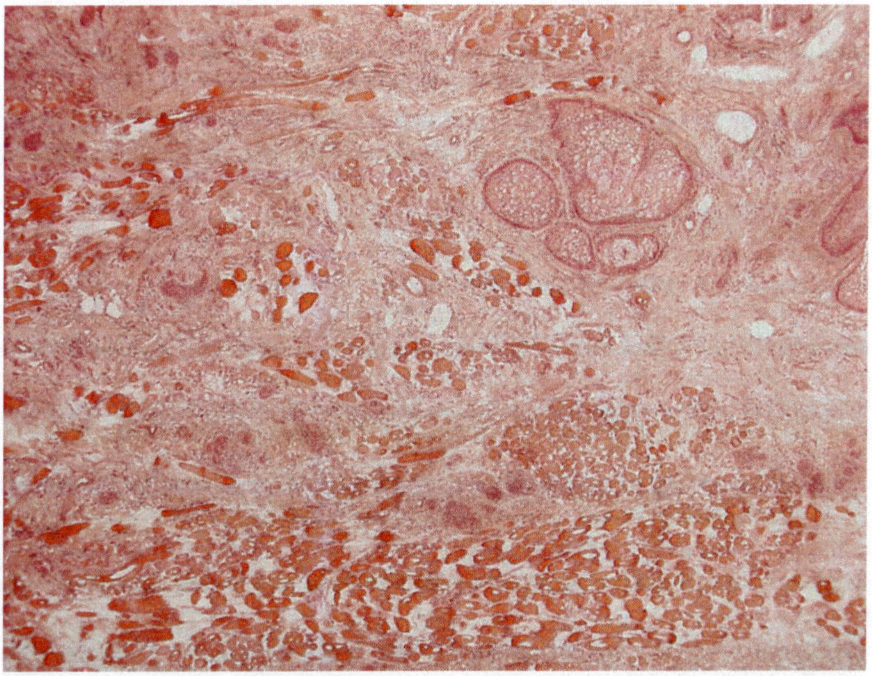

Fig. 20.4 Photomicrograph of a frozen section made during the Mohs excision of the tumor in Fig. 20.1. There are nests of epithelioid cells infiltrating the dermis. There is no associated inflammation, a characteristic feature of MAC which can contribute to small isolated islands of tumor being mistaken for normal eccrine apparatus (hematoxylin and eosin stain; original magnification ×40)

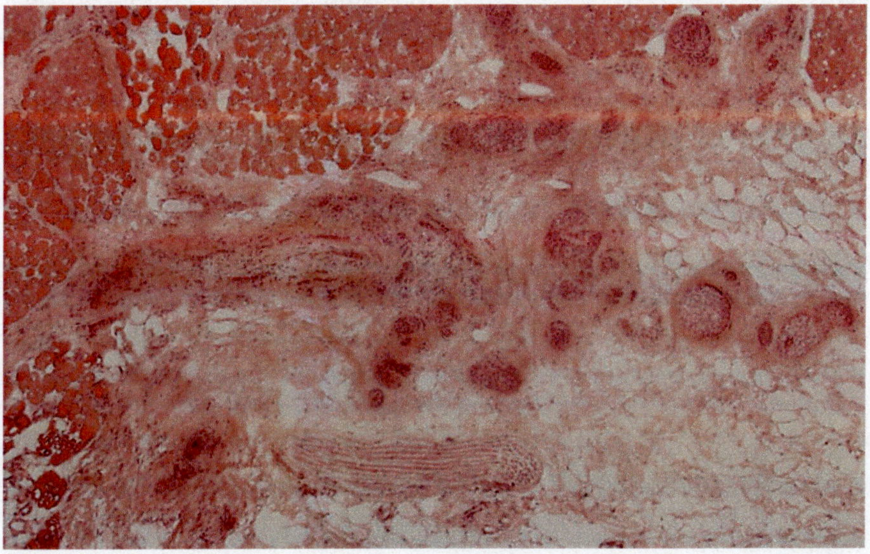

Fig. 20.5 Photomicrograph of a frozen section made during the Mohs excision of the tumor in Fig. 20.1. This shows a nerve, deep to muscle, invaded by epithelioid tumor strands without an associated inflammatory infiltrate (hematoxylin and eosin stain; original magnification×40)

mucopolysaccharides, and stains the perineural and intraneural involvement magenta.

Persistence of MAC seems to be more likely after previous incomplete excision when periocular skin is involved and when there is perineural infiltration. A previous incomplete excision will also reduce the likelihood of obtaining tumor-free margins when MMS is attempted subsequently [20, 34]. As in other situations, conventional excisions can fragment the tumor during attempted excision and during reconstruction [20]. One study reported that one of two recurrent tumors persisted despite MMS [16]. Two more studies reported persisting tumors following MMS in two out of six cases [34] and in two out of three cases [20], respectively.

Perineural invasion has also been linked with persistence of MAC following treatment. In three case series, the first reported perineural infiltration in six out of seven patients with persistent disease [17]; another, in three out of four [43]; and a third, in two out of three recurrent tumors [20].

Periocular MAC associated with perineural involvement is particularly likely to persist, including after MMS [20]. One possible reason for this is frequent failure to make an early correct diagnosis [35]. In a review study of 35 reported cases with periocular MAC, 5 out of 16 persisted after MMS, and 4 out of 10 after SSE. In the remaining nine patients, there was no available information on subsequent treatment [35]. Follow-up ranged from 2 months to 30 years. Two out of the three reported deaths directly related to MAC have occurred in periocular tumors with perineural infiltration. In view of the difficulty of tumor clearance at this site, some authors have suggested that enucleation should be considered in the management of this group of patients [35, 46]. Others disagree given the implications of this procedure [9, 20, 29, 47, 48].

Chemotherapy has been used as an adjuvant measure in two patients with complex MAC, both unsuccessfully. The first was administered cisplatinum and 5-fluorouracil, after several attempts at radiotherapy and then surgery for a lip tumor with local metastasis [47]. The second had a persistent lesion on the right nasolabial fold following surgery together with lung metastases which were treated with lobectomy. Chemotherapy with cisplatinum and 5-fluorouracil was attempted when further surgery was declined [43].

Summary: Prognosis and Follow-Up

- This is an indolent tumor, and the prognosis seems good, even in a number of inoperable cases reported in the literature. There have only been three reports in the literature of death directly attributable to MAC. A meta-analysis of 223 cases showed a 10-year overall survival rate of 86.4%.

20.7 Prognosis and Follow-Up

It is worth noting that two patients judged to have tumors too extensive for surgical intervention have been observed for several years without deterioration. One patient had involvement of the dura mater [47], and one had extensive facial infiltration [29].

MAC is an indolent and slow-growing tumor and the prognosis is usually good. Metastases are rare, and only five patients are reported to have had local spread (in-transit and lymph node) [47, 49–51] and three patients to have had distant metastases [43, 52, 53]. It is possible that in two of the patients reported to have had regional metastases, lymph node involvement may actually have been caused by occult contiguous infiltration along the neurovascular bundles [50, 51].

There are only three reports of death directly attributable to MAC [20, 53, 54]. One is thought to have been due to mediastinal metastases [53], and two others to intracranial extension of tumors on the face [20, 54]. In a meta-analysis of 223 patients with MAC from the database of the National Cancer Institute of the USA, the 10-year overall patient survival was calculated to be 86.4% (95% CI, 78–92%; standard error [SE], 3.3%) and 97.7% (SE, 5.2%) when matched with the US census population in 2000 [18].

Acknowledgments The authors would like to thank Dr. Alistair Robson, Consultant Dermatopathologist at St. John's Institute of Dermatology, for providing the photomicrograph of a diagnostic paraffin section and for photographing the frozen sections obtained during a Mohs excision.

References

1. Goldstein DJ, Barr RJ, Santa Cruz DJ. Microcystic adnexal carcinoma: a distinct clinicopathologic entity. Cancer. 1982;50(3):566–72.
2. LeBoit PE, Sexton M. Microcystic adnexal carcinoma of the skin. A reappraisal of the differentiation and differential diagnosis of an underrecognized neoplasm. J Am Acad Dermatol. 1993;29(4):609–18.
3. Brenn T, McKee PH. Tumors of the sweat glands. In: Calonje E, McKee PH, Granter SR, editors. Pathology of the skin with clinical correlations. 3rd ed. Mosby: Elsevier; 2005. p. 1649–53.
4. Wetter R, Goldstein GD. Microcystic adnexal carcinoma: a diagnostic and therapeutic challenge. Dermatol Ther. 2008;21(6):452–8.
5. Cooper PH, Mills SE, Leonard DD, Santa Cruz DJ, et al. Sclerosing sweat duct (syringomatous) carcinoma. Am J Surg Pathol. 1985;9(6):422–33.
6. Abenoza P, Ackerman AB, editors. Neoplasms with eccrine differentiation. Ackerman's histologic diagnosis of neoplastic skin disease: a method by pattern analysis. Philadelphia/London: Lea & Febiger; 1990. p. 373–412.

7. Yuh WT, Engelken JD, Whitaker DC, Dolan KD. Bone marrow invasion of microcystic adnexal carcinoma. Ann Otol Rhinol Laryngol. 1991;100(7):601–3.
8. Sebastien TS, Nelson BR, Lowe L, Baker S, et al. Microcystic adnexal carcinoma. J Am Acad Dermatol. 1993;29(5 Pt 2):840–5.
9. Page RN, Hanggi MC, King R, Googe PB. Multiple microcystic adnexal carcinomas. Cutis. 2007;79(4):299–303.
10. Ohtsuka H, Nagamatsu S. Microcystic adnexal carcinoma: review of 51 Japanese patients. Dermatology. 2002;204(3):190–3.
11. Park JY, Parry EL. Microcystic adnexal carcinoma. First reported case in a black patient. Dermatol Surg. 1998;24(8): 905–7.
12. Buhl A, Landow S, Lee YC, Holcomb K, Heilman E, Abulafia O. Microcystic adnexal carcinoma of the vulva. Gynecol Oncol. 2001;82(3):571–4.
13. Gardner ES, Goldberg LH. Neglected microcystic adnexal carcinoma: the second reported case in a black patient. Dermatol Surg. 2001;27(7):678–80.
14. Peterson CM, Ratz JL, Sangueza OP. Microcystic adnexal carcinoma: first reported case in an African American man. J Am Acad Dermatol. 2001;45(2):283–5.
15. Nadiminti H, Nadiminti U, Washington C. Microcystic adnexal carcinoma in African-Americans. Dermatol Surg. 2007; 33(11):1384–7.
16. Chiller K, Passaro D, Scheuller M, Singer M, et al. Microcystic adnexal carcinoma: forty-eight cases, their treatment, and their outcome. Arch Dermatol. 2000;136(11): 1355–9.
17. Leibovitch I, Huilgol SC, Selva D, et al. Microcystic adnexal carcinoma: treatment with Mohs micrographic surgery. J Am Acad Dermatol. 2005;52(2):295–300.
18. Yu JB, Blitzblau RC, Patel SC, Decker RH, Wilson LD. Surveillance, epidemiology, and end results (SEER) database analysis of microcystic adnexal carcinoma (sclerosing sweat duct carcinoma) of the skin. Am J Clin Oncol. 2010;33(2):125–7.
19. Salerno S, Terrill P. Will MAC be back? ANZ J Surg. 2003;73(10):830–2.
20. Palamaras I, McKenna JD, Robson A, Barlow RJ. Microcystic adnexal carcinoma: a case series treated with Mohs micrographic surgery and identification of patients in whom paraffin sections may be preferable. Dermatol Surg. 2010; 36(4):446–52. Epub February 17, 2010.
21. Smith KJ, Williams J, Corbett D, Skelton H. Microcystic adnexal carcinoma: an immunohistochemical study including markers of proliferation and apoptosis. Am J Surg Pathol. 2001;25(4):464–71.
22. Abbate M, Zeitouni NC, Seyler M, Hicks W, Loree T, Cheney RT. Clinical course, risk factors, and treatment of microcystic adnexal carcinoma: a short series report. Dermatol Surg. 2003;29(10):1035–8.
23. Wohlfahrt C, Ternesten A, Sahlin P, Islam Q, Stenman G. Cytogenetic and fluorescence in situ hybridization analyses of a microcystic adnexal carcinoma with del(6)(q23q25). Cancer Genet Cytogenet. 1997;98(2):106–10.
24. Stenman G, Sandros J, Mark J, Edström S. Partial 6q deletion in a human salivary gland adenocarcinoma. Cancer Genet Cytogenet. 1989;39(2):153–6.
25. Jin C, Martins C, Jin Y, et al. Characterization of chromosome aberrations in salivary gland tumors by FISH, including multicolor COBRA-FISH. Genes Chromosomes Cancer. 2001;30(2):161–7.
26. Hansen T, Kingsley M, Mallatt BD, Krishnan R. Extrafacial microcystic adnexal carcinoma: case report and review of the literature. Dermatol Surg. 2009;35(11):1835–9. Epub August 18, 2009.
27. Friedman PM, Friedman RH, Jiang SB, Nouri K, Amonette R, Robins P. Microcystic adnexal carcinoma: collaborative series review and update. J Am Acad Dermatol. 1999;41 (2 Pt 1):225–31.
28. Snow S, Madjar DD, Hardy S, et al. Microcystic adnexal carcinoma: report of 13 cases and review of the literature. Dermatol Surg. 2001;27(4):401–8.
29. Eisen DB, Zloty D. Microcystic adnexal carcinoma involving a large portion of the face: when is surgery not reasonable? Dermatol Surg. 2005;31(11 Pt 1):1472–7.
30. Brookes JL, Bentley C, Verma S, Olver JM, McKee PH. Microcystic adnexal carcinoma masquerading as a chalazion. Br J Ophthalmol. 1998;82(2):196–7.
31. Carroll P, Goldstein GD, Brown Jr CW. Metastatic microcystic adnexal carcinoma in an immunocompromised patient. Dermatol Surg. 2000;26(6):531–4.
32. Lupton GP, McMarlin SL. Microcystic adnexal carcinoma. Report of a case with 30-year follow-up. Arch Dermatol. 1986;122(3):286–9.
33. Burns MK, Chen SP, Goldberg LH. Microcystic adnexal carcinoma. Ten cases treated by Mohs micrographic surgery. J Dermatol Surg Oncol. 1994;20(7):429–34.
34. Thomas CJ, Wood GC, Marks VJ. Mohs micrographic surgery in the treatment of rare aggressive cutaneous tumors: the Geisinger experience. Dermatol Surg. 2007;33(3):333–9.
35. Clement CI, Genge J, O'Donnell BA, et al. Orbital and periorbital microcystic adnexal carcinoma. Ophthal Plast Reconstr Surg. 2005;21(2):97–102.
36. Fernández-Figueras MT, Montero MA, Admella J, de la Torre N, Quer A, Ariza A. High (nuclear) grade adnexal carcinoma with microcystic adnexal carcinoma-like structural features. Am J Dermatopathol. 2006;28(4):346–51.
37. Wang SQ, Goldberg LH, Nemeth A. The merits of adding toluidine blue-stained slides in Mohs surgery in the treatment of a microcystic adnexal carcinoma. J Am Acad Dermatol. 2007;56(6):1067–9.
38. Ongenae KC, Verhaegh ME, Vermeulen AH, Naeyaert JM. Microcystic adnexal carcinoma: an uncommon tumor with debatable origin. Dermatol Surg. 2001;27(11):979–84.
39. Vidal CI, Goldberg M, Burstein DE, Emanuel HJ, Emanuel PO. p63 Immunohistochemistry is a useful adjunct in distinguishing sclerosing cutaneous tumors. Am J Dermatopathol. 2010;32(3):257–61.
40. Thosani MK, Marghoob A, Chen CS. Current progress of immunostains in Mohs micrographic surgery: a review. Dermatol Surg. 2008;34(12):1621–36. Epub October 13, 2008.
41. Abbas O, Bhawan J. Expression of stem cell markers nestin and cytokeratin 15 and 19 in cutaneous malignancies. J Eur Acad Dermatol Venereol. 2010;25(3):311–6.
42. Stein JM, Ormsby A, Esclamado R, Bailin P. The effect of radiation therapy on microcystic adnexal carcinoma: a case report. Head Neck. 2003;25(3):251–4.
43. Gabillot-Carré M, Weill F, Mamelle G, Kolb F, et al. Microcystic adnexal carcinoma: report of seven cases

including one with lung metastasis. Dermatology. 2006; 212(3):221–8.
44. Barlow RJ, Ramnarain N, Smith N, et al. Excision of selected skin tumours using Mohs' micrographic surgery with horizontal paraffin-embedded sections. Br J Dermatol. 1996; 135(6):911–7.
45. Khachemoune A, Olbricht SM, Johnson DS. Microcystic adnexal carcinoma: report of four cases treated with Mohs' micrographic surgical technique. Int J Dermatol. 2005; 44(6):507–12.
46. Hoppenreijs VP, Reuser TT, Mooy CM, et al. Syringomatous carcinoma of the eyelid and orbit: a clinical and histopathological challenge. Br J Ophthalmol. 1997;81(8): 668–72.
47. Bier-Lansing CM, Hom DB, Gapany M, Manivel JC, et al. Microcystic adnexal carcinoma: management options based on long-term follow-up. Laryngoscope. 1995;105(11): 1197–201.
48. Lupton GP, McMarlin SL. Microcystic adnexal carcinoma. Report of a case with 30-year follow-up. Arch Dermatol. 1986;122(3):286–9.
49. Kirkland PM, Solomons NB, Ratcliffe NA. Microcystic adnexal carcinoma. J Laryngol Otol. 1997;111(7):674–5.
50. Ban M, Sugie S, Kamiya H, Kitajima Y. Microcystic adnexal carcinoma with lymph node metastasis. Dermatology. 2003;207(4):395–7.
51. Rotter N, Wagner H, Fuchshuber S, Issing WJ. Cervical metastases of microcystic adnexal carcinoma in an otherwise healthy woman. Eur Arch Otorhinolaryngol. 2003; 260(5):254–7.
52. Ohta M, Hiramoto M, Ohtsuka H. Metastatic microcystic adnexal carcinoma: an autopsy case. Dermatol Surg. 2004; 30(6):957–60.
53. Yugueros P, Kane WJ, Goellner JR. Sweat gland carcinoma: a clinicopathologic analysis of an expanded series in a single institution. Plast Reconstr Surg. 1998;102(3): 705–10.
54. Gomez-Maestra MJ, España-Gregori E, Aviñó-Martinez JA, Mancheño-Franch N, Peña S. Brainstem and cavernous sinus metastases arising from a microcystic adnexal carcinoma of the eyebrow by perineural spreading. Can J Ophthalmol. 2009;44(3):e17–8.

21 Atypical Fibroxanthoma

Richelle M. Knudson, Robert H. Cook-Norris, Jeremy S. Youse, and Randall K. Roenigk

Abstract

Atypical fibroxanthoma (AFX) is an uncommon neoplasm that typically involves sun-damaged areas of the head and neck; it is seen most frequently in elderly white men. UV radiation has been found to cause DNA damage in dermal fibroblasts and has been associated with the development of AFX. AFX typically presents as a rapidly growing, red, often ulcerated nodule on the ear, face, or scalp. AFX can resemble several other neoplasms, both clinically and histologically. Therefore, histologic examination, along with use of immunohistochemical stains, is essential in the diagnosis of AFX. Once a diagnosis of AFX is made, the treatment of choice is complete surgical removal. Treatment with Mohs micrographic surgery (MMS) has been found to be superior to treatment with wide local excision (WLE). MMS has the advantages of allowing for tissue conservation, which is especially important on the head and neck, and of achieving total microscopic margin control. Local recurrence, metastasis to regional lymph nodes, and distant metastasis have been reported; therefore, regular, long-term follow-up is recommended for at least the first 2 years after diagnosis of AFX.

Keywords

Atypical fibroxanthoma • Mohs micrographic surgery • Malignant fibrous histiocytoma • Treatment • Pleomorphic sarcoma

Abbreviations

AFX Atypical fibroxanthoma
MFH Malignant fibrous histiocytoma
MMS Mohs micrographic surgery
WLE Wide local excision

R.M. Knudson • R.H. Cook-Norris (✉) • J.S. Youse • R.K. Roenigk
Department of Dermatology, Mayo Clinic, Rochester, MN, USA
e-mail: cooknorris.robert@mayo.edu; youse.jeremy@mayo.edu

Summary: History

- Atypical fibroxanthoma is a soft-tissue neoplasm.
- Benign clinical course despite highly atypical cells.
- Aggressive potential has been controversial.

K. Nouri (ed.), *Mohs Micrographic Surgery*,
DOI 10.1007/978-1-4471-2152-7_21, © Springer-Verlag London Limited 2012

21.1 History

The term *atypical fibroxanthoma* was first used by Helwig [1] in 1961 to describe a soft-tissue neoplasm that generally followed a benign clinical course despite having highly atypical cells. Since that time, there has been controversy regarding the aggressive potential of this neoplasm. It has been described by some to be a benign entity or "pseudomalignancy" [2–4], by others to have a very low risk of recurrence or metastasis [5], and by others to be highly aggressive with high metastatic potential [6–19]. Several different terms, such as *pseudosarcoma, paradoxical fibrosarcoma, pseudosarcomatous reticulohistiocytoma*, and *cutaneous malignant fibrous histiocytoma*, have been used to describe the entity now commonly called atypical fibroxanthoma [1, 20–22].

Summary: Pathogenesis

- Origin is undifferentiated mesenchymal progenitor cell.
- UV radiation implicated in pathogenesis.

Table 21.1 Location of atypical fibroxanthoma by age at diagnosis in 93 patients

Location	All patients	Age at diagnosis <65 years (*n*=17)	≥65 years (*n*=76)
Face	64 (68.8)	10 (58.8)	54 (71.0)
Forehead	7	2	5
Temple	3	1	2
Suprabrow	1	0	1
Cheek	8	1	7
Chin	1	1	0
Lip	2	0	2
Nasal tip	4	1	3
Dorsal nose	2	0	2
Nasal ala	2	1	1
Postauricular	2	0	2
Ear	32	3	29
Scalp	14 (15.1)	2 (11.8)	12 (15.8)
Neck	1 (1.1)	0	1 (1.3)
Chest or back	2 (2.1)	2 (11.8)	0
Upper extremity	8 (8.6)	3 (17.6)	5 (6.6)
Lower extremity	2 (2.1)	0	2 (2.6)
Not documented	2 (2.1)	0	2 (2.6)

Adapted from Ang et al. [6]. Used with permission

[a] Values are no. of patients (%)

21.2 Pathogenesis

AFX is thought to originate from an undifferentiated mesenchymal progenitor cell that can differentiate into histiocytic, fibroblastic, or myofibroblastic phenotypes [23–25]. UV radiation, associated with the development of AFX [26], affects DNA molecules by causing the formation of cyclobutane pyrimidine dimers and pyrimidine-pyrimidone [4] photoproducts [27]. Specifically, single or double cytosine to thymine transitions are formed at dipyrimidine sites exclusively by UV photoproducts [28, 29]. Additionally, UV-induced p53 gene mutations at dipyrimidine sites have been demonstrated in AFX and have been implicated in its pathogenesis [30, 31].

Summary: Clinical Features

- Most common location is head and neck.
- Many different clinical presentations.

21.3 Clinical Features

AFX is an uncommon cutaneous tumor and generally occurs on the head or neck (Table 21.1) [6]. The male-to-female ratio has been reported to be 3:1, and older men of European descent are affected most often [5]. AFX tends to occur in patients with a previous history of skin cancer involving the head and neck. This distribution is thought to be a result of its association with UV radiation and sun exposure. Typically, patients initially have a red, often ulcerated, rapidly growing nodule on the ear, face, or scalp [5, 6, 32]. Clinical distinction of AFX from other neoplasms is difficult without histopathologic examination because it can resemble basal-cell carcinoma, squamous cell carcinoma, or keratoacanthoma (Fig. 21.1a–c). The average lesion size at diagnosis is 1.5–2.0 cm [6, 33–35]. Some reports suggest that patients younger than 65 years are more likely than older patients to have an AFX on a limb or areas other than the head and neck, but the data have been inconsistent [5, 6, 8, 36–39]. Involvement in areas of previous trauma and radiation therapy has

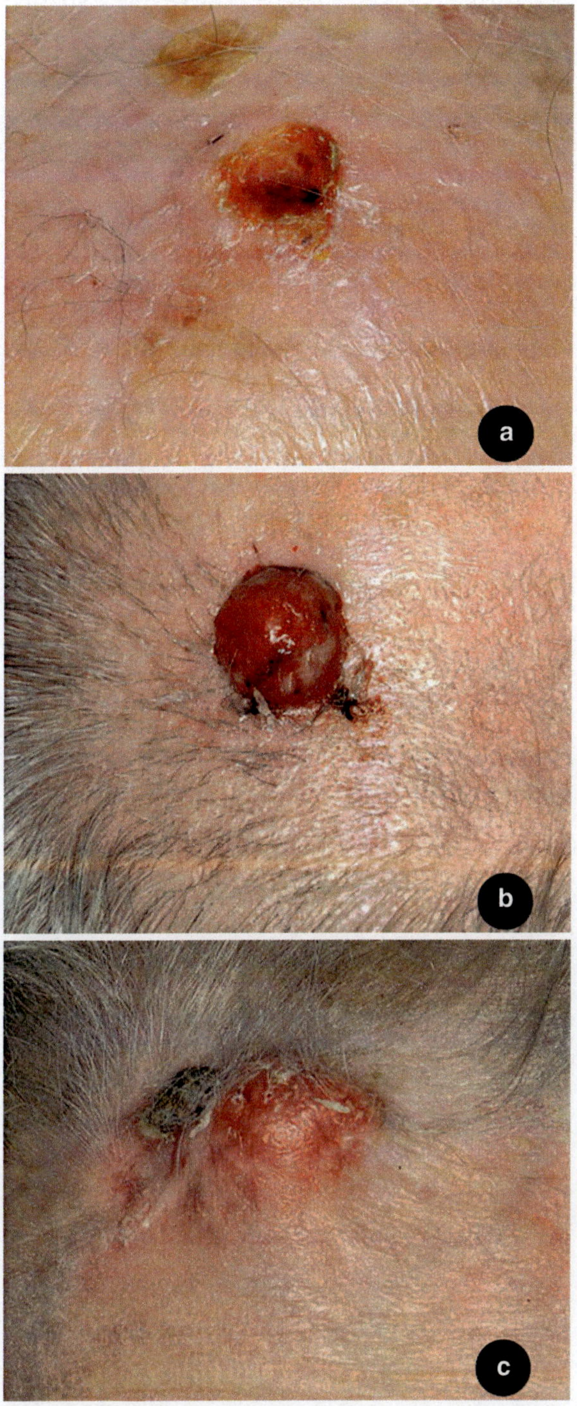

Fig. 21.1 Examples of atypical fibroxanthoma. (**a**) Superficially ulcerated plaque with overlying crust on the forehead. (**b**) Exophytic friable nodule on the scalp. (**c**) Red nodule with overlying crust on the forehead

been reported [4, 5]. Factors associated with a worse outcome include previous exposure to radiation, immunosuppression, and larger tumor size.

The metastatic potential of AFX has been a topic of controversy. Some consider it to be a benign process, whereas others regard it as a tumor with high metastatic potential [2–4, 6–19]. At least 22 cases of metastatic AFX have been reported in the literature, 12 involving regional lymph nodes [17]. Other sites of metastasis have included the parotid gland, peritoneum, liver, lung, soft tissue near the mastoid, and in-transit cutaneous metastases [7, 10, 11, 13, 15, 18]. A review of all the metastatic cases reported in the English-language literature showed that, of those with metastatic disease, 36% of cases (8/22) had a local recurrence at the primary tumor site, and the average time between diagnosis of the primary tumor and discovery of metastatic disease was 19.7 months [17]. At least five deaths due to metastasis have been reported in the literature [6, 7, 11, 37, 40].

Summary: Pathology

- Well-demarcated dermal proliferation of highly atypical, pleomorphic epithelioid, spindle, and multinucleated cells.
- Diagnosis made by excluding other malignant tumors (spindle cell melanoma, spindle cell squamous cell carcinoma, and leiomyosarcoma).
- Immunohistochemical stains are essential in making the diagnosis.
- AFX is negative for S100, cytokeratin stains, and desmin.

21.4 Pathology

Histologically, AFX is composed of a well-demarcated dermal proliferation of highly atypical, pleomorphic epithelioid, spindle, and multinucleated cells, generally within a surrounding background of solar elastosis (Fig. 21.2) [32]. Atypical mitoses are frequently present. Generally, involvement of the subcutaneous or deeper tissues is minimal. If involvement of the subcutaneous tissue is present, it is generally focal and limited. Several morphologic patterns have been described, including pleomorphic spindle and epithelioid cells, predominantly spindle cells, purely spindle cells, and

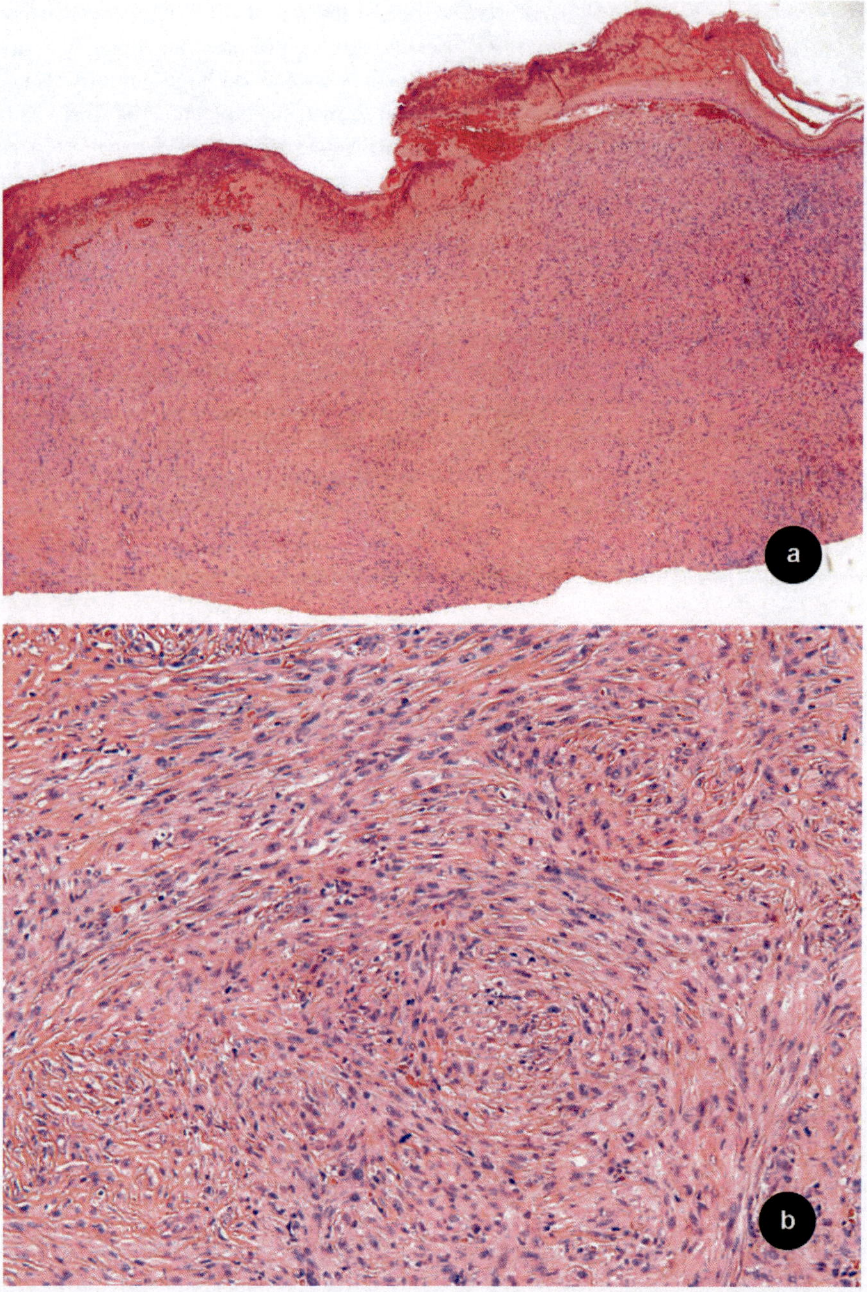

Fig. 21.2 Micrographs of atypical fibroxanthoma. Hematoxylin-eosin-stained biopsy specimens. (**a**) Original magnification, ×4. (**b**) Original magnification, ×20. Highly atypical pleomorphic epithelioid, spindle, and multinucleated cells are seen

predominantly epithelioid cells [32]. Various histologic variants also have been described, including keloidal, myxoid, clear cell, granular cell, and osteoclastlike giant cell variants; a spindle cell nonpleomorphic variant; variants with plaquelike changes; and tumors with hemorrhagic and pseudoangiomatous areas [5, 32].

Other entities have a similar histologic morphology to AFX, including spindle cell melanoma, leiomyosarcoma, and spindle cell squamous cell carcinoma. The diagnosis of AFX, therefore, is made by excluding other malignant neoplasms with a similar histologic appearance. The use of immunohistochemical stains

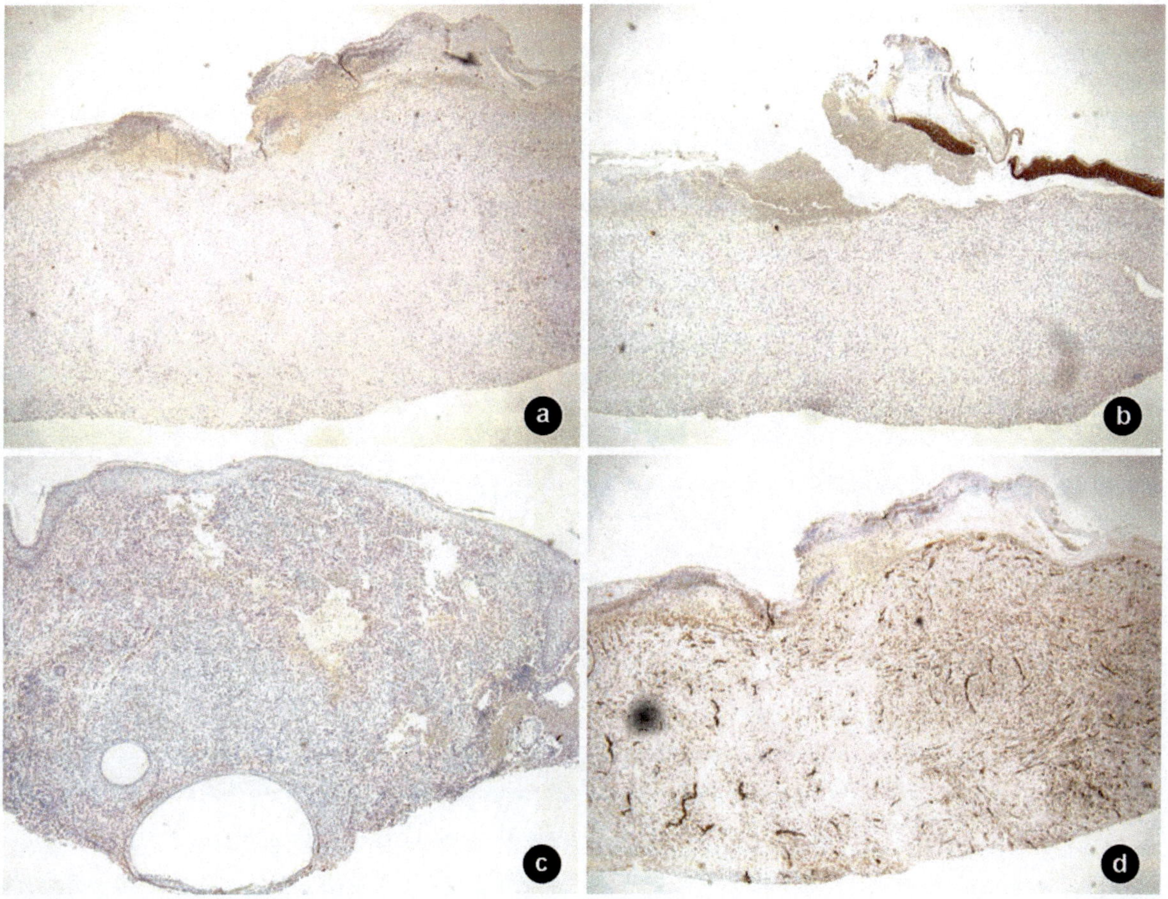

Fig. 21.3 Immunohistochemical staining in atypical fibroxanthoma. Staining with antibodies to various proteins shows that the tumor cells are negative for S100 (**a**), are negative for wide-spectrum keratin (**b**), are negative for desmin (**c**), and have focal positivity for CD31 (**d**). Original magnifications, ×4

is therefore essential in the diagnosis of AFX. AFX is negative for S100 protein (excludes spindle cell melanoma), high- and low-molecular-weight cytokeratins (generally exclude spindle cell squamous cell carcinoma), and desmin (excludes leiomyosarcoma) (Fig. 21.3). Scattered or grouped S100-positive Langerhans cells can be found in AFX, however; therefore, staining for CD1a can be useful in highlighting Langerhans cells in AFX. Use of stains for several other proteins has been reported in the literature, with variable results. Focal positivity has been reported for CD31 (Fig. 21.3); smooth muscle actin has been either focally positive or frequently positive; epithelial membrane antigen has been either negative or focally positive; and CD68 and vimentin were frequently found to be positive [5]. In some cases of spindle cell squamous cell carcinoma, keratin reactivity can be only focal or absent. Staining for high-molecular-weight cytokeratin 34βE12 and p63 has been found to be helpful in distinguishing poorly differentiated squamous cell carcinomas from AFX [3, 41–43]. Procollagen 1 staining also has been reported to be useful in the diagnosis of AFX but must be interpreted carefully because it can also be positive in desmoplastic malignant melanoma and desmoplastic squamous cell carcinoma [44].

Some have considered AFX to represent a superficial variant of malignant fibrous histiocytoma (MFH), which has recently been given the name *pleomorphic sarcoma* because the specific line of differentiation is unknown. Some consider these tumors to be on a spectrum, being classified as AFX when based in the dermis, superficial MFH when based in the subcutaneous tissue, and deep MFH when based in the deep soft tissue and skeletal muscle [39]. Typically, MFH lesions are larger, invade deeper,

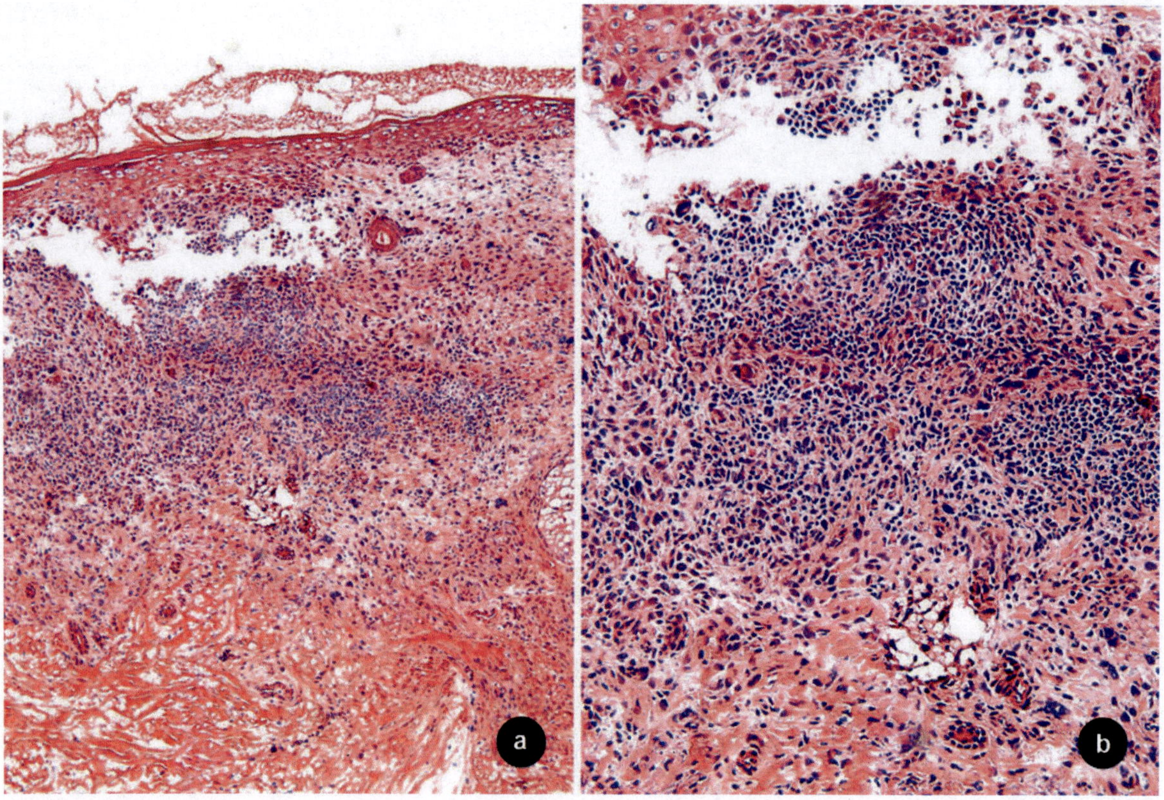

Fig. 21.4 Frozen section samples of atypical fibroxanthoma obtained by Mohs micrographic surgery. Hematoxylin-eosin staining. (**a**) Original magnification, ×10. (**b**) Original magnification, ×20

have frequent necrosis, and have vascular or perineural invasion. Staining for LN-2 (CD74) has been reported to be stronger in MFH than in AFX [45]. The relationship between UV radiation and lesion development has not been found with MFH as it has for AFX, which suggests that MFH and AFX have different mechanisms of molecular pathogenesis [30, 31]. MFH has been reported to be more aggressive than AFX, often with more-frequent recurrences and a greater propensity to metastasize, and therefore has a poorer prognosis than AFX.

Summary: Treatment

- Treatment of choice is complete surgical removal.
- Recently, Mohs micrographic surgery has been found to be superior to wide local excision.
- Recurrence rate has been reported to be 5%.
- Long-term follow-up is important to detect recurrence and/or metastasis.

21.5 Treatment

The treatment modality of choice for AFX is complete surgical removal. This is usually achieved using WLE, or total microscopic margin control is achieved using MMS (Fig. 21.4) [6, 33, 46, 47]. Historically, AFX has been treated with WLE because it was thought that complete, conservative, local excision was adequate treatment [4, 14, 48, 49]. A recommendation of 6-mm margins, similar to treatment recommendations for squamous cell carcinoma, was advocated [50]. However, no large studies have defined what constitutes *adequate* margins.

Many studies in recent decades have reported MMS to be superior to WLE for treatment of AFX, and therefore MMS is now the recommended treatment for AFX [6, 33–35, 46, 51–53]. The advantages of MMS are that it allows for both tissue conservation, which is especially important on the head and neck, and achievement of total microscopic margin control.

Two studies have compared WLE and MMS for the treatment of AFX. Davis et al. [33] reported their experience with 44 patients with AFX, of which 19 were treated with MMS and 25 were treated with WLE. There were no recurrences in patients treated with MMS after a mean follow-up of 29.6 months. In the 25 patients treated with WLE, there were 4 recurrences (16%) with a mean time to recurrence of 16 months [33, 53]. In a more recent study by Ang et al. [6] of patients with AFX, 59 of 88 tumors (67%) were treated with MMS, 23 (26.1%) were treated with WLE, and 6 (6.8%) were treated with other modalities (5 with electrodesiccation and curettage and 1 with shave excision). After a median follow-up of 4.5 years, there were no recurrences in those treated with MMS; there were 2 recurrences (8.7%) in patients treated with WLE after a median follow-up of 8.7 years.

Several other groups have reported their experience with the use of MMS for treatment of AFX [34, 35, 51, 54]. Of 13 cases of AFX treated with MMS reported by Seavolt et al. [35], follow-up data were available for 6 patients, and there were no recurrences after 2 years. Limmer et al. [51] reported treatment of AFX with MMS in six patients, and no recurrences were noted. In contrast to all previous studies reporting no recurrences after treatment with MMS, Huether et al. [34] reported 2 recurrences in 29 patients (6.9%) after a mean follow-up of 3.3 years.

The few data reported regarding the surgical margins necessary for tumor clearance have been conflicting. Limmer et al. [51] reported an average of 9-mm surgical margins for clearance of tumor. In contrast, Ang et al. [6] reported that the median margin needed for tumor clearance with MMS was 0.4 cm (range, 0–3.2 cm), but the margin was greater than 2.0 cm in two patients (3.4%). Therefore, if AFX is treated with WLE, a 2-cm margin would be necessary for clearance of 96.6% of tumors.

Because of the potential of AFX to metastasize to regional lymph nodes, sentinel lymph node biopsy has been suggested [7, 55]. However, there are essentially no data in the literature defining the role of sentinel lymph node biopsy after a diagnosis of AFX.

Adjuvant radiation therapy has been used both for locally recurrent AFX and for affected lymph nodes in metastatic disease [17, 50, 55]. The use of radiation therapy and/or adjuvant chemotherapy after surgical treatment of primary AFX, however, has not been reported.

The recurrence rate for AFX after removal has been reported to be 5% [19]. This rate is much different than the recurrence rates of 2–21% reported in the 1960s and 1970s [8, 48, 56, 57]. The true recurrence rate of AFX today is much lower than that reported in the past, most likely because more patients are being treated with MMS or because wider excision margins are being used with WLE. Because of the potential for recurrence, regular follow-up is necessary. Long-term follow-up including examination and palpation of the surgical site, palpation of regional lymph nodes, and possible evaluation for distant metastatic disease is also very important. This should be performed regularly for at least the first 2 years after diagnosis, because this is when most recurrences and metastases have been reported to occur [6, 17].

Summary: Conclusion

- AFX has the potential for regional and/or distant metastasis.
- Complete surgical removal of the primary tumor, ideally with MMS, is recommended.
- Long-term follow-up is important to detect recurrence and/or metastasis.

21.6 Conclusion

It is important to recognize the potential for regional and/or distant metastasis with a diagnosis of AFX. Therefore, complete surgical removal of the primary tumor, ideally with MMS, is recommended. MMS allows for total microscopic margin control and at the same time allows for tissue conservation. This is especially important for tumors on the head and neck, where AFX is most likely to occur. Long-term follow-up is essential for monitoring for the development of recurrence or metastasis.

References

1. Helwig EB. Atypical fibroxanthoma: proceedings of the 18th annual tumor seminar San Antonio Society of Pathologists, 1961. Tex State J Med. 1963;59:664–7.
2. Connors R, Ackerman A. Histologic pseudomalignancies of the skin. Arch Dermatol. 1976;112:1767–80.

3. Gleason BC, Calder KB, Cibull TL, et al. Utility of p63 in the differential diagnosis of atypical fibroxanthoma and spindle cell squamous cell carcinoma. J Cutan Pathol. 2009;36:543–7.
4. Starink TH, Hausman R, Van Delden L, Neering H. Atypical fibroxanthoma of the skin. Presentation of 5 cases and a review of the literature. Br J Dermatol. 1977;97:167–77.
5. Beer TW, Drury P, Heenan PJ. Atypical fibroxanthoma: a histological and immunohistochemical review of 171 cases. Am J Dermatopathol. 2010;32(6):533–40.
6. Ang GC, Roenigk RK, Otley CC, Kim Phillips P, Weaver AL. More than 2 decades of treating atypical fibroxanthoma at Mayo Clinic: what have we learned from 91 patients? Dermatol Surg. 2009;35:765–72.
7. Cooper JZ, Newman SR, Scott GA, Brown MD. Metastasizing atypical fibroxanthoma (cutaneous malignant histiocytoma): report of five cases. Dermatol Surg. 2005; 31:221–5.
8. Dahl I. Atypical fibroxanthoma of the skin: a clinico-pathological study of 57 cases. Acta Pathol Microbiol Scand A. 1976;84:183–97.
9. Grosso M, Lentini M, Carrozza G, Catalano A. Metastatic atypical fibroxanthoma of skin. Pathol Res Pract. 1987; 182:443–7.
10. Guiffrida TJ, Kligora CJ, Goldstein GD. Localized cutaneous metastases from an atypical fibroxanthoma. Dermatol Surg. 2004;30:1561–4.
11. Helwig EB, May D. Atypical fibroxanthoma of the skin with metastasis. Cancer. 1986;57:368–76.
12. Jacobs DS, Edwards WD, Ye RC. Metastatic atypical fibroxanthoma of skin. Cancer. 1975;35:368–76.
13. Kargi E, Gungor E, Verdi M, et al. Atypical fibroxanthoma and metastasis to the lung. Plast Reconstr Surg. 2003;111: 1760–2.
14. Kemp JD, Stenn KS, Arons M, Fischer J. Metastasizing atypical fibroxanthoma: coexistence with chronic lymphocytic leukemia. Arch Dermatol. 1978;114:1533–5.
15. Lum DJ, King AR. Peritoneal metastases from an atypical fibroxanthoma. Am J Surg Pathol. 2006;30:1041–6.
16. Muenster MR, Hoang MP. Left facial mass in an elderly man: metastasizing atypical fibroxanthoma of the skin. Arch Pathol Lab Med. 2006;130:735–6.
17. New D, Bahrami S, Malone J, Callen JP. Atypical fibroxanthoma with regional lymph node metastasis: report of a case and review of the literature. Arch Dermatol. 2010;146(12): 1399–404.
18. Sankar NM, Pang KS, Thiruchelvam T, Meldrum-Hanna WG. Metastasis from atypical fibroxanthoma of skin. Med J Aust. 1998;168:418–9.
19. Weedon D. Tumors and tumor-like proliferations of fibrous and related tissues. 2nd ed. London: Churchill Livingston; 2002.
20. Bourne RG. Paradoxical fibrosarcoma of the skin (pseudosarcoma): a review of 13 cases. Med J Aust. 1963;1:504–10.
21. Finlay-Jones LR, Nicoll P, ten Seldam RE. Pseudosarcoma of the skin. Pathology. 1971;3:215–22.
22. Gordon HW. Pseudosarcomatous reticulohistiocytoma. Arch Dermatol. 1964;90:319–25.
23. Alguacil-Garcia A, Unni KK, Goellner JR, Winkelmann RK. Atypical fibroxanthoma of the skin: an ultrastructural study of two cases. Cancer. 1977;40:1471–80.
24. Barr RJ, Wuerker RB, Graham JH. Ultrastructure of atypical fibroxanthoma. Cancer. 1977;40:736–43.
25. Longacre TA, Smoller BR, Rouse RV. Atypical fibroxanthoma. Multiple immunohistologic profiles. Am J Surg Pathol. 1993;17:1199–209.
26. Hall PA, McKee PH, Menage HD, Dover R, Lane DP. High levels of p53 protein in UV-irradiated normal human skin. Oncogene. 1993;8:203–7.
27. Moan J, Peak MJ. Effects of UV radiation of cells. J Photochem Photobiol B. 1989;4:21–34.
28. Larson KL, Strauss BS. Influence of template strandedness on in vitro replications of mutagen-damaged DNA. Biochemistry. 1987;26:2471–9.
29. Vogelstein B, Kinzler KW. Carcinogens leave fingerprints. Nature. 1992;355:209–10.
30. Dei Tos AP, Maestro R, Doglioni C, et al. Ultraviolet-induced p53 mutations in atypical fibroxanthoma. Am J Pathol. 1994;145:11–7.
31. Sakamoto A, Oda Y, Itakura E, et al. Immunoexpression of ultraviolet photoproducts and p53 mutation analysis in atypical fibroxanthoma and superficial malignant fibrous histiocytoma. Mod Pathol. 2001;14:581–8.
32. Luzar B, Calonje E. Morphological and immunohistochemical characteristics of atypical fibroxanthoma with a special emphasis on potential diagnostic pitfalls: a review. J Cutan Pathol. 2010;37:301–9.
33. Davis JL, Randle HW, Zalla MJ, Roenigk RK, Brodland DG. A comparison of Mohs micrographic surgery and wide excision for the treatment of atypical fibroxanthoma. Dermatol Surg. 1997;23:105–10.
34. Huether MJ, Zitelli JA, Brodland DG. Mohs micrographic surgery for the treatment of spindle cell tumors of the skin. J Am Acad Dermatol. 2001;44:656–9.
35. Seavolt M, McCall M. Atypical fibroxanthoma: review of the literature and summary of 13 patients treated with Mohs micrographic surgery. Dermatol Surg. 2006;32:435–41.
36. Evans HL, Smith JL. Spindle cell squamous carcinomas and sarcoma-like tumors of the skin: a comparative study of 38 cases. Cancer. 1980;45:2687–97.
37. Fretzin DF, Helwig EB. Atypical fibroxanthoma of the skin. A clinicopathologic study of 140 cases. Cancer. 1973;31: 1541–52.
38. Leong AS, Milios J. Atypical fibroxanthoma of the skin: a clinicopathological and immunohistochemical study and a discussion of its histogenesis. Histopathology. 1987;11: 463–75.
39. Weiss SW, Goldblum JR. Enzinger and Weiss's Soft Tissue Tumors, 5th edition, Mosby, 2008.
40. Rizzardi C, Angiero F, Melato M. Atypical fibroxanthoma and malignant fibrous histiocytoma of the skin. Anticancer Res. 2003;23:1847–51.
41. Dotto JE, Glusac EJ. p63 is a useful marker for cutaneous spindle cell squamous cell carcinoma. J Cutan Pathol. 2006;33:413–7.
42. Gray Y, Robidoux HJ, Farrell DS, Robinson-Bostom L. Squamous cell carcinoma detected by high-molecular-weight cytokeratin immunostaining mimicking atypical fibroxanthoma. Arch Pathol Lab Med. 2001;125: 799–802.
43. Greene LA, Cooper K. Atypical fibroxanthoma: an immunohistochemistry update. Adv Anat Pathol. 2008;15:374.

44. Jensen K, Wilkinson B, Wines N, Kossard S. Procollagen 1 expression in atypical fibroxanthoma and other tumors. J Cutan Pathol. 2004;31:57–61.
45. Lazova R, Moynes R, May D, Scott G. LN-2 (CD74). A marker to distinguish atypical fibroxanthoma from malignant fibrous histiocytoma. Cancer. 1997;79:2115–24.
46. Brown MD, Swanson NA. Treatment of malignant fibrous histiocytoma and atypical fibrous xanthomas with micrographic surgery. J Dermatol Surg Oncol. 1989;15:1287–92.
47. Dzubow LM. Mohs surgery report: spindle cell fibrohistiocytic tumors: classification and pathophysiology. J Dermatol Surg Oncol. 1988;14:490–5.
48. Kempson RL, McGavran MH. Atypical fibroxanthomas of the skin. Cancer. 1964;17:1463–71.
49. Poleksic S, Kalwaic HJ, Bialas RF. Benign atypical fibroxanthoma or a malignant tumor? A warning. Case reports. Plast Reconstr Surg. 1976;58:501–5.
50. Wylie J, Hampton N, Telfer MR, Clarke AM. Atypical fibroxanthoma: case series of 16 patients. Br J Oral Maxillofac Surg. 2010;48:466–8.
51. Limmer BL, Clark DP. Cutaneous micrographic surgery for atypical fibroxanthoma. Dermatol Surg. 1997;23:553–8.
52. Nouri K, Rivas MP. A primer of Mohs micrographic surgery: uncommon indications. Skin Med. 2004;3:259–65.
53. Zalla MJ, Randle HW, Brodland DG, Davis JL, Roenigk RK. Mohs surgery vs. wide excision for atypical fibroxanthoma: follow up. Dermatol Surg. 1997;23:1223–4.
54. Anderson PJ, McPhaden AR, Ratcliffe RJ. Atypical fibroxanthoma of the scalp. Head Neck. 2001;23:399–403.
55. Sahn RE, Lang PG. Sentinel lymph node biopsy for high-risk nonmelanoma skin cancers. Dermatol Surg. 2007;33:786–93.
56. Kroe DJ, Pitcock JA. Atypical fibroxanthoma of the skin: report of ten cases. Am J Clin Pathol. 1969;51:487–92.
57. Vargas-Cortes F, Winkelmann RK, Soule EH. Atypical fibroxanthomas of the skin: further observations with 19 additional cases. Mayo Clin Proc. 1973;48:211–8.

Extramammary Paget Disease

22

Bradley G. Merritt and David G. Brodland

Abstract

EMPD is an intraepidermal adenocarcinoma most often limited to the epidermis, with typical cases affecting genital skin in women and men. In patients with invasive disease, prognosis is based on the degree of invasion, with tumors less than 1 mm deep having very low mortality. Careful evaluation for an underlying malignancy should be carried out to exclude life-threatening disease, but the association of many coexistent malignancies is controversial. Reported underlying adnexal adenocarcinoma may, at least in some patients, represent invasive spread of primary epidermal disease. Mohs surgery has proven effective in the treatment of EMPD, and the implementation of CK7 immunostaining shows promise in further reducing the recurrence rate. Alternative treatments, including topical treatment with imiquimod and 5-fluorouracil as well as photodynamic therapy, may be effective in select cases of EMPD.

Keywords

Extramammary Paget disease • Adnexal adenocarcinoma • Apocrine glands • Mohs surgery • CK7 Immunostaining

Summary: Introduction

- EMPD is an intraepidermal adenocarcinoma usually limited to the epidermis, typically involving genital skin in women and men.
- Careful evaluation for an underlying malignancy should be carried out to exclude life-threatening disease, but the association of many coexistent malignancies is controversial.
- EMPD often shows dramatic subclinical spread. Recommended margins range from 1 to 5 cm.

B.G. Merritt (✉)
Department of Dermatology, UNC – Chapel Hill, Chapel Hill, NC, USA
e-mail: bgm2705@yahoo.com

D.G. Brodland
Departments of Dermatology and Otolaryngology, Shadyside Medical Center, University of Pittsburgh Medical Center, Pittsburgh, PA, USA

K. Nouri (ed.), *Mohs Micrographic Surgery*,
DOI 10.1007/978-1-4471-2152-7_22, © Springer-Verlag London Limited 2012

- EMPD demonstrates high rates of recurrence with standard excision.
- Mohs surgery has proven effective in the treatment of EMPD, and the implementation of CK7 immunostaining shows promise in further reducing the recurrence rate.

22.1 Introduction

Extramammary Paget disease (EMPD) is a rare, intraepithelial adenocarcinoma that affects anatomic regions with abundant apocrine sweat glands. The disease exists most commonly in a primary form, originating in the epidermis or cutaneous adnexa. Less often, EMPD occurs in a secondary form, associated with an underlying internal malignancy, usually of the lower gastrointestinal or urinary tract. Secondary EMPD is also reported to occur in association with underlying adnexal adenocarcinoma, though it is impossible in many cases to determine if epidermal disease leads to subsequent deeper, dermal adnexal involvement or epidermal disease results from epidermotropic spread of underlying adnexal adenocarcinoma. Adnexal adenocarcinoma can also develop as a separate neoplastic process, difficult to distinguish from EMPD. It is likely that EMPD represents the clinical manifestation of a variety of neoplastic processes.

When limited to the epidermis, primary EMPD is not life-threatening, but invasive disease can occur and may portend a poor prognosis, depending on depth of invasion, the degree of dermal adnexal involvement, as well as the presence of lymphovascular invasion. Patients with primary EMPD have a better prognosis than those with secondary EMPD due to the association of the latter with internal malignancy, so it is important to perform a full evaluation to exclude coexistent malignancy. Not only do patients with secondary EMPD have a significantly higher mortality rate up to 50% that is related to underlying internal malignancy; the presence of secondary EMPD signifies a worse prognosis compared to patients without EMPD who have the same coexistent malignancy.

Recent advances in immunohistochemistry have improved our understanding of the potential etiology of EMPD and allowed for more accurate diagnosis. Immunohistochemistry has been explored as a tool to aid in differentiating primary from secondary EMPD. The addition of CK7 staining to Mohs surgery has led to improved surgical margin control for a disease notorious for indistinct clinical margins, high rates of recurrence, and significant morbidity.

Surgical excision remains the mainstay of treatment for EMPD, and Mohs micrographic surgery is considered the treatment of choice in many cases, allowing for precise margin control with reduced recurrence rates. Alternative treatment regimens continue to be explored, including topical treatment with 5-fluorouracil and imiquimod, photodynamic therapy, laser vaporization, chemotherapy, and radiation therapy.

Summary: History of EMPD and Epidemiology

- EMPD is a disease of apocrine gland-bearing areas.
- EMPD most commonly affects Caucasian women ages 64–75.
- Primary and secondary EMPD are important to distinguish.
- Between 4% and 42% of patients with EMPD have or develop coexistent malignancy, though the association is not always clear. The affected age group is at higher baseline risk for malignancy, and causality is difficult to establish.
- Lower gastrointestinal and genitourinary malignancies are the most common associated underlying internal cancers.
- EMPD originating in deeper adnexal structures is sometimes present and may lead to epidermal disease by upward spread, though invasive disease originating in the epidermis secondarily affecting adnexa may be impossible to distinguish. In many cases, therefore, reportedly associated underlying adnexal adenocarcinoma may be a misnomer.

22.2 History of EMPD and Epidemiology

22.2.1 History of EMPD

Paget published the first series of cases of mammary Paget disease in 1874, describing 15 women with an intraepithelial adenocarcinoma associated with underlying breast cancer [1]. Fifteen years later, Crocker described an intraepithelial adenocarcinoma of the penis and scrotum with histopathologic features indistinguishable from Paget disease [2]. As case reports have accumulated in the medical literature, EMPD is now known to occur in areas rich in apocrine glands, including the vulvar, perianal, penoscrotal, and axillary areas, with rare involvement of the auditory canal, umbilicus, extramammary chest, thighs, tongue, eyelids, and cheek. Since Crocker's initial report over 100 years ago, the natural history of EMPD is better understood, but much about the etiology and pathogenic mechanism of the neoplasm remains a mystery.

22.2.2 Epidemiology

EMPD is rare, with an incidence estimated to be 0.11 per 100,000 person years [3]. Of all cases of Paget disease (both mammary and extramammary), EMPD accounts for 7–14% [3]. One of the largest registries including patients with mammary and extramammary Paget disease documents EMPD patients having invasive disease 21% of the time, compared to 44% of patients with invasive mammary Paget disease [3].

The age of onset of EMPD is typically 64–75 years, with no significant difference for patients with in situ versus invasive disease. Caucasian women and Asian men are affected at disproportionately high rates. Reasons for this discrepancy are unclear. In Caucasian patients, women predominate with a ratio ranging from 1.4:1 to 3.2:1, whereas in Asian patients, men predominate 2.2:1 to 14:1 [4]. EMPD with internal malignancy is less common in Asian patients when compared to Caucasian patients [4]. It has been speculated that this is due to the lower overall prevalence in the Asian population of cancers associated with secondary EMPD, including rectal cancer and urinary tract adenocarcinoma.

22.2.3 Associated Malignancies

Of patients with EMPD, 5–42% are reported to have an additional malignancy documented either before or after development of EMPD. These range from extragenital skin cancer to distant internal malignancies. The wide range of published percentages of second malignancy as well as the spectrum of different cancers has led to significant controversy regarding the true association between internal malignancies and EMPD. The baseline risk of cancer in the aged population typically affected by EMPD may account for many of the reported second malignancies. Nevertheless, the rate of internal malignancy is higher in patients with EMPD with a standardized incidence ratio of 1.7 [3]. The presence of EMPD should prompt a search for internal malignancy, especially of the lower gastrointestinal or genitourinary tract.

Of those patients with EMPD and a second malignancy, slightly more than half present with a second malignancy prior to their diagnosis of EMPD with a median time from diagnosis of primary malignancy until the diagnosis of EMPD ranging from 2.8 to 10.9 years. For patients diagnosed with EMPD prior to the diagnosis of a second malignancy, the median time to diagnosis of the second malignancy is 2.9–3.8 years [3]. The wide range noted in these patients further calls into question the likelihood of any true association of EMPD and a second malignancy in many cases.

In cases of EMPD with coexistent internal cancer, the location of EMPD is often correlated with site of the underlying internal malignancy. Perianal EMPD is associated with lower gastrointestinal malignancy, and penoscrotal EMPD is associated with urinary tract malignancy.

Distant internal malignancies reported in association with EMPD include breast carcinoma, ovarian carcinoma, bile duct carcinoma, hepatocellular carcinoma, renal cell carcinoma, lung carcinoma, stomach carcinoma, and pancreatic carcinoma [5, 6]. Whether a true association exists between distant primary neoplasms and EMPD or the tumors are coincidental remains to be proven. However, it is possible that there is a common yet undefined subcellular mechanism that leads to an increased incidence of diverse and distant synchronous or metachronous malignancy, a so-called oncogenic stimulus.

Though recent authors consider secondary EMPD to be a disease only related to underlying internal malignancy, some also classify EMPD related to local, deeper adnexal adenocarcinoma as secondary EMPD. Many EMPD cases labeled as secondary to underlying adnexal adenocarcinoma may actually be primary EMPD with deeper spread and subsequent adnexal involvement. It may be impossible to distinguish the initial site of malignancy as epidermal with invasive spread into deeper structures, or adnexal with upward, Pagetoid spread into the epidermis. Nevertheless, vulvar EMPD is reportedly associated with cutaneous adnexal adenocarcinoma 4–8% of the time and an internal malignancy documented 20% of the time [7]. Perianal EMPD is reported to be associated with cutaneous adnexal adenocarcinoma 7% of the time, with internal malignancy documented 14% of the time [7]. These numbers should be interpreted with caution, however, given the difficulty in assessing whether an underlying adnexal adenocarcinoma is truly a separate process.

The phenomenon of potential tumor spread from epithelial lining of internal organs locally contiguous to the skin has also been described, especially in vulvar EMPD. EMPD in association with endometrial, endocervical, vaginal, Bartholin's gland, urethral, and bladder neoplasms may arise by this mechanism [5].

22.2.4 Affected Areas: Sites with Apocrine Glands

EMPD is primarily a disease of apocrine gland-bearing skin. Apocrine glands are thought to function as a scent gland, primarily a form of sweat gland with secretions rich in sialomucin. At birth, apocrine glands are located in abundance in the axillary and anogenital areas. The glands become active in these regions during puberty. Modified apocrine glands are found in the eyelids (Moll's glands), external auditory canal, and nipple, where the glands contribute lipid secretions to tears, cerumen (ear wax), and milk, respectively. Apocrine glands are also found in the periumbilical region.

Given the abundance of apocrine glands in the vulvar area, it is not surprising that this is the most common site for EMPD in women, with about 67% of all cases presenting in female genital skin [3]. In men, EMPD most frequently affects genital skin. Rare cases have been reported in other apocrine gland-bearing areas, including the eyelids, auditory canal, and periumbilical skin.

Ectopic EMPD, disease occurring in skin without apocrine glands, has been reported on the sternum, buttock, back, chest, scalp, hypochondrium, upper abdomen, and face. The germinative milk line is a possible source for the origination of ectopic EMPD. It has been reported primarily in the Asian population [8, 9].

Summary: Clinical Presentation and Natural History

- EMPD is often diagnosed 2–4 years after onset of symptoms.
- Erythematous plaques with pruritus are the most common clinical presentation.
- Primary EMPD has an excellent overall survival but high local recurrence rate.
- The prognosis of invasive EMPD is related to depth of dermal invasion from the dermoepidermal junction.
- The prognosis of patients with secondary EMPD is poor and related to underlying malignancy.
- Though distinguishing EMPD arising in the epidermis with subsequent adnexal adenocarcinoma and EMPD secondary to adnexal carcinoma may be impossible, the presence of deeper adnexal adenocarcinoma signifies a worse prognosis.

22.3 Clinical Presentation and Natural History

22.3.1 Clinical Presentation

The diagnosis of EMPD is usually made after multiple other diagnoses have been considered and their typical treatment regimens failed. The differential diagnosis includes Bowen's disease, tinea cruris, contact dermatitis, lichen simplex chronicus, lichen planus, cutaneous T-cell lymphoma, psoriasis, and seborrheic dermatitis [10]. The average time from the onset of symptoms to diagnosis of EMPD is 2–4 years, but protracted courses of over 10 years prior to the final diagnosis are not uncommon. Onset is often insidious, and a high degree of clinical suspicion should be present in any vulvar, perianal, genital, or axillary dermatosis that does not respond to typical therapies.

EMPD presents with a variety of clinical manifestations. Erythematous plaques and pruritus are the most common clinical findings. Figure 22.1 shows an example of the typical clinical presentation. Patients may later develop erosions and ulcerative lesions, with a burning sensation as well as frank pain associated with more advanced lesions, especially in

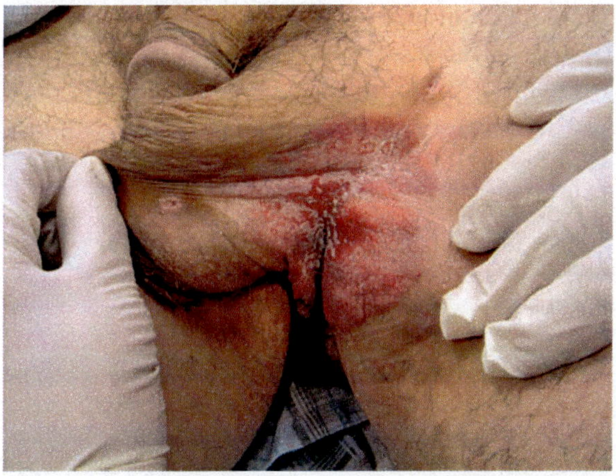

Fig. 22.1 EMPD typically presents with erythematous plaques, sometimes with erosions and ulcerations

anogenital areas. The disease can also present with scale, nodules, verrucous lesions, and hypopigmentation to depigmentation.

22.3.2 Prognosis

Patients with primary EMPD have a significantly better prognosis than those with secondary EMPD because of coexistent malignancy in the latter group. In terms of overall survival, primary EMPD confined to the epidermis has an excellent prognosis. Though evidence is limited and firm conclusions are difficult to make, primary EMPD restricted to the epidermis with no dermal involvement is reported to have no risk of metastasis [4]. Prognosis of invasive EMPD is closely related to depth of invasion from the dermoepidermal junction, with tumors <1 mm carrying zero to minimal risk of nodal involvement. Microscopic invasive disease (<1 mm) is also believed to have no adverse impact on survival. EMPD >1 mm depth has an increased risk of nodal involvement and metastasis. Overall, patients with primary invasive EMPD have a 5-year survival around 72%. In cases with palpable lymph node involvement, however, the prognosis is significantly worse, with 5-year survival reportedly 0% [5].

Though associated adnexal adenocarcinoma is controversial in terms of its pathogenesis and relationship to EMPD, the presence of adnexal adenocarcinoma signifies a worse prognosis. Patients with EMPD and adnexal adenocarcinoma have a mortality rate of 28–48%, compared to 3.8–18% for patients with EMPD and no associated adnexal adenocarcinoma.

Patients with secondary EMPD have mortality rates exceeding 50%, related to internal malignancy. Of patients with secondary EMPD, those who have a known internal malignancy prior to developing EMPD have a relative excess risk of death of 3.2 compared to EMPD patients without an underlying tumor. Patients who are diagnosed with a secondary malignancy after their diagnosis of EMPD have a relative excess risk of 2.5.

Summary: Clinical Subtypes

- EMPD most commonly affects vulvar, penoscrotal, perianal, and axillary regions.
- The vulva is the most commonly affected site in women, the penoscrotal/pubic area in men.
- Perianal and penoscrotal EMPD are more commonly associated with coexistent internal malignancies.
- Perianal EMPD is more likely to be associated with lower gastrointestinal malignancy.
- Penoscrotal EMPD is more likely to be associated with genitourinary malignancy.

22.4 Clinical Subtypes

22.4.1 Vulvar EMPD

The vulva is the most common site for women to be affected by EMPD. Primary EMPD is far more prevalent, but secondary vulvar EMPD has been described in association with endometrial, endocervical, vaginal, urethral, and bladder neoplasms [5]. The mean age of diagnosis of vulvar EMPD is 69 years of age, with 92% of women presenting postmenopause. Pruritus is the most common presenting symptom, affecting 91% of women. It is often accompanied by a burning sensation. Erythematous-white plaques appear in almost all (98%) patients [11]. Pain is a less common complaint, affecting around 11%. The disease is unilateral in 54% of women. The labia majora are most commonly involved (68%), while the labia minora are involved in 57% of patients. Less frequently, the disease involves the clitoris (20%), the perianal skin (18%), and the perineum (18%) [11].

Diagnosis of vulvar EMPD is delayed by an average of 20 months, with most patients treated for fungal infection or postmenopausal vulvovaginitis prior to diagnosis of EMPD. Delayed diagnosis leads to a statistically significant increase in lesion size but not tumor depth. In a series of 56 patients, invasive disease was reported in 18% [11]. Interestingly, in this series, recurrence rate was not related to size of the tumor or positive margins on excision. The only factor found to be predictive of recurrence was perineal involvement. Women with involvement of the perineum experienced recurrence both more often and in a shorter time frame compared to those without.

22.4.2 Perianal EMPD

Perianal EMPD (PPD) is less common than other subtypes, representing about 20% of cases of EMPD [12]. Its presence, however, is correlated more often than other subtypes with underlying malignancy, especially cancer of the anus or colorectum. Reports suggest a rate ranging from 33% to 86%, with the interesting exception of Chinese male patients who have a rate of underlying malignancy reported to be as low as 4.5% [12].The largest literature review to date revealed that in 58% of cases of PPD, the disease was cutaneous only, while in 10% of cases there was an associated synchronous or metachronous internal neoplasm, 28% of cases were reported to demonstrate intraepidermal spread of rectal carcinoma, and 1% of cases were associated with a cutaneous adnexal carcinoma [13]. The authors conclude that PPD exists in several clinical scenarios: primary EMPD, EMPD associated with adenocarcinoma of adnexal structures (either retrograde skin invasion by an adnexal carcinoma or an adenocarcinoma involving the epidermis and adnexal structures), and anorectal carcinoma with pagetoid spread [13]. The last scenario may include cases of adenocarcinoma mislabeled as EMPD.

Most patients with PPD who have underlying internal malignancy present with synchronous visceral malignancy and cutaneous disease. Internal malignancies reported in association include colon adenocarcinoma, prostate cancer, esophageal cancer, and lung cancer, though many of these may represent spurious reports of unclear significance. Perianal EMPD should prompt careful evaluation for a coexistent tumor, however, especially of the lower gastrointestinal tract.

22.4.3 Penoscrotal EMPD

Penoscrotal EMPD is often misdiagnosed, with reports documenting a rate up to 90% [14]. The most common diagnoses made prior to the correct identification of EMPD are chronic eczema and tinea cruris [14]. The average age at diagnosis is 64 years old. Average time from onset of symptoms to accurate diagnosis is about 4 years [15]. In a large case series of patients, lesion size at presentation ranged from 3 to 250 cm^2. Disease was limited to the scrotum in 59.2% of patients, whereas in 36.2% of patients, EMPD involved the scrotum, penis, and/or suprapubic skin [14].

Penoscrotal EMPD, like perianal EMPD, is more commonly associated with an underlying neoplasm in locally adjacent organs and structures, including cancer of the prostate, urethra, bladder, and testicles. Presence of EMPD on the penis or scrotum should lead to a thorough investigation for underlying internal malignancy.

22.4.4 Triple EMPD

EMPD involving the genital region as well as the bilateral axillae has been reported, primarily in Japanese men [16]. In all reported cases, the genital lesions preceded axillary involvement. Any patient with genital EMPD should undergo a thorough examination to exclude additional cutaneous involvement.

22.4.5 Unifocal or Multifocal Disease?

With multiple cases of triple EMPD reported and the well-documented tendency of EMPD to have significant subclinical extension with recurrence despite apparently clear margins, much has been written and speculated about the possible multifocal nature of at least some cases of EMPD. Uncertainty exists as to whether the tumor grows in a contiguous pattern or is the result of a field of cancerization with multiple foci [17]. Multifocal disease has been defined as the absence of tumor cells at the surgical margins of two clinically distinct, excised lesions. Many reports exist describing this phenomenon, most of which rely on standard hematoxylin and eosin for diagnosis and margin evaluation [17].

With immunostaining using CK7, EMPD has been found to have significant involvement undetectable on routine hematoxylin and eosin staining. Precise margin control of the tumor with Mohs surgery using CK7 has elucidated the digitate, often haphazard growth pattern that EMPD can demonstrate [17]. With standard excision and even Mohs surgery without the use of CK7 immunostaining, these haphazard extensions may be missed, giving the impression of multicentric disease [18]. Authors have recently questioned the likelihood of truly multicentric EMPD [17]. Other theories raise the possibility of multiple foci of spontaneous tumor regression, leaving behind islands of normal skin that lead to a false negative margin on excision of EMPD [18].

Summary: Diagnosing EMPD/Disease Pathophysiology

- Biopsy should be performed for any genital or extragenital dermatosis that fails to respond to the typical treatment for other possible diagnoses.
- Histology demonstrates Paget cells, which typically have centrally located nuclei; abundant, finely granular cytoplasm; and are usually located in the lower epidermis.
- Coexistent malignancy should be ruled out by performing a complete history and physical exam, review of systems, and appropriate diagnostic testing.

22.5 Diagnosing EMPD/Disease Pathophysiology

22.5.1 Histology

A skin biopsy should be performed for any genital or extragenital lesion(s) that are suspicious for EMPD or fail to respond to a reasonable course of the typical treatments for other possible diagnoses. The diagnosis of EMPD must be confirmed by histology, and overly superficial biopsies should be avoided in order to prevent diagnostic confusion. Typical findings include intraepidermal aggregates of pale-staining cells that are larger than keratinocytes and contain pleomorphic nuclei with pronounced atypia, prominent nucleoli, and mitotic figures [5, 19]. Paget cells typically have centrally located nuclei and abundant, finely granular cytoplasm [5]. Signet ring cells are not an uncommon finding. Reactive epidermal changes can be seen, including parakeratosis, hyperkeratosis, epidermal hyperplasia, and acantholysis. Most Paget cells are concentrated in the lower portion of the epidermis, in association with the pilosebaceous unit, but upward spread is not uncommon [5]. Paget cells may also be seen extending into sweat ducts, leading to uncertainty as to whether the neoplasm originates intraepidermally or from underlying cutaneous adnexal adenocarcinoma. Chronic inflammation with small capillary proliferation is also a common finding [11]. Over 90% of cases of EMPD demonstrate cytoplasmic mucin, staining positively with mucicarmine and PAS reagent.

22.5.2 Histologic Differential Diagnosis

Pagetoid spread, the upward migration of cells in the epidermis singly or in clusters, can also be seen in Bowen's disease, superficial spreading melanoma, mycosis fungoides, Langerhans cell histiocytosis, sebaceous carcinoma, and Spitz nevus [5, 14]. Longstanding Bowen's disease can demonstrate significant hyperkeratosis, elongation of the rete ridges, and reactive keratinocyte atypia. EMPD can occasionally be difficult to distinguish from Bowen's disease, but mucin, signet cells, and glandular structures are useful features to distinguish EMPD [8]. Melanoma demonstrates a greater degree of nesting at the dermoepidermal junction, there is no acinar formation, and mucin is absent [7].

Immunohistochemical analysis can be helpful in difficult cases, using a panel of CK7, CEA, EMA, S100, HMB-45, and Cam5.2. One series reports that in 25% cases of EMPD, immunohistochemistry for low-molecular weight cytokeratins, CEA, and S-100 protein was required to exclude Bowen's disease and superficial spreading melanoma from the differential diagnosis [7].

22.5.3 Evaluation for Internal Malignancy

After confirmation of the diagnosis of EMPD by histology, a workup to exclude underlying gastrointestinal, genitourinary, and other less commonly associated distant malignancies is prudent. A comprehensive review of systems should be performed with this in mind, and a complete physical exam should be carried out, including genital and rectal exams, and a thorough skin exam to assess the degree of involvement. Careful palpation of lymph nodes is mandatory. Bilateral "underpants pattern" erythema has been associated with pronounced lymphovascular invasion and should alert the clinician to the likelihood of nodal disease [20].

In cases where extent of the tumor is questionable, multiple biopsies may be helpful to establish a more accurate estimate of the margins. If the anal area is involved, examination for anorectal or colon cancer could include fecal occult blood testing as well colonoscopy. Urine cytology and cystoscopy should be considered to screen for uroepithelial cancers. Women should also undergo breast and pelvic examination, Papanicolaou smear, as well as mammograms and pelvic imaging studies. Men should be screened for underlying malignancy through physical examination of the prostate and testicles and by prostate-specific antigen assay.

CEA has been used to screen for systemic disease in patients with EMPD [20]. Its sensitivity for detecting EMPD metastasis has been reported as 70% and specificity 93.8%. The marker has demonstrated utility in predicting prognosis, with elevated levels associated with higher likelihood of death from EMPD. Although the sensitivity of CEA is lower than ideal for a screening test, serum CEA level may be useful as a marker of systemic metastasis and response to treatment [20].

22.5.4 Sentinel Lymph Node Biopsy

The value of sentinel lymph node biopsy in EMPD is controversial. No large studies exist to provide an evidence-based approach. Results from a small series of patients with primary genital EMPD who underwent sentinel node biopsy found positive nodes in 4 of 23 patients, and 3 of the 4 patients with positive nodes developed distant disease [21]. None of the patients with a negative sentinel lymph node biopsy developed distant disease. None of the patients with intraepidermal disease had a positive lymph node biopsy. Complete node dissection was not carried out in all patients, and no conclusion could be reached about any potential benefit of complete dissection. Further studies are needed to clarify the role of sentinel lymph node biopsy in EMPD.

22.5.5 Pathophysiology

There has been much debate about the pathophysiology of EMPD. Comparisons between mammary Paget disease and EMPD have been made in an effort to better understand the pathogenic mechanism. Mammary Paget disease is most often associated with underlying in situ or invasive ductal carcinoma of the breast, leading to the hypothesis that epidermotropic spread of neoplastic cells is responsible for cutaneous disease. The rare cases of mammary Paget disease without underlying breast carcinoma are referred to as primary Paget disease, and in these cases, the epidermis is felt to be the site of origin.

EMPD, on the other hand, is much less likely to be associated with an underlying neoplasm. Accordingly, it is believed that most cases of EMPD arise in the epidermis and have no association with an underlying cutaneous adnexal adenocarcinoma or internal malignancy.

Ackerman and colleagues reviewed the histology and clinical history of a series of cases of EMPD and concluded that EMPD is likely more than one disease, with the most common form originating in the epidermis and the less common subtypes originating in underlying glandular structures or contiguous internal organs with epidermotropic spread [22]. EMPD is now believed to exist in four clinical scenarios: first, disease originating in and contained within the epidermis; second, disease originating in the epidermis with secondary invasion of the dermis; third, epidermal disease secondary to underlying adnexal adenocarcinoma with epidermotropic spread (a controversial entity due to the difficulty in assessing origin of the tumor); and fourth, epidermal disease secondary to internal malignancy. In more recent classification schemes, the first three scenarios are classified as primary EMPD, while the fourth is classified as secondary EMPD [23].

22.5.6 Cell of Origin

The cell of origin of EMPD remains controversial. Theoretical candidate cells include epidermal/follicular stem cells, Toker cells, and apocrine gland cells. Recent immunohistochemical analysis has led to the theory that Toker cells may play a role as the benign precursor to the neoplastic cells, giving rise to at least some cases of vulvar EMPD [24]. Clear cells of Toker are thought to be germinative cells of the lactiferous duct, identifiable by routine hematoxylin & eosin staining in approximately 10% of normal nipples, and also present in accessory nipples along the milk line. They have also been identified using CK7 staining in mammary-like glands found in normal genital skin and are felt to be an interface between the epidermis and the epithelium of lactiferous ducts of the breast, ectopic breast tissue, and mammary-like glands of the vulva [24].

The finding of Toker cells in genital skin of females has led to the hypothesis that the pathogenesis of EMPD may be similar to that of mammary Paget's disease. Following this line of thinking, EMPD may arise by three mechanisms: first as a primary, intraepithelial neoplasm originating in the epidermis from Toker cells, with the potential for invasive spread; second as a neoplastic process arising from carcinoma of anogenital mammary like glands; and third as carcinoma arising from skin appendages, Bartholin glands, or other organs like the anus, rectum, urethra, or cervix [25].

22.5.7 Distinguishing Primary and Secondary EMPD by Immunohistochemical Techniques

At present, distinguishing primary from secondary EMPD is possible only by extensive medical evaluation to exclude underlying malignancy. Given the significant difference in prognosis between patients with primary and secondary EMPD related to underlying malignancy, interest has been increasingly focused on utilizing immunohistochemistry to distinguish primary and secondary EMPD, with the goal of gaining a reproducible and rapid method of establishing the likelihood for the presence or absence of an underlying malignancy.

Multiple immunostains have been examined in EMPD, including CK7, CK20, HER-2/neu, BRST-2, CDX2, androgen receptor, and cyclin D1. Some studies have suggested that a CK7+, CK20–, and BRST-2+ immunohistochemical phenotype is consistent with primary EMPD, while a CK7+, CK20+, and BRST-2– phenotype is consistent with secondary EMPD.

CK7 is a cytokeratin found in apocrine glands, sebaceous glands, secretory coils of eccrine glands, and in the epithelium of breast, lung, and genitourinary tract, but not the gastrointestinal tract. CK7 staining has been found to be near universally positive in cases of both primary and secondary EMPD. CK20 is a cytokeratin found in Merkel cells as well as most colorectal adenocarcinomas. BRST-2 is a monoclonal antibody that detects a glycoprotein expressed by apocrine glands, some eccrine glands, and minor salivary glands. Breast adenocarcinomas with apocrine features also express the BRST-2 antigen. HER-2/neu is a transmembrane growth factor receptor that is overexpressed in 25–30% of primary breast carcinomas, with high staining sensitivity for mammary Paget's disease and variable staining for both primary and secondary EMPD [19]. CDX2, a transcription factor that regulates the development of intestinal epithelium, has shown value in differentiating primary EMPD from EMPD secondary to anorectal malignancy. In the majority of cases, CDX2 stains positive in EMPD secondary to anorectal malignancy and is negative in primary anogenital EMPD [19].

A recent evaluation of a series of EMPD cases examined using CK7, CK20, HER-2/neu, BRST-2, CDX2, androgen receptor (AR), and cyclin D1 found CK7+ staining in 100% of cases (both primary and secondary EMPD) [19]. CK20 was positive in 22% of primary EMPD and 50% of secondary EMPD, while BRST-2 showed 48% positivity in primary EMPD and 25% in secondary EMPD. The authors conclude that the panel consisting of CK7, CK20, and BRST-2 has limited utility in distinguishing primary and secondary EMPD due to the variable staining pattern of CK20 and BRST-2. They also conclude that adding HER-2/neu and CDX2 may help differentiate primary anogenital EMPD from anogenital EMPD associated with anorectal adenocarcinoma, but fails to distinguish primary EMPD from EMPD secondary to uroepithelial or prostatic malignancy. Ber-EP4 is another immunohistochemical marker that has shown promise in distinguishing primary and secondary EMPD, but more research must be done to establish its utility as well as the overall value of immunostains in the diagnosis of EMPD.

Summary: EMPD Treatment

- Surgical excision is the standard treatment for EMPD.
- Wide local excision results in high recurrence rates.
- Mohs surgery has become the preferred method of managing many cases of EMPD due to the ability to evaluate 100% of the margin and conserve normal tissue, but has a higher recurrence rate than is seen for other cutaneous malignancies.
- The addition of CK7 immunostaining to Mohs surgery shows promise in providing more accurate margin control and lower recurrence rates.
- Scouting biopsies may be useful for preoperative estimation of margins prior to Mohs surgery.

22.6 EMPD Treatment

Surgical excision of EMPD remains the mainstay of treatment. Mohs micrographic surgery has become the preferred method of managing EMPD by many practitioners due to the ability to evaluate 100% of the margin while minimizing tissue loss and morbidity.

EMPD of the vulva has been treated surgically with methods ranging from vulvectomy (partial or total) to wide local excision with margins of 1–3 cm. Vulvectomy, the most extensive and morbid procedure, has the lowest reported recurrence rate in some series (15%), compared with 43% recurrence for wide local excision. Perianal and scrotal EMPD have an even higher rate of recurrence after wide local excision, some series reporting a rate up to 50%, though some authors have achieved a recurrence rate of 9.9% using a combination of 3-cm margins and intraoperative frozen sections [7, 14].

Some studies conclude that margin status is predictive of recurrence, with positive margins leading to higher rates of recurrence [15]. While this conclusion seems intuitive, many series document recurrence of EMPD that occurs independent of margin status, with patients who have reportedly clear margins going on to develop recurrent disease. This observation may be a testament to the importance of en face evaluation of 100% of the margins of excision of EMPD, as it is likely that many of the previously reported negative margins were falsely negative, evidenced by the recent incorporation of CK7 into Mohs surgery and the striking margin involvement not detected with routine hematoxylin and eosin staining.

22.6.1 Wide Local Excision and Recommended Margin

Wide local excision of EMPD leads to widely ranging reported recurrence rates of 9.9–60%. Given the rare occurrence of EMPD and lack of randomized trials, establishing an evidence-based margin of excision is difficult. Utilizing margin control with Mohs surgery, authors have concluded that a margin of 5 cm would successfully excise EMPD in 97% of patients [26]. In this study, margins of 2 cm would have completely excised tumor in only 59% of patients. The authors recommend 5 cm margins or Mohs surgery.

Other authors have concluded that the rate of recurrence does not differ when using margins >2 cm compared to margins <2 cm [20]. Their conclusion does not entirely contradict the findings mentioned above; however, suggesting that any margin less than 5 cm may be inadequate for the excision of many cases of EMPD. Examination of a series of patients with scrotal EMPD found that with 1–2 cm margins, 36% of the tumors were excised with a positive margin [20].

The introduction of intraoperative frozen sections has allowed better margin control and a significant reduction in recurrence rates to 9.9–25% [10, 14, 15, 20] Intraoperative frozen sections, however, do not typically allow en face evaluation of 100% of the margin, in contrast to Mohs surgery. Standard cross-sectional processing, utilized in most excisions including those employing intraoperative frozen sections in a non-Mohs surgery setting, allows examination of around 0.1% of the total margin, leading to the potential for a high false negative rate.

It is clear that when standard excision is used to treat EMPD, relying on visual exam to determine the extent of tumor prior to excision has proven to be inaccurate, validating the significant invisible extension present in EMPD as well as the potential value of Mohs surgery in the treatment of EMPD.

22.6.2 Time to Recurrence

In a large series of patients with scrotal EMPD, the average time from surgery to diagnosis of recurrence

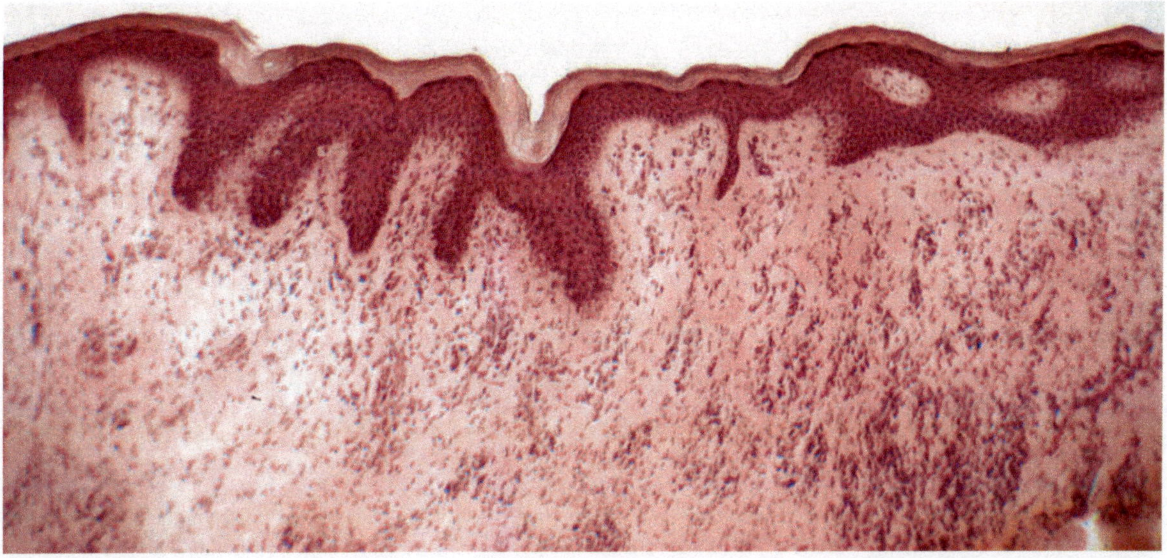

Fig. 22.2 Histologic illustration of normal-appearing skin on H & E frozen section staining, confirmed by CK7 staining to be affected by EMPD. 20× power

was 3 years and 5 months (range 3 months to 10 years) [15]. For vulvar EMPD, the mean time to recurrence was shorter after surgery with positive margins (49 months) than negative margins (73 months) [11]. These studies suggest that long-term follow-up is mandatory in patients with EMPD.

22.6.2.1 Mohs Surgery for EMPD

In 1979, Fred Mohs wrote that "the microscopically oriented histographic surgery technique offers the most reliable means of removing all neoplastic disease in EMPD and preserves as much normal tissue as possible" [27]. Since his writing, multiple case series have been published that confirm the efficacy of Mohs surgery for EMPD. Published series using Mohs surgery with hematoxylin and eosin staining demonstrate a recurrence rate ranging from 0% to 28%, with varying duration of follow-up [26, 28, 29]. In a survey of Mohs surgeons, Coldiron et al. reported cumulative recurrence rates of 27%, 17%, and 28% after using Mohs surgery to treat EMPD of the female genitalia, male genitalia, and perianal skin, respectively [18]. Hendi et al. reported treating 19 primary tumors with Mohs surgery with a 16% recurrence rate [26]. They also treated 8 recurrent tumors with Mohs surgery and reported a 50% recurrence rate. These series were published prior to the incorporation of CK7 immunostaining into Mohs surgery.

A recent comparison of men and women with genital EMPD treated with Mohs surgery or a variety of alternatives including wide local excision with margins up to 3 cm, vulvectomy, and hemivulvectomy found a recurrence rate of 18% in the Mohs surgery group versus 36% in the collective group treated with wide local excision, vulvectomy, or hemivulvectomy [4].

The average number of stages for patients with EMPD treated with Mohs surgery is 3 [28, 29]. EMPD also demonstrates one of the largest discrepancies between initial estimate of the clinical extent of tumor and final defect size. A series of ten patients with EMPD treated at one institution found a difference of 75 cm^2 between mean lesion size at presentation and mean defect size after completion of Mohs surgery, with a ratio of defect to lesion size of 3.2 [29].

22.6.3 Mohs Surgery with CK7 Immunostaining

As previously discussed, CK7 has proven to be a sensitive marker for detecting the presence of neoplastic cells in EMPD, with near 100% positivity in primary and secondary EMPD. Over the past decade, CK7 has been increasingly implemented in Mohs surgery, improving the detection of subtle disease that would otherwise go unseen. Figures 22.2 and 22.3 demonstrate an example where EMPD is unapparent on hematoxylin and eosin stained frozen section (Fig. 22.2) but apparent on CK7 stained frozen section (Fig. 22.3). In cases treated with

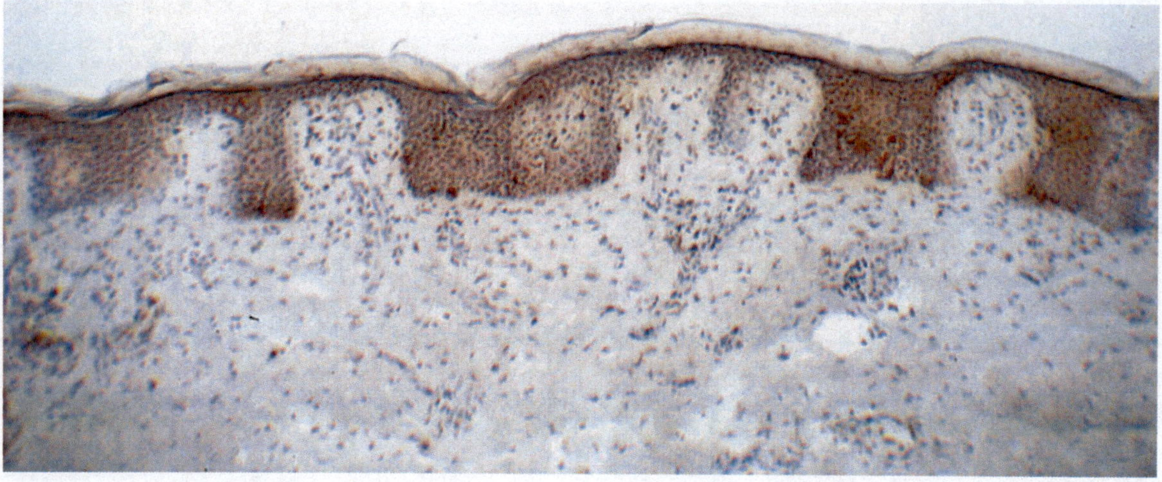

Fig. 22.3 Same frozen section specimen as seen in Fig. 22.2, but stained with CK7. This margin was confirmed by CK7 to be affected by EMPD. 20× power

Mohs surgery using CK7 in addition to hematoxylin and eosin, hematoxylin and eosin negative but CK7 positive foci are visualized in about 65% of cases (authors' experience). This suggests that the false negative rate may be as high as 65% when not using Mohs surgery with CK7, a possible explanation for the higher recurrence rate of EMPD compared to basal-cell and squamous-cell carcinomas treated with Mohs surgery. The recurrence rate of EMPD after Mohs surgery with the addition of CK7 has not yet been published, but preliminary data suggest a significant reduction in recurrence rates (authors' experience).

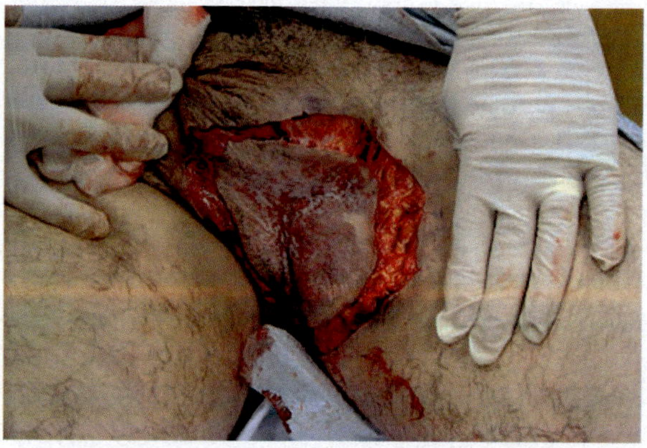

Fig. 22.4 The peripheral Mohs surgery technique allows for effective and time-saving treatment of histologically confirmed non-invasive EMPD

22.6.4 Peripheral Mohs Surgery

Peripheral Mohs surgery, as seen in Fig. 22.4, has been used for large tissue areas, >8 cm, with superficial/intraepidermal involvement and no histologic or clinical evidence of invasive disease [26]. In this modification, the peripheral margin of the tumor is initially excised using Mohs surgery to remove 2–3-mm-wide strips of epidermis, dermis, and subcutaneous tissue. These peripheral pieces are processed and evaluated using CK7 immunostaining to augment hematoxylin and eosin staining. After clearing the margin peripherally, the remaining central island of tumor, containing skin, adnexa, and superficial subcutaneous tissue, is excised at the level of the mid-subcutaneous tissue. This assures removal of the epidermal tumor, along with any tumor that may extend down the adnexa. Histologic evaluation of the entire deep margin of these superficial lesions is not undertaken. This modification has been performed as an alternative to save time and expense of microscopic examination of extremely large tissue areas. This method is not suitable for EMPD with histologic or clinical evidence of invasive disease [26].

22.6.5 Scouting Biopsies

Scouting biopsies have been proposed as an alternative method to improve the accuracy of the first stage of Mohs surgery, potentially reducing the number of stages needed to clear EMPD, shortening the total duration of the procedure, and reducing operative morbidity for patients [30]. Other benefits include a more accurate estimate of the size and type of reconstruction, allowing for a more informed preoperative consultation.

The technique consists of performing multiple punch biopsies, shave biopsies, or scissor biopsies between 1 and 5 cm from the clinically apparent margin, prior to initiating Mohs surgery. Specimens are examined microscopically. CK7 staining may be performed, improving the sensitivity of scouting biopsies. Photographs are used to carefully map the involved margins. This approach has been proposed to be especially useful in situations where the degree of involvement may have a significant impact on disease management. For example, urethral involvement is found suggesting that collaboration with a urologist might benefit the patient, or substantial tumor size leads to the consideration of general anesthesia [30].

Interestingly, false negative results have been reported using the scouting biopsy approach; hence the utility of this method remains to be determined.

Summary: Alternative Treatment Options

- Topical treatment of EMPD with imiquimod and 5-fluorouracil has shown variable success.
- Caution is advised when using topical treatment that may lead to the appearance of clinical cure but persistent subclinical, microscopic disease.
- Topical treatments may also fragment tumor, rendering Mohs surgery less effective.
- Radiation therapy may have a role in select cases of non-invasive EMPD.
- There is no consistently effective chemotherapeutic regimen for metastatic disease.

22.7 Alternative Treatment Options

22.7.1 Topical Therapies: Imiquimod and 5-Fluorouracil

Imiquimod has received considerable attention as a topical immunomodulator, FDA approved for the treatment of actinic keratoses and select non-facial superficial basal-cell carcinomas. Imiquimod has been used off-label for the treatment of in situ EMPD, with reports of successful treatment of primary and recurrent tumor both clinically and histologically. Authors propose the use of 5% imiquimod cream at least three times weekly for 8–16 weeks, but case reports exist that demonstrate multiple treatment regimens with varying efficacy [31]. Application of 5% imiquimod cream can be accompanied by a localized inflammatory response that can limit the frequency of application, and some studies have found that higher frequency of application leads to higher cure rates.

Imiquimod cream has also been used in the pre-Mohs surgery setting as a method of reducing the tumor burden prior to excision. Caution should be exercised when using a topical treatment that may partially treat a clinically indistinct tumor, leading to discontinuous growth. Using this approach may unintentionally render Mohs surgery less efficacious at achieving clear margins due to fragmentation of the tumor.

Because of the short duration of follow-up of most reported cases treated with 5% imiquimod, no definitive conclusion can be reached regarding the long-term efficacy and recurrence rate. Once long-term recurrence rates after treatment with imiquimod are better characterized, the topical treatment may prove to be a viable alternative to surgery in select patients. Presently, its use may best be reserved for patients who refuse or are unable to tolerate surgical treatment.

5-Fluorouracil has also been explored as a potential surgery-sparing treatment in EMPD. While reports suggest clinical clearance of tumor after 5-fluorouracil treatment, histologic persistence has been noted. Thus caution should be used when considering treatment with a topical therapy that may lead to masking of persistent tumor including deeper, potentially invasive disease [32].

22.7.2 Photodynamic Therapy

Photodynamic therapy (PDT) with topical ALA or intravenous porfimer sodium followed by treatment with a 632.8-nm argon-pumped dye laser has been used for non-invasive EMPD. Results of a recent retrospective series found 78% (7/9) of patients treated with intravenous porfimer photosensitization and argon laser disease free at follow-up (12–96 months) [33]. Eight of 16 patients treated with PDT using topical ALA had a complete clinical response, and 38% were disease free at follow-up (9–88 months). Larger series are needed to firmly establish the role of PDT in the treatment of non-invasive EMPD.

22.7.3 Laser Vaporization

Destruction of EMPD with carbon dioxide laser vaporization has been documented. While treatment of vulvar EMPD with laser vaporization preserves vulvar anatomy, there is a significant association with postoperative pain and a high recurrence rate [11].

22.7.4 Radiation Therapy

Radiation therapy has been used as a treatment for primary EMPD, following surgical excision of EMPD with the aim of reducing local recurrence, and as a treatment for recurrent disease. Intraepidermal and invasive EMPD have both been treated with radiation therapy, primarily disease located in the anogenital region. Patients in published series have generally been considered poor surgical candidates, and therefore, recurrence rates likely reflect a higher risk subset of patients with a worse prognosis.

Radiation therapy has proven to have acceptable cure rates for primary EMPD. Patients with secondary EMPD have an extremely poor prognosis, regardless of treatment with radiation therapy. In a 2002 review of the existing literature on radiation therapy for perianal Paget's disease, 43 cases were analyzed [34]. The overall outcome was progressive disease in 56%, no sign of recurrent disease in 37%, and unknown in three cases (7%). Of the patients with primary EMPD, recurrence after radiation therapy was 35%, compared to a recurrence of 77% in patients with secondary EMPD. In this review, 5-year survival was 20% for invasive perianal EMPD and 94% for non-invasive PPD, demonstrating a statistically significant difference in the survival curves.

Typical regimens consist of treating a field including 3 cm surrounding visible disease with 40–50 Gy. Photon, electron, and brachytherapy have all been used with success. Lower doses of radiation therapy are associated with a higher risk of recurrence, however [35, 36].

Radiation therapy has been successful in treating EMPD of the vulva, in many cases leading to a recurrence-free state [12]. Radiation therapy, like topical treatments, is most applicable in patients who are unsuitable candidates for surgical intervention. In cases where surgery for intraepidermal disease would result in significant loss of function (abdominoperineal resection and colostomy formation), reserving surgery for salvage treatment for cases of radiation therapy failure may be an acceptable alternative [34]. Chronic radiation toxicity is a potential concern, with pigmentary changes and atrophy as noted complications.

22.7.5 Chemotherapy for EMPD: Local and Systemic

Systemic chemotherapy has shown little efficacy in the treatment of metastatic disease. 5-fluorouracil, docetaxel, and cisplatin-based chemotherapy have been used in multiple patients with mixed results [35, 36].

Axillary EMPD has been treated with local chemotherapy using doxorubicin incorporated in large liposomes and paclitaxel incorporated in albumin nanoparticles [37]. Complete cure has not been obtained, but improved quality of life has been achieved with minimal treatment-related morbidity.

Summary: Conclusion

- EMPD most commonly presents as an intraepidermal adenocarcinoma with indistinct margins, affecting genital skin.
- EMPD is reported to sometimes occur in association with internal malignancy, though the true relationship is unclear in many cases.
- Distinguishing underlying adnexal carcinoma from spread of epidermal disease may be difficult.
- Mohs surgery is effective in treating EMPD. The addition of CK7 staining shows promise in improving the accuracy of margin control and reducing recurrence rates.

22.8 Conclusion

EMPD is an intraepidermal adenocarcinoma most often limited to the epidermis, with typical cases affecting genital skin in women and men. In patients with invasive disease, prognosis is based on the degree of invasion, with tumors less than 1 mm deep having very low mortality. Careful evaluation for an underlying malignancy should be carried out to exclude life-threatening disease, but the association of many coexistent malignancies is controversial. Reported underlying adnexal adenocarcinoma may, at least in some patients, represent invasive spread of primary epidermal disease. Mohs surgery has proven effective in the treatment of EMPD, and the implementation of CK7 shows promise in further reducing the recurrence rate. Alternative treatments, including topical treatment with imiquimod and 5-fluorouracil as well as photodynamic therapy, may be effective in select cases of EMPD.

References

1. Paget J. On disease of the mammary areola preceding cancer of the mammary gland. St Bartholomew Hosp Res Lond. 1874;10:87–9.
2. Crocker HR. Paget's disease affecting the scrotum and penis. Trans Pathol Soc Lond. 1888–1889;40:187–91.
3. Siesling S, Elferink MA, van Dijck JA, Pierie JP, Blokx WA. Epidemiology and treatment of extramammary Paget disease in the Netherlands. Eur J Surg Oncol. 2007;33:951–5.
4. Lee KY, Roh MR, Chung WG, Chung KY. Comparison of Mohs micrographic surgery and wide excision for extramammary Paget's Disease: Korean experience. Dermatol Surg. 2009;35:34–40.
5. Ekwueme KC, Zakhour HD, Parr NJ. Extramammary Paget's disease of the penis: a case report and review of the literature. J Med Case Reports. 2009;3:4.
6. Shaco-Levy R, Bean SM, Vollmer RT, Jewell E, Jones EL, Valdes CL, et al. Paget disease of the vulva: a study of 56 cases. Eur J Obstet Gynecol Reprod Biol. 2010;149(1): 86–91.
7. Zollo JD, Zeitouni NC. The Roswell Park Cancer Institute experience with extramammary Paget's disease. Br J Dermatol. 2000;142:59–65.
8. Cohen MA, Hanly A, Poulos E, Goldstein GD. Extramammary Paget's disease presenting on the face. Dermatol Surg. 2004;30:1361–3.
9. Sawada Y, Bito T, Kabashima R, Yoshiki R, Hino R, Nakamura M, et al. Ectopic extramammary Paget's disease: case report and literature review. Acta Derm Venereol. 2010;90(5):502–5.
10. Kyriazanos ID, Stamos NP, Miliadis L, Noussis G, Stoidis CN. Extra-mammary Paget's disease of the perianal region: a review of the literature emphasizing the operative management technique. Surg Oncol. 2011;20(2):e61–71.
11. Minicozzi A, Borzellino G, Momo R, Steccanella F, Pitoni F, de Manzoni G. Perianal Paget's disease: presentation of six cases and literature review. Int J Colorectal Dis. 2010;25:1–7.
12. Wang Z, Lu M, Dong GQ, Jiang YQ, Lin MS, Cai ZK, et al. Penile and scrotal Paget's disease: 130 Chinese patients with long-term follow-up. BJU Int. 2008;102:485–8.
13. Xu K, Fang Z, Zheng J, Lu Y, Li B, Sun C, et al. Intraoperative frozen biopsy in wide surgical excision of Paget's disease of the scrotum. Urol Oncol. 2009;27:483–5.
14. Kitajima S, Yamamoto K, Tsuji T, Schwartz RA. Triple extramammary Paget's disease. Dermatol Surg. 1997;23: 1035–8.
15. Hendi A, Perdikis G, Snow JL. Unifocality of extramammary Paget disease. J Am Acad Dermatol. 2008;59:811–3.
16. Coldiron BM, Goldsmith BA, Robinson JK. Surgical treatment of extramammary Paget's disease. A report of six cases and a reexamination of Mohs micrographic surgery compared with conventional surgical excision. Cancer. 1991; 67:933–8.
17. Perrotto J, Abbott JJ, Ceilley RI, Ahmed I. The role of immunohistochemistry in discriminating primary from secondary extramammary Paget disease. Am J Dermatopathol. 2010;32:137–43.
18. Hatta N, Yamada M, Hirano T, Fujimoto A, Morita R. Extramammary Paget's disease: treatment, prognostic factors and outcome in 76 patients. Br J Dermatol. 2008;158:313–8.
19. Hatta N, Morita R, Yamada M, Echigo T, Hirano T, Takehara K, et al. Sentinel lymph node biopsy in patients with extramammary Paget's disease. Dermatol Surg. 2004;30:1329–34.
20. Jones Jr RE, Austin C, Ackerman AB. Extramammary Paget's disease. A critical reexamination. Am J Dermatopathol. 1979;1:101–32.
21. Wilkinson EJ, Brown HM. Vulvar Paget disease of urothelial origin: a report of three cases and a proposed classification of vulvar Paget disease. Hum Pathol. 2002;33:549–54.
22. Willman JH, Golitz LE, Fitzpatrick JE. Vulvar clear cells of Toker: precursors of extramammary Paget's disease. Am J Dermatopathol. 2005;27:185–8.
23. Belousova IE, Kazakov DV, Michal M, Suster S. Vulvar toker cells: the long-awaited missing link: a proposal for an origin-based histogenetic classification of extramammary Paget disease. Am J Dermatopathol. 2006;28:84–6.
24. Hendi A, Brodland DG, Zitelli JA. Extramammary Paget's disease: surgical treatment with Mohs micrographic surgery. J Am Acad Dermatol. 2004;51(5):767–73.
25. Mohs FE, Blandchard L. Microscopically controlled surgery for extramammary Paget's disease. Arch Dermatol. 1979; 115:706–8.
26. O'Connor WJ, Lim KK, Zalla MJ, Gagnot M, Otley CC, Nguyen TH, et al. Comparison of Mohs micrographic surgery and wide excision for extramammary Paget's disease. Dermatol Surg. 2003;29:723–7.
27. Thomas CJ, Wood GC, Marks VJ. Mohs micrographic surgery in the treatment of rare aggressive cutaneous tumors: the Geisinger experience. Dermatol Surg. 2007;33:333–9.
28. Appert DL, Otley CC, Phillips PK, Roenigk RK. Role of multiple scouting biopsies before Mohs micrographic surgery for extramammary Paget's disease. Dermatol Surg. 2005;31:1417–22.
29. Cohen PR, Schulze KE, Tschen JA, Hetherington GW, Nelson BR. Treatment of extramammary Paget disease with topical imiquimod cream: case report and literature review. South Med J. 2006;99:396–402.
30. Brown RS, McCormack M, Lankester KJ, Spittle MF. Spontaneous apparent clinical resolution with histologic persistence of a case of extramammary Paget's disease: response to topical 5-fluorouracil. Cutis. 2000;66:454–5.

31. Housel JP, Izikson L, Zeitouni NC. Noninvasive extramammary Paget's disease treated with photodynamic therapy: case series from the Roswell Park Cancer Institute. Dermatol Surg. 2010;36:1718–24.
32. Brown RS, Lankester KJ, McCormack M, Power DA, Spittle MF. Radiotherapy for perianal Paget's disease. Clin Oncol (R Coll Radiol). 2002;14:272–84.
33. Brierley JD, Stockdale AD. Radiotherapy: an effective treatment for extramammary Paget's disease. Clin Oncol (R Coll Radiol). 1991;3:3–5.
34. Dilmé-Carreras E, Iglesias-Sancho M, Márquez-Balbás G, Sola-Ortigosa J, Umbert-Millet P. Radiotherapy for extramammary Paget disease of the anogenital region. J Am Acad Dermatol. 2011;65(1):192–4.
35. Zhu Y, Ye DW, Yao XD, Zhang SL, Dai B, Zhang HL, et al. Clinicopathological characteristics, management and outcome of metastatic penoscrotal extramammary Paget's disease. Br J Dermatol. 2009;161:577–82.
36. Kariya K, Tsuji T, Schwartz RA. Trial of low-dose 5-fluorouracil/cisplatin therapy for advanced extramammary Paget's disease. Dermatol Surg. 2004;30:341–4.
37. Damascelli B, Ticha V. Successful intra-arterial chemotherapy for extramammary Paget's disease of the axilla in a patient with Parkinson's disease. Cardiovasc Intervent Radiol. 2009;34 Suppl 2:S167–70.

Leiomyosarcoma

23

Marc Rubenzik, Boonyapat Limthongkul,
and Tatyana R. Humphreys

Abstract

Leiomyosarcoma (LMS) is an uncommon soft tissue malignancy that may arise in the skin or subcutis. LMS occurs most frequently on the head and neck followed by the trunk, arms, and legs. LMS is a spindle cell neoplasm with an infiltrative growth pattern that stains positively with immunohistochemistry for vimentin, desmin, smooth muscle actin, and H-caldesmon. LMS is characterized by a high local recurrence rate with conventional wide excision (up to 45%). While metastasis has been reported in up to 30% of subcutaneous tumors, the metastatic potential of superficial cutaneous tumors is thought to be minimal. The overall cure rate of LMS treated by Mohs micrographic surgery is 87% which compares favorably to wide excision and offers the advantage of tissue sparing.

Keywords

Leiomyosarcoma • Spindle cell • Cutaneous • Neoplasm • Mohs micrographic surgery

Summary: Introduction

- Leiomyosarcoma (LMS) is a malignant spindle cell neoplasm. Cutaneous LMS is a superficial variant of this uncommon soft tissue sarcoma.

23.1 Introduction

Leiomyosarcoma (LMS) is a rare malignant spindle cell neoplasm. Whereas the most common locations are uterine and retroperitoneal, LMS of the skin accounts for only about 2% of all soft tissue sarcomas [1]. LMS of the skin and subcutaneous tissue is usually designated as "superficial" in contrast to deep soft tissue sarcomas [2]. While cutaneous LMS can be a either primary or metastatic, the scope of this chapter is limited to treatment of primary cutaneous tumors. Primary skin LMS have been further divided histologically into cutaneous and subcutaneous based on the observed biological potential and prognostic values of each designation.

M. Rubenzik • B. Limthongkul • T.R. Humphreys (✉)
Department of Dermatology, Thomas Jefferson University, Philadelphia, PA, USA
e-mail: tatyana.humphreys@jefferson.edu

K. Nouri (ed.), *Mohs Micrographic Surgery*,
DOI 10.1007/978-1-4471-2152-7_23, © Springer-Verlag London Limited 2012

Summary: Clinical Features

- Cutaneous LMS typically presents as a firm subcutaneous nodule on the head, neck, extremities, or trunk that is relatively nonspecific in appearance. Erythema and ulceration may be present.

23.2 Clinical Features

In a recent large review of cutaneous soft tissue sarcomas, LMS was reported to occur most frequently on the head and neck (32%), followed by the trunk, arms, and legs (20%) [1]. Because they are derived from arrector pili, cutaneous leiomyosarcoma can theoretically occur on any hair-bearing skin surface, whereas the vascular-derived subcutaneous LMS can occur on any body site. Recent studies suggest that subcutaneous LMS predominantly occurs on the lower extremities, whereas the cutaneous variant presents more frequently on the head and neck (48%), followed by the extremities (31%), then the trunk (21%) [2]. Men are more commonly affected (74%) as are Caucasians (91%) [1]. The incidence of LMS increases linearly with patient age [1].

Primary LMS is typically a solitary indolent neoplasm that presents as a cutaneous nodule. Overlying erythema or discoloration occurs frequently [3, 4] while ulceration is uncommon. Like its benign leiomyoma counterpart, pain may be a presenting symptom [5]. In a recent study, the size at diagnosis ranged from 6 to 38 mm [6]. The clinical differential diagnosis includes any cutaneous or subcutaneous nodule such as a cyst, fibroma, lipoma, pseudolymphoma, lymphoma, neurofibroma, dermatofibroma, granuloma, and various subcutaneous malignancies [3].

While the etiology of LMS is unclear, it has been anecdotally associated with various types of trauma, including ionizing radiation, tick bite, inoculation site, venous stasis, and cutaneous tuberculosis [3]. Malignant transformation of benign leiomyomas has not been reported to date [3].

Summary: Histologic Features

- LMS is a spindle cell neoplasm with an infiltrative growth pattern. The tumor cells are blunt-ended with tapered nuclei, characteristic of smooth muscle morphology. While cytologic atypia is variable, an infiltrating pattern with subcutaneous extension supports a diagnosis of LMS rather than leiomyoma. LMS typically stains positively for vimentin, desmin, smooth muscle actin, and H-caldesmon.

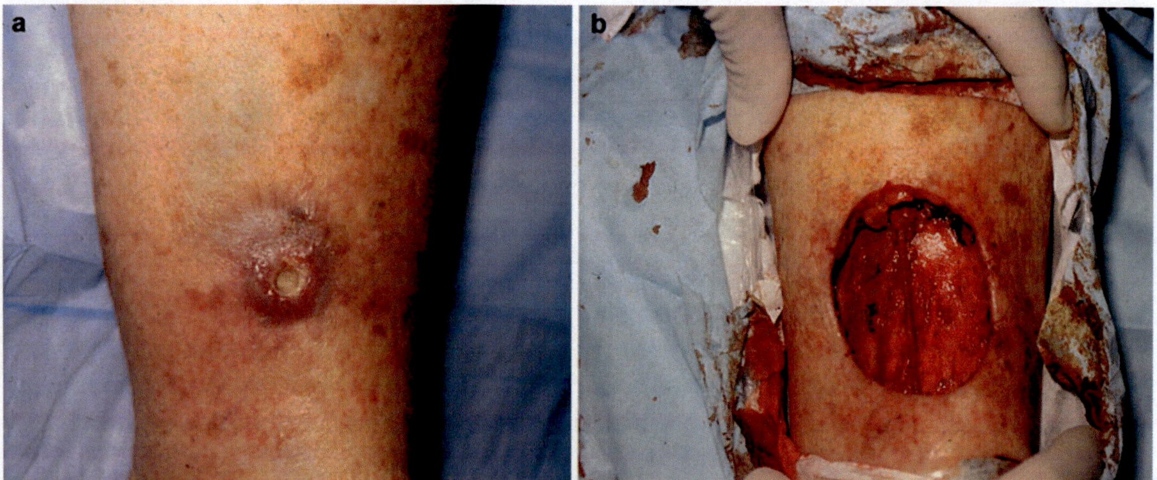

Fig. 23.1 (**a**) Primary cutaneous leiomyosarcoma on the lower leg. (**b**) Defect extending through subcutaenous fat following Mohs micrographic surgery

23.3 Histologic Features

The accepted derivation of cutaneous LMS is from arrector pili, dartoic, or breast smooth muscle, and the subcutaneous variant from vascular mural muscle. While a definitive derivation has not been conclusively proven, the frequency of cutaneous LMS on sites with greatest hair density supports this hypothesis. The vast majority of cutaneous LMS exhibit nodular aggregates and densely packed bundles of spindled smooth muscle cells (Fig. 23.2a, b). The superficial cutaneous variant tends to exhibit a diffuse infiltrative growth pattern with neoplastic cells splaying collagen bundles [3].

Subcutaneous LMS displays a characteristic circumscription and compressed collagen pseudocapsule [3]. Often, localized "hot spots" within the tumor demonstrate aggregates of atypical myocytes with bizarre mitotic figures interweaving chaotically between the more benign-appearing areas. Myxoid changes are not uncommon. Large thin-walled vessels may be noted within the neoplasm, and vascular invasion represents a poor prognostic indicator, as does involvement of deeper tissue planes, such as fascia and skeletal muscle [7].

Differentiating leiomyosarcoma from leiomyoma can be difficult; minimum criteria for malignancy include crowding, hyperchromatic nuclei, cellular atypia, irregular or asymmetric growth pattern with extension into the dermis, and mitoses (>1/hpf) [3]. Multinucleated giant cells with bizarre nuclei may be noted. Tumor depth, more so than grade, is correlated with metastases, local recurrence, and poor prognosis [2, 8–10]. A three-level grading system for soft tissue sarcomas has been developed by the French National Cancer Center, which takes into account differentiation (mature, certain, or uncertain), mitoses (0–9, 10–19, or 20+), and necrosis (<50% or >50%), though the unpredictable biological behavior of LMS based on grade alone limits the utility of this classification system [11].

The histologic differential diagnosis of LMS also includes other cutaneous and subcutaneous spindle cell neoplasms: atypical fibroxanthoma, malignant fibrous histiocytoma, hemangiopericytoma, fibrosarcoma, rhabdomyosarcoma, dermatofibroma, dermatofibrosarcoma protuberans, malignant schwannoma, nodular fasciitis, and synovial sarcoma [7]. The more common atypical fibrous xanthoma and malignant fibrous histiocytoma lack thin blunt-ended cells with tapered nuclei characteristic of smooth muscle. Due to its vascularity, the subcutaneous variant may resemble a hemangiopericytoma, but close inspection should reveal cells with characteristic smooth muscle morphology.

While phosphotungstic acid hematoxylin or Masson's trichrome staining can reveal the presence of muscle. LMS typically stains positively for vimentin, desmin, and smooth muscle actin (Fig. 23.2c). Subcutaneous and high-grade tumors may stain poorly or not at all. Staining for H-caldesmon, a regulatory protein specific for smooth muscle, has been shown to be positive in 60–73% of LMS [6]. Rare S-100 and cytokeratin positivity may make differentiating these tumors from melanoma and squamous cell carcinoma difficult [3]. Other reported variants include epithelioid, granular, and osteoclast-like giant cell predominant [3].

> **Summary: Prognosis**
>
> - LMS is characterized by a high local recurrence rate, which is greater for deeper subcutaneous tumors. While metastasis has been reported in up to 30% of subcutaneous tumors, the metastatic potential of superficial cutaneous tumors is thought to be minimal.

23.4 Prognosis

Due to the paucity of large studies and lack of consistent subtyping by histologic depth in the existing literature, the biological behavior of LMS is difficult to accurately assess. The prognosis of patients with superficial LMS depends on whether the tumor is cutaneous or subcutaneous in origin and whether the tumor is primary or recurrent. Early case reports suggested local recurrence rate for cutaneous LMS was 30–50% while up to 70% of subcutaneous tumors recurred [12–14]. The recurrent lesions tend to be larger, deeper, and more mitotically active than their primary lesions [13, 15].

In recent large case series, recurrence (or persistence of the tumor) following conventional wide excision has been shown to occur in about 16% of superficial LMS overall (6% for cutaneous and 18% for subcutaneous) [6, 16]. Recurrences of subcutaneous tumors after local excision are significantly greater than those limited to the dermis [3, 13, 14, 17], and greater tumor thickness is significantly associated with decreased disease-free survival [16]. Early literature suggested metastatic rates as

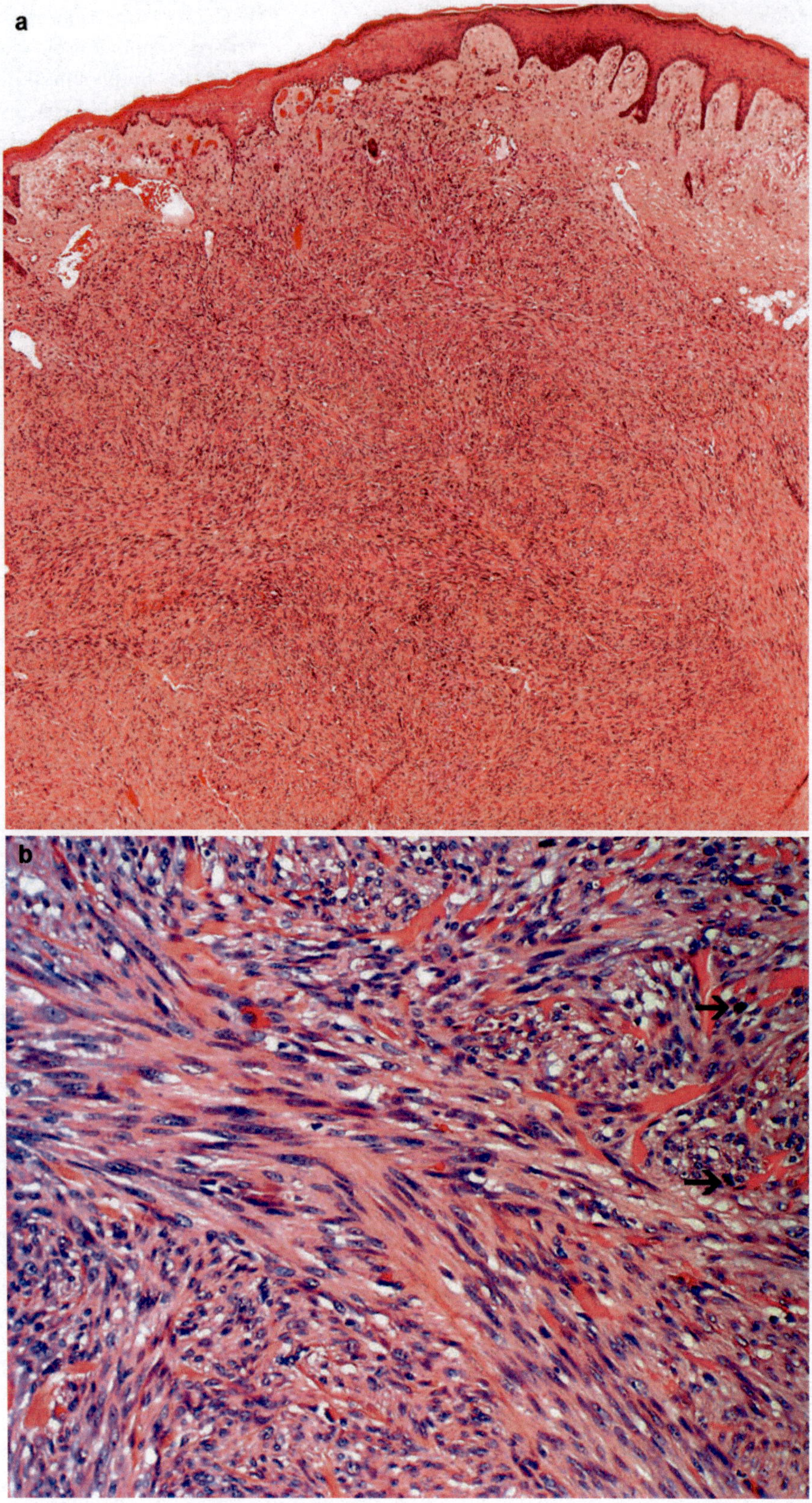

Fig. 23.2 (**a**) Low-power view of leiomyosarcoma. Note depth of tumor involving entire reticular dermis and extending into the subcutis. (**b**) High-power view (200×). Fascicles of elongated cells with blunt-tipped nuclei. (**c**) Positive immunohistochemical staining with actin (200×)

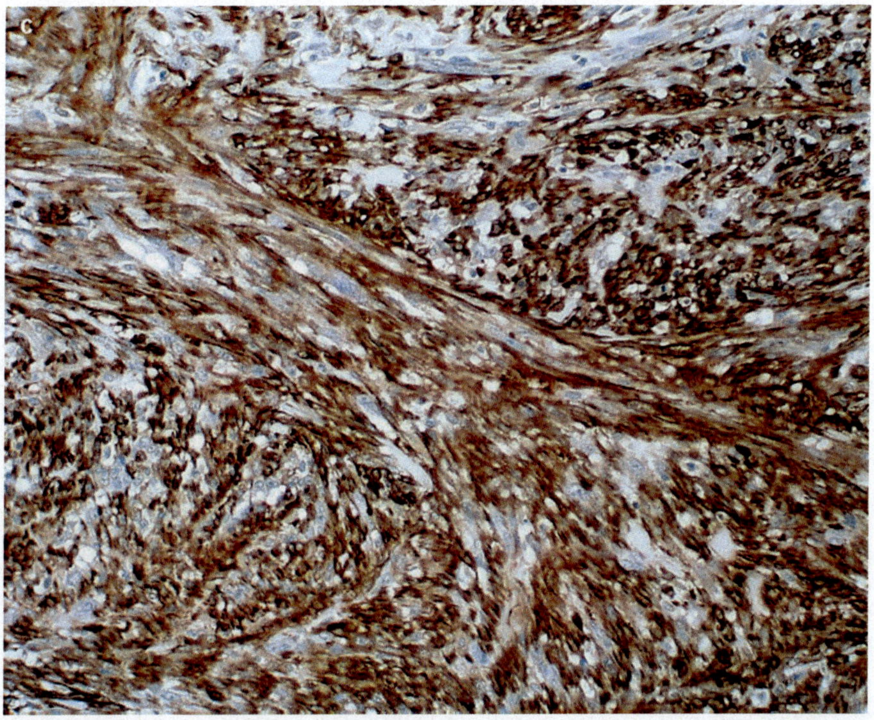

Fig. 23.2 (continued)

Table 23.1 Local recurrence rates with wide excision of LMS

Series	Cases	Recurrence rate[a] (%)	Cutaneous (%)	Subcutaneous (%)
Dahl and Angervall [12]	47	40		
Fields and Helwig [13]	67[b]	45	42	58
Bernstein and Roenigk [21]	34	30	14	48
Svarvar et al. [16]	206	16[c]		

[a]Combined overall recurrence rate
[b]Cases for which follow-up information is available
[c]Includes cases treated by local excision and radiotherapy

high as 60% for subcutaneous LMS [12, 18], though this figure has been attenuated by larger, more recent investigations. These later studies suggest that subcutaneous LMS may metastasize to distant sites in up to 30% of cases, whereas the strictly cutaneous variant is considered to have very limited, if any, metastatic potential [2, 6, 9, 16]. The lungs are the most common site for metastases, liver and bone are following; however, lymphangitic spread may occur [3, 14, 19, 20].

23.4.1 Treatment

Owing to the rarity of LMS, standards for treatment have not been firmly established. Standard treatment for superficial LMS has been wide local excision despite local recurrence rates of up to 45% (Table 23.1) [13]. While standard excisional margins have not been established, published margins range from 3.0 to 5.0 cm down to subcutaneous tissue or fascia [10, 13, 22, 23]. As stated above, recurrence rates correlate with the depth of invasion.

23.4.2 Mohs Micrographic Surgery (MMS)

A growing body of evidence supports the utility of Mohs micrographic surgery in reducing local recurrences. MMS has played a part in the treatment of LMS since 1987 [24]. Because of the ill-defined margins and infiltrative histology of LMS, conventional wide excision is not ideal. Since standard histological

Table 23.2 Leiomyosarcomas treated by MMS

References	Number of cases	Number of recurrences
Iacobucci et al. [24]	1	0
Brown et al. [26]	1	0
Davidson et al. [27]	1	0
Bernstein and Roenigk [21]	2	0
Huether et al. [28]	7	1
Humphreys et al. [29]	3	1
Vujevich et al. [25]	1	0
Total	16	2 (12.5%)

serial sectioning using a "bread-loafing" technique provides a very limited examination of the surgical margins, and false negative histologic reporting may contribute to the high recurrence rate of LMS with conventional excision. Wide excisional margins may also lead to greater tissue destruction resulting in profound functional, cosmetic, psychological, and social consequences [25]. Mohs micrographic surgery theoretically provides complete peripheral and deep margin evaluation, which prevents both inadequate and excessive tissue removal. While there are only 16 documented cases of LMS treated by Mohs micrographic surgery, only 2 cases have recurred (Table 23.2) [21, 24–29]. The aggregate recurrence rate of 12.5% for Mohs micrographic surgery compares favorably to that reported for wide excision.

MMS also has the advantage of tissue sparing when compared with the wide excision. The large LMS on the shin was excised using MMS. Sparing of the tibial nerve was possible in this particular case using Mohs surgery to assess the deep margins rather than a deep en bloc resection. Limiting the defect size while obtaining clear margins can significantly reduce postoperative morbidity especially on areas of the body such as the leg characterized by delayed wound healing. Although preliminary studies show the benefits of MMS for LMS, additional cases and longer follow-up periods are required to establish its efficacy.

Cryotherapy may be an alternative for patients unable to undergo surgery. Montes et al. described two elderly patients that were treated with cryosurgery for LMS of the scalp [30]. Treatments were done with tissue temperature 40–50°C for a period of 5 min and repeated treatment every 2 weeks for a total of three to six treatments. Neither patient showed evidence of recurrence 2 years after treatment. Adjuvant radiation or chemotherapy has no proven benefit for superficial LMS [31–33].

Patients diagnosed with subcutaneous LMS should receive a chest radiograph because of the potential for lung metastasis. Close clinical follow-up for a minimum of 5 years is recommended, as tumors usually recur within 1–5 years of initial surgery [10, 32].

Summary: Conclusion

- *The overall cure rate of leiomyosarcoma treated by Mohs micrographic surgery is 87%* which compares favorably to wide excision and offers the advantage of tissue sparing. Immunosuppression may promote aggressive tumor behavior. Deeply invasive tumors may result in cutaneous or distant metastases regardless of the method of excision.

23.5 Conclusion

LMS is a rare spindle cell tumor of smooth muscle derivation that may originate in the skin or deeper soft tissue. Because of the locally aggressive nature and propensity for recurrence, Mohs micrographic surgery may result in superior local control of superficial LMS.

References

1. Rouhani P, Fletcher CD, Devesa SS, Toro JR. Cutaneous soft tissue sarcoma incidence patterns in the U.S.: an analysis of 12,114 cases. Cancer. 2008;113(3):616–27.
2. Annest NM, Grekin SJ, Stone MS, Messingham MJ. Cutaneous leiomyosarcoma: a tumor of the head and neck. Dermatol Surg. 2007;33(5):628–33.
3. Holst VA, Junkins-Hopkins JM, Elenitsas R. Cutaneous smooth muscle neoplasms: clinical features, histologic findings, and treatment options. J Am Acad Dermatol. 2002; 46(4):477–90; quiz 491–474.
4. Altinok G, Dogan AI, Aydin SO, Gedikoglu G. Primary leiomyosarcomas of the skin. Scand J Plast Reconstr Surg Hand Surg. 2002;36(1):56–9.
5. De Giorgi V, Sestini S, Massi D, Papi F, Alfaioli B, Lotti T. Superficial cutaneous leiomyosarcoma: a rare, misleading tumor. Am J Clin Dermatol. 2008;9(3):185–7.
6. Massi D, Franchi A, Alos L, et al. Primary cutaneous leiomyosarcoma: clinicopathological analysis of 36 cases. Histopathology. 2010;56(2):251–62.
7. Ragsdale BD. Tumors with fatty, muscular, osseous, and/or cartilaginous differentiation. In: Elder DE, Elenitsas R, Johnson BL, Murphy GF, Xu X, editors. LEVER'S histopathology of

the skin. 10th ed. Philadelphia: Lippincott Williams & Wilkins; 2004. p. 781–2.
8. Pijpe J, Broers GH, Plaat BE, et al. The relation between histological, tumor-biological and clinical parameters in deep and superficial leiomyosarcoma and leiomyoma. Sarcoma. 2002;6(3):105–10.
9. Miettinen M, Fetsch JF. Evaluation of biological potential of smooth muscle tumours. Histopathology. 2006;48(1): 97–105.
10. Porter CJ, Januszkiewicz JS. Cutaneous leiomyosarcoma. Plast Reconstr Surg. 2002;109(3):964–7.
11. Brown FM, Fletcher CD. Problems in grading soft tissue sarcomas. Am J Clin Pathol. 2000;114(Suppl):S82–9.
12. Dahl I, Angervall L. Cutaneous and subcutaneous leiomyosarcoma. A clinicopathologic study of 47 patients. Pathol Eur. 1974;9(4):307–15.
13. Fields JP, Helwig EB. Leiomyosarcoma of the skin and subcutaneous tissue. Cancer. 1981;47(1):156–69.
14. Wascher RA, Lee MY. Recurrent cutaneous leiomyosarcoma. Cancer. 1992;70(2):490–2.
15. Oliver GF, Reiman HM, Gonchoroff NJ, Muller SA, Umbert IJ. Cutaneous and subcutaneous leiomyosarcoma: a clinicopathological review of 14 cases with reference to antidesmin staining and nuclear DNA patterns studied by flow cytometry. Br J Dermatol. 1991;124(3):252–7.
16. Svarvar C, Bohling T, Berlin O, et al. Clinical course of nonvisceral soft tissue leiomyosarcoma in 225 patients from the Scandinavian Sarcoma Group. Cancer. 2007;109(2): 282–91.
17. Tsujimoto M, Aozasa K, Ueda T, Morimura Y, Komatsubara Y, Doi T. Multivariate analysis for histologic prognostic factors in soft tissue sarcomas. Cancer. 1988;62(5):994–8.
18. Ueda T, Aozasa K, Tsujimoto M, et al. Multivariate analysis for clinical prognostic factors in 163 patients with soft tissue sarcoma. Cancer. 1988;62(7):1444–50.
19. Spencer JM, Amonette RA. Tumors with smooth muscle differentiation. Dermatol Surg. 1996;22(9):761–8.
20. Cook TF, Fosko SW. Unusual cutaneous malignancies. Semin Cutan Med Surg. 1998;17(2):114–32.
21. Bernstein SC, Roenigk RK. Leiomyosarcoma of the skin. Treatment of 34 cases. Dermatol Surg. 1996;22(7):631–5.
22. Chow J, Sabet LM, Clark BL, Coire CI. Cutaneous leiomyosarcoma: case reports and review of the literature. Ann Plast Surg. 1987;18(4):319–22.
23. Fish FS. Soft tissue sarcomas in dermatology. Dermatol Surg. 1996;22(3):268–73.
24. Iacobucci JJ, Stevenson TR, Swanson NA, Headington JT. Cutaneous leiomyosarcoma. Ann Plast Surg. 1987;19(6): 552–4.
25. Vujevich JJ, Goldberg LH, Kimyai-Asadi A, Law R. Recurrent nodule on the nasal columella: a good reason to re-biopsy. Int J Dermatol. 2008;47(7):728–31.
26. Brown MD, Zachary CB, Grekin RC, Swanson NA. Genital tumors: their management by micrographic surgery. J Am Acad Dermatol. 1988;18(1 Pt 1):115–22.
27. Davidson LL, Frost ML, Hanke CW, Epinette WW. Primary leiomyosarcoma of the skin. Case report and review of the literature. J Am Acad Dermatol. 1989;21(5 Pt 2):1156–60.
28. Huether MJ, Zitelli JA, Brodland DG. Mohs micrographic surgery for the treatment of spindle cell tumors of the skin. J Am Acad Dermatol. 2001;44(4):656–9.
29. Humphreys TR, Finkelstein DH, Lee JB. Superficial leiomyosarcoma treated with Mohs micrographic surgery. Dermatol Surg. 2004;30(1):108–12.
30. Montes LF, Ocampo J, Garcia NJ, et al. Response of leiomyosarcoma to cryosurgery: clinicopathological and ultrastructural study. Clin Exp Dermatol. 1995;20(1):22–6.
31. Hwang ES, Gerald W, Wollner N, Meyers P, La Quaglia MP. Leiomyosarcoma in childhood and adolescence. Ann Surg Oncol. 1997;4(3):223–7.
32. Guron G, Neugut AI. Soft tissue sarcomas. Is adjuvant chemotherapy indicated? N Y State J Med. 1993;93(3): 156–8.
33. Haffner AC, Zepter K, Fritz T, Dummer R, Lejeune FJ, Burg G. Complete remission of advanced cutaneous leiomyosarcoma following isolated limb perfusion with high-dose tumour necrosis factor-alpha and melphalan. Br J Dermatol. 1999;141(5):935–6.

Merkel Cell Carcinoma

24

Stephanie A. Diamantis and Victor J. Marks

Abstract

Merkel cell carcinoma (MCC) is a rare, aggressive tumor of neuroendocrine derivation mostly seen in elderly and immunosuppressed individuals. MCC has a propensity for local recurrence and regional and distant metastases. Because of the rarity of MCC, no evidenced-based unified treatment algorithm exists. Surgery is the mainstay of treatment for localized MCC. Mohs micrographic surgery (MMS) may be a tissue-sparing alternative to wide local excision. Radiation of the primary tumor site and/or regional lymph node basin may favorably improve recurrence rates. Chemotherapy is an option for inoperable or widespread disease. Prognosis is generally poor, especially if regional and distant metastases are present.

Keywords

Merkel cell carcinoma • Mohs micrographic surgery • Merkel cell polyomavirus • Trabecular cell carcinoma • Wide local excision

Summary: Overview of Merkel Cell Carcinoma

- Merkel cell polyomavirus may play a role in the development of Merkel cell carcinoma.
- Merkel cell carcinoma is more common in the elderly, white, and immunosuppressed populations.
- The most common location for Merkel cell carcinoma is the head and neck.

S.A. Diamantis (✉)
Department of Dermatology, Geisinger Medical Center, Danville, PA, USA
e-mail: sadiamantis@geisinger.edu

V.J. Marks
Department of Dermatologic Surgery, Geisinger Health System, Danville, PA, USA

24.1 Overview of Merkel Cell Carcinoma

Merkel cell carcinoma (also called trabecular cell carcinoma, primary cutaneous neuroendocrine carcinoma, and primary small cell carcinoma of the skin) was initially described by Toker in 1972 [1–3]. The cell of origin is the Merkel cell, a mechanoreceptor usually found in the basal layer of the epidermis [4, 5].

Recent work by Feng et al. describes a virus, the Merkel cell polyomavirus (MCV), integrated into Merkel cell carcinoma (MCC) tumor cell DNA. In 10 patients with MCC, 8 (80%) were found to have evidence of genomic sequences containing MCV in their tumors. The majority of these tumors showed a clonal pattern of integrated viral DNA in the MCC tumor genome, arguing for an oncogenic role of MCV. Only

K. Nouri (ed.), *Mohs Micrographic Surgery*,
DOI 10.1007/978-1-4471-2152-7_24,

8% of control tissues (16% of control skin tissues) showed MCV sequences [6, 7].

Merkel cell carcinoma is a rare tumor, but the incidence has tripled over the past two decades. The highest incidence rates are in the elderly population [8, 9]. Mean age at diagnosis is 67.9 years, but reports in the literature range from age 15 to 97 years old [10, 11]. Immunosuppression is a risk factor for developing MCC [12, 13]. MCC is more common in patients with organ transplantation, HIV, B-cell lymphoma, or other immunosuppressed conditions [8, 14]. White individuals are more frequently affected than black individuals [11, 12]. MCC also typically occurs in sun-exposed areas, although the exact role of ultraviolet light exposure in the pathogenesis of MCC remains unknown [10, 15]. Areas of the head and neck are most often affected followed by the trunk and extremities [10, 15–17].

Summary: Diagnosis of Merkel Cell Carcinoma

- Merkel cell carcinoma presents as a rapidly growing nodule on sun-exposed skin of elderly individuals.
- Clinical presentation is nonspecific, and biopsy is necessary to establish a diagnosis.
- Merkel cell carcinoma is characterized by a dense dermal infiltrate of small blue atypical cells, staining positive with CK-20 and negative with TTF-1.

24.2 Diagnosis of Merkel Cell Carcinoma

24.2.1 Clinical Features

Patient evaluation should begin with a history of the lesion in question, addressing its duration, evolution, symptoms, and previous treatment. The clinical presentation of MCC is non-specific, and diagnosis requires pathologic evaluation. Typically, MCC presents as a rapidly growing, blue, or violaceous solitary nodule on sun-exposed skin of elderly individuals [11]. The surface is usually smooth but can rarely ulcerate. Most primary tumors are <2 cm on presentation [18].

24.2.2 Pathology

Histologic exam reveals a poorly circumscribed, diffuse dermal infiltrate of densely packed atypical small blue cells with scant cytoplasm. The epidermis is usually not involved, and a grenz zone is often present (see Fig. 24.1). Mitotic figures are common, and vascular/lymphatic invasion can also be seen. Three pathologic subtypes are described in the literature based on cellular pattern: trabecular (rare, less aggressive), intermediate (more common), small cell (most aggressive, can mimic other small cell tumors) [4, 11].

Immunostains are often helpful in differentiating merkel MCC from other small, round blue cell tumors. The most widely used immunostains for MCC include cytokeratin 20 (CK-20) and thyroid transcription factor 1 (TTF-1). MCC stains positive with CK-20 with a sensitivity ranging from 89% to100% [19]. Staining with TTF-1 is negative in MCC which differentiates it from small cell lung carcinoma (SCLC) which can be very similar histologically (SCLC stains positive with TTF-1) [20]. Other neuroendocrine markers positive in MCC include chromogranin A, synaptophysin, neuron-specific enolase, and neurofilament protein (see Fig. 24.2). Leukocyte-common antigen, S-100, and pancytokeratin are useful markers to rule out other diagnoses such as melanoma, squamous cell carcinoma, and leukemia [20]. Staining with cytokeratin or neurofilament protein produces a pattern of perinuclear dot positivity which is specific for MCC [5, 19]. Electron microscopy is also useful in diagnosing MCC as electron dense granules are noted in the cytoplasm [2].

24.2.3 Differential Diagnosis

Since MCC is rarely suspected on initial evaluation, the clinical differential diagnoses are numerous and include other benign and malignant tumors such as adnexal neoplasms, pyogenic granuloma, keratoacanthoma, squamous cell carcinoma, basal-cell carcinoma, atypical fibroxanthoma, melanoma, leukemia, lymphoma, and metastatic carcinoma to the skin. The histologic differential includes other small, round blue cell processes such as small cell lung cancer, leukemia, lymphoma, Ewing's sarcoma, melanoma, and neuroblastoma.

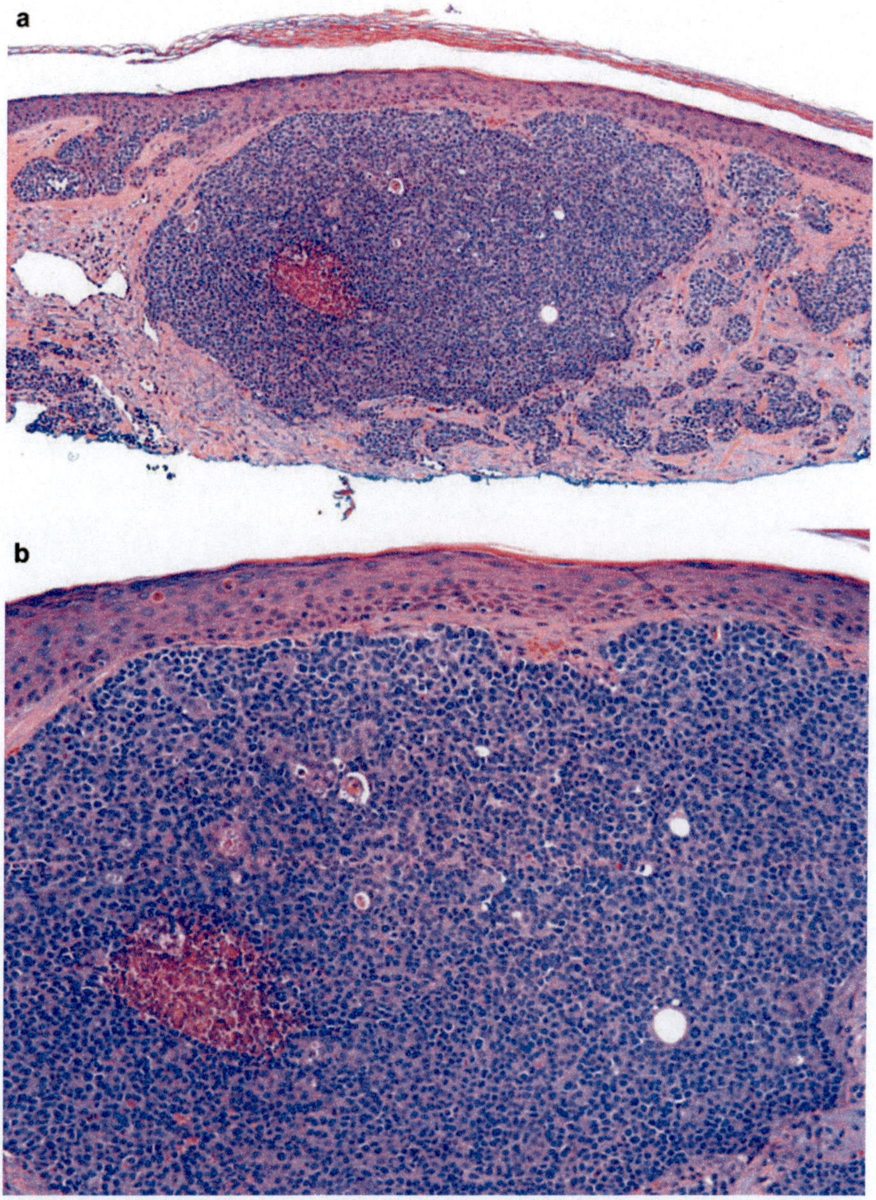

Fig. 24.1 Histopathology of Merkel cell carcinoma on hematoxylin and eosin (10× and 40×)

Summary: Management of Merkel Cell Carcinoma

- Complete skin and lymph node exam is important in initial evaluation of a patient with Merkel cell carcinoma and subsequent staging.
- Prognosis in Merkel cell carcinoma is largely determined by tumor stage.
- Surgery is the treatment of choice for localized disease.
- Merkel cell carcinoma has an overall poor prognosis, with a high propensity for recurrence, especially with lymph node involvement or widespread disease.

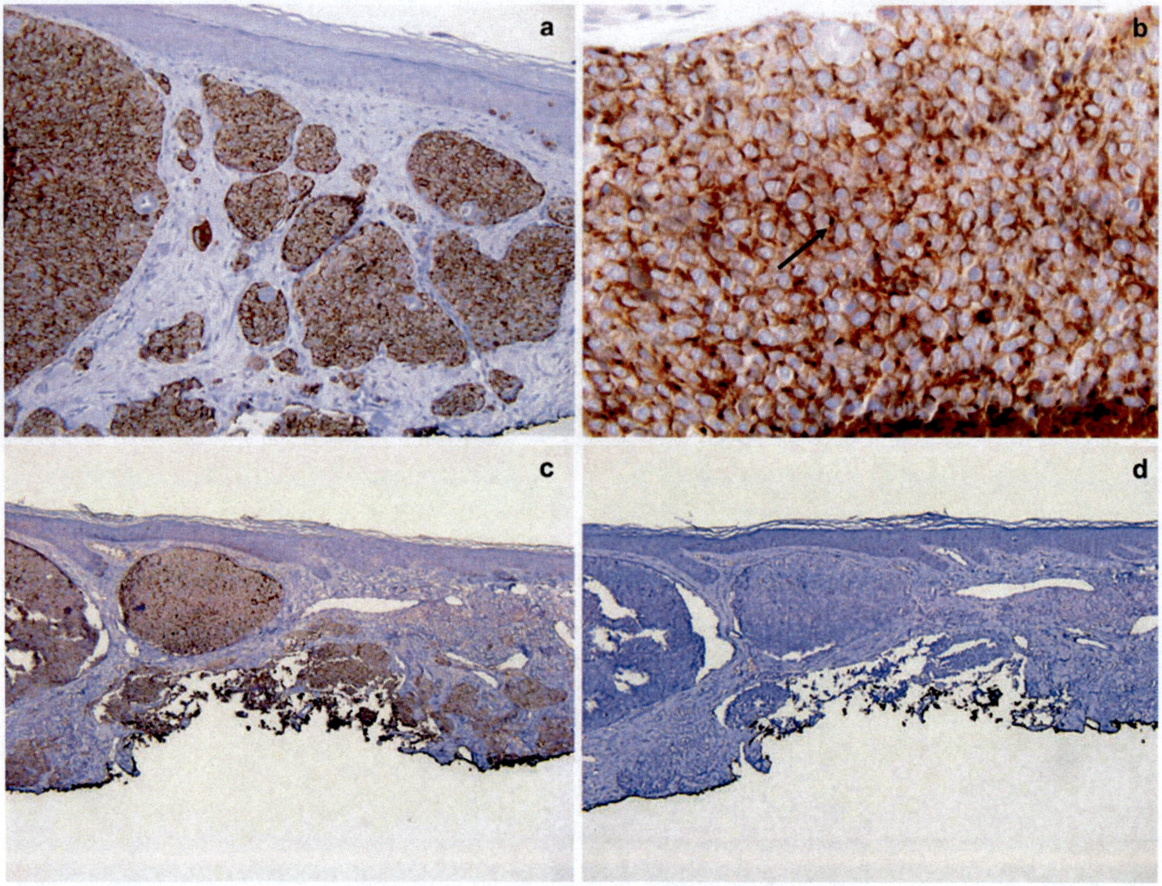

Fig. 24.2 Immunostains and Merkel cell carcinoma. **a** and **b** show perinuclear dot positivity with CK-20 (refer to *arrow* on **b**). Positive synaptophysin stain in **c**. Negative TTF-1 stain in **d**

24.3 Management of Merkel Cell Carcinoma

24.3.1 Patient Evaluation and Staging

Patient evaluation begins with assessment of the primary tumor and correct histopathologic diagnosis using hematoxylin and eosin as well as immunostains. Once the diagnosis of MCC is established, a complete skin and clinical lymph node exam is recommended to evaluate for regional and/or distant spread. If clinically indicated, imaging should be performed for staging purposes. Useful imaging modalities include computed tomography (CT), magnetic resonance imaging (MRI), and positron emission tomography–computed tomography (PET-CT) [20].

Multiple competing staging systems have been proposed in the past [21–24]. Given the heterogeneity of these systems, the American Joint Committee on Cancer (AJCC) developed Merkel cell-specific guidelines using the primary tumor, regional lymph node involvement, and distant metastasis (TNM system) [25]. In summary, stage I and II define patients with local disease based on tumor size (I is <2 cm; II is >2 cm). If patients are pathologically node-negative they are substaged as A (substaged as B if only clinical evaluation of nodes was performed). Patients with lymph node involvement are stage III (substaged as A for pathologically positive, clinically occult nodes and B for clinically evident nodes). Stage IV defines patients with distant metastasis [25].

Sentinel lymph node (SLN) evaluation has been advocated in the evaluation of patients with melanoma, and a similar approach has been proposed for MCC. Studies have shown MCC spreads in an orderly fashion, and metastasis occurs via lymphatic spread to regional lymph nodes prior to systemic spread [21].

Lymph node involvement appears to be important in staging and prognosis. The use of immunostains on sentinel lymph nodes may improve detection of occult disease [26]. Some authors report 19–40% of sentinel lymph nodes sampled are positive [12, 27]. Sentinal lymph node evaluation is best performed prior to wide local excision to preserve draining patterns of the primary tumor. SLN biopsy is less reliable on the head/neck because of the complex draining pattern which increases the likelihood of false negative results [20].

The National Comprehensive Cancer Network (NCCN) also recently published guidelines for evaluation and management of patients with MCC based on lower-level evidence and panel consensus. Patients are stratified into three groups at the outset: those with no clinical nodal involvement, those with clinical nodal involvement, and those with metastatic disease. These guidelines can be used in conjunction with the AJCC recommendations for staging in determining prognosis and management strategies in patients with MCC [20].

24.3.1.1 No Clinical Nodal Involvement

The following are recommendations based on clinical nodal involvement:

- If a patient has already undergone wide local excision, options are to observe *or* consider radiation therapy to the primary tumor site, in transit lymphatics, and draining nodal basins.
- If no prior excision has been done, one may consider sentinel lymph node biopsy with immunostains (especially CK-20 and pancytokeratins AE1/AE3) followed by observation *or* radiation as above. Note that sentinel lymph node (SLN) biopsy is less reliable on the head and neck because of a less predictable draining pattern.
- If SLN biopsy is performed and is *positive*, consider the following: consultation with tumor board, node dissection ± radiation, adjuvant chemotherapy (although the benefit of chemotherapy is controversial).

24.3.1.2 Clinical Nodal Involvement

The panel recommends fine needle aspiration (FNA) of the clinically involved lymph node. If FNA is positive, image to assess for distant metastases. If FNA is negative, do an open biopsy. If the open biopsy is negative, refer to guidelines listed above for node-negative patients.

24.3.1.3 Metastatic Disease

If widespread disease is found on imaging, consider consultation with a tumor board and treatment with a combination of surgery, radiation, and chemotherapy. More common sites of distant metastatic disease include liver, bone, brain, lung, and skin [11, 18].

24.3.2 Treatment

Appropriate treatment of MCC depends on accurate diagnosis and staging. The treatment of choice for localized disease is surgical [10]. Different surgical approaches have been described in the literature. Some support wide local excision with 1–2-cm margins down to fascia, but most studies agree that wide local excision with 2.5–3-cm margins has lower rates of recurrence [10, 16, 18, 20]. Additional approaches include Mohs surgery or a modified Mohs technique where an additional final layer is sent for permanent sectioning after tumor extirpation [20].

Merkel cell carcinoma is a very radiosensitive tumor, but the indications for radiation are unclear given the lack of prospective studies. Multiple retrospective studies show a decreased local recurrence rate with adjuvant radiation [28–32]. A larger retrospective analysis of 1,254 patients showed statistically significant reduction in local and regional recurrence in patients who received adjuvant radiation, but no reduction in rate of metastatic disease or survival benefit [30].

Systemic chemotherapy has also been used in metastatic Merkel cell carcinoma even though little evidence is available regarding its benefit. Most studies agree there is no survival advantage [10, 15].

Regardless of the stage at diagnosis, patients with a history of MCC need close follow-up to detect recurrence. Patients should be followed regularly with history and physical, complete skin exam, lymph node exam and imaging if clinically indicated as follows: every 1–3 months for 1 year, 3–6 months for the second year, then annually [20].

24.3.3 Prognosis

Merkel cell carcinoma is an aggressive tumor with a high propensity for local recurrence (25–30%), regional lymph node involvement and distant metastasis. Regional lymph node involvement is present in 52–66%, and is usually noted within 2 years of diagnosis. Distant metastatic disease is noted in 34–36% or patients who almost always have preceding or concurrent nodal disease. Five-year survival rates range from

30% to 64%, depending on lymph node or systemic involvement [20, 21, 30].

A recent study published by Lemos et al. addressed staging and survival in 5,823 patients from the National Cancer Data Base with MCC. They note an overall 5-year survival rate of 40% and relative survival of 54% (when patients were compared with age and sex-matched controls). Patients with localized disease and pathologically negative lymph nodes had the best overall survival (76% at 5 years) [25].

Factors associated with a poor prognosis include: tumor size greater than 2 cm, metastatic disease at presentation, vascular or lymphatic invasion noted on pathology, small cell histologic pattern, greater than 10 mitoses per high-power field [18]. Other studies note poor prognosis if the primary tumor is on located on the head and neck. This may be secondary to incomplete excision as highest recurrence rates are on the head and neck [18]. Lymph node status is particularly important in prognostication and correlates with survival. Lack of lymph node involvement improves survival rate [21].

Summary: Mohs Micrographic Surgery and Merkel Cell Carcinoma

- Mohs micrographic surgery is an alternative to wide local excision in the treatment of primary Merkel cell carcinoma.
- Mohs micrographic surgery offers the advantage of circumferential complete margin assessment with sparing of normal tissue.

24.4 Mohs Micrographic Surgery and Merkel Cell Carcinoma

Mohs micrographic surgery (MMS) is an effective alternative to wide local excision for local control of disease [33]. The Mohs technique is commonly used in the treatment of non-melanoma skin cancers, but its use is increasing in rare tumors such as MCC. Two major advantages of MMS include circumferential margin assessment (including the deep margin) and sparing of uninvolved tissue. In areas where excess tissue is lacking (i.e., the head and neck), the Mohs technique is especially useful. For example, one patient developed a MCC on the left upper eyelid margin requiring three stages for clear margins, and the patient is without recurrence or metastasis 2 years later [34]. Merkel cell carcinoma has an extensive vertical growth phase, and complete evaluation of the deep margin is imperative because of the high risk of recurrence with incomplete excision [12]. In general, MMS is associated with higher success rates because of the extent of margin assessment, and the high rate of complete tumor extirpation minimizes the risk of local recurrence [35]. Disadvantages of MMS include length of the procedure and interpretation of frozen sections rather than permanent sections (the surgeon needs excellent slide quality from the technician/lab).

Few retrospective studies and no prospective studies evaluate the use of MMS in the treatment of MCC. Gollard et al. performed a retrospective analysis of 22 patients with MCC, and 8 patients were treated with MMS (with permanent sections). Tumor size ranged from 0.7 to 1.9 cm (average 1.2 cm). An average of 1.4 layers was needed to get a clear margin. Average margin for clearance was 1.5 cm (1.2 cm on face, 1.9 cm on extremities). Five of the eight patients treated with MMS also got radiation (three local to the tumor bed, two to lymph node basin as well). Average follow-up was 37 months, and none of the patients treated with MMS had a local recurrence. However, two patients developed distant metastatic disease 8 and 10 months after surgery [10].

O'Conner et al. retrospectively evaluated 86 patients with MCC to determine rates of local recurrence and development of metastatic disease after surgical treatment. A total of 41 patients with clinically localized disease were treated with wide local excision (WLE), and 13 patients were treated with MMS (only 12 of which were included in analysis because the tumor persisted in the 13th case). In patients treated with wide local excision: mean preoperative size was 1.57 cm, no adjuvant radiation was used, local recurrence rate was 32%, regional metastatic rate was 49%, and 26% of patients MMS: mean preoperative size was 2.98 cm (notably larger than those in the WLE group), 4 patients were also treated with radiation, local recurrence rate was 8.3%, regional metastatic rate was 33%, and no patients died of metastatic disease [16].

Boyer et al. performed a retrospective analysis to determine the effect of adjuvant radiation when combined with MMS. Forty-five patients with Stage I disease were treated with MMS, and 20 also received adjuvant postoperative radiation (to primary site ± regional lymph node basin). In the MMS alone group, mean preoperative size was 14 mm, with a 13.7 mm mean margin post-Mohs. Local (marginal) recurrence was 4%. Regional recurrence (defined as marginal + in transit lesions) was 16%. Lymph node metastatic rate was 16%, and distant metastatic rate was 8%. In the MMS + radiation group, the mean preoperative size was 18.4 mm, with a 20.6 mm mean margin. Local recurrence was 0%. Lymph node metastatic rate was 15%, and distant metastatic rate was 5%. There was no significant difference in local recurrence or metastatic pattern between the two groups. Five year survival rate was 79% in MMS alone and 80% in the MMS + radiation group. The authors conclude MMS is an effective alternative to WLE, and the most important step in managing MCC is complete removal of the primary tumor. The higher marginal recurrence rate seen with WLE may be secondary to inadequate excision of primary tumor (infiltrating border not clinically evident, narrow margin) or incomplete evaluation of pathologic margin [17]. Notably, no difference in recurrence or survival was observed with tumor bed/draining lymph node basin radiation [17].

Another retrospective study looked at MCC of the extremities. Thirty-two patients were treated with WLE and six patients were treated with MMS with primary endpoints of overall survival and recurrence. No difference was observed in local recurrence rates. Lymph node status was noted to be important in the risk of regional recurrence, which is in agreement with other studies. Radiation reduced local recurrence rate but had no overall survival benefit [12].

Not all case reviews have shown a favorable outcome when MMS is used as a treatment modality for MCC. Hanke et al. treated four patients with MMS. Three developed local recurrence, one had regional metastasis to lymph nodes, and two patients had distant metastases. No data was available regarding stage at presentation [3]. Similarly, a chart review of 22 patients with MCC revealed the best survival in patients who underwent wide local excision (with 2–3 cm margins) and elective/prophylactic dissection of the lymphatic drainage basin [15]. It is this author's opinion that the risk/benefit ratio and morbidity associated with complete lymph node dissection may be unfavorable, especially with the availability of sentinel lymph node biopsy.

Wide local excision with 2–3-cm margins is the standard of care for primary MCC, but local recurrence rates reported in literature range from 27% to 32% [16–18]. In those studies looking at MMS for the treatment of MCC, margins after Mohs surgery ranged from 1.2 to 3.3 cm, sparing centimeters of normal skin in the majority of cases [10, 16, 17]. Overall, MMS compares favorably with WLE and usually is tissue-sparing, but may have less effect when in transit and nodal metastasis present. Postoperative radiation may be considered in patients with large or recurrent tumors, or in patients where excision is incomplete or impossible [17].

Summary: Conclusion

- Merkel cell carcinoma is a rare tumor with a high likelihood of regional involvement and metastatic spread.
- Sentinal lymph node biopsy is important in prognosis and management.
- Complete surgical excision with margin control is the mainstay of management for primary Merkel cell carcinoma.

24.5 Conclusion

Merkel cell carcinoma is a rare tumor with a propensity for local recurrence, regional, and distant metastatic spread. Staging is based on the tumor size and involvement of lymph nodes and/or distant organs. Lymph node involvement is an important prognostic indicator and predictor of survival. The mainstay of management for primary Merkel cell carcinoma is complete excision with clear surgical margins. Mohs micrographic surgery is an effective alternative to wide local excision. Mohs surgery has the advantage of circumferential margin assessment and sparing of uninvolved tissue. The role of adjuvant radiation to the postoperative tumor bed and/or draining lymph node basin is unclear. Radiation may lower the rate of local recurrence, although no survival benefit has been noted. Patients with a history of Merkel cell carcinoma need close follow up to detect recurrence.

References

1. Toker C. Trabecular carcinoma of the skin. Arch Dermatol. 1972;105(1):107–10.
2. Roenigk RK, Goltz RW. Merkel cell carcinoma – a problem with microscopically controlled surgery. J Dermatol Surg Oncol. 1986;12(4):332–6.
3. Hanke WC, Conner AC, Temofeew RK, Lingeman RE. Merkel cell carcinoma. Arch Dermatol. 1989;125(8):1096–100.
4. Weedon D. Neural and neuroendocrine tumors. In: Skin pathology. 2nd ed. New York: Churchill Livingstone; 2002. p. 989.
5. Su W, Kheir SM, Berberian B, Cockerell CJ. Merkel cell carcinoma in situ arising in a trichilemmal cyst: a case report and literature review. Am J Dermatopathol. 2008;30(5):458–61.
6. Feng H, Shuda M, Chang Y, Moore PS. Clonal integration of a polyomavirus in human merkel cell carcinoma. Science. 2008;319(5866):1096–100.
7. Viscidi RP, Shah KV. Cancer. A skin cancer virus? Science. 2008;319(5866):1049–50.
8. Hodgson NC. Merkel cell carcinoma: changing incidence trends. J Surg Oncol. 2005;89(1):1–4.
9. Lemos B, Nghiem P. Merkel cell carcinoma: more deaths but still no pathway to blame. J Invest Dermatol. 2007;127(9): 2100–3.
10. Gollard R, Weber R, Kosty MP, Greenway HT, Massullo V, Humberson C. Merkel cell carcinoma: review of 22 cases with surgical, pathologic, and therapeutic considerations. Cancer. 2000;88(8):1842–51.
11. Taylor G, Mollick D, Hellman E. Merkel cell carcinoma. In: Rigel D, editor. Cancer of the skin. 1st ed. Philadelphia: Elsevier; 2005. p. 323.
12. Senchenkov A, Barnes SA, Moran SL. Predictors of survival and recurrence in the surgical treatment of merkel cell carcinoma of the extremities. J Surg Oncol. 2007;95(3):229–34.
13. Ruan JH, Reeves M. A merkel cell carcinoma treatment algorithm. Arch Surg. 2009;144(6):582–5.
14. An KP, Ratner D. Merkel cell carcinoma in the setting of HIV infection. J Am Acad Dermatol. 2001;45(2):309–12.
15. Brissett AE, Olsen KD, Kasperbauer JL, et al. Merkel cell carcinoma of the head and neck: a retrospective case series. Head Neck. 2002;24(11):982–8.
16. O'Connor WJ, Roenigk RK, Roenigk RK, Brodland DG. Merkel cell carcinoma. Comparison of mohs micrographic surgery and wide excision in eighty-six patients. Dermatol Surg. 1997;23(10):929–33.
17. Boyer JD, Zitelli JA, Brodland DG, D'Angelo G. Local control of primary merkel cell carcinoma: review of 45 cases treated with mohs micrographic surgery with and without adjuvant radiation. J Am Acad Dermatol. 2002;47(6):885–92.
18. O'Connor WJ, Brodland DG. Merkel cell carcinoma. Dermatol Surg. 1996;22(3):262–7.
19. Schmidt U, Muller U, Metz KA, Leder LD. Cytokeratin and neurofilament protein staining in merkel cell carcinoma of the small cell type and small cell carcinoma of the lung. Am J Dermatopathol. 1998;20(4):346–51.
20. Miller Sea. Practice guidelines in oncology: Merkel cell carcinoma. www.nccn.org (2010). Accessed November 20, 2010.
21. Yiengpruksawan A, Coit DG, Thaler HT, Urmacher C, Knapper WK. Merkel cell carcinoma. Prognosis and management. Arch Surg. 1991;126(12):1514–9.
22. Allen PJ, Zhang ZF, Coit DG. Surgical management of merkel cell carcinoma. Ann Surg. 1999;229(1):97–105.
23. Allen PJ, Bowne WB, Jaques DP, Brennan MF, Busam K, Coit DG. Merkel cell carcinoma: prognosis and treatment of patients from a single institution. J Clin Oncol. 2005;23(10): 2300–9.
24. Clark JR, Veness MJ, Gilbert R, O'Brien CJ, Gullane PJ. Merkel cell carcinoma of the head and neck: is adjuvant radiotherapy necessary? Head Neck. 2007;29(3):249–57.
25. Lemos BD, Storer BE, Iyer JG, et al. Pathologic nodal evaluation improves prognostic accuracy in merkel cell carcinoma: analysis of 5823 cases as the basis of the first consensus staging system. J Am Acad Dermatol. 2010;63(5): 751–61.
26. Allen PJ, Busam K, Hill AD, Stojadinovic A, Coit DG. Immunohistochemical analysis of sentinel lymph nodes from patients with Merkel cell carcinoma. Cancer. 2001;92(6): 1650–5.
27. Zeitouni NC, Cheney RT, Delacure MD. Lymphoscintigraphy, sentinel lymph node biopsy, and Mohs micrographic surgery in the treatment of merkel cell carcinoma. Dermatol Surg. 2000;26(1):12–8.
28. Boyle F, Pendlebury S, Bell D. Further insights into the natural history and management of primary cutaneous neuroendocrine (merkel cell) carcinoma. Int J Radiat Oncol Biol Phys. 1995;31(2):315–23.
29. Meeuwissen JA, Bourne RG, Kearsley JH. The importance of postoperative radiation therapy in the treatment of merkel cell carcinoma. Int J Radiat Oncol Biol Phys. 1995;31(2): 325–31.
30. Lewis KG, Weinstock MA, Weaver AL, Otley CC. Adjuvant local irradiation for merkel cell carcinoma. Arch Dermatol. 2006;142(6):693–700.
31. Suntharalingam M, Rudoltz MS, Mendenhall WM, Parsons JT, Stringer SP, Million RR. Radiotherapy for merkel cell carcinoma of the skin of the head and neck. Head Neck. 1995;17(2):96–101.
32. Wilson LD, Gruber SB. Merkel cell carcinoma and the controversial role of adjuvant radiation therapy: clinical choices in the absence of statistical evidence. J Am Acad Dermatol. 2004;50(3):435–7. discussion 437–8.
33. Brown TJ, Jackson BA, Macfarlane DF, Goldberg LH. Merkel cell carcinoma: spontaneous resolution and management of metastatic disease. Dermatol Surg. 1999;25(1):23–5.
34. Pathai S, Barlow R, Williams G, Olver J. Mohs' micrographic surgery for merkel cell carcinomas of the eyelid. Orbit. 2005;24(4):273–5.
35. Pennington BE, Leffell DJ. Mohs micrographic surgery: established uses and emerging trends. Oncology (Williston Park). 2005;19(9):1165–71. discussion 1171–2, 1175.

25 Selected Sweat Gland Carcinomas

Howard A. Oriba and Stephen N. Snow

Abstract

This chapter will discuss rare sweat gland tumors that occur in the skin primarily. We have limited our discussion to porocarcinoma, hidradenocarcinoma, malignant cylindroma, spiradenocarcinoma, cutaneous adenoid cystic carcinoma, and mucinous carcinoma of the skin.

Each tumor is presented with a brief summary of clinical presentation, natural history, histopathology, and treatment. Mohs micrographic surgery experience is also discussed.

Keywords

Porocarcinoma • Hidradenocarcinoma • Malignant cylindroma • Spiradenocarcinoma • Cutaneous adenoid cystic carcinoma • Mucinous carcinoma of the skin

Summary: Porocarcinoma

- A rare sweat gland carcinoma that usually arises de novo, but can develop from malignant transformation of benign poroma.
- Potential for epidermotropic metastases.
- Patients developing metastatic disease have a high mortality.
- Histological factors that may predict behavior include mitoses per high power field greater than 14, lymphovascular invasion, and tumor depth greater than 7 mm.

25.1 Porocarcinoma

Porocarcinoma (PC) is an uncommon carcinoma originally described in 1963 as epidermotropic eccrine carcinoma [1]. Other terms used to describe this lesion include malignant eccrine poroma, malignant porosyringoma, malignant hidroacanthoma simplex, eccrine adenocarcinoma, and poroepithelioma. This tumor is of eccrine origin, arising from the acrosyringeum, which is the intraepidermal portion of the eccrine duct.

H.A. Oriba (✉)
Department of Mohs Surgery, The Skin Cancer Center, Sun City Center, FL, USA
e-mail: horiba@pol.net

S.N. Snow
Department of Dermatology, University of Wisconsin School of Medicine & Public Health, Madison, WI, USA

K. Nouri (ed.), *Mohs Micrographic Surgery*,
DOI 10.1007/978-1-4471-2152-7_25, © Springer-Verlag London Limited 2012

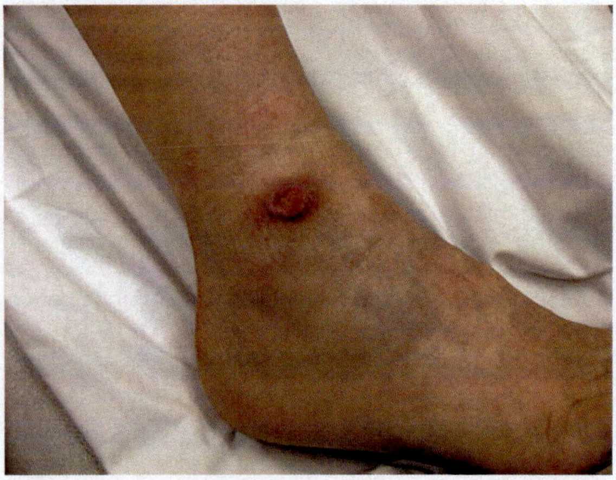

Fig. 25.1 Porocarcinoma. A 54-year-old man with a hyperpigmented, non-healing tumor of the right ankle. The central ulceration was the result of the biopsy (Courtesy of Thomas Rozum M.D., Berlin)

PC usually presents as a verrucous nodule, or plaque, mostly on acral areas of the lower extremities [2–6] (see Fig. 25.1). They appear moist and tend to bleed with minor trauma. Other reported sites included head and neck, trunk, vulva, breast, and upper extremity. In contrast, benign eccrine poromas occur mostly on palms and soles. Clinical lesion size is variable, ranging from less than 1 to 10 cm. Most patients are older than 50 years of age, but PC is known to present in all age groups. Interestingly, PC can arise in preexisting poroma that has clinically become symptomatic, suggesting that PC arise via malignant transformation which may be manifested by bleeding, ulceration, increase in size, or pain. Spontaneous cases are also known to exist as well [6, 7]. PC has also arisen in organoid nevus [8], and seborrheic keratosis [9–11]. There appears to be no sexual or ethnic predisposition.

Clinically, PC initially is a slow-growing lesion, and then enters a proliferative, vertical growth phase with propensity to metastasize to regional lymph nodes. Several large review series report a frequency of about 20% [5, 6]. However, other series have reported less-frequent lymph node metastasis [2, 3, 12]. Visceral metastases can occur in about 10–12% of the cases [5, 6], and invariably lead to fatal outcome [5, 13–16]. Parameters for sentinel lymph node biopsy of PC have not been defined; nevertheless, it is clear that dissemination to lymph node or visceral organs portends high morbidity and tends to lead to a fatal outcome.

The histopathology of PC can consist solely of an intraepidermal component or with dermal invasion. The intraepidermal tumor cells are small basaloid cells that are arranged in nests and islands that abruptly contrast with eosinophilic keratinocytes. Single pagetoid spread is not seen. Dermal invasion occurs with broad anastomosing columns of tumor cells to varying levels of the dermis (see Fig. 25.2). The cells appear clear because they contain varying amounts of glycogen, hence PAS positive, diastase labile. Cytologic atypia is manifested by hyperchromasia, atypical mitotic figures. Ductal structure can be present, helpful in the histological diagnosis, and can be highlighted with immunohistochemical staining with carcinoembryonic antigen and epithelial membrane antigen [17]. Other histological features that may be present include foci of squamous differentiation [18, 19] (see Fig. 25.3), clear cell areas [18], and melanin pigment [20]. Perineural involvement has been reported [6]. One study found features associated with aggressive clinical behavior and poor prognosis that included mitoses per high power field greater than 14, lymphovascular invasion, and tumor depth greater than 7 mm [5]. Tumors with an infiltrative or pushing border had increased risk of local recurrence [5].

An important distinction is warranted when PC presents as an in situ form [21]. This histological presentation can represent in situ PC, epidermotropic porocarcinoma, or a cutaneous metastasis of PC. Epidermotropic porocarcinoma is a pattern seen adjacent to PC and metastatic PC. Cutaneous metastasis of PC demonstrates small epidermotropic deposits of PC, and clinically appears as multiple cutaneous deposits in a lymphangitic pattern. Separating these similar histological presentations can be difficult and impossible without clinical correlation. The epidermotropic porocarcinoma presentation may represent a field effect in which the neoplasia is multifocal. Epidermotropism may not be an independent risk for aggressive clinical behavior [6]. The histological differential diagnosis of epidermotropic PC includes Bowen's disease, extramammary Paget disease, and melanoma in situ. Special stains are needed to delineate these entities.

Surgical excision is the main therapeutic approach. The role of prophylactic lymphadenectomy is controversial. Sentinel lymph node biopsy has been used to stage PC [22], and should be considered for histologically aggressive lesions. PC does not respond primarily to radiotherapy [23] or chemotherapy. Chemotherapy may play a role in treating metastatic

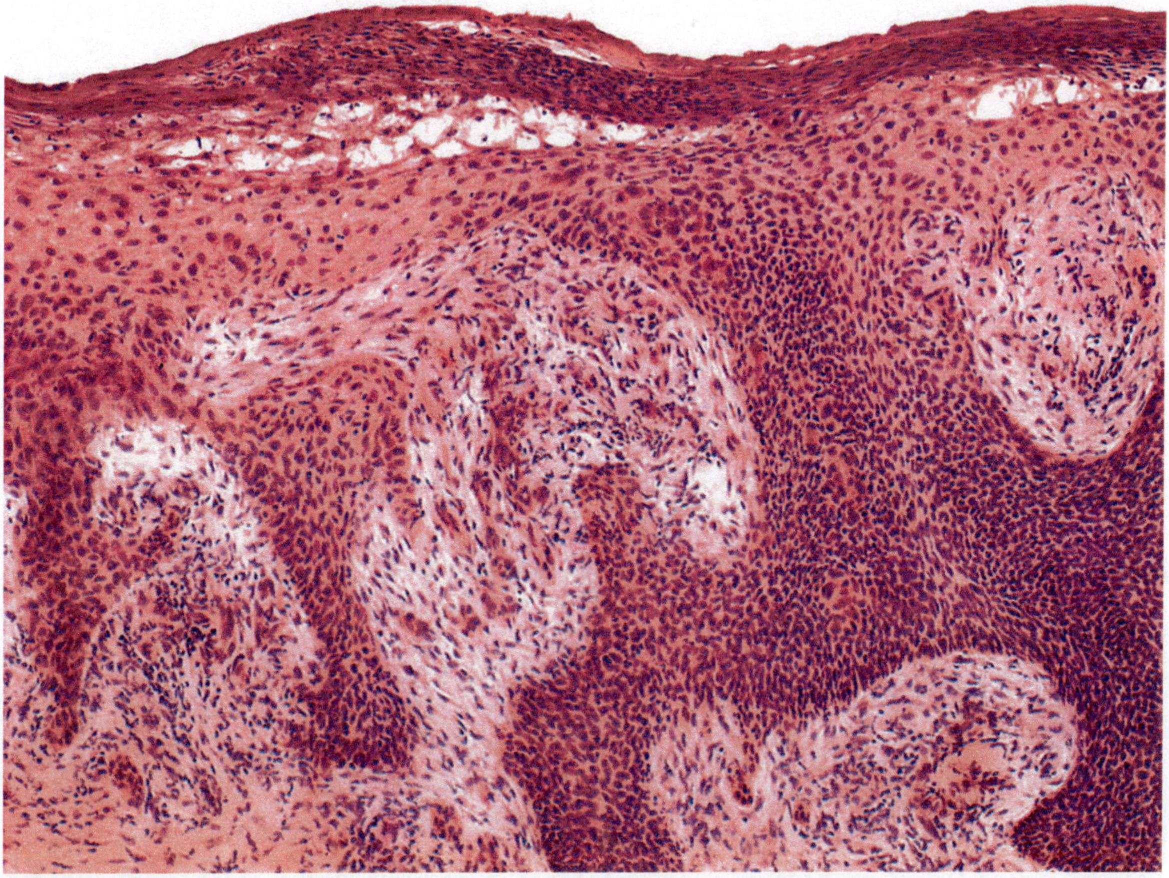

Fig. 25.2 Porocarcinoma. Basaloid cells extending from the epidermis in broad anastomosing columns. Frozen, 100× [143]

eccrine porocarcinoma [24, 25]. Since there is limited experience with Mohs micrographic surgical treatment of PC, its role in treatment remains unresolved. A total of 15 cases have been reported in English literature with favorable outcomes [11, 26–30] (see Table 25.1). No signs of recurrence were noted with a mean follow-up period of 23 months. Due to potential metastatic spread of PC, early intervention with Mohs micrographic surgery maybe a suitable approach. Other indications could include treating in situ lesion, or PC in non-proliferative growth phase where metastasis have not occurred. Care must be taken when evaluating Mohs layer since pagetoid extension of PC cells may be in a noncontiguous, multifocal pattern. Extra Mohs layer may be indicated after initial clear layer is obtained. Toluidine blue stain may aid in some cases; however glycogen-containing cell in PC can be variable. Further studies are needed to validate this therapeutic approach.

Summary: Hidradenocarcinoma

- Is a highly aggressive neoplasm, which may metastasize widely, and is fatal.
- Can occur in a wide range of age group, and has been seen children.
- Most cases arise de novo.
- Tumor can have foci of bland-appearing histology; hence all areas of tumor need to be extirpated.

25.2 Hidradenocarcinoma

Hidradenocarcinomas (HC) are an extremely rare form of sweat gland carcinomas that have an aggressive, potentially fatal course. It was originally described in 1949 [31], but the literature is strewn with synonyms

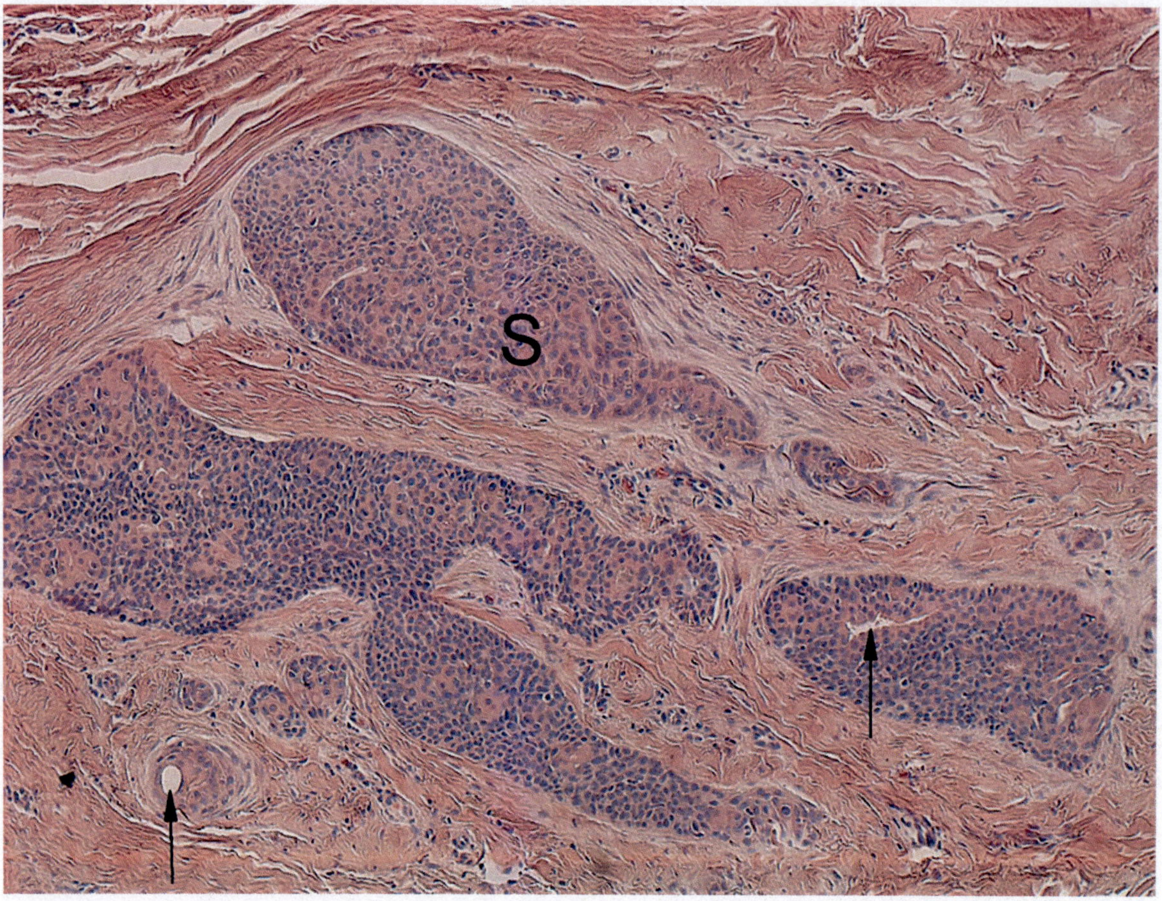

Fig. 25.3 Porocarcinoma. Infiltrative pattern of invasion showing ducts (*arrows*) and squamous proliferation (S). Paraffin, 100× [143]

Table 25.1 Mohs surgery experience with porocarcinoma

Reference	Location	Age/sex	Metastasis	Recurrence to date	FU (months)
[4]	Chin	36/M	–	–	60
[27]	Antihelix	71/F	–	–	12
[26]	Foot	79/F	–	–	36
	Scalp	74/M	–	–	48
	Shin	67/F	–	–	12
	Foot	39/F	–	–	5
	Temple	63/F	–	–	12
[11]	Back	78/F	–	–	12
[29]	Chest	36/M	–	–	30
	Shin	74/F	–	–	31
	Thigh	77/F	–	–	29
	Ankle	54/M	–	–	15
[28]	Eyelid	71/M	NA	NA	NA
[30]	Back	56/M	NA	NA	NA
	Heel	71/F	–	–	2

NA data not available, – none

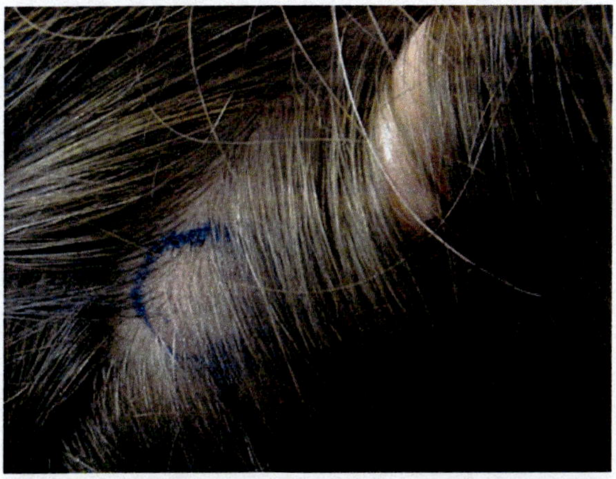

Fig. 25.4 Hidradenocarcinoma. A 45-year-old man with a biopsy-proven HAC of the scalp. When the patient presented for Mohs surgery, another subcutaneous tumor (*purple circle*) developed on the right postauricular scalp. Biopsy confirmed a metastatic lymph node metastasis [143]

such as malignant acrospiroma, malignant hidradenoma, clear cell eccrine carcinoma, malignant clear cell myopepithelioma, and clear cell papillary carcinoma. It may represent both apocrine and eccrine derivation [32].

HC can present in patients of any age, though favor older patients, but cases have been reported in children [33] and at birth [34]. They can present as a solitary flesh-colored nodule, erythematous or ulcerated nodule of variable size [35] (see Fig. 25.4). Most occur on the head and neck region, and less commonly on extremities or trunk [34, 36]. Other sites of presentation include hands, feet, eyelids, axilla, and vulva [3]. The natural history of this lesion is varied [34, 36]. Rarely, some lesions remain localized; however, most have an aggressive course, metastasizing to lymph nodes, bones, and other visceral organs. Malignant transformation has been reported [3, 37–39].

The histopathology of HC is distinguished from its benign counterpart by displaying features of infiltrative pattern, loss of circumscription, and asymmetry at low power magnification. Solid and cystic spaces are present; however, the cystic spaces and ducts may be irregularly shaped. Cytologically, the tumor cells are composed of round and polygonal cells with biphasic cytoplasmic content. One type of cells has a clear cytoplasm with eccentric nuclei, and the second cell type has eosinophilic cytoplasm with a round or oval vesicular nuclei (see Fig. 25.5). As in the benign counterpart, the biphasic cellular population ratio can vary. The clear cells contain glycogen, some PAS-positive, diastase-resistant material as well. Lipid is not present. Mitotic figures are usually present; however, lack of them does not signify benignity. Both benign and malignant counterparts of hidradenoma can have mitoses in varying ratios. Cellular pleomorphism may be minimal or absent. Melanocytes can occasionally be found as well. Therefore, with diminished clear cell changes, bland appearance, a specimen can pose a challenging interpretation. At times, distinction from benign hidradenoma cannot be made. The histological differential diagnosis can include a benign hidradenoma, malignant eccrine spiradenoma, and malignant chondroid syringoma. Adequate tissue sampling is critical aspect to making the correct diagnosis. Immunohistochemical studies are not helpful in differentiating benign from malignant hidradenoma.

Surgery is treatment of choice. All patients should be staged prior to treatment. The literature advocates wide excision with consideration of prophylactic lymph node dissection [33, 40, 41]. Margins have not been defined. Sentinel lymph node biopsy could aid in staging due to HC's potential to metastasize [42] There are reports that postoperative radiation may be helpful [43–45], and chemotherapy may play an adjunctive role [46, 47]. Adjunctive hormonal therapy may also be helpful, particularly targeting estrogen receptors [42, 48], and Her-2/neu protein [49].

The Mohs micrographic surgical experience is limited for this carcinoma. Seven cases have been treated to date with Mohs micrographic surgery [29, 50–53]. A review of the limited cases suggests adequate local control, but there was limited follow-up (see Table 25.2). No recurrences were observed with a mean follow-up time of 26 months. Patients should have a thorough physical examination and staging with imaging studies prior to treatment. Sentinel lymph node biopsy should also be considered. One should consider obtaining tumor marker studies such as estrogen and Her-2/neu.

If Mohs micrographic surgery is contemplated, a number of potential issues come to mind. First, frozen section artifacts may come into play. Clear cell changes and ducts may be difficult to visualize. Since this tumor can extend to the subcutis, one should consider taking a deeper layer, possibly into adipose. Complete removal of the tumor would

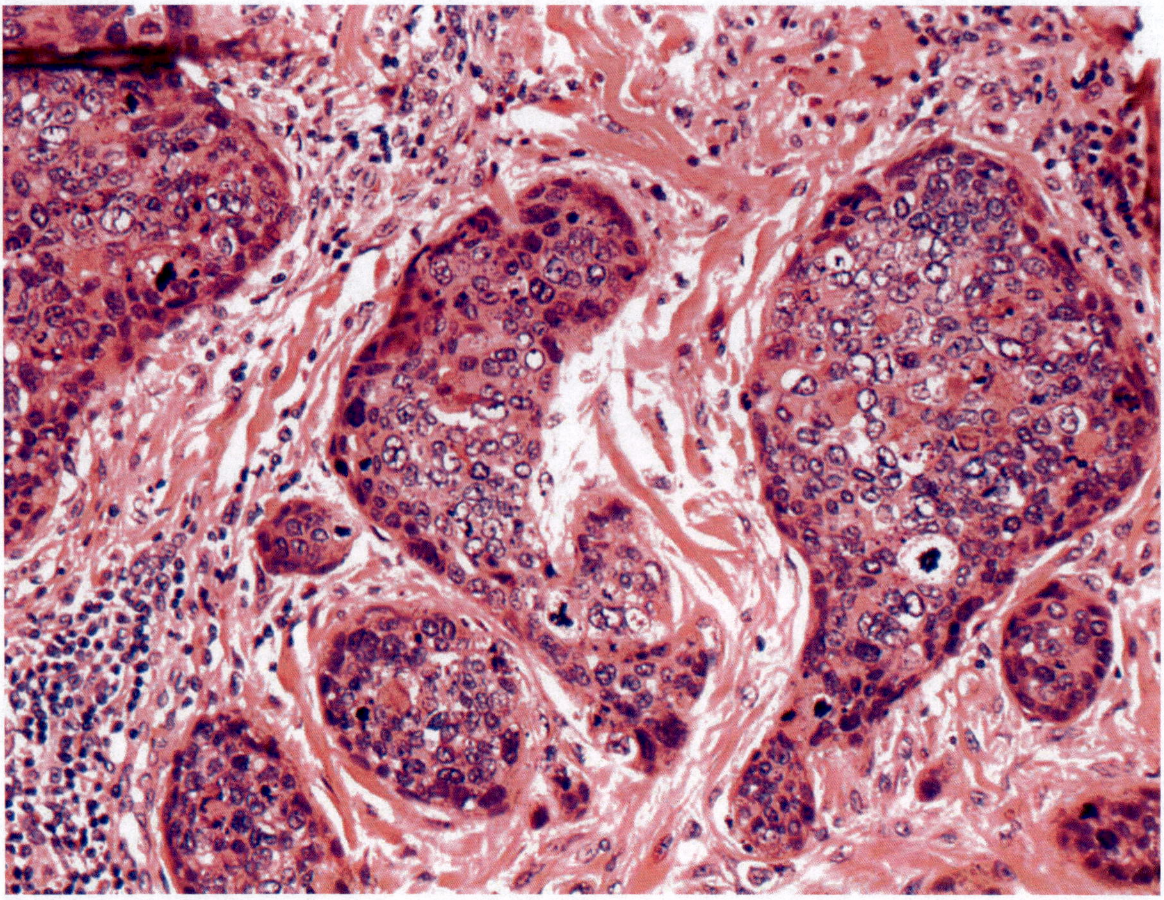

Fig. 25.5 Hidradenocarcinoma. There are irregular-shaped islands containing two-cell-type population and atypical mitotic figures. Paraffin, 200× [143]

Table 25.2 Mohs surgery experience with hidradenocarcinoma

Reference	Location	Age/sex	Metastasis	Recurrence to date	FU (months)
[52]	Scalp	74/F	[b]	NA	NA
[50][a]	Chin	63/F	–	–	18
[51][a]	Foot	40/M	–	–	11
[29]	Back	12/M	–	–	44
[29]	Groin	60/M	–	–	41
[29]	Scalp	74/F	–	–	30
[53]	Scalp	45/M	–	–[c]	12

NA data not available, – none
[a]Recurrent hidradenoma
[b]Metastatic on presentation
[c]Received postoperative radiotherapy

include bland-appearing areas, since HC can have bland areas and potential for malignant transformation if left behind. Perhaps, the last layer should include permanent H&E sections. The role of immunohistochemistry in Mohs sections of HC has not been studied. At present it plays a limited role, but in the future, could help in evaluating Mohs sections.

Summary: Cutaneous Adenoid Cystic Carcinoma

- Is a rare appendageal tumor that occurs mostly on face, head, and neck region.
- Metastatic disease must be excluded from other visceral organs such as salivary gland, breast, and lung.
- Is a locally destructive neoplasm, low potential for metastasis, and rarely fatal.
- Perineural invasion is a common feature.

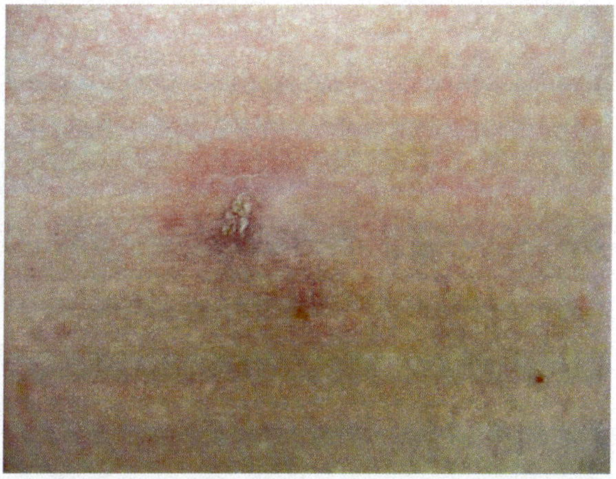

Fig. 25.6 CACC. A 54-year-old woman with a recurrent erythematous plaque of the sternum (Courtesy of Xu et al. [79])

25.3 Cutaneous Adenoid Cystic Carcinoma

Cutaneous adenoid cystic carcinoma (CACC), originally described by Boggio [54], is a rare sweat gland carcinoma with approximately 150 reported cases to date [55–59]. There also exists a more common, non-cutaneous form of the neoplasm that arises from salivary glands and oral cavity. The cutaneous and non-cutaneous adenoid cystic carcinoma (NACC) forms share similar histological features, but because they can behave biologically quite differently, need to be distinguished.

CACC is a neoplasm that presents as a slow-growing nodule, most commonly on the scalp and chest (see Fig. 25.6). Other reported sites include external auditory canal [60], eyelid, trunk, and perineum. The NACC sites of origin include salivary glands, respiratory tract, lacrimal glands, breast, uterus, cervix, vulva, thymus, prostate, and esophagus [61]. The typical age of presentation for CACC ranged from 14 to 90 years of age, with mean age of onset of 59 years of age [54]. No sexual or racial predisposition has been observed.

CACC can manifest in two means: one as primary lesion, second as progression of neoplasm form underlying glandular structure to skin, or less likely as a metastatic lesion. Since the salivary form of ACC is a highly malignant neoplasm that can result in fatal metastasis, it is important to distinguish the nature of lesion. Treatment and management is quite different for metastatic ACC and non-cutaneous ACC. CACC can be locally destructive but has potential for metastasis. However, there is high chance of local recurrences, occurring as late as 35 years [62]. Of the available reported cases, potential sites of metastasis for CACC are lymph nodes [62–67] or lung [55, 68–70]. Since CACC and non-cutaneous NACC can be histologically indistinguishable, the diagnosis of CACC is based on histological and clinical correlation. Exclusion of a non-cutaneous source must be verified to make a diagnosis of CACC.

The histopathology of CACC consists of basaloid cells in islands and cords in reticular dermis, forming cribiform, tubular, and solid areas [71] (see Fig. 25.7). There is lack of epidermal connection as well as peripheral palisading. Basophilic mucin (hyaluronic acid) is present in the small cyst and interspersed between tumor cells. The stroma may appear fibrous. Often a thickened basement membrane that is PAS positive, diastase resistant, surrounds the tumor islands and tubular areas. Perineural invasion is common and a hallmark of this neoplasm, present up to 76% of the cases [57] (see Fig. 25.8). Immunohistochemical staining reveals positivity to epithelial membrane antigen and mildly positive to carinoembryonic antigen [55, 72]. There is also variable staining to S-100, vimentin, and cytokeratin [71]. The nosology remains controversial, although apocrine derivation is favored.

CACC can be confused with adenoid BCC. Both lesions can have a cribiform pattern; however, BCC should have epidermal connection, peripheral palisading, and retraction artifact. If necessary, immunohistochemical staining can assist in the diagnosis. Another entity in the histological differential diagnosis is mucinous carcinoma. The islands of epithelial cells can form cribiform pattern, but appear to float in pools of mucin, separated by thin fibrovascular septa. The mucin is sialomucin, PAS positive, hyaluronidase resistant, and sialidase labile.

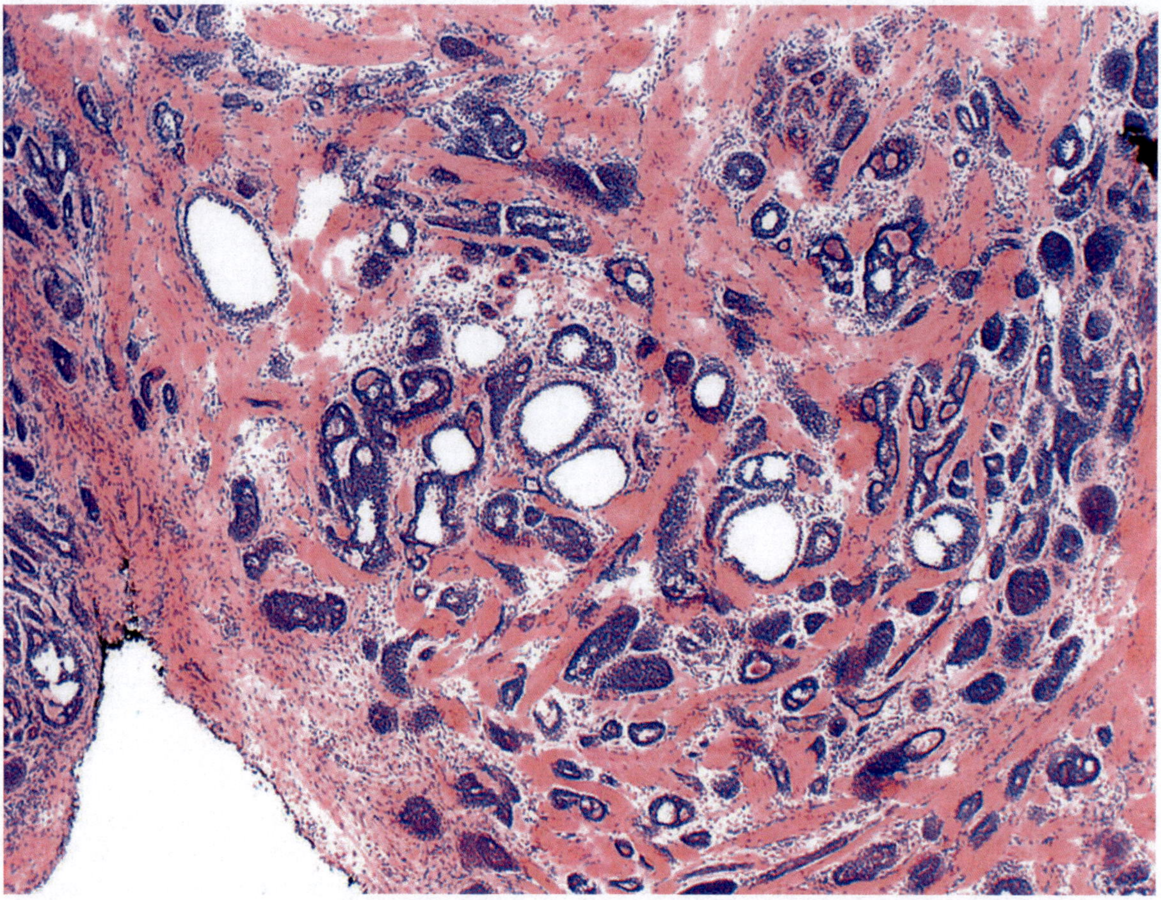

Fig. 25.7 CACC. There are islands of basaloid cells some of which have cystic spaces in desmoplastic stroma. However, peripheral palisading and artifactual retraction are absent. Frozen, 40× (Courtesy of Xu et al. [79])

Treatment for CACC is surgical excision. Due to high local recurrence (up to 44%) with wide excision surgery [58], Mohs micrographic surgery offers a sensible approach. There have been seven reported cases of ACC treated by Mohs micrographic surgery [73–79] (see Table 25.3). There were no recurrences with a mean follow-up of 16 months. Many authors have recommended obtaining additional tumor-free layer with fresh frozen or permanent sections. This is prudent advice in view of the highly perineural behavior of this neoplasm. Toluidine blue frozen sections might aid some Mohs surgeon who prefer this to hematoxylin and eosin method because mucin is present. There has been limited use of postoperative radiotherapy as adjunctive modality [63]. Metastatic disease has been treated with chemotherapy [80].

Due to the limited number of cases, it is difficult to assess the optimal therapeutic choice of treatment. Mohs micrographic surgery would seem to offer the best choice in managing this neoplasm with high predilection for perineural invasion and local destructive effects in cosmetic sensitive areas. Reported cases of pulmonary metastasis appear to be less than 10%; nevertheless, these patients need close surveillance.

Summary: Spiradenocarcinoma (Malignant Spiradenoma)

- Usually arises from malignant transformation of spiradenoma.
- Can be an aggressive neoplasm with fatal outcomes occurring with disseminated disease.
- Predictive factors for its biology are not available.

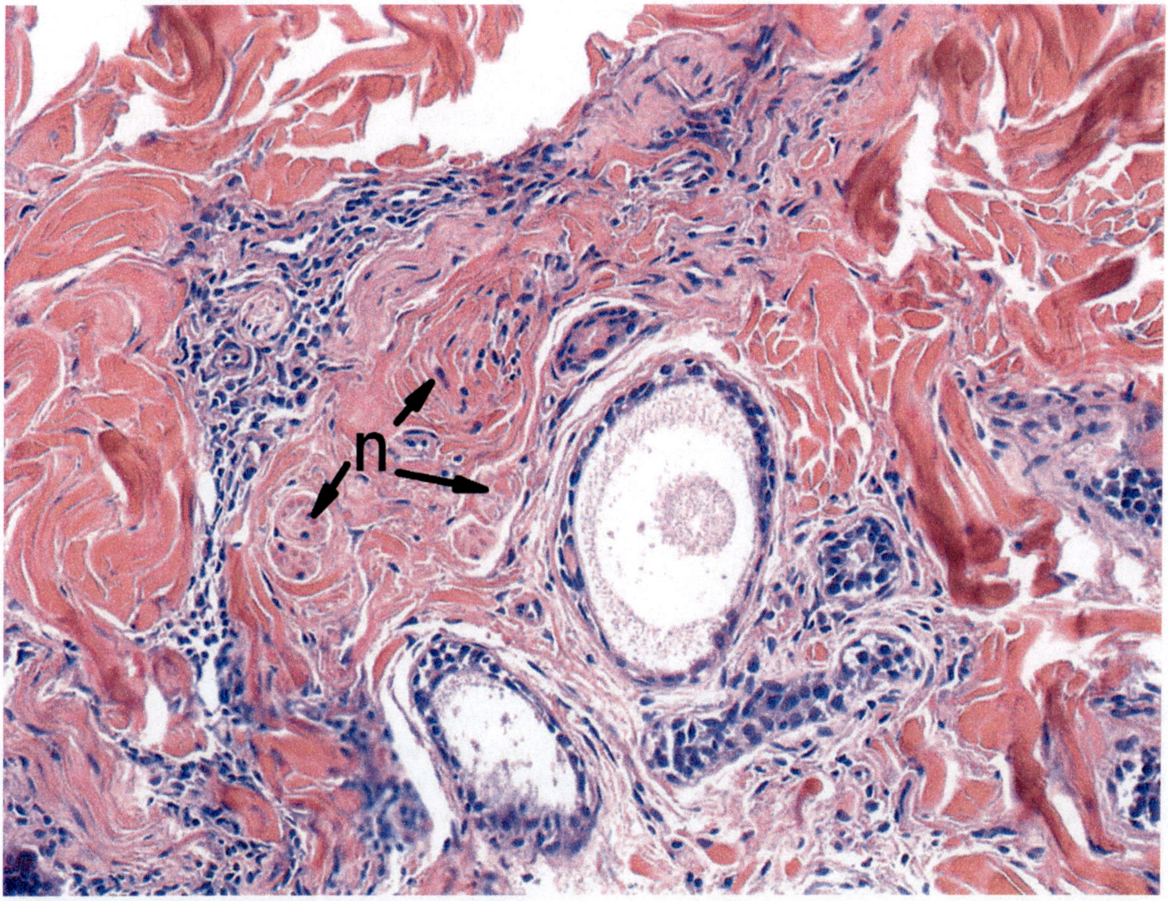

Fig. 25.8 Perineural CACC (*arrows* indicate nerve). Paraffin, 200× (Courtesy of Xu et al. [79])

Table 25.3 Mohs surgery experience with cutaneous adenoid cystic carcinoma

Reference	Location	Age/sex	PNI	Metastasis	Recurrence to date	FU (months)
[73]	Back	68/F	–	–	–	18
[74]	Scalp	65/M	–	–	–	10
[75]	Scalp	45/F	–	–	–	18
[76]	Scalp	57/F	–	–	–	28[a]
[74]	Scalp	62/F	+	–	–	6
[78]	Eyelid	59/M	+	–	–	12
[79]	Chest	58/F	+	–	–	24

PNI perineural, *FU* follow-up in months, – none
[a]received post-op radiation therapy

25.4 Spiradenocarcinoma (Malignant Spiradenoma)

Spiradenocarcinomas (SC) are rare, aggressively growing tumors that arise mostly from the malignant transformation of a benign spiradenoma [81–88], originally described by Dabska in 1972 [89]. Rarely de novo lesions have been known to arise [85, 90–92]. They usually present as enlarging cutaneous nodule of long-standing duration, with a mean period of at least 20 years. Lesions have ranged in size from 0.8 to 13 cm. Other changes noted include increasing

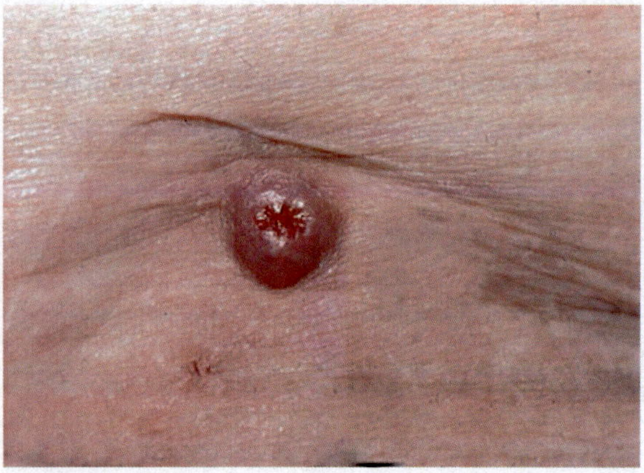

Fig. 25.9 Spiradenocarcinoma. A 78-year-old woman with a recurrent tumor erupting through a previously placed skin graft from popliteal fossa. Clinically, lesion looked like a nodular basal cell carcinoma [143]

tenderness and/or color changes. Most lesions are found on the extremities and trunk, but can occur on the head and neck (see Fig. 25.9). SC has been reported to occur in patients ranging in age from 22 to 85 years, without any ethnic or gender inclination.

A comprehensive review of SC cases has documented nearly 100 cases [91, 92]. SC has the ability to metastasize with a fatal outcome. Metastasis has mostly occurred to lymph nodes and lungs, followed by brain, bone, and liver. The actual frequency of metastasis and its effect on survival are difficult to ascertain with the limited and inadequate data collection. Furthermore, because of its rarity, predictive factors for its biological behavior cannot be arrived at this point in time. Histological grading of SC is not entirely predictive [93]. Further study analyzing tumor depth, angiolymphatic invasion, and histological patterns may be of importance. p53 and Ki-67 immunohistochemical staining might provide clues to malignant potential [94].

Histologically, the diagnosis is based on presence of benign spiradenoma, with areas adjacent to it undergoing malignant transformation. The areas of transformation may be focal or widespread, exemplified by cellular pleomorphism, nuclear hyperchromasia, and atypia with frequent mitoses, necrosis, and hemorrhage. Atypical mitoses are present. Also, one may see adjacent to spiradenoma with areas of basaloid and squamoid pattern [82], clear cell [85], and histiocytic-like and sarcomatous changes with rhabdomyoblastic and osteosarcomatous differentiation [84]. Lower power magnification may demonstrate infiltrative borders and sheet-like growth pattern (see Fig. 25.10). Absence of features of a benign spiradenoma in a specimen can pose a diagnostic challenge. The differential diagnosis includes malignant cylindroma, spiradenocylindrocarcinoma, metastatic adenocarcinoma, squamous cell carcinoma, melanoma, ductal carcinoma of the breast, and carcinosarcoma. Immunohistochemistry is not helpful for separating benign and malignant forms of spiradenoma. SC reveal variable staining to epithelial membrane antigen, cytokeratin, S-100, and CEA [95]. Any changing spiradenoma deserves examination of multiple profiles and adequate tissue sampling to evaluate for malignant transformation. The histogenesis of SC is believed to be apocrine, not eccrine [96].

The mainstay of treatment for therapy for SC is wide excision with clear margins, and lymph node dissection if indicated. Strong consideration of sentinel lymph node biopsy should be entertained. The use of Mohs micrographic surgery has been limited [97], and its role has not been delineated. At least, it seems appropriate for local control of the disease. Postoperative radiotherapy [82, 98], and systemic chemotherapy [99] are of limited use at the present. Estrogen-receptor-positive SC have been treated postoperatively with tamoxifen [98].

Summary: Malignant Cylindroma

- Is a very rare adnexal carcinoma that arises from malignant transformation.
- Is locally aggressive, with potential erosion into bone, but rarely metastasizes.
- Genetic cases of multiple cylindromas are linked to CYLD.
- Treatment is surgical, usually requiring removal of significant amounts of tissue.

25.5 Malignant Cylindroma

Malignant cylindroma (MC) is a very rare tumor, with less than 40 cases reported in the literature, originally described by Wiedemann [100] in 1929. Despite its rarity, some features appear to be consistent. Most lesions arise from preexisting cylindroma, and in patients with multiple cylindromas [101, 102].

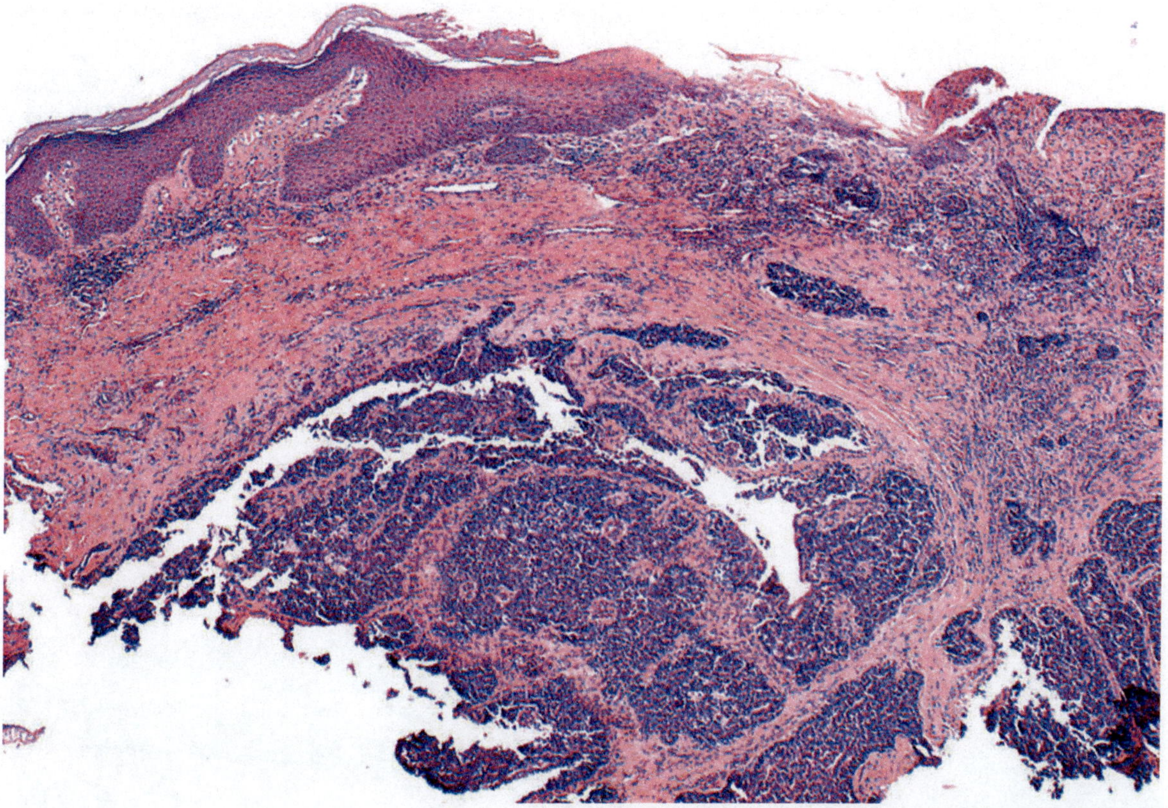

Fig. 25.10 Spiradenocarcinoma. Tumor lobule containing small basaloid cell with some larger cells, with infiltrative growth pattern. Paraffin, 40× [143]

Clinically, MC is similar to benign form of cylindroma, but malignant transformation is heralded by ulceration, bleeding, change in size, or change in color. MC tends to occur in middle-aged individuals, usually on the scalp, but can occur in other regions of the head and neck (see Fig. 25.11). The limited number of MC cases reviewed [103] demonstrate the range of MC presentation from 50 to 96 years of age, mean of 71. There may be a slight female preponderance. Malignant transformation occurred in range of several months to 60 years, with mean of 27 years. MC are locally aggressive, some capable of boney erosion [104]. Metastasis is rare; however MCs have been reported to disseminate to lymph nodes, bone, liver, and other organs which can lead to a fatal outcome [105–108].

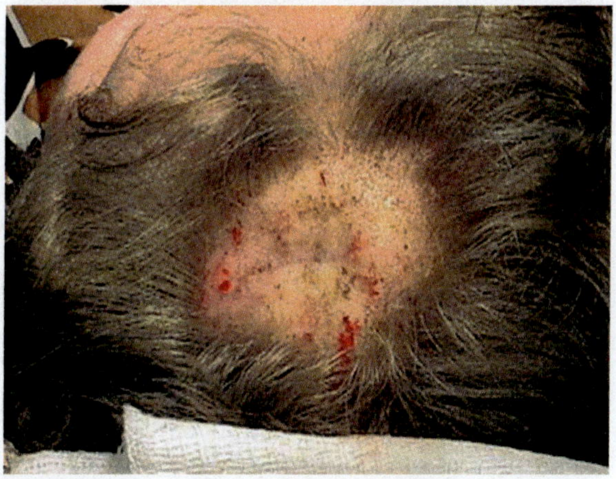

Fig. 25.11 Malignant cylindroma. A 79-year-old woman status post-excisional biopsy-proven MC of the parietal scalp [143]

One should be aware of genetic predisposition to develop multiple cylindromas in familial cylindromatosis, multiple familial trichoepitheliomas, and Brooke-Spiegler syndrome (BSS), which share a genetic mutation in the tumor regulatory gene CYLD [109]. In BSS, there can be simultaneous occurrence of trichoepitheliomas, spiradenoma, and cylindroma. More molecular studies are needed to evaluate CYLD role in MC.

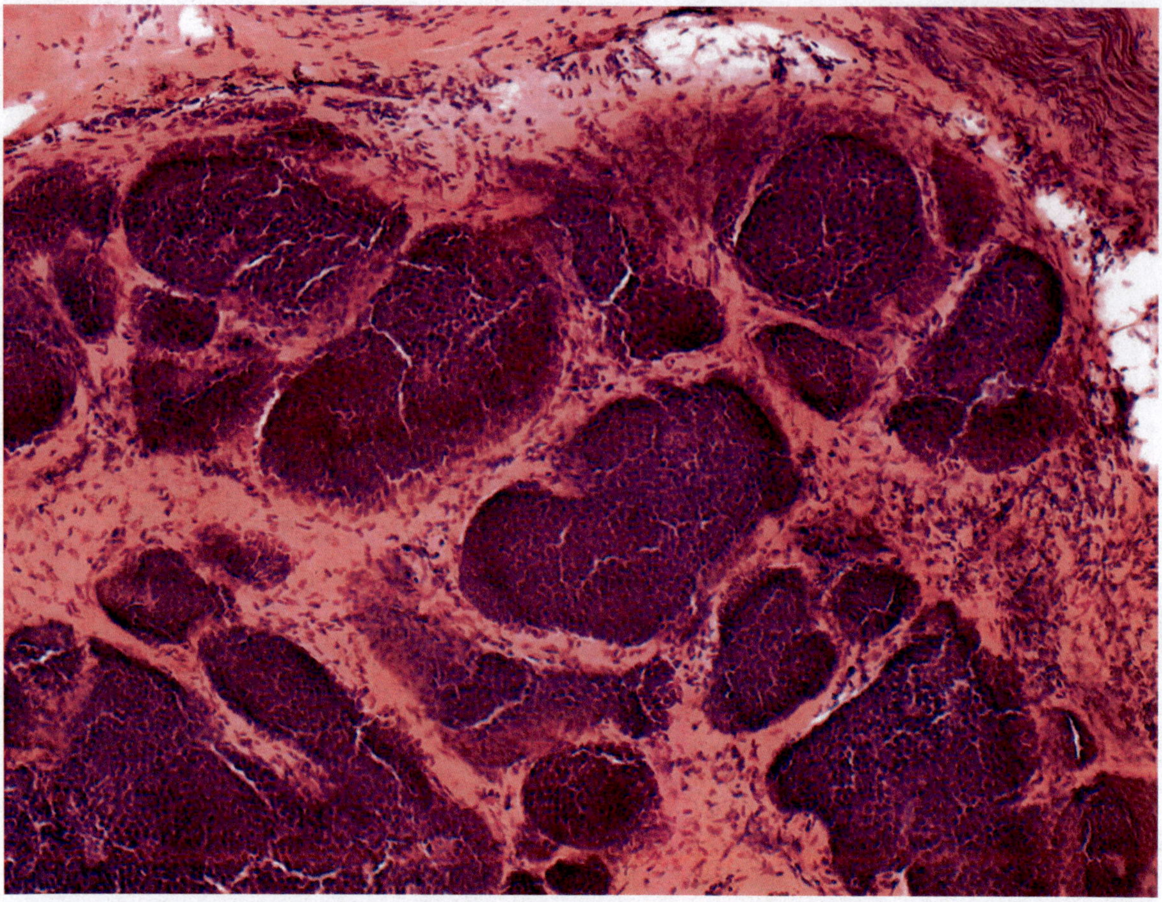

Fig. 25.12 Malignant Cylindroma. Irregularly shaped islands of basaloid cell varying in size and shape with disruption of classic jigsaw puzzle pattern. Note loss of two cell population, and hyaline sheath. Frozen section, 100× [143]

The histopathology of MC demonstrates disruption of the organized jigsaw pattern, typical of cylindroma (see Fig. 25.12). The scanning magnification often demonstrates sheets of atypical cells with infiltrative growth pattern. The two cell population is lost and replaced by larger pleomorphic cells with mitoses. The peripheral palisading seen in the periphery of the tumor lobules is often lost. Necrosis is seen in the tumor islands. There is loss or thinning of the PAS-positive hyaline membrane. Interestingly, partial preservation of the hyaline membrane may have a good prognosis [110]. Focal squamous differentiation may occur. Occasionally, a benign cylindroma may be bordering an MC, which aids in the diagnosis. In its absence, the histological diagnosis can be challenging, invoking differential diagnosis of malignant spiradenoma (MS). Some areas of MC cannot be separated from MS. Spiradenocylindrocarcinoma, a malignant hybrid tumor of spiradenoma and cylindroma, is also in the differential diagnosis [94, 111]. Clinical correlation is needed in most cases. Classically, cylindromas are thought to be of apocrine origin. Enzyme histochemistry and immunohistochemistry have not been conclusive. At this point, there are two competing theories on the histogenesis of cylindromas [112]. One concept believes in a pluripotent stem cell of the abortive adnexal anlagen, and another believes origin lies in folliculo-sebaceous-apocrine unit.

Treatment for the limited number of cases has been surgical. Surgical margins have not been defined. Radiotherapy has been used as palliative, adjunctive therapy [106]; however, data are insufficient to evaluate its efficacy. There are reports of radiotherapy possibly inducing malignant transformation in a benign [106].

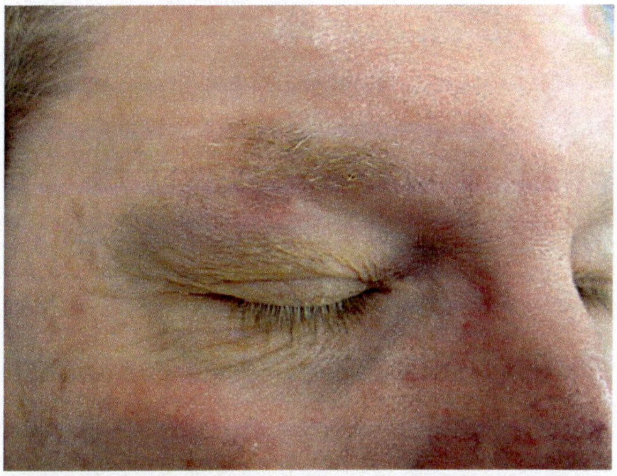

Fig. 25.13 Mucinous carcinoma. A 59-year-old man with an erythematous biopsy site on the right upper lid below the brow

Only one case of MC treated by the Mohs micrographic surgical method has been reported [113]. In a case involving the external auditory canal, wide excision was followed by Mohs micrographic surgery to remove an MC [114]. Wide excision approach has a local recurrence rate of 41% [101]. These rare tumors could be ideal Mohs surgery cases due to low chance of metastasis. Its local aggressive behavior should call attention to potential boney involvement of scalp cases. Furthermore, since some MCs can involve significant portions of the scalp, the Mohs technique may aid in salvaging the remaining normal tissue. Cylindromas have been treated by Mohs micrographic surgery [115, 116]. More cases of MC are needed to establish Mohs micrographic surgery as a treatment modality.

Summary: Mucinous Carcinoma of the Skin

- Most common site is head, favoring eyelids.
- Is a low-grade-malignancy, slow-growing tumor that has a high local recurrence with low metastatic rate, and fatal outcomes are rare.
- Imperative to evaluate for metastatic source.

25.6 Mucinous Carcinoma of the Skin

Mucinous carcinoma (MuC) of the skin is a rare cutaneous malignancy that was originally described by Lennox et al. in 1952 [117]. The tumor usually arises on the face [118–121], particularly the eyelids (see Fig. 25.13). Other sites of involvement include scalp, axilla, trunk, perianal, vulva, and foot. Most lesions arise on older individuals, mean age of 63 years, with range of 8–87 years [120]. They present as asymptomatic nodules, growing for months to years, ranging in size from 0.4 to 12 cm [121]. Ulceration is rare. Although complete data are not available, there is a slight predisposition for males. Interestingly, there is a higher than usual frequency in African-American individuals, compared to other sweat gland carcinomas of the skin [122]. MuC rarely metastasizes, but due to incomplete excision have a high local recurrence rate. Metastases are usually regional to lymph nodes [123] at a frequency of about 10%, and distant metastases are rare [124–127], Death is unusual, but has occurred in patients with distant metastases.

Of significance, mucinous carcinoma can arise in other organs, and may metastasize to the skin from breast, gastrointestinal tract, lacrimal and salivary glands in vicinity of the paranasal sinuses/nose, lung (bronchi), renal pelvis, ovaries, and prostate [128]. Metastatic lesions are most commonly from breast and colon cancer. One must thoroughly evaluate for a source of metastasis, prior to arriving at the diagnosis of primary cutaneous MuC. Clinically, most metastatic lesions are within vicinity of the organ. Breast carcinoma rarely metastasizes to the eyelid or facial area, but favors chest region. Colorectal carcinoma tends to metastasize to the abdomen wall. Therefore, most mucinous carcinomas located on the facial area are likely to be primary lesions. However, it is imperative a thorough physical examination, appropriate blood work, and imaging studies be performed.

Histologically, MuC is a dermal tumor that is unencapsulated and can extend into the deep subcutaneous tissue. One finds collections of epithelial cells in large pools of basophilic mucin, separate by fibrous septae (see Fig. 25.14). The epithelial cells are small and cuboidal with eosinophilic or vacuolated cytoplasm. Mitoses are rare. Pleomorphism is variable. The epithelial cells may have a cribiform or duct-like appearance. The mucin is sialomucin, PAS positive, hyaluronidase resistant. It is also reacts to mucicarmine, alcian blue at pH 2.5, and colloidal iron. MuC can have local neuroendocrine differentiation [129] or resemble infiltrating breast carcinoma [130]. Immunohistochemistry reveals reactivity to

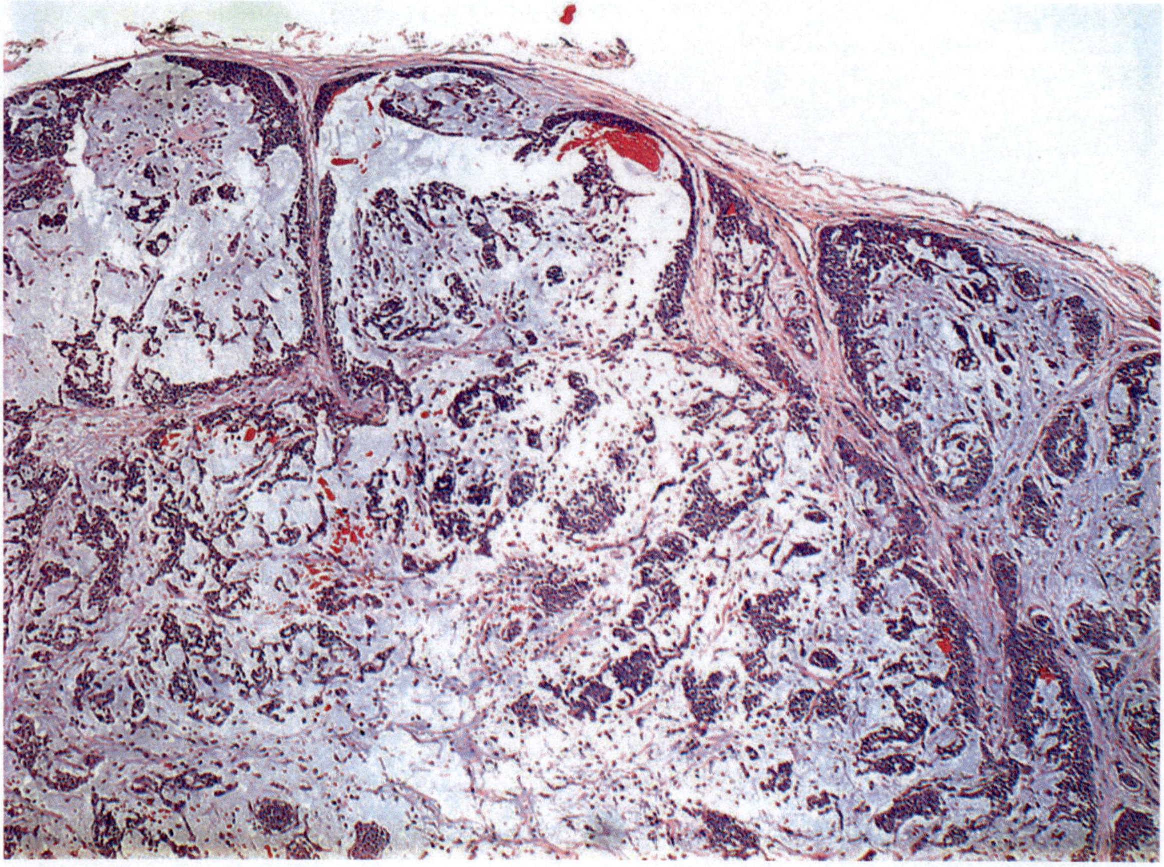

Fig. 25.14 Mucinous carcinoma. There are islands of basaloid cells forming tubular and solid areas in a fibrous stroma. The tumor resembles a cystic basal cell carcinoma. However, peripheral palisading and artifactual retraction are absent. Paraffin, 40×

low molecular weight cytokeratins, epithelial membrane antigen, carcinoembryonic antigen, vimentin, and occasionally to S-100 [131, 132]. On histological grounds, separating MuC of the skin from metastatic tumor can be indistinguishable. Some factors in favor of primary cutaneous origin are presence of an in situ component and absence of CK20 staining [131, 133] (exclude colorectal carcinoma). One study suggests the combination of dirty cell necrosis and presence of epithelial cells with absorptive/goblet cell differentiation favors intestinal origin [134]. The histogenesis of MuC has not been established definitively; however, most favor an apocrine origin [135].

Treatment for MuC is wide excision with clear margins. Recurrences after surgical excision have been reported as high as 28% [120]. Since MuC is derived from the secretory coil of sweat glands in the deep dermis and subcutaneous fat, these tumors tend to be deep-seated, which may partially explain inadequate margins. They tend to be widest at the deepest portion of tumor. The tumor can grow in a noncontiguous fashion, with tumor satellites occurring away from the main tumor. Often as one excises or takes a Mohs layer, you will encounter a thick, clear viscous material extruded from the lesion, which represents sialomucin. The use of Mohs micrographic surgery has been limited [136–142]. In our opinion, it would seem best suited for periocular MuC cases due to the technique's tissue-sparing capacity to preserve anatomical function and aesthetics. There are 11 published cases describing the use of Mohs micrographic surgery (see Table 25.4). Most of the cases occurred in ocular region, and with a mean follow up of 33 months, had no recurrences. In one paper, immunohistochemistry was utilized to aid in examining the Mohs layer [140]. Radiation and chemotherapy regimens have not been successful [124].

Table 25.4 Mohs surgery experience with mucinous carcinoma of the skin

Reference	Location	Age/sex	Metastasis	Recurrence to date	FU (months)
[136]	Eyelid	65/M	–	–	60
[136]	Scalp	69/F	–	–	48
[121]	Scalp	54/F	–	–	9
[120]	Eyelid	50/F	–	–	60
[137]	Eyelid	55/F	–	–	24
[138]	Scalp	61/F	–	–	30
[139]	Eyelid	54/M	–	–	12
[140]	Canthus	64/F	–	–	36
[141]	Eyelid	54/M	–	–	12
[142]	Eyebrow	72/F	–	–	42
[142]	Eyelid	66/F	–	–	26

– none

Summary: Conclusion

- Chapter contains noninclusive discussion of very rare sweat gland carcinomas.
- Neoplasm can arise from malignant transformation or arise de novo with varying biological behavior.
- Histopathology can be challenging in frozen sections.
- Nosology of sweat gland carcinomas is controversial.
- Mohs surgical experience is limited, but can play a vital role in controlling and eradicating some of the neoplasm.

25.7 Conclusion

This chapter has discussed rare sweat gland carcinomas that may confront dermatologist and Mohs micrographic surgeon. These tumors are quite rare, and a limited number of cases have been collected, often with different nomenclature. They do not have any distinctive clinical features, and often the initial clinical impression is incorrect. Some of the neoplasms represent malignant transformations of benign counterpart; others arose de novo. Hence, all lesions should be completely removed, including benign appearing areas. They have varying biological behavior from locally destructive tumors to ones that can metastasize. Histopathology of CACC and MuC can be indistinguishable from metastatic lesion; hence, care must be taken to thoroughly evaluate for a primary malignancy. The lineage of these sweat gland carcinomas is controversial and remains unsettled. The Mohs micrographic surgical experience is limited. It is clear that the Mohs technique can play a role in controlling and eradicating these adnexal carcinomas. More cases need to be reported and collected.

References

Porocarcinoma

1. Pinkus H, Mehregan AH. Epidermotropic eccrine carcinoma: a case combining features of eccrine poroma and Paget's disease. Arch Dermatol. 1973;88:597–607.
2. Shaw M, McKee PHG, Lowe D, et al. Malignant eccrine poroma: a study of twenty seven cases. Br J Dermatol. 1982;107:675–80.
3. Mehregan AH, Hashimoto K, Rahbari H. Eccrine adenocarcinoma. A clinicopathologic study of 35 cases. Arch Dermatol. 1983;119:104–14.
4. Akiyoshi E, Nogita T, Yamaguchi R, et al. Eccrine porocarcinoma. Dermatologica. 1991;182:239–42.
5. Snow SN, Reizner GT. Eccrine porocarcinoma of the face. J Am Acad Dermatol. 1992;27(Pt 2):306–11.
6. Robson A, Greene J, Ansari N, et al. Eccrine porocarcinoma. A clinicopathological study of 69 cases. Am J Surg Pathol. 2001;25:710–20.
7. Pascual A, Ackerman AB. Porocarcinoma. In: Neoplasms with eccrine differentiation. Philadelphia: Lea & Febiger; 1990. p. 415–31.
8. Tarkhan II, Domingo J. Metastasizing eccrine porocarcinoma developing in a sebaceous nevus of Jadassohn. Report of a case. Arch Dermatol. 1985;121:413–5.
9. Orella JAL, Penalba AV, Juan CCS, et al. Eccrine porocarcinoma. Report of nine cases. Dermatol Surg. 1997;23: 925–8.

10. Madan V, Cox NH, Gangopadhayay M. Porocarcinoma arising in a broad clonal seborrheic keratosis. Clin Exp Dermatol. 2007;33:350–1.
11. Johr R, Saghari S, Nouri K. Eccrine porocarcinoma arising in a seborrheic keratosis evaluated with dermoscopy and treated with Mohs' technique. Int J Dermatol. 2003;42: 653–7.
12. Baptista AP, Tellechea O, Reis JP. Eccrine porocarcinoma: a review of 24 cases. Ann Dermatol Venereol. 1993;120: 107–15.
13. Huet P, Danduran M, Pignodel C, et al. Metastasizing eccrine porocarcinoma: a report of a case and review of the literature. J Am Acad Dermatol. 1996;35:860–4.
14. Kolde G, Macher E, Grundmann E. Metastasizing eccrine porocarcinoma. Report of two cases with fatal outcome. Pathol Res Pract. 1991;187:477–81.
15. Barzi AS, Ruggeri S, Recchia F, et al. Malignant metastatic eccrine poroma. Dermatol Surg. 1997;23:267–72.
16. Grimme H, Petres A, Begen E, et al. Metastasizing porocarcinoma of the head with lethal outcome. Dermatology. 1999;198:298–300.
17. Swanson PE, Cherwitz DL, Neumann MP, et al. Eccrine sweat gland carcinoma: a histological and immunohistochemical study of 32 cases. J Cutan Pathol. 1987;4:65–86.
18. Gschnait F, Horn F, Lindlbauer R, et al. Eccrine porocarcinoma. J Cutan Pathol. 1980;7:349–53.
19. Mohamed F, Blok J, Grayson W. The squamous variant of eccrine porocarcinoma: a clinicopathological study of 21 cases. J Clin Pathol. 2008;61:361–5.
20. Hara K, Kamiya S. Pigmented eccrine porocarcinoma: a mimic of malignant melanoma. Histopathology. 1995;27: 86–8.
21. Miyashima M, Suzuki H. In situ porocarcinoma: a case with malignant expression in clear tumor cells. Int J Dermatol. 1993;32:749–50.
22. Bogner PN, Fullen DR, Lowe L, et al. Lymphatic mapping and sentinel lymph node biopsy in the detection of early metastasis from sweat gland carcinoma. Cancer. 2003;97: 2285–9.
23. Harari PM, Shimm DS, Bangert J, et al. The role of radiotherapy in the treatment of malignant sweat gland neoplasms. Cancer. 1990;65:1727–41.
24. Dummer R, Becker JC, Boser B, et al. Successful therapy of metastatic eccrine poroma using perilesional interferon-alpha and interleukin-2. Arch Dermatol. 1992;128:1127–8.
25. Gutermuth J, Audring H, Voit C, et al. Antitumor activity of paclitaxel and interferon-alpha in a case of metastatic eccrine porocarcinoma. J Eur Acad Dermatol Venereol. 2004;18: 477–9.
26. Wittenberg GP, Robertson DB, Solomon AR, et al. Eccrine porocarcinoma treated with Mohs micrographic surgery: a report of five cases. Dermatol Surg. 1999;25:911–3.
27. McMichael AJ, Gay J. Malignant eccrine poroma in an elderly African-American woman. Dermatol Surg. 1999;25: 733–5.
28. D'Ambrosia R, Ward H, Parry E, et al. Eccrine porocarcinoma of the eyelid treated with Mohs micrographic surgery. Dermatol Surg. 2004;30(Pt 1):570–1.
29. Wildemore JK, Lee JB, Humphreys TR. Mohs surgery for malignant eccrine neoplasms. Dermatol Surg. 2004;30(Pt 2):1574–9.
30. Cowden A, Dans M, Militello G, et al. Eccrine porocarcinoma arising in two African American patients: distinct presentations both treated with Mohs micrographic surgery. Int J Dermatol. 2006;45:146–50.

Hidradenocarcinoma

31. Liu Y. The histogenesis of clear cell papillary carcinoma of the skin. Am J Pathol. 1949;25:93–103.
32. Ko CJ, Cochran AJ, Eng W, et al. Hidradenocarcinoma: a histological and immunohistochemical study. J Cutan Pathol. 2006;23:726–30.
33. Chow CW, Campbell PE, Burry AE. Sweat gland carcinomas in children. Cancer. 1984;53:1222–7.
34. Hernandez-Perez E, Cestoni-Parducci R. Nodular hidradenoma and hidradenocarcinoma. A ten year review. J Am Acad Dermatol. 1985;12:15–20.
35. Chung CK, Heffernan AH. Clear cell hidradenoma with metastasis. Case report with a review of the literature. Plast Reconstr Surg. 1971;48:177–9.
36. Berg JW, McDivitt RW. Pathology of sweat gland carcinoma. Pathol Annu. 1968;3:122–44.
37. Mambo NC. The significance of atypical nuclear changes in benign eccrine acrospiromas: a clinical and pathological study of 18 cases. J Cutan Pathol. 1984;11:35–44.
38. Biddlestone LR, McLaren KM, Tidman MJ. Malignant hidradenoma: a case report demonstrating insidious histological and clinical progression. Clin Exp Dermatol. 1991; 16:474–7.
39. Hunt SJ, Santa Cruz DJ, Kerl H. Giant eccrine acrospiroma. J Am Acad Dermatol. 1990;23:663–8.
40. Wong TY, Suster S, Nogita T, et al. Clear cell eccrine carcinoma of the skin: a clinicopathologic study of nine patients. Cancer. 1994;73:1631–43.
41. Massad LS, Bitterman P, Clarke-Pearson DL. Metastatic clear cell eccrine hidradenocarcinoma of the vulva: survival after primary surgical resection. Gynecol Oncol. 1996;61: 287–90.
42. Tolland JP, Brenn T, Guldbakke KK, et al. Mohs micrographic surgery, sentinel lymph node mapping, and estrogen receptor analysis for the treatment of malignant nodular hidradenoma. Dermatol Surg. 2006;32:1294–301.
43. Harari PM, Shimm DS, Bangert JL, et al. The role of radiotherapy in the treatment of malignant sweat gland neoplasms. Cancer. 1990;65:1737–40.
44. Messing MJ, Richardson MS, Smith MT, et al. Metastatic clear cell hidradenocarcinoma of the vulva. Gynecol Oncol. 1993;48:264–8.
45. Souvatzidis P, Sbano P, Mandato F, et al. Malignant nodular hidradenoma of the skin: report of seven cases. J Eur Acad Dermatol Venereol. 2008;22:549–54.
46. Long WP, Dupin C, Levine EA. Recurrent malignant acrospiroma. Dermatol Surg. 1998;24:908–12.
47. Jouary T, Kaiafa A, Lipinski P, et al. Metastatic hidradenocarcinoma: efficacy of capecitabine. Arch Dermatol. 2006; 142:1366–7.
48. Obaidat NA, Alsaad KO, Ghazarian D. Skin adnexal neoplasm. J Clin Pathol. 2007;60:145–59.

49. Nash JW, Barrett TL, Kies M, et al. Metastatic hidradenocarcinoma with demonstration of Her-2/neu gene amplification by fluorescence in situ hybridization: potential treatment implications. J Cutan Pathol. 2007;34:49–54.
50. House NS, Helm KE, Maloney ME. Management of a hidradenoma with Mohs micrographic surgery. J Dermatol Surg Oncol. 1994;20:619–22.
51. Will R, Coldiron B. Recurrent clear cell hidradenoma of the foot. Dermatol Surg. 2000;26:685–6.
52. Dzubow LM, Grossman DJ, Johnson B. Eccrine adenocarcinoma – report of a case, treatment with Mohs surgery. J Dermatol Surg Oncol. 1986;12:1049–53.
53. Yavel R, Hinshaw M, Rao V, et al. Hidradenoma and a hidradenocarcinoma of the scalp managed using Mohs micrographic surgery and a multidisciplinary approach: case reports and review of the literature. Dermatol Surg. 2009;35:273–81.

Cutaneous Adenoid Cystic Carcinoma

54. Boggio R. Adenoid cystic carcinoma of the scalp. Arch Dermatol. 1975;111:793–4.
55. Seab JA, Graham JH. Primary cutaneous adenoid cystic carcinoma. J Am Acad Dermatol. 1987;17:113–8.
56. Van der Kwast TH, Vuzevski VD, Ramaekers F, et al. Primary cutaneous adenoid cystic carcinoma: a case report, immunohistochemistry, and review of the literature. Br J Dermatol. 1988;118:567–78.
57. Urso C. Primary cutaneous adenoid cystic carcinoma. Am J Dermatopathol. 1999;21:400.
58. Naylor E, Sarkar P, Perlis C, et al. Primary cutaneous adenoid cystic carcinoma. J Am Acad Dermatol. 2008;5(4): 636–41.
59. Dores GM, Huycke MM, Devesa SS, et al. Primary cutaneous adenoid cystic carcinoma in the United States: incidence, survival, and associated cancers, 1976 to 2005. J Am Acad Dermatol. 2010;63:71–8.
60. Perzin KH, Gullane P, Conley J. Adenoid cystic carcinoma involving the external auditory canal. A clinicopathologic study of 16 cases. Cancer. 1982;50:2873–83.
61. Lawrence JB, Mazur MT. Adenoid cystic carcinoma: a comparative pathological study of tumors in the salivary gland, breast, lung, and cervix. Human Pathol. 1982;13: 916–24.
62. Beck HG, Lechner W, Wunsch PH. Adenoid cystic sweat gland cancer. Hautarzt. 1986;37:405–9.
63. Kato N, Yasukawa K, Onozuka T. Primary cutaneous adenoid cystic carcinoma with lymph node metastasis. Am J Dermatopathol. 1998;20:571–7.
64. Fordice J, Kershaw C, El-Naggar A, et al. Adenoid cystic carcinoma of the head and neck: predictors of morbidity and mortality. Arch Otolaryngol Head Neck Surg. 1999;125: 149–52.
65. Weekly M, Lydiatt DD, Lydiatt WM, et al. Primary cutaneous adenoid cystic carcinoma metastatic to cervical lymph nodes. Head Neck. 2000;22:84–6.
66. Chu SS, Chang YL, Lou PJ. Primary cutaneous adenoid cystic carcinoma and regional lymph node metastasis. J Laryngol Otol. 2001;115:673–5.
67. Doganay L, Bilgi S, Aygit C, et al. Primary cutaneous adenoid cystic carcinoma with lung and lymph node metastases. J Eur Acad Dermatol Venereol. 2004;18:383–5.
68. Sanderson KV, Batten JC. Adenoid cystic carcinoma of the scalp with pulmonary metastasis. Proc R Soc Med. 1975;68:649–50.
69. Pappo O, Gez E, Cracium I, et al. Growth analysis of lung metastases appearing 18 years after resection of cutaneous adenoid cystic carcinoma. Cases report and review of the literature. Arch Pathol Lab Med. 1992;116:76–9.
70. Chang SE, Ahn SJ, Choi JH, et al. Primary adenoid cystic carcinoma of skin with lung metastasis. J Am Acad Dermatol. 1999;40:640–2.
71. Bergman R, Lichtig C, Moscana RA, et al. A comparative immunohistochemical study of adenoid cystic carcinoma of the skin and salivary glands. Am J Dermatopathol. 1991;13: 162–8.
72. Wick MR, Swanson PE. Primary adenoid cystic carcinoma of the skin. Am J Dermatopathol. 1986;8:2–11.
73. Lang PG, Metcalf JS, Maize JC. Recurrent adenoid cystic carcinoma of the skin managed by microscopically controlled surgery (Mohs surgery). J Dermatol Surg Oncol. 1986;12:395–8.
74. Chesser RS, Bertler DE, Fitzpatrick JE, et al. Primary cutaneous adenoid cystic carcinoma treated with Mohs micrographic surgery toluidine blue technique. J Dermatol Surg Oncol. 1992;18:175–6.
75. Krunic AL, Kim S, Medenica M, et al. Recurrent adenoid cystic carcinoma of the scalp treated with Mohs micrographic surgery. Dermatol Surg. 2003;29:647–9.
76. Fueston JC, Gloster HM, Mutasim DF. Primary cutaneous adenoid cystic carcinoma: a case report and literature review. Cutis. 2006;77:157–60.
77. Barnes J, Garcia C. Primary cutaneous adenoid cystic carcinoma: a case report and review of the literature. Cutis. 2008;81:243–6.
78. Sammour R, Lafaille P, Joncas V, et al. Adenoid cystic carcinoma of the eyelid: a rare cutaneous tumor treated with Mohs micrographic surgery. Dermatol Surg. 2009;35: 997–1000.
79. Xu YG, Hinshaw M, Longley BJ, et al. Cutaneous adenoid cystic carcinoma with perineural invasion treated by Mohs micrographic surgery – a case report with literature review. J Oncol. 2010. doi:115/2010/469049.
80. Ikegawa S, Saida T, Obayashi H, et al. Cisplatin combination chemotherapy in squamous cell carcinoma and adenoid cystic carcinoma of the skin. J Dermatol. 1989;16: 227–30.

Spiradenocarcinoma

81. Evans HL, Su WPD, Smith JL, et al. Carcinoma arising in eccrine spiradenoma. Cancer. 1979;43:1881–4.
82. Cooper PH, Fierson HF, Morrison AG. Malignant transformation of eccrine spiradenoma. Arch Dermatol. 1985;121: 1445–8.
83. Wick MR, Swanson PE, Kaye VN, et al. Sweat gland carcinoma ex eccrine spiradenoma. Am J Dermatopathol. 1987;9: 90–8.

84. McKee PH, Fletcher CD, Starvrinos P, et al. Carcinosarcoma arising in eccrine spiradenoma. A clinicopathologic and immunohistochemical study of two cases. Am J Dermatopathol. 1990;12:335–43.
85. Argenyi ZB, Nguyen AV, Balogh K, et al. Malignant eccrine spiradenoma. A clinicopathologic study. Am J Dermatopathol. 1992;14:381–90.
86. Biernat W, Wozniak L. Spiradenocarcinoma. A clinicopathologic and immunohistochemical study of three cases. Am J Dermatopathol. 1994;16:377–82.
87. Tay JS, Tapen EM, Solari PG. Malignant eccrine spiradenoma: case report and review of the literature. Am J Clin Oncol. 1997;20:552–5.
88. Beekley AC, Brown TA, Porter C. Malignant eccrine spiradenoma: a previously unreported presentation and review of the literature. Am Surg. 1999;65:236–40.
89. Dabska M. Malignant transformation of eccrine spiradenoma. Pol Med J. 1972;11:388–96.
90. Yildirim S, Akoz T, Akan M, et al. De novo malignant eccrine spiradenoma with an interesting and unusual location. Dermatol Surg. 2001;27:417–20.
91. Fernandez-Acenero MJ, Mazarbeitia F, Mestre de Juan MJ, et al. Malignant spiradenoma: a report of two cases and literature review. J Am Acad Dermatol. 2001;44: 395–8.
92. Hantash BM, Chan JL, Egbert BM, et al. De novo malignant eccrine spiradenoma: a case report and review of the literature. Dermatol Surg. 2006;32:1189–98.
93. Granter SR, Seeger K, Calonje E, et al. Malignant eccrine spiradenoma (spiradenocarcinoma). A clinicopathologic study of 12 cases. Am J Dermatopathol. 2000;22:97–103.
94. Carlsten JR, Lewis MDJ, Saddler K, et al. Spiradenocylindrocarcinoma: a malignant hybrid tumor. J Cutan Pathol. 2005;32:166–71.
95. Mirza I, Kloss R, Sieber SC. Malignant eccrine spiradenoma. Arch Pathol Lab Med. 2002;126:591–4.
96. McCalmont TH. A call for logic in classification of adnexal neoplasms. Am J Dermatopathol. 1996;18:103–9.
97. Russ BW, Meffert J, Bernert R. Spiradenocarcinoma of the scalp. Cutis. 2002;69:455–8.
98. Sridhar KS, Benedetto P, Otrakji CL, et al. Response of eccrine adenocarcinoma to tamoxifen. Cancer. 1989;64:366–70.
99. Yaremchuk MJ, Elias LS, Graham RR, et al. Sweat gland carcinoma of the hand: two cases of malignant eccrine spiradenoma. J Hand Surg Am. 1984;9A:910–4.

Malignant Cylindroma

100. Wiedemann A. Weitere beitrage zur kenntnis der sogenannten zylindrome der kopfhaut. Arch Dermatol. 1929;159:180–7.
101. Gerretsen AI, van der Putte SCJ, Deenstra W, et al. Cutaneous cylindroma with malignant transformation. Cancer. 1993;72:1618–23.
102. Biernat W, Biernat S. Cutaneous adnexal carcinoma arising within a solitary cylindroma-spiradenoma. Am J Dermatopathol. 1996;18:77–82.
103. Cho C, Lo JS, Snow SN, et al. Malignant cylindroma. In: Miller SJ, Maloney ME, editors. Cutaneous oncology: pathophysiology, diagnosis, and treatment. Oxford: Blackwell; 1998.
104. Urbanski SJ, Fromm L, Abramowicz A, et al. Metamorphosis of dermal cylindroma: possible relation to malignant transformation. J Am Acad Dermatol. 1985;12:188–95.
105. Bondenson L. Malignant dermal eccrine cylindroma. Acta Derm Venereol. 1979;59:92–4.
106. Hammond DC, Grant KF, Simpson WD. Malignant degeneration of dermal cylindroma. Ann Plast Surg. 1990;24:176–8.
107. Lotem M, Trattner A, Kahanovick S. Multiple dermal cylindroma undergoing a malignant transformation. Int J Dermatol. 1992;31:642–4.
108. Durani BK, Kurzen H, Jaeckel A, et al. Malignant transformation of multiple dermal cylindromas. Br J Dermatol. 2001;145:653–6.
109. Young AI, Kellermayer R, Szigeti R, et al. CYLD mutations underlie brooke-spiegler, familial cylindromatosis, and multiple familial trichoepitheliomas syndromes. Clin Genet. 2006;70:246–9.
110. Donner LR, Ruff T, Diaz JA. Well differentiated malignant cylindroma with partially preserved hyaline sheaths. A locally invasive neoplasm? Am J Dermatopathol. 1995;17:169–73.
111. Michal M, Lamovec J, Mukensnabl P, et al. Spiradenocylindromas of the skin: tumors with morphological features of spiradenoma and cylindroma in the same lesion: report of 12 cases. Pathol Int. 1999;49:419–25.
112. Maybehm M, Fischer HP. Spiradenoma and dermal cylindroma: comparative immunohistochemical analysis and histogenetic considerations. Am J Dermatopathol. 1997;19: 154–61.
113. Lo JS, Peschen M, Snow SN, et al. Malignant cylindroma of the scalp. J Dermatol Surg Oncol. 1991;17:897–901.
114. Mashkevich G, Undavia S, Iacob C, et al. Malignant cylindroma of the external auditory canal. Otol Neurotol. 2005; 27:97–101.
115. Lo JS, Snow SN, Mohs FE. Cylindroma treated by Mohs micrographic surgery. J Dermatol Surg Oncol. 1991;17: 871–4.
116. Behrozan DS, Goldberg LH, Glaich AS, et al. Mohs micrographic surgery for deeply penetrating, expanding benign cutaneous neoplasms. Dermatol Surg. 2006;32:958–65.

Mucinous Carcinoma of the Skin

117. Lennox B, Pearse AGE, Richard HGH. Mucus secreting tumors of the skin with special reference to the so called mixed salivary tumor of the skin and its relations to hidradenoma. J Pathol Bacteriol. 1952;64:865–80.
118. Mendoza S, Helwig EB. Mucinous (adenocystic) carcinoma of the skin. Arch Dermatol. 1971;103:68–78.
119. Wright JD, Font RL. Mucinous sweat gland adenocarcinoma of eyelid. A clinicopathologic study of 21 cases with histochemical and electron microscopic observations. Cancer. 1979;44:1757–68.
120. Snow SN, Reizner GT. Mucinous eccrine carcinoma of the eyelid. Cancer. 1992;70:2099–104.

121. Karimpour DJ, Johnson TM, Kang S, et al. Mucinous carcinoma of the skin. J Am Acad Dermatol. 1996;36:323–6.
122. Hurt MA, Santa Cruz DJ. Tumors of the skin. In: Fletcher CDM, editor. Diagnostic histopathology of tumors. Edinburgh: Churchill Livingstone; 1995.
123. Pilgrim JP, Wolfish PS, Kloss SG, et al. Primary mucinous carcinoma of the skin with metastases to the lymph node. Am J Dermatopathol. 1985;7:461–9.
124. Yeung KY, Stinson JC. Mucinous (adenocystic) carcinoma of the sweat glands with widespread metastasis. Cancer. 1997;39:2556–62.
125. Ajithkumar TV, Nileena N, Abraham EK, et al. Bone marrow relapse in primary mucinous carcinoma of skin. Am J Clin Oncol. 1999;22:303–4.
126. Jih MH, Friedman PM, Kimyai-Asadi A, et al. A rare case of fatal primary cutaneous mucinous carcinoma of the scalp with multiple in transit and pulmonary metastases. J Am Acad Dermatol. 2005;52S:76–80.
127. Rao KV, Tikku I, Kapur BM, et al. Invasive primary mucinous of the skin. Int Surg. 1978;63:168–70.
128. Fukamizu H, Tomita K, Inoue K, et al. Primary mucinous carcinoma of the skin. J Dermatol Surg Oncol. 1993;19: 625–8.
129. Rahilly MA, Beattie GJ, Lessells AM. Mucinous eccrine carcinoma of the vulva with neuroendocrine differentiation. Histopathology. 1995;27:82–6.
130. Yamamoto O, Nakayama K, Asahi M. Sweat gland carcinoma with mucinous and infiltrating duct-like patterns. J Cutan Pathol. 1992;19:334–9.
131. Eckert F, Schmid U, Hardmeier T, et al. Cytokeratin expression in mucinous sweat gland carcinomas: an immunohistochemical analysis of four cases. Histopathology. 1992;21: 161–5.
132. Carson HJ, Gattuso P, Raslan WF, et al. Mucinous carcinoma of the eyelid. An immunohistochemical study. Am J Dermatopathol. 1995;17:494–8.
133. Qureshi JS, Salama ME, Chitale D, et al. Primary cutaneous mucinous carcinoma: presence of myoepithelial cells as a clue to cutaneous origin. Am J Dermatopathol. 2004;26:353–8.
134. Dmitry VK, Suster S, LeBoit P, et al. Mucinous carcinoma of the skin, primary, and secondary. A clinicopathologic study of 63 cases with emphasis on morphologic spectrum of primary cutaneous forms: homologies with mucinous lesions in the breast. Am J Surg Pathol. 2005;29:764–82.
135. Requena L, Kiryu H, Ackerman AB. Mucinous carcinoma. In: Requena L, Kiryu H, Ackerman AB, editors. Neoplasms with apocrine differentiation. Philadelphia: Lippincott-Raven; 1998.
136. Weber P, Hevia O, Gretzula J, et al. Primary mucinous carcinoma. J Dermatol Surg Oncol. 1988;14:170–2.
137. Bertagnoli R, Cook DL, Goldman GD. Bilateral primary mucinous carcinoma of the eyelid treated with Mohs surgery. Dermatol Surg. 1999;25:566–8.
138. Ortiz KJ, Gaughan MD, Bang RH, et al. A case of primary mucinous carcinoma of the scalp treated with Mohs surgery. Dermatol Surg. 2002;28:751–4.
139. Cabell CE, Helm KF, Sakol PJ, et al. Primary mucinous carcinoma in a 54 year old man. J Am Acad Dermatol. 2003;49:941–3.
140. Marra DE, Schanbacher CF, Torres A. Mohs micrographic surgery of primary cutaneous mucinous carcinoma using immunochemistry for margin control. Dermatol Surg. 2004;50:799–802.
141. Tannous ZS, Afram MM, Zembowicz A, et al. Treatment of synchronous mucinous carcinoma and endocrine mucin-producing sweat gland carcinoma with Mohs micrographic surgery. Dermatol Surg. 2005;51:564–7.
142. Cecchi R, Rapicano V. Primary cutaneous mucinous carcinoma: report of two cases treated with Mohs micrographic surgery. Australas J Dermatol. 2006;47:192–4.
143. Snow S, Longley J, Stewart D. Atlas of Mohs Surgery Frozen Sections Madison: Do-It Digital Printing; 2010

Sebaceous Carcinoma

26

Stephen N. Snow and Yaohui Gloria Xu

Abstract

Ocular sebaceous carcinoma (SC) is an uncommon adnexal tumor that typically occurs on the upper eyelids, in white women at an average age of 72. The best outcome is achieved when the tumor status is primary, present on the central lid, less than 6 months duration, less than 6 mm in size, and devoid of pagetoid conjunctival spread. Pagetoid spread is present in about 50–80% of primary tumors.

Classic Mohs surgery uses frozen sections to recognize pagetoid cells. These can be supplemented with paraffin sections especially for assessment of epithelial margins. The Mohs surgery local success rate for primary and recurrent SC is 88% and 70%, respectively.

Our updated review accumulated 57 patients; the overall local recurrence rate following Mohs surgery was 12.3% (7 of 57), regional metastasis 8.8% (5 of 57), and no deaths. These results compare favorably to standard wide excision with local recurrence of 18%, regional metastasis of 8%, and 6% deaths.

Keywords

Sebaceous carcinoma, ocular • Sebaceous carcinoma, extraocular • Meibomian gland carcinoma • Mohs micrographic surgery • Frozen sections • Oil Red O

Summary: Introduction

- Sebaceous carcinoma is an uncommon malignant neoplasm of sebaceous glands most frequently found on the eyelids (meibomian gland > glands of Zeis).
- It accounts for 4% of ocular skin malignancies and is the most malignant primary tumor of the eye.
- About 1 in 100 clinical chalazion is a sebaceous carcinoma on biopsy.

S.N. Snow (✉)
Department of Dermatology, University of Wisconsin School of Medicine & Public Health, Madison, WI, USA
e-mail: snsnow@dermatology.wisc.edu

Y.G. Xu
Department of Dermatology, University of Wisconsin, Madison, WI, USA

K. Nouri (ed.), *Mohs Micrographic Surgery*,
DOI 10.1007/978-1-4471-2152-7_26,

- Poor prognosis occurs when lesions are recurrent, greater than 10 mm in size, longer than 6 months of duration, involving both lids, involving canthus, and having aggressive histologic features.

26.1 Introduction

Sebaceous carcinoma (SC) is a rare adnexal skin cancer that challenges the abilities of all physicians and surgeons. Although it comprises about 4% of ocular skin malignancies, SC is one of the most malignant primary tumors of the eye with a 5-year death rate of 15% [1]. Most tumors originate from the meibomian gland, and about 10% arise from the glands of Zeis. SC typically presents in Caucasian women between the ages of 60 and 80 years. It is rare under 40 years of age unless there is a history of previous irradiation. It is usually unilateral and involves the upper lid twice as frequently as the lower. It has been reported to occur disproportionately in Asians and East Indians [2]. It mimics more common entities like a sty, chalazion, or unilateral conjunctivitis. After a well-defined therapeutic trial period, refractory lesions should be biopsied to rule out an incipient SC. In one study, about 1 in 100 clinical chalazion was a SC on biopsy [3]. Every effort should be made to diagnose and treat SC before 6 months duration. Mohs surgeons and dermatologists have an opportunity for early diagnosis because about 25% of the cases have a contemporaneous history of skin cancer. Lesions that are greater than 10 mm in size, present for more than 6 months, and involve both lids and intervening canthus have a poor prognosis.

26.1.1 Origin

Sebaceous carcinoma is a malignant neoplasm derived from cells that comprise sebaceous glands. In the orbital region, these are the meibomian glands of the tarsus and the Zeis glands associated with the lid margin cilia, caruncle, and eyebrow. Sebaceous glands are usually associated with hair follicles and the hairy parts of the body [4]. Sebaceous glands not associated with hair follicles are found also in the mucosa of the mouth (Fordyce granule) [5] and vulva regions [6] where sebaceous carcinoma is known to occur [7, 8].

26.1.2 History

Mohs micrographic surgery (MMS) for eyelid cancers was first performed by Frederic Mohs using a local anesthetic in 1953 [9]. Two decades later, two dermatologists and trainees of Dr. Mohs, Ted Tromovitch and Sam Stegeman, presented their successful series of 102 basal and squamous cell carcinomas using frozen sections (including periorbital cancers) managed by MMS [10]. The first reported case of sebaceous carcinoma of the lid treated by MMS was presented by Dixon, Mikhail, and Slater in 1980 in the Journal of the American Academy of Dermatology [11, 12]. They reported a case in an 84-year-old woman with a primary sebaceous carcinoma of the upper lid of 6 months duration. The patient was followed for 2.5 years without a recurrence. Other early Mohs surgery pioneers include Harvey and Anderson [13], Dzubow [14], Folberg et al. [15], and Ratz et al. [16]. In 1994, Yount et al. [17] presented their favorable series of 8 cases using mainly paraffin sections in close collaboration with pathology and oculoplastic service.

26.1.3 Extraorbital Sites

Sebaceous carcinoma occurs in other sites of the body. Recently, the National Cancer Institute‘s database known as the Surveillance, Epidemiology, and End Results (SEER) reported a total of 1349 cases of sebaceous carcinoma in the USA accumulated from 1974 to 2004. This database represented 26% of the population from 12 states. There were 522 cases of the eyelids; 549 cases involving the scalp, ear, lip, neck and other facial sites; and 278 cases of the trunk, extremity, genitalia, and other sites. The clinical course, pathology, management, and prognosis are similar for extraorbital and periorbital sebaceous carcinoma. Survival analysis for orbital and periorbital versus nonorbital sites supports a similar prognosis with a 5-year survival of 75.2% versus 68% [7]. Sawyer et al. [18] accumulated 130 cases of extraorbital SC from the medical literature. The metastatic rate was 18% (23 of 130). The death rate from visceral metastasis was 7% (9 of 130).

26.1.4 Incidence

Sebaceous carcinoma accounts for about 4% of malignant tumors of the periorbital region. Basal cell carcinoma accounts for about 90%, squamous cell carcinoma

5%, and melanoma and other malignancies account for 1% [19, 20]. For all SC sites, the SEER database shows that the median age was 73 years. The sex distribution for SC was about equal with men numbering 729 (52%) and women 620 (46%). The most frequent site for SC was the eyelid (38.7%). In the USA, the degree of previous radiation and ultraviolet exposure may play a larger role than racial factors. The SEER reports suggest that the incidence of SC is increasing possibly due to increased awareness, referrals to tertiary centers, and increased radiation exposure [7]. The SEER database did not break out the periorbital survival data.

Summary: Demographics

- Sebaceous carcinoma typically occurs on the upper eyelids in older Caucasian females with mean age of 72.
- Muir–Torre syndrome is associated more with sebaceous adenoma than sebaceous carcinoma.
- Risk factors for sebaceous carcinoma include older age, female sex, ethnicity (Caucasian, Asian, and Indians), irradiation, ultraviolet exposure, preexisting nevus sebaceous, Muir–Torre syndrome, and immunosuppression.

26.2 Demographics

26.2.1 Age, Sex, Irradiation, Race

Sebaceous carcinoma is generally a disease of older individuals. The mean age is 72 (range 50–92) [19]. White women are predominantly affected, and the upper lid is affected twice as frequently as the lower lid. However, it can occur in children and young adults within 11 years after radiation for retinoblastoma [21]. Bilateral SC has been reported in a patient who had prior whole face irradiation for eczema [22]. Internationally, SC is reported as more prevalent in the Asia and India [2, 23]. In the USA, the SEER race distribution was Caucasian > Asian/Pacific Islander > African American [7].

26.2.2 Muir–Torre Syndrome (MTS)

The Muir–Torre syndrome is an autosomal dominant condition in which patients develop cutaneous adenomas, keratoacanthomas, and internal malignancies mainly of the stomach and duodenum and urinary tract. MTS is associated with microsatellite instability and mismatch repair genes. Occasional patients with the Muir–Torre syndrome have developed periocular sebaceous carcinoma. MTS is associated more with sebaceous adenomas than sebaceous carcinomas [24]. Cohen et al. [25] showed that 24.2% of 120 MTS patients had an SC.

26.2.3 Human Papillomavirus (HPV)

A study from Japan showed that 13 of 21 tumors (62%) were positive for HPV DNA using in situ hybridization techniques [26].

26.2.4 Other Risk Factors

Risk factors for sebaceous carcinoma include older age, female sex, ethnicity (Caucasian, Asian, and Indians), irradiation, preexisting nevus sebaceous [27, 28], Muir–Torre syndrome [29], and immunosuppression. There is no convincing data to support thiazide diuretics [30].

Summary: Clinical Presentation

- Sebaceous carcinoma can mimic both a neoplastic process and an inflammatory condition.
- It typically presents with multiphasic growth pattern: papular nodular tumor; in situ invasion of the epithelia; and multicentric lesions.
- It can resemble a sty, chalazion, pyogenic granuloma of the lid margin, or unilateral conjunctivitis.

26.3 Clinical Presentation

Sebaceous carcinoma is known widely as the great masquerader because it can mimic both a neoplastic process and an inflammatory condition. Sebaceous carcinoma typically presents as a malignancy with multiphasic growth pattern: (1) papular nodular tumor, (2) in situ invasion of the epithelia, and (3) multicentric lesions. The most common presentation is a localized papular-nodular subcutaneous growth, resembling a sty, chalazion, or pyogenic granuloma of the lid margin. The color is usually yellow due to lipids (Figs. 26.1–26.4). About 40–80%

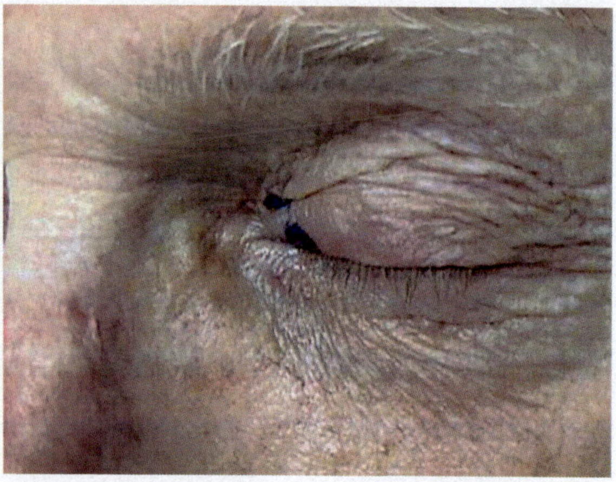

Fig. 26.1 Sebaceous carcinoma. An 82-year-old man with a lesion on the left inner canthus. The original biopsy was a chalazion. When it recurred, it was re-biopsied to be a sebaceous carcinoma. The patient was then referred to Mohs surgery for treatment (With permission, Snow et al. [31]. John Wiley & Sons)

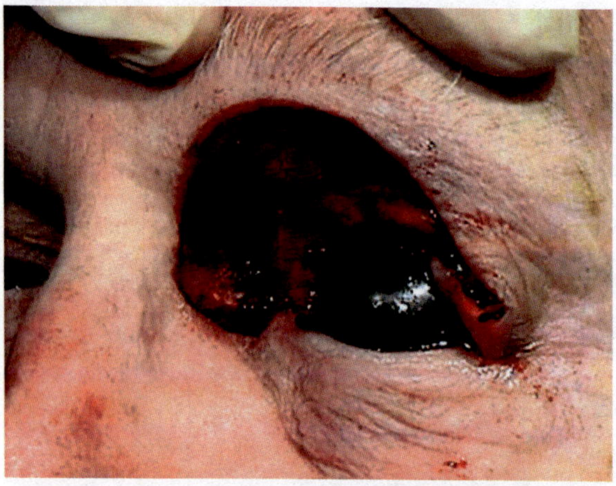

Fig. 26.2 Sebaceous carcinoma. The tumor was excised in four stages of excision. The defect extended from the inner canthus and bridge to the lateral orbital commissure. The medial excision removed the upper and lower lid puncta and canaliculi. The overall size was 22 by 50 mm. About two-thirds of the upper lid was removed (With permission, Snow et al. [31]. John Wiley & Sons)

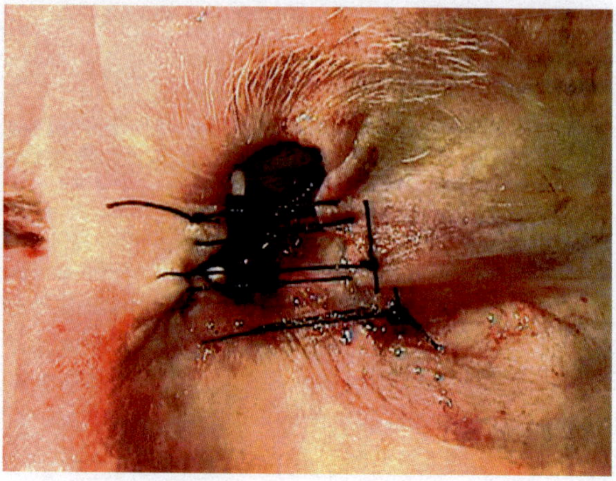

Fig. 26.3 Sebaceous carcinoma. Advancement of the upper lid margin medially to partially close the defect and provide corneal protection (With permission, Snow et al. [31]. John Wiley & Sons)

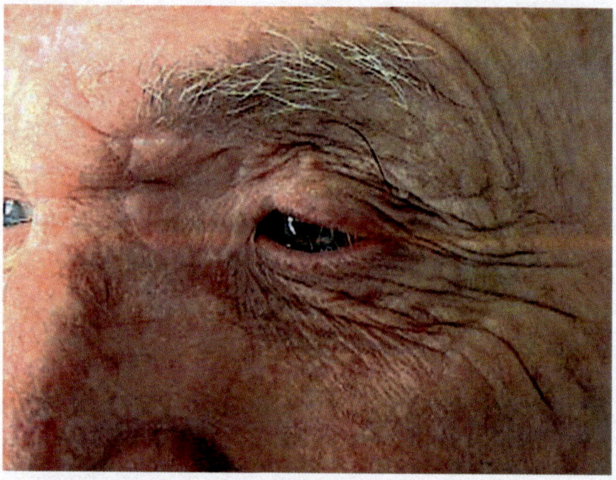

Fig. 26.4 Sebaceous carcinoma. The defect was repaired by oculoplastic service. This is the follow photo at 1 year postoperatively. The patient is tumor free for 10 years (With permission, Snow et al. [31]. John Wiley & Sons)

of SCs will also demonstrate invasion of the adjacent conjunctiva and/or epidermis [17, 31]. Perhaps 5% of SC will present as unilateral conjunctivitis showing only superficial changes in the epithelium. These lesions grow insidiously within the surface epithelium and have been confused with chronic conjunctivitis and/or squamous cell carcinoma in situ. A pattern of yellow "tigroid" streaks of lipid may be observed on the conjunctiva [32]. Involvement of the fornices or caruncle is the sign that is more consistent with sebaceous carcinoma [29, 33]. Lastly, a small percentage of SC are multicentric being derived from meibomian gland, glands of Zeis (Fig. 26.5), or other orbital sebaceous gland.

Summary: Histopathology

- There are four classic invasive architectural patterns: (1) lobular, (2) comedocarcinoma, (3) papillary, and (4) mixed.

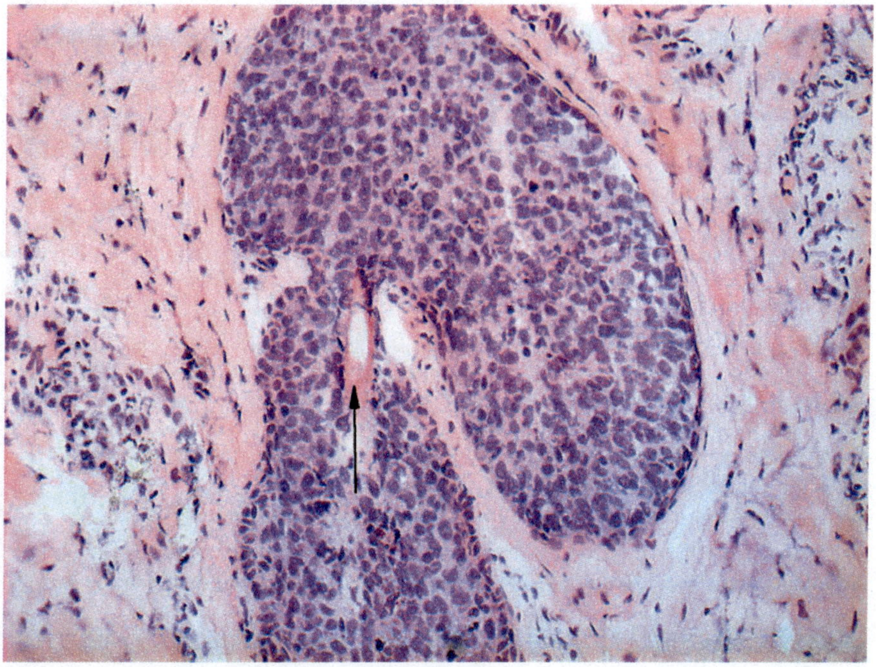

Fig. 26.5 Sebaceous carcinoma. Sebaceous carcinoma cells surrounding a hair follicle (*arrow*) indicating Zeis gland origin. Frozen 200× (Copyrighted by Steven N. Snow. Used with permission)

- Sebaceous carcinoma is grouped into well-differentiated, moderately differentiated, and poorly differentiated tumors.
- SC invades adjacent structures by three mechanisms: (1) direct invasion, (2) pagetoid spread, and (3) multicentric discontinuous spread. There is a concern of "skip" areas.
- Certain clinicopathologic features predict a poor prognosis and metastasis.

26.4 Histopathology

SC is classified by pattern of differentiation, degree of differentiation, and mechanism of invasion [4].

26.4.1 Pattern of Differentiation

There are four classic invasive architectural patterns: (1) lobular, (2) comedocarcinoma, (3) papillary, and (4) mixed. Lobular pattern is observed in 40% of the cases and mimics the normal sebaceous gland architecture with less differentiated cells at the periphery and more differentiated cells together with the accumulation of lipids centrally. About 32% display the comedocarcinoma pattern with lobules and large central necrosis surrounded by viable peripheral cells (Fig. 26.6) [34]. The papillary type shows papillary projections and sebaceous differentiation. The mixed pattern shows combinations of the three types. Basal cell carcinoma with sebaceous differentiation is negative for EMA and pagetoid spread, but has peripheral palisading of basal cells and clefting [35].

26.4.2 Degree of Differentiation

Sebaceous carcinoma is grouped into well-differentiated, moderately differentiated, and poorly differentiated tumors. Well differentiated shows cells that resemble well developed lobular pattern. The atypical sebocytes possess large atypical nuclei that contain foamy cytoplasm. Moderate well-differentiated SC still shows a recognizable lobular pattern and frothy sebocytes [4]. In poorly differentiated SC, the lobular

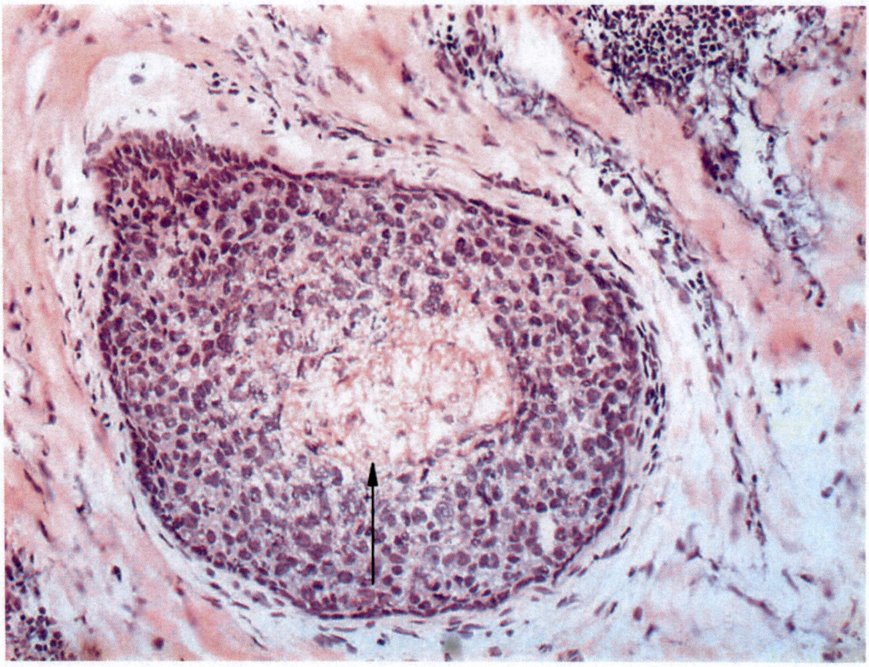

Fig. 26.6 Sebaceous carcinoma. Comedocarcinoma type showing central necrosis (*arrow*). Frozen 200× (Copyrighted by Steven N. Snow. Used with permission)

pattern is absent and there are many mitotic figures and pyknotic nuclei [4]. Special stains, such as Oil Red O, that stain lipid globules (Fig. 26.7), and immunochemistry (EMA, Cam 5.2) are usually helpful for identifying poorly differentiated SC [36, 37].

26.4.3 Mechanisms of Invasion

SC invades adjacent structures by three mechanisms: (1) direct invasion, (2) pagetoid spread, and (3) multicentric discontinuous spread. The concept of "skip" areas is discussed. Additionally, the clinicopathologic parameters of poor prognosis are listed.

26.4.3.1 Direct Invasion

Direct invasion of local tissue by SC cells consists of lobules and cords of cells with sebaceous differentiation and is the most common mechanism of spread. Mohs surgeons are familiar with this infiltrative type of invasion as observed in nodular and infiltrative basal cell carcinoma, and infiltrative squamous cell carcinoma. Perineural invasion was observed in 7% [17, 34].

26.4.3.2 Pagetoid Spread

Pagetoid spread of atypical sebocytes within the epidermal or epithelial layers is present in about 50% of the reported cases and 100% of advanced cases (Figs. 26.8, 26.9). The atypical sebocytes possess large nuclei with foamy cytoplasm and may be interspersed singly or in nests (pagetoid) or occupy the full thickness (bowenoid) of the epithelia [29]. For three decades, Mohs surgeons have been familiar with these clear cell characteristics as observed in cutaneous Bowen's disease, squamous cell carcinoma in situ, melanoma, extramammary Paget's disease [38], and other epidermotropic neoplasms. Multicentric pagetoid foci are considered unlikely because light and ultrastructural studies have revealed a lack of gradual transition of the overlying epithelia into pagetoid cells, indicating secondary spread (from below) rather than an in situ transformation [4].

26.4.3.3 Multicentric Origin

Historically, multicentric tumors have been observed in 19–36% of advanced cases and associated with the highest fatalities [4, 39, 40]. Multicentricity implies that there are different sebaceous gland cell types (e.g., meibomian, Zeis) [4] or different sites not previously involved with tumor. In a Zeis gland derived tumor, SC cells typically surround a hair shaft [4]. In this updated review, there were 57 cases of SC treated by Mohs surgery (see Table 26.1). There were seven local recurrent tumors. Multicentric SC was suspected in 5.3% (3 of 57).

Fig. 26.7 Sebaceous carcinoma. Oil red O (*orange*) showing staining the cytoplasmic lipid of the atypical sebocytes. The cells have invaded the hair follicle infundibulum. Notice, that some of the atypical sebocytes are stained inconsistently. Eosin counter stain has been omitted. Frozen 200× (With permission, Snow et al. [59])

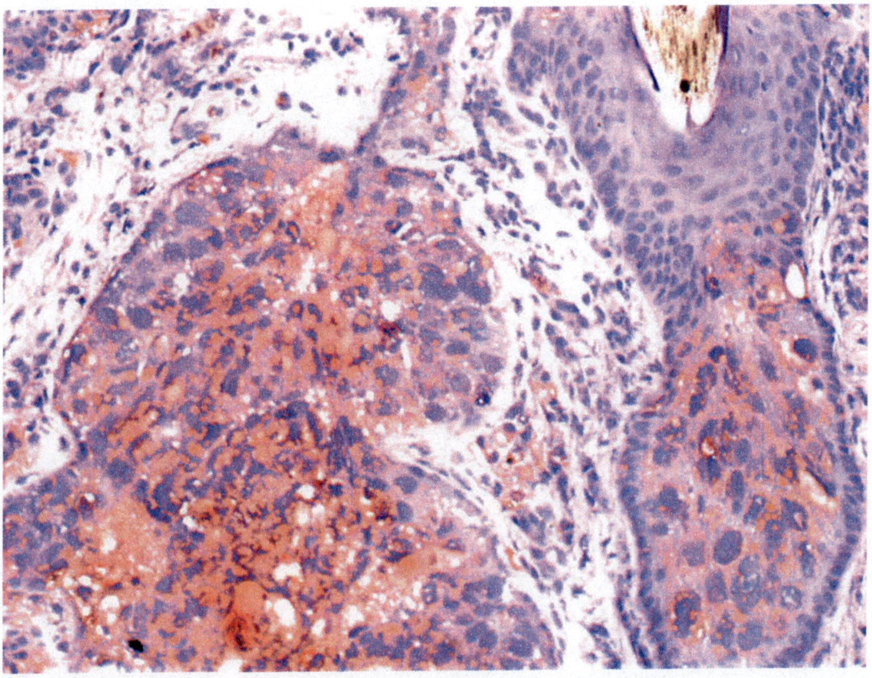

Fig. 26.8 Sebaceous carcinoma. This shows intraepithelial sebaceous carcinoma expanding to involve the full-thickness epithelium. Frozen 100× (With permission, Snow et al. [59])

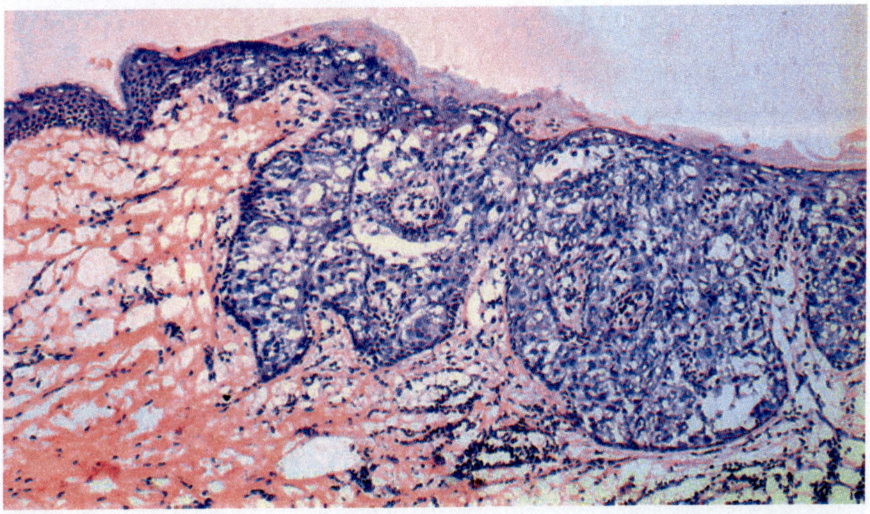

By contrast, Shields et al. [45] reported that in their series of 60 cases, that 3 of 11 (27%) recurrences were multifocal because they recurred in new sites that were previously not involved with tumor. Pereira et al. [34] reviewed 44 cases of SC for degree of sebaceous differentiation, vacuoles, growth pattern, atypical mitoses, multicentricity, lymphatic, perineural invasion, and others. Of the 11 parameters evaluated, no cases were classified as multicentric. From the Mohs surgery perspective, isolated multicentric foci do not negate the validity of applying Mohs surgery to these cancers because each individual focus will be followed to its microscopic termination. Multicentric tumors, however, do confuse the surgeon into thinking that the tumor recurred after treatment rather than representing a separate new tumor. Mohs surgeons have an opportunity to assess this phenomenon through expert mapping of recurrent tumor and reexamination of recurrent SC and comparison of the

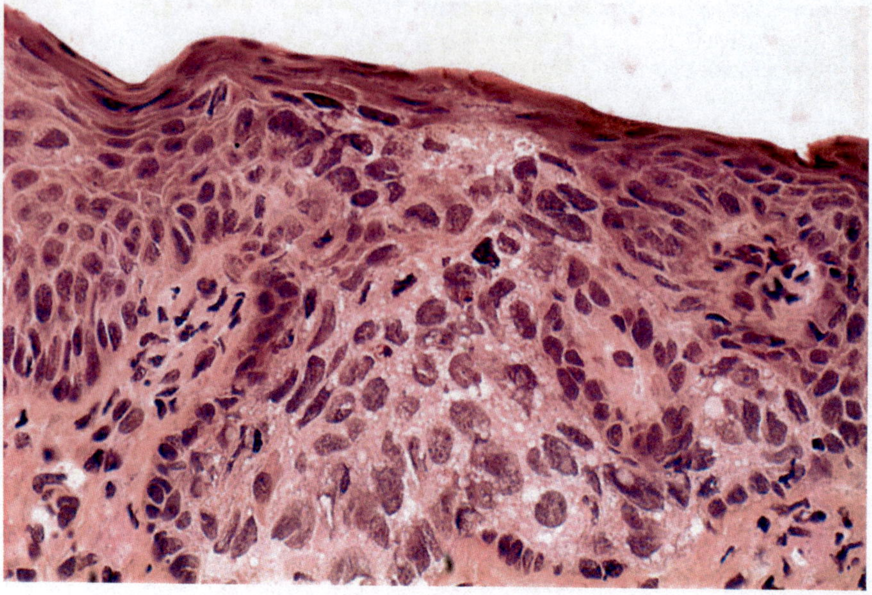

Fig. 26.9 Sebaceous carcinoma. Pagetoid spread of atypical sebocytes above the basal layer of the epithelium. The atypical sebocytes have large nuclei and pale-staining cytoplasm. Frozen 400× (With permission, Snow et al. [59])

Table 26.1 Updated results for selected categories of ocular sebaceous carcinoma treated by MMS[a]

	2002 review	2010 review updated	Total
Total number of cases reported	49	8	57
Local recurrence	6	1	7
Number without recurrence	43	7	50
Success rate	87.8% (43 of 49)		87.7% (50 of 57)
Tumor status[b]			
Primary: number without recurrence	14	4	18
Total cases	16	5	21
Success rate			85.7% (18 of 21)
Recurrent: number without recurrence	7	3	10
Total cases	10	3	13
Success rate			76.9% (10 of 13)
Multicentric tumors	3	0	3
Incidence rate	6.1% (3 of 49)		5.3% (3 of 57)

[a]Eight cases were added from Arora et al. (1 case) [41], Callahan et al. (2 cases) [42], Lai et al. (2 cases) [29], Thomas et al. (2 cases) [43], and Hwang et al. (1 case) [44]

[b]Excludes 24 cases in which tumor status was not stated

histopathology of the primary and recurrent SC tumors. Theoretically, different histopathology supports the thesis of multicentricity, while similar pathology to the original tumor suggests a local recurrence.

26.4.3.4 "Skip" Areas

The concept of a "skip" or "patchy" area of tumor is sometimes mentioned as a possible mechanism for local persistence of pagetoid SC [14, 19]. An example would be the evaluation of the surgical margins on frozen sections that was read as negative and later found to have residual tumor on paraffin sections [15]. A discontinuous focus may occur in a recurrent tumor treated by curettage [14]. Every Mohs surgeon knows that deeper cuts are made into the tissue block when thawed frozen sections are submitted for paraffin sections, thereby increasing the likelihood of finding tumor. To avoid the possibility of a narrow Mohs margin, excising an extra layer for paraffin sections may be judicious.

26.4.4 Clinicopathologic Features of Poor Outcomes

Rao et al. [4] listed the clinicopathologic features of a poor prognosis and metastasis. In ascending order of metastasis, these are (1) duration of symptoms of more than 6 months, (2) tumor larger than 10 mm, (3) multicentric origin, (4) highly infiltrative pattern, (5) upper and lower lid involvement, (6) pagetoid invasion, (7) orbital invasion, and (8) vascular and lymphatic invasion. In general, upper lid SC metastasizes to the preauricular and parotid nodes. Lower lid SC metastasizes usually to the submandibular and cervical neck nodes [19]. Historically, regional node metastasis occurred in about 30% of the cases [19]. Standard therapy is parotidectomy, neck dissection, and radiation [17, 41].

Summary: Treatment

- A diagnostic biopsy should be considered for any lesion on eyelids that is suspicious for sebaceous carcinoma. Scouting biopsy might be needed for multicentric lesions.
- Traditional wide local excision is the main method that oculoplastic surgeons use to excise sebaceous carcinoma. Exenteration might be needed for patients with orbital spread.
- Mohs micrographic surgery is an efficient method to remove sebaceous carcinoma using frozen sections. Oil Red O stain that highlights lipid on frozen sections is useful.
- Mohs micrographic surgery can be supplemented with paraffin sections especially for assessment of epithelial margins.

26.5 Treatment

The following paragraphs focus on surgical management. Other methods of management include radiation [42, 46], cryosurgery [42], mitomycin C [47].

26.5.1 Biopsy Procedure

The most common presentation for SC is a sty or chalazion. When the patient is examined, there is usually moderate swelling with or without discomfort. An incisional biopsy is a relatively simple procedure that provides drainage, and promotes healing. A partial-thickness biopsy is typically performed. A full-thickness skin and conjunctiva biopsy is indicated where a previous incisional biopsy was inconclusive. When there is severely inflamed tissue, several additional scouting biopsies are taken. For advanced tumors that have "skip" areas or have multiple foci that may be missed with a single biopsy, therefore, several biopsies may be necessary [42]. One should be wary if a biopsy of the conjunctiva, fornix, and caruncle returns a diagnosis of SCC in situ [29, 33].

26.5.2 Conjunctiva Mapped Biopsies

Extension of the tumor to the fornix may require conjunctival map scouting biopsies that are excised with scissors, submitted to ocular pathology, and sectioned vertically. Ideally, between 12 and 16 biopsies are performed – 3–4 conjunctival biopsies each on upper palpebrum, upper bulbar, lower bulbar, and lower palpebrum [48, 49]. Extensive conjunctival involvement and/or orbital invasion portends a poor prognosis resulting in exenteration [19].

26.5.3 Oil Red O and Sudan Black Stains

If the diagnosis of SC is known to the Mohs surgeon and/or dermatopathologist in advance, Oil Red O may be used to highlight lipid. This stain is used only on frozen sections in which the solvent and alcoholic steps that dissolve lipid vacuoles are omitted. The frozen slides lack eosin counter stain. When SC comes into a pathology lab as an unknown, the tissue is placed in the automated tissue processor. There are more than 6 alcoholic steps that dissolve lipid making interpretation difficult (e.g., pagetoid SC looks like SCC in situ) [34, 50]. In a series of 20 cases, the initial clinical diagnosis was incorrect in all cases, and half the cases were misdiagnosed by the pathologists interpreting the initial biopsy [51]. Reengineering the protocols for lipid staining is not always practical because in many cases the diagnosis is not suspected until after the tissue is embedded in paraffin [52]. Sudan IV stains lipid black [17, 42]. Also, both stains may not stain every atypical sebocyte because the sebocytes may be too poorly differentiated to contain any lipid [52]. Still, use of Oil Red O may be useful for pagetoid SC [14].

26.5.4 Traditional Wide Local Excision (WLE)

Traditional excision with a wide tumor margin is the main method that oculoplastic surgeons employ to excise SC. The tumor margin is then checked by general or ocular pathologists using frozen and/or paraffin sections cut vertically. The local recurrence rate with a 1–3-mm margins is 36%. Reportedly, 5-mm margins had no local recurrences [53]. Shields et al. reported that, following standard wide excision, there was local recurrence rate of 18%, regional metastasis of 8%, and 6% deaths [45].

26.5.5 Mohs Micrographic Surgery

If the cancer is a primary tumor, of short duration, less than 5 mm in size, and clinically confined to a single lid, a 3-mm margin is an acceptable starting point for Mohs surgery. Tumors that originate near the canthi and potentially involve both lids probably require more extensive Mohs surgery with at least a 5-mm margin, providing there is oculoplastic availability. In Yount's series [17], their initial Mohs layer was 5 mm around the primary tumor. This margin cleared the tumor in six of seven primary tumors. One case required three layers. Fast-track, 24-hour paraffin sections were used in nearly all cases. There were no recurrences with a follow-up range from 34 to 84 months. The case that required extra Mohs stages was a 15-mm primary SC that involved the lateral canthus and more than half of both lids. The single failure was a recurrent tumor of the inner canthus. The tumor was treated twice before Mohs surgery. At 3 years post Mohs, the tumor recurred locally with a neck node metastasis. The patient was treated by exenteration, maxillectomy, and neck dissection and was tumor free for another 3 years.

In a preliminary report by Ilyas et al. [54], at the University of Wisconsin, Mohs Surgery Clinic, there were 16 patients with SC of the eyelid treated from 1987 to 2008. The local success rate was 93% with a follow of 7 months to 14 years.

26.5.6 Surgical and Tissue Processing Issues

Mohs surgeons who regularly operate on the lids for BCC and SCC know that the evaluation of the conjunctival epithelial margin is critical for a successful outcome. The epithelium is thin, fragile, and easily destroyed by rubbing, curettage, and/or electrocautery. The epithelium shrinks after removal, and it is difficult to section 100% of the epithelial margin. To obtain good horizontal sections, the epithelium should be attached to a tissue lattice such as dermis or submucosa to provide structure and prevent the epithelium from folding over itself during the flattening procedure.

26.5.7 Frozen Sections

Mohs surgery is an efficient method to remove SC using frozen sections. Both the invasive and epithelial components of SC are recognizable by frozen sections. A disadvantage of frozen sections is that it may contain freeze artifact that hinders tumor cell recognition in the epithelial conjunctiva. Taking an extra epithelial layer is helpful to provide assurance, or referral to a tertiary center may be considered.

26.5.8 Paraffin Sections

Submission for paraffin sections should be planned beforehand with a dermatopathologist, so s/he knows what to look for in the sections. Paraffin sections have two advantages. First, when surgery is performed over two or more days, there is usually an inflammatory infiltrate that may hide atypical sebocytes. Second, SC is a difficult cancer, and the extra margin allows the Mohs surgeon/pathologist an opportunity double check their findings. The disadvantage is that most non-Mohs technicians who only work in paraffin labs have trouble in getting a complete horizontal layer, resulting in an incomplete margin check. Oil red O and Sudan black can not be performed on paraffin sections.

26.5.9 Exenteration

Exenteration is the removal of the eye (and lids) and other orbital contents within the bony walls of the orbit and neighboring sinuses [1]. The accepted indications for exenteration are involvement of the globe or anterior third of the orbit by infiltrative tumor, and widespread irreparable involvement of the bulbar conjunctiva [17]. In our review, the rate of exenteration was 10.5% (6 of 57). The overall rate of exenteration in SC ranges from 13% (8 of 60) [45] to 23% [55].

26.5.10 Mohs Surgery, Practical Points

In the typical Mohs surgery practice, the treatment of a sebaceous carcinoma is intercalated among other Mohs cases. Schedule a presurgical consult to assess the tumor and coordinate dermatopathology and oculoplastic care, with a 1-week delay for paraffin sections with possible immunohistochemistry stains. A primary SC tumor of short duration that is limited to either the upper lid or lower lid usually can be excised in one to two Mohs layers without disruption of the clinic schedule. A recurrent tumor or a SC that involves the either canthus or conjunctiva requires more detailed planning. Frequently, frozen sections are used to determine the preliminary margin, followed by a final layer for paraffin sections to double check the epithelial margin. If possible, a complex SC case should not be scheduled on a very busy day. Ocular cases require time to excise tumor and carefully read microscopic slides. Do not hurry microscopic analysis for the sake of a reconstruction deadline. If there are confusing inflammatory cells, double check results with another layer, or send defrosted specimen for paraffin sections. Delay repair if needed because a recurrence can lead to orbital involvement and exenteration. After excision, take time to orient and flatten tissue specimens properly. Mucous epithelium folds over easily, and pagetoid cells are more difficult to recognize through folded tissue sections. Hand-deliver specimens to the technician and indicate the mucous epithelium site that needs to be sectioned. If dermatopathology service is available, consider taking an additional epithelial layer for fast-track paraffin sections. Similarly, escort the specimens into the lab and indicate the mucosal side so that the technician can flatten the specimens in the cassette. The Mohs surgeon should be prepared to perform corneal protective repair.

26.5.11 Corneal Protection Measures

Since reconstruction is often delayed while waiting for paraffin section results, the cornea may be protected from injury in several ways. These protective measures include: (1) sterile ophthalmic ointment, nonirritating contact layer, and eye pad; (2) a moist plastic chamber to cover the eye; and (3) temporary tarsorrhaphy [17].

Summary: Follow-Up Considerations

- Traditional wide local excision resulted in local recurrence of 18%, regional metastasis of 8%, and 6% deaths.
- Our updated review accumulated 57 patients treated with Mohs micrographic surgery; the overall local recurrence rate following Mohs surgery was 12.3% (7 of 57), regional metastasis 8.8% (5 of 57), and no deaths. The Mohs surgery local success rate for primary and recurrent sebaceous carcinoma was 88% and 70%, respectively. These results compare favorably to traditional wide local excision.
- Sentinel lymph node has been used in some patients of sebaceous carcinoma.
- Long-term follow-up is warranted for patients treated with either traditional wide local excision or Mohs surgery.

26.6 Follow-Up Considerations

Mohs surgery for SC has not yet achieved the high cure rate of basal and squamous cell carcinoma. Local recurrence is about 12% and if not recognized early is attended with exenteration and lymph node metastasis [31]. All SC patients should be followed at least 5 years, longer if possible (see below).

26.6.1 Local Recurrence

Table 26.1 updates the previous 2002 review that accumulated 49 cases of SC treated by Mohs surgery [31]. Eight additional cases were added yielding a total of 57 cases. There were 17 males, 39 females, and 1 not stated. Age range was 31–94, mean 70.4 years. The eyelid distribution was upper ($n=35$), lower ($n=17$), canthi ($n=4$), and caruncle ($n=1$). There were seven local recurrences achieving a local success rate of 87.7%. The local success

Table 26.2 Cumulative results of 57 cases of ocular sebaceous carcinoma treated by Mohs micrographic surgery

Source	Number of cases treated by Mohs surgery	Number of local recurrences	Number with regional node metastases	Number Mohs cases treated by exenteration	Number of deaths
Yount [17]	8	1	1	1	0
Spencer [56]	18	2	1	1	0
Snow [31]	9	1	1	1	0
Series[a] 1980–2001	14	2	1	2	0
Cases[b] 2004–2007	6	0	1	0	0
Callahan [42]	2 of 14 cases	1	0[c]	1	0[d]
Ilyas [54][e]	7				
Total	57	7	5	6	0
%		12.3% (7 of 57)	8.8% (5 of 57)	10.5% (6 of 57)	

[a]Total of 14 cases from Dixon et al. (1 case) [11], Harvey and Anderson (3 cases) [13], Dzubow (2 cases) [14], Folberg et al. (3 cases) [15], Ratz et al. (3 cases) [16], Coldiron et al. (1 case) [57], and Zurcher et al. (1 case) [55], follow-up mean of 2.3 years, range 0.1–7 years

[b]Total of 6 cases from Lai et al. (2 cases) [29], Thomas et al. (2 of 3 cases; 1 lip and 2 lid cases) [43], Hwang et al. (1 case) [44], and Arora et al. (1 case with metastasis) [41]. Fifty-seven-year-old woman, recurrent chalazion of the upper lid, paraffin sections, with regional metastasis at time of repair treated by total parotidectomy, neck dissection, and radiation. NED after 3 years of follow-up

[c]An 82-year-old woman with primary SC lower lid developed recurrent lesion at 71 months post Mohs, underwent exenteration, total parotidectomy, and neck dissection; however, the patient had no positive regional node metastases

[d]A 92-year-old woman with a high-grade primary SC of the upper lid treated by WLE, recurred at 47 months. Tumor was refractory to cryotherapy, exenteration, and debulking. No regional lymph nodes. The patient presumably died of disease through direct extension and/or complications of incompletely resected SC

[e]Reported 16 cases, 7 new cases, and 9 previously reported by Snow et al. [31]

rate for primary and recurrent tumors was 86% and 77%, respectively. This case updates the multicentric incidence of 5.4% in Mohs surgery cases. In total, six of seven local recurrences were treated by exenteration. The average time for local recurrence was 10 months, range from 1 to 19 months. However, recently, Callahan [42] reported a local recurrence at 71 months post Mohs (see Table 26.2). Using WLE, Shields et al. [45] reported a local recurrence of 18% (11 of 60) at 16 months, and of these 3 of 11 (27%) were assessed to be of multifocal origin, developing in new sites not previously involved with tumor.

26.6.2 Metastasis

Following Mohs surgery, there were five regional node metastases, yielding a metastatic rate of 8.8% (5 of 57). Four of these metastases from the 2002 paper are reviewed here. Since 2002, a single case was added from Arora et al. [41]. This was a 57-year-old woman with a recurrent chalazion of the upper lid treated by curettage for about 1.5 years. The tumor was excised using paraffin sections. At the time of reconstruction, a preauricular cheek lymph node was noted. A fine need aspiration confirmed metastatic SC. The patient had a total parotidectomy, neck dissection, and radiation. The patient was NED for 3 years. From the 2002 review, there were 4 other patients with regional metastases: (1) a primary SC of the caruncle (a high risk anatomic site) metastasized to the submandibular and neck nodes at 1 month post Mohs [15]; (2) a recurrent tumor of the upper lid of 4 years duration, metastasized to the neck at 10 months, and was treated by surgery and radiation [17]; (3) a tumor that involved both lids, metastasized to the parotid nodes at 9 months [56]; and (4) a patient with long-standing chronic blepharitis was misdiagnosed as SCC in situ and developed a submandibular lymph node while undergoing Mohs surgery [31]. Mohs surgery confirmed orbital spread requiring exenteration. The patient was followed for 1 year then lost to follow-up [31]. Shields et al. [45] reported a regional metastasis rate of 8% (5 of 60) and death rate of 6%.

26.6.3 Distant Metastasis

In this updated series, after Mohs surgery, there were no deaths and no patient developed distant metastasis. In Callahan's combined study of Mohs and WLE [42], there was one patient who was treated initially with WLE who probably died of direct extension into the brain. Hematogenous dissemination is to lung, liver, bone, and brain [4].

26.6.4 Sentinel Lymph Node (SLN)

In a recent study, ten patients with eyelid sebaceous carcinoma were investigated with SLN evaluation. The SLN status was negative in all ten patients. During the study period, two patients developed regional metastasis. One of the patients previously had a false-negative reading for SLN biopsy which was later reinterpreted as positive for micrometastasis. The authors concluded that SLN evaluation is a feasible and safe procedure for high-risk patients [58].

Summary: Conclusion

- Management of sebaceous carcinoma is challenging given the nature of the cancer and possible technical errors during Mohs surgery.
- While Mohs surgery is 88% successful in the removal of the presenting lesion, one must be vigilant in recognizing new lesions, and close and long-term follow-up is necessary.

26.7 Conclusion

Sebaceous carcinoma is a versatile tumor that challenges the abilities of all Mohs surgeons. Technical factors such as mapping the excision and flattening the epithelial margin for frozen (as well as paraffin) sections are difficult, and incomplete sectioning and inaccurate reading are possible. A brief section on the practical points of treating these cancers is presented to help avoid technical errors. This chapter also contains updated information for SC treated by MMS. The Mohs surgery local recurrence rate was 12%, regional metastasis 9%, and no deaths. These results compare favorably to standard wide excision with local recurrence of 18%, regional metastasis of 8%, and 6% deaths [45]. The management of SC tests the fundamental principles of the Mohs method that depend on (1) tumor cell contiguity and (2) long-term presence without metastasis. Current reviews report that perhaps 6% of primary tumors and 27% of recurrent tumors have a multicentric origin. Isolated multicentric tumors do not negate the validity of applying Mohs surgery to these cancers because each individual focus will be followed to its microscopic termination. Multicentric tumors rarely occur simultaneously and present at different times and at different sites. "Skip" areas represent noncontiguous SC discovered when frozen sections are thawed and submitted for paraffin confirmation of tumor margins. Taking a separate, additional Mohs layer may solve this technical problem. While Mohs surgery is 88% successful in the removal of the presenting lesion, Mohs surgeons must be vigilant in recognizing new lesions, and close follow-up is necessary.

References

1. Nassab RS, Thomas SS, Murray D. Orbital exenteration for advanced periorbital skin cancers: 20 years experience. J Plast Reconstr Aesthet Surg. 2007;60:1103–9.
2. Maheshwari R. Review of orbital exenteration from an eye care centre in Western India. Orbit. 2010;29:35–8.
3. Ozdal PC, Codere F, Callejo S, Caissie AL, Burnier MN. Accuracy of the clinical diagnosis of chalazion. Eye (Lond). 2004;18:135–8.
4. Rao NA, Hidayat AA, McLean IW, Zimmerman LE. Sebaceous carcinomas of the ocular adnexa: a clinicopathologic study of 104 cases, with five-year follow-up data. Hum Pathol. 1982;13:113–22.
5. Wang H, Yao J, Solomon M, Axiotis CA. Sebaceous carcinoma of the oral cavity: a case report and review of the literature. Oral Surg Oral Med Oral Pathol Oral Radiol Endod. 2010;110:e37–40.
6. Escalonilla P, Grilli R, Canamero M, et al. Sebaceous carcinoma of the vulva. Am J Dermatopathol. 1999;21:468–72.
7. Dasgupta T, Wilson LD, Yu JB. A retrospective review of 1349 cases of sebaceous carcinoma. Cancer. 2009;115:158–65.
8. Dowd MB, Kumar RJ, Sharma R, Murali R. Diagnosis and management of sebaceous carcinoma: an Australian experience. ANZ J Surg. 2008;78:158–63.
9. Mohs FE. Chemosurgery: microscopically controlled surgery for skin cancer. Springfield: Charles C Thomas; 1978. p. 107.

10. Tromovitch TA, Stegeman SJ. Microscopically controlled excision of skin tumors. Arch Dermatol. 1974;110:231–2.
11. Dixon RS, Mikhail GR, Slater HC. Sebaceous carcinoma of the eyelid. J Am Acad Dermatol. 1980;3:241–3.
12. Pelachyk JM, Mikhail GR. In: Mikhail G, editor. Mohs micrographic surgery. Philadelphia: WB Saunders; 1991. p. 119–20.
13. Harvey JT, Anderson RL. The management of meibomian gland carcinoma. Ophthalmic Surg. 1982;13:56–61.
14. Dzubow LM. Sebaceous carcinoma of the eyelid: treatment with Mohs surgery. J Dermatol Surg Oncol. 1985;11:40–4.
15. Folberg R, Whitaker DC, Tse DT, Nerad JA. Recurrent and residual sebaceous carcinoma after Mohs' excision of the primary lesion. Am J Ophthalmol. 1987;103:817–23.
16. Ratz JL, Luu-Duong S, Kulwin DR. Sebaceous carcinoma of the eyelid treated with Mohs' surgery. J Am Acad Dermatol. 1986;14:668–73.
17. Yount AB, Bylund D, Pratt SG, Greenway HT. Mohs micrographic excision of sebaceous carcinoma of the eyelids. J Dermatol Surg Oncol. 1994;20:523–9.
18. Sawyer AR, McGoldrick RB, Mackey S, Powell B, Pohl M. Should extraocular sebaceous carcinoma be investigated using sentinel node biopsy? Dermatol Surg. 2009;35:704–8.
19. Shields JA, Demirci H, Marr BP, Eagle Jr RC, Shields CL. Sebaceous carcinoma of the ocular region: a review. Surv Ophthalmol. 2005;50:103–22.
20. Deprez M, Uffer S. Clinicopathological features of eyelid skin tumors. A retrospective study of 5504 cases and review of literature. Am J Dermatopathol. 2009;31:256–62.
21. Kivela T, Asko-Seljavaara S, Pihkala U, Hovi L, Heikkonen J. Sebaceous carcinoma of the eyelid associated with retinoblastoma. Ophthalmology. 2001;108:1124–8.
22. Rumelt S, Hogan NR, Rubin PA, Jakobiec FA. Four-eyelid sebaceous cell carcinoma following irradiation. Arch Ophthalmol. 1998;116:1670–2.
23. Saito A, Tsutsumida A, Furukawa H, Saito N, Yamamoto Y. Sebaceous carcinoma of the eyelids: a review of 21 cases. J Plast Reconstr Aesthet Surg. 2008;61:1328–31.
24. Rishi K, Font RL. Sebaceous gland tumors of the eyelids and conjunctiva in the Muir-Torre syndrome: a clinicopathologic study of five cases and literature review. Ophthal Plast Reconstr Surg. 2004;20:31–6.
25. Cohen PR, Kohn SR, Kurzrock R. Association of sebaceous gland tumors and internal malignancy: the Muir-Torre syndrome. Am J Med. 1991;90:606–13.
26. Hayashi N, Furihata M, Ohtsuki Y, Ueno H. Search for accumulation of p53 protein and detection of human papillomavirus genomes in sebaceous gland carcinoma of the eyelid. Virchows Arch. 1994;424:503–9.
27. Matsuda K, Doi T, Kosaka H, et al. Sebaceous carcinoma arising in nevus sebaceus. J Dermatol. 2005;32:641–4.
28. Kazakov DV, Calonje E, Zelger B, et al. Sebaceous carcinoma arising in nevus sebaceus of Jadassohn: a clinicopathological study of five cases. Am J Dermatopathol. 2007;29:242–8.
29. Lai TF, Huilgol SC, Selva D, James CL. Eyelid sebaceous carcinoma masquerading as in situ squamous cell carcinoma. Dermatol Surg. 2004;30:222–5.
30. Buitrago W, Joseph AK. Sebaceous carcinoma: the great masquerader: emerging concepts in diagnosis and treatment. Dermatol Ther. 2008;21:459–66.
31. Snow SN, Larson PO, Lucarelli MJ, Lemke BN, Madjar DD. Sebaceous carcinoma of the eyelids treated by Mohs micrographic surgery: report of nine cases with review of the literature. Dermatol Surg. 2002;28:623–31.
32. Song A, Carter KD, Syed NA, Song J, Nerad JA. Sebaceous cell carcinoma of the ocular adnexa: clinical presentations, histopathology, and outcomes. Ophthal Plast Reconstr Surg. 2008;24:194–200.
33. Leibovitch I, Selva D, Huilgol S, et al. Intraepithelial sebaceous carcinoma of the eyelid misdiagnosed as Bowen's disease. J Cutan Pathol. 2006;33:303–8.
34. Pereira PR, Odashiro AN, Rodrigues-Reyes AA, et al. Histopathological review of sebaceous carcinoma of the eyelid. J Cutan Pathol. 2005;32:496–501.
35. Misago N, Suse T, Uemura T, Narisawa Y. Basal cell carcinoma with sebaceous differentiation. Am J Dermatopathol. 2004;26:298–303.
36. Borczuk AC, Sha KK, Hisler SE, Mann JM, Hajdu SI. Sebaceous carcinoma of the lung: histologic and immunohistochemical characterization of an unusual pulmonary neoplasm: report of a case and review of the literature. Am J Surg Pathol. 2002;26:795–8.
37. Thosani MK, Marghoob A, Chen CS. Current progress of immunostains in Mohs micrographic surgery: a review. Dermatol Surg. 2008;34:1621–36.
38. Mohs FE, Blanchard L. Microscopically controlled surgery for extramammary Paget's disease. Arch Dermatol. 1979;115:706–8.
39. Doxanas MT, Green WR. Sebaceous gland carcinoma. Review of 40 cases. Arch Ophthalmol. 1984;102:245–9.
40. Wolfe 3rd JT, Yeatts RP, Wick MR, Campbell RJ, Waller RR. Sebaceous carcinoma of the eyelid. Errors in clinical and pathologic diagnosis. Am J Surg Pathol. 1984;8:597–606.
41. Arora A, Barlow RJ, Williamson JM, Olver JM. Eyelid sebaceous gland carcinoma (SGC) treated with 'slow' Mohs' micrographic surgery. Eye (Lond). 2004;18:854–5.
42. Callahan EF, Appert DL, Roenigk RK, Bartley GB. Sebaceous carcinoma of the eyelid: a review of 14 cases. Dermatol Surg. 2004;30:1164–8.
43. Thomas CJ, Wood GC, Marks VJ. Mohs micrographic surgery in the treatment of rare aggressive cutaneous tumors: the Geisinger experience. Dermatol Surg. 2007;33:333–9.
44. Hwang FS, Neekhra A, Lucarelli MJ, et al. Sebaceous cell carcinoma of the eyelid: a rapidly enlarging lesion with massive xanthogranulomatous inflammation. Ophthal Plast Reconstr Surg. 2010;26:208–10.
45. Shields JA, Demirci H, Marr BP, Eagle Jr RC, Shields CL. Sebaceous carcinoma of the eyelids: personal experience with 60 cases. Ophthalmology. 2004;111:2151–7.
46. Yen MT, Tse DT, Wu X, Wolfson AH. Radiation therapy for local control of eyelid sebaceous cell carcinoma: report of two cases and review of the literature. Ophthal Plast Reconstr Surg. 2000;16:211–5.
47. Russell HC, Chadha V, Lockington D, Kemp EG. Topical mitomycin C chemotherapy in the management of ocular surface neoplasia: a 10-year review of treatment outcomes and complications. Br J Ophthalmol. 2010;94:1316–21.

48. Putterman AM. Conjunctival map biopsy to determine pagetoid spread. Am J Ophthalmol. 1986;102:87–90.
49. Koreen IV, Flint A, Nelson CC, Frueh BR, Elner VM. Nondiagnostic conjunctival map biopsies for sebaceous carcinoma. Arch Ophthalmol. 2009;127:961–3.
50. O'Neal ML, Brunson A, Spadafora J. Ocular sebaceous carcinoma: case report and review of the literature. Compr Ther. 2001;27:144–7.
51. Tan KC, Lee ST, Cheah ST. Surgical treatment of sebaceous carcinoma of eyelids with clinico-pathological correlation. Br J Plast Surg. 1991;44:117–21.
52. Sinard JH. Immunohistochemical distinction of ocular sebaceous carcinoma from basal cell and squamous cell carcinoma. Arch Ophthalmol. 1999;117:776–83.
53. Dogru M, Matsuo H, Inoue M, Okubo K, Yamamoto M. Management of eyelid sebaceous carcinomas. Ophthalmologica. 1997;211:40–3.
54. Ilyas H, Kim N, Yavel RM, Lucarelli MJ, Rose JG, Snow SN. Abstract: sebaceous carcinoma of the eyelids treated with Mohs micrographic surgery. Mohs College 40th annual meeting. Canada: Vancouver; 2008.
55. Zurcher M, Hintschich CR, Garner A, Bunce C, Collin JR. Sebaceous carcinoma of the eyelid: a clinicopathological study. Br J Ophthalmol. 1998;82:1049–55.
56. Spencer JM, Nossa R, Tse DT, Sequeira M. Sebaceous carcinoma of the eyelid treated with Mohs micrographic surgery. J Am Acad Dermatol. 2001;44:1004–9.
57. Coldiron B, Smoller BR. Neoplasms of the pilosebaceous unit. In: LeBoit PE, Arndt KA, Robinson JK, Wintroub BU, editors. Cutaneous medicine and surgery. Philadelphia: WB Saunders; 1996. p. 1464–75.
58. Ho VH, Ross MI, Prieto VG, et al. Sentinel lymph node biopsy for sebaceous cell carcinoma and melanoma of the ocular adnexa. Arch Otolaryngol Head Neck Surg. 2007;133:820–6.
59. Snow SN, Longley J, Stewart D, Fish F. Atlas of Mohs Surgery Frozen Sections 2010.

Mohs Micrographic Surgery for the Eyelid

27

Michael P. McLeod, Marilyn Zabielinski
Sonal Choudhary, and Keyvan Nouri

Abstract

The eyelid protects the eye from environmental insults and assists in keeping the cornea moist. At only 0.6 mm thick, the periorbital skin is one of the thinnest cutaneous surfaces of the body. Mohs micrographic surgery (MMS) offers advantages over other resection techniques for this area because it attempts to conserve tissue and preserve function. A thorough understanding of the anatomy of this area is paramount to avoid permanently damaging vital structures. The patient's eye must be protected at all times.

Basal cell carcinoma (BCC) is the most common malignancy in the periorbital region and accounts for 90–95% of all periorbital malignancies. Although BCCs are not likely to metastasize, they can locally grow to destroy the eye, orbit, nose, and sinuses. A number of histologic subtypes of periorbital BCCs are associated with a higher likelihood of recurrence including: multicentric, desmoplastic, basosquamous, keratotic, morpheaform, and micronodular. Dr. Mohs published the largest series using Mohs micrographic surgery (MMS) to treat periorbital BCC, and out of 1,124 cases of primary BCC and 290 recurrent BCCs, the 5-year cure rates were 99.4% and 92.4%, respectively!

The second most common periorbital malignancy is squamous cell carcinoma (SCC), accounting for approximately 5–10% of all periorbital malignancies. Similar to BCC, SCC presents more commonly on the lower eyelid but not to the same extent as BCC. Unlike periorbital BCC, the metastatic rates of periorbital SCC have been reported to be as high as 21%. Unfortunately, SCC of the eyelid is much more likely to recur and metastasize when compared to other anatomical locations.

M.P. McLeod • S. Choudhary
Department of Dermatology and Cutaneous Surgery,
University of Miami Leonard M. Miller School of Medicine,
Miami, FL, USA

M. Zabielinski
University of Miami, Miami,
FL, USA

K. Nouri (✉)
Department of Dermatology and Cutaneous Surgery,
University of Miami Leonard M. Miller School of Medicine,
Miami, FL, USA

Sylvester Comprehensive Cancer Center, University of Miami
Hospital and Clinics, Miami, FL, USA
e-mail: knouri@med.miami.edu

K. Nouri (ed.), *Mohs Micrographic Surgery*,
DOI 10.1007/978-1-4471-2152-7_27,

Keywords

Mohs micrographic surgery • Eyelid • Periorbital • Basal cell carcinoma • Squamous cell carcinoma • Melanoma • Merkel cell carcinoma • Microcystic adnexal carcinoma • Sebaceous carcinoma

Summary: Introduction

- The eyelids protect the eye from environmental insults and assist in keeping the cornea moist.
- Small growths in the tumor size can significantly derange tissue planes.
- A thorough understanding of the anatomy of this area is paramount to avoid permanently damaging vital structures.

27.1 Introduction

The eyelid protect the eyes from environmental insults and assist in keeping the cornea moist. The tissue surrounding the eyelid is very thin, and consequently, small tumors can significantly derange tissue planes. To complicate matters, wide resections can have serious implications to the eye's function. A thorough understanding of the anatomy of this area is paramount to avoid permanently damaging vital structures. Mohs micrographic surgery (MMS) is one technique used to remove tumors from this area. It offers advantages over other resection techniques in this area because it attempts to conserve tissue, and hence preserve function. It was originally for skin cancers in the periorbital region that the fresh frozen tissue technique detailed in Chap. 8 of this text became popular.

Summary: Review of the Relevant Anatomy

- The periorbital skin is one of the thinnest cutaneous surfaces of the body.
- The main function of the eyelid is to protect the eye from both desiccation and foreign matter.
- The orbital septum acts as a cover over the orbital contents and prevents the spread of cancer into these structures.
- The eyelid consists of two lamellae: the anterior lamella consists of skin and orbicularis oculi muscle, and the posterior lamella consists of the tarsi and conjunctiva.

27.2 Review of the Relevant Anatomy

At only 0.6 mm thick, the periorbital skin is one of the thinnest cutaneous surfaces of the body. The eyelids lack subcutaneous fat and the subcutaneous fascia is thinner than that found in the neck, thorax, and abdomen. The main function of the eyelid is to protect the eye from both desiccation and foreign matter. The eyelids assist in distributing lacrimal fluid across the eye's surface to the medial canthus where it is collected into the nasolacrimal sac, then into the nasolacrimal duct, and finally into the nasal cavity. Each orbit is framed by the circular orbicularis oculi muscle. The eyelid, from superficial to deep, consists of the cutaneous surface, orbicularis oculi muscle, ciliary glands, palpebrae muscles, tarsal muscles and glands, and the palpebral conjunctiva. The orbital septum is a slender, fibrous, multilayered membrane that is considered the anterior orbital boundary and lies between the orbital rim and the tarsus, therefore serving as a barrier between the orbit and the lid. The septum thickens as it inserts onto the orbital rim. This thickening is referred to as the arcus marginalis. It inserts at about 3–5 mm above the tarsal plate. The orbital septum fuses with the capsulopalpebral fascia approximately 5 mm below the tarsus, and this common fascia inserts into the inferior tarsal angle in the lower eyelid. The orbital septum is found approximately at the same level as the tarsal muscles. It covers the orbital contents and acts as a barrier to prevent the spread of skin cancer into these strucutres. Fortunately, skin cancers tend to proliferate over it, rather than through it. From a surgical perspective, the eyelid consists of two lamellae. The anterior lamella consists of skin and orbicularis oculi muscle, while the posterior lamella is comprised of the tarsi and conjunctiva [1].

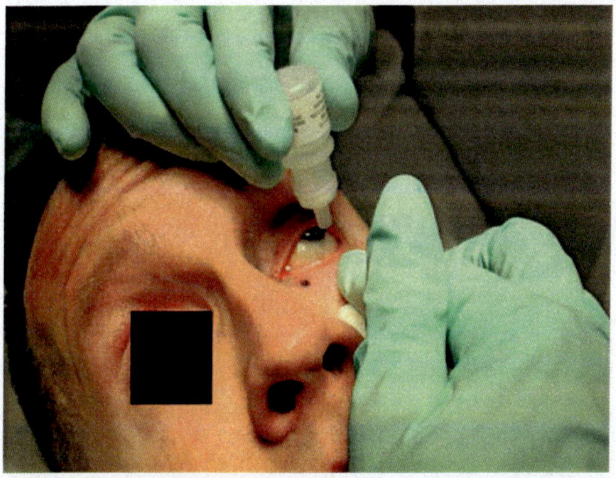

Fig. 27.1 Application of lubricating eye drops prior to eye guard insertion

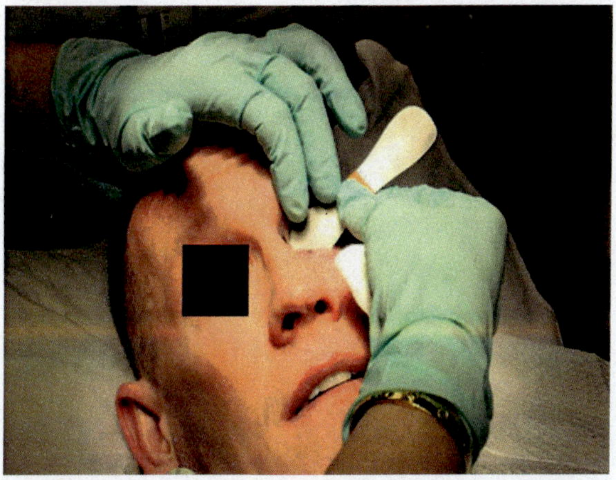

Fig. 27.2 Insertion of an eye shield used to protect the eye from unintentional injury

Summary: Anatomical Considerations When Using Mohs Micrographic Surgery in the Periorbital Region

- The medial canthal area contains the draining system of the lacrimal apparatus and is a highly vascularized area; therefore, a cutaneous tumor has the ability to proliferate deeply in this area and cause significant impairment of the eye function.
- The patient's eye must be protected at all times.
- Anesthetic eye drops are used along with eye shields whenever operating close to the eyeball itself.
- Due to the complex nature of surgery in the periorbital region, an oculoplastic reconstructive surgeon may be required to appropriately repair a Mohs defect.

27.3 Anatomical Considerations When Using Mohs Micrographic Surgery in the Periorbital Region

The medial canthal area is considered an embryonic fusion plane. Therefore, skin cancers have a propensity to proliferate deeply along that plane. The eye utilizes a specialized tearing system, which is located in the medial canthal area. Tearing fluid is produced in the lacrimal gland, which is located in the anterior upper temporal segment of the orbit and the superior conjunctival fornix. The tearing fluid is collected in the inferior medial puncta. From the puncta, the tearing fluid travels through the vertical canaliculi, then through the horizontal canaliculi to the common canaliculi and into to the lacrimal sac. From there, the fluid goes into the nasolacrimal duct and drains into the nose underneath the inferior turbinate. An invasive skin cancer can penetrate into these richly vascularized areas and damage tearing functions of the eyes.

Due to the complex nature of Mohs surgery of the eye, often times, an oculoplastic reconstructive surgeon is required to appropriately repair a Mohs defect. The patient's eye must be protected at all times. Anesthetic eye drops are used along with eye shields whenever operating close to the eyeball itself. A chalazion eyelid clamp may be useful to assist in electrocautery. Besides removing the tumor, the goals of eye surgery include maintaining visual acuity, tear flow, sufficient orbital lubrication, and minimizing corneal exposure [2, 3].

When performing Mohs surgery on the eyelid, it is important to use an eye guard to protect the eye itself. Additionally, care must be taken when using electrocautery so as not to transmit electricity through the eye guard. Lubricating eye drops should be used to protect the eye from injury secondary to the eye guard. (See Fig. 27.1). The eye guard should not be moved quickly when in place so that the conjunctiva and /or cornea is not injured. (See Fig. 27.2)

Summary: Periorbital BCC

- Basal cell carcinoma is the most common malignancy in the periorbital region and accounts for 90–95% of all periorbital malignancies.
- Although BCC is not likely to metastasize, it can locally grow large enough to destroy the eye, orbit, nose, and sinuses.
- The lower eyelid is the most common periorbital location for skin cancer.
- Dr. Mohs published the largest series using MMS to treat periorbital BCC: out of 1,124 cases of primary BCCs and 290 recurrent BCCs, 5-year cure rates were 99.4% and 92.4%, respectively.
- The other standard approach to removing periorbital BCC is conventional frozen section excision.
- Glatt and colleagues demonstrated a 99.2% clearance rate for periorbital BCC treated by conventional frozen excision with 3–4 mm margins taken during each stage involving 236 cases and a 5-year cure rate of 97.5%.

27.4 Periorbital BCC

Basal cell carcinoma (BCC) is the most common malignancy in the periorbital region, accounting for 90–95% of all skin cancers in this region [4–6]. Periorbital BCC most commonly presents in patients during their sixth to eighth decades of life [7, 8]. Only 15% of periorbital BCC occurs in children or young adults. Although BCCs are not likely to metastasize, they can locally grow large enough to destroy the eye, orbit, nose, and sinuses [9].

The lower eyelid is the most common periorbital location for skin cancer [1, 10–13], with the medial canthus being the second most common location [11, 13]. It is hypothesized that the lower eyelid is the most common periorbital location for skin cancer because this area is exposed to a higher amount of ultraviolet radiation compared to other periorbital locations [11, 13].

Even after removing a BCC through Mohs surgery or conventional frozen excision, it can still recur. A number of BCC tumor characteristics are associated with recurrence including size >2 cm, prior recurrent tumors, medial or upper eyelid location involvement, a history of radiation to the lesion, involvement of multiple eyelid segments, immunosuppression, ill-defined clinical borders, tarsal invasion, and invasion into the orbit, nose, or sinuses [5, 8, 14–18]. A number of histologic subtypes and tumor characteristics of periorbital BCCs are associated with a higher likelihood of recurrence including desmoplastic, basosquamous, keratotic, morpheaform, micronodular, multicentric tumors, and poorly differentiated tumors, as well as those with perineural invasion [3, 14, 15, 18, 19].

Dr. Mohs published the largest series using Mohs micrographic surgery (MMS) to treat periorbital BCC. Out of 1,124 cases of primary BCC and 290 recurrent BCCs, 5-year cure rates were 99.4% and 92.4%, respectively [11]. Periorbital BCCs less than 3 cm have 5-year cure rates of 97.5–100%, while BCCs greater than 3 cm have 5-year cure rates of 80% [11]. Dr. Mohs reported that lower eyelid BCCs have a 98.6% cure rate. Upper eyelid lesions clear 98.5% of the time, while medial canthus BCCs clear in 97.2% of cases, and lateral canthus BCCs are cleared 91% of the time. Remarkably, eyebrow lesions cleared 100% of the time [11].

Robins and colleagues used MMS on 631 cases of periocular BCC and reported a 98.1% success rate for primary lesions and a 93.6% for recurrent lesions [20]. Callahan and colleagues used MMS on 109 cases of periocular BCC and reported a 100% success rate. Drs. Monheit and Callahan demonstrated similar results as Drs. Mohs and Robins. Their study involved 283 cases of periorbital BCC tumors from a total of 315 periorbital cutaneous tumors treated by MMS. They reported that the 5-year cure rate was above 98% for all of the tumors combined [21]. Unfortunately, there was one fatality in their series from a metastatic BCC. In 2004, the Australian MMS database (the largest prospective database), part 1, looked at high-risk periocular BCC in 1,295 patients that were managed by MMS [22]. The most common reason for referral for MMS was the fact that the tumor was located in a periocular area (55%) [22]. Twenty-four percent of the patients were referred because of recurrence, which was the second most common reason for referral [22]. The most common site for periocular BCC was the medial canthus or lower eyelid [22]. Those on the lower eyelid were more common in males, and those on the medial canthus more common in females [22].

Patients with lower eyelid BCC were older than those with medial canthus BCC (the mean difference was 4.7 years) [22]. The most common histologic subtypes were nodulocystic and infiltrating (34.8%). The majority of the lower lid tumors were infiltrating BCCs, and the majority of the upper lid and medial canthus tumors were nodulocystic BCCs [22]. Infiltrating BCCs were significantly larger than nodulocystic or superficial subtypes, and as a consequence, had larger defect sizes [22]. Twelve cases (1%) had histologically confirmed perineural invasion [22]. Seven of these were medial canthal and five were lower eyelid BCCs [22]. Interestingly, there was no association between tumor size and site. In this study, 32% of the periocular tumors were recurrent, and of these, the superficial BCCs were more likely to be recurrent [22]. Compared to the primary BCCs, these recurrent tumors were larger in size and resulted in larger defects as well [22]. Out of the 415 recurrent BCCs, only 15/415 cases had recurred after primary MMS, of which 7/15 had undergone MMS only. There was no association between the site of the tumor and the number of levels required for complete excision, although morphea BCCs and recurrent cases required more levels, as did recurrent cases [22]. The Mohs surgeon managed 915/1,295 cases. Out of the remaining 380 cases referred for repair, 314 were managed by an oculoplastic surgeon and 63 by a plastic surgeon. It was noted that after 1996, there was an increase in the referrals to oculoplastic surgeons instead of plastic surgeons [22].

The Mohs Australian database, part 2, included a 5-year follow-up of 819 patients treated by MMS for periocular BCC [23]. Forty-two percent had a 5-year follow-up, and out of these, 2% had recurrences [23]. All of these 7/346 patients with recurrences had been previously recurrent, with up to three recurrences before MMS had been performed. As noted above, prior recurrence was the main predictor of recurrence following MMS, as were infiltrating and superficial histologic subtypes [23].

The other standard approach to removing periorbital BCC is by conventional frozen section excision. Glatt and colleagues demonstrated a 99.2% clearance rate for 236 cases involving periorbital BCC treated by conventional frozen excision with 3–4 mm margins taken during each stage [24]. Out of the 236 patients, 81 were followed for 5 years, and the 5-year cure rate was 97.5% [24]. Older and colleagues reported a 100% success rate with conventional frozen section control in 113 cases [25].

Nemet et al. investigated 485 cases of periocular BCC and SCC [26]. BCCs were surgically excised with 3 mm, and SCCs with a 5 mm margin. Frozen section or MMS were used for incompletely excised cases and those located in the medical canthus or close to the lacrimal drainage system [26]. Excision was incomplete in 54.4% of the cases, and 84.6% chose to have reexcision guided by either frozen section or MMS and 10.6% chose radiation therapy [26]. Patients with morpheaform-type BCC had a significantly higher rate of incomplete excision compared with nodular-type BCC (43.6–23.5%, respectively) [26]. The rate of incomplete excision was also significantly higher at the medial canthal region compared with other tumor locations [26]. Notably, there were no recurrences in any of the 19 cases in which MMS technique was used for reexcision compared to 4.7% recurrences in which frozen section was used [26]. The average time to recurrence was reported to be 32 ± 17 months [26].

Summary: Periorbital SCC

- The second most common periorbital malignancy is squamous cell carcinoma, accounting for approximately 5–10% of all periorbital malignancies.
- Similar to BCC, SCC also presents more commonly on the lower eyelid but not to the same extent as BCC.
- Periorbital SCC metastatic rates have been reported to be as high as 21%.
- Factors which are associated with a higher rate of periorbital SCC metastasis include: perineural invasion, recurrence following treatment, large tumor size, and poor differentiation.
- Dr. Mohs used MMS for 213 cases of periorbital SCC and reported an overall 98.1% 5-year cure rate. Primary periorbital SCCs had a 98.5% cure rate versus 95.8% for recurrent SCCs.
- Using conventional surgical excision, the recurrence rate is approximately 18% for periorbital SCC.

27.5 Periorbital SCC

The second most common periorbital malignancy is squamous cell carcinoma [4]. SCC accounts for approximately 5–10% of all periorbital malignancies and has an incidence of 0.09–2.42 per 100,000 [5, 6, 27, 28]. The mean age of presentation is during the seventh decade of life [29]. Similar to BCC, SCC also presents more commonly on the lower eyelid but not to the same degree as BCC [30]. SCC has the following periorbital distribution: lower eyelid (48.6–68%), medial canthus (30–36%), upper eyelid (22.5%), and lateral canthus (16.2%) [31, 32]. SCC of the eyelid is much more likely to recur and metastasize when compared to other anatomical locations. Periorbital SCC metastatic rates have been reported to be as high as 21% [28]. Factors which are associated with a higher rate of periorbital SCC metastasis include: perineural invasion, recurrence following treatment, large tumor size, and poor differentiation [30].

Dr. Mohs used MMS for 213 cases of periorbital SCC and reported an overall 98.1% 5-year cure rate. Primary periorbital SCCs had a 98.5% cure rate versus 95.8% for recurrent SCCs [11].

Another large multicenter trial demonstrated that MMS had the lowest recurrence rate at 3.6% when compared to other modalities of treatment [32]. For periorbital SCC in situ, the overall recurrence rate was 8.3%, with a primary SCC in situ recurrence rate of 5% and a recurrent SCC in situ recurrence rate of 12% [32]. Using conventional surgical excision, the recurrence rate is approximately 18% for periorbital SCC [4, 33].

Moul and colleagues feel that "MMS should be a consideration especially for large or poorly delineated tumors, recurrent tumors, those with perineural involvement or moderately to poorly differentiated subtypes, and those close to important anatomic structures." [4]

Another important clinical point to keep in mind when dealing with SCC is that demonstrated by a study conducted by Doxanas and colleagues who demonstrated the importance of accurate histopathologic diagnosis of SCC of the eyelid [34]. Forty-four tumors were originally diagnosed as squamous cell carcinoma, but in fact, only 31 of the tumors were squamous cell carcinomas of the eyelid, 75% occurring in patients over the age of 60 [34]. The incorrect initial pathologic diagnosis was most commonly sebaceous gland carcinoma, followed by basal cell carcinoma [34]. Others were incorrectly diagnosed as seborrheic keratosis, inverted follicular keratosis, and papilloma [34]. This study also demonstrated the risk factors associated a likelihood of developing SCC, as three of the patients had a history of prolonged exposure to radiation therapy for acne, eczema, and SCC of the limbus 10–20 years prior to their diagnosis [34]. Squamous cell carcinoma presented in some patients as a lesion with rolled up margins and a central crater with or without intermittent bleeding, and in other patients as a chronic, scaly erythematous lesion. Three patients reported chalazion as their presenting symptom [34]. This study conveys the importance of performing biopsies on lesions that appear suspicious or as persistent benign lesions do not heal, especially because SCC has a higher metastatic potential.

Summary: Other Tumors

- It can be difficult to distinguish the surgical borders of melanoma on frozen sections, especially in the setting of chronic sun damage.
- Lentigo maligna is the most common type of melanoma to present in the periocular region.
- Frozen sections of melanoma are subject to artifact.
- Sebaceous carcinoma is most commonly located on the upper eyelid, and approximately 8% of these tumors metastasize.
- Spencer and colleagues have reported the largest series involving periorbital sebaceous carcinoma with 18 cases, of which 13 were primary and 5 recurrent. Two out of the 18 cases recurred over an average follow-up time of 37 months.
- Most cases of reported periorbital microcystic adnexal carcinoma have been located on the lower eyelid, and MMS or conventional frozen section excisions have become the standard of care.
- In general, Merkel cell carcinoma is associated with a very poor prognosis, and the current National Comprehensive Cancer Network guidelines recommend wide local excision with 2 cm or greater margins, MMS with permanent section technique, or MMS with frozen sections, along with appropriate lymph node biopsy and adjuvant radiation therapy.

27.6 Other Tumors

Recently, there has been much investigation into the use of MMS for melanoma; however, very few of the studies specifically examined its use for periorbital melanoma [4]. Lentigo maligna is the most common type of melanoma to present in the periocular region, likely due to chronic sun exposure [4]. In general, melanoma presents some difficulties for MMS in that it can be problematic to accurately distinguish surgical borders when using frozen sections, especially in the setting of chronic sun damage. Frozen sections of melanoma are subject to artifact, making it nearly impossible in some instances to determine the surgical borders of the tumor. Modifications of MMS, such as rush permanent sections and immunostains attempt to minimize those artifacts or "highlight" the melanoma cells. Using a variation of MMS known as Mapped Serial Excision, Malhotra and colleagues demonstrated a recurrence rate of 7.4% with a mean follow-up time of 32 months for periorbital lentigo maligna and lentigo maligna melanoma [35]. For a deeper discussion of MMS for melanoma please refer to Chap. 17 and for a discussion of immunostaining melanoma cells in the setting of MMS, please refer to Chap. 13.

More studies should be carried out to examine the efficacy of MMS for melanomas located in the periorbital region. Lentigo maligna is a slowly growing lesion, and therefore the follow-up times for studies should be in excess of 5 years.

Sebaceous carcinoma is most commonly located on the upper eyelid [12]. It can resemble a chalazion or even blepharitis; however, care should be taken not mistake it for these benign conditions, as the metastatic rate is about 8% [4, 36]. Spencer and colleagues have reported the largest series involving periorbital sebaceous carcinoma with 18 cases, of which 13 were primary and five recurrent [37]. Two of the 18 cases recurred over an average follow-up time of 37 months. Snow and colleagues reviewed the literature and determined that out of 49 reported cases of sebaceous carcinoma, 12% recurred over a 3.1 mean follow-up period [36]. Sebaceous carcinoma is known to have "skip" areas and some experts have suggested using oil red O, CAM 5.2, or permanent sections to more clearly define the surgical tumor margins [38–40]. For an in depth discussion of Mohs micrographic surgery for sebaceous carcinoma, please refer to Chap. 2.

Another uncommon tumor encountered in the periorbital region is microcystic adnexal carcinoma (MAC). Of the 15 cases found in the literature of periorbital MAC, ten were on the lower eyelid and five on the medial canthus [41–43]. For periorbital MAC, MMS or conventional frozen section excision has become the standard of care [4]. For a discussion of MAC in general, please refer to Chap. 19.

On rare occasions, Merkel cell carcinoma (MCC) can present in the periorbital region. The current National Comprehensive Cancer Network guidelines recommend wide local excision with two centimeter or greater margins or MMS with permanent or frozen sections [4]. The prognosis for MCC is very poor, with only a 30–64% 5-year survival rate [44, 45].

Summary: Conclusion

- Both BCC and SCC account for almost all of the periocular cutaneous tumors.
- It is important to consider Mohs surgery as a treatment option for periocular BCC and SCC to excise completely with conservation of the delicate tissue.

27.7 Conclusion

In conclusion, both basal cell and squamous cell carcinoma account for almost all of the periocular cutaneous tumors. Periocular BCC and SCC have very high 5-year cure rates when using both MMS and the conventional frozen section technique. However, it appears that MMS tends to have a slightly higher 5-year cure rate, which is important to take into consideration because of the location of these tumors. Periocular tumors are located in an area such that a diagnosis needs to be make quickly and precisely so that the tumor can be excised quickly and completely to prevent recurrence which can cause significant damage to such a delicate tissue as the eye.

References

1. Monheit GD, Callahan MA, Callahan A. Mohs micrographic surgery for periorbital skin cancer. Dermatol Clin. 1989;7(4):677–97.
2. Poulsen M, Burmeister B, Kennedy D. Preservation of form and function in the management of head and neck skin cancer. World J Surg. 2003;27:868–74.
3. Margo CE, Waltz K. Basal cell carcinoma of the eyelid and periocular skin. Surv Ophthalmol. 1993;38:169–92.

4. Moul DK, Chern PL, Shumaker PR, Zelac DE, Greenway HT. Mohs micrographic surgery for eyelid and periorbital skin cancer. Int Ophthalmol Clin. 2009;49(4):111–27.
5. Francis IC, Benecke PS, Kappagoda MB. A ten-year hospital survey of eyelid cancer. Aust J Ophthalmol. 1984;12: 121–7.
6. Cook BE, Bartley GB. Epidemiologic characteristics and clinical course of patients with malignant eyelid tumors in an incidence cohort in Olmsted county, Minnesota. Ophthalmology. 1999;106:746–50.
7. Keramidas DC, Anagnostou D. Basal-cell carcinoma of the lower lid in a 27-month-old child. Z Kinderchir. 1987;42: 250–1.
8. Nerad JA, Whitaker DC. Periocular basal cell carcinoma in adults 35 years of age and younger. Am J Ophthalmol. 1988;106:723–9.
9. Shah HA, Lee HB, Nunery WR. Neglected basal cell carcinoma in a schizophrenic patient. Ophthal Plast Reconstr Surg. 2008;24:495–7.
10. Cook BE, Bartley GB. Treatment options and future prospects for the management of eyelid malignancies: an evidence-based update. Ophthalmology. 2001;108:2088–100.
11. Mohs FE. Micrographic surgery for the microscopically controlled excision of eyelid cancers. Arch Ophthalmol. 1986;104:901–9.
12. Swanson MW, Cloud G. A retrospective analysis of primary eye cancer at the University of Alabama 1958–1988 part 2: eyelid tumors. J Am Optom Assoc. 1991;62:820–3.
13. Wong VA, Marschall JA, Whitehead KJ, Williamson RM, Sullivan TJ. Management of periocular basal cell carcinoma with modified en face frozen section controlled excision. Ophthal Plast Reconstr Surg. 2002;18(6):430–5.
14. Older JJ, Grostern RJ. Eyelid tumors: clinical diagnosis and surgical treatment. New York: Thieme; 2003.
15. Weber RS, Miller MJ, Goepfert J. Basal and squamous cell skin cancers of the head and neck. Baltimore: Williams & Wilkins; 1996.
16. Cunneen TS, Yong JL, Benger R. Lung metastasis in a case of metatypical basal cell carcinoma of the eyelid: an illustrative case and literature review to heighten vigilance of its metastatic potential. Clin Experiment Ophthalmol. 2008;36:475–7.
17. Howard GR, Nerad JA, Carter KD, Whitaker DC. Clinical characteristics associated with orbital invasion of basal cell and squamous cell tumors of the eyelid. Am J Ophthalmol. 1992;113(2):123–33.
18. Leibovitch I, McNab A, Sullivan T, Davis G, Selva D. Orbital invasion by periocular basal cell carcinoma. Ophthalmology. 2005;112(4):717–23.
19. Spencer WH. Ophthalmic pathology: an atlas and textbook. Philadelphia: W.B. Saunders; 1986. p. 2169–78.
20. Robins P, Rodríguez-Sains R, Rabinovitz H, Rigel D. Mohs surgery for periocular basal cell carcinomas. J Dermatol Surg Oncol. 1985;11(12):1203–7.
21. Callahan MA, Monheit OD, Callahan A. Cancer excision from eyelids and ocular adnexa. The Mohs' fresh tissue technique and reconstruction. A 5-year study of 109 patients. Ala J Med Sci. 1983;20:289–94.
22. Malhotra R, Huilgol SC, Huynh NT, Selva D. The Australian Mohs database, part I: periocular basal cell carcinoma experience over 7 years. Ophthalmology. 2004;111(4):624–30.
23. Malhotra R, Huilgol SC, Huynh NT, Selva D. The Australian Mohs database, part II: periocular basal cell carcinoma outcome at 5-year follow-up. Ophthalmology. 2004;111(4):631–6.
24. Glatt HJ, Olson JJ, Putterman AM. Conventional frozen sections in periocular basal-cell carcinoma: a review of 236 cases. Ophthalmic Surg. 1992;23(1):6–8.
25. Older JJ, Quickert MH, Beard C. Surgical removal of basal cell carcinoma of the eyelids utilizing frozen section control. Trans Sect Ophthalmol Am Acad Ophthalmol Otolaryngol. 1975;79:658–63.
26. Nemet AY, Deckel Y, Martin PA, et al. Management of periocular and squamous cell carcinoma: a series of 485 cases. Am J Ophthalmol. 2006;142(2):293–7.
27. Shulman J. Treatment of malignant tumours of the eyelids: a clinicopathological study. Surv Ophthalmol. 1962;15:37–47.
28. Marks R, Rennie G, Selwood TS. Malignant transformation of solar keratoses to squamous cell carcinoma. Lancet. 1988;1:795–7.
29. Limawararut V, Leibovitch I, Sullivan T, Selva D. Periocular squamous cell carcinoma. Clin Experiment Ophthalmol. 2007;35(2):174–85.
30. Reifer DM, Hornblass A. Squamous cell carcinoma of the eyelid. Surv Ophthalmol. 1986;30:1930–2.
31. Faustina M, Diba R, Ahmadi MA, Esmaeli B. Patterns of regional and distant metastasis in patients with eyelid and periocular squamous cell carcinoma. Ophthalmology. 2004;111(10):1930–2.
32. Malhotra R, James CL, Selva D, Huynh N, Huilgo SC. The Australian Mohs database: periocular squamous intraepidermal carcinoma. Ophthalmology. 2004;111(10):1925–9.
33. Sullivan TJ, Boulton JE, Whitehead KJ. Intraepidermal carcinoma of the eyelid. Clin Experiment Ophthalmol. 2002;30:23–7.
34. Doxanas MT, Lliff WJ, Lliff NT, Green WR. Squamous cell carcinoma of the eyelids. Ophthalmology. 1987;94(5): 538–41.
35. Malhotra R, Chen C, Huilgol S, Hill DC, Selva D. Mapped serial excision for periocular lentigo maligna and lentigo maligna melanoma. Ophthalmology. 2003;110(10):2011–8.
36. Snow SN, Larson PO, Lucarelli MJ, Lemke BN, Madjar DD. Sebaceous carcinoma of the eyelids treated by Mohs micrographic surgery: report of nine cases with review of the literature. Dermatol Surg. 2002;28(7):623–31.
37. Spencer JM, Nossa R, Tse DT, Sequeira M. Sebaceous carcinoma of the eyelid treated with Mohs micrographic surgery. J Am Acad Dermatol. 2001;44(6):1004–9.
38. Ni C, Searl SS, Kuo PK, Chu FR, Chong CS, Albert DM. Sebaceous cell carcinomas of the ocular adnexa. Int Ophthalmol Clin. 1982;22(1):23–61.
39. Sinard JH. Immunohistochemical distinction of ocular sebaceous carcinoma from basal cell and squamous cell carcinoma. Arch Ophthalmol. 1999;117:776–83.
40. Yount AB, Bylund D, Pratt SG, Greenway HT. Mohs micrographic excision of sebaceous carcinoma of the eyelids. J Dermatol Surg Oncol. 1994;20(8):523–9.
41. Leibovitch I, Huilgol SC, Richards S, Paver R, Selva D. Periocular microcystic adnexal carcinoma: management and outcome with Mohs' micrographic surgery. Ophthalmologica. 2006;220(2):109–13.
42. Hoppenrejis VP, Reuser TT, Mooy CM, deKizer RJ, Mouritis MP. Syringomatous carcinoma of the eyelid and orbit: a

clinical and histopathological challenge. Br J Ophthalmol. 1997;81(8):668–72.
43. Duffy MT, Harrison W, Sassoon J, Hornblass A. Sclerosing sweat duct carcinoma of the eyelid margin: unusual presentation of a rare tumor. Ophthalmology. 1999;106(4):751–6.
44. Bichakjian CK, Lowe L, Lao CD, et al. Merkel cell carcinoma: critical review with guidelines for multidisciplinary management. Cancer. 2007;110(1):1–12.
45. Allen PJ, Bowne WB, Jaques DP, Brennan MF, Busam K, Coit DG. Merkel cell carcinoma: prognosis and treatment of patients from a single institution. J Clin Oncol. 2005; 23(10):2300–9.
46. Auw-Haedrich C, Frick S, Boehringer D, Mittelviefhaus H. Histologic safety margin in basal cell carcinoma of the eyelid: correlation with recurrence rate. Ophthalmology. 2009;116(4):802–6.

Mohs Surgery for Periungual and Subungual Skin Cancer

28

Steven Chow and Richard G. Bennett

Abstract

Mohs surgery for a malignancy in the periungual and subungual location is advantageous because it is a tissue-sparing technique that preserves maximum function and normal appearance. Traditional surgical treatment for such tumors is wide local excision and closure; in some cases, amputation of the digit is considered. The amount of tissue removed with these standard surgical treatments may be quite debilitating for the patient. Often, Mohs surgery will preserve a significant amount of nail matrix so that an almost normal-appearing nail regrows.

Keywords

Mohs surgery • Nails • Nail unit • Digit

Summary: Introduction

- Traditional surgical treatment for malignancy in the periungual and subungual is wide local excision.
- Mohs surgery is advantageous because it is a tissue sparing technique and preserves a significant amount of nail matrix.

S. Chow
Department of Dermatology, University of Southern California, Santa Monica, CA, USA

R.G. Bennett (✉)
Department of Dermatology, UCLA and USC, Santa Monica, CA, USA
e-mail: drrgb@ucla.edu

28.1 Introduction

Mohs surgery for a malignancy in the periungual and subungual location is advantageous because it is a tissue-sparing technique that preserves maximum function and normal appearance. Traditional surgical treatment for such tumors is wide local excision and closure; in some cases, amputation of the digit is considered. The amount of tissue removed with these standard surgical treatments may be quite debilitating for the patient. Often, Mohs surgery will preserve a significant amount of nail matrix so that an almost normal-appearing nail regrows.

K. Nouri (ed.), *Mohs Micrographic Surgery*,
DOI 10.1007/978-1-4471-2152-7_28, © Springer-Verlag London Limited 2012

Summary: Anatomy

- The nail unit can be divided into several components: nail matrix, nail plate, supporting structures (nail bed and phalangeal bone), nail folds, cuticle, and hyponychium.
- Main arteries and nerves run longitudinally along both sides of the digit and have dorsal and ventral branches.

28.2 Anatomy

Knowledge of nail unit anatomy is critical for management of tumors beside and underneath the nail. The nail unit and adjacent structures important for Mohs surgery will be summarized.

28.2.1 Nail Matrix

The nail matrix generates the nail plate and is the most proximal portion of the nail unit. The nail matrix connects to the ventral surface of the proximal nail fold, and a portion of the nail matrix can be seen by the clinician as the lunula. The nail matrix can be divided into proximal, intermediate, and distal components. The proximal matrix produces the superficial nail plate. The intermediate matrix produces the majority of the nail body. The distal matrix produces a portion of the nail bed epidermis. Laterally, the matrix continues proximally to form a "horn" on either side.

28.2.2 Nail Plate

The nail plate is formed by the nail matrix and is composed of a hard multilayered keratin sheet.

28.2.3 Supporting Portion: Nail Bed and Phalangeal Bone

The nail bed lies beneath the nail plate and begins from the distal edge of the nail matrix and continues to the hyponychium. The nail bed's pink color is due to its vascularity, and the space between the nail bed and the underlying phalanx is only a few millimeters thick, without any underlying subcutaneous tissue or fat [1, 2].

28.2.4 Nail Folds

The nail folds surround the nail plate on three sides, and consist of a proximal nail fold and two lateral nail folds. The proximal nail fold has a dorsal and ventral surface. The dorsal surface is seen as the skin along the nail unit's proximal border. The ventral surface of the proximal nail fold lies beneath the dorsal surface and becomes contiguous with the proximal nail matrix. The lateral nail folds frame the lateral edges of the nail plate.

28.2.5 Cuticle

The cuticle, also known as the eponychium, sheaths the most proximal nail plate. The cuticle seals the pocket between the dorsal proximal nail fold and the nail plate. By doing so, pathogens are prevented from entering this region.

28.2.6 Hyponychium

The hyponychium is the most distal component of the nail unit and is located under the free edge of the nail plate and seals the nail bed along the distal groove.

28.2.7 Arteries and Nerves of the Digit

The main digital nerves run longitudinally on both the radial and ulnar sides of the digit and have both dorsal and ventral branches. The main digital arteries (the volar and dorsal digital arteries) run adjacent to the nerves and provide contralateral circulation via their many anastomoses [3]. The volar digital arteries reach the pulp of the fingers and originate from the superficial palmer arch to provide the primary arterial supply of the digit. The dorsal digital arteries primarily supply the proximal region of the fingers and branch off the dorsal metacarpal artery of the dorsal carpal arch. The thumb has aberrant arterial connections resulting from a lack of a direct bilateral blood supply. Therefore, when operating in this region, caution is recommended [3].

28.2.8 Extensor Tendon

The extensor tendon attaches onto the dorsal proximal end of the distal phalanx just proximal to the nail matrix. This tendon thins out as it attaches onto the bone.

Summary: Tumors

- Nail unit tumors are rare entities, with Bowen's disease carcinomas, in our experience, being the most frequent tumor of the nail unit.
- Involvement of the bone by the tumor precludes Mohs surgery. When there is tumor invasion into the bone, the patient should be evaluated for management by a hand surgeon.
- For tumors of the nail unit without bone involvement, their removal by Mohs surgery is ideal. Mohs surgery removes affected tissue and allows for maximum normal tissue preservation.

28.3 Tumors

28.3.1 Squamous Cell Carcinoma

Among the nail unit malignancies in the upper and lower extremities, squamous cell carcinoma is the most frequently reported. A squamous cell carcinoma of the nail unit is considered a low-grade malignancy with a good prognosis. While this carcinoma rarely metastases [4], it can invade the distal phalanx. Extensive disease, which can be due to poor differentiation of the primary tumor or increased depth of tumor invasion, may require amputation and lymph node dissection [5].

Squamous cell carcinoma of the nail unit most commonly affects the thumb, which can result in significant hand disability if amputation of the affected digit is required. Polydactylous disease is commonly due to an environmental exposure, as the condition must develop independently in each digit [6, 7]. Some causes of squamous cell carcinoma of the digits include: solar radiation, arsenic, x-ray radiation, tar, or warts (particularly human papillomavirus 16 exposure) [6, 8, 9]. Besides surgery, treatment modalities for squamous cell carcinoma of the nail unit include: radiation [10, 11], photodynamic therapy [12], or the CO_2 laser [13].

Squamous cell carcinoma of the digit and nail unit often present as a nonspecific irritation and may be misdiagnosed as onychomycosis, paronychia, or eczema. Skin ulceration, onycholysis, and nail plate destruction may occur over time due to the delayed diagnosis. Keratoacanthomas of the nail bed or matrix are typically diagnosed early, as compression of this rapidly growing tumor between the nail plate and the bone causes great pain. A radiograph of the affected digit may be useful prior to Mohs surgery, as the radiograph can inform the surgeon whether there is tumor invasion into bone. Caution is warranted, however, as inflammation and infection create a radiologic image suggestive of tumor invasion when true tumor invasion is not present [8, 9, 14]. Additionally, some authors have noted periosteal tumor invasion despite a normal radiograph [8, 9]. De Berker et al. described the removal of a portion of the distal phalanx and decalcification of the bone for 48 h and then embedding the tissue in permanent paraffin blocks to rule out tumor invasion into the bone [9]. If definitive bone involvement has occurred, amputation of the affected digit by a hand surgeon along the metacarpal-phalangeal joint is recommended, or amputation at the interphalangeal joint proximal to bone invasion as seen by radiograph [2, 14]. For squamous cell carcinomas not involving the bone, Mohs surgery is a preferred treatment option and provides the highest cure rate along with the greatest amount of tissue preservation compared to other treatment modalities (see Fig. 28.1a–c).

28.3.2 Bowen's Disease

Due to its distinct histologic appearance, Bowen's disease is categorized separately from squamous cell carcinoma by some, but not all authors. Dysplastic changes consisting of cellular atypia, loss of epidermal polarity, and large bowenoid cells may be seen within the entire thickness of the epidermis. Sometimes these changes are more subtle and do not involve the entire epidermal thickness. However, Bowen's disease may also invade the dermis, and Mohs surgery can be quite useful in determining such invasion (see Fig. 28.2). Thus when using Mohs surgery to excise Bowen's disease carcinoma in this area, high slide quality is extremely important. As opposed to squamous cell carcinomas, keratin pearls are absent. It is also felt that the keratinizing variants of squamous cell carcinomas may be more aggressive than the bowenoid variants [6]. Bowen's disease generally presents as a scaly path of the nail folds (see Fig. 28.5c), but has also been reported to present as mel-

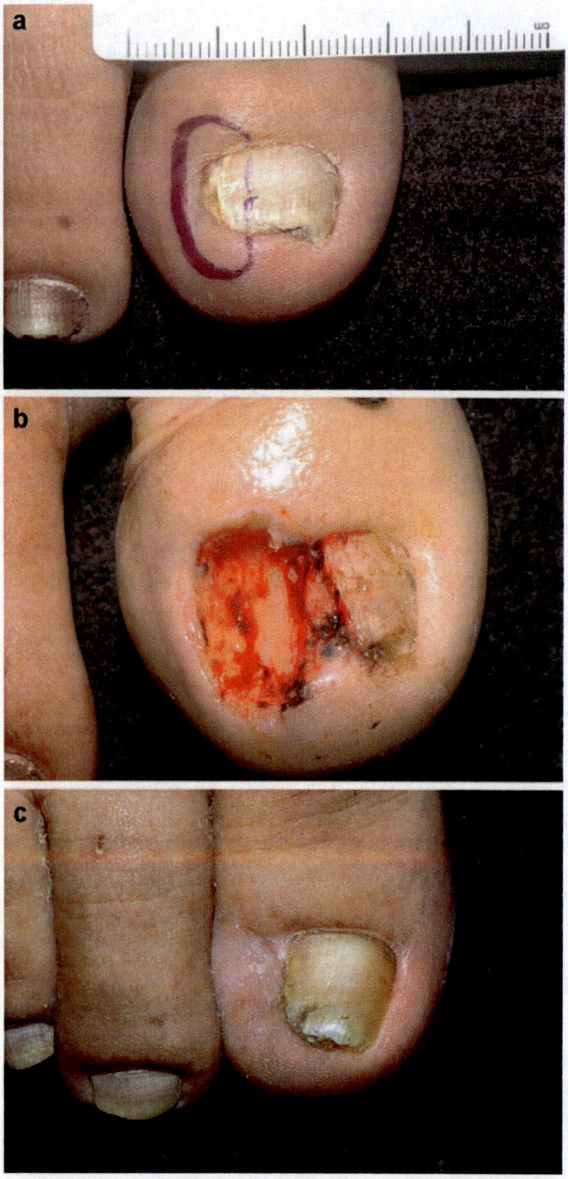

Fig. 28.1 (**a**) Squamous cell carcinoma along lateral nail fold of the right first toe. (**b**) Wound after final Mohs surgery stage. Note bone exposure in center of wound. (**c**) Healed result 1 year postoperatively

anonychia [15]. It has been treated by CO_2 laser vaporization by some investigators [13]. However, we feel Mohs surgery offers the patient the highest likelihood of cure, because as previously stated, these tumors can be quite subtle, histologically (see Fig. 28.3a–d). Unlike non-Bowen's squamous cell carcinoma, Bowen's disease carcinoma in the periungual location is frequently associated with oncogenic human papillomavirus.

28.3.3 Melanoma

Malignant melanoma of the subungual location is uncommon and accounts for 2–3% of all cutaneous melanomas in Caucasian populations and 20% in African and Asian populations [16–19]. Patient prognosis depends on early detection, and this is particularly true of subungual melanomas. Blessing evaluated 100 cases of subungual melanomas; the mean Breslow depth of the patients was 4.7 mm, and greater than 70% of the cases were staged Clark IV or V at onset [16]. Metastases to the epitrochlear and axillary nodes are common because of delayed diagnosis [20]. Due to the aggressiveness of this disease and its delayed diagnosis averaging 2 years after the initial presentation, the 5-year survival for a subungual melanoma is 50% or less [21]. Moehrle et al. evaluated 73 patients with subungual melanomas and found that at the time of diagnosis, 4.1% (3 patients) had in-transit metastasis and 11% (8 patients) had regional lymph node metastasis [22].

Subungual melanoma most commonly occurs between the sixth and seventh decades of life [19] and is often misdiagnosed as a subungual hematoma, pyogenic granuloma, chronic paronychia, or onychomycosis. When diagnosed, subungual melanomas are more often located on the thumb (58%) compared to the other fingers and the hallux (86%) compared to the other toes [18, 23]. The prevalence of subungual melanomas on the thumbs and great toes can be devastating for patient, as these are the most used digits [22]. Unfortunately, 20% of subungual melanomas are amelanotic, which can make diagnosis difficult [21]. The classic presentation of a melanoma involving the nail matrix is seen with "Hutchinson's sign," which is pigmentation along the proximal nail fold at the end of a pigmented nail streak [20]. With time, melanoma may become darker, nodular, and even ulcerate. If the melanoma is localized, traditional surgery is a wide local excision, which can result in complete amputation of the affected digit. Green's 20th edition of *Operative Hand Surgery* recommends amputation for a subungual melanoma 1 joint more proximal to the joint closest to the melanoma [24]. Amputations have also been recommended at the level of the metacarpal/metatarsal bones or at the metatarsophalangeal or metacarpophalangeal joints and possible lymph node dissection [17, 19].

The application of Mohs surgery has been used for melanomas involving the nail unit. Brodland presented

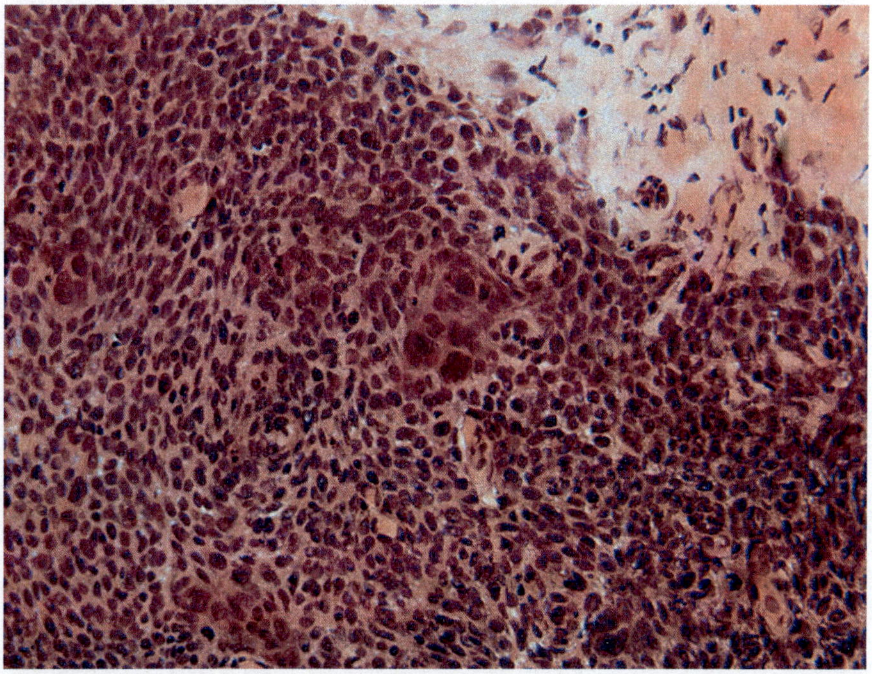

Fig. 28.2 Invasive Bowen's disease carcinoma. Note large bowenoid cells and a general lack of keratinization of the atypical cells

14 cases of a nail apparatus treated with Mohs surgery [25]. One particular benefit of Mohs surgery in the treatment of melanomas is that more tissue is examined than with standard surgical excision; thus subtle areas of melanoma invasion may be identified. For example, in the case reported by Do et al., a biopsy-proven melanoma in situ was treated with Mohs surgery. During surgery, an invasive component was identified that resulted in a partial amputation of the digit [26]. We believe melanoma in situ of the nail bed is easily treated with Mohs surgery and can avoid amputation for the patient, which may occur with traditional surgery (see Fig. 28.4a–c). However, melanoma in situ of the nail bed can be subtle in its histologic appearance, and thus high-quality frozen sections are necessary to provide the patient with the best possible cure rate.

28.3.4 Basal Cell Carcinoma

Nail unit basal cell carcinomas are rare and more commonly occur on the fingers than on the toes [27, 28]. The rarity of basal cell carcinomas on the fingernail unit, despite the amount of sun exposure on the hands, is attributed to the lack of pilosebaceous units in this region. Ultraviolet radiation is still felt to be a contributing factor, however, along with chronic trauma and arsenic [29].The variable clinical presentation of nail unit basal cell carcinomas makes diagnosis difficult, and patients may be misdiagnosed for many months until a biopsy is performed. Prior to the diagnostic biopsy, common clinical diagnoses include: an eczematous process, chronic paronychia, pyogenic granuloma, psoriasis, chronic ulcer, onychomycosis, longitudinal melanonychia, or even acral melanoma.

Treatment for basal cell carcinomas involving the nail unit has included radiation, curettage followed by salicyclic acid and podophyllin application [30], curettage with grenz rays [31], Mohs surgery, wide local excision, and amputation.

28.3.5 Warts

Warts are benign tumors induced by human papilloma virus. The most common site for ungual warts is along the lateral nail fold [4]. When the wart grows beneath the nail plate, onycholysis and nail dystrophy can occur. Periungual warts are felt to be inoculated by trauma and may be mistaken for other conditions, such as Bowen's disease or squamous cell carcinoma [4]. For treatment of subungual warts, care must be made to avoid damaging the nail matrix; otherwise nail plate dystrophy can

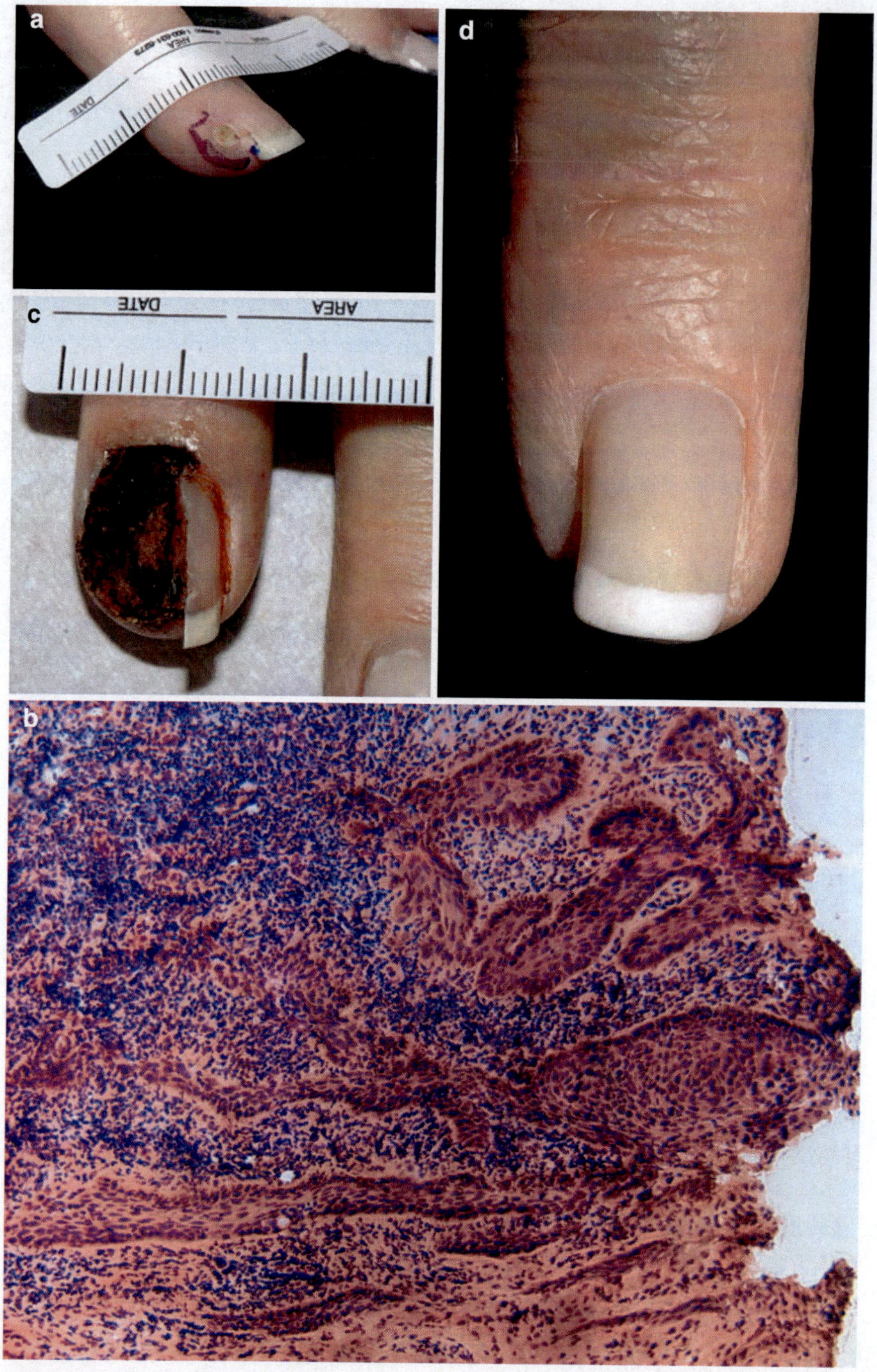

Fig. 28.3 (**a**) Bowen's disease carcinoma of left medial (radial) lateral nail fold of the fourth finger. (**b**) Bowen's disease carcinoma of the nail bed. Note the atypical cells longitudinally arranged corresponding to the nail bed ridges. (**c**) Postoperative appearance after Mohs surgery. Note bone exposure in center of wound. (**d**) Healed result 1 year postoperatively

occur. Although benign, periungual warts can be persistent, painful, and recurrent despite meticulous treatment attempts. We have treated such warts successfully with Mohs surgery and feel this treatment modality has a place in the management of periungual warts.

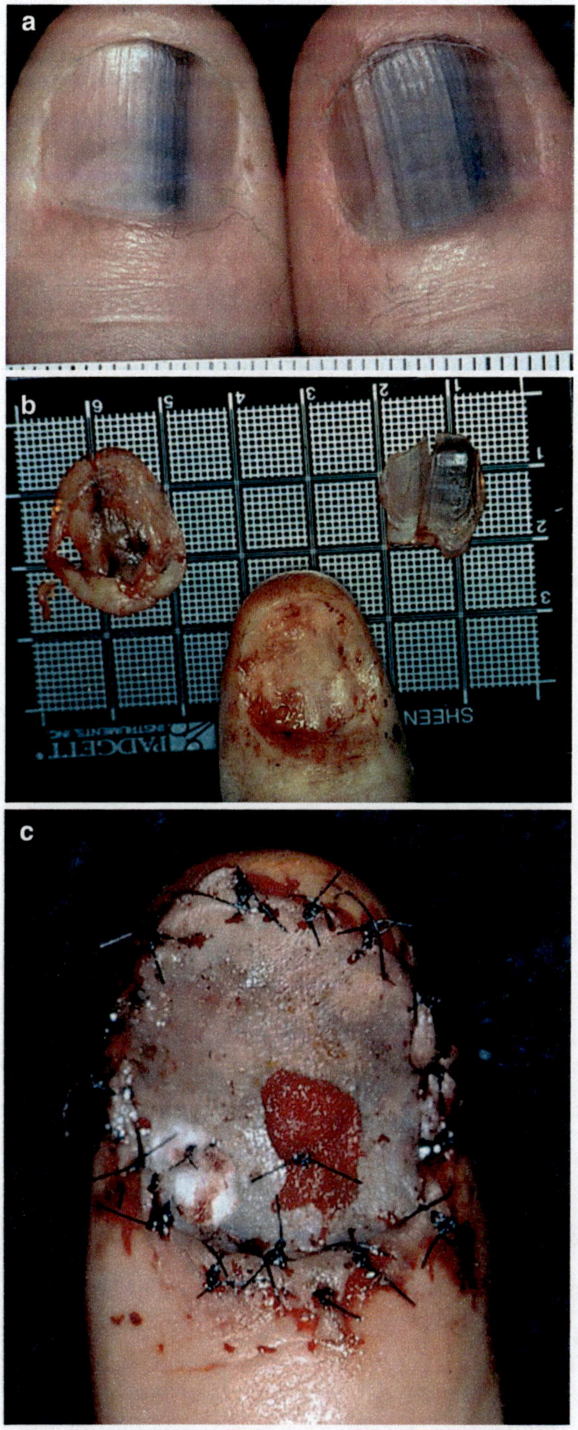

Fig. 28.4 (**a**) Bilateral melanoma in situ of the thumbnail nail beds. (**b**) Removal of nail plate (*upper right*) and first stage Mohs layer (*upper left*). (**c**) Split-thickness skin graft of nail bed

Summary: Mohs Technique

- Preoperative Evaluation
  - Imaging of the affected digit should be done preoperatively to detect for bone invasion by tumor.
- Anesthesia
  - A proximal digital block at the base of the digit is commonly used to anesthetize the digit and nail unit. Lidocaine 2% without epinephrine is recommended.
- Instruments
  - Additional instrumentation may be necessary when performing Mohs surgery on the nail unit: a nail splitter and a tourniquet.
- Preoperative Preparation
  - A penrose drain may be utilized as a tourniquet.
- Dressings and postoperative care
  - When applying a dressing around the digit, the bandage should be designed as to not compromise the blood supply.

28.4 Mohs Technique

28.4.1 Preoperative Evaluation

A thorough medical and surgical history, knowledge of the patient's current medications, and a physical examination are necessary prior to beginning any procedure. Pertinent information that should always be obtained includes a list of medication allergies, whether the patient requires preoperative antibiotics, knowing if the patient has a pacemaker and/or defibrillator, and whether the patient currently takes a blood thinner. Due to the increase prevalence of methicillin-resistant *Staphylococcus aureus* (MRSA), the patient should also be asked regarding a history of MRSA infections. If there is a positive prior history of a MRSA infection, the surgeon should consider appropriate antibiotic therapy with either doxycycline (Vibramycin^{Rx}) or trimethoprim and sulfamethoxazole (Bactrim^{Rx}) during the postoperative period.

Working in conjunction with the patient's primary care physician may be necessary prior to the patient undergoing surgery. For instance, if working on a diabetic patient's foot, the patient's blood glucose should be well controlled prior to any surgical work. Additionally, patients on a blood thinner like warfarin (Coumadin^{Rx}) may need their International Normalized Ratio (INR) adjusted prior to Mohs surgery. Also prior to Mohs surgery, radiographic imaging of the affected digit should be obtained to evaluate for possible bone invasion by tumor. If bone involvement by the tumor is seen on the radiographs, then a hand surgeon should be consulted to consider partial digit amputation. We usually recommend obtaining simple x-ray radiographs with PA, lateral and oblique views.

The surgical site should be inspected, measured, and photographed prior to Mohs surgery. Any unusual clinical features along the nail and adjacent regions should be evaluated. In nail surgery, additional effort should also be made to evaluate the palms and soles for additional pathology. For instance, if pitting on the palms is noted, the patient may have basal cell nevus syndrome and require additional evaluation by his primary care physician after the completion of Mohs surgery. If, for example, multiple palmar and/or planter keratoses are identified, the patient may have had significant arsenic exposure in the past, and additional work-up is necessary [20]. Examination for epitrochlear and axillary lymph nodes should be done preoperatively. Finally, the risks, benefits, and alternatives of the surgical procedure must be discussed with the patient in order to obtain informed consent.

28.4.2 Anesthesia

A proximal digital block at the proximal lateral sides of the digit is the most common technique used for anesthetizing the region surrounding the nail unit. This procedure minimizes pain and the number of injections required to anesthetize the digit. The main nerves to be anesthetized have both dorsal and ventral branches and run along the radial and ulnar sides of the digit. This distribution results in overlapping sensory innervations at the digit tip; thus, all four nerves should be anesthetized prior to any procedure. Using a 30-gauge needle, the anesthesia should initially be inserted in the region between the dorsal and ventral nerve pathways. After insertion, the needle may be angled dorsally and ventrally to anesthetize each specific nerve branch. The same technique is repeated for the other side of the digit. It is the opinion of the authors that anesthetizing a longitudinal section of a nerve, as opposed to injecting the anesthesia in a "ring" configuration, provides a more effective nerve block. For a proximal digital block, a maximum of 2–3 mL of 2% plain lidocaine is recommended for each side of the digit. Recent literature suggests that lidocaine with epinephrine may be locally infiltrated into a digit without complications, even if the patient has several comorbidities [32]. However, we feel that lidocaine with epinephrine should be avoided in diabetics, especially when working on the feet. The problem arises that unless one obtains a fasting blood glucose prior to surgery, one cannot be sure the patient is not a diabetic. In some cases, local anesthesia must also be injected into the distal digit to supplement a digital nerve block to provide for patient comfort during surgery. An important aspect of digital blocks is to wait an adequate time for nerve block anesthesia to occur. Usually it takes at least 20 min for nerve block anesthesia to become adequate.

28.4.3 Instruments

For Mohs surgery, our standard instrument trays include: an Adson Dressing Forceps, Bard-Parker #15 scalpel blade on a Bard-Parker #3 standard handle, a Fox 4-mm curette, blunt-tipped Stevens straight tenotomy scissors, a curved hemostat, a skin hook, a nail splitter, and a penrose drain.

When working on a finger, a latex glove fitted over the patient's hand with the operative fingertip cut and rolled isolates the surgical field and also creates a tourniquet for surgery.

28.4.4 Preoperative Preparation

The digit is cleaned by the patient with soap and water prior to surgery to remove any gross contaminants. The additional application of an antibacterial such as alcohol or povidone-iodine to the surgical site is done prior to Mohs surgery. After anesthetizing the digit, a sterile towel is placed beneath and around the surgical region to delineate the surgical field.

If working on a finger, a latex surgical glove can be used to provide a tourniquet (see Fig. 28.5a–c). After applying a correctly sized surgical glove onto the patient's hand, the glove fingertip on the operative

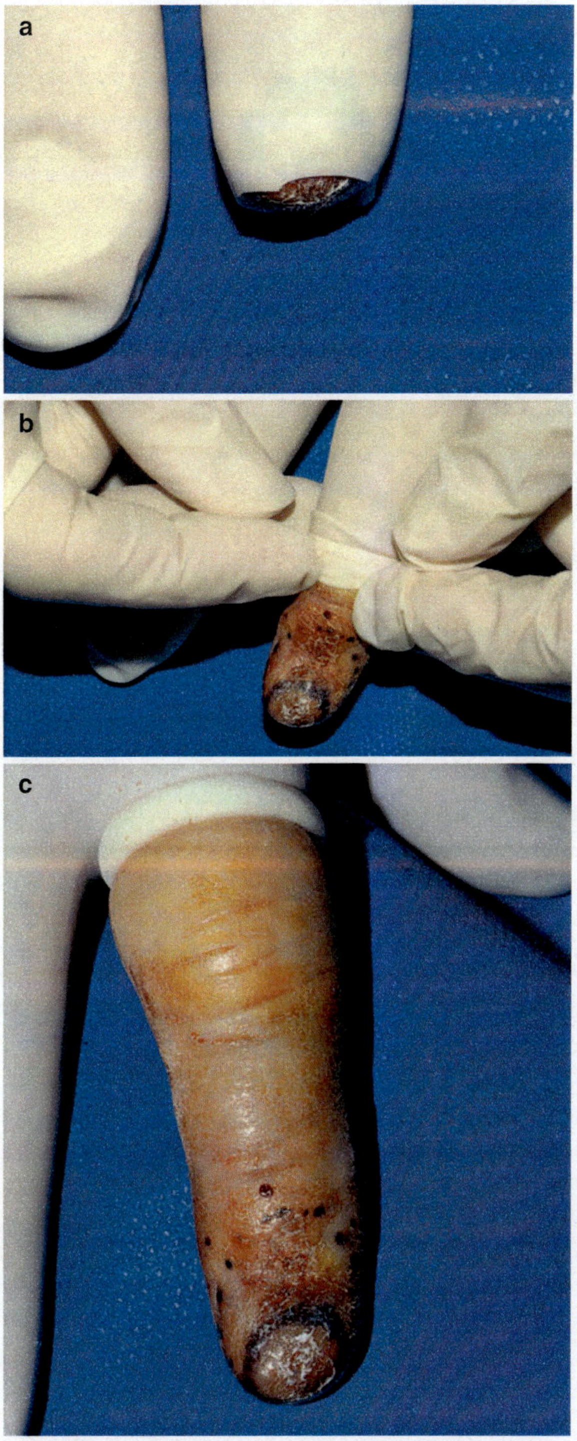

Fig. 28.5 (**a**) Finger tip cut off of latex glove. (**b**) Latex glove finger rolled back proximally to base of finger. (**c**) Rolled latex glove finger at base of finger provides tourniquet. Note poorly defined scaly patch of distal phalanx. This lesion is a recurrent Bowen's disease carcinoma that was previously removed by surgery by a plastic surgeon. Prior surgery excised the total nail unit, including the nail matrix, nail bed, and nail folds

finger is removed with a scissors. Then the cut latex glove finger is rolled proximally to the finger base where the constriction of the latex ring around the digit creates a tourniquet. The latex glove used as a tourniquet also serves to isolate the surgical field.

An alternative tourniquet may be made from a 3/8″ penrose drain (see Fig. 28.6a–c). The Penrose drain is placed around the base of the digit and its two ends pulled upward; the two ends are then clamped with a hemostat just above the digit. Then the hemostat is turned 360° to increase the pressure as needed to stop the bleeding. Regardless of whether a penrose drain or a surgical glove tourniquet is utilized, the tourniquet should only remain in place for as short a time as possible. While a rubber band has been utilized as a digit tourniquet in some offices, the narrow surface area of the rubber band can result in great focal pressure on blood vessels and nerves which can lead to injury.

28.4.5 Mohs Technique

Removal of all or part of the nail plate is necessary prior to Mohs surgery. A nail splitter is used to cut the nail prior to removal. The wider shaft of this instrument is inserted between the nail and its bed. It is then slid toward the nail cuticle where the tapered blade of the nail splitter on the top of the nail slips underneath the proximal nail fold. The nail is then cut, and in doing so, split. A hemostat is used to securely grasp the side of the nail plate to be removed, and the nail plate is removed from the digit with a twisting motion. Then, the abnormal tissue in the nail bed or nail fold is curetted to delineate the tumor-involved area. We place the curettings onto the gauze on the Mohs card to be processed as a separate slide with the subsequent Mohs layer. A 2-mm margin of tissue around the curetted region is cut with a scalpel blade cutting tangentially to the tissue. Usually, 3-score marks are then made outward from the Mohs layer onto the surrounding skin to help maintain specimen orientation. The Mohs layer is removed with a scalpel, and care is taken to ensure that the base of the Mohs layer is smooth and complete. The Mohs layer is placed onto the gauze adjacent to the curettings, and Mohs card is brought to the laboratory for processing.

In the laboratory, the tissue is subsectioned and its non-epidermal edges colored by at least two different dyes, and a map is drawn onto the Mohs card to

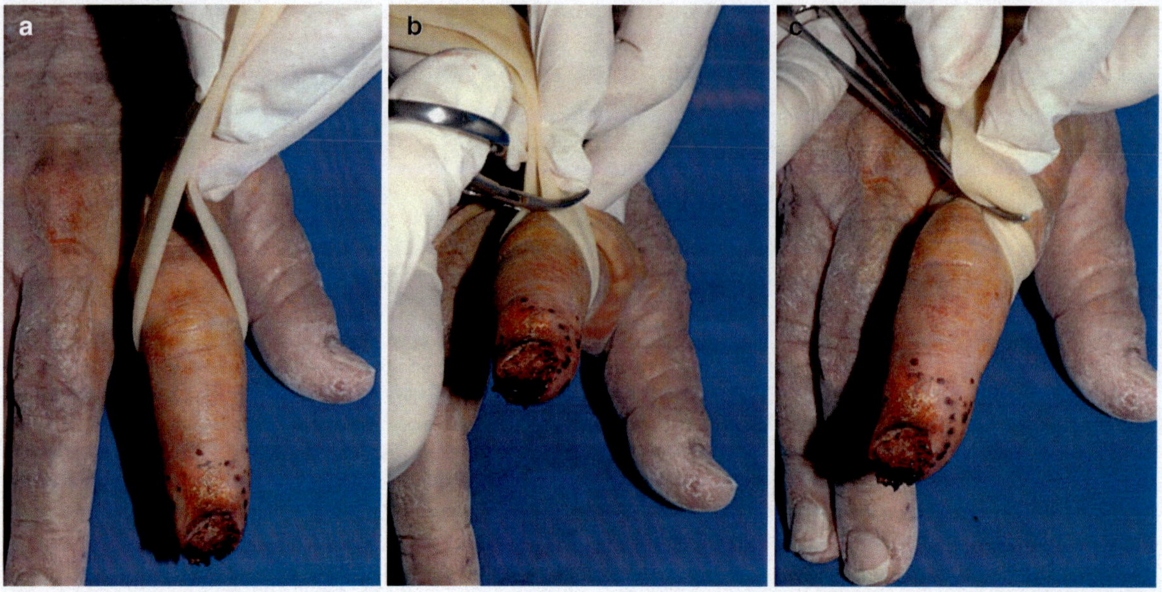

Fig. 28.6 (**a**) Ends of penrose drain being pulled upward at base of finger. (**b**) Penrose drain being clamped at base of finger. (**c**) Penrose drain turned 360° to tighten the tourniquet

delineate the location of each removed subsection in relation to the surgical defect. The different color dyes are indicated on the map by colored inks whose colors match the colors of the dyes on the tissue. We feel this reduces the error rate when indicating on the map the location of tumor as seen under the microscope. The tissue is fixed onto glass slides and stained. In our laboratory, the primary stain utilized is hematoxylin and eosin, while a toluidine blue stain is reserved for the management of basal cell carcinomas. The slides are then reviewed by the surgeon. The processing of the frozen sections allows for evaluation of the skin margins as well as the undersurface of the tissue. Any remaining tumor identified on the slides is marked onto the corresponding section of the diagram on the Mohs card. If tumor is identified on the initial stage, a second layer of tissue is removed from the patient at the affected area. These steps are repeated until a tumor-free margin is obtained.

A special problem that occurs when removing tumor that involves the nail matrix is that once the final Mohs layer has been taken, a lateral horn of the matrix must be removed along with the matrix. If this is not done, the lateral matrix horn will regrow as a small spicule which will be a nuisance for the patient.

28.4.6 Dressings and Postoperative Care

Between each Mohs layer, the surgical site is bandaged with a temporary dressing. A piece of nonadherent dressing is cut to fit the defect. Gauze is then cut and folded over the nonadherent dressing. Paper tape is applied in an oblique fashion to secure the temporary dressing, as the vascular supply may theoretically be impeded by winding tape circumferentially around the digit. The tape is also cut so that it does not totally encircle the digit. Tube dressings are another modality that provides a simple pressure dressing. Unfortunately, such dressings may cause complications if not properly used. Ersek demonstrated finger necrosis after the application of an elastic net bandage applied in many layers. The use of the elastic net dressing increased the pressure on the patient's finger and impeded blood flow after each successive layer [33].

In our experience, postoperative wounds of the periungual/subungual area often go in depth to bare bone and involve a variable amount of matrix. Because it is difficult to always determine the extent of matrix remaining, our bias is to let wounds in this area heal by granulation and epidermization. Second intention healing often produces excellent functional and cosmetic results. Rarely, if the whole matrix has been excised, a split-thickness skin graft may be considered.

After completion of the Mohs surgery without a repair, a pressure dressing is applied. The pressure dressing is used to facilitate hemostasis by applying constant pressure along the surgical site. Vaseline or an antibiotic ointment is initially applied to the surgical site to promote wound healing. A non-stick dressing is placed over the site, and then gauze is cut and then applied. Paper tape may be used to secure the bandage. For exudative wounds, Kerlix may be applied to wrap the entire digit. This dressing is removed by the patient after 24 hours. Oral antibiotics and pain-alleviating medications may also be given depending on the situation. Prescribing a sling for the patient to elevate the arm helps reduce postoperative edema and pain. For work on a patient's toes, sandals, or a special boot that exposes the toes and laces along the dorsum of the foot, are useful.

Summary: Complications

- Extensor tendon rupture can occur when excising tissue proximal to the nail matrix.

28.5 Complications

Primary complications with nail unit surgery include pain, infection, and swelling of the digit. Pain-alleviating medications such as hydrocodone and acetaminophen (Vicodin^{Rx}) or codeine and acetaminophen (Tylenol #3^{Rx}) are useful for alleviating patient discomfort. Oral antibiotics effective against *Staphylococcus aureus* and/or methicillin-resistant *Staphylococcus aureus* should be considered. Edema of the digit and hand is a complication that may cause temporary tenderness and stiffness along the digit. This problem will resolve gradually with time, and elevation of the extremity will expedite the recovery process.

Transection of the extensor tendon has occurred in one of our cases. If not repaired immediately, the patient will not be able to dorsiflex the finger.

Summary: Conclusions

- Mohs surgery is particularly useful in removing tumors of the nail unit because this technique preserves as much normal tissue as possible, especially nail matrix.

28.6 Conclusions

While tumors of the nail unit are relatively rare, traditional surgical techniques of wide local excision or amputation can be debilitating for the patient. Mohs surgery offers many advantages compared to traditional surgical methods. Because Mohs surgery requires the mapping of the tumor, complete clearance of the disease may be obtained. As unaffected tissue (especially the matrix, either in part or totally) is spared, Mohs surgery assures maximal preservation of the surrounding noncancerous tissue. The ultimate benefit to the patient is that Mohs surgery provides an alternative surgical method that leads to a more cosmetically and functionally acceptable result for the patient.

References

1. Zaiac MN, Weiss E. Mohs micrographic surgery of the nail unit and squamous cell carcinoma. Dermatol Surg. 2001; 27:246–51.
2. Goldminz D, Bennett RG. Mohs micrographic surgery of the nail unit. J Dermatol Surg Oncol. 1992;18(8):721–6.
3. Bennett RG. Fundamentals of cutaneous surgery. St. Louis: Mosby; 1988. A. p134, B. p134.
4. Salasche SJ, Garland LD. Tumors of the nail. Dermatol Clin. 1985;3:501–19.
5. Virgili A, Rosaria Zampino M, Bacilieri S, Bettoli V, Chiarelli M. Squamous cell carcinoma of the nail bed: a rare disease or only misdiagnosed? Acta Derm Venereol. 2001;81:306–7.
6. Baran RL, Gormley DE. Polydactylous disease of the nail. J Am Acad Dermatol. 1987;17:201–4.
7. Porembski MA, Rayan GM. Subungual carcinomas in multiple digits. J Hand Surg Eur Vol. 2007;32(5):547–9.
8. Peterson SR, Layton EG, Joseph AK. Squamous cell carcinoma of the nail unit with evidence of bony involvement: a multidisciplinary approach to resection and reconstruction. Dermatol Surg. 2004;30(2 Pt 1):218–21.
9. de Berker DA, Dahl MG, Malcolm AJ, Lawrence CM. Micrographic surgery for subungual squamous cell carcinoma. Br J Plast Surg. 1996;49(6):414–9.

10. Conill C, Verger E, Vilalta A, Palou J. Case report: squamous cell carcinoma of the nail bed. Br J Radiol. 1993;66:163–4.
11. Yaparpalvi R, Mahadevia PS, Gorla GR, Beitler JJ. Radiation therapy for the salvage of unresectable subungual squamous cell carcinoma. Dermatol Surg. 2003;29:294–6.
12. Wong TW, Sheu HM, Lee JY, Fletcher RJ. Photodynamic therapy for Bowen's disease (squamous cell carcinoma in situ) of the digit. Dermatol Surg. 2001;27(5):452–6.
13. Goron KB, Garden JM, Robinson JK. Bowen's disease of the distal digit: outcome of treatment with carbon dioxide laser vaporization. Dermatol Surg. 1996;22:723–8.
14. Lumpkin LR, Rosen T, Tschen JA. Subungual squamous cell carcinoma. J Am Acad Dermatol. 1984;11:735–8.
15. Baran RL, Simon C. Longitudinal melanonychia: a symptom of Bowen's disease. J Am Acad Dermatol. 1988; 18:1359.
16. Blessing K, Kernohan NM, Park KG. Subungual malignant melanoma: clinicopathological features of 100 cases. Histopathology. 1991;19:425–9.
17. Pack GT, Oropeza R. Subungual melanoma. Surg Gynecol Obstet. 1967;124:571–82.
18. Takematsu H, Obata M, Tomita Y, et al. Subungual melanoma: a clinicopathologic study of 16 Japanese cases. Cancer. 1985;55:2725–31.
19. Lingam MK, McKay AJ, Mackie RM, Aitchison T. Single-centre prospective study of isolated limb perfusion with melphalan in the treatment of subungual malignant melanoma. Br J Surg. 1995;82:1343–5.
20. James WD, Berger TG, Elston DM. Andrews' diseases of the skin. 10th ed. Philadelphia: Saunders; 2006. 695, 859.
21. Scher RK, Daniel CR. Nails: therapy, diagnosis, surgery. Philadelphia: Saunders; 1990. p. 209.
22. Moehrle M, Metzger S, Schippert W, Garbe C, Rassner G, Breuninger H. "Functional" surgery in subungual melanoma. Dermatol Surg. 2003;29(4):366–74.
23. Moehrle M, Haefner HM. Is subungual melanoma related to trauma? Dermatology. 2002;204:259–61.
24. Green DP. Green's operative hand surgery. 5th ed. Philadelphia: Elsevier/Churchill Livingstone; 2005. 2204pp.
25. Brodland DG. The treatment of nail apparatus melanoma with Mohs micrographic surgery. Dermatol Surg. 2001;26:269–73.
26. Do AN, Goleno K, Geisse JK. Mohs micrographic surgery and partial amputation preserving function and aesthetics in digits: case reports of invasive melanoma and digital dermatofibrosarcoma protuberans. Dermatol Surg. 2006;32(12): 1516–21.
27. Herzinger T, Flaig M, Diederich R, Röcken M. Basal cell carcinoma of the toenail unit. J Am Acad Dermatol. 2003;48(2):277–8.
28. Martinelli PT, Cohen PR, Schulze KE, Dorsey KE, Nelson BR. Periungual basal cell carcinoma: case report and literature review. Dermatol Surg. 2006;32(2):320–3.
29. Guanna AL, Kolbusz R, Goldberg L. Basal cell carcinoma on the nailfold of the right thumb. Int J Dermatol. 1994;33:204–5.
30. Nelson LM, Hamilton CF. Primary carcinoma of the nail bed. Arch Dermatol. 1970;101:63–7.
31. Hoffman S. Basal cell carcinoma of the nail bed. Arch Dermatol. 1973;108:828.
32. Firoz B, Davis N, Goldberg LH. Local anesthesia using buffered 0.5% lidocaine with 1:200,000 epinephrine for tumors of the digits treated with Mohs micrographic surgery. J Am Acad Dermatol. 2009;61(4):639–43.
33. Ersek RA. Ischemic necrosis and elastic net bandages. Tex Med. 1982;78:47.

Genitalia

29

Irene Vergilis-Kalner and Arash Kimyai-Asadi

Abstract

Although tumors of the external genitalia are not as common as those occurring in sun-exposed skin, a wide variety of carcinomas and other tumors occur in the male and female external genitalia. The incidence of these tumors is both significant and rising, and due to their location and aggressiveness may carry significant functional, anatomic, and psychosexual morbidities as well as the risk of mortality secondary to tumor metastasis. Mohs micrographic surgery is the treatment of choice for most tumors in this anatomic region because of reduced recurrence rates, maximum sparing of histologically uninvolved tissue, and improved feasibility of anatomically and functionally sensitive reconstruction.

Keywords

Genitalia • Skin cancer • Mohs micrographic surgery • Reconstruction • Squamous cell carcinoma • Extramammary Paget's disease

Summary: Introduction

- Major advantages of Mohs micrographic surgery (MMS) in management of mucocutaneous neoplasms of the male and female external genitalia include:
  - MMS allowing for margin control, which enables complete removal of the tumor and subsequently leads to reduced recurrence rates in the treatment of a variety of neoplasms

29.1 Introduction

The advantages of total microscopic control of excision margins that are provided by Mohs micrographic surgery (MMS) often justify consideration of this modality in the management of neoplasms of the male and female external genitalia. MMS has three major advantages in the management of mucocutaneous neoplasms of the genital region. First, MMS has been shown to reduce recurrence rates in the treatment of a variety of cutaneous neoplasms. The excision in successive layers with complete microscopic examination of the entire surgical margin of each excisional specimen assures eradication of any subclinical outgrowths that may extend beyond the clinically visible and palpable borders of a cancer, thereby reducing postsurgical recurrences.

I. Vergilis-Kalner
Assistant Professor of Dermatology, Department of Dermatology, UMDNJ, New Jersey

A. Kimyai-Asadi (✉)
DermSurgery Associates,
Houston, TX, USA
e-mail: akimyai@yahoo.com

K. Nouri (ed.), *Mohs Micrographic Surgery*,
DOI 10.1007/978-1-4471-2152-7_29,

Second, MMS reduces the amount of normal tissue that is removed around a tumor. Upon histologically confirmed elimination of the entire tumor, the excisions are ceased, and the surgical removal of a potentially significant additional margin of normal tissue is obviated. Thus, significantly reduced recurrence rates do not come at the expense of unnecessary removal of additional tissue around a tumor site as is typically the case in surgical oncology. As such, MMS allows for maximal conservation of normal tissue in critical anatomic structures such as the genitalia, while yielding higher cure rates than other conventional methods of treatment.

Third, with complete histologic control of the surgical margins, the surgeon can be confident that the tumor is no longer present, and therefore feels free to pick the optimal reconstructive method without particular concern regarding tumor recurrence and without the need to delay reconstruction or alter reconstructive choices while awaiting delayed histopathology results or while monitoring the local area for tumor recurrence.

Further advantages of MMS include the absence of need for general anesthesia, the fact that surgery is performed on an outpatient basis, and the fact that patients remain ambulatory. As such, Mohs micrographic surgery should be considered the technique of choice in the management of most cutaneous malignancies of the genital region.

Summary: Surgical Technique

- Steps during Mohs micrographic surgery (MMS):
  - Clinical margins of the tumor are evaluated and marked with a surgical pen.
  - The patient is asked to verify the location of the tumor.
  - Local anesthesia is obtained with an injection of lidocaine mixed with epinephrine and buffered with sodium bicarbonate to reduce injection site pain.
  - Bulky tumors may be curetted prior to taking the first stage to debulk the tumor and to delineate possible subclinical tumor spread.
  - The first stage is removed, and subsequently, the tissue is mapped.

29.2 Surgical Technique

The effectiveness of the Mohs technique is dependent on the individual steps that constitute the surgical procedure. These steps include preoperative physical examination, skin tumor extirpation, tissue mapping, histologic processing, and microscopic examination. The procedure is repeated until histologically clear margins are obtained. The postoperative defect is subsequently repaired by an optimal reconstructive technique.

When initially examining a patient, the clinical margins of the tumor are evaluated and marked with a surgical marking pen (Fig. 29.1a). The patient is then asked to verify the location of the tumor with a mirror, and the patient's identity is again confirmed. Local anesthesia is obtained with an injection of lidocaine mixed with epinephrine buffered with sodium bicarbonate. A curette may be used prior to excision to debulk and delineate possible subclinical tumor spread, although the utility of preoperative curettage is debatable and may result in larger surgical defects. Furthermore, the loose tissue of the penile shaft and prepuce, scrotum, and female genitalia are not easily amenable to preoperative curettage, making this modality best reserved for bulky genital tumors requiring preoperative debulking.

Classical MMS advocates that the blade be beveled at a 45° angle to the skin surface when excising the tumor margin. This allows the epidermis, dermis, and deeper tissue to be cut on the cryostat in a straight line and to be examined in one plane. However, this does not guarantee a complete epidermal edge for histologic evaluation in every case due to difficulties in tissue flattening and sectioning sections composed of epidermis, dermis, and fat. A more complete epidermal and dermal edge may be obtained by using a peripheral 90° vertical incision all around a neoplasm and separately examining horizontal sections from the tumor's base to evaluate the deep margin and vertical sections from the tumor's periphery to evaluate the peripheral margin (Fig. 29.1b). The 90° removal approach may also speed up the procedure by obviating the need for incising the margins vertically at 90° and excising the beveled edge to facilitate subsequent closure.

After tumor excision, the excised tissue must be accurately mapped and marked with ink for proper orientation. Despite a unified concept of margin control for tumor extraction, there are several variations in each step of this technique. Most Mohs micrographic

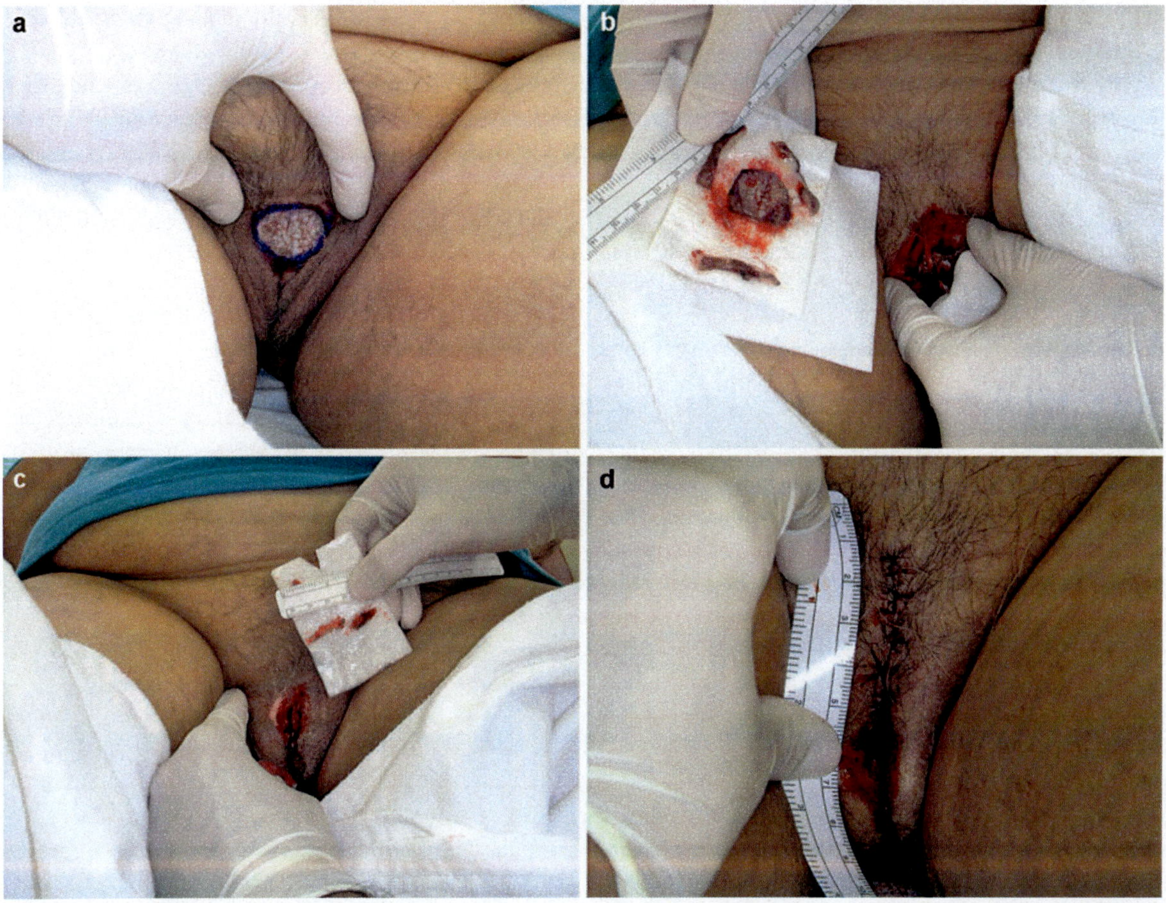

Fig. 29.1 (**a**) Bowen's disease of the vulva; image depicts clinical margins of the tumor being evaluated and marked with a surgical marking pen in preparation for taking an MMS layer. (**b**) MMS surgery layer demonstrated next to its respective defect. (**c**) MMS surgery layer taken after the previous stage has shown involvement of the lateral margin. (**d**) Reconstruction of the surgical defect following removal of skin cancer with MMS

surgeons map their tissue using hand-drawn sketches to orient the specimens. This method is inexpensive, simple, and quick and gives the surgeon artistic freedom to illustrate the size and shape of removed neoplastic tissue and the surgical defect. Some Mohs micrographic surgeons use preprinted maps or sketches of anatomic sites. It is as simple and rapid as drawing a picture by hand, except that the size and shape of the anatomic regions are fixed. Digital and Polaroid photographs produce the most accurate representations of the excised tissue, defects, and their interrelationship. They may also provide dimensions and archival information for follow-up. Currently, this approach is used by a minority of Mohs surgeons, but it may increase with the more widespread use of digital photography and electronic medical records.

Preparing tissue specimens for processing involves inking, flattening, freezing, sectioning, and staining, followed by microscopic examination. The Mohs histotechnologist plays a crucial role in this process and must consistently orient the tissue so that the correct surface is sectioned. Mohs surgeons should be familiar with the processes of flattening, freezing, sectioning, and staining tissue in order to efficiently communicate and troubleshoot quality issues with their histotechnologists.

Flattening the tissue in order to section the complete undersurface and the epidermal margin is critical for the complete en face examination of the outer margin of a tissue specimen. Heat-extractor flattening in the cryostat with or without preceding relaxing tissue cuts or slits is the most common method used for tissue flattening. Relaxing cuts are particularly useful when thick specimens are obtained for processing or when the tissue is inelastic. Aerosol or liquid nitrogen freezing on a glass slide, plastic or metal plate, or X-ray film is another technique commonly used to flatten tissue. More than one method is frequently utilized depending on the particular specimen.

The flattened tissue is then embedded in optimal cutting temperature compound so that the specimen may be sectioned and slides may be prepared for histologic evaluation. Thinner sections are necessary for proper evaluation of epithelial involvement. As such, epidermal and dermal specimens should be sectioned at 4–6 μm, whereas fatty subcutaneous tissue may be sectioned at a thickness of 15–25 μm. Sections that are too thick are difficult to evaluate and can lead to inaccurate interpretation. While thinner sections enhance cellular detail, they require more deeply frozen specimens. Furthermore, fatty tissue tends to fray when the sections are very thin. Obtaining several serial sections of each tissue specimen allows one to further differentiate normal adnexal structures or artifact from tumor nests. Although more processing time is required for serial sections, it may reduce the number of erroneous or equivocal interpretations of the surgical margins.

Subsequent to sectioning, the tissue slides are stained. Hematoxylin-eosin is the most commonly used tissue stains in MMS, and it can be used for all cutaneous neoplasms including squamous cell carcinoma, basal cell carcinoma, and malignant melanoma. Toluidine blue is an alternative stain that is particularly useful when evaluating basal cell carcinoma and is preferred by some Mohs surgeons. Toluidine blue highlights islands of basal cell carcinoma by metachromatically staining the mucopolysaccharides surrounding tumor nests a vibrant purple-pink color. The use of both toluidine blue and hematoxylin-eosin for different sections of the same specimen has occasionally been advocated when the histologic assessment of a tumor is not straightforward. For malignant melanoma, the concomitant use of MART-1 immunostains with hematoxylin-eosin stained sections may improve the sensitivity and specificity of detection of melanoma in frozen sections performed from the surgical margins.

The surgeon then evaluates the slides to determine if the surgical margins are involved with tumor. One of the major advantages of MMS is its potential to allow the surgeon maximal conservation of normal tissue. If tumor is present in the surgical margins, the corresponding location is marked on the Mohs map. Similarly, the presence of dense inflammation, fibrosis, or stromal changes at the margins may require additional excision to ensure that the margins are truly free of tumor. If the lateral margin is involved, an additional excision of 1–2 mm of tissue is performed (Fig. 29.1c). If tumor is present in the deep margin, an incision is made along the inside of the defect's edge, and a thin strip of tissue is removed from the depth of the defect for additional histologic evaluation. These stages are repeated until the margins are found to be histologically clear, and reconstruction, when required, is then performed. Once the histologically examined margins are free of tumor, the surgical defect is reconstructed regardless of how narrow the surgical margins utilized were (Fig. 29.1d).

Summary: Reconstruction

- Most Mohs micrographic surgery (MMS) defects on the genitalia can be repaired with primary linear closure

29.3 Reconstruction

Most lesions on the penile shaft, female genitalia, and scrotum can be repaired with a primary linear closure. On the glans penis, which is a richly vascularized area, skin grafts allow for preservation of structure and function and are a great option for reconstruction of most defects. If the urethral meatus is involved, the insertion of a Foley catheter may be necessary to reduce the risk of meatal stenosis.

In general, if the surgical defect is extensive and cannot be closed with a primary linear closure, a variety of advancement, rotation, and transposition flaps, as well as skin grafts, may be used to reconstruct such defects. When there is no available skin for closure, penile burial with subsequent surgical release in the scrotum or in the suprapubic region may be performed. Posterior scrotal skin may be used for primary closure of the scrotum, as posterior scrotal skin can usually be stretched to cover most scrotal defects. Moreover, any subsequent defect from the expansion of the posterior scrotal skin to cover the injured area can be grafted. Other reconstruction techniques include abdominal pedicled fascial flaps and paraumbilical island flaps. Furthermore, genital skin has frequently been reconstructed with grafts from the inner arms which provide a good match in color and texture and allow for inconspicuous closure of the donor site. Skin from the lateral external portion of the lower limb could also be used to reconstruct defects on the genitalia resulting in satisfactory color and texture match in the recipient site. Significant urethral involvement may be managed utilizing mucosal grafts from the buccal epithelium.

Summary: Common Genital Lesions Treated with Mohs Micrographic Surgery
- Basal cell carcinoma
- Squamous cell carcinoma in situ, including erythroplasia of Queyrat, Bowen's disease (intraepithelial carcinoma), and cutaneous horn
- Invasive squamous cell carcinoma
- Malignant melanoma in situ
- Malignant melanoma
- Extramammary Paget's disease
- Dermatofibrosarcoma protuberans
- Granular cell tumor
- Kaposi's sarcoma
- Leukemias (including lesions of cutaneous T cell lymphoma) and lymphoblastomas
- Langerhans cell histiocytosis
- Hemolymphangioma
- Localized metastases

29.4 Common Genital Lesions Treated with Mohs Micrographic Surgery

29.4.1 Basal Cell Carcinoma

Although basal cell carcinoma (BCC) is the most common human malignancy, BCCs arising on non-sun-exposed genitalia are rather uncommon and have an unclear pathogenesis [1]. A delay in diagnosis can result in larger and more invasive tumors and increased potential for scarring, anatomic deformity, functional compromise, and tumor recurrence. There have been several reports in the literature of BCCs arising in the vulvar region, with some tumors presenting with characteristic BCC-like lesions and others presenting with non-specific symptoms such as unilateral pruritus [2]. BCCs have also been reported on the scrotum, perineum, and perianal regions. Scrotal BCCs often present as persistent ulcerations or plaques without identifiable predisposing factors. These lesions are often poorly circumscribed with relatively high recurrence rates when treated with standard excisions. Furthermore, metastatic disease may be more common as compared to BCCs arising from non-genital locations. Therefore, MMS, which offers the highest cure rate while sparing tumor-free surrounding tissue, is considered the gold standard of treatment for BCCs in the genital region and is the most appropriate initial therapeutic approach.

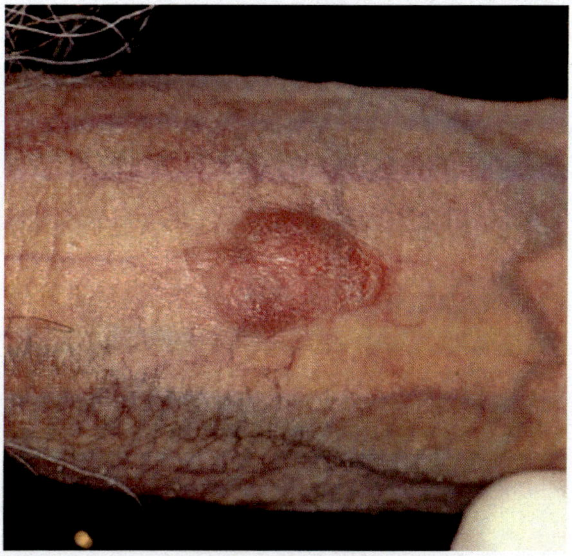

Fig. 29.2 SCC on the shaft of the penis

29.4.2 In Situ and Invasive Squamous Cell Carcinoma (Including Verrucous Carcinoma)

By far, the most common form of penile and vulvar carcinoma is SCC (Fig. 29.2 and 29.3). The incidence of penile carcinoma is significantly higher in some emerging countries as compared to developed nations. This is thought to be due to socioeconomic disparities and religious behaviors that contribute to the different incidence rates, as poor local hygiene has been recognized as unfavorable risk factor, while circumcision shortly after birth has been recognized as favorable risk factor. Ritual practice of circumcision seems to influence the prevention of penile cancer statistically, as early circumcision seems to be associated with a lower

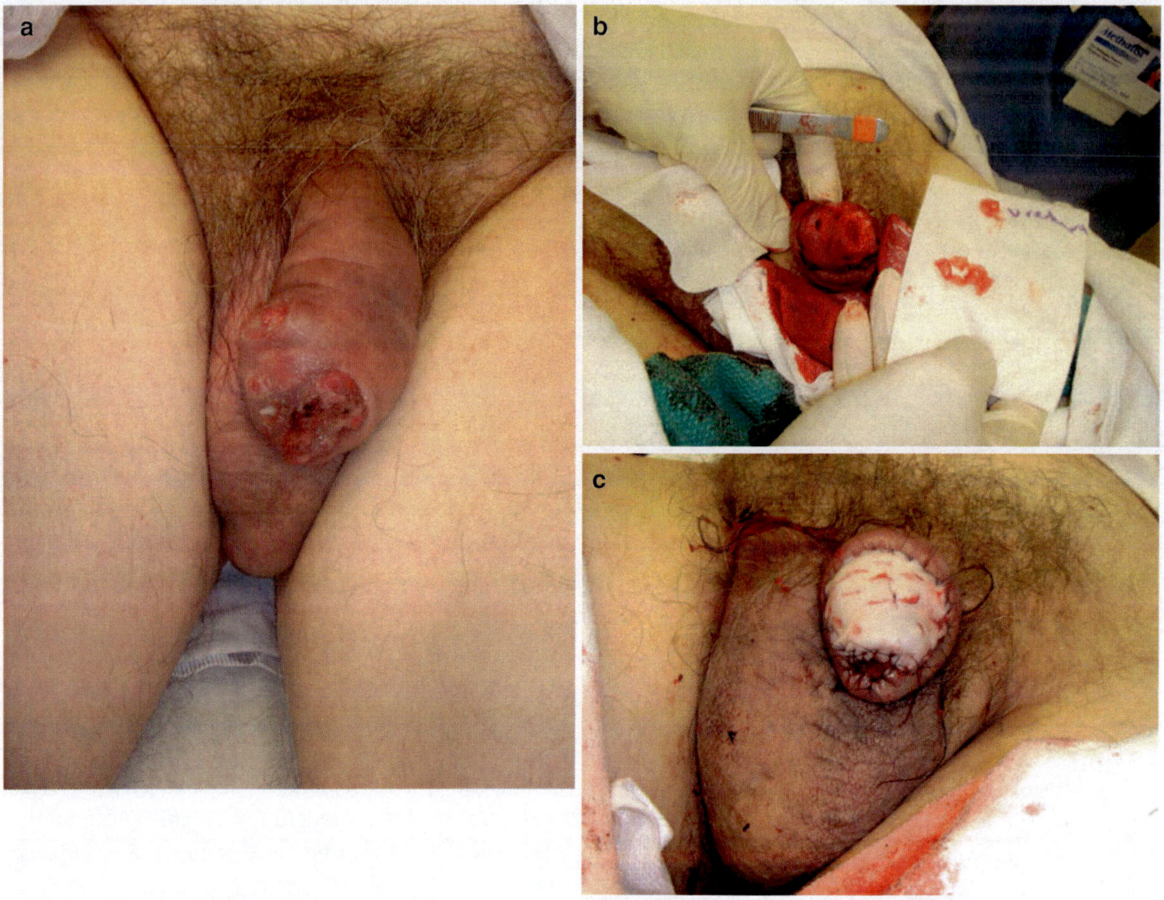

Fig. 29.3 Invasive squamous cell carcinoma of the penis measuring 6.0 x 5.0 x 5.0 cm (**a**) involving the prepuce, glans penis, and urethral meatus, cleared after 5 stages of MMS (**b**), and repaired with a combination of advancement of the penile shaft to repair the prepuce and ventral surface of the distal penis, as well as a full-thickness skin graft from the inner arm for reconstruction of the dorsolateral glans penis (**c**)

incidence of penile cancer compared to later circumcision. Most often, penile SCCs develop in patients over the age of 50. The common presentation for penile cancer is balanoposthitis, followed by an ulcerated lesion, and the most common site where penile cancer occurs is on the glans, followed by the prepuce [3].

Squamous cell carcinomas (SCCs) in the non-sun-exposed genital region have been reported to occur most commonly in the setting of human papilloma virus infection and preexisting chronic inflammatory conditions, such as lichen sclerosus et atrophicus and lichen planus. Balanitis xerotica obliterans (penile lichen sclerosus et atrophicus) may precede, coexist with, or develop after the development of SCC. Non-verruciform low-grade squamous carcinomas, which are strongly associated with lichen sclerosus, are more frequent in the foreskin of elderly men. These lesions are often multicentric, and subsequent independent tumors may show some verrucous features. Likewise, balanitis has a chance of progressing to squamous cell carcinoma, and if not adequately treated, may lead to invasion.

Premalignant lesions associated with SCC include cutaneous horn, pseudoepithelioma, keratotic and micaceous balanitis, balanitis xerotica obliterans, giant condyloma, and bowenoid papulosis. SCC in situ of the penis includes erythroplasia of Queyrat and Bowen's disease, which can progress to invasive SCC, with the potential for metastasis to local lymph nodes and distant sites. Risk factors include poor hygiene, being uncircumcised, smoking, and phimosis.

Additionally, HPV coinfection is present in a significant percentage of patients with penile carcinoma. Clinically, invasive SCCs may be either papillary or cauliflower-like, or sclerosing and infiltrating. The prognosis is somewhat better for the former variant.

Penile carcinoma is an aggressive disease with significant treatment-associated urologic and psychosexual morbidity, particularly when partial or complete penectomies are performed instead of tissue-sparing techniques such as MMS. For this reason, MMS is optimal in order to minimize interference with functional anatomy without compromising local cancer control. As a surgical treatment that allows for the highest possible cure rate, maximum tissue sparing, and complete margin control, MMS is considered the treatment of choice for in situ and invasive SCCs of the penis. Due to its ability to metastasize to the lymph nodes, MMS may help minimize the risk of recurrence and ensuing metastasis, with multiple reports in the literature substantiating the successful use of MMS for invasive SCCs of the penis.

Penile SCCs affecting the urethral meatus have a significant propensity for tracking along the urethral epithelium (Fig. 29.3), and the extent of this involvement may be difficult to estimate clinically. MMS is the optimal treatment in this case, as only involved urethral mucosa is removed, without risking missing subclinical urethral spread.

Microscopically, carcinoma of the scrotum (chimney sweeps' disease) is most often Bowen's intraepithelial carcinoma or invasive squamous cell carcinoma. Originally, soot and tar products were suspected as factors. Today, this occupational disease is seen also in persons working with mineral oil, paraffin, and tar. Early recognition of chronic warty or eczematous-appearing growths on the scrotum is critical.

Vulvar SCCs arising on the labia minora, majora, and at the vaginal vestibule, as with the lesions mentioned above, are all also best treated by MMS.

Intraepithelial carcinoma (Bowen's disease) of the anus is diagnosed with increasing frequency, as is in situ carcinoma of the vulva, which is also now diagnosed in younger patients than in the past. The reason for this apparent increase in frequency is unknown. Infection by herpes simplex virus type 2 and human papilloma virus are prime suspects in carcinomas arising in the anus and the female lower genital tract. The extensive involvement of the anal mucosa by Bowen's disease and its potential to become invasive carcinoma necessitate a surgical approach that is concerned with both cure as well as preservation of anal function. Of note, squamous cell carcinoma in situ of the vulva frequently involves the perianal skin and anal mucosa. Furthermore, the anogenital region, comprising the cervix, vagina, vulva, perineum, and anus, has the potential for the development of multicentric and multiple primary malignancies. All of these tumors are best treated with MMS, which allows complete control of the margin and gives the best results in terms of the cure and sparing tissue in these regions, often with good cosmetic and functional results.

29.4.3 In Situ and Invasive Malignant Melanomas

Although uncommon, melanoma of the male and female genitalia is not very rare. The potentially higher incidence of malignant melanoma arising in the nevi on the genitalia has led some to advocate that pigmented nevi of the genitalia be excised when discovered. Metastasis occurs rapidly from malignant melanoma of the anogenital region, possibly due to delayed diagnosis as compared to cutaneous melanomas.

The results of multiple investigators have confirmed the value of MMS in the treatment of malignant melanoma. The success of MMS confirms that melanoma grows in a contiguous fashion before it spreads systemically. It is known that once tumor metastasizes from the primary site, trying to improve survival by increasing the extent of conventional surgery is typically fruitless. Therefore, the goal of surgery is to remove the entirety of the primary tumor, including any subclinical extensions. The value of MMS is the ability to identify these extensions microscopically and to excise tumor-bearing tissue while sparing normal skin. Furthermore, MMS may spare a significant diameter of normal skin that may be removed with fixed-margin standard surgical excisions for melanoma, a distinct advantage to patients whose melanomas are on the genitalia and in patients whose melanomas have indistinct clinical margins and who would require an even wider margin of normal skin when using standard surgical techniques and who are at substantial risk of tumor recurrence and subsequent metastasis.

In recent years, techniques have been developed to enhance the ability to detect melanoma cells on frozen section slides. During MMS for melanoma, tyrosine and silver stains, in addition to more commonly used Melan-A and MART-1 immunohistochemical stains, can be used to highlight premelanin, melanin, and melanocytes. The use of these stains during MMS allows for improved clearance of malignant melanoma while preserving as much of the healthy surrounding tissue as possible by improving the sensitivity and specificity of the microscopic examination of the excised margins.

29.4.4 Extramammary Paget's Disease

Extramammary Paget's disease (EMPD) is an uncommon intraepithelial neoplasm typically occurring in apocrine-gland-rich regions. EMPD usually involves the epidermis but may extend into the dermis, and deeper invasion can occur. The anogenital region is a very common site of occurrence, with the most commonly involved anatomical sites being the vulvar, perianal, perineal, scrotal, and penile regions. Its peak incidence is in patients between 65 and 70 years of age, and postmenopausal Caucasian women are most commonly affected. However, in some populations, such as the Asian population, EMPD seems to affect more men than women, and the scrotum and perianal areas are the most commonly involved sites. The onset of EMPD is insidious. Clinically, the lesions typically present as well-defined, moist, and erythematous plaques usually accompanied by pruritus or other nonspecific symptoms such as bleeding, edema, burning, or pain. EMPD tends to carry a good prognosis because the spread of atypical cells is usually limited to the epidermis.

Histopathological examination shows epidermal acanthosis and elongated rete ridges. Paget's cells are large, mucin-containing intraepidermal cells with a large nucleus and abundant pale cytoplasm (Fig. 29.4). Recent studies of perianal and vulvar EMPD have described distinct immunohistochemical subtypes termed cutaneous and endodermal. Cutaneous EMPD is characteristically positive for cytokeratin 7, negative for cytokeratin 20, and positive for gross cystic disease fluid protein 15, whereas endodermal EMPD is positive for cytokeratins 7 and 20, while it stains negative for gross cystic disease fluid protein 15. Consequently, intraoperative cytokeratin-7 immunostaining may be used with MMS for EMPD. In addition, to facilitate identification of involved tissue, a rapid carcinoembryonic antigen stain has also been reported to have been used as an adjunct to conventional H&E-stained slides to enhance the ability to obtain clear margins with MMS [4]. This technique was particularly useful in highlighting involvement in areas of marked dysplasia and artifact where discrimination is often difficult. Specifically, in anal epithelium, the presence of goblet cells may complicate discrimination of EMPD from normal epithelium.

Since it is a malignant lesion, surgery remains the treatment of choice. Wide surgical excision is currently the standard treatment for EMPD. However, EMPD almost always extends well beyond its clinically apparent borders. Consequently, standard excision is often insufficient to achieve complete remission, with EMPD having a notoriously high rate of recurrence after wide local excision. Recurrence is often associated with invasion. Therefore, MMS should be considered the gold standard of treatment for nonmetastatic EMPD.

Effective clearance of EMPD with Mohs micrographic surgery was first reported in 1979 [5]. It has since been suggested that this malignancy may be multifocal, particularly as reports of recurrences after resection with MMS have appeared. However, investigators have found the tumor to be unifocal with thin, long, and finger-like projections extending from the main body of tumor [6]. As such, if there are any doubts, an additional resection of a margin of tissue may be considered even after clear surgical slides are obtained. Overall, MMS has been shown to achieve a significantly lower recurrence rate for EMPD as compared to standard wide excision [7].

The alternative to MMS is wide local excision with a 4-cm surgical margin. In comparison, MMS is a tissue-sparing technique that not only minimizes the size of the surgical defect in comparison to wide local excision but also provides the best cure rates. Furthermore, multiple scouting biopsies, which can be processed as either permanent or frozen sections prior to initiating MMS, can be a beneficial adjuvant technique and can be used to guide the extent of the initial Mohs layer, allowing for MMS to more rapidly clear tumors with the best preservation of the healthy surrounding tissue [8]. In addition, there have been reports of 5-fluorouracil being applied topically for 10 days prior to MMS, resulting in a sharply delineated, erythematous patch of biopsy-proven EMPD well beyond the original clinical borders [9].

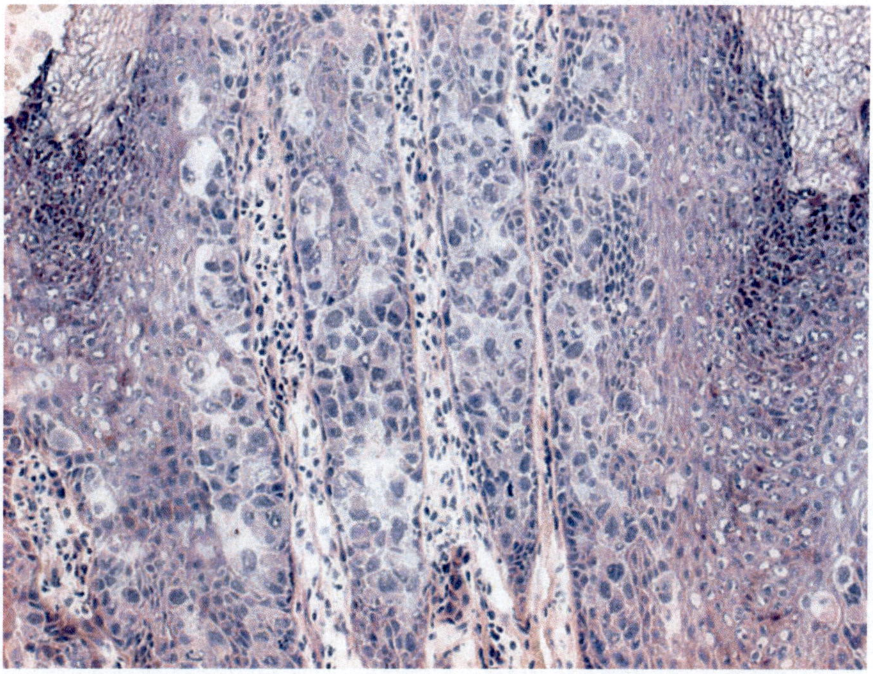

Fig. 29.4 Histologic depiction of EMPD on an MMS layer showing epidermal acanthosis and elongated rete ridges, as well as the large, mucin-containing intraepidermal Paget's cells with their large nucleoli and abundant pale cytoplasm

29.4.5 Dermatofibrosarcoma Protuberans

Dermatofibrosarcoma protuberans (DFSP) is a tumor of intermediate malignancy characterized by its aggressive local growth due to pseudopodium-like outgrowths and marked propensity to recur after surgical excision. To achieve complete cure with conventional surgery, surgical margins up to 5 cm are required, leading to wide scars and significant deformity. Nonetheless, wide local excision for DFSP suffers a high recurrence rate due to the significant subclinical growth seen with these tumors, particularly in terms of subcutaneous spread. MMS is the optimal treatment for DFSP, both ensuring complete excision by examination of all margins as well as minimizing normal tissue loss. MMS is generally advocated for treatment of DFSP lesions on the genitalia to ensure precise margin control and allow sparing of the surrounding healthy tissue.

29.4.6 Granular Cell Tumor

MMS has also been reported to successfully treat granular cell carcinoma in situ of the glans penis, thus establishing MMS as a tissue-sparing option for patients with perineal granular cell carcinoma [10].

29.4.7 Kaposi's Sarcoma

Kaposi's sarcoma can occur on the genitalia, with several cases in the literature reporting lesion presenting on glans penis and scrotum. As a tissue-sparing technique, MMS may be considered in the management of these lesions.

29.4.8 Leukemias and Lymphoblastomas

Leukemias and lymphoblastomas occurring on the male genitalia and solitary lesions may be treated using MMS.

29.4.9 Langerhans Cell Histiocytosis

Lesions of Langerhans cell histiocytosis may occur on the genital region, and Mohs micrographic surgery may be used for the treatment of solitary lesions.

29.4.10 Haemolymphangioma

There is also a report in the literature of haemolymphangioma, an atypical presentation of giant cell fibroblastoma, in the perineoscrotal area, originating from the posterior border of the left scrotum to the anal margin, successfully treated with Mohs micrographic surgery [11].

Summary: Conclusions

- Mohs micrographic surgery (MMS) should be considered the treatment of choice for the majority of malignant cutaneous neoplasms on the genital region.

29.5 Conclusions

Tumors of the genital region are common and occur with increasing frequency in both men and women. In order to best preserve locoregional anatomy, to minimize the risk of recurrence, and to reduce the risk of metastasis and death associated with tumor recurrence, MMS should be considered the treatment of choice for the majority of malignant cutaneous neoplasms on the genital region.

References

1. Nehal KS, Levine VJ, Ashinoff R. Basal cell carcinoma of the genitalia. Dermatol Surg. 1998;24:1361–3.
2. Saini R, Sarnoff DS. Basal cell carcinoma of the vulva presenting as unilateral pruritus. J Drugs Dermatol. 2008;7: 288–90.
3. Rando Sous A, P'erez-Utrilla P'erez M, et al. A review of penile cancer. Adv Urol 2009:1–3.
4. Harris DW, Kist DA, et al. Rapid staining with carcinoembryonic antigen aids limited excision of extramammary Paget's disease treated by Mohs surgery. J Dermatol Surg Oncol. 1994;20:260–4.
5. Coldiron BM, Goldsmith BA, Robinson JK. Surgical treatment of extramammary Paget's disease. A report of six cases and a reexamination of Mohs micrographic surgery compared with conventional surgical excision. Cancer. 1991;67: 933–8.
6. Hendi A, Perdikis G, Snow JL. Unifocality of extramammary Paget disease. J Am Acad Dermatol. 2008;59:811–3.
7. Lee KY, Roh MR, et al. Comparison of Mohs micrographic surgery and wide excision for extramammary Paget's disease: Korean experience. Dermatol Surg. 2009;35:34–40.
8. Appert DL, Otley CC, et al. Role of multiple scouting biopsies before Mohs micrographic surgery for extramammary Paget's disease. Dermatol Surg. 2005;31:1417–22.
9. Eliezri YD, Silvers DN, Horan DB. Role of preoperative topical 5-fluorouracil in preparation for Mohs micrographic surgery of extramammary Paget's disease. J Am Acad Dermatol. 1987;17:497–505.
10. Nash PA, Bihrle R, et al. Mohs' micrographic surgery and distal urethrectomy with immediate urethral reconstruction for granular carcinoma in situ with significant urethral extension. Urology. 1996;47:108–10.
11. Buche S, Delasalle EM, et al. Atypical presentation of giant cell fibroblastoma. Ann Dermatol Venereol. 2010;137:381–5.

30 Deep Structures of the Head and Neck

Sarah G. Baker, Douglas M. Sidle, and Simon Yoo

Abstract

The skin and subcutaneous tissue is an intricate and dynamic network with many key components contributing to its overall structural and functional integrity. Precise knowledge of the individual components that make up this vital organ as well as the manner by which they interact with one another is a critical tool for the cutaneous surgeon. This chapter explores the deep subcutaneous structures of the head and neck including motor and sensory nerves, muscles of facial expression, soft tissue structures (fatty layers and fascia), mucosa, and bony and cartilaginous skeletons.

Keywords

Facial nerve • Trigeminal nerve • Facial fat • Facial fascia • Muscles of facial expression • Bony skeleton • Cartilage

Summary: Introduction

- Comprehensive knowledge of cutaneous and subcutaneous anatomy is critical for the dermatologic surgeon.

30.1 Introduction

Adequate understanding of regional cutaneous and subcutaneous anatomy is critical for the dermatologic surgeon. It allows one to perform procedures more confidently, providing the best possible functional and cosmetic result for the patient. This knowledge also enables surgeons to adequately counsel their patients

S.G. Baker (✉)
Department of Dermatology, Northwestern University, Chicago, IL, USA
e-mail: baker.sarah.g@gmail.com

D.M. Sidle
Department of Otolaryngology – Head & Neck Surgery, Northwestern Feinberg School of Medicine, Chicago, IL, USA

S. Yoo
Department of Dermatology, Otolaryngology, Surgery, Northwestern University, Chicago, IL, USA

K. Nouri (ed.), *Mohs Micrographic Surgery*,
DOI 10.1007/978-1-4471-2152-7_30,

regarding potential complications. One must be familiar with all aspects of cutaneous anatomy including cosmetic subunits, skin tension lines, underlying blood supply, fascial planes, nerves, musculature, and other vital structures to avoid adverse and potentially devastating structural and functional consequences.

Summary: Innervation of the Face and Scalp

- The facial nerve (cranial nerve VII) provides motor innervation to the muscles of facial expression.
- The facial nerve possesses five main branches: the temporal, zygomatic, buccal, mandibular, and cervical rami.
- The temporal and marginal mandibular branches of the facial nerve are particularly susceptible to injury given their superficial locations.
- The trigeminal nerve (cranial nerve V) provides sensory innervation to the face and anterior scalp as well as motor innervation to the muscles of mastication.
- Prior to exiting the skull, the trigeminal nerve divides into three main branches: the ophthalmic (V1), maxillary (V2), and mandibular (V3) divisions.
- The sensory innervation of the external ear is complex and comprised of contributions from the trigeminal, facial, glossopharyngeal, and vagus nerves as well as the cervical plexus (C2 and C3).

30.2 Innervation of the Face and Scalp

30.2.1 Motor Innervation of the Face and Scalp

The facial nerve (cranial nerve VII) provides motor innervation to the muscles of facial expression. In addition, it also provides sensory innervation to a portion of the external auditory canal, soft palate, and pharynx as well as taste to the anterior two-thirds of the tongue. Precise knowledge of the anatomy of this structure is critical for the cutaneous surgeon. Permanent injury to this nerve may lead to significant cosmetic and functional deficits [1].

The facial nerve originates in the pons and subsequently enters the internal acoustic meatus, coursing through the temporal bone and emerging through the stylomastoid foramen. Following its exit from the stylomastoid foramen, the facial nerve gives rise to the posterior auricular nerve which innervates the occipitalis and posterior auricular muscles [2, 3]. The site of entry of the facial nerve into the parotid gland may be approximated at the center of a line connecting the superior tragus with the angle of the mandible. After exiting the stylomastoid foramen, the facial nerve is protected by the mastoid process. Children under the age of five do not have a fully developed mastoid process; therefore the facial nerve may be particularly vulnerable to injury at this site [4].

Within the deeper substance of the parotid gland, the facial nerve first divides to form superior (temporofacial) and inferior (cervicofacial) divisions. It then presumes a more superficial location anteriorly within the parotid gland, dividing into its five main branches: the temporal, zygomatic, buccal, mandibular, and cervical rami (Figs. 30.1 and 30.2). A small percentage of patients may present with aberrations in this branching pattern [5]. Within the parotid gland, one must also be mindful of the parotid duct, which drains secretions from the parotid gland into the oral cavity. This structure courses superiorly to the masseter muscle, then deep to the buccinator muscle, opening into the oral cavity in the vicinity of the second upper molar. Its course can be plotted by drawing an imaginary line from the notch of the ear, inferior to the tragus, to the center of a vertical line from the alar rim to the oral commissure. Injury to the parotid gland itself may lead to the formation of a draining sinus which often heals spontaneously. If the parotid duct is injured, however, a chronic, nonhealing sinus tract may form requiring surgical repair [1].

Following their exit from the parotid gland, divisions of the facial nerve are covered by superficial fascia until they reach their respective muscle of facial expression, which they enter at the posterolateral aspect. The most superior branch of the facial nerve is the temporal branch. This branch exits the parotid gland superiorly, coursing over the zygomatic arch and temporal fossa and further divides into four rami innervating the orbicularis oculi, corrugator supercilii, frontalis, and temporoparietalis muscles [4].

The area of greatest risk of injury to the temporal branch can be estimated by connecting the endpoints

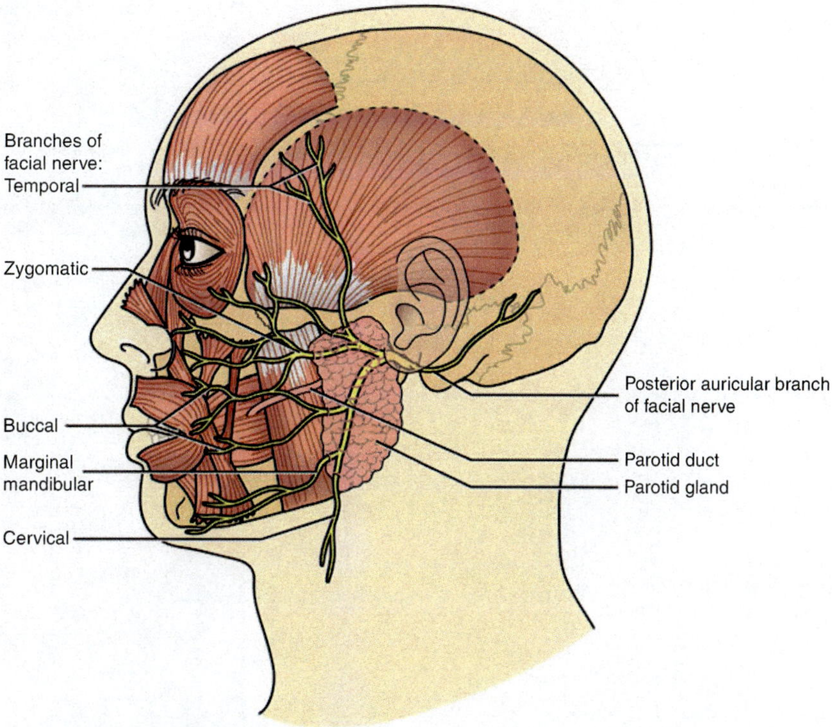

Fig. 30.1 Branches of the facial nerve

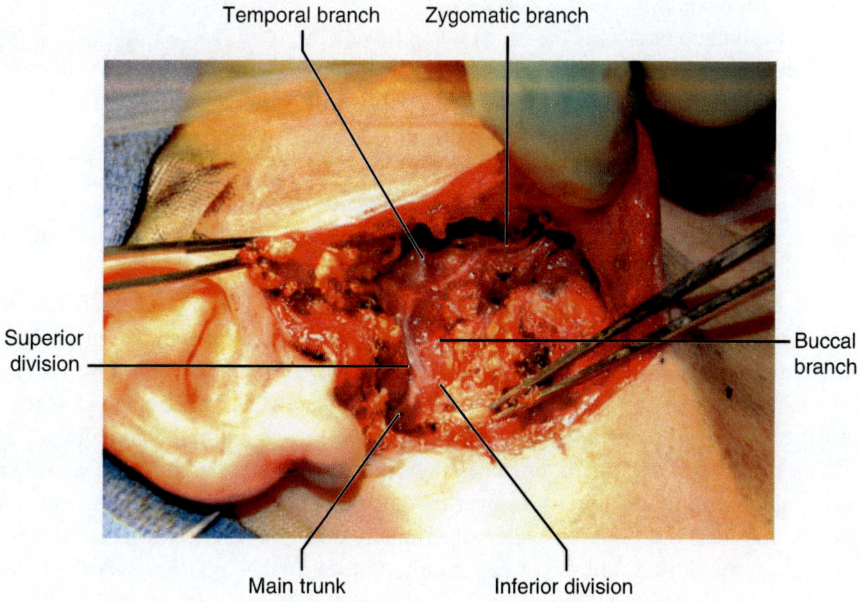

Fig. 30.2 Facial nerve dissection

of the lines drawn from the earlobe to a point just superiorly and laterally to the highest forehead crease and from the earlobe to the lateral eyebrow (Fig. 30.3) [5]. Damage to the temporal branch of the facial nerve may lead to paralysis of the frontalis muscle and resultant flattening of the forehead and inability to elevate the brow (Fig. 30.4a, b). Compensatory wrinkling of the contralateral forehead and elevation of the contralateral brow also occurs, leading to quizzical appearance. Muscle atrophy may ensue over time, causing ptosis and redundant eyelid skin, and the visual field may be obstructed. Procedures such as browplasty or

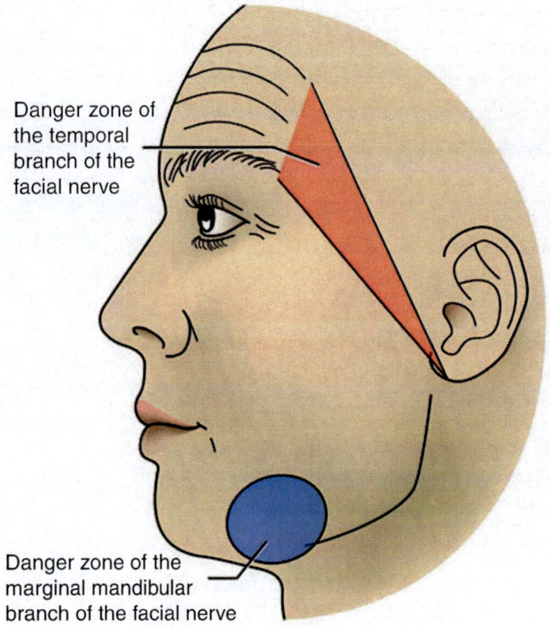

Fig. 30.3 Danger zones of the face

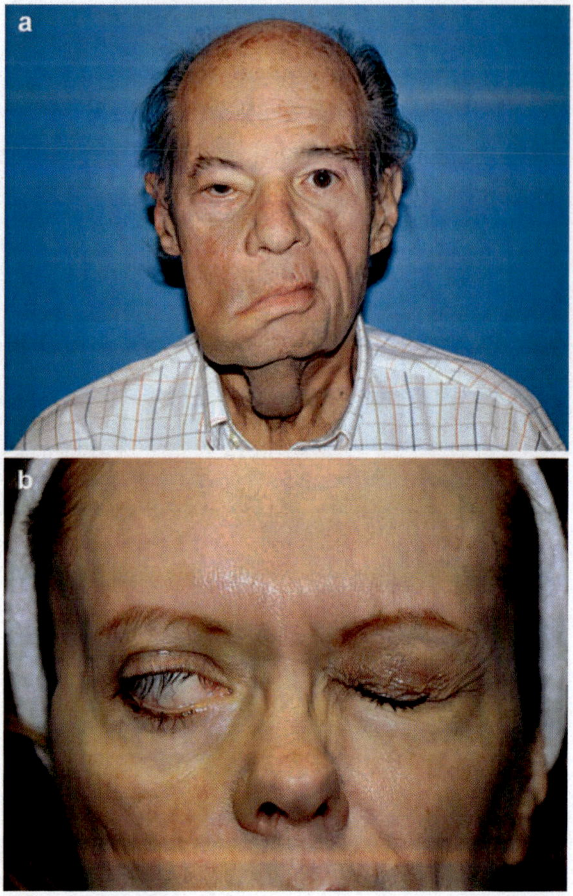

Fig. 30.4 (**a**) Right facial nerve paralysis (right brow ptosis, right lower lid eversion and ectropion, asymmetric smile). (**b**) Patient with facial paralysis who developed severe lagophthalmos and Bell's phenomenon to protect the cornea

blepharoplasty may lessen the functional and cosmetic deficits following injury to this nerve [6].

The zygomatic branch of the facial nerve travels in the direction of the lateral canthus and provides innervation to the lower portion of the orbicularis oculi, procerus, and nasalis muscles. Muscles of the midface and lip elevators, specifically the depressor septi, nasalis, levator labii superioris alaeque nasi, levator labii superioris, zygomaticus major/minor, buccinator, orbicularis oris, and levator anguli oris muscles, are supplied by the buccal division of the facial nerve [2, 4]. It should be noted that the exact muscles supplied by the buccal and zygomatic divisions of the facial nerve may vary among individuals, and these branches arborize and anastomose with one another.

The buccal and zygomatic branches may be more susceptible to injury as they travel over the buccal fat pad. In this location, they run rather superficially and are only covered by a thin fascia and risorius muscle which may be of variable thickness or even absent in some individuals [4]. If the zygomatic branch is disrupted, one may experience difficulty tightly closing the lower eyelid. Weakness of the lip elevators, buccinators, or nasal muscles is less common due to significant anastomoses with the buccal branch of the facial nerve.

Another branch of the facial nerve particularly susceptible to injury is the marginal mandibular ramus due its superficial location as well as its lack of anastomoses with other branches. It is responsible for innervating the risorius, orbicularis oris, depressor anguli oris, depressor labii inferioris, mentalis, and platysma muscles. This branch exits the inferior aspect of the parotid gland and maintains a superficial course as it travels over the masseter muscle near the angle of the mandible. In this location, it is only covered by skin, subcutaneous fat, and fascia. The marginal mandibular nerve then courses over the body of the mandible where it is covered superficially by platysma muscle (Fig. 30.3). The thickness of the platysma muscle is relatively unpredictable and may only present as a layer of fascia. In approximately 20% of individuals, the marginal mandibular nerve travels 1–2 cm and rarely up to 4 cm below the mandible [5]. The nerve may also be translocated below the angle of the mandible in surgical positioning if the head is hyperextended and rotated contralaterally [1]. Marginal mandibular nerve injury

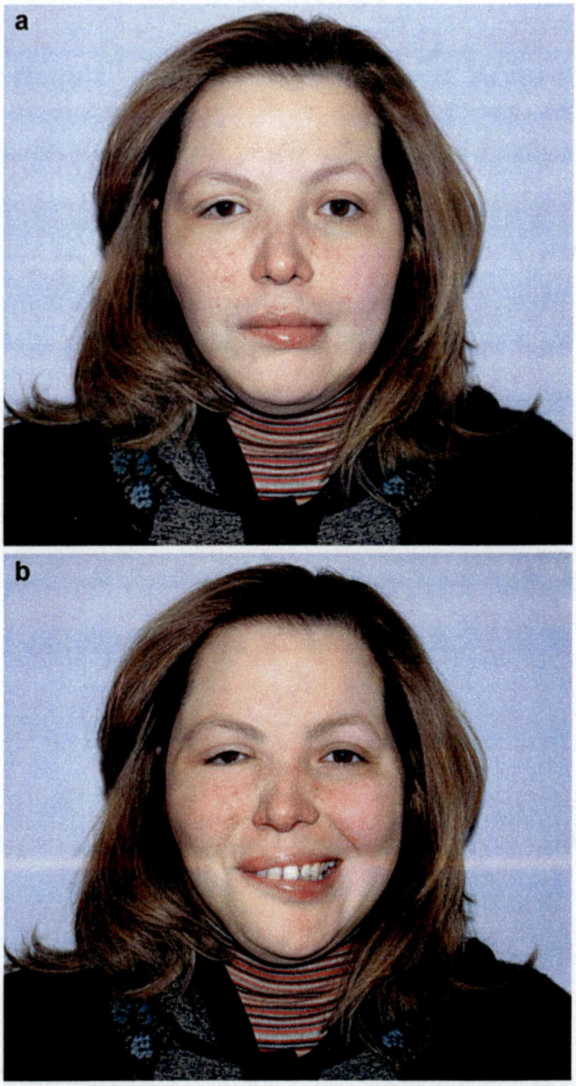

Fig. 30.5 (a and b) Marginal mandibular nerve injury (a – at rest, b – full smile)

results in an asymmetric smile (Fig. 30.5a, b). When smiling is attempted, there is an inability to pull down the ipsilateral lip or evert the vermillion border, creating the appearance of a smirk. At rest, there may be little obvious deformity. The final branch of the facial nerve is the cervical division which innervates the platysma muscle and is of little functional significance [4].

Motor nerve injury may lead to permanent anatomic defects, especially if a nerve root or a large, proximal, or non-anastomosing nerve branch is transected. Generally, nerves located medially to a line from the lateral canthus to the angle of the mouth are relatively protected from permanent damage either by overlying musculature or sufficient anastomoses. Temporary motor nerve paralysis from local anesthesia may last several hours following injection. Neuropraxia, or injury to a nerve secondary to stretching, is reversible but may take up to 6 months to recover. Permanent nerve injury may be differentiated from temporary nerve injury by inability to mount adequate muscle contraction on nerve stimulation test [4].

30.2.2 Sensory Innervation of the Face and Scalp

The trigeminal nerve (cranial nerve V) provides sensory innervation to the face and anterior scalp as well as motor innervation to the muscles of mastication. Prior to exiting the skull, it divides into three main branches: the ophthalmic (V1), maxillary (V2), and mandibular (V3) divisions (Fig. 30.6). Several branches of the trigeminal nerve exit the skull through foramina located along the midpupillary line, providing specific locations for effective regional nerve blocks. Sensory nerves are located more superficially than the motor branches of the facial nerve; hence, they are more susceptible to trauma [6].

Prior to exiting the orbit, the first branch of the trigeminal nerve, the ophthalmic nerve (V1), divides into three rami: the frontal, nasociliary, and lacrimal nerves. The frontal branch is the largest branch and a continuation of V1. Within the skull, it subdivides, giving off the supratrochlear and supraorbital nerves. The supratrochlear nerve exits the orbit approximately 1 cm lateral to the midline, piercing the corrugator muscle and traveling superiorly. This branch innervates the medial aspects of the forehead, scalp, conjunctiva, and upper eyelid. The supraorbital nerve exits via the supraorbital foramen at the superior orbital rim approximately 2.5 cm lateral to the midline. It provides innervation to the scalp, forehead, conjunctiva, and upper eyelids [4, 6]. The nasociliary branch bifurcates to give rise to the infratrochlear nerve as well as the anterior ethmoidal nerve, which innervates the upper nasal and septal mucosa and terminates as the external nasal nerve. The infratrochlear branch leaves the skull superiorly to the medial canthus and supplies sensation to the nasal root and medial canthal region. The external nasal branch of the anterior ethmoidal nerve exits onto the nose between the nasal bone and superior lateral nasal cartilage and provides sensory innervation to the nasal dorsum, supra-tip, tip, and columella. The lacrimal nerve exits at the superolateral aspect of the orbital

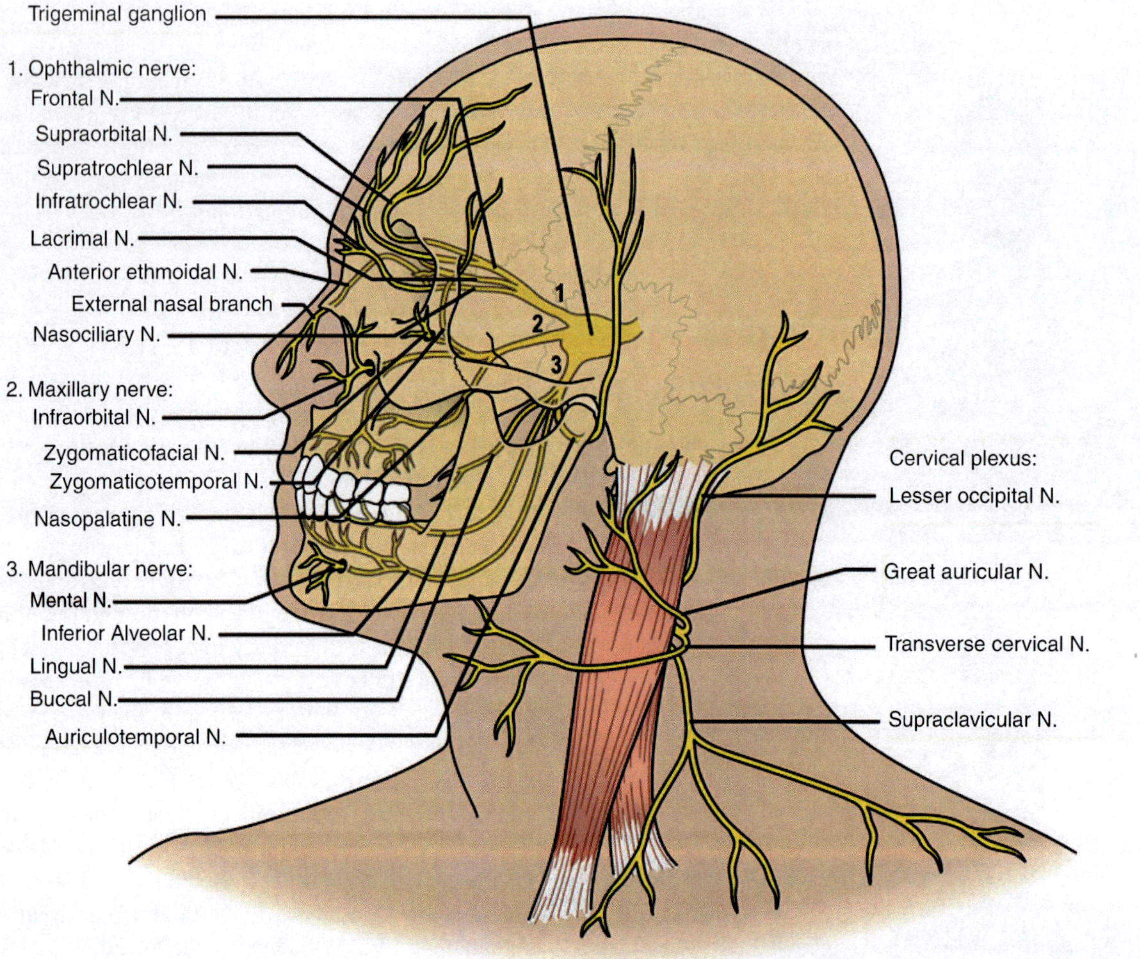

Fig. 30.6 Branches of the trigeminal nerve

rim and supplies sensation to the lateral upper lid, conjunctiva, and lateral forehead (Fig. 30.7) [6, 7].

The sensory innervation of the midface is supplied by the maxillary (V2) division of the trigeminal nerve. This nerve exits the middle cranial fossa via the foramen rotundum, giving off two small branches, the zygomaticotemporal and the zygomaticofacial nerves. The zygomaticotemporal nerve exits the skull near the lateral orbital margin and provides sensory innervation to the anterior temple and supratemporal scalp, and the zygomaticofacial nerve emerges from the zygomatic bone, lateral to the infraorbital foramen, to innervate the malar eminence and a portion of the lateral canthus. The maxillary division of the trigeminal nerve then courses through the infraorbital canal at the floor of the orbit, giving off branches to the upper alveolus, gingival mucosa, palate, and nasal floor and finally exits the skull through the infraorbital foramen. These terminal branches supply sensory innervation to the lower eyelid, conjunctiva, medial cheek, nasal ala, upper lip, and superior labial mucosa (Fig. 30.7) [2, 4]. The infraorbital foramen is located at the midpupillary line 2.5 cm lateral to the midline and 1 cm inferior to the lower orbital rim. A regional nerve block may be performed at this location either through a percutaneous or an intraoral approach.

The mandibular nerve (V3) is the largest and most complex branch of the trigeminal nerve. It not only provides sensory innervation but is also responsible for motor innervation of the muscles of mastication (the temporalis, masseter, and medial and lateral pterygoid muscles), the tensor tympani, and the tensor veli palatini. There are three main branches of the mandibular nerve: the auriculotemporal, buccal, and inferior alveo-

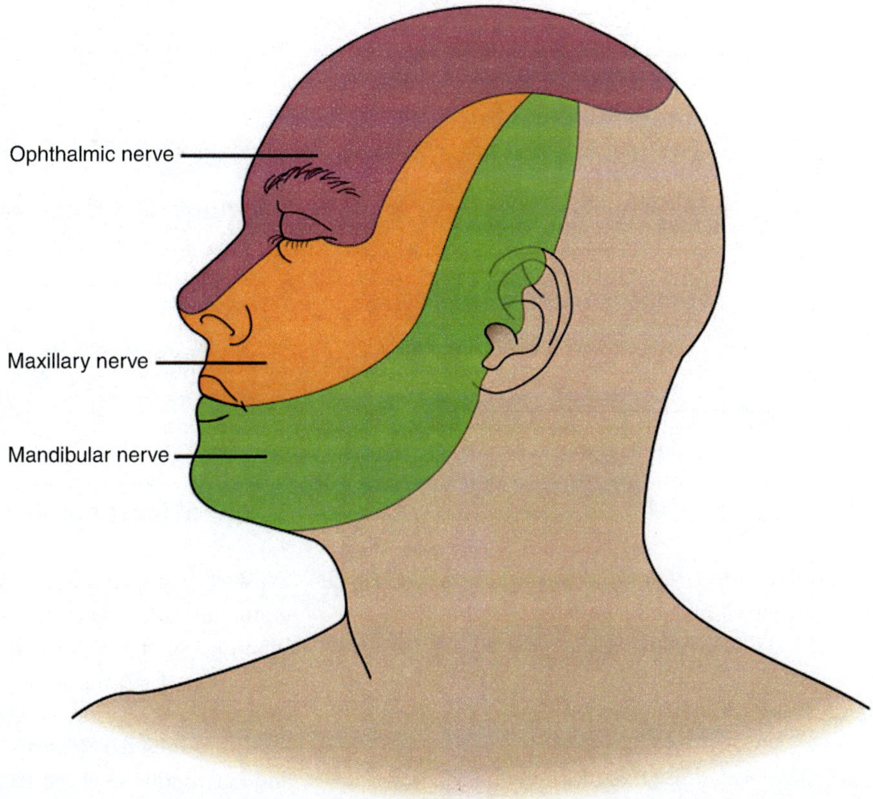

Fig. 30.7 Sensory distribution of the trigeminal nerve

lar branches. The auriculotemporal nerve is a branch of the posterior trunk of the mandibular nerve which emerges inferiorly to the zygomatic arch to course superficially, just deep to the superficial temporal artery. It travels superiorly over the zygomatic arch and anterior to the ear, providing innervation to the posterior temple, temporoparietal scalp, upper one-third of the auricle, tympanic membrane, and the anterior portion of the external ear and external auditory canal (Fig. 30.7). Interestingly, the auriculotemporal nerve also possesses parasympathetic secretomotor fibers which innervate the parotid gland. Disruption and misdirection of these fibers to sweat glands may lead to Frey syndrome [5].

The buccal branch of the mandibular nerve initially courses deep to the parotid gland then travels more superficially over the surface of the buccal fat pad and buccinator muscle. It provides sensation to the skin of the mid-cheek then pierces the buccinator, traveling inferiorly to supply the buccal and gingival mucosa. The inferior alveolar branch terminates as the mental nerve after coursing through the mandible to supply sensation to the lower teeth. The mental nerve exits the mandible through the mental foramen, innervating the skin of the chin, the lower lip, and the inferior labial mucosa. A mental nerve block may be performed by locating the mental foramen, which is approximately 2.5 cm lateral to the midline in the center of the mandible or inferior to the second premolar if the intraoral approach is preferred [6].

Sensory innervation to the scalp is provided by branches of the trigeminal nerve as well as the cervical plexus. These nerves course through the scalp at the level of the subcutaneous fat and travel centripetally. Caution must be taken in this region as transections of these nerve branches may lead to large areas of permanent hypoesthesia. Several branches of the trigeminal nerve are responsible for sensory innervation to the scalp. The supratrochlear and supraorbital nerves, branches of V1, supply the central scalp extending anteriorly from the forehead as far as the vertex. The temporal scalp is innervated by the zygomaticotemporal nerve, a division of V2, as well as the auriculotemporal branch of V3. The lesser occipital nerve is a branch of the cervical plexus (C2) which emerges posterior to the sternocleidomastoid muscle and travels superiorly to supply sensation to the lateral scalp posterior to the ear. The greater occipital nerve is a branch of C2 and C3 which supplies the occipital scalp to the

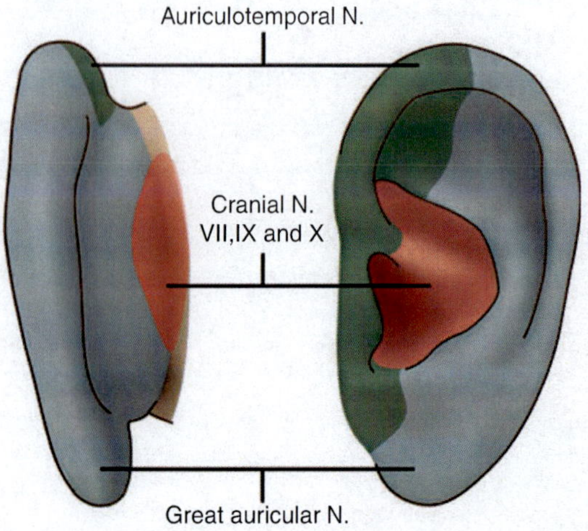

Fig. 30.8 Innervation of the auricle

level of the vertex. The third occipital nerve, a branch of C3, supplies the midline occipital scalp [8].

30.2.3 Innervation of the Ear

Extrinsic muscles of the ear include the anterior, superior, and posterior auricular muscles. They are innervated by branches of the facial nerve but possess little functional importance. The sensory innervation of the external ear is quite complex and comprised of contributions from several different nerves including the trigeminal, facial, glossopharyngeal, and vagus nerves as well as the cervical plexus (C2 and C3). Anteriorly, the auriculotemporal nerve, a branch of V3, supplies sensation to the skin overlying the tragus, anterior helix, anterior and superior external auditory canal, and a portion of the external surface of the tympanic membrane. A majority of the anterior auricle as well as the posterolateral auricle is innervated by the great auricular nerve, a branch of C2 and C3. The lesser occipital nerve also provides sensory innervation to the skin overlying the mastoid process. The conchal bowl, posterior external auditory meatus, posterior tympanic membrane, and the posterior auricular sulcus are supplied by the sensory fibers from the seventh, ninth, and tenth cranial nerves (Fig. 30.8) [4, 9, 10]. Adequate local anesthesia of the auricle, with the exception of the conchal bowl, may be obtained by injecting a ring of anesthesia circumferentially around the base of the ear including the posterior auricular sulcus. The conchal bowl and external auditory canal must be anesthetized separately.

Summary: Muscles of Facial Expression

- Muscles of facial expression enable human beings to communicate nonverbally and aid in functions such as lacrimation, mastication, and speech.
- Muscles of facial expression are encased by an interconnected, unified layer of fascia, forming the superficial musculoaponeurotic system (SMAS) which allows them to work synergistically or antagonistically with one another.

30.3 Muscles of Facial Expression

Muscles of facial expression enable human beings to communicate nonverbally. In addition, they aid in functions such as lacrimation, mastication, speech, and protection of vital structures such as the mouth and eye (Fig. 30.9a, b). Injury to the motor nerves that supply these muscles can lead to devastating consequences, and knowledge of these structures is of utmost importance to the cutaneous surgeon. Unlike muscles of the body, which originate and insert on the bony structures which they act upon, the muscles of facial expression may originate on bone but insert directly onto the skin, other soft tissue structures, or adjoining muscles [1, 4]. This unique characteristic allows for the formation of skin tension lines. Muscles of facial expression are encased by an interconnected, unified layer of fascia, forming the superficial musculoaponeurotic system (SMAS) which allows them to work synergistically or antagonistically with one another.

30.3.1 Muscles of the Forehead

The muscles of the forehead include the frontalis, the corrugator supercilii, and the procerus muscles. The frontalis muscle originates at the frontal hairline where it is directly connected to the galea aponeurotica, a fibrous band of connective tissue that spans across the length of the scalp, connecting to the occipitalis muscle posteriorly. Collectively, this muscle may be termed the "occipitofrontalis" muscle. The frontalis muscle serves to raise the forehead and eyebrows and contributes to horizontal wrinkling of the forehead (Table 30.1).

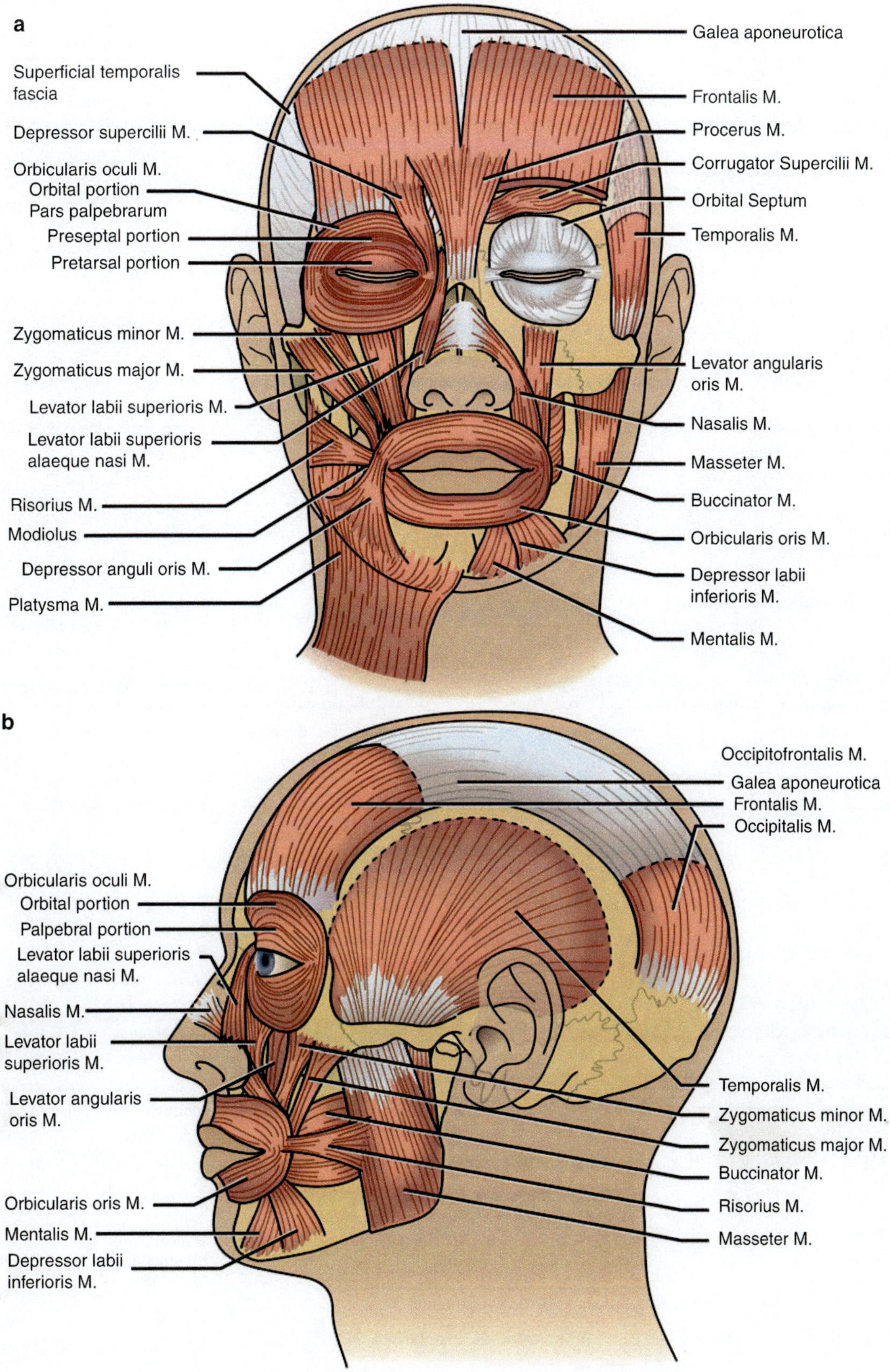

Fig. 30.9 (**a**) Muscles of facial expression (*frontal view*). (**b**) Muscles of facial expression (*lateral view*)

Table 30.1 Action and innervation of the muscles of facial expression [1, 4, 6, 13]

Muscle	Action	Innervation
I. Muscles influencing the forehead and eyebrow		
1. Frontalis m.	Raises forehead and eyebrow	Temporal branch of CN VII
2. Corrugator supercilii m.	Pulls brows medially and downward	Temporal branch of CN VII
3. Procerus m.	Pulls medial brows and central forehead downward	Zygomatic branch of CN VII
II. Muscles influencing the eyelid		
1. Orbicularis oculi m.	Palpebral portion – voluntary gentle closure of the eyelids, involuntary blink reflex	Superiorly – Temporal branch of CN VII
	Orbital portion – voluntary tight closure of the eyelids	Inferiorly – Zygomatic branch of CN VII
2. Levator palpebrae superioris m.	Eyelid elevation	Oculomotor nerve
3. Frontalis m.	Opens the eyelid widely	Temporal branch of CN VII
III. Muscles influencing the ear (rudimentary in most individuals)		
1. Posterior auricular m.	Draws ear posteriorly	Posterior auricular branch of CN VII
2. Anterior auricular m.	Draws ear anteriorly and superiorly	Temporal branch of CN VII
3. Superior auricular m.	Draws skin of temples posteriorly	Temporal branch of CN VII
IV. Muscles influencing the nose		
1. Procerus m.	Shortens the nose	Zygomatic branch of CN VII
2. Nasalis m.	Tightens skin over nasal bridge, flares nostrils, opens nasal aperture during deep inspiration	Zygomatic branch of CN VII – alar portion Buccal branch of CN VII – transverse portion
3. Levator labii superioris alaeque nasi m.	Flares nostrils	Buccal branch of CN VII
4. Depressor septi m.	Pulls columella inferiorly	Buccal branch of CN VII
V. Muscles influencing the mouth		
1. Orbicularis oris m.	Purses and puckers the lips, draws corners of the mouth inward, aids in speech and pronunciation	Buccal branch of CN VII Marginal mandibular branch of CN VII
2. Buccinator m.	Presses cheek to teeth while chewing, preventing food accumulation, prevents overdistension of cheeks in instances of increased intraoral pressure	Buccal branch of CN VII
3. Lip elevators		
(a) Levator labii superioris alaeque nasi m.	Elevates upper lip	Buccal branch of CN VII
(b) Levator labii superioris m.	Elevates upper lip	Buccal branch of CN VII
(c) Zygomaticus major m.	Elevates upper lip and pulls it laterally	Buccal branch of CN VII
(d) Zygomaticus minor m.	Elevates upper lip and pulls it laterally	Buccal branch of CN VII
(e) Levator anguli oris m.	Draws the corner of the mouth laterally	Buccal branch of CN VII
(f) Risorius m.	Draws the corner of the mouth laterally	Buccal branch of CN VII
4. Lip depressors		
(a) Depressor anguli oris m.	Depresses lower lip and pulls mouth laterally and downward	Marginal mandibular branch of CN VII
(b) Depressor labii inferioris m.	Depresses and retracts lower lip	Marginal mandibular branch of CN VII
(c) Platysma m.	Tenses the skin of the neck	Cervical branch of CN VII
5. Lower lip elevator		
(a) Mentalis m.	Elevates lower lip and wrinkles chin	Marginal mandibular branch of CN VII

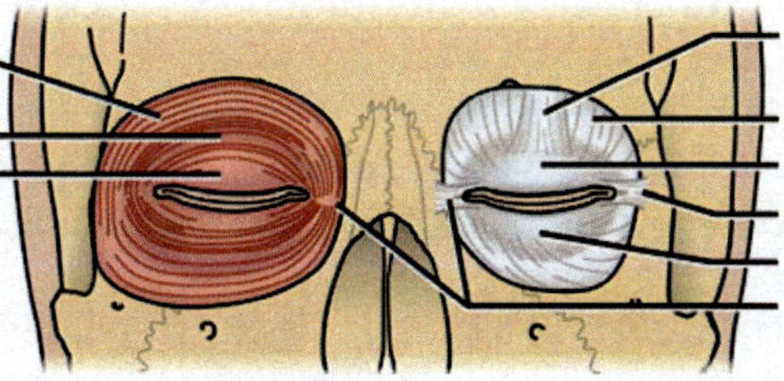

Fig. 30.10 Periocular musculature and connective tissue structures

It is divided into left and right bellies, which insert into the skin of the forehead as well as the corrugator, procerus, and orbicularis oculi muscles. Motor innervation of the frontalis muscle is provided by the temporal branch of the facial nerve [6].

The corrugator supercilii is a "V"-shaped muscle that originates on the frontal bone medial to the eyebrows. It travels superior to the brow, running deep to the frontalis, procerus, and orbicularis muscles and eventually inserts into the skin of the medial brow. It is responsible for pulling the brows medially and downward and creates a scowl and vertical rhytides overlying the glabella. The procerus muscle is a solitary muscle, originating from the superior nasal bones and lateral cartilage and inserting into the skin overlying the nasal root as well as the aponeurosis of the nasalis muscle [4]. It pulls the medial brows and forehead skin downward, creating horizontal furrows overlying the nasal root and bridge [6].

30.3.2 Muscles of the Periorbital Region

The orbicularis oculi muscle is the most important muscle governing eyelid function. It is subdivided into orbital, preseptal, and pretarsal segments based on their relationship to the orbit, septum, and tarsal plates. The pretarsal and preseptal components collectively comprise the pars palpebrarum, which is involved in involuntary blinking and voluntary gentle closure of the eyelid (Fig. 30.10). When tight closure of the eyelid is necessary, the orbital component of the muscle may be elicited voluntarily.

The preseptal and pretarsal portions of the orbicularis oculi muscle arise from two heads. The superficial heads converge to form the medial canthal tendon, and the deep heads pass posterior to the lacrimal sac, attaching to the lacrimal diaphragm and lacrimal crest, respectively. Contraction of these muscles with blinking augments the pumping mechanism and tear flow in the lacrimal apparatus. Both the pretarsal and preseptal segments insert into the ligamentous attachments at the lateral canthus [11]. The orbital portion of the orbicularis oculi muscle originates from the medial orbital margin and medial canthal tendon. Superiorly, this muscle intertwines with the procerus, frontalis, and corrugator supercilii muscles. Laterally, it connects to the superficial temporalis fascia, and it extends variable distances inferiorly on the cheek [4, 12].The levator palpebrae superioris, although not considered a muscle of facial expression, is vital to proper eyelid function. This muscle originates within the inner orbit and serves to open the eyelid. It receives its motor innervations from the oculomotor or third cranial nerve. If the motor innervation to the orbicularis oculi muscle is disrupted, the levator palpebrae superioris muscle acts unopposed leading to chronic lid elevation [1].

30.3.3 Muscles of the Nose

The muscles of the nose are highly variable in their development among different individuals. The procerus muscle, as discussed previously, extends inferiorly from the paired frontalis muscle to insert in the skin overlying the nasal root and the aponeurosis of the nasalis muscle. Upon contraction, it shortens the nose and creates horizontal "bunny lines" overlying the nasal root. The nasalis muscle is the deepest muscle of the nose, originating on the maxillary bone. This muscle consists of a transverse and alar component. The transverse component travels over the nasal bridge where it inserts into an aponeurosis, decussating with fibers from the contralateral side. It serves to tense the skin over the dorsal nose. The alar portion of the nasalis muscle inserts into the lateral crus of the alar cartilage and assists in flaring the nostril [4]. The depressor septi muscle inserts at the septal cartilage and lies deep to the orbicularis oris muscle. It is thought to displace the nasal septum inferiorly upon deep inspiration as well as draw the columella downwards [13].

30.3.4 Muscles of the Cheek and Perioral Region

The muscles of the mouth constitute an intricate framework of interconnected synergistic and antagonistic muscle groups that enable individual to communicate both verbally and nonverbally with the world. These muscles may be further subdivided into muscles that function to elevate or depress the mouth. The lip elevators and depressors typically insert into the orbicularis oris, a large muscle surrounding the circumference of the mouth which does not possess attachments to bony or cartilaginous structures, allowing for a significant amount of mobility [4, 13].

The muscles of the upper mouth consist of six structures that serve to elevate the lips or retract and elevate the angle of the mouth. The buccal branch of the facial nerve provides motor innervation to these muscles. The four lip elevators in this group consist of the levator labii superioris alaeque nasi, the levator labii superioris, the zygomaticus minor, and the zygomaticus major muscles. Two muscles that function to retract and raise the oral commissures are the levator anguli oris and risorius muscles [4, 6].

The levator labii superioris alaeque nasi muscle originates on the medial maxillary bone and divides into two heads. The medial portion of the levator labii superioris alaeque nasi inserts into the alar cartilage and skin overlying the alar rim and aids in flaring the nostril. The lateral division of this muscle inserts at the medial aspect of the orbicularis oris muscle as well as the skin of the upper cutaneous lip and aids in elevation of the upper lip. The levator labii superioris arises at the infraorbital portion of the maxilla and inserts more laterally into the orbicularis oris muscle and the skin of the upper lip. It also functions to raise the upper lip. The zygomaticus major muscle originates laterally on the zygoma beneath the orbicularis oculi muscle. It travels inferiorly and medial over the masseter and buccinator muscles to insert at the lateral orbicularis oris muscle and skin at the oral commissure. It not only elevates the lip but also draws it laterally, enabling one to smile. The zygomaticus minor muscle originates at the zygomatic bone inferiorly and medially to the zygomaticus major. It travels superiorly and parallel to this muscle to insert medially to the angle of the mouth at the orbicularis oris muscle and overlying skin and functions identically to its counterpart. The zygomaticus muscles are also predominately responsible for creation of the nasolabial fold [6].

The levator anguli oris muscle lies more deeply than the remaining lip elevators, originating from the canine fossa of the maxilla and inserting at the orbicularis oris and overlying skin just inferior to the angle of the mouth. The risorius muscle is a thin, poorly developed muscle which is occasionally absent in individuals, especially African-Americans. It originates in the soft tissue overlying the parotid gland and inserts at the corner of the mouth. It may also be continuous with the platysma. These muscles draw the corner of the mouth laterally. The modiolus is formed from the convergence of the lip elevators, depressors, and the orbicularis oris muscles, and it is typically located approximately 1 cm lateral to the oral commissure [13].

The buccinator muscle spans across a large portion of the cheek, originating posterior and medially to the last molar at the alveolar process of the maxilla and the medial mandible at the convergence of the body and ramus. This muscle inserts into the orbicularis oris muscle as well as the skin of the lips and the labial mucosa and functions to press the cheek against the teeth while chewing, preventing food accumulation. It also acts to prevent overdistension of the cheeks in situations of increased intraoral pressure (i.e., playing a musical instrument). The buccinator and orbicularis oris muscle act synergistically, allowing one to whistle [4].

The orbicularis oris is a large, circumferential muscle surrounding the mouth. It serves as a sphincter, allowing for pursing and puckering of the lips and pulling the corners of the mouth inward. It is also important in speech and annunciation, aiding in the pronunciation of the letters M, V, F, P, B, and O. This muscle originates from and interdigitates with numerous muscles surrounding the mouth as well as the modiolus [4, 14].

The muscles of the lower lip include the depressor labii inferioris, the depressor anguli oris, and the mentalis muscles. The depressor labii inferioris originates from the mandible medial to the mental foramen and inserts into the orbicularis oris as well as the skin and labial mucosa. It functions to depress and retract the lower lip [2]. The depressor anguli oris originates from the mandible, lateral to the mental foramen and inferior to the canine tooth and first and second premolars, and inserts into the orbicularis oris and skin. This muscle acts by depressing the lower lip and pulling the corner of the mouth laterally. Over time, this muscle may contribute to the formation of marionette lines. The mentalis muscle originates from the mandible, traveling inferiorly to insert on the skin of the lower chin. It enables wrinkling

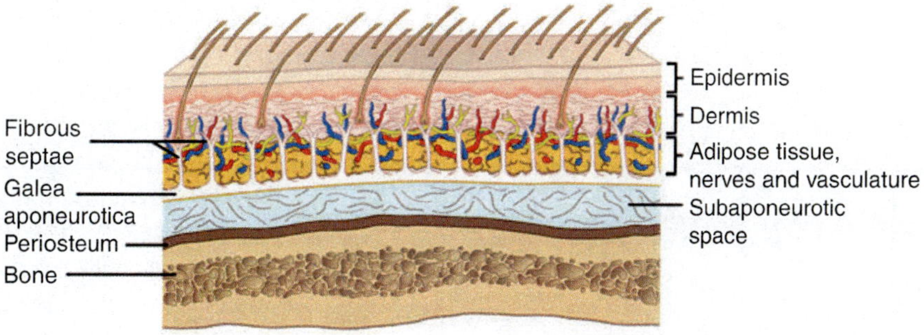

Fig. 30.11 Layers of the scalp

of the chin and chin elevation. There may be a small separation between the left and right bodies of this muscle, causing a dimpled or clefted appearance of the chin. The platysma muscle extends from the superficial fascia of the chest inferior to the clavicle and travels over the anterolateral neck and mandible to insert with the muscles of the lower lip. It is also continuous with the SMAS of the lower face. Contraction of the platysma leads to tensing of the skin of the neck, and it derives its innervation from the cervical branch of the facial nerve [1, 13].

Summary: Soft Tissue Components of the Scalp and Face

- The scalp consists of five soft tissue layers including the skin, connective tissue (fat), aponeurosis (galea aponeurotica), loose connective tissue (subgaleal compartment), and periosteum.
- The soft tissue structures of the face include the skin, the superficial and deep subcutaneous fat, superficial fascia, and deep fascia.
- The superficial musculoaponeurotic system, or SMAS, is a fibromuscular layer which connects to the overlying skin via vertically oriented fibers, allowing the muscles and soft tissues of the face to move together as a unit.

30.4 Soft Tissue Components of the Scalp and Face

30.4.1 Scalp

The scalp consists of five soft tissue layers which can be easily remembered using the pneumonic "SCALP." This denotes the skin (epidermis and dermis), connective tissue (fat), aponeurosis (galea aponeurotica), loose connective tissue (subgaleal compartment), and periosteum (Fig. 30.11). The fatty layer of the scalp consists of collections of fat lobules separated by fibrous septae which connect the skin to the underlying galea, creating a dense, compact structure. Blood vessels, nerves, and lymphatics travel within the fibrous septae in the subcutaneous layer. The septae bind tightly to scalp blood vessels, inhibiting vasospasm and rapid hemostasis in the event of scalp injury. The galea of the scalp is a strong, dense, inelastic connective tissue layer and is contiguous with the SMAS of the face. It also serves as an aponeurosis between the frontalis and occipitalis muscles as described previously. Anteriorly, the galea inserts into the supraorbital ridge, and posteriorly, it attaches to the highest nuchal line. Laterally, it envelops the temporoparietalis muscle and is contiguous with the temporalis fascia. Dissection and undermining beneath the galea is relatively simple given the loose, relatively avascular areolar tissue in the subgaleal space, allowing for increased scalp mobility for closures [1, 8].

30.4.2 Face

The soft tissue structures of the face include the skin, the superficial and deep subcutaneous fat, superficial fascia, and deep fascia. The superficial facial fat lies superiorly to the SMAS and is composed of distinct compartments including the central, middle, and lateral temporal-cheek fat of the forehead and cheek and the jowl fat of the lower face [15]. Fibrous septae divide fatty lobules and compartments. These septae are extensions of superficial fascia, and nerves and blood vessels course within them. The superficial fatty layer tends to vary in thickness depending on region and the

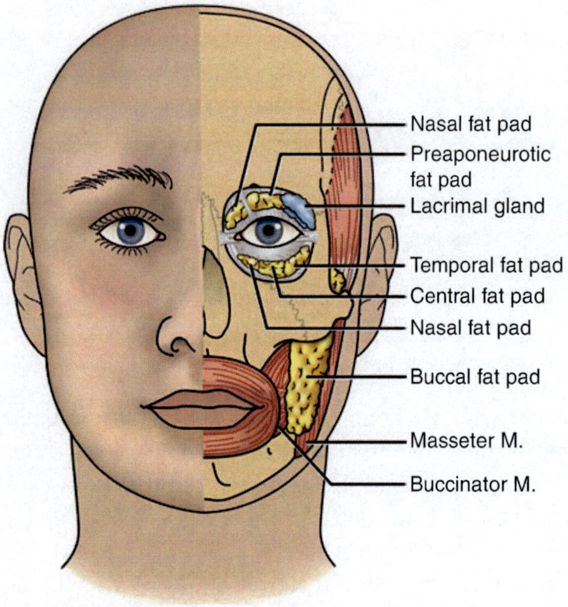

Fig. 30.12 Deep fatty structures of the face

individual. It is most prominent over the temples, concavities of the cheeks, and the neck region and negligible over the eyelid and post-auricular region [1, 16].

The deeper fatty layers of the face include the buccal fat pad as well as the sub-orbicularis oculi and retro-orbicularis oculi fat. This tissue runs deep to the SMAS and is comprised of more loosely arranged fat, lacking the distinct fibrous septae of the superficial fat. Loss of deep facial fat with aging is thought to lead to alteration in facial shape and contour [16]. The buccal fat pad overlies the posterolateral portion of the maxillary bone lateral to the buccinator muscle. It functions to provide volume to the cheek as well as augment the actions of the muscles of mastication by acting as a smooth gliding surface. The deep fatty layers of the orbit are separated from the anterior portion of the eyelid by the orbital septum. This septum atrophies with age, leading to anterior displacement and "pseudoherniation" of fat pads within the orbit. The superior orbit contains two distinct fat pads, the nasal and preaponeurotic fat pads, and the lacrimal gland occupies the lateralmost compartment. Inferiorly, there are three separate fat pads including the nasal, central, and temporal fat pads (Fig. 30.12). Each structure is separated by a thin layer of fascia. Care must be taken to distinguish the lacrimal gland at the lateral aspect of the superior orbit as this may be confused with fatty tissue [5, 15, 16, 17].

The superficial musculoaponeurotic system, or SMAS, is a fibromuscular layer which connects to the overlying skin via vertically oriented fibers, allowing the muscles and soft tissues of the face to move together as a unit [18, 19]. The SMAS extends superiorly from the platysma to the temporalis and frontalis muscles and from the orbicularis oculi muscle to the trapezius muscle posteriorly [6, 20]. It becomes thin and discontinuous in the central face and develops a thicker, inelastic consistency in areas without underlying musculature, forming the superficial temporalis fascia and galea aponeurotica. Sensory nerves and axial arteries typically lie within the SMAS whereas motor nerves travel deep to this layer. The deep fascia of the face is derived from the deep cervical fascia. It forms a continuous immobile layer consisting of periosteum, perichondrium, and the investing fascia of the muscles of mastication [13].

Summary: Bony and Cartilaginous Structures of the Face and Scalp

- The structure of the face is largely determined by the underlying bony structures which serve as important anatomic landmarks.
- The structure and functional support of the nose is provided by its bony and cartilaginous skeleton. The superior one-third of the nose consists of two paired nasal bones whereas the structural support for the distal portion of the nose is comprised of cartilage and fibrofatty tissue.
- With the exception of the earlobe, which does not contain cartilage, the structure of the auricle is created by a single fragment of elastic cartilage.

30.5 Bony and Cartilaginous Structures of the Face and Scalp

30.5.1 Bony Landmarks

The shape of the face is largely determined by the underlying bony structures (Fig. 30.13). These structures may also serve as important landmarks, and

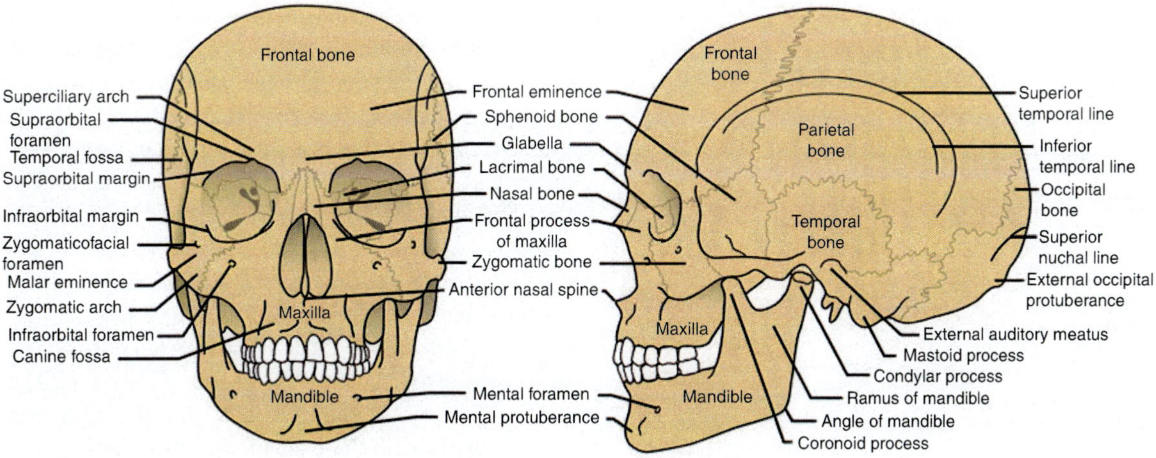

Fig. 30.13 Bony landmarks of the skull

knowledge of the bony topography is invaluable to the cutaneous surgeon. The external calvarium is comprised of the frontal, sphenoid, parietal, and occipital bones which are separated by cranial sutures. These bones, with the exception of the sphenoid, dictate the nomenclature by which the various regions of overlying scalp are referred. The occipital bone possesses a medial prominence termed the occipital protuberance. Lateral to this structure are two ridges termed the highest and superior nuchal lines. The highest nuchal line serves as the bony attachment of the occipitofrontalis muscle. The frontal and parietal bones possess two slightly elevated ridges called the inferior and superior temporal lines. These prominences serve as the superior attachment points for the temporalis muscle and temporalis fascia, respectively, which overly the temporal fossa. The mastoid process is the inferiormost portion of the temporal bone, and it protects the facial nerve as it emerges from the skull. It also serves as an attachment point for the occipitalis muscle [1, 4].

The frontal bone comprises the forehead and anterior scalp. Inferiorly, it also forms the orbital roof and supraorbital margin. The supraciliary arches are rounded prominences deep to the eyebrows which meet centrally to form the glabella. Inferiorly to these prominences lies the superior orbital rim which terminates laterally at the zygomatic process. The supraorbital notch may be palpated along the superior orbital rim, approximately 2.5 cm from the midline [20]. The lateral orbit is formed by the zygomatic process of the frontal bone and the frontal process of the zygomatic bone. Medially, the orbital rim is formed by the maxillary process of the frontal bone, the frontal process of the maxillary bone, and the lacrimal bone. A fossa formed by the lacrimal and maxillary bones houses the lacrimal sac. Much of the infraorbital margin and the orbital floor are comprised of the maxillary bone [20].

The maxillary bone also forms the upper jaw, lateral nasal sidewall, and the roof of the mouth. It is further subdivided into the body as well as the zygomatic, frontal, alveolar, and palatine processes. Anteriorly, the body of the maxilla houses the infraorbital foramen. The zygomatic process forms the medial cheekbone and connects laterally to the zygomatic bone. The zygomatic bone forms the zygomatic arch and lateral cheekbone as well as a portion of the lateral orbital rim and orbital floor. The frontal process of the maxilla contributes to the lateral nasal sidewall and the medial orbital rim. The alveolar process houses the upper teeth, and the palatine process comprises the hard palate [20].

The mandible constitutes the chin and jawbones and is the only mobile bone of the skull. It is made up of a body which houses the lower teeth and is connected by the angle of the mandible to a posterior ramus. The posterior ramus gives off the anterior, coronoid, and posterior condylar processes. The condylar process serves as a point of articulation of the mandible with the temporal bone. The mandible fuses centrally at the mandibular symphysis. The mental foramen is typically situated lateral to the midline, and inferior to the first and second premolars [20]. The masseter muscle attaches to the inferior aspect of the mandibular

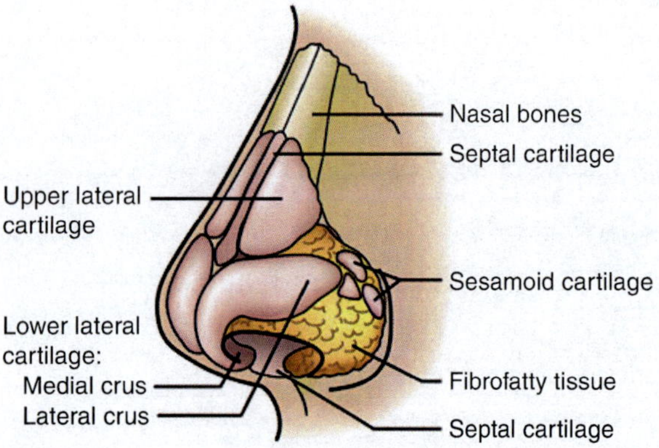

Fig. 30.14 Bony and cartilaginous structures of the nose

ramus. Anterior to the masseter, there is a shallow groove that houses the facial artery, which should be palpable at this point.

30.5.2 Cartilaginous Structures

The structure and functional support of the nose is provided by its bony and cartilaginous skeleton (Fig. 30.14). The superior one-third of the nose consists of two paired nasal bones that articulate proximally with the nasal processes of the frontal bone, laterally with the maxillary frontal processes, and inferiorly with the ethmoid bone which also forms the perpendicular plate of the nose. The perpendicular plate of the ethmoid, along with contributions from the vomer, forms the bony septum which articulates with the cartilaginous septum distally [20]. The pyriform aperture, or the opening of the nose into the skull, is formed superiorly by the nasal bones and inferolaterally by the maxilla. The proximal portions of the nasal bones are thicker, becoming progressively thin and more prone to fracture as they approach the nasal cartilage. The middle one-third of the nose consists of the paired upper and lower lateral cartilages which are continuous with one another and the septal cartilage. Proximally, lateral nasal cartilage overlaps and articulates with the nasal bone via ligamentous attachments. Laterally and distally, these cartilages connect to the nasal ala via fibrofatty tissue. The cartilaginous nasal septum is fused dorsally to the lateral cartilages with the exception of its distal portion, the septal angle, which contributes to the columella. The lobule is the most distal, mobile portion of the nose and derives its structural support from the lower lateral cartilages. The medial crura of the lower lateral cartilages comprise the columella, while the lateral crura provide structural support to the nasal ala. The point where the crura meet one another is termed the dome which forms the nasal tip. Although the lateral crura provide structural support for the nasal ala, the majority of the ala is composed of dense fibrofatty tissue without a cartilaginous component [20, 21].

With the exception of the earlobe which does not contain cartilage, the structure of the auricle is created by a single fragment of elastic cartilage (Fig. 30.15). The conchal cartilage abuts the mastoid bone, anchoring the auricle to the skull. This cartilaginous network extends to the distal portion of the external auditory meatus formed by the temporal bone [5].

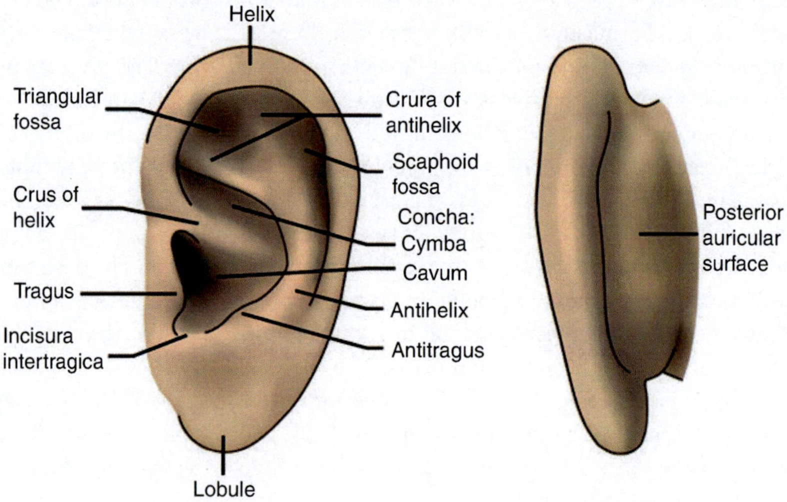

Fig. 30.15 External topography of the auricle

Summary: Muscosa of the Lip, Nose, and Conjunctiva

- It is important to close each tissue layer of the lip individually in full-thickness defects to maintain proper lip function and to prevent dead space formation.
- The eyelid is divided into an anterior lamellar division comprised of skin and orbicularis muscle and a posterior lamellar division comprised of the tarsal plate, orbital septum, and conjunctival mucosa.

30.6 Muscosa of the Lip, Nose, and Conjunctiva

The cutaneous lip is divided from the vermilion lip by the white roll, a soft tissue prominence augmented by the underlying orbicularis oris muscle. At this point, there is a conversion to a dry mucosal surface, lacking normal keratinization, follicular units, or glandular tissue. Posteriorly, the vermilion lip then transitions to form a wet mucosal surface or buccal mucosa (Fig. 30.16). It is important to close each tissue layer (skin, muscle, mucosa) individually in full-thickness lip defects to maintain proper lip function and to prevent dead space formation [4, 14].

The anterior inner naris is comprised of the vestibule lined by modified squamous epithelium. The vestibule possesses many small hairs termed vibrissae which function to filter dust and debris, inhibiting entry into the respiratory tract. Posterior to the vestibule, the inner naris becomes the nasal cavity proper, and there is a transition from stratified squamous epithelium to ciliated pseudostratified columnar epithelium. The superior, middle, and inferior nasal turbinates, ensheathed by a layer of periosteum and overlying highly vascularized epithelium, are attached to the lateral walls of the nasal cavity. The superior, middle, and inferior meatuses are crevices which run below their respective turbinates (Fig. 30.17) [22].

The eyelid is typically divided into an anterior lamellar division comprised of skin and orbicularis muscle and a posterior lamellar division made up of the tarsal plate, orbital septum, and conjunctival mucosa (Fig. 30.18). These lamellae are partitioned by a layer of

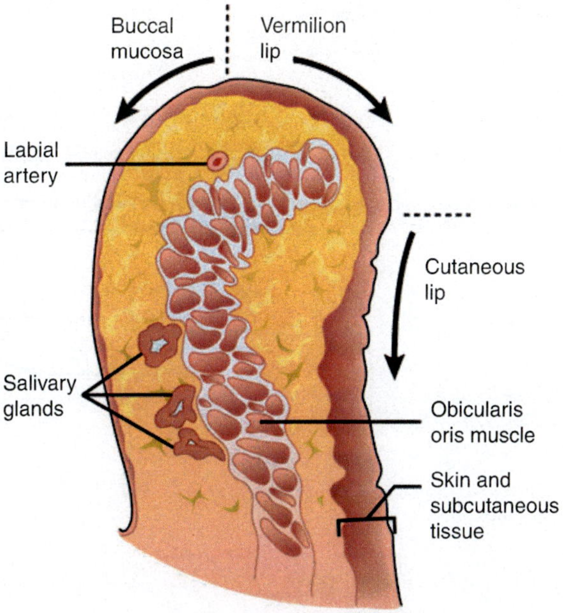

Fig. 30.16 Cross-sectional anatomy of the lip

fascia, also termed the gray line, at the lid margin. The tarsi are thick collections of fibrous tissue important for lid structure and stability. These structures also house the Meibomian (sebaceous) glands. The conjunctiva is a thin layer of mucosa that spans from the posterior aspect of the lid and is reflected inferiorly at the fornix to adhere to the anterior surface of the globe [4, 11].

Summary: Musculature, Innervation, and Bony Structures of the Neck

- The sternocleidomastoid muscle is an important anatomic landmark of the neck. It divides the neck into anterior and posterior triangles, functions to flex the neck and rotate the head contralaterally, and is innervated by the spinal accessory nerve (cranial nerve 11).
- The anterior triangle of the neck may be subdivided into the submental, submandibular, carotid, and muscular triangles.
- The spinal accessory nerve is especially susceptible to injury within the posterior triangle. Injury to this nerve leads to difficulty abducting the arm, chronic shoulder pain, and difficulty shrugging the shoulders.

Fig. 30.17 Nasal mucosal anatomy

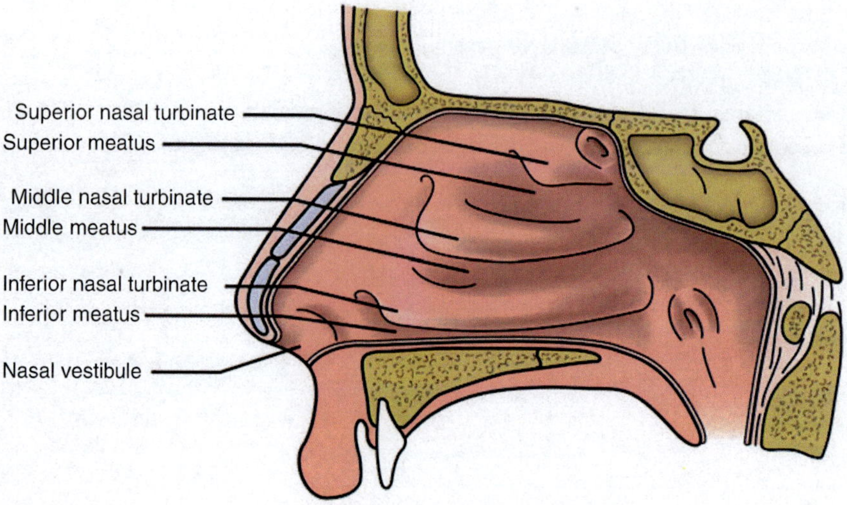

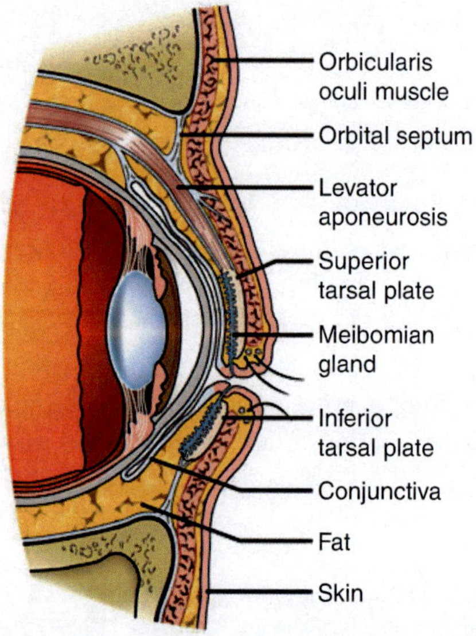

Fig. 30.18 Cross-sectional anatomy of the eyelid

30.7 Musculature, Innervation, and Bony Structures of the Neck

The neck is bounded by the clavicle and sternum inferiorly and the mandible superiorly. The hyoid bone is located just inferiorly to the mandible at the midline if the anterior neck. The thyroid cartilage, cricoid cartilage, and tracheal rings, respectively, rest below the hyoid bone. Posteriorly, the cervical vertebrae provide stability to the neck [22].

The platysma, as discussed previously, is considered a muscle of facial expression. It originates in the superficial fascia of the upper chest, covering the neck and extending over the body of the mandible to intercalate with the muscles of the lower lip. It is ensheathed by a layer of superficial fascia that is continuous with the SMAS and innervated by the cervical division of the facial nerve. There are also layers of deep cervical fascia which cover the superficial and deep muscles of the neck, brachial plexus, and laryngotracheal structures. The sternocleidomastoid muscle is an important anatomic landmark of the neck. It has two heads that attach inferiorly to the sternum and medial clavicle and travel obliquely to insert at the mastoid process of the temporal bone and lateral to the superior nuchal line of the occipital bone, respectively. This muscle divides the neck into anterior and posterior triangles, functions to flex the neck and rotate the head contralaterally, and is innervated by the spinal accessory nerve (cranial nerve 11) [4, 22].

The anterior triangle of the neck is bordered posteriorly by the sternocleidomastoid muscle, which spans from the mastoid process to the sternum, superiorly by a line extending from the mastoid process along the base of the mandible to the anterior chin, and medially by a line extending from the chin to the jugular notch. It is further subdivided into submental, submandibular, carotid, and muscular triangles (Fig. 30.19). Particular areas of concern within the anterior triangle include the facial artery within the submandibular triangle. The internal and external carotid arteries, the internal jugular vein, and the vagus nerve travel within the carotid sheath in the carotid triangle and are protected

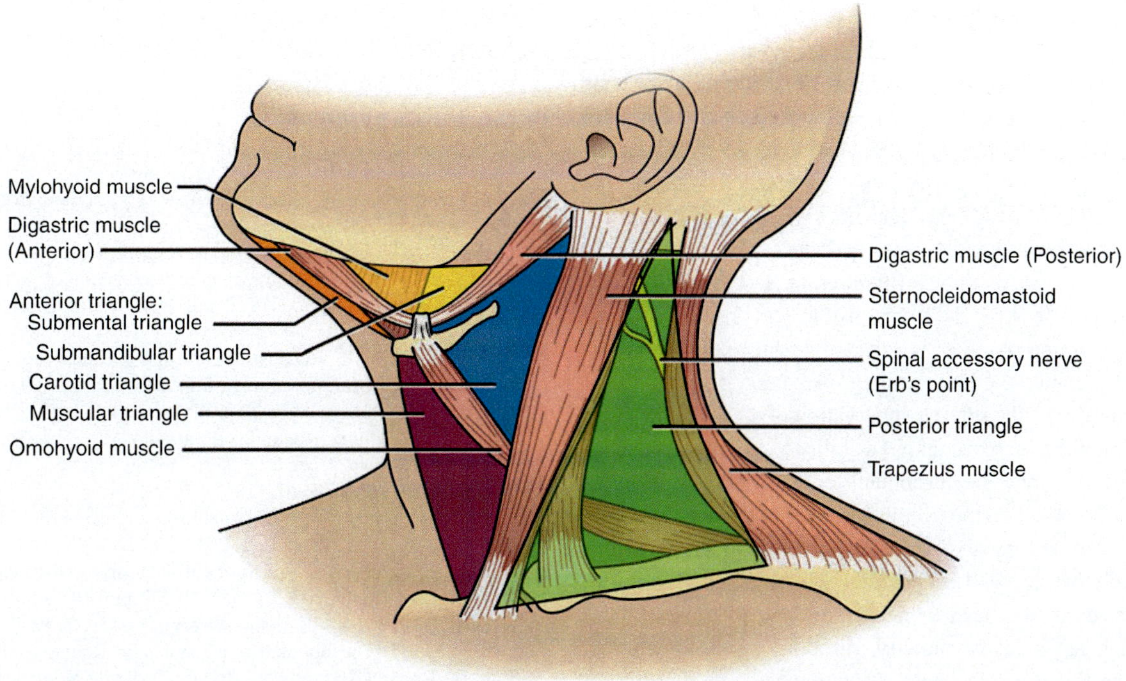

Fig. 30.19 Triangles of the neck

only by skin, platysma, and deep cervical fascia. The hypoglossal nerve is also located within the carotid triangle [4, 22].

The posterior triangle of the neck is bounded anteriorly by the sternocleidomastoid muscle, posteriorly by the anterior trapezius muscle, and inferiorly by the clavicle. Deep to the posterior triangle lay the splenius capitus, levator scapulae, and scalene muscles in addition to the brachial plexus. These structures are invested by deep cervical fascia. The spinal accessory nerve is especially susceptible to injury within this triangle. It exits the skull via the jugular notch, traveling deep to the sternocleidomastoid muscle and emerges at Erb's point, traveling over the posterior triangle to innervate the trapezius muscle. Erb's point may be estimated by drawing a horizontal line from the thyroid notch to the posterior border of the sternocleidomastoid muscle. The region spanning 2 cm above and 2 cm below this point and running the horizontal length of the posterior triangle denotes the danger zone where the nerve is most likely to be injured. Clinically, if the spinal accessory nerve is injured, the patient will have difficulty abducting the arm, chronic shoulder pain, and difficulty shrugging the shoulder. It should also be noted that the transverse cervical nerve, a branch of C2 and C3 which provides sensory innervation to the anterolateral neck, as well as lesser occipital and great auricular nerves, exits from beneath the sternocleidomastoid muscle near Erb's point and is relatively susceptible to injury within the posterior triangle [1, 22].

Summary: Conclusion

- Cranial nerve VII is responsible for providing motor innervation for the muscles of facial expression.
- Cranial nerve V contributes sensory innervation to the face and a portion of the scalp.
- Muscles of facial expression allow mankind to communicate nonverbally.
- Injury to motor nerves in the head or neck may lead to consequences such as facial asymmetry, difficulty in pronunciation, inability to protect vital structures such as the eye, or restricted limb movement.

30.8 Conclusion

In conclusion, the anatomy of the head and neck is an intricate, complex network, and adequate knowledge of anatomic structures is critical for anyone performing surgical or cosmetic procedures in these regions. The deeper structures of the head and neck were reviewed in this section including the motor and sensory nerves, muscles, bony and cartilaginous structures, fat, fascia, and mucosa. Cranial nerve VII is responsible for providing motor innervation for the muscles of facial expression. The fifth cranial nerve, or trigeminal nerve, contributes a majority of the sensory innervation of the face and a portion of the scalp. Mankind's ability to communicate nonverbally may be attributed to the muscles of facial expression, and the overall structure of the face is largely determined by the underlying bony and cartilaginous skeletons as well as subcutaneous fat. Injury to motor nerves in the head or neck may lead to consequences such as facial asymmetry, difficulty in pronunciation, inability to protect vital structures such as the eye, or restricted limb movement. Loss of adipose tissue may have various cosmetic implications. Familiarity with these structures will allow one to more adequately counsel patients about risks and benefits of procedures.

References

1. Robinson JK. Anatomy for procedural dermatology. In: Robinson JK, Hanke CW, Siegel DM, Fratila A, editors. Surgery of the skin: procedural dermatology. 2nd ed. St. Louis: Mosby; 2004. p. 3–27.
2. Bentsianov B, Blitzer A. Facial anatomy. Clin Dermatol. 2004;22:3–13.
3. Hiatt JL, Gartner LP. Textbook of head and neck anatomy. 4th ed. Philadelphia: Lippincott, Williams and Wilkins; 2010.
4. Salasche SJ, Bernstein G, Senkarik M. Surgical anatomy of the skin. Norwalk: Appleton and Lange; 1988.
5. Larrabee WF, Makielski KH, Henderson JL. Surgical anatomy of the face. Philedelphia: Lippincott, Williams and Wilkins; 2004.
6. Meine JG, Moosally AJ. The face (forehead, cheeks and chin). In: Roenigk RK, Ratz JL, Roenigk HH, editors. Roenigk's dermatologic surgery: current techniques in procedural dermatology. 3rd ed. New York: Informa; 2006. p. 239–46.
7. Meirson DH. Nasal anatomy and reconstruction. Dermatol Clin. 1998;16(1):91–108.
8. Brewer JD, Roenigk R. The scalp. In: Roenigk RK, Ratz JL, Roenigk HH, editors. Roenigk's dermatologic surgery: current techniques in procedural dermatology. 3rd ed. New York: Informa; 2006. p. 187–96.
9. Ceilley RI. The ear. In: Roenigk RK, Ratz JL, Roenigk HH, editors. Roenigk's dermatologic surgery: current techniques in procedural dermatology. 3rd ed. New York: Informa; 2006. p. 197–205.
10. Reddy LV, Zide MF. Reconstruction of skin cancer defects of the auricle. J Oral Maxillofac Surg. 2004;62:1457–71.
11. Robinson JK. The eye and eyelid. In: Roenigk RK, Ratz JL, Roenigk HH, editors. Roenigk's dermatologic surgery: current techniques in procedural dermatology. 3rd ed. New York: Informa; 2006. p. 207–18.
12. Ridgway JM, Larrabee WF. Anatomy for blepharoplasty and brow-lift. Facial Plast Surg. 2010;26:177–85.
13. Flowers FP, Zampogna JC. Surgical anatomy of the head and neck. In: Bolognia JL, Jorizzo JL, Rapini RP, editors. Dermatology. 2nd ed. St. Louis: Mosby; 2008. p. 2159–71.
14. Greenway HT. The lips and oral cavity. In: Roenigk RK, Ratz JL, Roenigk HH, editors. Roenigk's dermatologic surgery: current techniques in procedural dermatology. 3rd ed. New York: Informa; 2006. p. 231–8.
15. Rohrich RJ, Pessa JE. The fat compartments of the face: anatomy and clinical implications for cosmetic surgery. Plast Reconstr Surg. 2007;119:2219–27.
16. Kahn DM, Shaw RB. Overview of current thoughts on facial volume and aging. Facial Plast Surg. 2010;26:350–5.
17. Kahn JL, Wolfram-Gabel R, Bourjat P. Anatomy and imaging of the deep fat of the face. Clin Anat. 2000;13:373–82.
18. Gardetto A et al. Does a superficial musculoaponeurotic system exist in the face and neck? an anatomical study by the tissue plastination technique. Plast Reconstr Surg. 2003;111:664–72.
19. Ghassemi A et al. Anatomy of the SMAS revisited. Aesthetic Plast Surg. 2003;27:258–64.
20. Bennett RG. Fundamentals of cutaneous surgery. St. Louis: Mosby; 1988.
21. Menick FJ. Nasal reconstruction. Plast Reconstr Surg. 2010;125:138–50.
22. Moosally AJ, McGillis T. The neck. In: Roenigk RK, Ratz JL, Roenigk HH, editors. Roenigk's dermatologic surgery: current techniques in procedural dermatology. 3rd ed. New York: Informa; 2006. p. 247–53.

Complications of Mohs Micrographic Surgery

31

Adam A. Ingraffea and Hugh M. Gloster Jr.

Abstract

The incidence of non-melanoma skin cancer is increasing rapidly in the United States. The rapid rise in the number of cases of NMSC has lead to an increasing demand for Mohs micrographic surgery. Along with this dramatic rise in the number of procedures being performed comes the risk of increased complications. However, with careful planning, good judgment, and proper techniques the risk of complications can be minimized. The primary goal of this chapter is to review the current recommendations and evidence for the prevention of the common complications in the setting of Mohs surgery. More serious, but thankfully rare, complications, as well as several recently described complications will also be reviewed.

Keywords

Mohs surgery • Complications • Bleeding • Infection • Nerve injury

Summary: Bleeding Complications

- Serious bleeding complications are rare in Mohs surgery.
- Discontinuation of anticoagulant medication is not necessary and is not generally recommended.
- Serious and even fatal thrombotic complications have been reported to occur after the discontinuation of medically necessary blood thinners.

A.A. Ingraffea (✉) • H.M. Gloster Jr.
Department of Dermatology, University of Cincinnati, Cincinnati, OH, USA
e-mail: ingrafam@ucmail.uc.edu

K. Nouri (ed.), *Mohs Micrographic Surgery*,
DOI 10.1007/978-1-4471-2152-7_31, © Springer-Verlag London Limited 2012

31.1 Bleeding Complications

Bleeding complications can take the form of excessive or undesired bleeding as well as the opposite problem of unintended thrombosis. As many of our patients are elderly and are routinely prescribed multiple anticoagulants (e.g., aspirin, clopidogrel, coumadin, and heparin), it is important to be aware of the current recommendations for anticoagulant management as it relates to Mohs surgery. In addition, more and more patients are taking over the counter medicines which may also increase the risk for surgical bleeding. Therefore, the first step to successfully preventing a bleeding complication is a thorough medical history with specific emphasis on the patient's medications.

Most surgical bleeds occurring during Mohs surgery are relatively minor and easily controlled with pinpoint electrocoagulation or primary ligation of a transected vessel. In order to avoid unnecessary sectioning of a larger artery it is important to be familiar with the major arteries which may be encountered during a surgical procedure. The most commonly transected major vessels in the face are the superficial temporal artery and branches of the facial artery. The superficial temporal artery is the terminal branch of the external carotid artery, and it is easily palpated superior and anterior to the tragus. As it travels in an ascending course over the zygoma it bifurcates into an anterior and parietal branch. Above the zygoma it lies within the thin subcutaneous fat of the anterior scalp.

The facial artery branches off the external carotid artery and crosses over the mandible anterior to the masseter muscle where it can be palpated. As it crosses the mandible the facial artery is covered by the platysma and risorius muscles. The artery then courses in a diagonal and superior direction, giving off the inferior and superior labial arteries. The artery travels up towards the medial canthus where it anastamoses with the dorsal nasal artery, a branch of the internal carotid artery. When transected, most named arteries should be clamped and ligated (Fig. 31.1).

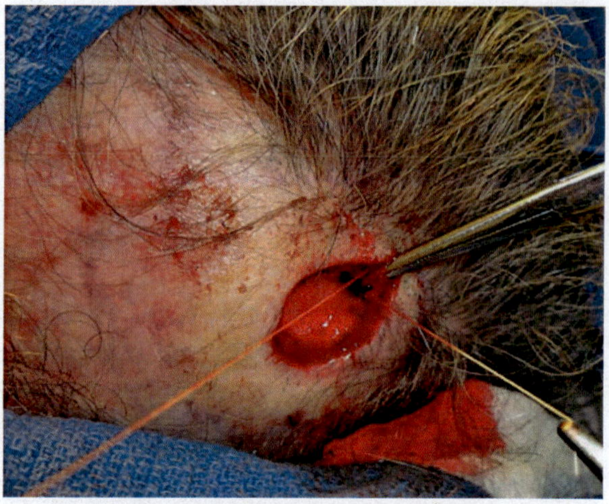

Fig. 31.1 Large transected vessels should be clamped and ligated

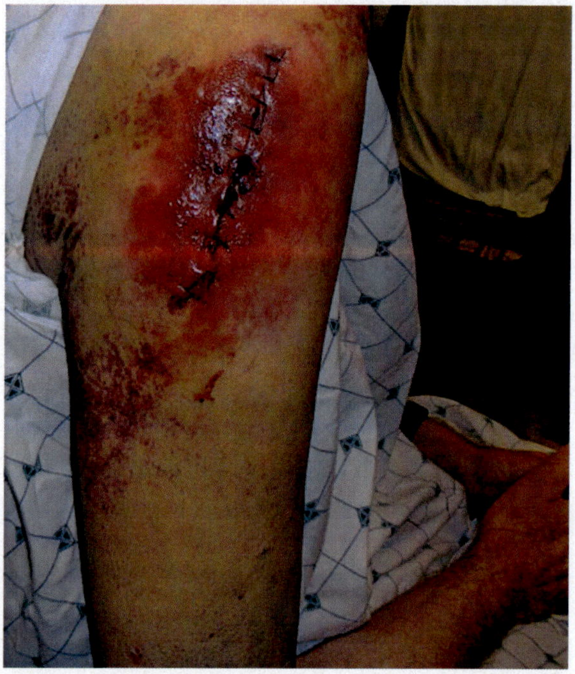

Fig. 31.2 Hematoma on the arm of a patient taking Plavix and aspirin

In addition to the brisk bleeding of a transected artery, the Mohs surgeon must also deal with the oozing of small vessels and capillaries. This oozing can be especially frustrating when surgery is performed on patients taking anticoagulants, especially aspirin. Anticoagulant use is the most common cause of persistant intraoperative bleeding, if the surgeon fails to respond adequately with meticulous hemostasis this can lead to the formation of a postoperative hematoma (Fig. 31.2). The list of anticoagulants encountered continues to grow, including both prescription and over-the-counter medications.

While it is tempting from a convenience point of view to have patients discontinue their anticoagulant medications, in most cases, this is not to be recommended. Patients taking aspirin for pain or inflammation may safely stop taking the medications for 7 days prior to surgery and restart several days after surgery, nonsteroidal anti-inflammatory drugs (NSAIDs) can be stopped 3 days prior to surgery since they have less profound effects on platelet aggregation. In addition, herbal supplements such as Vitamin E, the four G's (ginko, ginseng, ginger, garlic), and fish oil, among others, should be stopped prior to surgery. The most important question remains, should patients stop taking medically indicated anticoagulants prior to Mohs surgery? There have been seven published studies which have investigated this issue. The largest study to evaluate the effect of taking a single anticoagulant agent involved 653 patients [1]. This study found a small, 1.6% versus 0.7%, but statistically insignificant increase in serious bleeding in the group taking either aspirin, warfarin, or NSAIDs when compared to controls. The largest study to date examined 760 consecutive patients in an academic Mohs practice and compared the bleeding complications between patients taking no anticoagulants, one anticoagulant, and two or more anticoagulants [2]. The study concluded that the use of two or more anticoagulants increased the risk of serious bleeding when compared to one or no anticoagulant. However, the study reported only four events of serious bleeding so it may be underpowered to detect differences between the three groups. In another study of 96 patients taking either warfarin or no warfarin there was significantly more minor bleeding in the warfarin group (26%) versus the no-warfarin group (6%); however there were no serious bleeding events in either group [3].

Kargi et al. evaluated 102 patients taking either aspirin, warfarin or no anticoagulant and found that aspirin was not associated with an increased risk of bleeding complications [4]. However, an increased risk of serious bleeding complications was noted in patients taking warfarin. The definition of serious complication in this study may have been too broad as it included wound infection and loss of skin graft as well as hematoma and persistent bleeding. This article reported five serious complications in the warfarin group and none in the aspirin or control groups. The authors did not provide detailed information on the type of serious complication encountered, so it is difficult to attribute all these to the use of warfarin. For example, a skin graft may fail due to a poor wound bed or improper suturing technique, and wound infections may occur for many reasons that have nothing to do with the use of warfarin. Finally, in a prospective study of 322 patients taking aspirin, warfarin, NSAIDs, or no anticoagulant, Billingsly et al. found no statistically significant increase in patients taking anticoagulants [5].

In order to ascertain what can be learned from the currently available studies, Lewis et al. performed a meta-analysis of studies published between 1966 and 2005 [6]. A total of 1,373 patients met the criteria for study inclusion. The analysis revealed that patients taking warfarin were seven times more likely to suffer a moderate to severe complication than the control group. However, this conclusion is not entirely beyond reproach. In the warfarin group of the meta-analysis, there were a total of 122 patients, with 7 experiencing severe complications. Of these 7 patients, 5 were from the previously described study by Kargi et al. which failed to limit severe complications to bleeding alone, but also included infection and loss of skin graft. The meta-analysis also concluded that patients taking aspirin or NSAIDs were twice as likely to suffer serious bleeding complications, but this finding did not meet statistical significance. The study did not evaluate the effects of taking multiple anticoagulants on bleeding complications. It seems likely, therefore, that the risks of serious bleeding complications in patients, who undergo Mohs surgery, are small but may be slightly increased especially when taking warfarin.

In spite of the apparent low risk associated with continuing anticoagulant therapy, many surgical dermatologists still discontinue medically necessary anticoagulants. A survey of Mohs surgeons performed in the year 2005 found that 37% discontinue medically necessary aspirin and 44% discontinue medically necessary Coumadin [7].

If it is accepted that anticoagulants pose a small but manageable risk to the patient undergoing a Mohs procedure, what are the risks associated with the discontinuation of these medicines? Kovich et al. surveyed 168 members of the American College of Mohs Micrographic Surgery about thrombotic events occurring in the perioperative period in patients who had discontinued their anticoagulation [8]. A total of 46 thrombotic events were reported, of these 54% occurred after discontinuing warfarin and 39% after discontinuing aspirin. The most common thrombotic event reported was stroke, followed by TIA and MI. A total of three deaths were reported. The authors were able to estimate to incidence of thrombotic events and calculate the risk of thrombosis associated with discontinuation of anticoagulant medications. Overall, the risk was estimated to be 1 event for 12,816 operations, for warfarin it was 1 in 6,219 and for aspirin 1 in 21,448. The authors concluded that based on these low but significant risks for severe complications following discontinuation of anticoagulants, and due to the lack of studies showing significant risks of severe complications from the continuation of anticoagulants, there is compelling evidence for patients to continue medically necessary anticoagulants during Mohs surgery.

In summary, the best way to prevent serious bleeding is through avoidance of larger vessels, if a vessel is transected it should be cauterized completely or tied-off. The issue of anticoagulants, while somewhat controversial, is probably best handled on a case-by-case basis with a bias towards the continuation of medically necessary anticoagulation due to the risk of potential severe thrombotic events if these medications are discontinued.

Summary: Infectious Complications

- Mohs surgery has a very low rate of infectious complications.
- Prophylactic antibiotics are rarely necessary before Mohs surgery and should not be routinely prescribed.
- MRSA infections are increasing in incidence and all wound infections should be cultured and treated appropriately.

31.2 Infectious Complications

Surgical procedures of the skin in general and Mohs surgery in particular are both remarkably free of infectious complications. The very low incidence of infections reported is all the more remarkable considering that the majority of these procedures are not carried out under strictly sterile conditions. Mohs surgery is traditionally characterized as a clean procedure since there are often multiple dressing changes during the procedure and patients often get up to use the bathroom or spend time in the waiting room. The low risk of surgical site infections associated with Mohs surgery makes the routine use of prophylactic antibiotics unnecessary and is not recommended. In addition, due to the very low risk of bacteremia during Mohs surgery, antibiotic prophylaxis to prevent bacterial endocarditis, and hematogenous total joint infections is not indicated under routine conditions. However, there are certain instances when antibiotic prophylaxis should be considered for the prevention of surgical site infections as well as bacterial endocarditis and joint infections. The most recent guidelines on the prevention of bacterial endocarditis where published by the American Heart Association (AHA) in 2007 [9]. These new guidelines provided a dramatic departure from earlier guidelines and greatly reduced the number of situations in which antibiotic prophylaxis is recommended. It should be noted from the outset that the AHA guidelines are not specific to dermatology or skin surgery and are based on recommendations regarding dental procedures. These recommendations relate to Mohs only when a procedure involves the oral mucosa. The highlights of the last AHA update included several important statements: (1) An extremely small number of cases of infective endocarditis (IE) might be prevented by antibiotic prophylaxis for dental procedures even if such prophylactic therapy were 100% effective. (2) Infective endocarditis prophylaxis for dental procedures is reasonable only for patients with underlying cardiac conditions associated with the *highest risk* of adverse outcome from IE. (3) For patients with these underlying cardiac conditions, prophylaxis is reasonable for all dental procedures that involve manipulation of gingival tissue or the periapical region of teeth or *perforation of the oral mucosa*. The cardiac conditions presenting the highest risk for IE are summarized below (adapted from the AHA guidelines [9]) (Table 31.1).

It is clear from these updated guidelines that the risks of IE occurring after Mohs surgery are very low, and prophylactic antibiotic therapy should be limited to very specific situations. The only circumstance where prophylactic antibiotic treatment would definitely be recommended for Mohs surgery would be a patient with a high risk cardiac condition undergoing a perforating procedure of the oral mucosa, (e.g., a lip wedge removal, flap or a linear closure extending into the oral mucosa). If Mohs surgery is to be undertaken on high risk patients with clinical signs of an infected surgical site, then aggressive antibiotic therapy should be considered.

Table 31.1 Cardiac conditions associated with the *highest risk* of endocarditis for which prophylaxis for dental procedures is reasonable

Prosthetic cardiac valve or prosthetic material used for cardiac valve repair
Previous IE
Congenital heart disease (CHD)[a]
Unrepaired cyanotic CHD, including palliative shunts and conduits
Completely repaired congenital heart defect with prosthetic material or device, whether placed by surgery or by catheter intervention, during the first 6 months after the procedure[b]
Repaired CHD with residual defects at the site or adjacent to the site of a prosthetic patch or prosthetic device (which inhibit endothelialization)
Cardiac transplantation recipients who develop cardiac valvulopathy

[a]Except for the conditions listed above, antibiotic prophylaxis is no longer recommended for any other form of CHD
[b]Prophylaxis is reasonable because endothelialization of prosthetic material occurs within 6 months after the procedure

Table 31.2 Patients at potential increased risk of experiencing hematogenous total joint infection

All patients during first 2 years following joint replacement
Immunocompromised/immunosuppressed patients
Inflammatory arthropathies such as rheumatoid arthritis, systemic
Lupus erythematosus
Patients with comorbidities
Drug- or radiation-induced immunosuppression
Previous prosthetic joint infections
Malnourishment
Hemophilia
HIV infection
Insulin-dependent (type 1) diabetes
Malignancy

In 2003 the American Dental Association (ADA) and the American Academy of Orthopaedic Surgeons issued an updated consensus statement regarding the prevention of hematogenous total joint infections in patients undergoing dental procedures [10]. The major conclusions of the statement are as follows: (1) Antibiotic prophylaxis is not indicated for patients with pins, plates, or screws. (2) Antibiotic prophylaxis is not routinely advisable in most patients with total joint replacement. (3) It is advisable to consider premedication for a small number of patients with high-risk indications undergoing dental procedures. Patients at high risk for joint infection are indicated in the table below (Adapted from the 2003 consensus statement) (Table 31.2).

The recent guidelines suggest it is rarely necessary to prophylaxis patients for the prevention of bacterial endocarditis and hematogenous total joint infection, what about for the prevention of surgical site infections?

In a recently published study, Maragh and Brown, reviewed the infection rate in 1,000 consecutive patients who underwent Mohs surgery and were not treated with prophylactic antibiotics [11]. The overall infection rate was 8/1115 or 0.7%. All the cases were performed on an outpatient basis and were a mixture of sterile and clean technique. The authors found the highest risk of infection was associated with surgery on the nose (5/8 infections, 1.7% rate) and with flap closure (7/8 infections, 2.4% rate). The authors concluded that due to the exceedingly low rate of infections following Mohs surgery, the routine use of antibiotic prophylaxis, is not recommended, even in cases involving the nose or flap closure.

In another study, 5,091 lesions were treated in 2,424 patients over a 3-year period with a variety of procedures including curettage, Mohs surgery, simple excisions, and wedge excisions [12]. None of the patients were given prophylactic antibiotics and none ceased taking aspirin or warfarin. The surgeons followed sterile operative techniques. The overall infection rate was an impressively low 1.47%. The authors reported several circumstances that lead to unacceptably high, (>5%), infection rates: procedures below the knee, wedge excisions of the lip or ear, skin grafts, and lesions in the groin. They recommended that prophylactic antibiotics be reserved exclusively for patients in one of the above groups. Interestingly, they reported no increased rate of infection in diabetic patients, smokers or those on anticoagulants. However, in a follow-up study by the same authors involving 7,224 lesions in 4,197 patients, diabetes was shown to increase the risk of wound infection by 66%. Diabetes did not lead to an increase in any other complication [13].

Methicillin Resistant Staphylococcus Aureus (MRSA) infections, both community- and hospital-acquired, have been increasing in incidence recently. It is important to consider an individual patients risk for

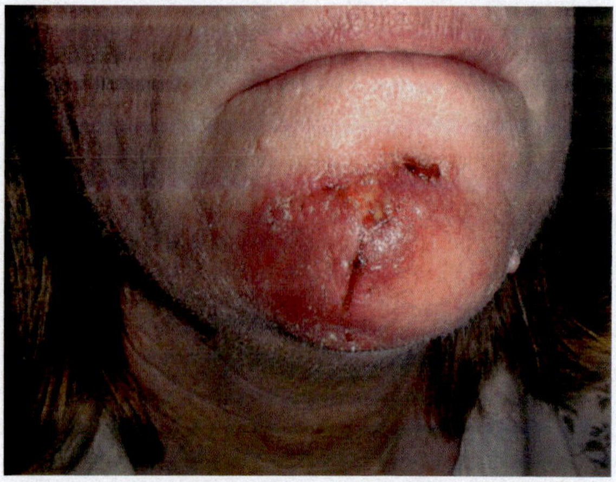

Fig. 31.3 This wound cultured positive for MRSA

MRSA infection on a case-by-case basis (Fig. 31.3). The increasing incidence of MRSA infection highlights the importance of obtaining wound cultures in all suspected infections. If a high index of suspicion exists for an MRSA wound infection, treatment with appropriate antibiotics (i.e., trimethoprim sulfamethoxysole (TMP-SMX), Clindamycin or Doxycycline) should be considered while cultures are pending. A recent publication recommended preoperative MRSA screening and decontamination which included mupirocin ointment for 5–7 days to the nares and 5–7 days of TMP-SMX, starting the day before surgery, to reduce the rate of postoperative infection [14]. The authors were able to reduce the rate of MRSA infection from 0.3% before screening to 0% after the screening and decontamination procedure began.

The issue of whether sterile technique need be followed during Mohs surgery has been evaluated in several recent publications. In one study, 1,400 Mohs cases were performed either with clean or sterile gloves [15]. No statistical difference in infection rates were found between the group treated with sterile gloves and the group treated with clean gloves. The authors concluded that utilizing clean versus sterile gloves could save $0.95 per pair without increasing the risk of infection. In another study an upgraded sterility program including the use of sterile gloves during all phases of the Mohs procedure, along with other changes lead to a decrease in infection rate from 2.5% to 0.9% [16]. The authors concluded that the additional material costs associated with the prevention of one infection were $672.50.

Summary: Nerve Injury

- A thorough understanding of facial anatomy is needed to avoid unnecessary nerve injury.
- The temporal and marginal mandibular branches of the facial nerve are most likely to be injured during Mohs surgery.
- Many nerve injuries will improve spontaneously over a 6-month period, if significant deficit is still present then treatment should be considered.

31.3 Nerve Injury

In order to avoid potentially disfiguring motor nerve damage, the Mohs surgeon must be aware of the danger zones encountered in the head/neck regions. There are four important danger zones where motor nerves are relatively superficial and may be at risk for injury.

Three of the danger zones relate to branches of the seventh cranial nerve (facial nerve), the fourth danger zone involves the eleventh cranial nerve (spinal accessory nerve).

The facial nerve exits the skull via the stylomastoid foramen and penetrates the parotid gland. After exiting the parotid gland, it divides into the five facial motor nerve branches: from superior to inferior, temporal, zygomatic, buccal, and marginal mandibular and cervical nerves. The first danger zone frames the temporal branch as it courses superiorly. The temporal branch exits the parotid gland, crosses the zygomatic arch then dips below the frontalis muscle. The danger zone is identified by a triangle covering the area where the nerve is most at risk for damage (Fig. 31.4). The first side of triangle is composed of a line drawn from a point 0.5 cm inferior to the tragus up to a point 2.0 cm lateral and superior to the tail of the eyebrow. The second side is drawn down through the eyebrow to the lateral orbital rim. The triangle is completed by drawing a line horizontally from the lateral orbital rim back to the first side of the triangle. The facial nerve is at greatest danger as it crosses over the zygomatic arch due to its superficial position just below the subcutaneous fat between the superficial and deep temporalis fascia. In order to avoid injuring the temporal nerve, the plane of undermining in the first danger zone

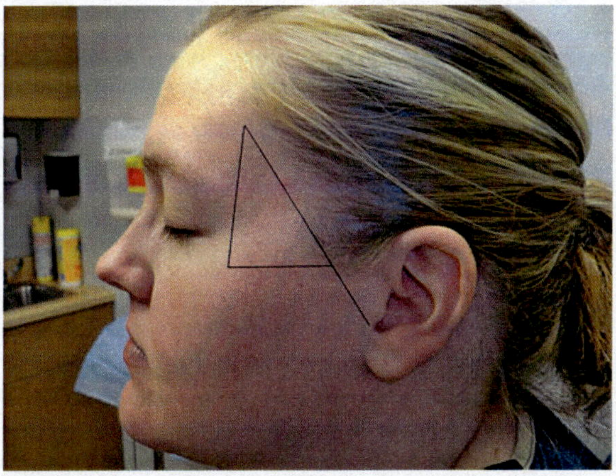

Fig. 31.4 Danger zone 1 outlined. The temporal branch is most in danger as it passes over the zygoma

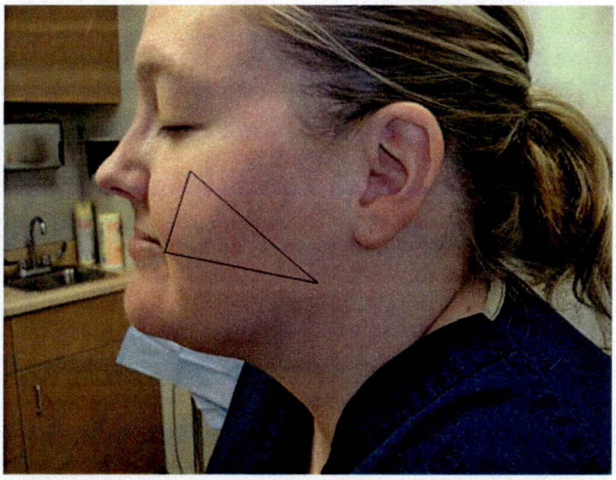

Fig. 31.5 Danger zone 2 is outlined by the triangle

should be in the superficial subcutaneous fat. Injury to the facial nerve results in ipsilateral brow ptosis, diminished forehead rhytids, and a weak frown.

Management of facial nerve injury should include watchful waiting for the first 6 months following surgery, since many motor nerve deficits will improve spontaneously over this time period [17]. Neuropraxia, a temporary conduction deficit due to stretching or trauma of the nerve, resolves spontaneously. If the brow ptosis is mild and the patient is most bothered by a flat forehead, contralateral injection of botulinum toxin can help improve the facial asymmetry [18]. If, after 6 months, significant brow ptosis persists, referral to a facial plastic surgeon should be considered. Techniques which may improve the patients function and appearance include an ipsilateral brow lift or a nerve graft.

The second danger zone involves the zygomatic and buccal branches of the facial nerve. The limits of the second danger zone are defined by a triangle drawn from the angle of the mandible up to the mid zygoma then down to the oral commissure and back to the angle of the mandible (Fig. 31.5). Undermining in this area should be performed above the level of the SMAS. Nerve damage is more likely to occur to the buccal branch and results in ipsilateral lip droop, difficulty eating and an asymmetrical smile.

The third danger zone follows the marginal mandibular branch as it crosses over the mandible proximal to the masseter muscle and travels medially to innervate the depressors of the mouth. The limits of the third danger zone are defined by a circular area centered on the mandible, approximately 2 cm lateral and 2 cm inferior to the oral commissure (Fig. 31.6). In this area, the SMAS is very thin and offers little protection to the marginal mandibular nerve. The facial artery is also in jeopardy at the lateral edge of this danger zone. Damage to the marginal mandibular nerve can cause serious functional speech and cosmetic deficits to the patient. The ipsilateral lip tends to be elevated due to weakness of the lip depressors, the patient may also have difficulty fully showing the teeth on the affected side.

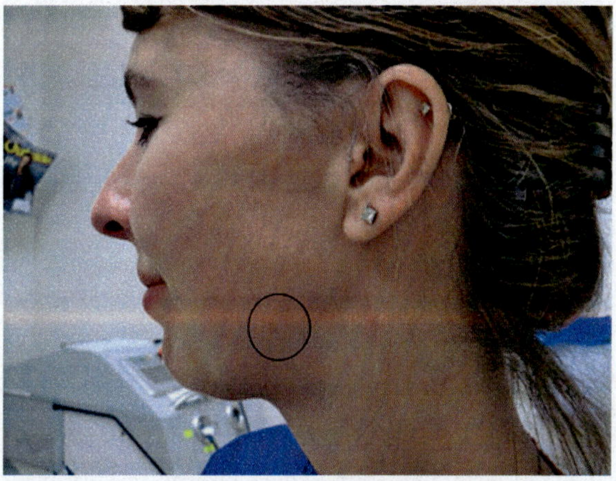

Fig. 31.6 Danger zone 3 is shown by the circle

The fourth and final danger zone involves the spinal accessory nerve (cranial nerve XI), which is located on the lateral neck in an area known as Erb's point. Erb's point, an important landmark in the posterior triangle of the neck, can be located by having the patient turn

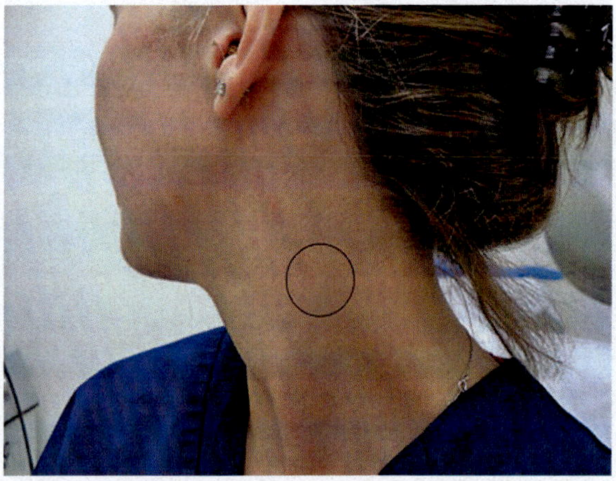

Fig. 31.7 Danger zone 4 is outlined by the circle. Erb's point is found in the center of the circle

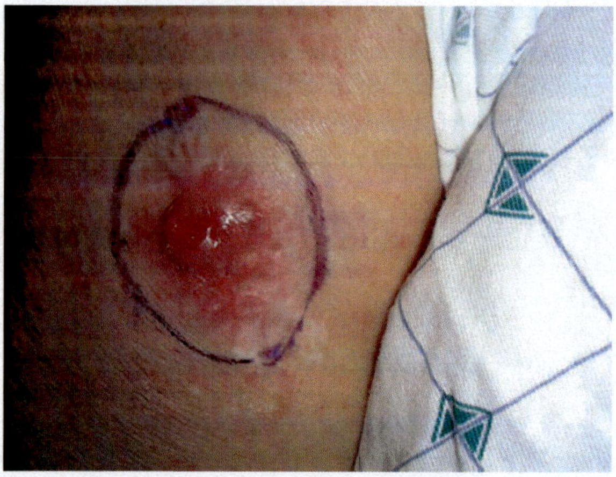

Fig. 31.8 A recurrent basal cell carcinoma

their head in the opposite direction and then drawing a vertical line down from the mastoid process approximately 6 cm to the posterior border of the sternocleidomastoid muscle. A 3-cm circle at this point delineates the fourth danger zone (Fig. 31.7). The spinal accessory nerve, which courses within the fascia investing the sternocleidomastoid and trapezius muscles, may be avoided by staying within the subcutaneous fat when performing sugery in Erb's point. In addition to the spinal accessory nerve, which supplies motor innervation to the neck and shoulder, the greater auricular nerve (C2 and C3) is also located in the Erb point and provides sensory innervation to the neck and ear. Damage to the greater auricular nerve results in loss of sensation to the periauricular area, while damage to the spinal accessory nerve results in a "winged scapula" and weakness in the neck and shoulder, an unfortunate result which is often permanent and requires nerve grafting to restore function.

Summary: Tumor Recurrence

- Mohs surgery offers the lowest possible recurrence rates for BCC and SCC.
- Factors associated with increased tumor recurrence include: large size, poor differentiation, delay in treatment, tumor location in the central face, and the presence of chronic lymphocytic leukemia.

31.4 Tumor Recurrence

It is generally accepted that Mohs surgery provides the lowest possible recurrence rates of any treatment modality for Basal Cell and Squamous Cell carcinoma (Fig. 31.8). The 5-year recurrence rate of BCC treated with Mohs surgery has been reported to range between 1% and 3% for primary tumors and 5% and 7% for recurrent tumors [19–22]. For SCC, the 5-year recurrence rate has been variously reported to range from 3% to 5% for primary tumors and 6% to 10% for recurrent lesions [19, 20, 23]. The largest of these studies reported by Dr. Mohs himself showed a 1% 5-year recurrence rate in 8,643 tumors treated by Mohs chemosurgery [19]. Two recent publications from Australia prospectively evaluated the 5-year recurrence rates of BCC and SCC treated by Mohs surgery. For BCC, the authors found that the factors associated with a higher risk of recurrence were prior recurrence, longer time before surgery, and more stages of Mohs for tumor clearance [24]. Prior studies had identified large tumor size, aggressive histology, and location in the facial "H-zone" to be risk factors for recurrence. For SCC, the risk factors were larger size, poor differentiation, and prior recurrence [25]. The reported overall recurrence rate for BCC was 1.4% for primary and 4% for recurrent tumors, while for SCC, the recurrence rate was 2.6% for primary and 5.9% for recurrent lesions. Other factors associated with a higher risk of recurrence of SCC include tumor depth greater than 4 mm (Clark level IV), tumor location in previous areas treated by radiation, thermal injury, Bowen's disease, chronic ulcers, as well as specific sites such as the ear, lips, and genital area.

Another risk factor for recurrence of both BCC and SCC which has received significant attention recently is the concomitant presence of chronic lymphocytic leukemia (CLL) [25, 26]. Patients with CLL undergoing Mohs surgery have been reported to have a sevenfold higher risk of recurrence of SCC and a 14-fold higher increase in recurrence of BCC when compared to controls. The reasons for this increased risk are not completely clear but may include an impaired host immune response as well as positive Mohs margins being obscured by dense lymphocytic infiltrates. It has been suggested that dense peri-tumoral infiltrates may be a marker for patients with undiagnosed CLL, and further work-up should be done in these cases. In summary, Mohs surgery offers the lowest possible rates of tumor recurrence. Risk factors for tumor recurrence include, large size, poor differentiation, a prior recurrence, a long delay in treatment, and the presence of CLL.

Summary: Medication Complications

- Medication complications are rarely encountered in Mohs surgery.
- True lidocaine allergy is very rare.
- Lidocaine with epinephrine may be used safely on the digits.
- Allergy contact dermatitis to topical antibiotics is very common

31.5 Medication Complications

The most commonly employed medicines in Mohs surgery are lidocaine and epinephrine. They are both remarkably safe and free of serious complications, yet there are several possible side effects that should be considered when employing these medications. Lidocaine, along with bupivacaine and mepivacaine, belong to the amide class of local anesthetics. Due to an improved safety profile and decreased allergic potential the amide anesthetics have largely replaced the earlier ester class, which includes procaine, tetracaine, and benzocaine. True lidocaine allergy is very rare and most patients reporting an allergy to lidocaine actually experienced a prior vasovagal reaction. Lidocaine hypersensitivity can be either type I immediate hypersensitivity or type IV delayed hypersensitivity. Both are very rare, with type I reported more often. A French study re-challenged 199 patients with reported lidocaine allergies, of these, only 1 developed an allergic reaction [27]. In an Israeli study of 236 patients referred for evaluation of local anesthetic allergy, skin prick and intradermal testing failed to demonstrate a single reaction [28]. In another study, 183 patients with supposed lidocaine allergy were patched tested, 4 positive reactions were reported, 2 of these patients also positive reactions to intradermal injection [29].

The maximum recommended dose for plain lidocaine is 4.5 mg/kg, whereas the maximum recommended dose for lidocaine with epinephrine is 7.0 mg/kg. The maximum dose should not be administered to the patient for at least 2 h. Alam et al. measured the peak lidocaine serum concentrations during and after Mohs surgery in 19 patients, the maximum reported concentration in any patients was 0.3 μg/ml [30]. This level is well below the minimal concentration of 5 μgml needed for objective signs of lidocaine toxicity to develop. At the 5 μg/ml level, signs of lidocaine toxicity include paresthesias, muscle fasciculations, and tinnitus. The authors conclude that even relatively large volumes of 1% lidocaine with epinephrine are associated with serum levels well below toxic levels.

Epinephrine is also a very safe medication. Historically there has been controversy as to the safety of using epinephrine in the digits. Several recent reviews failed to detect any reported cases of finger necrosis or gangrene with commercial preparations of lidocaine with epinephrine [31, 32]. All the reported cases were reported with earlier ester anesthetics or with noncommercial preparations of unknown concentration. Additional evidence for the safety of low concentration 1:100,000 epinephrine comes from a review of 59 cases of accidental auto-injection with high concentration 1:1,000 epinephrine (Epi-Pen) [33]. The review found no reported cases of tissue necrosis even in 32 patients who received no treatment. It seems that there is no doubt, that dilute epinephrine is safe for use in the fingers and toes. One situation in which the use of plain lidocaine may be considered is when performing surgery on a pregnant patient. Although small doses are probably safe, epinephrine is a category C medication, whereas plain lidocaine is category B.

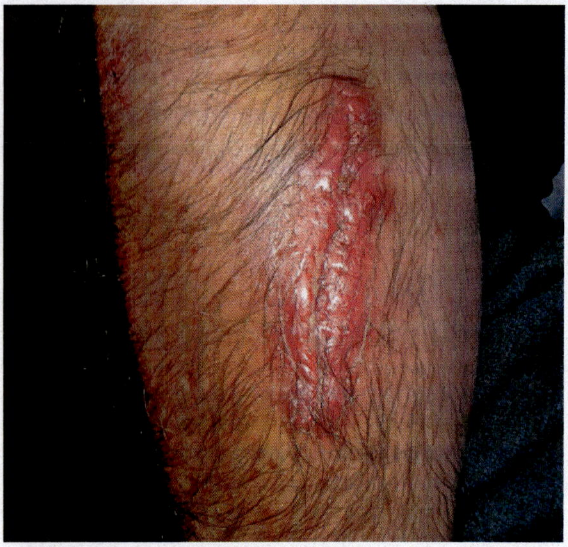

Fig. 31.9 Allergic contact dermatitis to Neosporin

Other medications which may cause side effects include topical antiseptics. Chlorhexidine may cause an acute keratitis if it enters the eye, so care must be taken when using this antiseptic in the periocular area. Chlorhexidine is also toxic to the inner ear and should not be used for procedures in the periauricular area. Hexachlorophene, another topical antiseptic, has been associated with seizures and neurotoxicity, especially in small children. Povidone-iodine is the most commonly used disinfectant in skin surgery. Rare reports of contact dermatitis to this agent have been reported, so patients with known iodine allergy should avoid exposure. A recent publication demonstrated that chlorhexidine/alcohol was superior to povidone-iodine in preventing wound infection in clean-contaminated surgeries [34].

"Should I apply Neosporin to the wound?" is a frequent question asked by patients after surgery. Neomycin and bacitracin along with polymyxin b are the active ingredients in Neosporin or triple antibiotic. In the years 2005–2006, neomycin and bacitracin were the fifth and sixth most common reported allergens in the patch test results of the North American Contact Dermatitis group [35]. In a landmark study published in 1996, Smack et al. showed there was no statistical difference in wound infection rates among patients undergoing dermatological surgery who were given either white petrolatum or bacitracin ointment [36]. The authors concluded that bacitracin offered no advantage over white petrolatum in preventing infection and increased the risk for contact dermatitis (Fig. 31.9).

In conclusion, toxic levels of lidocaine are very rarely encountered during Mohs surgery, lidocaine with epinephrine is safe to use on the digits, chlorhexidine/alcohol may offer improved efficacy over povidone-iodine as a surgical scrub, and white petrolatum is an ideal postoperative ointment.

Summary: Recently Described Complications

- Eruptive SCCs and keratoacanthomas may develop in areas of prior surgery.
- Treatment of these lesions is difficult and often requires repeated Mohs surgeries and systemic retinoids.
- Cerebral air emboli may occur during Mohs sugery of the scalp and skull when the patient is placed in the seated position.

31.6 Recently Described Complications

Numerous reports have detailed the development of eruptive keratoacanthomas and squamous cell carcinomas after skin cancer surgery [37–39]. The mechanism behind the development of this pathergy type of reaction is not known but may be due to field cancerization. The stimulus of postsurgical wound healing may be sufficient to drive the development of subsequent tumors in an area of mutated epithelium. Thankfully, this is a rarely reported phenomenon as treatment is often challenging and may require multiple Mohs procedures as well as oral retinoids to control the development of new lesions.

The development of cerebral air emboli following Mohs surgery has also been reported in two patients [40]. Both patients underwent outpatient Mohs surgery for SCCs of the scalp, both were placed in the seated position, and both had extensive resections including removal of periosteum. Both patients developed neurological dysfunction and were rapidly transported to the emergency room. Luckily, the first patient recovered without sequelae; unfortunately the second patient suffered severe impairment to his language and a left hemiplegia and died shortly thereafter. After reviewing the literature, the authors concluded that having the patient in the seated position is a risk factor for the development of cerebral air emboli as it lowers the hydrostatic pressure within the cerebral vessels. The authors therefore recommend placing the patient in the recumbent position during surgery of the scalp involving the outer layers of the skull.

Summary: Conclusion

- Mohs surgery is an extremely safe procedure.
- Most patients should continue their anticoagulants during Mohs surgery.
- Antibiotic prophylaxis is rarely required and in general not recommended.
- Nerve damage can be avoided by a thorough knowledge of the relevant anatomy.

31.7 Conclusion

Mohs surgery is an extremely safe and effective treatment for cancers of the skin. Serious complications are, in general, very rare and most all can be avoided by a careful and conscientious approach to the individual patient. Most patients can safely continue their anticoagulants during Mohs surgery and thus avoid the risk of serious thrombotic complications. Antibiotic prophylaxis is rarely required thus avoiding the risks of antibiotic allergy and resistance. Nerve damage can usually be avoided by a detailed knowledge of facial anatomy, and when it does occur spontaneous improvement can often be expected. Tumor recurrence is rare after Mohs surgery. Increased surveillance for recurrence may be indicated in certain patients with large tumors, poorly differentiated tumors, long neglected tumors, and with CLL. Medication complications are not common in Mohs surgery and most can be avoided by limiting the use of topical antibiotics after surgery. It is our hope that Mohs surgery can continue to set the standard of excellence for safety and efficacy in skin cancer surgery.

References

1. Otley CC, Fewkes JL, Frank W, et al. Complications of cutaneous surgery in patients who are taking warfarin, aspirin, or nonsteroidal anti-inflammatory drugs. Arch Dermatol. 1996;132:161–6.
2. Shimizu I, Jellinek NJ, Dufresne RG, et al. Multiple antithrombotic agents increase the risk of postoperative hemorrhage in dermatologic surgery. J Am Acad Dermatol. 2008;58:810–6.
3. Sayed S, Adams BB, Liao W, et al. A prospective assessment of bleeding and international normalized ratio in warfarin-anticoagulated patients having cutaneous surgery. J Am Acad Dermatol. 2004;51:955–7.
4. Kargi E, Babuccu O, Hosnuter M, et al. Complications of minor cutaneous surgery in patients under anticoagulant treatment. Aesthetic Plast Surg. 2002;26:483–5.
5. Billingsley EM, Maloney ME. Intraoperative and postoperative bleeding problems in patients taking warfarin, aspirin, and nonsteroidal antiinflammatory agents: a prospective study. Dermatol Surg. 1997;23:381–5.
6. Lewis KG, Dufresne RD. A meta-analysis of complications attributed to anticoagulants among patients following cutaneous surgery. Dermatol Surg. 2008;34:160–5.
7. Kirkorian AY, Moore BL, Siskind J, Marmur ES. Perioperative management of anticoagulant therapy during cutaneous surgery: 2005 Survey of Mohs Surgeons. Dermatol Surg. 2007;33:1189–97.
8. Kovich O, Otley CC. Thrombotic complications related to discontinuation of warfarin and aspirin therapy perioperatively for cutaneous operation. J Am Acad Dermatol. 2003;48:233–7.
9. Wilson W, Taubert KA, Gewitz M, et al. Prevention of infective endocarditis guidelines from the American Heart Association a guideline from the American Heart Association Rheumatic Fever, Endocarditis, and Kawasaki Disease Committee, Council on Cardiovascular Disease in the Young, and the Council on Clinical Cardiology, Council on Cardiovascular Surgery and Anesthesia, and the Quality of Care and Outcomes Research Interdisciplinary Working Group. Circulation. 2007;116:1736–54.
10. American Dental Association; American Academy of Orthopedic Surgeons. Antibiotic prophylaxis for dental patients with total joint replacements. J Am Dent Assoc. 2003;134(7):895–9.
11. Maragh SL, Brown MD. Prospective evaluation of surgical site infection rate among patients with Mohs micrographic surgery without the use of prophylactic antibiotics. J Am Acad Dermatol. 2008;59(2):275–8.
12. Dixon AJ, Dixon MP, Askew DA, et al. Prospective study of wound infections in dermatologic surgery in the absence of prophylactic antibiotics. Dermatol Surg. 2006;32(6):819–26; discussion 826–7.
13. Dixon AJ, Dixon MP, Dixon JB. Prospective study of skin surgery in patients with and without known diabetes. Dermatol Surg. 2009;35(7):1035–40.
14. Cordova KB, Grenier N, Chang KH, et al. Preoperative methicillin-resistant *Staphylococcus aureus* screening in Mohs surgery appears to decrease postoperative infections. Dermatol Surg. 2010;36(10):1541–3.
15. Rhinehart MB, Murphy MM, Farley MF, et al. Sterile versus nonsterile gloves during Mohs micrographic surgery: infection rate is not affected. Dermatol Surg. 2006;32(2):170–6.
16. Martin JE, Speyer LA, Schmults CD. Heightened infection-control practices are associated with significantly lower infection rates in office-based Mohs surgery. Dermatol Surg. 2010;36(10):1529–36.

17. Flynn TC, Emmanouil P, Limmer B. Unilateral transient forehead paralysis following injury to the temporal branch of the facial nerve. Int J Dermatol. 1999;38(6):474–7.
18. Hendi A. Temporal nerve neuropraxia and contralateral compensatory brow elevation. Dermatol Surg. 2007;33:114–6.
19. Mohs FE. Chemosurgery: microscopically controlled surgery for skin cancer – past, present and future. J Dermatol Surg Oncol. 1978;4:41–54.
20. Mohs FE. Chemosurgery for the microscopically controlled excision of cutaneous cancer. Head Neck Surg. 1978;1:150–63.
21. Robins P. Chemosurgery: my 15 years of experience. J Dermatol Surg Oncol. 1981;7:779–89.
22. Julian CG, Bowers PW. A prospective study of Mohs' micrographic surgery in two English centers. Br J Dermatol. 1997;136:515–8.
23. Robins P, Dzubow LM, Rigel DS. Squamous-cell carcinoma treated by Mohs' surgery: an experience with 414 cases in a period of 15 years. J Dermatol Surg Oncol. 1981;7:800–1.
24. Leibovitch I, Huilgol S, Selva D, et al. Basal cell carcinoma treated with Mohs surgery in Australia II. Outcome at 5-year follow-up. J Am Acad Dermatol. 2005;53:452–7.
25. Mehrany K, Weenig RH, Pittelkow MR. High recurrence rates of basal cell carcinoma after Mohs surgery in patients with chronic lymphocytic leukemia. Arch Dermatol. 2004;140(8):985–8.
26. Mehrany K, Weenig RH, Pittelkow MR. High recurrence rates of squamous cell carcinoma after Mohs surgery in patients with chronic lymphocytic leukemia. Dermatol Surg. 2005;31(1):38–42.
27. Amsler E, Flahault A, Mathelier-Fusade P, et al. Evaluation of re-challenge in patients with suspected lidocaine allergy. Dermatology. 2004;208(2):109–11.
28. Berkun Y, Ben-Zvi A, Levy Y, et al. Evaluation of adverse reactions to local anesthetics: experience with 236 patients. Ann Allergy Asthma Immunol. 2003;91(4):342–5.
29. Mackley CL, Marks Jr JG, Anderson BE. Delayed-type hypersensitivity to lidocaine. Arch Dermatol. 2003; 139(3):343–6.
30. Alam M, Ricci D, Havey J, et al. Safety of peak serum lidocaine concentration after Mohs micrographic surgery: a prospective cohort study. J Am Acad Dermatol. 2010;63(1):87–92.
31. Denkler K. A comprehensive review of epinephrine in the finger: to do or not to do. Plast Reconstr Surg. 2001;108(1): 114–24.
32. Krunic AL, Wang LC, Soltani K, et al. Digital anesthesia with epinephrine: an old myth revisited. J Am Acad Dermatol. 2004;51(5):755–9.
33. Fitzcharles-Bowe C, Denkler K, Lalonde D. Finger injection with high-dose (1:1,000) epinephrine: does it cause finger necrosis and should it be treated? Hand. 2007;2(1):5–11.
34. Darouiche RO, Wall Jr MJ, Itani KM, et al. Chlorhexidine-alcohol versus povidone-iodine for surgical-site antisepsis. N Engl J Med. 2010;362(1):18–26.
35. Zug KA, Warshaw EM, Fowler Jr JF, et al. Patch-test results of the North American Contact Dermatitis Group 2005–2006. Dermatitis. 2009;20(3):149–60.
36. Smack DP, Harrington AC, Dunn C, et al. Infection and allergy incidence in ambulatory surgery patients using white petrolatum vs bacitracin ointment. A randomized controlled trial. JAMA. 1996;276(12):972–7.
37. Bangash SJ, Green WH, Dolson DJ, et al. Eruptive postoperative squamous cell carcinomas exhibiting a pathergy-like reaction around surgical wound sites. J Am Acad Dermatol. 2009;61(5):892–7.
38. Goldberg LH, Silapunt S, Beyrau KK, et al. Keratoacanthoma as a postoperative complication of skin cancer excision. J Am Acad Dermatol. 2004;50(5):753–8.
39. May JT, Patil YJ. Keratoacanthoma-type squamous cell carcinoma developing in a skin graft donor site after tumor extirpation at a distant site. Ear Nose Throat J. 2010; 89(4):E11–3.
40. Goldman G, Altmayer S, Sambandan P, et al. Development of cerebral air emboli during Mohs micrographic surgery. Dermatol Surg. 2009;35(9):1414–21.

Eyelid Reconstruction After Mohs Micrographic Surgery

32

Jennifer I. Hui and David T. Tse

Abstract

The eyelid consists of the anterior and the posterior lamellae. During reconstruction, both must be repaired to achieve optimal eyelid function, globe protection, and cosmesis. The method of reconstruction is dependent upon the depth/thickness of the defect, the state of the eyelid margin, and the overall size of the wound. Regardless of which method is chosen, a key principle remains: there must be an inherent blood supply for either the anterior or the posterior lamella (pedicle flap). An inherent vascular supply will ensure tissue survival and optimize the functional and cosmetic outcome. Additional principles of reconstruction include provision of maximal horizontal stabilization and minimization of vertical tension. There must be proper fixation of the eyelid at the lateral canthal angle, and the globe must face an epithelialized eyelid surface. Lastly, in the upper eyelid, the levator must be identified and necessary repairs addressed during reconstruction to ensure proper opening and function.

Keywords

Eyelid reconstruction • Eyelid defect • Tarsoconjunctival graft • Myocutaneous advancement flap • Skin graft • Hard palate graft

Summary: Anterior Lamellar Defects – Summary Statement

- Anterior lamellar defects may be closed in numerous ways, including: (1) primary closure, (2) full-thickness skin graft, or (3) local tissue flap. The posterior lamella must first be examined closely to ensure it is intact. Anterior lamellar repair should not induce eyelid malposition or distortion.

J.I. Hui (✉) • D.T. Tse
Department of Ophthalmic Plastic, Orbital Surgery and Oncology service, Bascom Palmer Eye Institute, Miami, FL, USA
e-mail: jhui@med.miami.edu

K. Nouri (ed.), *Mohs Micrographic Surgery*,
DOI 10.1007/978-1-4471-2152-7_32, © Springer-Verlag London Limited 2012

32.1 Anterior Lamellar Defects: Summary Statement

The anterior lamella consists of the thin eyelid skin and the orbicularis oculi. At times, only these tissues are removed during the excision of the malignant tumor. The posterior lamella must be examined closely to ensure that it is intact.

32.1.1 Upper Eyelid

Upper eyelid defects after Mohs micrographic surgery can range in depth. Regardless of wound depth, the levator muscle is the key structure. The levator is responsible for the upper eyelid's opening movement, and the areas surrounding it must be examined prior to initiation of any reconstructive procedure. Any defect within the muscle must be repaired in order to achieve proper eyelid function and globe protection. Prior to closure, the deeper tissues within the wound must be evaluated. If the orbital septum has been opened during the Mohs excision, the surgeon should gently explore the orbital fat and levator complex. Bleeding points and disruption of the tissues are key factors that need to be addressed. All bleeding points must be controlled to decrease the risk of retrobulbar hemorrhage. Next, the levator's course and attachment are examined; any defects must be resolved prior to anterior lamellar closure. If the levator has been disinserted, it should be repositioned. Vertical lamellar 5-0 Merseline sutures may be used to reinsert the aponeurosis. Lamellar (partial-thickness) bites are key in eyelid reconstruction as full-thickness bites will cause corneal epithelial defects. Lastly, the lid height and contour should be compared to the other side for symmetry.

32.1.1.1 Primary Closure

A small defect may be closed primarily if lid distortion will not be induced. To avoid distortion, tension should be directed along a horizontal plane. This requires a vertical incision with undermining of the skin and subcutaneous tissues adjacent to the wound. Undermining should continue a short distance along the horizontal plane. The anterior lamella is undermined from the tarsal plate. Care should be taken to keep the septum intact. Undermining should be sufficient to allow for a tension-free closure. If needed to improve wound stability, the orbicularis is closed with buried, interrupted 7-0 Vicryl sutures. The skin is then closed with interrupted 7-0 nylon or Vicryl sutures.

If insufficient anterior lamella remains to allow for an undistorted closure, a full-thickness pentagonal wedge, including the anterior lamella defect, may be excised. A relative excess of posterior lamella will induce buckling of the margin so that the lid will no longer be in apposition to the globe. A pentagonal wedge procedure will prevent this relative excess. Additionally, a layered, primary closure provides the best tissue match, smooth lid margin, and continuous lash line.

To begin, a chalazion clamp is placed over the wound prior to incision to provide stability, hemostasis, and protection of the eye. Care must be taken to avoid trauma to the underlying globe. The wound edges are freshened and fashioned with a #15 blade into a pentagonal-shaped defect with the apex oriented inferiorly. The tarsal borders incisions should be sharp and perpendicular to the lid margin. The resulting full-thickness defect is closed primarily. Three interrupted 5-0 Vicryl sutures are placed at partial-thickness (lamellar) depth through the tarsal plate. Next, the lid margin is closed with a 4-0 or 5-0 silk vertical mattress suture through the meibomian gland orifices to provide anteroposterior alignment. This vertical lid margin suture induces puckering of the wound edges to prevent postoperative notching of the margin. The orbicularis layer is closed with interrupted, buried 7-0 Vicryl sutures, and the skin edges are closed with interrupted 7-0 Vicryl sutures. The ends of the silk sutures are left long and secured away from the wound on the lid skin with a 7-0 Vicryl suture.

If needed, a lateral canthotomy will provide 5–6 mm of medial advancement of the temporal eyelid margin if tension precludes proper lid margin reapproximation [1, 2]. To begin the canthotomy, a 4–5-mm horizontal incision through skin and orbicularis muscle is made with Stevens or Wescott scissors from the lateral canthal angle and directed toward the orbital rim. The tips of the scissors are used to identify the lateral attachment of the lid. The superior crus of the lateral canthal tendon is cut with a vertical incision. The incision allows for medial mobilization of the wound without excess tension. The conjunctiva should not be disrupted during the cantholysis. The incision is then closed with interrupted 7-0 Vicryl sutures.

32.1.1.2 Myocutaneous Advancement Flap

A third option for the closure of an anterior lamella defect of the upper eyelid with an intact lid margin is the myocutaneous advancement flap. It is ideal for larger defects as well as those that involve the medial canthal area because it provides the best tissue match and, most importantly, an autonomous blood supply. To maximize cosmesis, incisions should be hidden in natural skin creases when possible. Second, the flap must be of adequate size to prevent distortion of the eyelid. Lastly, the flap must be anchored to minimize tension on the final closure.

The flap is outlined with a marking pen. Local tissues may be recruited with sufficient undermining in some cases. For larger defects, the advancement should be harvested in either a semicircular manner or as a cheek flap extending 1–2 cm beyond the lateral commissure. The skin is incised with a #15 blade. Wescott scissors are used to cut down to the orbital rim through the orbicularis muscle. Stevens scissors are used to undermine the temporal eyelid and skin and muscle of the cheek, allowing for medial movement of the myocutaneous flap. Buried, interrupted, tension-bearing 4-0 or 5-0 Vicryl sutures are placed in the muscular layer, and the skin is closed with interrupted and running 7-0 Vicryl sutures.

32.1.1.3 Full-Thickness Skin Graft

Some defects will be too large to close primarily. For those defects that do not involve the eyelid margin, a free full-thickness skin graft may be employed [3, 4]. Split-thickness skin grafts are generally not recommended in eyelid reconstruction [5].

A full-thickness graft may be harvested from multiple possible sites, including the *contralateral* upper eyelid, the preauricular area, the retroauricular area, the supraclavicular region, and the upper inner arm. The donor skin graft should be hairless and of similar coloring to achieve the best outcome. If there is any concern for skin cancer on areas of the face, it is advisable to avoid using the contralateral upper eyelid in case it will be needed for future reconstructive procedures.

The skin graft should be about 10–15% larger than the defect. Once the area is outlined in the donor area, it can be harvested with a #15 blade and Stevens scissors. The graft is then thinned of subcutaneous fat and connective tissue (unless eyelid skin is used), trimmed to the appropriate dimensions, and sutured to the edges of the defect with interrupted 7-0 and running Vicryl sutures. Two to three buttonholes should be made in the central portion of the graft to allow for egress of blood during healing.

32.1.2 Lower Eyelid

With the exception of the levator, anterior lamellar defects of the lower eyelid are addressed in a fashion similar to that of the upper eyelid.

32.1.2.1 Primary Closure

Anterior lamella defects without lid margin involvement are closed primarily if distortion is not induced. Closure is achieved in the same manner as outlined for the upper eyelid. The primary distinction is that the vertical height of the tarsus is 33–50% of that in the upper eyelid. If necessary, lateral canthotomy with lysis of the inferior crus may be used to provide 3–5 mm of medial mobilization of the remaining lateral eyelid margin.

32.1.2.2 Myocutaneous Advancement Flap

Myocutaneous advancement flaps are also an option for the closure of a lower eyelid anterior lamella defect with an intact lid margin. As with the upper lid, it is ideal for larger defects as well as those that involve the medial canthal area.

This skin-muscle flap is advanced to fill the anterior lamellar defect and is ideal for a medial defect. The creation of the flap begins with an infralash incision that extends toward the lateral canthus and arches superiorly. The laxity of the periocular tissues determines the degree of lateral extension of the incision. The incision is made with a #15 blade and the skin-muscle flap is undermined with Stevens scissors anterior to the orbital septum. Undermining is extended into the temporal region and inferiorly toward the cheek and continued until the temporal edge of the flap can be advanced nasally to the medial edge of the defect without tension. The most important step in the execution of a myocutaneous advancement flap is the strategic placement of a tension-bearing permanent suture (4-0 Prolene) at the zygoma or the lateral orbital rim. Closure is begun at the tip of the advancement flap with deep, interrupted 5-0 Vicryl sutures followed by superficial, interrupted 7-0 Vicryl skin sutures.

32.1.2.3 Ellipse Sliding Flap

Another option for the closure of anterior lamella defects is the elliptical sliding flap [3]. The tissue around the defect is undermined in the suborbicularis fascial plane, advanced, and then closed primarily. A circular or ovoid defect can be converted into an ellipse to prevent dog-ear formation. Distortion of the surrounding tissue and the size of the resulting scar are minimized by orienting the ellipse parallel to the relaxed skin tension lines. Anterior lamella defects near the lid margin should not be reconstructed with this flap because ectropion or retraction may be induced by excessive perpendicular tension.

The defect should be incorporated into the ellipse with its long axis parallel to rhytids. The ellipse angle should be 30° with the long axis four times longer than the short axis. The skin and subcutaneous tissue are incised with a #15 blade and then undermined with Wescott scissors along the edges of the flap. Undermining is performed until the edges of the elliptical defect may be closed without tension. The subcutaneous tissue is closed with deep, interrupted 5-0 Vicryl sutures and the skin with interrupted 7-0 Vicryl sutures.

32.1.2.4 Unipedicle Flap

Another fruitful option for closing anterior lamellar defects of the lower eyelid is a unipedicle flap from the upper eyelid. The flap is hinged laterally overlying the canthus. Excess upper lid skin and orbicularis are harvested and then rotated into the lower lid defect. First, a flap based at the lateral canthus is outlined with a marking pen. The skin is incised with a #15 blade, and skin-orbicularis flap is dissected free from the underlying intact orbital septum. The flap is rotated inferiorly to fill the lower anterior lamella defect and secured with deep, interrupted 6-0 or 7-0 Vicryl sutures. The skin is closed with interrupted and running 7-0 Vicryl sutures. The unipedicle flap may leave the patient with a prominent area of tissue at the lateral canthus. If necessary, a second stage procedure 6–8 weeks later is undertaken to thin the base of the flap and remove this excess tissue.

32.1.2.5 Skin Graft

Full-thickness skin grafting is one option used to repair defects that are too large for primary closure. Split-thickness skin grafts are also not recommended in reconstruction of the lower eyelid [5]. The *ipsilateral* upper eyelid is an excellent donor site (with similar caveats as previously discussed). Other sites include those discussed in the upper eyelid section. For very large defects, a combination of myocutaneous advancement flap and full-thickness skin grafting may be employed.

Summary: Full-Thickness Eyelid Defects

- Full-thickness defects may be closed primarily or with a combination of local tissue advancement and graft. The key principle in the repair of a full-thickness eyelid defect is that either the anterior or posterior lamella must have an inherent vascular supply. Two free grafts will not survive.

32.2 Full-Thickness Eyelid Defects

Full-thickness eyelid defects involve the skin, orbicularis oculi, tarsal plate, and conjunctiva. The anterior and posterior lamellae must be addressed as two separate units, and one must have an inherent blood supply.

32.2.1 Upper Eyelid

32.2.1.1 Primary Closure

As described above, full-thickness eyelid defects may be closed primarily. The wound must be fashioned into a pentagonal wedge with the apex directed superiorly. Defects up to 30% of the central lid and up to 50% in older patients may be closed using this technique. Even, uniform wound closure requires that the tarsal defect extend perpendicular to the lid margin for its full length. The levator aponeurotic attachments should be preserved to minimize postoperative ptosis. If necessary, lateral canthotomy with superior crus cantholysis may be used to provide 3–5 mm of medial mobilization of the remaining lateral eyelid margin.

32.2.1.2 Free Tarsal Graft + Flap

Larger defects of the eyelid will require reconstruction of the anterior and posterior lamella separately.

Upper lid posterior lamellar defects may be addressed with a free tarsal graft from the contralateral upper eyelid. A large chalazion clamp is placed, and the donor lid is everted. A marking pen is used to outline a graft of appropriate length on the conjunctival surface. The inferior border should be parallel to and no more than 4 mm from the lid margin. The vertical height of the graft is determined by the vertical height of the tarsus. A #15 blade is used to incise the conjunctiva and full-thickness tarsal plate. The tarsus and its conjunctiva are dissected free from the overlying levator aponeurosis. Conjunctiva and Mueller's muscle attachments are severed from the superior tarsal border with scissors so 2 mm of conjunctiva remains attached to the graft. The donor site is then allowed to heal secondarily.

The graft is soaked in antibiotic solution and then placed into the contralateral upper eyelid defect with the conjunctival surface in apposition to the globe. The superior edge of the graft with the conjunctival remnant lies along the new lid margin. The lateral edge of the graft is sutured to the tarsal remnant or the stump of the superior crus of the lateral canthal tendon with lamellar 5-0 Vicryl sutures. If there is insufficient tissue remaining laterally, the graft is secured to the lateral orbital rim at the level of the lateral orbital tubercle with interrupted 4-0 Vicryl sutures. The medial edges are then secured with interrupted lamellar 5-0 Vicryl sutures. The superior edge is attached to the superior forniceal conjunctiva and edges of Mueller's muscle and levator aponeurosis with interrupted and running 7-0 Vicryl sutures.

If the free tarsal graft is insufficient to address the horizontal extent of the defect, it may be flanked by hard palate grafts (see below).

The anterior lamella may then be repaired with an advancement flap as outlined above. A free skin graft cannot be used; either the anterior or the posterior lamella must have an inherent blood supply to ensure tissue survival. Once the flap is in place, the conjunctival remnant is then advanced anteriorly and secured to the inferior flap skin edge with a running 7-0 Vicryl suture. This step is needed to reestablish the mucocutaneous junction along the newly reconstructed eyelid margin. To minimize postoperative retraction, the superior eyelid must be immobilized and kept on stretch. This is best accomplished with a temporary 4-0 silk suture tied over bolsters with traction directed inferiorly.

32.2.1.3 Hard Palate Graft + Flap

Various other tissues have been used to replace deficient posterior lamella if a free tarsal graft is not available or insufficient. These include hard palate grafts, nasal or ear cartilage grafts, donor sclera, and synthetic materials. Hard palate grafts are the method of choice to address deficient posterior lamella [6, 7]. The gingival surface of the roof of the mouth is an excellent donor site [8]. They provide a long lasting, rigid, and epithelialized surface. Hard palate grafts may be used in conjunction with free tarsal grafts if the entire upper eyelid must be reconstructed. In this case, the free tarsal graft should be placed centrally. Hard palate grafts should flank the tarsus medially, laterally, and superiorly.

When harvesting a hard palate graft, the central palatine raphe, anterior palatine rugae, and the area overlying the greater palatine foramen where the anterior palatine artery exits should be avoided. A graft of appropriate size and shape is outlined with a marking pen. The midline of the hard palate should be avoided. In most cases, rectangular-shaped grafts are harvested with a #15 or #64 blade. It is very difficult to thin the graft once it is free from the donor bed, thus the graft thickness should be taken into consideration during the initial dissection. The palatal periosteum is left intact to enhance healing of the donor site. Oxidized regenerated cellulose or microfibrillar collagen hemostat may be used to achieve hemostasis.

The graft is then soaked in antibiotic solution and trimmed to the appropriate dimensions. It is placed into the defect and secured to the tarsal remnants (or canthal tissue remnants or free tarsal graft) with interrupted partial-thickness 5-0 Vicryl sutures.

32.2.2 Lower Eyelid

32.2.2.1 Primary Closure

Primary closure with or without lateral canthotomy/cantholysis is achieved as outlined in the previous sections. Closure must not induce tension as this will cause lower eyelid retraction.

32.2.2.2 Hughes Tarsoconjunctival Flap + Graft/Flap

In the lower lid, deficient posterior lamella not amenable to primary closure may be addressed with a Hughes tarsoconjunctival flap [2]. A Hughes flap provides excellent structural support and an inherent blood supply. The main disadvantage is obscuration of the pupil by the tarsoconjunctival bridge for 4–8 weeks.

To begin the flap formation, the inferior border of the defect is squared off with a #15 blade to create a rectangular defect with the lateral and medial edges perpendicular to the lid margin. The edges are advanced centrally with forceps, and the horizontal defect is measured. A lateral canthotomy may be employed to increase horizontal movement and reduce the width of the defect.

The ipsilateral upper lid is everted over a chalazion clamp. A three-sided flap is harvested on the central tarsal conjunctival surface of the upper lid with a #15 blade. The incision should be at least 4 mm from the lid margin to minimize postoperative entropion, contour deformities, loss of lashes, and trichiasis. Vertical incisions through the tarsus and conjunctiva are directed superiorly in a plane perpendicular to the lid margin. The flap is undermined from the overlying levator aponeurosis and orbicularis muscle with Wescott scissors. Dissection is continued above the superior tarsal border between the conjunctiva and Mueller's muscle toward the superior fornix. The tarsoconjunctival flap is then mobilized into the lower lid defect so that the upper lid superior tarsal border is aligned with the lower lid margin remnant. Interrupted partial-thickness 5-0 Vicryl sutures are passed through the tarsus to secure the lateral and medial edges of the flap to the tarsal stumps. Finally, interrupted and running 7-0 Vicryl sutures are used to secure the inferior edge of the flap to the cut edge of the inferior forniceal conjunctiva and lower eyelid retractors.

The second stage of the Hughes procedure is undertaken 4–8 weeks later. It is delayed until the reconstructed lower lid has established its new blood supply and sufficient time has passed to counteract the downward contractile forces of scar maturation and gravity. The flap is incised 0.5–1.0 mm above the new lower lid margin with blunt Wescott or Stevens scissors. Care is taken to avoid traumatizing the underlying cornea. The excess mucosa from the lower portion of the flap is left to retract or sutured to a skin incision made along the new lid margin with a running 7-0 Vicryl suture. This process establishes the new mucocutaneous border. The superior portion of the flap is allowed to retract under the upper lid.

The anterior lamella may be addressed with either a full-thickness skin graft or an advancement flap. A tarsoconjunctival graft will serve as a vascular source for a skin graft.

32.2.2.3 Free Tarsal Graft/Hard Palate Graft + Flap

The posterior lamella may be repaired with a free tarsal graft or a hard palate graft. The anterior lamella may be repaired with a myocutaneous advancement flap, an ellipse sliding flap, or a unipedicle flap. The newly reconstructed eyelid should be kept on stretch to prevent retraction during the healing process. A 4-0 silk suture should be placed through the newly created lid margin. The suture is secured to the forehead with Benzoin and paper tape and kept in place for 2 weeks.

Summary: Special Circumstances

- Medial canthal defects may be closed with a glabellar flap. This advancement of local tissue not only provides wound closure but allows for repair with tissue of adequate depth. Other special circumstances include the use of a galeal or pericranial flap in cases of an insufficient vascularized pedicle and the use of a tissue expander in patients with deficient anterior lamella.

32.3 Special Circumstances

32.3.1 Medial Canthal Defect

Defects of the medial canthus have additional considerations. First, the lacrimal system must be evaluated. If there is uncertainty regarding the state of the canaliculi, a 00-Bowman probe may be used to check for defects. The punctum is first dilated. For the upper lid, the Bowman probe is placed into the punctum and directed superiorly (inferiorly for the lower lid) for approximately 2 mm. It is then angled toward the medial canthus through the canaliculus until a hard stop is felt. If the canaliculus is intact, the Bowman probe that has been placed into the lacrimal system should not be visible. If canalicular defects are encountered, they must first be repaired.

One option is to place a mini Monoka stent into the lacerated canalicular lumen. The stent is first trimmed to the appropriate length. After placement, the edges of the lacerated canaliculus are reapproximated with a few interrupted 7-0 Vicryl sutures.

If the canalicular defect is too medial for a Monoka stent, a donut silicone stent may be placed. A pigtail lacrimal probe is passed through the intact opposing canaliculus and into the proximal portion of the lacerated canaliculus. It is then threaded through the severed distal portion. A 6-0 Prolene is threaded through the eyelet at the tip of the probe. The probe's path is reversed and separated from the Prolene which alone now maintains the canalicular system. Next, a piece of silicone stent (~26–27 mm in length) is guided over the Prolene. The suture ends are then tied together and the knot is trimmed. The knot is then rotated to face the common canaliculus. Reconstruction is now directed toward the soft tissues.

32.3.1.1 Glabellar Flap

A glabellar flap is an excellent method of reconstructing an anterior lamellar defect of the medial canthal region. It is a modified V- to Y-rotation flap [3]. First, an inverted V incision is outlined from the midpoint of the glabella just above the brow at an angle less than 60°. Both segments of the flap should extend below the brow with the longer portion joining the lateral aspect of the defect. The previously outlined skin and subcutaneous tissue are incised with a #15 blade and then undermined extensively with Stevens scissors. It is then rotated into the defect. The apex of the flap is placed at the lateral edge. Once the tip of the flap is trimmed to fit the defect, the flap is secured with buried anchoring, interrupted 5-0 Vicryl sutures. The skin is then closed with interrupted and running 7-0 Vicryl sutures. The donor site is sutured in a V- to Y-closure in two layers. The donor site closure may induce a shortening of the interbrow distance. Occasionally, the flap requires a secondary debulking 6–8 weeks later at its base if the tissue from the donor forehead glabellar region is thicker than that of the recipient medial canthus.

32.3.2 Insufficient Vascularized Pedicle

Some flaps are too large to close primarily or with local tissue recruitment. Because two free grafts overlying each other will not survive, additional methods of repair must be employed to provide an inherent blood supply. Galeal and pericranial flaps provide well-vascularized tissue beds upon which further reconstruction may be based [9]. Skin is not transposed with a galeal or pericranial flap. Bunching over the nasal bridge is less of concern secondary to the thinner nature of these flaps when compared to a glabellar flap. The galeopericranial flap is thought to be superior to the pericranial flap because of its increased vascularity.

The five layers of scalp's soft tissue are the skin, subcutaneous soft tissue, galea aponeurotica, subgaleal loose areolar tissue, and periosteum. The pericranium consists of the periosteum and the overlying subaponeurotic loose connective tissue. It is contiguous with the deep temporal fascia in the temporal region. The pericranium also has a dual blood supply, which ensures the viability of a pericranial flap. The galea aponeurotica is composed of dense fibrous tissue.

The posterior lamella is first reconstructed prior to the repair of large upper eyelid defects. The soft tissue defect is then filled with a galeopericranial or pericranial flap. To begin, a standard bicoronal incision is made over the vertex of the skull. A transcoronal incision provides access to the pericranium of the forehead. The plane of dissection is between the subcutaneous tissue and the galea for a galeopericranial flap. The plane for pericranial flaps is subgaleal. The loose areolar tissue and periosteum of the frontal bone are left intact. Dissection proceeds toward the supraorbital rim while care is taken to leave the supraorbital and supratrochlear neurovascular bundles undisturbed. Dissection stops where the vessels enter the base of the flap. The pericranium and galea are incised and elevated from the frontal bone with an elevator. The flap is mobilized and turned down anteriorly through the skin defect. It may be turned in multiple arcs for reconstructive purposes. The length, width, angle, and shape are tailored for the specific deformity to allow for adequate rotation and coverage. It is important to avoid a transverse incision of the flap 2 fingerbreadths above the superior orbital rim because the frontalis nerve enters the frontalis muscle in this area. Once the flap is in place, it serves as a well-vascularized bed for a full-thickness skin graft.

32.3.3 Insufficient Anterior Lamella

Very large anterior lamellar defects may require additional methods beyond skin grafts and flaps. Tissue expansion has been used in periocular reconstruction in patients with extensive defects [10]. The posterior lamella is first reconstructed with a free tarsal or hard palate graft. Tissue expansion is an ideal method to provide vascularized skin that is similar in appearance, thickness, and texture to the skin adjacent to the defect while preserving the maximal amount of normal tissue. It also allows for more rapid vascularization of any free grafts beneath the flap. The non-hair-bearing nature and pliability of the created tissue are additional advantages. The main disadvantage is the creation of temporary disfigurement.

Reconstructive tissue is recruited in a staged fashion from the adjacent skin, such as the forehead, temporalis, and preauricular regions, and the lid. Care should be taken with expansion of the lid proper to avoid pressure on the underlying globe. First, a skin incision is made along the hairline, brow, or a preexisting incision line. The incision site should not be located over the subsequently placed expander or interfere with the vascular supply or subsequent rotation of the flap.

The recipient pocket is dissected in the subcutaneous tissues. In the forehead region, a large pocket is dissected between the periosteum and the galea or deep fascia of the frontalis muscle. In the temporal region, a pocket is dissected in a plane between the subdermal fatty layer and the superficial temporal fascia. Complete hemostasis is an absolute requirement to prevent the formation of a hematoma.

Next, the expander is soaked in an antibiotic solution. The deflated device is tested for leaks and placed into the recipient pocket. All remaining air is expressed from the device, and the expander is filled with a sufficient amount of saline to flatten its folds and remove any dead space within the pocket. The expander is deflated until the tension on the skin is adequate to provide hemostasis. A remote expander is placed into the pocket through the same skin incision. The wound is closed in two layers.

Serial expansion ensues 2–3 weeks after placement. A 27-gauge needle is used to percutaneously inject saline through the port. Inflation is carried out until the expander feels taut. In general, 10–15% of the total expander volume is injected at any one time. The expander is reinjected two times per week with approximately 1 mL of saline in the remote expander and 10 mL in the larger expander. Expansion is usually complete in 6–8 weeks. The expander is removed, and the newly created skin now provides a local skin flap for eyelid reconstruction. In most cases, serial expansion also allows for sufficient thinning of the dermal tissue so the final flap is of appropriate thickness to fill the defect and match the adjacent tissue.

Summary: Postoperative Care and Follow-up

- Postoperatively, a pressure patch is usually placed over the eyelids to prevent bleeding and excessive movement of reconstructed tissues.

32.4 Postoperative Care and Follow-up

A pressure patch is usually placed over the reconstructed eyelids immediately postoperatively. The patch reduces postoperative bleeding and acts as a splint to prevent excessive movement of the reconstructed tissues. The patch is angled inferolaterally, beginning at the central forehead. Benzoin or Mastisol should be used on the skin in the forehead and cheek areas to secure the patch. Following installation of ophthalmic antibiotic ointment over the cornea, two sterile eyepads are placed over the *closed* eyelid. Next, two 4×4 gauze pads are unfolded, gently reformed into a round configuration, and placed over the eyepads. Lastly, 2-in. paper tape is layered firmly over the dressings and anchored to the Benzoin/Mastisol. The patient is instructed to keep the patch in place and dry for 1 week.

Summary: Conclusion

- The key principle in eyelid reconstruction is the need for either the anterior or the posterior lamella to have an inherent vascular supply.

32.5 Conclusion

Eyelid reconstruction must achieve optimum function, globe protection, and aesthetics. The choice of reconstructive method is dependent upon the state of the eyelid margin. Defects involving the lid margin require reconstruction of both the anterior and posterior lamellae. The key principle of eyelid reconstruction is the need for the anterior or the posterior lamella to have an inherent blood supply (pedicle flap). A robust, inherent vascular supply ensures tissue survival and the most favorable surgical outcome for the patient.

References

1. Kersten RC et al. Section 7: Orbit, eyelids, and lacrimal system. In: American Academy of Ophthalmology, editor. Basic and clinical science course. San Francisco: American Academy of Ophthalmology; 2003.
2. Kronish J. Eyelid reconstruction. In: Tse DT, editor. Color atlas of ophthalmic surgery: oculoplastic surgery. Philadelphia: J.B. Lippincott Company; 1992. p. 260–70.
3. Kronish J. Eyelid reconstruction. In: Tse DT, editor. Color atlas of ophthalmic surgery: oculoplastic surgery. Philadelphia: J.B. Lippincott Company; 1992. p. 245.
4. Nerad JA. Eyelid reconstruction. In: Krachmer JH, editor. The requisites in ophthalmology oculoplastic surgery. St. Louis: Mosby; 2001. p. 282.
5. Cook Jr BE, Bartley GB. Treatment options and future prospects for the management of eyelid malignancies: an evidence-based update. Ophthalmology. 2001;108: 2088.
6. Bartley GB, Kay PP. Posterior lamellar eyelid reconstruction with a hard palate mucosal graft. Am J Ophthalmol. 1989;107:609–12.
7. Beatty RL, Harris G, Bauman GR, Mills MP. Intraoral palatal mucosal graft harvest. Ophthal Plast Reconstr Surg. 1993;9:120–4.
8. Beatty RL et al. Intraoral palatal mucosal graft harvest. Ophthal Plast Reconstr Surg. 1997;13(2):90.
9. Tse DT et al. Use of galeal and pericranial flaps for reconstruction of orbital and eyelid defects. Arch Ophthalmol. 1997;115:932.
10. Tse DT, McCafferty LR. Controlled tissue expansion in periocular reconstructive surgery. Ophthalmology. 1993;100: 260.

Flaps

33

Jessica M. Sheehan and Thomas E. Rohrer

Abstract

When simple primary closure is not ideal, a tissue-movement procedure, such as a flap, should be considered. The planning and execution of a flap repair following Mohs surgery vary from case to case. A skilled surgeon evaluates the risks and benefits of various options in each individual patient and anticipates potential complications. The elements to successful flap execution include proper patient selection and preparation, comprehension of risks and necessary precautions, use of sterile or clean technique, informed procedure design and meticulous suture technique, as well as good postoperative wound care and patient education. Flaps are commonly classified according to their primary movement – advancement flaps, rotation flaps, transposition flaps, and interpolation flaps – and each has its benefits and drawbacks. Meticulous postoperative wound care is necessary to ensure an optimal outcome. Patients should be seen for follow-up to evaluate outcomes and any necessary interventions.

Keywords

Defect repair • Flap • Advancement • Rotation • Transposition • Interpolation

Summary: Introduction

- The planning and execution of a flap repair following Mohs surgery vary from case to case. A skilled surgeon evaluates the risks and benefits of various options in each individual patient and maximizes repair success by weighing risks and benefits.

33.1 Introduction

While flap design and successful implementation is as much an art form as it is a science, there are many principles to keep in mind when planning the closure.

J.M. Sheehan (✉)
Northshore Center for Medical Aesthetics,
Northbrook, IL, USA
e-mail: Jessicasheehan09@gmail.com

T.E. Rohrer
SkinCare Physicians, Chestnut Hill, MA, USA

K. Nouri (ed.), *Mohs Micrographic Surgery*,
DOI 10.1007/978-1-4471-2152-7_33, © Springer-Verlag London Limited 2012

As with all surgical repairs, wounds should be closed under minimal tension without distorting critical anatomic structures and landmarks (eyelid, eyebrow, nose, lip, hairline, etc.). Scars should be placed within cosmetic units, along cosmetic unit junctions, or along skin tension lines. The flap must be executed such that the mobilized skin and associated adnexal structures are viable, and there is maximal preservation of sensory and motor nerve function.

The planning and execution of a flap repair following Mohs surgery vary from case to case. A skilled surgeon evaluates the risks and benefits of various options in each individual patient and anticipates potential complications. The elements to successfully perform any dermatologic surgery include proper patient selection and preparation, comprehension of risks and necessary precautions, use of sterile or clean technique, informed procedure design and meticulous suture technique, and postoperative wound care and patient education.

Summary: Risks and Precautions

- There are many risks to dermatologic surgery and flap repair, including pain, bleeding, bruising, infection, dehiscence, and undesirable scar. These risks should be explained to the patient and/or family before surgery. Steps should be taken to minimize these risks.

33.2 Risks and Precautions

It is important that both the patient and practitioner be aware of the risks of dermatologic surgery. In fact, it is required by law in all 50 states that these risks be documented for proper patient consent [1]. The main risks of dermatologic surgery and flap repair include the following.

Pain from the procedure itself is mitigated by the use of local anesthesia, although the delivery of lidocaine in and of itself is painful. Postoperative pain is typically minimal and controlled with over-the-counter analgesics such as acetaminophen. Meticulous operative technique will also help minimize postoperative pain. More severe pain may require the prescription of narcotics.

Excessive bleeding, subsequent bruising, and possible hematoma formation are also risks. A hematoma is a particularly undesirable complication as it can interfere with flap viability. Most dermatologic surgeons now recommend that medically necessary anticoagulation, including aspirin, clopidogrel, heparin, and warfarin, be continued perioperatively [2]. Herbal supplements such as ginseng or garlic, vitamin E, aspirin, and nonsteroidal anti-inflammatory agents that are not prescribed by a physician should be discontinued 2 weeks prior to surgery if possible [2]. The consumption of alcohol should also be restricted immediately before and after the procedure. Meticulous hemostasis with electrocautery or coagulation, arterial ligation of larger arteries, and the application of a compression bandage minimize the risk of bleeding.

Risk of infection exists whenever the barrier of the skin is breached. Wound infection is relatively uncommon [3] and occurs more frequently in particular patient populations, such as those who are diabetic, smokers, or immunosuppressed, and at certain surgical sites, such as the ear or lower leg [4]. Sterile technique and atraumatic tissue handling minimize this risk. Prophylactic antibiotics may be administered for high-risk patients or if the wound base or suture perforates into non-sterile areas, such as the nasal or oral cavities.

Wound dehiscence or flap necrosis occurs in wounds with high tension, in poorly vascularized flaps, or in cases of poor wound healing or infection. Tobacco smoking considerably increases this risk. This risk is reduced by proper design of the flap, which includes a broad pedicle, minimal torsion of the tissue, and minimal tension. The use of buried subcutaneous sutures is paramount, and at times fascial plication is required to relieve tension on wound edges. Patients should be advised in minimizing activity and immobilization of the wound edges for 1–2 weeks after surgery.

Undesirable scars are always a possibility. While many steps can be taken to minimize the appearance of the final scar, it is important for the patient to understand that all dermatologic surgery will result in the formation of a scar. Free margins must be respected and never distorted. Closures are best hidden when they are placed on along cosmetic unit junctions and contained in as few cosmetic units as possible. The long axis of the excision and/or design of a repair should be placed in the direction of rhytides or relaxed skin tension lines. Remove standing cones of redundant tissue. Buried vertical mattress sutures should be placed to attain good wound eversion and minimize the tension on the wound edges as it heals. Wounds heal best under the optimal conditions of a clean, occluded environment.

Summary: Flap Design and Execution

- The design and execution of a cutaneous flap require attention to multiple factors. These include functional and cosmetic surgical outcomes and the comprehension of tissue perfusion forces affecting the viability of transferred tissue. Flaps are either based on a large, named artery or on unnamed arterioles and capillaries of the subdermal vascular plexus. They are commonly classified by their primary movement.

33.3 Flap Design and Execution

When simple primary closure is not the ideal repair (i.e., because a wound is too large, there is too much tension on the wound edges, or an unacceptable functional or cosmetic result would ensue), a tissue-movement procedure, such as a flap, should be considered. A local skin flap is a portion of full-thickness skin and variable subcutaneous tissue transferred from an adjacent donor site into the surgical defect. The flap maintains its blood supply via a vascular pedicle that remains connected to the donor site.

The vascular perfusion pressure, the force of blood flow through a vessel, is greatest at the proximal end of a vessel and decreases steadily as it travels more distal into the flap. To ensure flap survival, the perfusion pressure must be great enough to keep the distal capillaries of the flap patent. If the pressure falls below a certain critical level, the capillaries close leading to an insufficient blood supply to the distal end of the flap.

For years, it was believed that the viable length of a flap was directly proportional to the width of the pedicle. In 1970, Milton discovered that axial flaps in a pig model under the same conditions of blood supply only survive to a finite length regardless of width [5]. Daniel and Williams, as well as Stell, confirmed Milton's findings and concluded that there was an upper limit of flap length that cannot be increased by increasing the pedicle width [6, 7]. The maximal flap length is determined by vascular supply, not simply pedicle width. The greater the perfusion pressure in the flap pedicle, the longer the flap can be without undergoing necrosis [8]. In addition, the greater the perfusion pressure in the pedicle, the narrower the pedicle may be.

Random pattern flaps, the most widely used in dermatologic surgery, are supported by the small arterioles and capillaries of the subdermal vascular plexus found in the mid to superficial fat. Therefore, undermining and flap mobilization must be performed at or below this level to ensure adequate blood supply. If undermining occurs too superficially, the intradermal vasculature alone will often not be able to support a flap. In general, random pattern flaps on the face should have a maximal length to width ratio of 3:1 [9, 10]. This is however only a rough guideline, and individual patient characteristics such as tobacco use, sebaceous nature of skin, prior radiation or surgical procedures, and precise location all affect vascular perfusion. To help ensure flap survival, the pedicle length to width ratios should not exceed 2:1 on the trunk and extremities.

Axial pattern flaps, with few exceptions, are supported by a large, named artery. They have the highest perfusion pressure at the base and therefore can support very narrow, long flaps (generally greater than 4:1 length to width ratio). Musculocutaneous flaps have the next greatest vascular perfusion pressure, followed by fasciocutaneous flaps, and finally random pattern flaps. Stell discovered that the greatest length of a viable axial flap was 60% greater than that of a random pattern flap [7].

The two movements involved in repairing a defect with a flap are the primary movement, which is the action of placing the flap into the defect, and the secondary movement of tissue in the donor area, which closes the secondary defect and facilitates primary flap movement. Both movements are important in terms of distributing tension in the proper direction and over a larger area so as to minimize tension on the flap itself which might compromise its survival [11]. Flaps are commonly classified according to their primary movement – advancement flaps, rotation flaps, transposition flaps, and interpolation flaps. This classification underplays the reality that many flaps have more than one primary movement, e.g., a rotation flap usually has a component of advancement to fill the distal portion of a wound. Therefore another way to classify flaps is by whether the primary movement is "sliding," which displaces tissue redundancy at a site distant from the defect (advancement and rotation) or "lifting," where a flap is moved over intact skin, reorienting wound tension (transposition and interpolation).

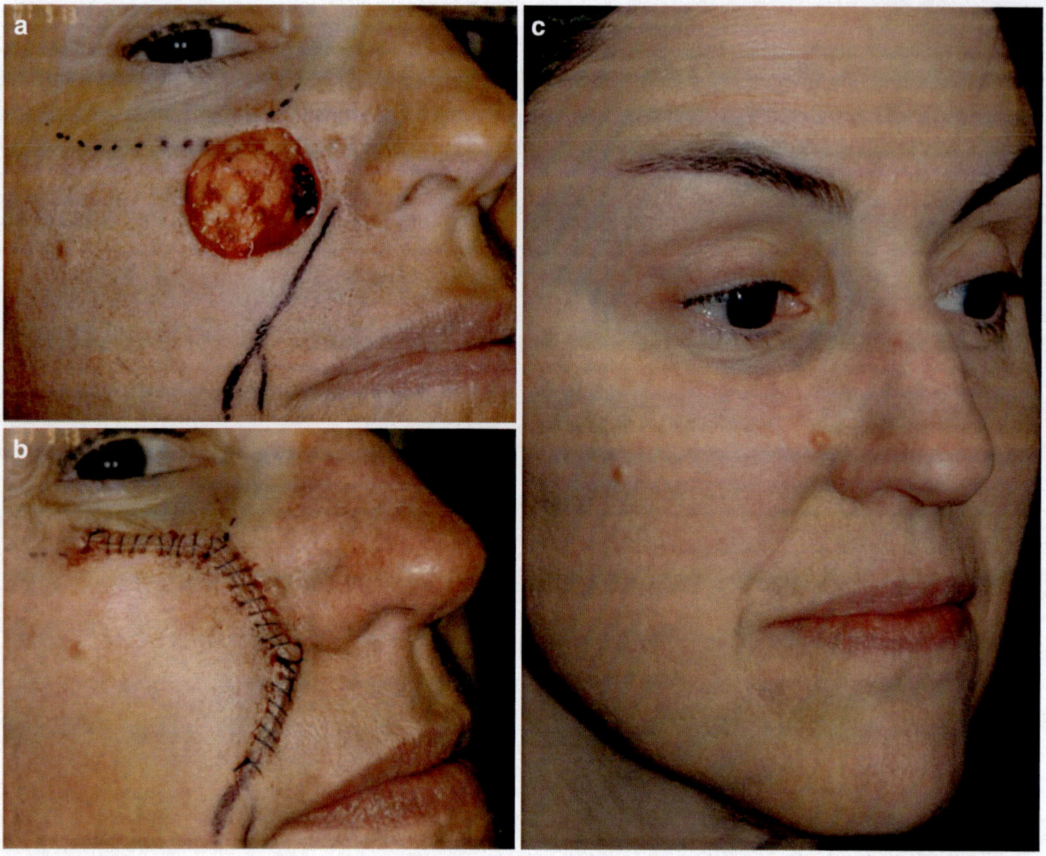

Fig. 33.1 Single advancement flap, U-plasty of right cheek, (**a**) after Mohs; (**b**) immediately afer repair; (**c**) 3 months post-operative

> **Summary: Advancement Flaps**
> - A rotation flap is a random pattern flap. The primary movement of an advancement flap is the one-dimensional sliding of tissue directly into a defect, redistributing tissue redundancy. There are several variations, including single and bilateral advancement flaps and island pedicle flaps.

33.4 Advancement Flaps

The primary movement of an advancement flap is the one-dimensional sliding of tissue directly into a defect. In essence, incisions are made tangentially to the defect to free up neighboring tissue. With the wound edge acting as the free margin of the flap, the tissue is advanced into place, displacing tissue cones. While some adjacent tissue laxity may be tapped into with an advancement flap, the tension vectors of the closure remain the same, and therefore the primary advantage of an advancement flap is the displacement of closure lines into more cosmetically acceptable locations.

33.4.1 Single Advancement

The simplest example of a pure advancement flap is the U-plasty, whereby double, non-parallel incisions are made tangential to the Mohs defect. The flap is undermined, advanced into the defect, and secured with sutures, creating a U-shaped scar (Fig. 33.1). Redundant tissue cones may be sewn out using the rule of halves or removed as Burow's triangles at the base of the flap. The U-plasty is often used in the repair of a forehead, placing scars horizontally and running with the natural skin tension lines. However, the tension vectors are unchanged, and therefore this flap does not significantly free up tissue, limiting its utility.

An L-plasty or O to L advancement is a single tangent flap where an incision is made at one end of a defect extending outward for some length, and the tissue mobilized is then advanced into the defect (Fig. 33.2). Tissue redundancy is created on the side

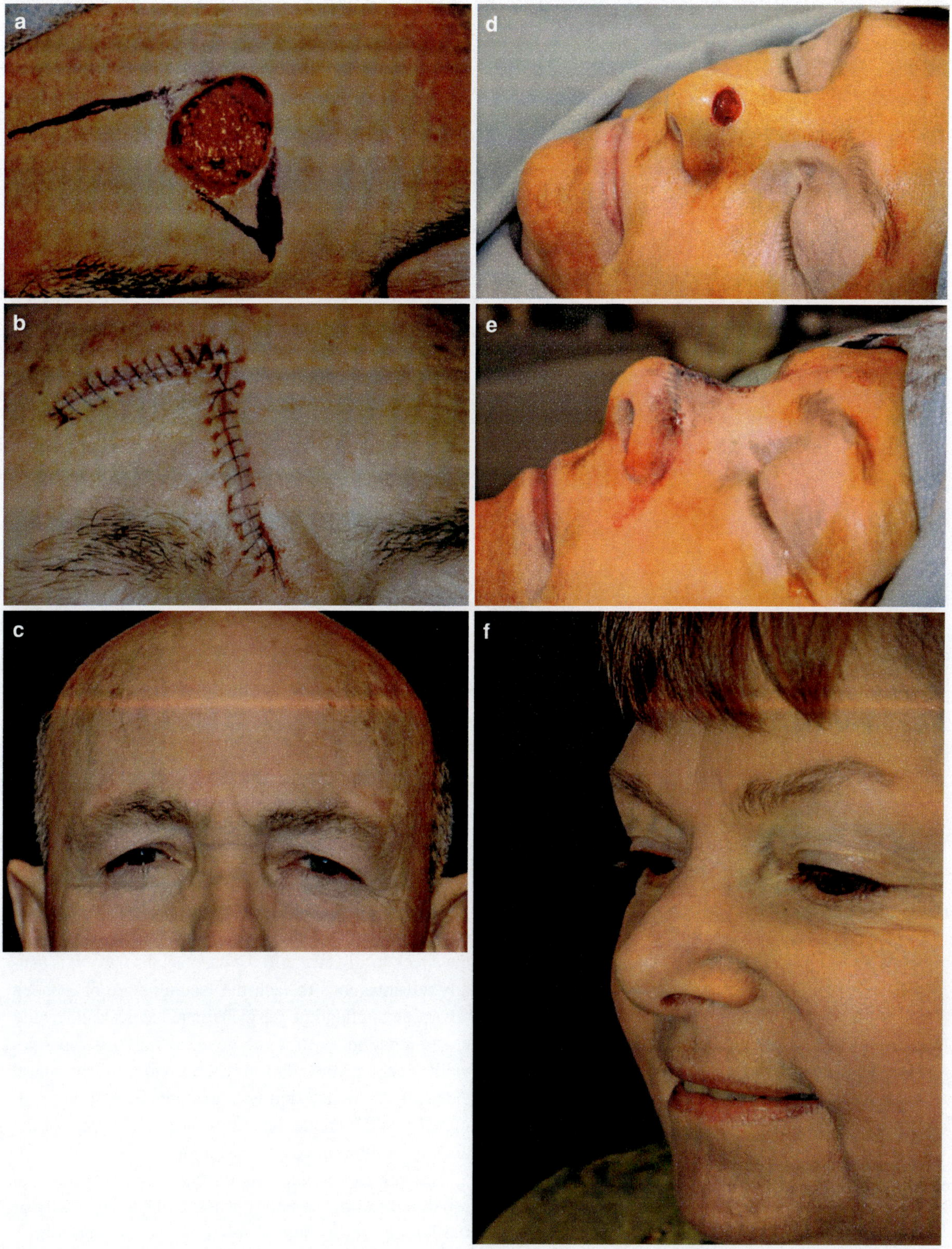

Fig. 33.2 O to L advancement flap. (**a**)After Mohs on forehead; (**b**) immediately after repair; (**c**) 6 weeks post-operative; (**d**) After Mohs on nasal supratip; (**e**) immediately after repair; (**f**) 3months post-operative

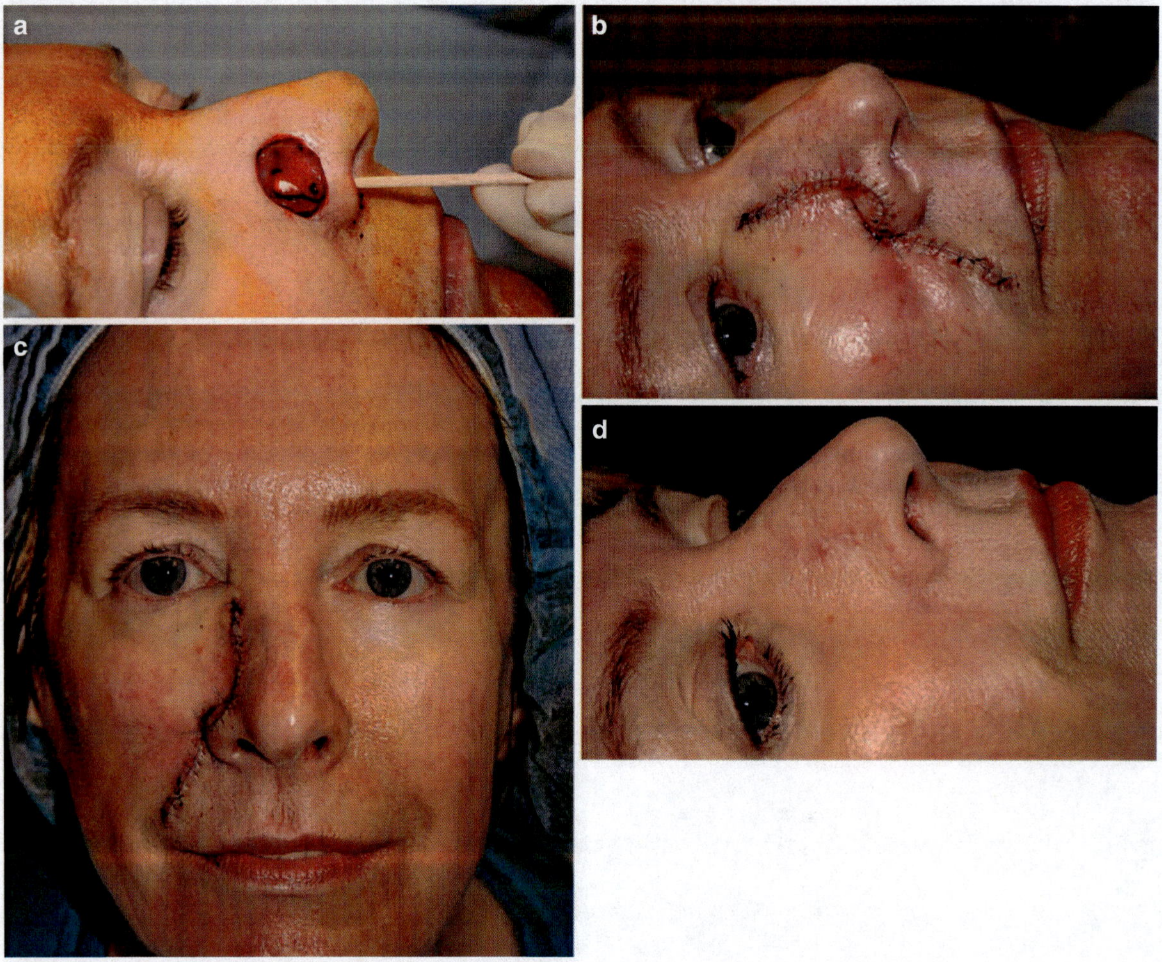

Fig. 33.3 Cheek advancement flap (with conchal bowl full thickness skin graft on ala)

of the defect opposite the flap incision and must be removed or carefully sewn out. While this type of advancement flap may tap into some distant laxity, it is generally minimal. Advancement flaps spread the tension out over a longer distance and offer some of the closure line to be perpendicular to the vector of tension. O to L advancement flaps are particularly useful with defects where the limb of the flap may be incorporated into RSTLs or cosmetic unit junctions or where a linear closure may otherwise cross a free margin or cosmetic unit junction, as may be the case on the eyebrow, nose, or upper lip.

A larger single advancement flap is the cheek advancement flap, used to repair medium to large defects of the medial cheek and/or lateral nose (Fig. 33.3). The incision may placed in the alar crease or nasolabial fold by removing tissue above and below the defect to allow the cheek to advance into the nasofacial sulcus. It is usually advantageous to tack the leading edge of a cheek advancement flap into periosteum at the nasal sidewall–cheek junction, even if the defect is on the nasal sidewall. Tacking the flap to periosteum at the nasal sidewall–cheek junction will take pressure off the leading edge and recreate the natural concave surface of the area, preventing unnatural webbing.

Helical rim advancement flaps may be used to repair defects of the helix, utilizing the tissue laxity of the lobule. Traditionally, this flap was created with a through-and-through incision inferior to the defect along the scaphoid fossa, terminating in the lobule and

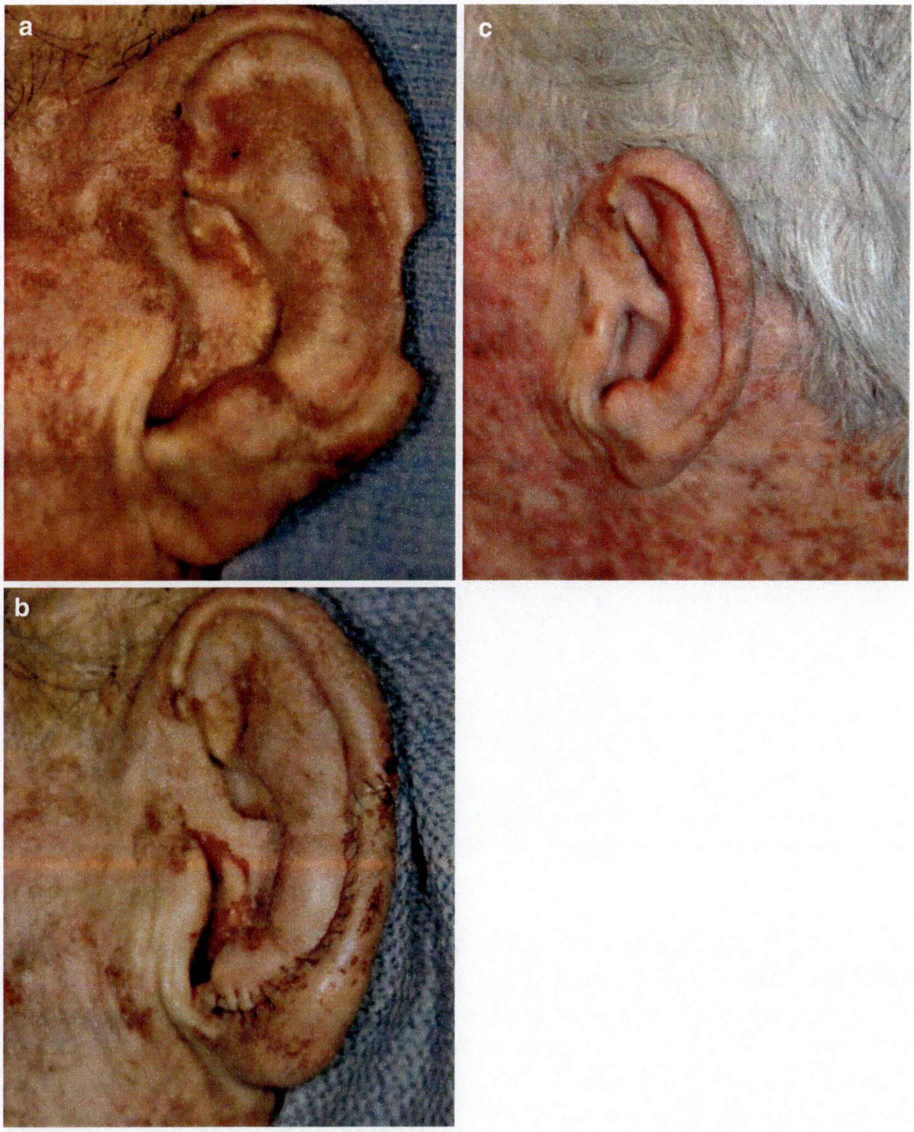

Fig. 33.4 Helical rim advancement flap

creating a narrow pedicle to be advanced (conceptually similar to the U-plasty). The survivability of this flap is proportional to the length to width ratio and could only be performed on inferior helical defects where this ratio will not exceed 3–4:1. A more popular modification of this flap is to use a single tangent incision along the scaphoid fossa, leaving the posterior auricular skin intact [12] (conceptually analogous to the L-plasty) (Fig. 33.4). This allows for the maintenance of a more reliable blood supply via the tissue inferiorly and posteriorly and permits the repair of defects more distant from the lobule. It is important to have good eversion when closing this flap at the helical rim as forces of contraction during healing will tend to invert the wound edge and create an aesthetically unpleasant notch.

33.4.2 Bilateral Advancement

If two sets of parallel incisions are made symmetrically on both edges of the defect, a bilateral advancement flap, termed an H-plasty, has been created. This flap is essentially a bilateral U-plasty and is occasionally used

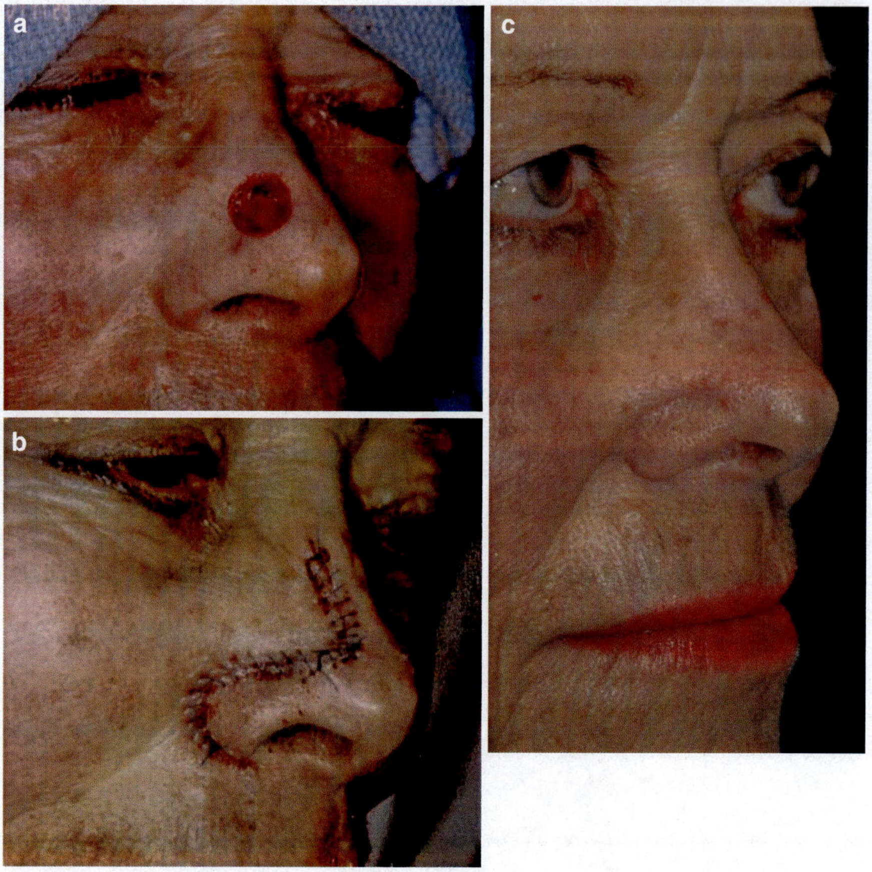

Fig. 33.5 Crescentic advancement flap, nasal sidewall

on the forehead and upper lip to hide incision lines along relaxed skin tension lines and cosmetic unit junctions.

Another commonly employed bilateral advancement flap is an O-to-T flap, also termed on A-to-T or a T-plasty, analogous to a bilateral L-plasty. The standing cone is removed from one end of the defect, creating a triangle or transforming on "O" into an "A." Single incisions extend from the base of this triangular defect, and the two sides of the triangle slide together along this baseline. The T-plasty is best performed with the broad base along a free margin or cosmetic unit junction (e.g., lip, eyebrow).

33.4.3 Crescentic Advancement

The crescentic advancement flap utilizes the removal of a small crescent of tissue along an advancement flap to either better hide the scar line or increase the length of the line to prevent distortion. This flap is particularly useful for the repair of upper lip and perialar defects. The superior standing cone is removed in a crescentic shape around the ala such that the superior scar line is placed in the perinasal sulcus (Fig. 33.5) [13]. For defects on the upper cutaneous lip, the inferior cone is removed along relaxed skin tension lines (Fig. 33.6) of the upper lip. If the inferior cone approaches the vermillion border, it is best to extend the cone through the vermillion border and terminate it in the wet mucosa to prevent downward distortion of the vermillion. A modification of the crescentic advancement includes the repair of a small, perialar defect of the medial cheek where both cones are removed around the ala, and the entire scar line is placed in the nasal sulcus, similar to the cheek advancement. Another modification of this type of flap is the East–West flap or modified Burow's advancement flap of Dzubow [14]. This flap is used in nasal tip and supratip defects that are off midline. The Burow's triangle is designed to extend inferiorly down the midline of the nose into the columella, and the flap is advanced horizontally into place (Fig. 33.7).

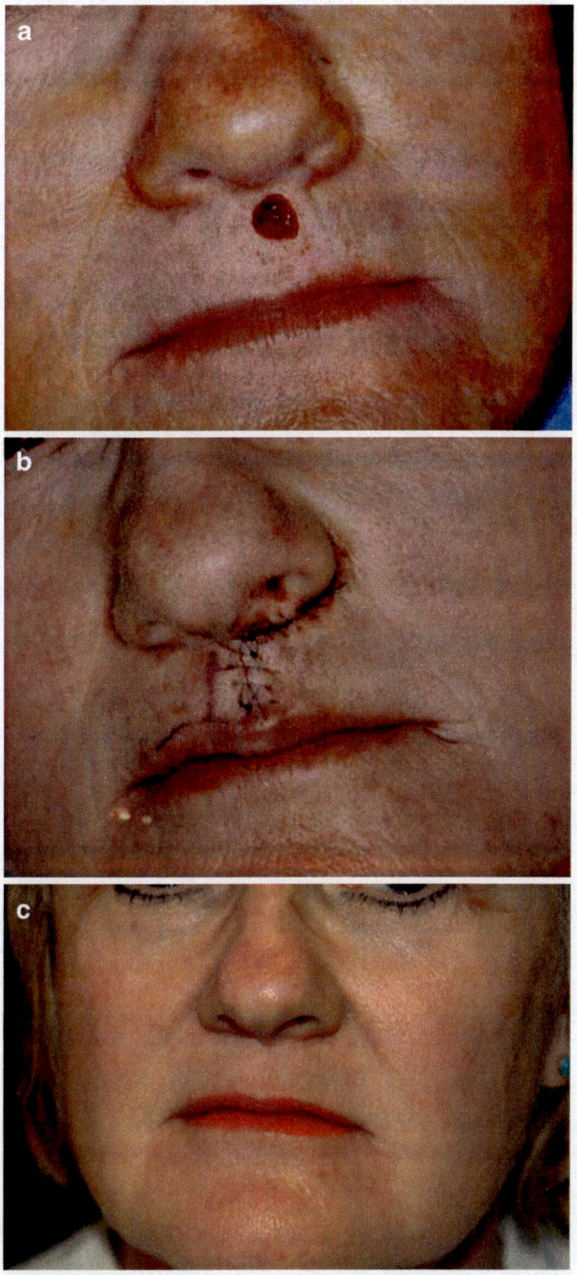

Fig. 33.6 Crescentic advancement flap upper lip

33.4.4 Island Pedicle

A subcutaneous island pedicle flap, also referred to as a V–Y advancement flap, may be considered as a variation of an advancement flap that has had all of its connections to the epidermis and dermis severed, maintaining its blood supply through a subcutaneous tissue pedicle (Fig. 33.8) [15]. The flap is designed within cosmetic units when possible and, as with all repairs, it is optimal for the incision lines to run along cosmetic junctions. The island pedicle flap is frequently used on nasal and perioral closures where free margins are at risk for distortion. The tension vectors of an island pedicle flap are primarily in the same direction as that of a primary closure; however, they are displaced distal to the wound (i.e., superior to the nasal tip, superior or lateral to the vermillion border) and help avoid distortion of the area around the defect.

An island pedicle flap is created by extending two non-parallel tangential incisions to meet at an approximate 30° angle, similar to when planning a Burow's triangle. The difference is that the incision lines stay essentially parallel for a short distance before converging, creating a slightly larger triangle than would be created with a Burrow's triangle. This extra length gives tissue that more closely approximates the size of the defect and minimizes local distortion. The triangle may be designed larger or smaller depending on how much tension sharing is desired. Incisions are made into the superficial subcutaneous tissue. The tip and sides of the flap are undermined widely extending outward from the flap in the subcutaneous plane. The triangular flap is also undermined slightly to help mobilize it. The flap is then advanced into the defect and sutured into place. In order for the flap to fit properly into a circular defect, either the corners of the flap must be trimmed or the defect squared off. The flap must be undermined with attention both to the mobility of the tissue as well as to the maintenance of a subcutaneous vascular pedicle. While the initial design should have a broad pedicle, if mobility is limited, the pedicle may be progressively diminished (particularly at the trailing tip of the flap).

When closing defects on the nasal dorsum and tip, a muscular flap is often created laterally on one or both sides. For this musculocutaneous island pedicle flap, undermining is performed both above and below the nasalis muscle. If there is not enough laxity to close the defect without upward tension on the nasal tip, the muscular flap is released horizontally at the superior and inferior edge to create a muscular sling that advances with the flap into place. The muscular attachment gives a robust blood supply to the flap and helps ensure its survival.

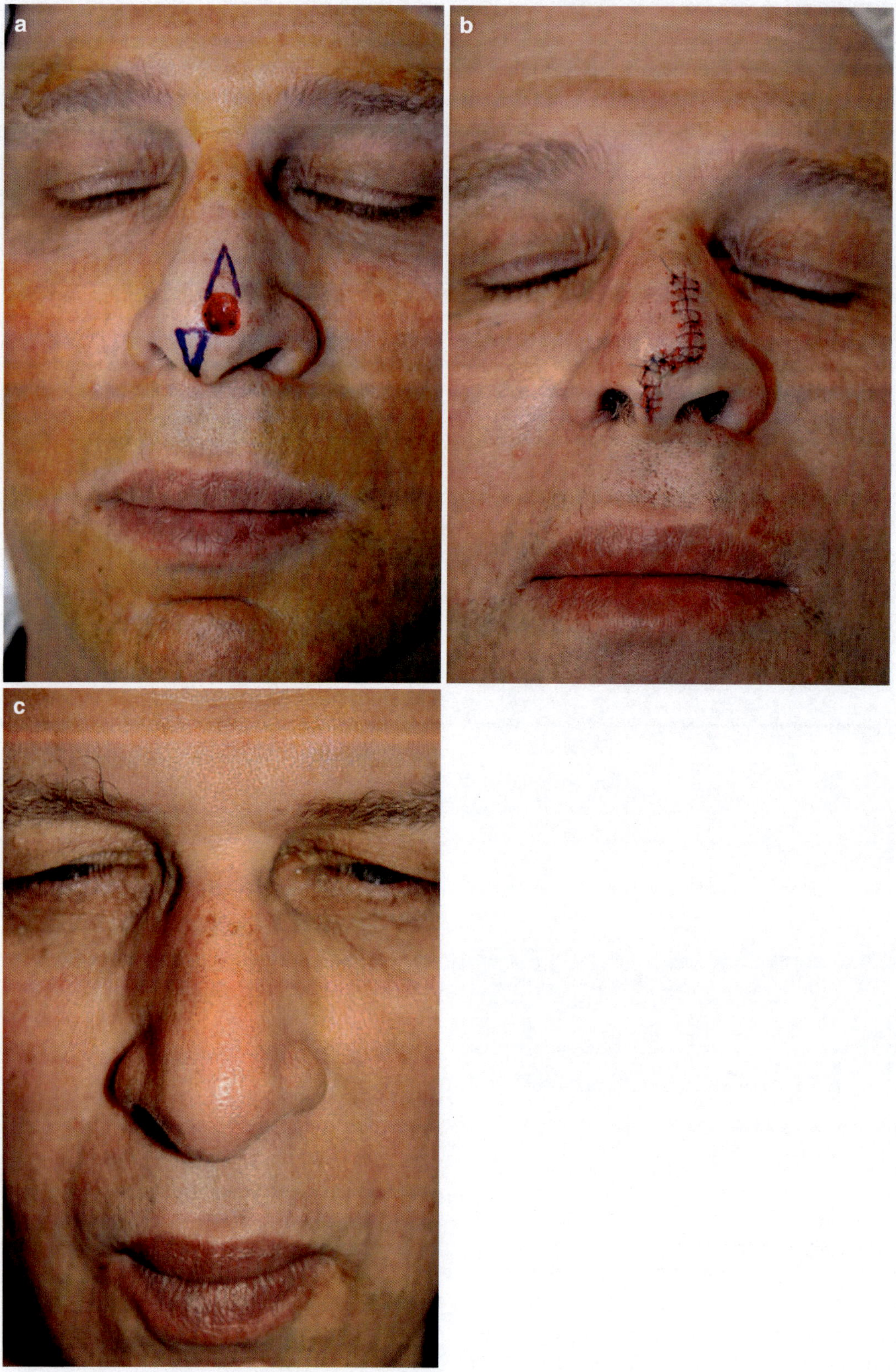

Fig. 33.7 East–West advancement flap/Dzubow modified Burow's advancement flap, left nasal tip

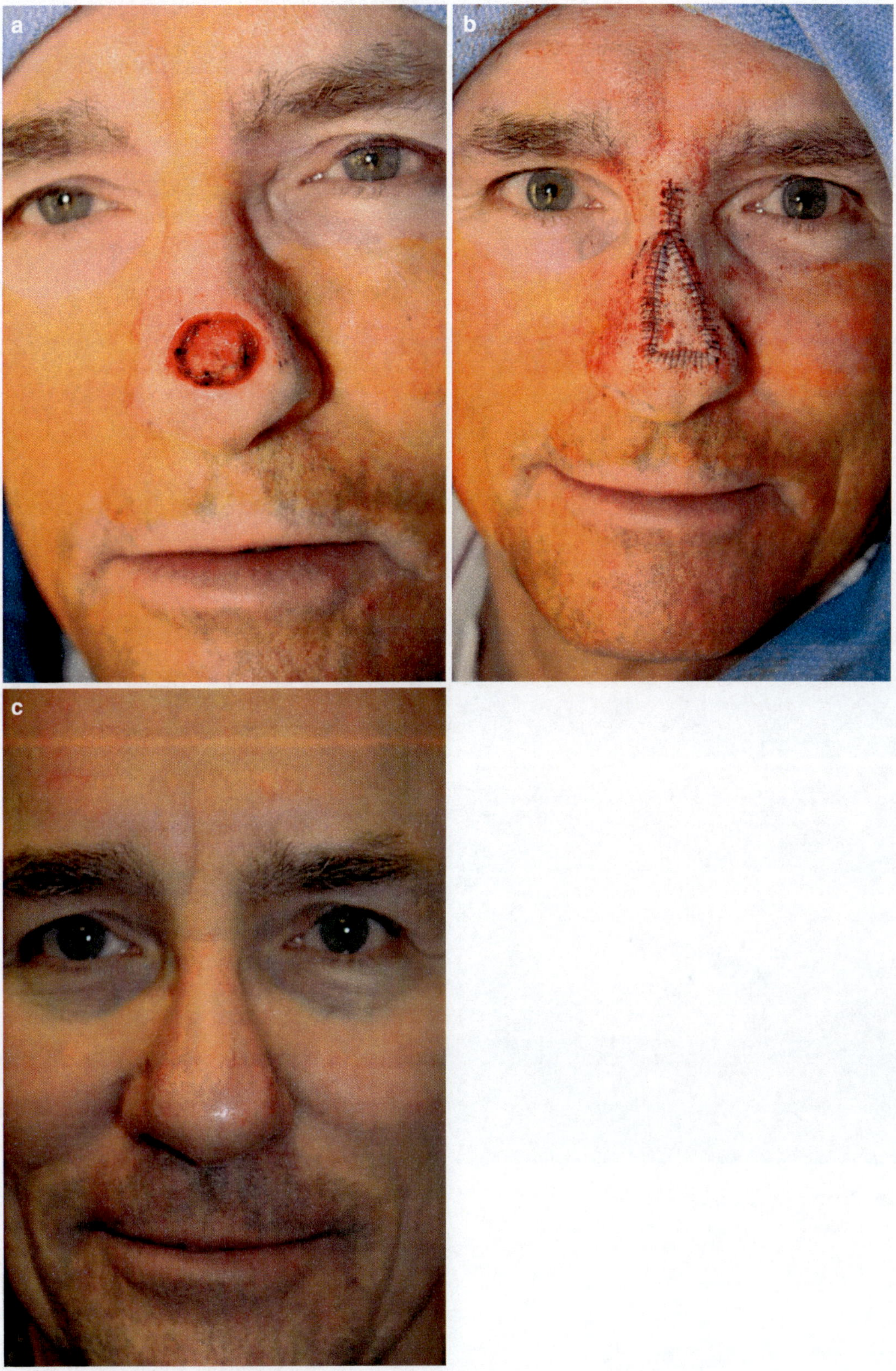

Fig. 33.8 Island pedicle flap, nasal dorsum

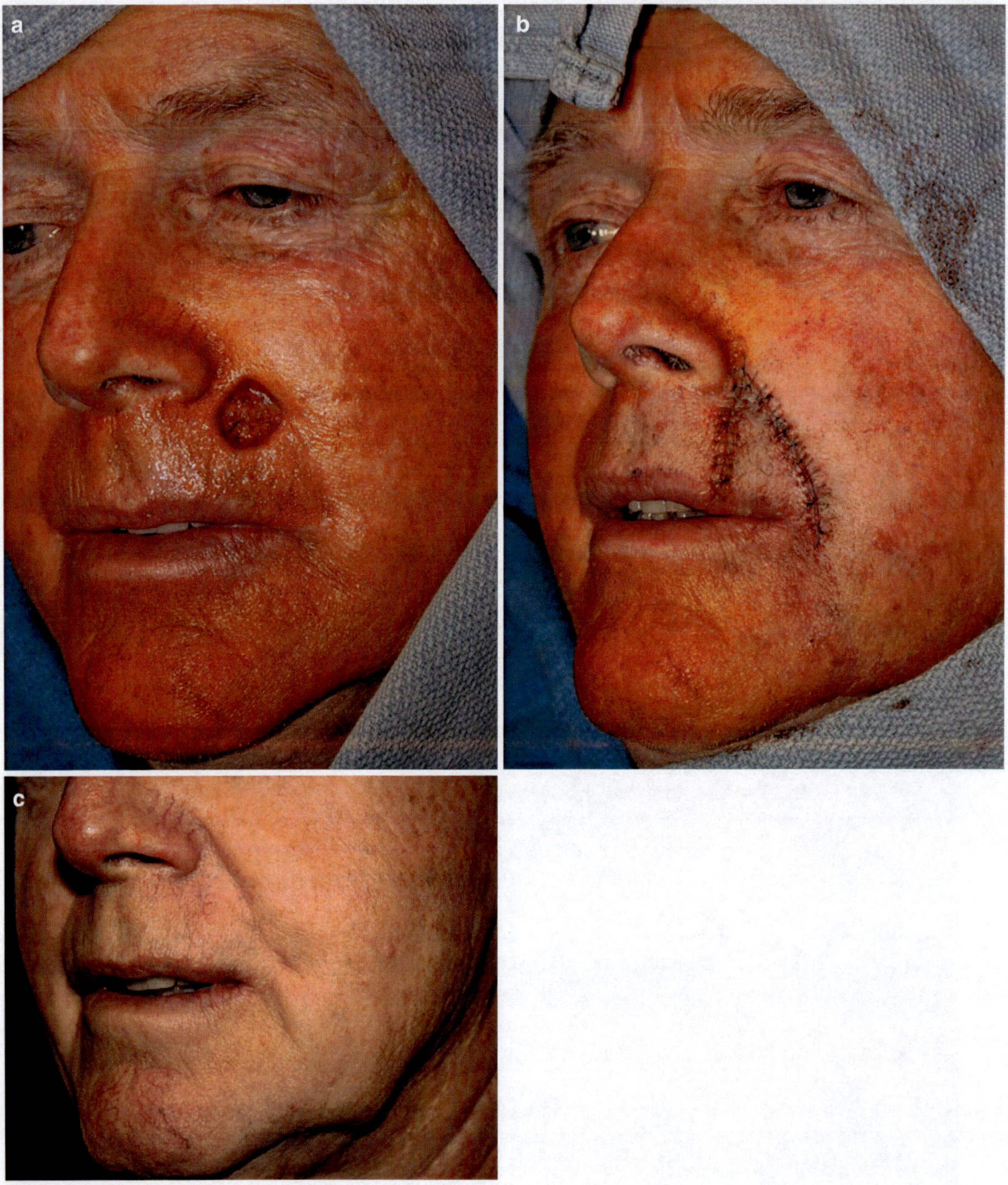

Fig. 33.9 Rotation flap, upper cutaneous lip

Summary: Rotation Flaps

- A rotation flap is a random pattern flap. The primary movement of a rotation flap is the sliding of tissue about a pivot point into a defect, redistributing wound tension as well as tissue redundancy. There are several variations including single and bilateral rotation flaps and dorsal nasal flaps.

33.5 Rotation Flaps

In a rotation flap, skin moves into the defect by rotating around a pivot point (Fig. 33.9). This is classically used to close relatively large defects on the cheek, temple, or scalp. The design of the traditional rotation flap uses a curvilinear incision along an arc adjacent to the primary defect. Adjacent lax tissue is recruited while the closure tension is redirected in multiple directions away from the primary defect. The flap is designed with attention to its length and curvature [16]. Rotation flaps often require long incision lines, as a larger arc of the rotation vector allows closure with minimal tension on the flap's tip while simultaneously decreasing the width of the secondary defect. The ideal arc of a rotation flap extends up to five times the width of the defect and makes up approximately one-quarter of the circumference of a circle.

As the flap is raised and undermined, the adjacent tissue laxity allows the flap to rotate into the primary defect. The stiffness about the pivot point may hinder the flap's movement [16], and undermining the area of pivotal restraint improves flap mobility. If restraint of motion keeps the tip from moving into the distal defect, a back-cut can increase tissue movement in areas of limited tissue laxity, such as the nose. The back-cut cannot extend so far across the base of the flap that it interferes with blood flow into the flap.

33.5.1 Dorsal Nasal Rotation

Also known as the Rieger flap, this flap is employed to repair nasal defects involving the nasal dorsum or tip [17]. The tissue reservoir of the nasal root and glabella allows for the movement of the dorsal nasal skin superior to the defect. A long, sweeping arc is created that extends into the nasofacial sulcus and terminates in the glabella. A back-cut in the glabella improves the rotational mobility of this flap and is termed a hatchet flap (Fig. 33.10). If the arc of this flap is not long enough or there is too much tension on the leading edge of the flap, elevation of the nasal tip will result. Wide undermining at the level of the perichondrium is required.

33.5.2 Bilateral Rotation

At times, the size of the defect or the tension on the flap mandates a bilateral rotation flap, in which tissue is rotated into a defect from two opposite sides. The vectors of rotation may be mirror images of each other, recapitulating the premise of the A–T advancement flap. This may be utilized for large defects on the scalp and larger defects on the lower mucosal lip (Fig. 33.11). The vectors of movement may also be in opposition, creating an O–Z flap, often used for large defects of the scalp.

Summary: Transposition Flaps

- A transposition flap is a random pattern flap. The primary movement of a transposition flap is not merely sliding but rather the lifting of the flap over intervening tissue, redistributing tension vectors. There are several variations of the rhombic, banner, and bilobed flaps.

33.6 Transposition Flaps

A transposition flap is a random pattern flap that borrows skin laxity from an adjacent area in order to fill a defect in an area with little or no skin laxity. In its migration from the donor site to the recipient site, the flap is lifted over, or "transposed" with, a segment of intervening tissue. When the secondary defect is closed, the transposition flap pushes tissue into a defect rather than pulling it, as with the advancement and rotation flaps. The flap is rotated as it is transposed, and it must be designed so that it is not forced to rotate to such a degree that will result in too much tension/torsion on its pedicle.

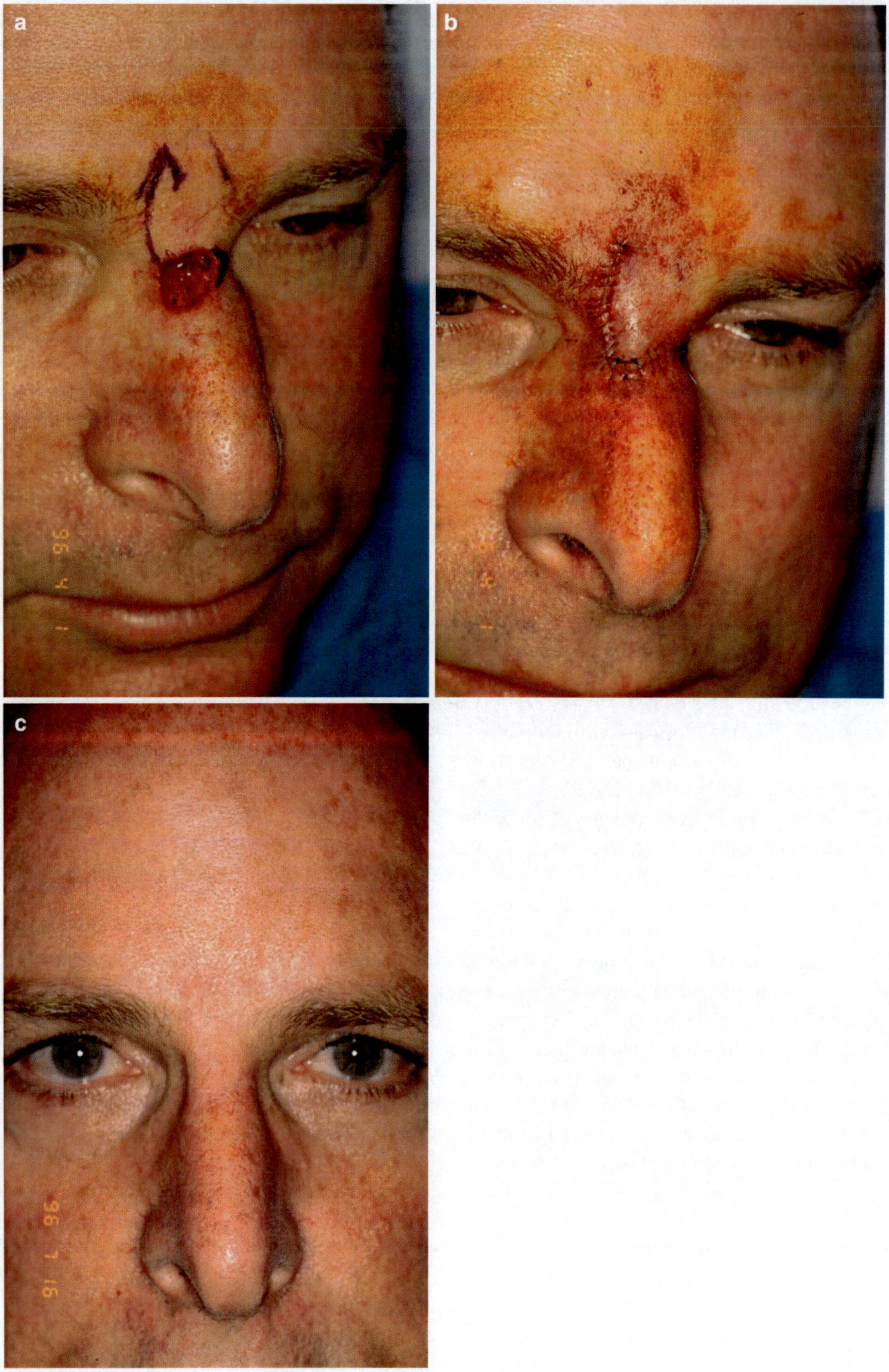

Fig. 33.10 Hatchet flap

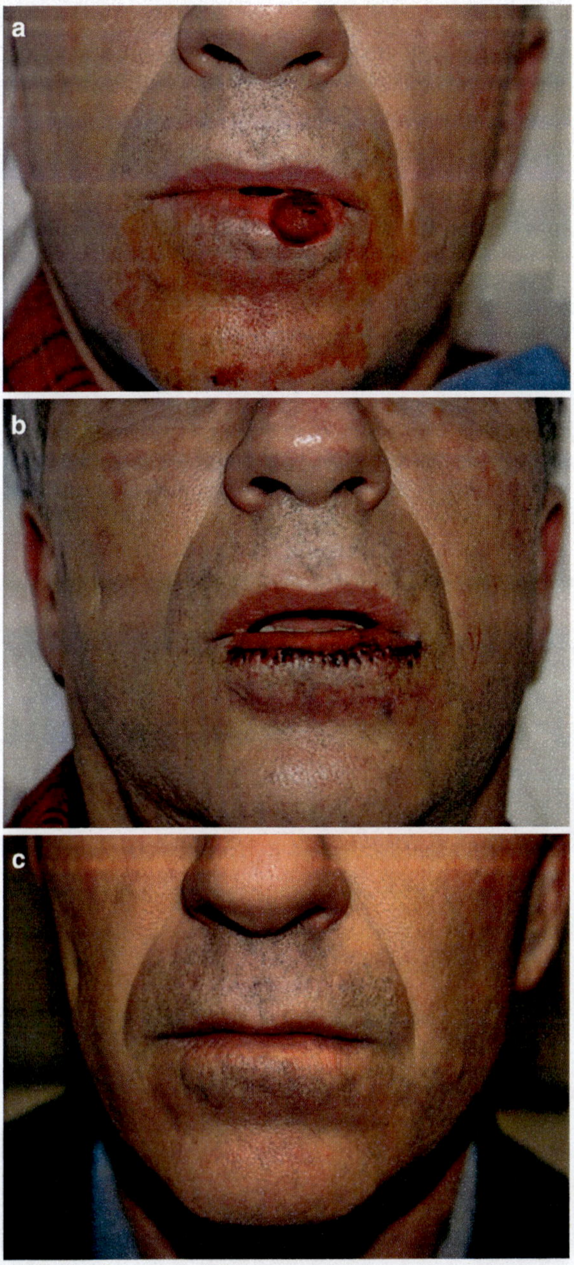

Fig. 33.11 Bilateral rotation flap mucosal lip

Transposition flaps have several advantages over other closures. Their primary function is to redistribute and redirect tension. This is useful in the closure of defects which would otherwise close under high tension or distort a nearby anatomical structure leading to functional or aesthetic impairment. Transposition flaps are usually smaller than advancement and rotation flaps. The resulting scars are geometric broken lines that may be less noticeable than longer linear closures in certain areas. This geometric broken line scar, however, may also be thought of as a disadvantage because such a scar is difficult to completely place along a relaxed skin tension line or cosmetic unit junction. One of the biggest advantages of transposition flaps are that they utilize adjacent skin and provide an excellent color and textural match.

The most common transposition flaps in cutaneous surgery include rhombic flaps (and their variations), bilobed flaps, and banner flaps such as the nasolabial flap. Knowledge of the tissue dynamics used in these three basic transposition flaps can be carried over to the planning and execution of the numerous variations of these flaps.

33.6.1 Rhombic

First described by Lindberg in 1963, the classic rhombic flap was designed to create a secondary defect perpendicular to the primary defect [18]. When closed, it would not only provide tissue to the primary defect but also redirect the tension vector by 90°. This allowed the primary defect to be closed under almost no wound edge tension. Subsequent modifications by Dufourmental and Webster provide more tension sharing between the primary and secondary defects. These modifications are useful in situations where some laxity around the primary defect is available [19]. (Fig. 33.12)

The classic Lindberg rhombic flap is designed by conversion of the primary defect into a four-sided parallelogram with each side of equal length and tip angles of 60° and 120° [18]. This rhombus forms the recipient site for the flap as well as the template on which to plan the flap incisions. In its classic configuration (Fig. 33.13), the incisions are designed by extending a line outward from one of the obtuse tips for a length equal to that of one side of the rhombus. From the free end of the extending line a second line is drawn parallel to one of the near sides of the rhombus, equal in length to that side. The tip angle in this configuration is 60°. The flap is lifted and transposed into place. The tension vector is redirected from that of closing the primary defect to that of closing the new secondary defect created in the design of the flap. This allows the tension vector to be shifted and redirected by 90°.

There are four possible flap designs off of the short axis of any rhomboid defect (Fig. 33.13). Which of these four flap configurations is selected depends on several factors that affect the outcome. A surgeon must consider adjacent anatomic structures and skin type, as well as the optimal location to place a scar.

The triangle of tissue redundancy created by the rotation of the transposition flap is removed by trimming a Burrow's triangle at the pivot point. The transposed tissue may be rounded to fit the circular defect, or the defect may be squared off to accommodate the angular flap.

As with any closure, understanding the tension forces is essential to the planning, execution, and outcome of the repair. There are two main tension forces associated with the classic rhombic flap. The first set of tension forces are realized during the approximation and closure of the secondary defect. The second set of

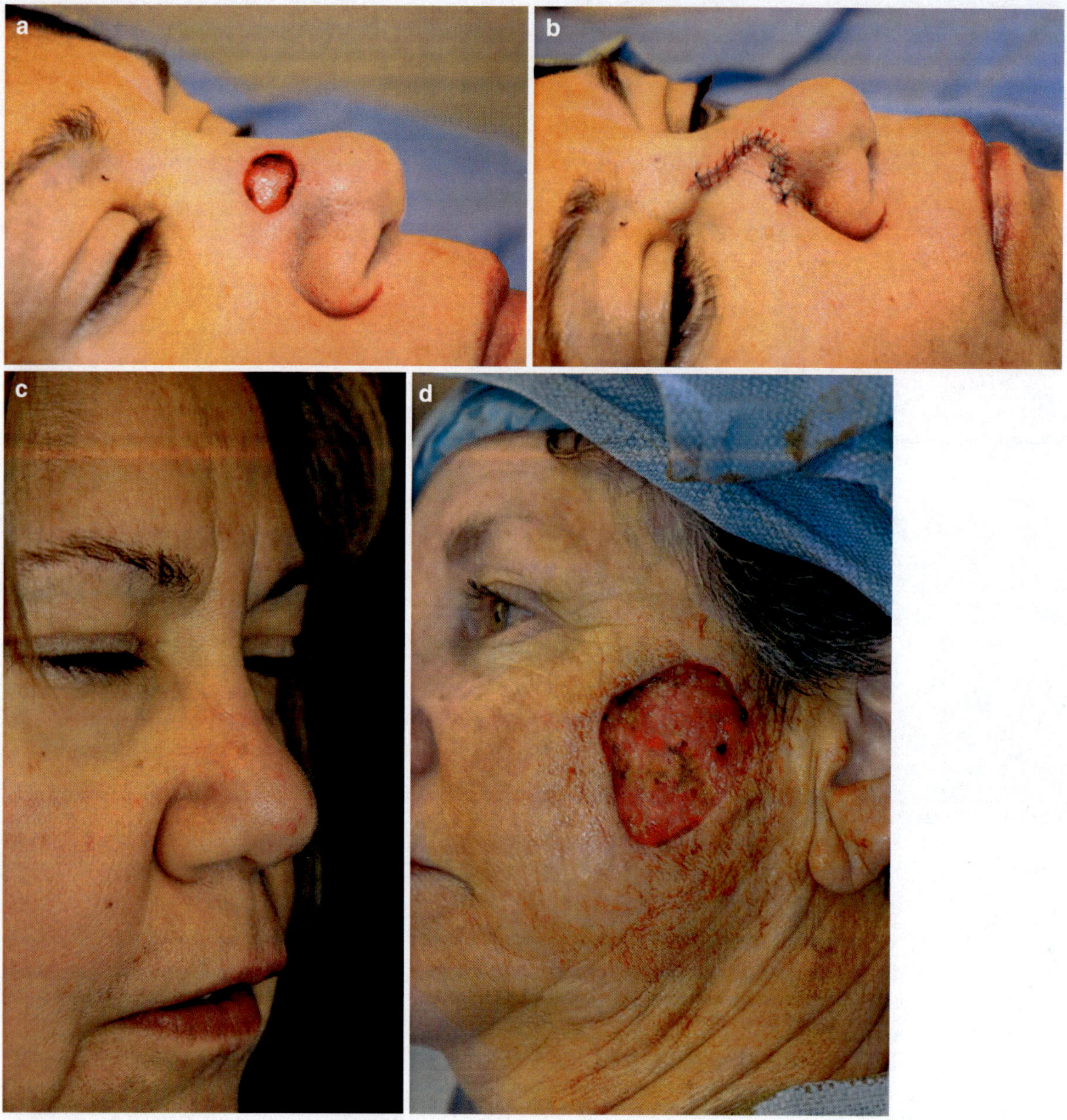

Fig. 33.12 Rhombic transposition flap, nasal sidewall; (**a**) After Mohs, right nasal sidewall; (**b**) immediately after repair; (**c**) 3 months post-operative; (**d**) after Mohs large defect of left lateral cheek; (**e**) Immediately after repair; (**f**) 6 weeks post-operative.

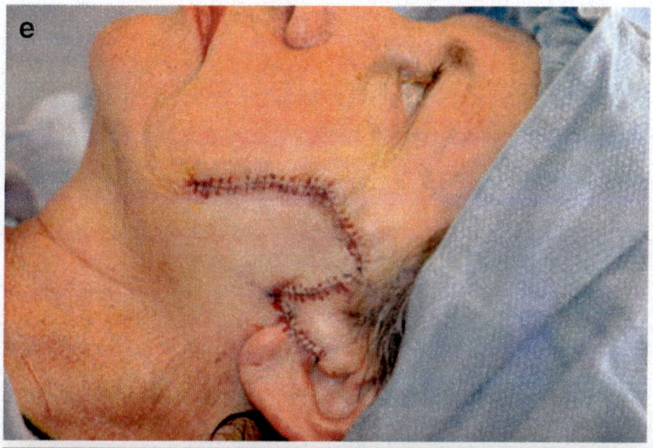

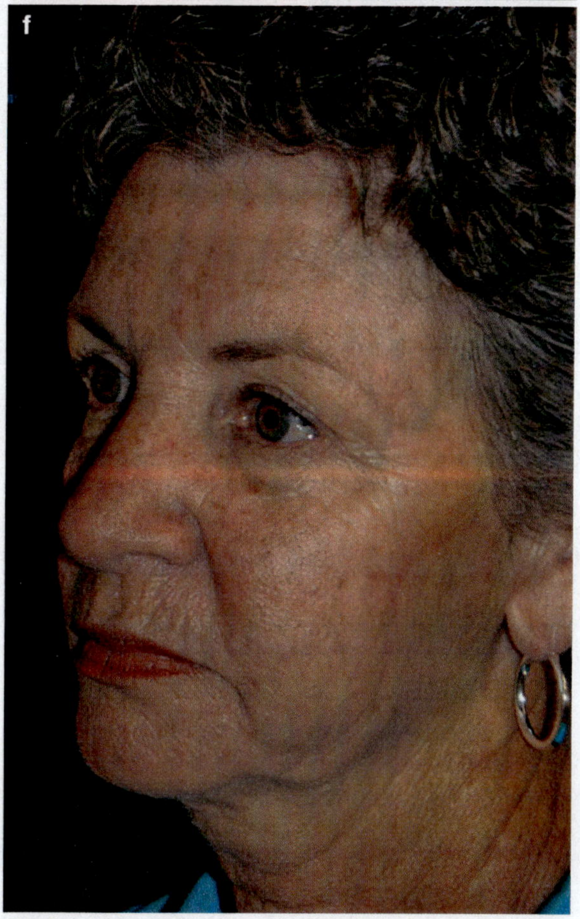

Fig. 33.12 (continued)

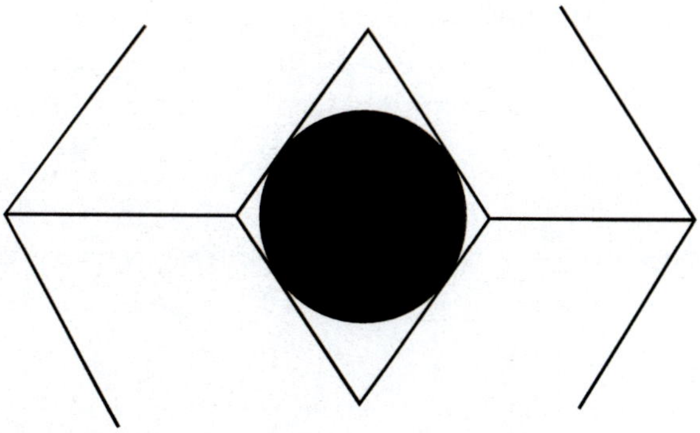

Fig. 33.13 Four possible designs of rhombic flap

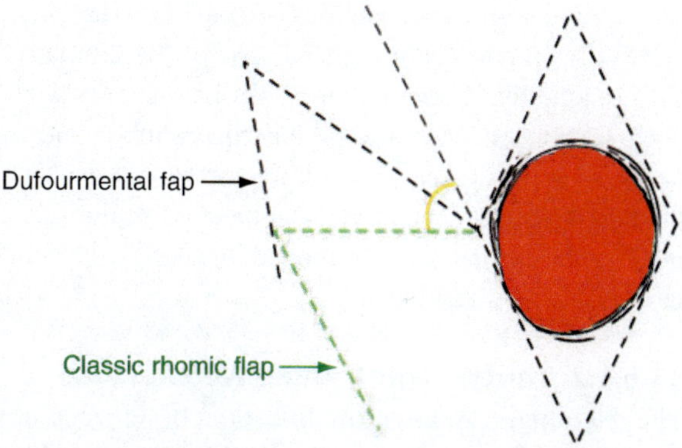

Fig. 33.14 Dufourmental modification of rhombic flap

tension forces are generated at the tip of the flap when moving it into the primary defect. These forces are due to the resistance to rotation at the flap's pedicle as well as shortening of the length of the flap during rotation into the recipient site. Dzubow describes these forces as pivotal restraint [16]. Securing the flap into the recipient site under high tension is not advised because it may lead to tip ischemia and necrosis.

33.6.1.1 Dufourmental

The Dufourmental flap modification differs from the classic rhombic transposition flap (Fig. 33.14) in that it utilizes a narrower flap tip angle and a shorter arc of rotation, allowing easier closure of the secondary defect, and some sharing of the tension between the primary and secondary defects.

As with the classic rhombic flap, it is designed by extending the first line from the short axis of the rhomboid defect. However, the angle at which the first line is extended differs from the classic rhombic flap in that it bisects the angle formed by the first line of the classic rhombic flap (which extends straight out from the short axis of the rhombic defect) and the line formed by extending one of the sides of the rhombus from the same corner of the rhombus. The length of the first line is equal to that of a side length of the rhombus. The

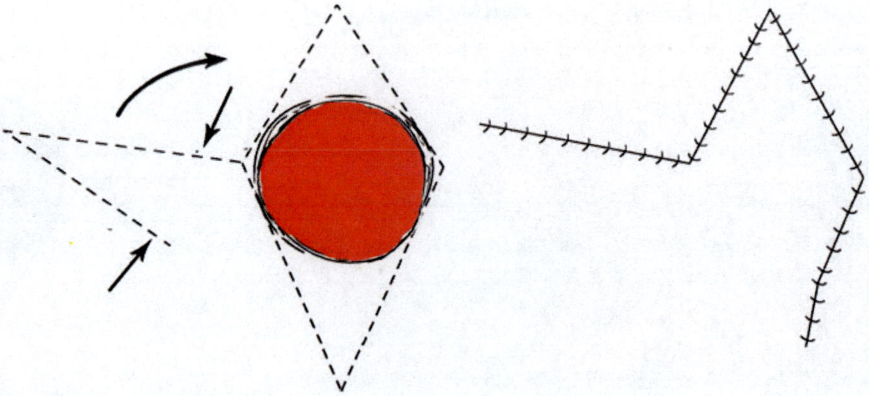

Fig. 33.15 Webster 30° modification of rhombic flap

second line originates from the free end of the first line and is drawn parallel to the long axis of the rhombus. This second line's orientation results in a slightly widened pedicle, a decrease in the tip volume, and a decrease in the degree of rotation necessary to execute the flap. The tissue redundancy at the base of the leading edge of the flap can be removed by taking a slightly larger Burrow's triangle.

33.6.1.2 Thirty-Degree Angle Webster Flap

The 30° angle Webster modification of the classic rhombic flap utilizes a more acute angle than other rhombic transposition flaps allowing for even greater tension sharing between the primary and secondary defects. A Webster 30° angle flap is planned similarly to the Dufourmental flap; however, its distal tip angle is designed to be 30° (Fig. 33.15). This gives the flap a slimmer design and narrower pedicle. The flap area is only 50% of the area of the primary defect; therefore, it only relieves half of the tension from the primary defect. This modification is used in situations where a fair amount of laxity exists in the horizontal axis of the rhombic-shaped defect. Since this design places more tension on the primary defect, care must be taken not to close with too much lateral tension or distort adjacent anatomic structures.

Rhombic transposition flaps are very versatile and may be used to reconstruct a variety of defects. Transposition flaps are generally used when there is insufficient laxity in the immediate surrounding area of closure and or the tension vectors need to be redirected. This is particularly important when repairing defects near free margins such as the eyelids and the nose. The most common areas where they are employed include the nasal dorsum, nasal sidewall, medial and lateral canthus, lateral forehead, temple, cheek, perioral region, inferior chin, and the dorsal hand.

33.6.2 The Banner Flap

Banner-type flaps are random pattern finger-shaped cutaneous flaps that, like other transposition flaps, tap into adjacent skin to borrow laxity and fill a defect [20]. This flap is most commonly planned as a melolabial transposition to repair defects of the nasal ala or from the pre- or postauricular area to close defects on the ear. For an optimal cosmetic result, the scar is generally placed at the junction of two cosmetic units, providing excellent camouflage (in the nasolabial fold or preauricular sulcus).

The fundamental design of the banner flaps consist of a finger-shaped flap drawn with a width that is equal to the width of the defect and a length equal to the distance from the pivot point to the far edge of the defect. The flap is transposed and rotated in an arc around the pivot point to fill the defect. Since this is a long random pattern flap with a narrow pedicle, the risk of vascular compromise may be high if the entire length of the flap is used and its pedicle originates from an area of minimal vascularity. To minimize risk of vascular compromise, the flap is typically designed to rotate through an angle of 60–120° instead of the originally described 180°. Typical locations for use of Banner-type flaps include the nasal ala, the superior helix of the ear, and the medial anterior ear.

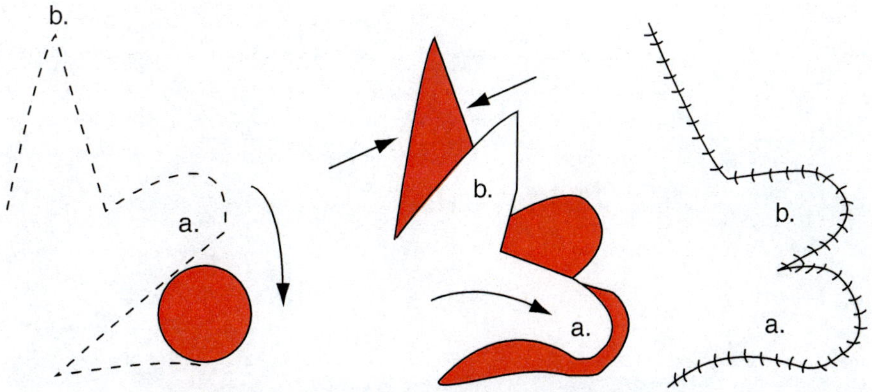

Fig. 33.16 Zitelli bilobed flap modification

33.6.3 Bilobed Flap

The bilobed flap used today is a highly evolved transposition flap. The bilobed flap was first described by Esser in 1918. It became a workhorse flap only after the modifications described by Zitelli were published in 1989 (Fig. 33.16) [21]. The design of the bilobed flap actually consists of two transposition flaps executed in succession which follow the same direction of rotation over intervening tissues. The basic premise of this flap is to fill the defect with the primary lobe, while filling the secondary defect with the secondary lobe, leaving a triangular-shaped tertiary defect to be closed primarily. This series of transposition flaps allow the surgeon to further the reach of the flap and borrow laxity from donor sites at a greater distance from the defect while decreasing the arc of rotation of the pedicle.

The Zitelli modification of the bilobed flap is designed by placing the lobes over a 90° arc from the center of the defect, with the primary lobe rotating from a pivot point that is created by removing a Burow's triangle at one pole of the defect [21]. The width of the primary lobe should be equal to the width of the defect and should be long enough to just extend past the edge of the defect. The secondary lobe must be trimmed to match the secondary defect left by the transposition of the primary lobe.

As with the rhombic flap, the bilobed flap redirects the principal tension vector and takes advantage of tissue laxity of the donor site. This flap is predominantly used for small- to medium-sized defects of the lower nose as the tension is redirected to a near vertical vector, preventing distortion of the alar rim (Fig. 33.17). The bilobed flap works especially well when the Burrow's triangle falls along the alar crease.

Summary: Interpolation Flaps

- Interpolation flaps import pedicled tissue from a site distant to the defect. These are axial flaps that can support a larger mass of tissue than random flaps. Because the flap is used to repair defects distant from the donor site, the vascular pedicle must temporarily be left in place to ensure adequate blood supply, requiring more than one stage to complete the repair. Types of interpolation flaps include paramedian forehead, nasolabial, Abbé, and retroauricular flaps.

33.7 Interpolation Flaps

Interpolation flaps are more complex repairs that import pedicled tissue from a site distant to the defect. They are typically utilized on defects that are either too wide or too deep to reconstruct with local flaps or grafts. Many interpolation flaps may be classified as axial flaps if their vascular pedicle is based on a large, named artery. They are also commonly referred to as staged flaps as more than one stage is required to complete the repair. Interpolation flaps require careful planning and significant, albeit temporary, disfigurement of the patient.

The first stage of on interpolation flap involves the design and creation of the flap, including repair of the secondary defect. The flap is designed around a substantial artery and therefore is able to support a larger mass

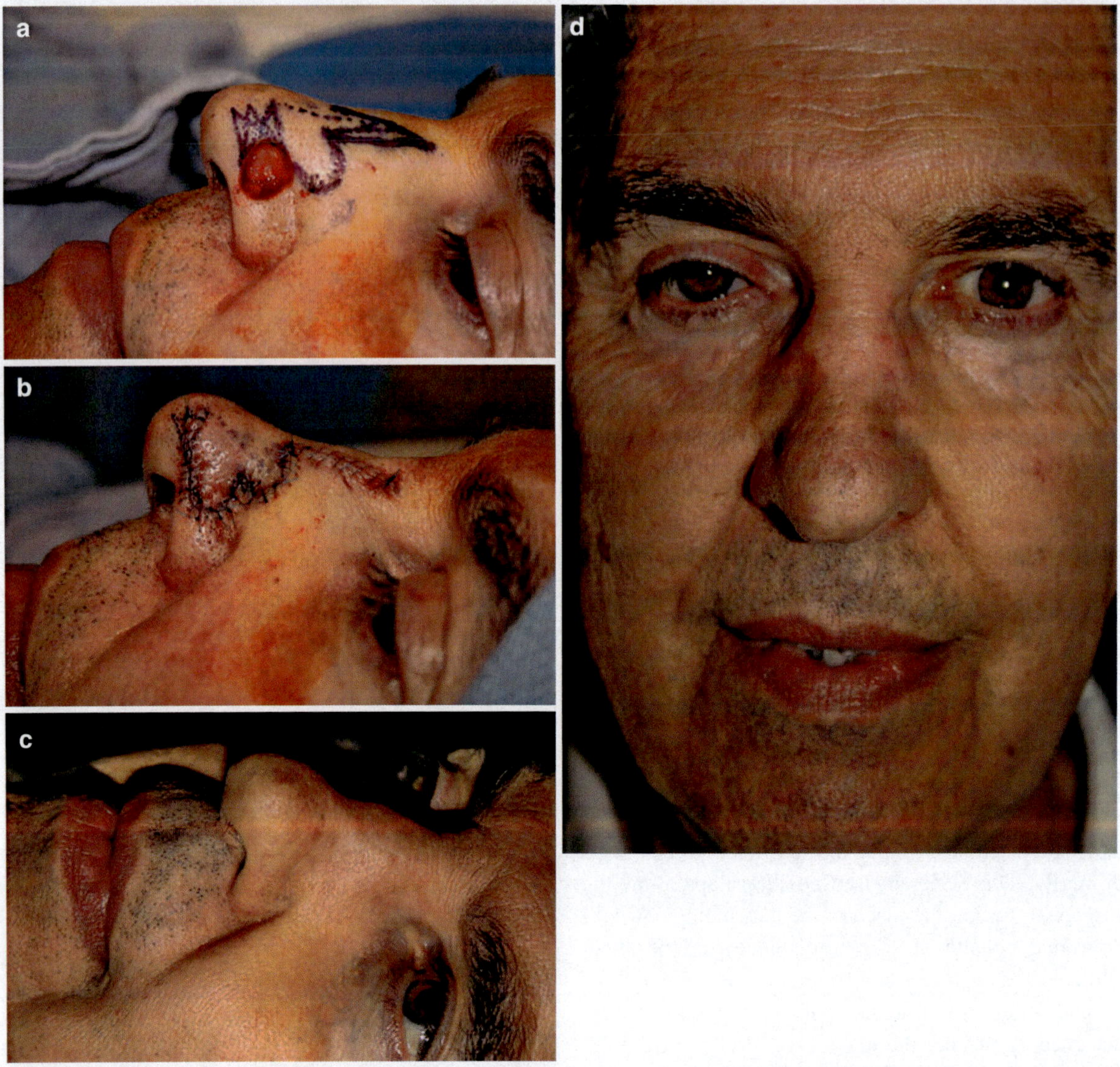

Fig. 33.17 Medially based bilobed flap. (**a**) after Mohs with flap design; (**b**) Immediately after repair; (**c** & **d**) 3 months post-oprative

of tissue than random flaps. Because the flap is used to repair defects distant from the donor site, the vascular pedicle must temporarily be left in place to ensure adequate blood supply. The distal end of the flap is thinned to match the depth of the defect and sutured in place. The area is bandaged and kept moist. The second stage generally takes place 2–3 weeks later, by which time the flap has established a local blood supply from the donor site. The pedicle is then divided from the donor site and the proximal portion of the flap is secured into the original defect. Due to granulation tissue formation, this portion of the flap may need to be thinned out subcutaneously to approximate the depth of the defect. The pedicle is also separated from the donor site which will then require further steps for complete repair.

33.7.1 Paramedian Forehead

The paramedian forehead flap is useful to repair large, deep nasal defects that may or may not require cartilage grafts. Tissue is mobilized from the forehead, based on one of the supratrochlear arteries, and transposed to repair large distal nasal defects with the pedicle remaining attached in the glabellar region (Fig. 33.18). The supratrochlear artery is located at the

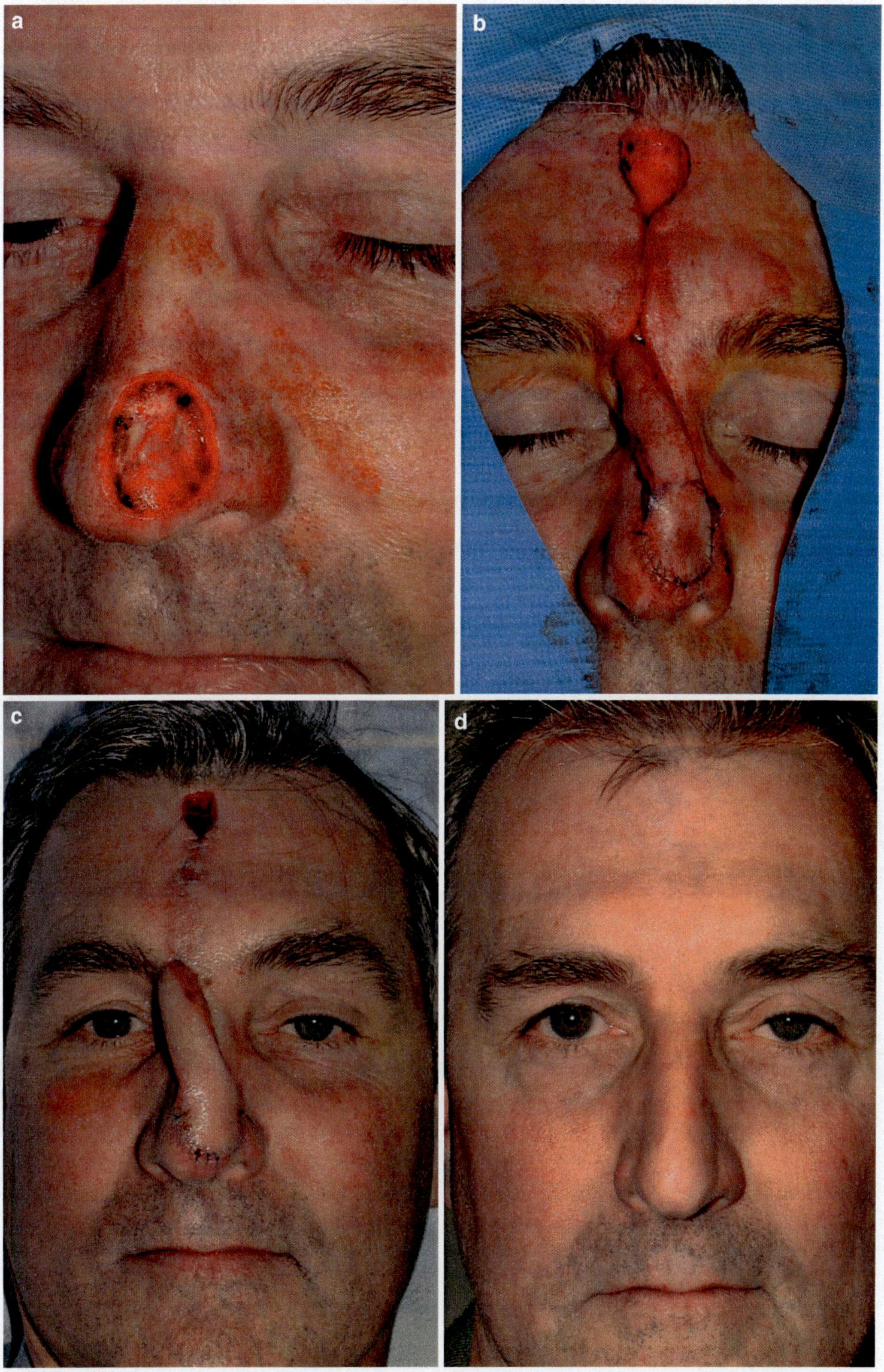

Fig. 33.18 Paramedian forehead flap for large deep defect of nasal tip and dorsum. (**a**) After Mohs; (**b**) Immediately after flap secured; (**c**) At flap take-down 3 weeks later; (**d**) 6 months post-operative

medial border of the eyebrow, approximately 1.5–2 cm from the midline.

The aesthetics of the repair is often improved when the defect is enlarged to include the total cosmetic subunit. The portion of the flap that will fill the defect is the superior portion closest to the hairline; the width here should be equal to the widest portion of the defect, although the pedicle itself need be no wider than 1–1.5 cm. Its height must be equal to the distance from the base of the flap to the distal edge of the defect. In designing the flap, it is important that the vertical height of the forehead be able to accommodate the necessary length of the flap. The tissue is rotated approximately 180° around its pedicle and should be rotated medially as to minimize obscuration of the medial visual field of the ipsilateral eye; therefore, the flap will require less rotation if it is harvested from the forehead supplied by the supratrochlear artery contralateral to the defect.

The donor site is undermined and closed primarily as far superiorly as it will close resulting in a long linear scar. The donor site is repaired with a side-to-side closure, The superior portion of the defect will be the widest, as it is here that the width of the defect must be accommodated, and thus, generally this portion of the wound is too tight to be closed and is left to heal by secondary intention. The distal aspect of the flap is debulked to the depth of the defect and secured at the distal margin with sutures. The proximal margin, by design, cannot be secured until the pedicle is divided. The pedicle should be circumferentially wrapped with Vaseline or Xeroform gauze or Surgicel to prevent desiccation.

The second stage takes place 3 weeks subsequently. The pedicle is separated from the brow, the wound edges are freshened, and the donor defect is closed. After the pedicle is separated from the defect, the tissue is further debulked and trimmed, and the remaining edge is secured.

33.7.2 Nasolabial Interpolation

This flap is utilized to repair complex defects of the ala, particularly in instances when cartilage grafting is also required to restore the structural integrity of the alar rim. The flap is harvested from the medial cheek and nasolabial fold and is based on branches of the angular artery (Fig. 33.19).

The aesthetics of the repair is often improved when the defect is enlarged to include the entire alar lobule. The flap is designed around a pedicle that will be placed at the alar groove, extending as an ellipse that will be easily closed in the nasolabial fold. Through-and-through nasal defects will require the repair of the mucosa, and thus, the width of the flap must take this into account. This myocutaneous flap is dissected from the donor site, rotated downwardly, debulked and trimmed, and secured to the widely undermined defect.

As with the paramedian forehead flap, the pedicle may be wrapped with Vaseline or Xeroform gauze or Surgicel. Three weeks later, the pedicle is separated, the wound edges are freshened, and the donor defect is closed. After the pedicle is separated from the defect, the tissue is further debulked and trimmed, and the remaining edge is secured.

The reverse nasolabial flap, also known as a Spear's flap, is employed when the defect involves the alar groove. The motion of this flap is an upward rotation, opposite of the traditional nasolabial interpolation flap.

33.7.3 Abbé

The Abbé flap is also known as the lip-switch flap and is reserved for repair of large, deep defects, typically of the upper lip. It is particularly useful for defects that involve up to half of the lip without crossing the midline and those that penetrate into the muscularis. The Abbé flap is harvested from the ipsilateral lower lip and is based on the inferior labial artery. This artery is located deep to or within the orbicularis oris muscle and runs along the mucosal aspect of the vermillion border [22].

The vermillion border and flap design must be properly marked out. The defect should be full thickness (including muscularis and oral mucosa) and may be enlarged to encompass the total cosmetic unit which includes the ipsilateral upper cutaneous lip. The flap, also designed to be full thickness to fill the enlarged defect, is rotated upon a vascular pedicle that makes up the lateral aspect of the flap. The inferior labial artery will be visualized as it is transected at the mobilized (medial) edge of the flap. The pedicle itself should be about 1 cm thick, containing the robust blood supply.

The donor site is undermined and closed first to facilitate the movement of the flap. It should be closed in layers as in the repair of a lip wedge resection: mucosa, muscularis, subcutaneous, then cutaneous. The flap is rotated superiorly and also inset with a layered closure. Careful attention should be given to aligning the vermillion borders at the donor site and defect.

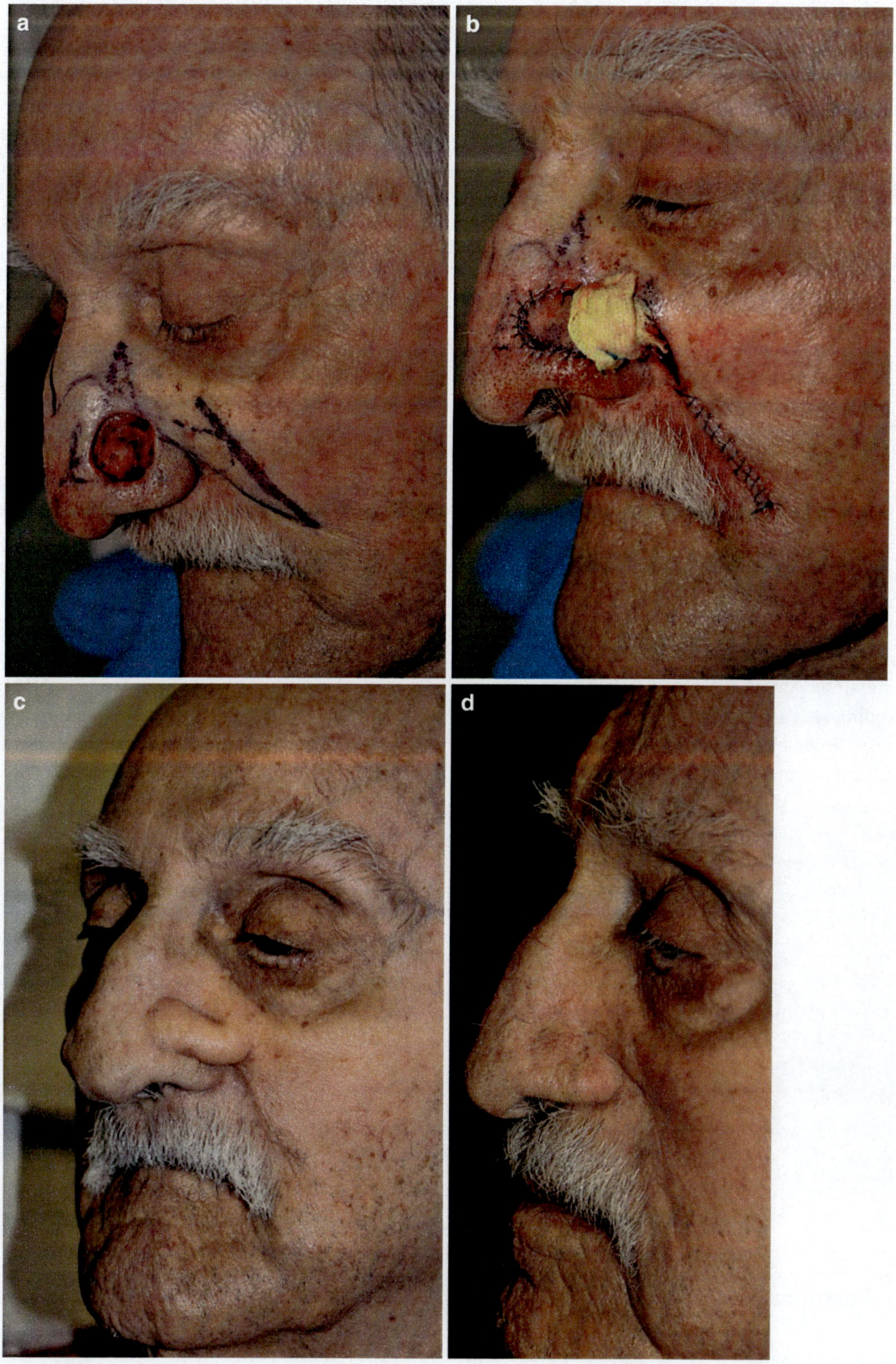

Fig. 33.19 Nasolabial interpolation flap. (**a**) after Mohs with flap design; (**b**) immediately after repair (note Xeroform gauze-unrapped pedicle); (**c**) At flap pedicle take down, 3 weeks later; (**d**) 6 weeks post-operative

The pedicle of the Abbé flap should not be circumferentially wrapped but kept moist with occlusive ointment. As with other interpolation flaps, the pedicle will remain in place for at least 3 weeks. During this time, the oral aperture will be significantly distorted, and the patient must be counseled. The pedicle is divided and the final repair takes place, again with careful attention to the placement of the vermillion borders.

33.7.4 Retroauricular

The retroauricular flap is a two-staged interpolation flap useful for large defects of the helix. Defects in this location typically involve the perichondrium and are not suitable for grafts. This flap is considered a random flap as it is not based on a large named artery. It is harvested from the richly vascularized skin of the postauricular scalp and is advanced over intervening intact skin to fill the helical defect; the pedicle remains attached to the posterior scalp. The flap should be thinned to match the depth of the defect and carefully sewn into place. The pedicle is circumferentially dressed, and the patient is warned of likely postoperative bleeding and discomfort. The donor site is not repaired until pedicle take-down and often, due to its inconspicuous location, is allowed to heal secondarily.

Summary: Postoperative Care

- Meticulous postoperative wound care is necessary to ensure an optimal outcome. Verbal and written instructions regarding home wound care should be reviewed and then provided in writing to the patient. A pressure dressing should be applied and left intact for 24–48 h. It is important that the wound be kept clean, moist, and covered until suture removal. This will eliminate desiccation, promote reepithelialization, reduce bacterial contamination, and aid in hemostasis.

33.8 Postoperative Care

Meticulous postoperative wound care is necessary to ensure an optimal outcome. Attention must be made to limit postoperative bleeding of all surgical wounds, particularly flaps, as hemorrhage or hematoma formation may jeopardize tissue survival and increase the risk of infection. Meticulous intraoperative hemostasis and good postoperative compression dressings are very important in minimizing postoperative bleeding. A pressure dressing should be applied and left intact for 24–48 hours This dressing includes a layer of ointment applied directly to the wound, nonstick bandage such as Telfa, gauze for pressure, and surgical tape. Finally, elastic dressing materials, such as Flexinet or Coban, may be helpful for wounds on the scalp or extremities.

For any type of aforementioned procedure or repair, it is important that the wound be kept clean, moist, and covered until suture removal. This will eliminate desiccation, promote reepithelialization [23], reduce bacterial contamination, and aid in hemostasis. Verbal instructions regarding home wound care should be reviewed and then provided in writing to the patient. After removal of the pressure dressing, the wound should be cleaned once or twice daily with attention to gentle removal of any crust and debris that may have formed. This is followed by a layer of ointment. A bland, non-medicated ointment, such as petrolatum or Aquaphor is preferred over bacitracin or Neosporin. The use of topical antibiotics following cutaneous surgery increases the risk of contact dermatitis [24] without imparting a significant reduction in infection rates [25].

The signs and symptoms of hemorrhage and wound infection should be reviewed as early intervention can reduce serious complications. To minimize nonemergency calls, however, it is helpful to educate the patient as to what to expect during normal wound healing. The patient should be provided with the physician's contact information and should be encouraged to call with any questions or concerns.

Summary: Complications

- Complications include bleeding and hematoma, discomfort and pain, infection, flap necrosis, trapdoor deformity, hypertrophic scar, atrophic scar, erythema, and telangiectasias. Precautions should be taken to minimize these risks, and treatment options exist.

33.9 Complications

Early complications of Mohs surgery and all types of closure are bleeding, pain, and infection. Bleeding typically occurs in the first 24 hours after surgery and must be addressed promptly. Low-flow ooze may be treated

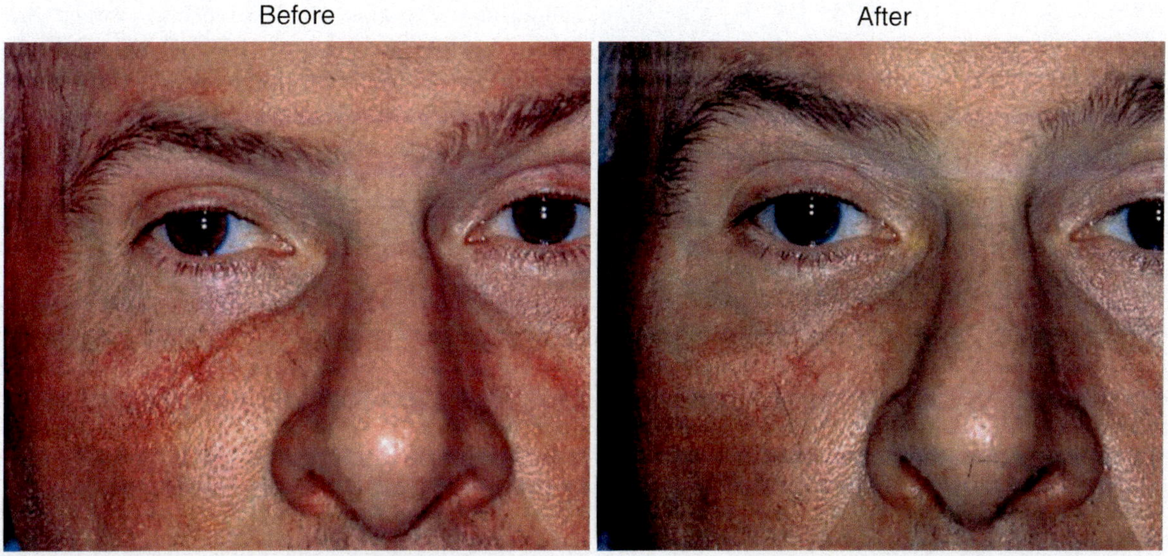

Fig. 33.20 (**a**) Post-operative erthema and telangiectasia after linear repair of right upper cheek; (**b**) after treatment with pulsed dye laser

by compression. Patients should be instructed to apply direct pressure for at least 20 minutes without peeking to see if it is working. Frank arterial hemorrhage or large hematoma formation will require partial or complete suture removal, evacuation of clot, and exploration of the wound to allow visualization and closure of the bleeding vessel. Patients should be instructed to call if they see an enlarging mass below or around the wound.

Signs of infection usually occur within the first week after surgery and include increased pain, erythema, and heat around the wound, purulent and sometimes foul-smelling drainage, and fever. When wound infection is suspected, a culture must be obtained for pathogen identification and antibiotic susceptibility, and treatment with a broad-spectrum antibiotic should be initiated. Methicillin-resistant *Staphylococcus aureus* (MRSA) infections are increasing dramatically in frequency and should always be considered in the case of wound infections [26].

In the early postoperative period, partial or complete flap necrosis may occur. This may be due to inadequate blood supply from the wound bed, which is more commonly encountered in smokers, or when an underlying hematoma is present. Flap design may also lead to vascular compromise and flap necrosis, as when the pedicle is too narrow to support the mass of the flap, when there is too much torque, or when there is too much tension at the flap's leading edge. Areas of partial necrosis will heal secondarily and may lead to a less appealing scar which can be revised after wound healing is complete.

Later in the postoperative period, a trapdoor deformity may occur in which the center of the flap becomes elevated and the suture line becomes depressed. It may resolve spontaneously over a period of 6–12 months. However, if the trapdoor effect or pin-cushioning persists, it may respond to intralesional steroids, flap elevation with flap thinning, and/or resurfacing. The trapdoor effect may be prevented with wide undermining around the primary defect, proper thinning of the flap, proper sizing of the flap, and the use of a geometric shape for the flap.

An expected consequence of surgery is the formation of a scar. While the goal of reconstructive surgery is to minimize the appearance of the resultant scar, at times they may widen or even become hypertrophic. With time, hypertrophic scars tend to flatten and soften. Their course may be hastened with the administration of intralesional steroids and laser treatment. In areas under tension and/or motion, such as the upper back and arms over the deltoids, scars may spread or become atrophic. While scar spread may become less noticeable with time as the initial dark-pink color fades, the width generally does not change significantly. Erythema and telangiectasia often form around scars during the healing phase and may persist for extended periods of time. Highly vascular areas (rosacea) and those under high tension are more likely to develop persistent erythema and telangiectasia. This can be effectively treated with lasers, such as the pulsed dye laser, KTP, or intense pulsed light (Fig. 33.20).

Summary: Monitoring and Follow-Up

- Follow-up is required for suture removal, as well as to evaluate outcomes and potential complications and to intervene as necessary.

33.10 Monitoring and Follow-Up

If nonabsorbable epidermal sutures are placed, the patient should return for suture removal at the appointed time. Typically, sutures on the face and neck are removed at postoperative day 7, while sutures elsewhere on the body are removed at 10–14 days. It is helpful to see the patient after 4–6 weeks for follow-up to evaluate outcomes and any necessary interventions.

Summary: Conclusion

- The elements to successful flap execution include proper patient selection and preparation, comprehension of risks and necessary precautions, as well as proper postoperative wound care and patient education. There are several subtypes and variations of each flap type, and each has an important role in dermatologic surgery.

33.11 Conclusion

The planning and execution of repair following Mohs surgery vary from case to case. The creation of a flap should be considered when simpler closures are not ideal. The elements to successful flap execution include proper patient selection and preparation, comprehension of risks and necessary precautions, use of sterile or clean technique, informed procedure design and meticulous suture technique, as well as proper postoperative wound care and patient education. Flaps are commonly classified according to their primary movement – advancement flaps, rotation flaps, transposition flaps, and interpolation flaps. There are several subtypes and variations of each flap type, and each has an important role in dermatologic surgery. Meticulous intraoperative technique and postoperative wound care are necessary to ensure an optimal outcome. Patients should be seen for follow-up to monitor for potential complications, evaluate outcomes, and employ necessary treatments or interventions.

References

1. Berg JW, Appelbaum PS, Lidz CW, Parker LS. Informed consent: legal theory and clinical practice. 2nd ed. New York: Oxford University Press; 2001.
2. Chang LK, Whitaker DC. The impact of herbal medicines on dermatologic surgery. Dermatol Surg. 2001;278:759–63.
3. Futoryan T, Grande D. Postoperative wound infection rates in dermatologic surgery. Dermatol Surg. 1995;21(6):509–14.
4. Dixon AJ, Dixon MP, Askew DA, Wilkinson D. Prospective study of wound infections in dermatologic surgery in the absence of prophylactic antibiotics. Dermatol Surg. 2006; 32(6):819–26; discussion 826–817.
5. Milton SH. Pedicled skin-flaps: the fallacy of the length: width ratio. Br J Surg. 1970;57(7):502–8.
6. Daniel RK, Williams HB. The free transfer of skin flaps by microvascular anastomoses. An experimental study and a reappraisal. Plast Reconstr Surg. 1973;52(1):16–31.
7. Stell PM. The pig as an experimental model for skin flap behaviour: a reappraisal of previous studies. Br J Plast Surg. 1977;30(1):1–8.
8. Chilukuri S, Leffell D. Basic principles of flap reconstruction. In: Cook JL, Rohrer TE, Nguyen TH, Mellette JR, editors. Flaps and grafts in dermatologic surgery. London: Elsevier; 2007.
9. Fazio MJ, Zitelli JA. Flaps. In: Ratz JL, Geronemus RG, Goldman MP, et al., editors. Textbook of dermatologic surgery. Philadelphia: Lippincott-Raven; 1998. p. 225–7.
10. Heniford BW, Bailin PL, Marsico Jr RE. Field guide to local flaps. Dermatol Clin. 1998;16(1):65–74.
11. Dzubow LM. Flap dynamics. J Dermatol Surg Oncol. 1991;17(2):116–30.
12. Antia NH, Buch VI. Chondrocutaneous advancement flap for the marginal defect of the ear. Plast Reconstr Surg. 1967; 39(5):472–7.
13. Mellette Jr JR, Harrington AC. Applications of the crescentic advancement flap. J Dermatol Surg Oncol. 1991;17(5): 447–54.
14. Dzubow LM, Lambert RW. A dorsal nasal advancement flap for off midline defects. J Am Acad Dermatol. 2004;50(3): 380–3.
15. Tomich JM, Wentzell JM, Grande DJ. Subcutaneous island pedicle flaps. Arch Dermatol. 1987;123(4):514–8.
16. Dzubow LM. The dynamics of flap movement: effect of pivotal restraint on flap rotation and transposition. J Dermatol Surg Oncol. 1987;13(12):1348–53.
17. Rieger RA. A local flap for repair of the nasal tip. Plast Reconstr Surg. 1967;40(2):147–9.
18. Limberg AA. Design of local flaps. Mod Trends Plast Surg. 1966;2:38–61.
19. Bray DA. Clinical applications of the rhomboid flap. Arch Otolaryngol. 1983;109(1):37–42.

20. Masson JK, Mendelson BC. The banner flap. Am J Surg. 1977;134(3):419–23.
21. Zitelli JA. The bilobed flap for nasal reconstruction. Arch Dermatol. 1989;125(7):957–9.
22. Schulte DL, Sherris DA, Kasperbauer JL. The anatomical basis of the Abbe flap. Laryngoscope. 2001;111(3):382–6.
23. Eaglstein WH. Moist wound healing with occlusive dressings: a clinical focus. Dermatol Surg. 2001;27(2):175–81.
24. Gette MT, Marks Jr JG, Maloney ME. Frequency of postoperative allergic contact dermatitis to topical antibiotics. Arch Dermatol. 1992;128(3):365–7.
25. Smack DP, Harrington AC, Dunn C, Howard RS, Szkutnik AJ, Krivda SJ, et al. Infection and allergy incidence in ambulatory surgery patients using white petrolatum vs bacitracin ointment. A randomized controlled trial. JAMA. 1996; 276(12):972–7.
26. Cruse PJ, Foord R. The epidemiology of wound infection. A 10-year prospective study of 62,939 wounds. Surg Clin North Am. 1980;60(1):27–40.

Skin Grafting

34

Susana M. Leal-Khouri and Sarah E. Grummer

Abstract

A skin graft may be necessary when closure of a wound is required, but primary closure or use of a flap is not feasible due to size or location of a wound. Skin grafts can have cosmetic, functional, and practical purposes. A defining characteristic of grafts is that they are completely separated from their original blood supply and depend entirely on the development of a blood supply with the recipient wound bed for survival. Full-thickness skin grafts (FTSG) and split-thickness skin grafts (STSG) are the two broad categories of skin grafts. While grafts do not have quite the cosmetic match as tissue adjacent to the primary wound, harvesting from anatomic locations that are similar in color and texture to the wound is beneficial and preferred. Proper patient selection, meticulous execution, and close follow-up are essential to ensuring a successful graft. Both cosmetic and functional outcome can be excellent.

Keywords

Skin graft • Skin grafts • Skin grafting • Full-thickness grafts • Split-thickness grafts • Graft harvesting • Wound care • Revascularization • Biologic skin substitutes

Summary: Introduction

- Skin grafts involve transfer of skin, which has been separated from its vascular supply, to a wound bed.
- May be classified based on origin: autografts, allografts, or xenografts.
- May be classified based on thickness: full-thickness grafts or split-thickness grafts.

S.M. Leal-Khouri (✉)
Department of Dermatology and Cutaneous Surgery, University of Miami, Key Biscayne, Dade, FL, USA

Florida International University School of Medicine, Key Biscayne, Dade, FL, USA
e-mail: susanalealkhouri@aol.com

S.E. Grummer
Department of Mohs Surgery, Dermatology and Plastic Surgery, Key Biscayne, Dade, FL, USA

K. Nouri (ed.), *Mohs Micrographic Surgery*,
DOI 10.1007/978-1-4471-2152-7_34,

34.1 Introduction

A skin graft may be necessary when closure of a wound is required, but primary closure or use of a flap is not feasible due to size or location of a wound. By definition, grafting involves the transfer of noncontiguous skin, which has been separated from its vascular supply, to a wound bed. Grafts may be categorized based on the origin or thickness of the donor tissue. In terms of origin, grafts may be classified as autografts, allografts, or xenografts. An autograft is derived from the patient's skin and is the most frequently used graft in dermatologic surgery. When the donor tissue is harvested from another person, then the graft is referred to as an allograft. Finally, a xenograft is one that is derived from another species, for example, a porcine graft. Allografts and xenografts are often used for chronic wounds or burn wounds. The utility of an allo- or xenograft is derived from the stimulation of wound healing, protection, and debridement.

The thickness of a graft can also be used as a method of categorization. Specifically, a full-thickness skin graft (FTSG) includes epidermis and the entire dermis. Adnexal structures are preserved. On the other hand, a split-thickness skin graft (STSG) contains epidermis and only a part of the dermis, with little or no preservation of adnexal structures. Finally, a composite graft includes not only skin but also another type of tissue, such as cartilage, perichondrium, or adipose tissue.

Summary: Physiology

- There are three distinct phases in which nutrition is supplied to the graft: plasmatic imbibition, inosculation/anastomosis, and capillary ingrowth/revascularization.
- Primary contraction of a graft occurs once the graft is harvested due to elastic fiber recoil. Secondary contraction occurs after graft placement and is due to contraction of myofibroblasts and contractile proteins.

34.2 Physiology

Of paramount importance to graft survival is the ability of the transferred tissue to revascularize with the wound bed. Investigation of graft wound healing has elucidated distinct phases in which nutrition is supplied to the graft, specifically, plasmatic imbibition, inosculation/anastomosis, and capillary ingrowth/revascularization [1].

Plasma imbibition is the first phase and occurs during the first 2 days after a graft has been performed. In this phase, the transferred tissue receives nutrition by imbibing exudate from the wound bed and can increase in weight by up to 40%. During imbibition, the graft and the wound bed are held together via a layer of fibrin [2]. The second phase, inosculation, is defined by an anastomosis of the preexistent vessels of the graft and the wound base [3]. This phase occurs during the second and third postoperative days. Revascularization involves the growth, proliferation, and connection of vessels from the recipient base and sidewalls [1, 4]. The rate of revascularization is dependent on the thickness of the graft and the vascularity of the recipient bed. During the fifth to seventh postoperative days, blood flow occurs. Lymphatic flow also reestablishes around postoperative day seven [5]. As a result, the graft often loses a significant amount of the weight that was gained during the imbibition phase. During the second to third postoperative months, sensory reinnervation commences and proceeds from the periphery to the center of the graft. It is important to note that the reinnervation is a slow process and full sensory capacity may not be regained at the graft site [6].

Primary contraction of a graft occurs once the graft has been harvested due to elastic fiber recoil. On the other hand, secondary contraction is due to contraction of myofibroblasts and contractile proteins and commences after graft placement. The thinner the graft is, the greater the amount of secondary contraction. STSG experience greater secondary contraction, while FTSG experience greater primary contraction.

Summary: Indications

- A skin graft can be used to address the cosmetic, functional, or practical needs of a patient's surgical defect or wound.

34.3 Indications

Skin grafts can have cosmetic, functional, and practical purposes. A graft can have cosmetic benefits by preventing contracture. On the other hand, grafts can be used to restore function, such as when used for wounds secondary to burns or for chronic ulcers. Often a graft may be used when healing by second intention, a primary closure, or utilization of a local flap are not feasible options.

Summary: Preoperative Assessment

- Review of a patient's medication list and medical and social history is important to ensure proper patient selection prior to performing a graft in a given clinical scenario.

34.4 Preoperative Assessment

There are many factors which must be taken into account prior to performing a graft. First, a thorough review of the patient's medical and social history must be performed. Pertinent information includes a history of coagulation abnormalities, alcohol consumption, arterial or venous insufficiency, collagen vascular disease, diabetes mellitus, poor nutrition, infections, need for antibiotic prophylaxis, use of tobacco, and/or prior radiation treatment [7]. Additionally, a review of the patient's medications (e.g., steroids, chemotherapeutic agents) is also of paramount importance [8]. The likelihood of graft revascularization and successful healing of the graft is in part predicated on the patient's medical history and medication list. One may advise patients to discontinue aspirin and nonsteroidal anti-inflammatory agents 1 week prior to the grafting procedure as excessive bleeding may cause blood to accumulate between the graft and wound bed, thereby leading to the potential for graft failure.

Summary: Site Selection

- Color and texture match are important factors to consider when choosing a harvest site so that cosmesis can be optimized.

34.5 Site Selection

While grafts do not have quite the cosmetic match as tissue adjacent to the primary wound, harvesting from anatomic locations that are similar in color and texture to the wound is beneficial and preferred. In order to maximize cosmesis, various factors must be taken into account when choosing a site to harvest, including photodamage, color, existing adnexal structures (e.g., hair), and the appearance of the donor site scar. Commonly used sites for FTSG are: pre- and postauricular regions, creases of the upper eyelids, nasolabial folds, supraclavicular region, lateral neck, antecubital fossa, and groin. Sites that can be concealed are often chosen as harvesting sites for STSG. These include: the abdomen, back, buttocks, anterior thighs, and upper inner arms.

Summary: Full-Thickness Skin Grafts

- Full-thickness skin grafts (FTSG) contain epidermis and dermis and retain adnexal structures.
- Given wound contraction upon harvesting donor tissue, a FTSG should be oversized ~10–20% to allow for contracture.
- It is important to defat the donor tissue after harvesting in order to improve contact between the graft and wound bed as well as to decrease the nourishment requirements.
- Close apposition of the graft to the wound bed promotes vascularization and minimizes risk of hematoma or seroma formation.
- Meticulous approximation of the wound edges to the graft is paramount to the optimal cosmesis of the graft. Bolsters are used to stabilize and protect the graft.

34.6 Full-Thickness Skin Grafts

By definition, full-thickness skin grafts (FTSG) contain both epidermis and dermis. Often, adnexal structures are preserved. FTSG are more durable than STSG. Additionally, FTSG provide a good cosmetic outcome, especially when the color and texture of the surrounding recipient site are taken into consideration. In dermatologic surgery, especially after the removal of a skin cancer, areas that are conducive to FTSG include nasal ala and tip, helix, medial canthus, lower eyelid, digits, and extremities [5]. When choosing a donor site, the surgeon must consider both the ease of closure and appearance of the resultant scar.

Placement of a FTSG directly onto bone or cartilage is not recommended as insufficient vascular supply at these sites can compromise graft survival. If it is necessary to immediately place a FTSG over cartilage devoid of perichondrium, a 2-mm punch biopsy instrument may be used to punch out cartilage, allowing for ingrowth of a blood supply via granulation tissue. Otherwise, a delayed graft may be optimal as granulation after 2–3 weeks can contribute to success of the graft [9]. Although FTSG do not experience the same degree of contraction as do STSG, the added thickness increases the metabolic demands and therefore contributes to the increased risk of graft failure. This factor is important to consider in patients with poor health, vascular disease, or tobacco use.

34.6.1 Graft Harvesting

Once the appropriate donor site has been chosen, anesthetized, cleansed, and prepared for harvest, a template of the recipient site is made in order to control for size and shape match. Given contracture of the donor tissue, one should harvest a greater amount (~10–20%) of tissue to allow for contracture [10]. When grafting eyelid defects, the harvested tissue should be oversized even more to allow for contraction and to avoid ectropion. Often a template is made with a blood imprint of the recipient site onto a nonadherent pad. Using the template, the donor site can be marked with a surgical marking pen. The use of an elliptical incision along the relaxed skin tension lines is beneficial. The graft should be large enough to align fully in the wound and should not be pulled tight as this can result in vascular compromise. FTSG should be limited to less than 5 cm to avoid necrosis as the new graft receives oxygen and nutrients via diffusion from the wound base for several weeks [5].

Once the graft has been harvested, it can be wrapped in sterile saline-soaked gauze and placed in a Petri dish. Hemostasis of the donor site is then achieved. The donor site is repaired later after the graft has been placed as it is important to allow nutrient diffusion to the graft to begin. Curved iris scissors are used to defat the graft until glistening white dermis is revealed (Fig. 34.1a, b). The amount of dermis that is removed varies according to the thickness of the tissue needed to fill the wound bed. It is important to remove the subcutaneous tissue in order to improve contact between the graft and wound bed as well as to decrease the nourishment requirements.

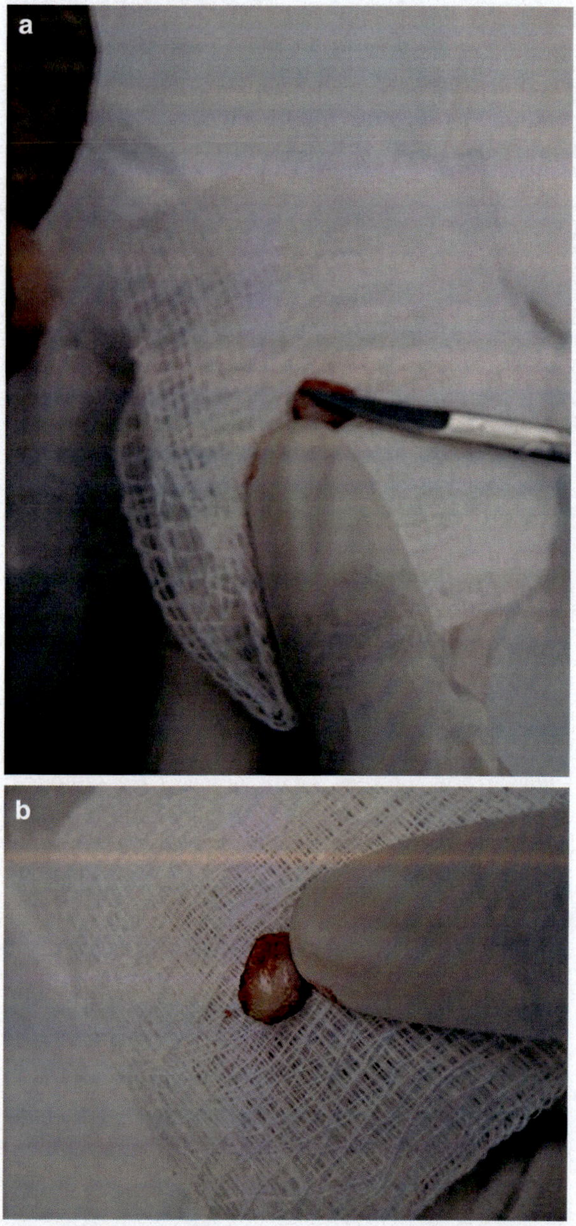

Fig. 34.1 (**a**, **b**) Curved iris scissors are used to defat the graft until glistening white dermis is revealed (All photos courtesy of Susana Leal-Khouri, M.D.)

34.6.2 Graft Fixation

Close apposition of the graft to the wound bed is necessary to promote vascularization and to minimize dead space that may lead to hematoma or seroma formation. Using a sterile smooth Adson forceps, the graft is placed onto the wound bed, and then the tissue is trimmed to fit the size of the defect. One should avoid using deep buried sutures to avoid the risk of puncturing underlying blood vessels and subsequent hematoma formation and because of the risk of the foreign material (i.e., suture material) decreasing the graft–bed contact.

Grafts should be placed as securely as possible in order to avoid shearing forces that may disrupt the contact between the graft and the wound bed, thus leading to failure. The corners of the graft should be anchored to the bed with interrupted nonabsorbable sutures. Next, running absorbable sutures should be used around the perimeter. Meticulous approximation of the wound edges to the graft is paramount to the optimal cosmesis of the graft. Large grafts may benefit from drainage slits and basting sutures, which are placed in the center of the graft in order to secure the graft to the recipient wound bed to increase contact [11]. Often, a 5-0 silk suture placed in a spiral fashion in the center of the graft is used.

Bolsters are used to stabilize and protect the graft and to provide a uniform pressure dressing to the grafted area. Bolster materials include saline-soaked dental rolls, saline- or iodine-soaked gauze, Xeroform (Johnson and Johnson Medical, Arlington, TX), and mineral oil–soaked cotton balls. The bolsters should have a nonstick surface and should be fitted to the size of the graft. Simple interrupted sutures using 4-0 silk are placed in pairs directly across from one another 2–3 mm from the graft margins. Depending on the size of the graft, approximately two to four pairs can be placed. In order for the pairs to be tied to secure the bolster material, the tails of the suture should be kept 6–8 cm long.

Once the sutures have been placed, antibiotic ointment or petrolatum is applied to the graft in order to create a moist environment to improve healing. Then, a nonadherent contact layer, such as Xeroform (Johnson and Johnson Medical, Arlington, TX) or Adaptic (Johnson and Johnson Medical, Arlington, TX), is attached to the graft followed by the bolster material. The bolster sutures are then tied into their respective pairs. After securing the bolster, fluffed gauze can be taped over the bolster to give added protection and security to the graft. The donor site is then closed, most often in a layered fashion, and an appropriate dressing is applied.

Delayed grafting should be considered in the following situations: when the risk of graft failure is high, such as in smokers and those with vascular disease; when there is exposed bone or cartilage; or when the wound is large or deep [9]. Granulation tissue that forms during 1–2 weeks of delay can contribute to a greater chance of graft survival.

Summary: Split-Thickness Skin Grafts

- Contain epidermis and variable amounts of dermis and are usually devoid of adnexal structures.
- Thin nature of the tissue allows for easier monitoring after removal of skin cancer with a high risk of recurrence.
- Extra tissue should be harvested in order to allow for contraction.
- Meshing of the graft allows for an increase in size of the harvested tissue, drainage to avoid hematoma or seroma formation, and decreased time needed for healing.

34.7 Split-Thickness Skin Grafts

Split-thickness skin grafts (STSG) contain epidermis and variable amounts of dermis. They are frequently devoid of adnexal structures; therefore, they do not grow hair or produce sweat or sebum. STSG are indicated for large defects (>5 cm), slow- or nonhealing chronic wounds, or painful wounds. STSG can be divided based on thickness: thin (0.125–0.275 mm), medium (0.275–0.4 mm), and thick (0.4–0.75 mm) [5]. Since they are thinner than FTSG and have less tissue to revascularize, the use of a STSG is preferred for chronic wounds. Additionally, this property makes them beneficial for wounds with a decreased vascular supply, such as irradiated tissue and fibrotic chronic ulcers. When there is a high risk of recurrence after skin cancer surgery, a STSG can be beneficial as the thin nature of the tissue allows for easier monitoring. STSG may be harvested using a dermatome or the freehand technique, depending on the size of graft needed and location of the recipient site.

A disadvantage of the STSG is fragility. Specifically, they are thinner and less resistant to trauma. Further, they do not prevent wound contracture, which is especially important to consider if used to repair defects around free anatomic margins. The cosmetic outcome is inferior to that of a FTSG as color and texture usually are not a good match. The technique of meshing the STSG further reduces cosmesis. Additionally, the donor site usually hypopigments.

34.7.1 Graft Harvest

Once the donor site is selected, it is anesthetized, cleansed, and prepared for harvesting. The wound to be grafted is measured in order to harvest the appropriate-sized donor skin. As with the FTSG, it is important to harvest extra tissue to allow for contracture. One may harvest a STSG with a dermatome or the freehand method [12]. A uniform width and depth can be achieved with the dermatome. Dermatomes are manually powered or powered by battery, electricity, gas, or air. A lubricant, such as mineral oil, is applied to the donor site to ensure easy movement of the dermatome over the donor skin. During harvesting, an assistant uses a sterile tongue depressor to apply countertraction to the area in front of the dermatome, while the surgeon applies traction behind the dermatome with his/her other hand. A slightly downward and forward motion is used to harvest the skin. Using forceps, the donor skin is removed from the dermatome as it is harvested in order to prevent damage to the graft. The donor skin is then detached by a fluid upward movement or by scissors or scalpel.

Once the graft is detached, it is placed in saline. The open donor site is dressed with gauze soaked in saline or 1:400,000 epinephrine solution to achieve hemostasis. The graft is transferred to a meshing plate with sterile saline to keep the graft moist. Attention to the orientation of the graft is important, and care should be taken to prevent rolling of the graft while it is guided slowly through the mesher in order to prevent wrinkling.

Meshing of the STSG has many purposes. First, meshing results in a graft that is larger than the size of the original tissue while still maintaining integrity. Second, the interstices created permit drainage of wound exudate and therefore help to avoid hematoma or seroma formation. Moreover, meshing decreases the time needed for complete healing and decreases morbidity. On the other hand, meshing diminishes the cosmetic appearance of the graft. There is also a higher incidence of wound contraction with meshing.

Punch grafts and pinch grafts are freehand STSG that are sometimes used to repair nonhealing ulcers [13]. Once the donor site has been anesthetized, cleansed, and prepped, the grafts are harvested with a 4-mm punch biopsy instrument (punch graft) or by scalpel or Weck knife (pinch grafts). The graft is then placed in saline-soaked gauze, and the donor site is covered with saline-soaked gauze. This method allows for several small grafts to be placed on the defect. The cosmetic result is often variable as the grafts are not of uniform thickness; however, overall take is good.

34.7.2 Graft Fixation

The three-dimensional flexibility of meshed, dermatome harvested grafts allows for ease in fitting and fixing irregular wounds with nonabsorbable superficial sutures or surgical staples. When stapling, one prong of the staple is hooked through the graft, then the other prong is placed on the skin surrounding the graft [14]. The stapler is squeezed and the staple placed. The staples should only be placed deep enough to secure the graft in place. The graft is then held in place with a pressure dressing consisting of several layers, including a nonstick petroleum jelly–impregnated gauze, nonadherent dressing, followed by a pressure and compression dressing (in the absence of arterial insufficiency). An occlusive dressing is used for the donor site, which allows for rapid healing, decreased pain, and control of acute wound exudate. The dressing on the recipient site should be changed weekly; however, those on the donor site should not be disturbed until the dressing begins to leak.

Freehand harvested grafts do not need to be sutured in place. The dressings and wound care described for the STSG from dermatome harvested grafts are sufficient to secure both the grafted and donor sites.

Summary: Composite Grafts

- Composite skin grafts are used principally to repair full-thickness skin defects in areas where cartilage must be replaced.
- Increased metabolic demands lead to higher risk of failure, and one should limit the size to less than 1.5 cm.

34.8 Composite Grafts

Composite grafts may include fat, perichondrium, or cartilage along with the epidermis and dermis; however, it is the cartilage-containing grafts that are most often used in dermatologic surgery. Composite skin grafts are used principally to repair full-thickness skin defects in areas where cartilage must be replaced. They also can be used to repair partial-thickness defects when contraction of a free margin or patency of key functional structures, such as the nasal valve, are needed. It should be noted that the composite graft is at a higher risk of failure secondary to increased metabolic demands and is also limited by size. Furthermore, any mechanism that interferes with revascularization, such as a shearing force, is a major threat to the survival of the graft [15].

The nasal ala and helical rim are the sites in which these grafts are frequently utilized. Donor sites include the conchal bowl, helical crus, or helical rim. However, one should limit the size to less than 1.5 cm as composite grafts are less viable than other grafts and have a higher rate of failure [15]. It is advisable to make the composite graft slightly larger than the defect, usually adding about 3–5 mm to the defect measured along the axis where the cartilage will be placed. The overlying skin and cartilage are harvested en bloc. The excess skin from the medial and lateral aspects of the graft is removed so that cartilage "pegs" remain [16]. The cartilaginous portion of the graft that extends beyond the margins of the defect will be used to stabilize the graft into pockets created with a blade at the medial and lateral aspects of the recipient site. This allows the graft to be anchored into the recipient site and allows the cartilage to contact fully vascularized tissue just beyond the defect margins. The graft should be sutured in place carefully so as to minimize strangulation of the vessels. Frequently, 6-0 mild chromic gut or fast-absorbing gut suture is used for the mucosal side, and 6-0 nonabsorbable suture is used for the skin side. The cartilage will heal on its own and does not need to be sutured in place. Application of a bolter, such as that for a FTSG, is recommended. Additionally, intranasal antibiotic-impregnated gauze should be used to stabilize the graft. Oral antibiotics are recommended given the nasal colonization of bacteria.

Summary: Postoperative Instructions

- Any activity that can disrupt the integrity of the graft or induce hematoma formation should be avoided.
- After 5–7 days, the bolster for a full-thickness skin graft should be removed by the physician.
- If the cosmetic outcome of the graft is not satisfactory, dermabrasion may be considered after 6–12 weeks.

34.9 Postoperative Instructions

The most important part of postoperative care is to minimize patient activity. Any activity that can disrupt the integrity of the graft or induce hematoma formation should be avoided. If a graft is on the head or neck region, the patient should be given instructions to elevate his/her head on a pillow when sleeping, and should not bend over. When a graft involves the cheek or lip, the patient should be instructed to avoid vigorous chewing. Patients with grafts on the extremities should be encouraged to elevate the extremity, and crutches or splints should be utilized as deemed necessary.

Many dermatologic surgeons prescribe a short course of antibiotics as prophylaxis against streptococcal and staphylococcal infections. In the case of a graft to the ear, antibiotics to cover *Pseudomonas* are often prescribed. Occasionally, pain medications are given to alleviate discomfort.

34.9.1 FTSG

After 5–7 days, the bolster should be removed by the physician. Bolster sutures are cut, and the bolster dressing is moistened with saline to prevent drying. The graft is held in place with saline-soaked cotton-tipped applicators. More often than not, the graft appears discolored at the time of bolster removal. Darker colors may indicate death of the epidermis. It is important to leave the graft in place, even if the epidermis is necrotic, as the dermis is often viable. If the dermis is necrotic as well, the graft will slough off in 2 weeks. A new graft may be placed at a later date.

34.9.2 STSG

The dressing should be changed weekly. At postoperative day 7, the petroleum jelly–impregnated gauze is removed from the STSG site by moistening with saline. The graft is held in place with saline-soaked, cotton-tipped applicators while the gauze is gently lifted. The STSG usually turns pink after 2 days. In the case of hematoma formation, the blood should be drained in order to reestablish proper graft to wound bed apposition, or the graft may fail. A large-bore needle or angiocatheter can be used for this purpose, and then the area can be flushed with saline. Grafts that are at a higher risk of failure should be examined sooner than 7 days. After 7 days, the sutures or staples holding the graft to the bed are removed. Protective and compression dressings should be continued for at least 2–3 weeks after complete healing.

The STSG donor site dressing is changed every 3 days or when the dressing leaks or falls off. The donor site may take several weeks to reepithelialize. Wound care should continue until the site is completely healed.

If a patient is not satisfied with the cosmetic outcome of the graft, dermabrasion may be considered after 6–12 weeks. This can allow for smoother graft edges and allow for blending of the graft with the surrounding skin.

Summary: Cultured Skin Substitutes

- Epidermal, dermal, and bilayered cultured skin substitutes can be useful for second intention healing and delayed grafts.

34.10 Cultured Skin Substitutes

Skin substitutes are grafts that have been processed or cultured prior to application. These may be: autologous, allogeneic, or xenogeneic; epidermal, dermal, or with elements of both; temporary or permanent; and biologic or synthetic [17].

34.10.1 Epidermal

Cultured epidermal autografts are obtained by first harvesting skin from the recipient. The culturing of the keratinocytes is then performed in the laboratory to create large sheets of graftable epidermis. The process takes about 3 weeks after which large sheets of keratinocytes are available for permanent coverage with acceptable cosmesis. The grafts are fragile and can blister easily secondary to the lack of a dermal component.

Cultured epidermal allografts are useful for immediate use. As they are allogeneic in origin, prolonged persistence does not occur; however, neither does graft rejection. Donor cells are slowly replaced by the patient's own cells. Therefore, these allografts serve as a temporary covering and stimulus for healing in acute and chronic wounds. It should be noted that these grafts are thin and are limited by their inherent fragility.

34.10.2 Dermal

Alloderm is a dermal, permanent skin substitute. Alloderm (LifeCell Corp., The Woodlands, TX) is derived from human allograft cadaver skin. Once the epidermis is removed, the dermal cells are removed prior to chemical processing to produce a nonantigenic acellular dermis. A complete intact basement membrane complex is present even though the epidermis is not. A meshed STSG can be layered over the Alloderm. Alternatively, cryopreserved Alloderm is hydrated prior to application and treated similar to a STSG, often being meshed prior to application [18].

Oasis (Cook Inc, Bloomington, IN) is porcine small intestine submucosa and is categorized as a bioactive dermal-like matrix. The freeze-dried cellular matrix retains its natural collagen and matrix structure and contains most of the bioactive matrix protein present in the human dermis. Advantages of Oasis are that it has a long shelf life and can be stored at room temperature. Wound bed incorporation occurs over about 7 days; therefore, it needs to be reapplied if the wound has not yet healed [19, 20].

34.10.3 Bilayered

Apligraf (Organogenesis, Canton, MA) is a bilayered, permanent human skin equivalent approved for venous leg ulcers and diabetic foot ulcers [21]. It is derived from bovine collagen and living allogeneic human skin keratinocytes and fibroblasts from neonatal foreskin. When examined histologically, Apligraf resembles human skin but lacks adnexal structures, Langerhans cells, or blood vessels, and its mechanism of action is unclear. Apligraf is useful for patients who need large areas grafted and who have little available donor tissue.

34.10.4 Graft Fixation

Prior to placement of the skin equivalent, the wound bed should be cleansed, debrided, and irrigated. If necessary, a hemostatic agent may be applied in order to control bleeding. It should be noted that these grafts should not be applied to an infected wound.

A pH color chart and expiration date ensure viability for Apligraf.

Using a forceps, the skin equivalent is gently loosened from the storage dish (note: the dermal side is down in the storage dish). The grafts should not be allowed to fold on themselves, and using saline to moisten the graft may help to avoid this. One may trim the graft to fit the wound bed. The graft is held in place, with direct contact to the wound bed, with nonstick petroleum jelly–impregnated gauze and a compression dressing. Nonabsorbable superficial sutures, Steri-Strips, or staples, followed by nonstick petroleum jelly–impregnated gauze and a compression dressing may also be used to fix the graft to the wound bed.

34.10.5 Postoperative Instructions

The secondary dressing/compression dressing should be changed after 3–5 days. The graft is examined by removing the primary dressing after 5–7 days. Using sterile saline to moisten the primary dressing is helpful so as not to remove the graft from the wound bed. Gently lifting the dressing off the graft while saline-soaked cotton-tipped applicators are used to hold the graft in place is helpful as well. These grafts undergo several color changes (translucent, white, or yellow) and typically do not take; however, they work by healing through cytokine release.

Summary: Graft Failure

- Graft failure can result from insufficient wound bed vascularity, hematoma or seroma formation, ischemia secondary to excess tension on the graft, improper dressings, infection, or noncompliance by the patient.

34.11 Graft Failure

Graft failure can result secondary to several factors. These include: insufficient wound bed or graft vascularity; lack of contact between the wound bed and graft secondary to hematoma or seroma formation; excess tension on the graft due to improper size of the graft or fixation, leading to ischemia; improper dressings; infection; and noncompliance with postoperative instructions or patient medications. Proper clinical and patient selection, meticulous execution, and close follow-up are essential to ensuring a successful graft. Cosmetic and functional outcome can be excellent.

Summary: Conclusion

- Meticulous attention to detail and identification of the proper patient and clinical scenario are paramount to the success of a graft and subsequently to a good cosmetic and functional outcome.

34.12 Conclusion

Skin grafting is a useful technique that should not be overlooked when the dermatologic surgeon is considering reconstructive options. While many defects and wounds can be closed via primary closure or use of a skin flap, there are situations when a skin graft is preferred. In addition to meticulous attention to detail, identification of the proper patient and clinical scenario is paramount to the success of a graft and subsequently to a good cosmetic and functional outcome. Advances in the production of skin substitutes continue to provide options with which to treat patients and will continue to be a dynamic component to skin grafting in the future.

References

1. Smahel J. The healing of skin grafts. Clin Plast Surg. 1977;4(3):409–24.
2. Converse JM, Uhlschmid GK, Ballantyne Jr DL. 'Plasmatic circulation' in skin grafts. The phase of serum imbibition. Plast Reconstr Surg. 1969;43:495–9.
3. Converse JM, Smahel J, Ballantyne Jr DL, Harper AD. Inosculation of vessels of skin graft and host bed: a fortuitous encounter. Br J Plast Surg. 1975;28:274–82.

4. Zarem HA, Zweifach BW, McGehee JM. Development of microcirculation in full thickness autogenous skin grafts in mice. Am J Physiol. 1967;212:1081–5.
5. Johnson TM, Ratner D, Nelson BR. Soft tissue reconstruction with skin grafting. J Am Acad Dermatol. 1992;27: 151–65.
6. Waris T, Rechardt L, Kyosola K. Reinnervation of human skin grafts: a histochemical study. Plast Reconstr Surg. 1983;72:439–47.
7. Goldminz D, Bennerr RG. Cigarette smoking and flap and full-thickness graft necrosis. Arch Dermatol. 1991;127: 1012–5.
8. Pollack SV. Wound healing: a review. IV. Systemic medications affecting wound healing. J Dermatol Surg Oncol. 1982;8(8):667–72.
9. Ceilley RI, Bumsted RM, Panje WR. Delayed skin grafting. J Dermatol Surg Oncol. 1983;9:288–93.
10. Hill TG. Contouring of donor skin in full-thickness skin grafting. J Dermatol Surg Oncol. 1987;13:883–8.
11. Adnot J, Salaache SJ. Visualized basting sutures in the application of full-thickness skin grafts. J Dermatol Surg Oncol. 1987;13:1236–9.
12. Snow SN, Stiff M, Lambert D, Tsoi C, Mohs FE. Freehand technique to harvest partial-thickness skin to repair superficial facial defects. Dermatol Surg. 1995;21:153–7.
13. Burns DA, Sarkany DI. Management of stasis ulcers by pinch grafts. Br J Dermatol. 1976;95 Suppl 14:82.
14. Tromovitch TA, Stegman SJ, Glogau RG. Split-thickness skin grafts. Flaps and grafts in dermatologic surgery. Chicago: Year Book Medical Publishers; 1989. p. 55–63.
15. Tromovitch TA, Stegman SJ, Glogau RG. Composite grafts. Flaps and grafts in dermatologic surgery. Chicago: Year Book Medical Publishers; 1989. p. 65–7.
16. Ratner D, Katz A, Grande DJ. An interlocking auricular composite graft. Dermatol Surg. 1995;21:789–92.
17. Bello YM, Falabella AF. Use of skin substitutes in dermatology. Dermatol Clin. 2001;19:555–61.
18. Druecke D, Steinstraesser L, Homann HH, Steinau HU, Vogt PM. Current indications for glycerol-preserved allografts in the treatment of burn injuries. Burns. 2002;28 Suppl 1:S26–30.
19. Brown-Estris M, Cutshall W, Hiles M. A new biomaterial derived from small intestinal submucosa and developed into a wound matrix device. Wounds. 2002;14:150–66.
20. Demling R, Niezgoda J, Haraway G, Mostow E. Small intestinal submucosa wound matrix and full thickness venous ulcers. Wounds. 2004;16:18–23.
21. Trent JT, Kirsner RS. Tissue engineered skin: Apligraf, a bilayered living skin equivalent. Int J Clin Pract. 1998;52: 408–13.

35 Side to Side Closure After Mohs Surgery

Michael P. McLeod, Katlein França, Sonal Choudhary, Yasser A. Alqubaisy, and Keyvan Nouri

Abstract

Side to side closure is defined as linear closure. Meticulous planning must be carried out so that inherent, vertical, and lateral restraints are optimized. Provided that function and form are conserved, then cosmetic appearance should be considered. The principles of tissue closure including free margins, aesthetic units, and relaxed skin tension lines should be carefully considered when performing side to side closures. This chapter discusses side to side closures as well as a number of complications that can occur when using this type of closure.

Keywords

Side to side closures • Tissue repair • Cosmetic subunits

M.P. McLeod • K. França • S. Choudhary
Department of Dermatology and Cutaneous Surgery, University of Miami Leonard M. Miller School of Medicine, Miami, FL, USA

Y.A. Alqubaisy
Department of Dermatology and Cutaneous Surgery, University of Miami Hospital, Miami, FL, USA

K. Nouri (✉)
Department of Dermatology and Cutaneous Surgery, University of Miami Leonard M. Miller School of Medicine, Miami, FL, USA

Sylvester Comprehensive Cancer Center, University of Miami Hospital and Clinics, Miami, FL, USA
e-mail: knouri@med.miami.edu

Summary: Introduction
- The simplest closure is generally the best one to use.
- Inherent restraint is the natural flexibility found in the tissue.
- Vertical restraint is a measure of how much a particular tissue is kept in place by its attachment to the underlying tissue.

35.1 Introduction

Essentially, a side to side closure is defined as linear closure [1].

Generally speaking, the simplest closure is usually the best one.

K. Nouri (ed.), *Mohs Micrographic Surgery*,
DOI 10.1007/978-1-4471-2152-7_35, © Springer-Verlag London Limited 2012

Meticulous planning must be carried out so that inherent, vertical, and lateral restraints are optimized [2]. Inherent restraint is the natural flexibility found in the tissue. A good example of a tissue that has more inherent restraint from the view point of the dermatologic surgeon is the cutaneous tissue of the scalp [2]. Vertical restraint is a measure of how much a particular tissue is kept in place by its attachment to the underlying tissue.

Summary: Side to Side Closures

- Side to side closures of wounds have aesthetic and functional purposes.
- Primary side to side closures have the advantage of simplifying the wound care for the patient, and generally a better cosmetic result is obtained.
- The wound should not be closed if there is active oozing of blood and foreign debris embedded in the tissue.

35.2 Side to Side Closures

The side to side closure of wounds must pay respect first to functionality and secondarily to aesthetic composition. The principal idea is to eliminate the dead space by approximating the subcutaneous tissues. The epidermis should be carefully aligned to minimize the scar formation. It is also important to avoid a depressed scar by precisely everting the skin edges.

Primary side to side closures have the advantage of simplifying wound care for the patient, who simply needs to keep suture line dry and clean. It heals much more quickly and with less pain and facilitates the biological event of healing by joining the wound edges compared to leaving the wound to heal by secondary intention.

This technique should be carried out in the acute wound as soon as possible to minimize the risk of infection. Active bleeding from the wound and foreign debris that cannot be completely removed are contraindications to closure.

Summary: Suturing of the Wounds

- The purpose of the ideal suture is to approximate the wound edges and reestablish the tissue closure with a functional yet aesthetically pleasing scar.
- The surgeon must also understand the wound healing process and the principles of tissue closure (aesthetic units, relaxed skin tension lines, and tensile strength) to perform an adequate skin approximation.
- The skin edges must be handled gently, and the wound edges approximated with as little tension as possible.

35.3 Suturing of the Wounds

The purpose of the ideally suture is to approximate the wound edges and reestablish the tissue closure with a functional and aesthetic scar. The use of good materials and methods of suturing are the determinant factor for a good technique. The surgeon must also understand the wound healing process and the principles of the tissue closure (aesthetic units, relaxed skin tension lines, and the tensile strength) to perform a good skin approximation.

The skin edges must be handled gently, and the wound approximated with as little tension as possible.

Summary: Cosmetic Subunits

- Provided that function and form are conserved, then cosmetic interests should be considered.
- Important contour lines for the face are the hairline, eyebrows, philtrum, alar crease, nasolabial fold, labiomental crease, and vermillion-cutaneous junction.
- Care should be taken to not cross multiple cosmetic units when carrying out a side to side closure.

35.4 Cosmetic Subunits

Provided that function and form are conserved, then cosmetic interests should be considered. Care should be taken to not cross multiple cosmetic units when performing a side to side closure. Important contour lines for the face are the hairline, eyebrows, philtrum, alar crease, nasolabial fold, labiomental crease, and vermillion-cutaneous junction. The forehead also has 3 units within itself: the glabella, temple, and suprabrow. The periorbital region also contains several subunits demarcated by the orbicularis oculi muscle: the palprebral (pretarsal, preseptal subunits) and orbital subunit. The nose itself has several subunits: the root, dorsum, lateral sidewalls, alae nasi, tip, and soft triangle. The lips contain two subunits: the cutaneous upper lip and cutaneous lower lip. The cutaneous upper lip is demarcated medially by the philtral crest, inferiorly by the vermilion-cutaneous junction, and laterally by the nasolabial fold. The cutaneous lower lip is bordered superiorly by the vermillion-cutaneous junction and laterally by either the labiomental crease or the infraoral crease. The philtrum lines are infranasal and care should be taken not to disrupt these lines because even small deviations can result in noticeable scars. The chin is bordered by the labiomental crease which actually continues underneath the jawline.

Summary: Complex Facial Defects

- Complex facial defects following Mohs micrographic surgery are often a concern for dermatologic surgeons.
- Reconstruction of these defects should follow the same principles used for the closure of simple or smaller defects.

35.5 Complex Facial Defects

Complex facial defects following Mohs micrographic surgery are often a concern for dermatologic surgeons. The reconstruction of these defects should follow the same principles used for the closure of simple or smaller defects. The specific anatomic area should be considered in choosing a method for closure. Flaps may be considered in some areas, including a tunneled pedicle flap and artificial skin substitute for large areas[3]. The reconstitution must preserve the cosmetic facial units and the function of the area [4]. Some cases may require general anesthesia and hospitalization.

Summary: General Considerations

- The wound care resulting from a side to side closure is not significantly different from a normal routine closure.
- A nonstick bandage can be left in place for a week, or if desired, can be changed daily or twice daily at least 1 day following suture placement.

35.6 General Considerations

The wound care resulting from a side to side closure is not significantly different from a normal routine closure. Generally, the wound is moisturized with daily sterile vaseline application. A nonstick pressure dressing can be left for 48 hours. Afterwards, the wound should be cleansed daily with soap and water or sterile saline followed by application of sterile vaseline and nonstick dressing.

Summary: Complications

- Anytime that a side to side closure is used, the surgeon should keep in mind the "terrible tetrad," consisting of "wound infection, dehiscence, bleeding, and necrosis."
- Dehiscence is defined as the reopening of a surgically closed wound.
- Dehiscence is often the result of high closure tension, too few or inappropriately placed dermal sutures, or patient factors including inappropriate activity, systemic corticosteroids, and smoking.
- Bleeding during the first 24 hours can be brisk, causing a hematoma, or lead to ecchymosis formation.

35.7 Complications

Anytime that a side to side closure is used, the surgeon should keep in mind the "terrible tetrad," consisting of "wound infection, dehiscence, bleeding, and necrosis" [5].

Wound infections occur approximately 6–7 days after surgery [5]. A mild erythematous reaction, which is considered normal, is usually present around the sutures and constitutes a foreign-body reaction against the sutures [5]. However, if the redness continues to worsen, marked swelling develops with pus and discharge; a wound infection may have developed. What may begin as cellulitis can move toward a systemic infection and eventually sepsis if not treated appropriately. Simple surgical wound infections can be treated with cephalexin, or if allergic to penicillin, the patient may take erythromycin. If MRSA is suspected, other antibiotics that cover this infection (i.e., Doxaciclin, Vancomicin, Bactrin) may be warranted [5].

Dehiscence is another possible complication when managing side to side closure and can be secondary to tissue necrosis or a wound infection [6]. It is defined as the reopening of a surgically closed wound [5]. It is often the result of high closure tension, too few or inappropriately placed dermal sutures, or patient factors including inappropriate activity, systemic corticosteroids, and smoking [5]. When dehiscence occurs within 48 h of the closure, it can simply be re-sutured; however, after that time, healing by secondary intention can be used [6]. If the wound was under excess tension, then a wider undermining may be required before closing the wound after dehiscence [5].

Bleeding during the first 24 hours can be brisk, cause a hematoma, or lead to ecchymoses. Brisk bleeding can occur when the epinephrine used in the local anesthetic wears off and vasodilation leads to rupture of the newly formed blood clot [5]. When hematomas form, they generally occur 3–4 days after surgery and present as a growing gelatinous mass that can be painful [5]. Due to their expansive nature and the limited space to expand into, hematomas can exert pressure on the wound and reduce perfusion to the lesion, resulting in necrosis and even dehiscence [5]. In addition, hematomas offer an excellent environment for bacteria to proliferate, leading to a wound infection [5]. Ecchymoses can be quite dramatic to the patient and tend to migrate toward where the gravity takes them. They are usually benign and do not significantly change the final outcome. The patient should be educated regarding their potential appearance so that it does not have psychological consequences for the patient. Bleeding should be treated with 20 min of firm pressure. If this is not successful and the bleed is significant, the wound should be reexplored, and the offending vessel or vessels, ligated or cauterized. In addition, a drain can be used to evacuate blood and prevent hematoma formation. If the hematoma is not rapidly expanding or expanding enough to apply enough pressure on the wound to result in necrosis, then watchful waiting may be used, and the hematoma should reabsorb after 3 or so months [5].

Summary: Conclusion

- The purpose of the ideal closure is to reestablish the function of the tissue with an aesthetic scar.
- This chapter discusses side to side closures as well as a number of complications that can occur when using this type of closure.

35.8 Conclusion

Side to side closures of wounds have aesthetic and functional purposes. Primary side to side closures have the advantage of simplifying wound care for the patient. The purpose of the ideal closure is reestablish the function of the tissue with an aesthetically appealing scare. The surgeon must also understand the wound healing process and the principles of the tissue closure (aesthetic units, relaxed skin tension lines, and the tensile strength) to perform an adequate skin approximation. This chapter discusses side to side closures as well as a number of complications that can occur when using this type of closure.

References

1. Lawrence N. Complex closures. In: Nouri K, Leal-Khouri S, editors. Techniques in dermatologic surgery. New York: Mosby; 2003. p. 135–9.
2. Chen TM, Wanitphakdeedecha R, Nguyen TH. Flaps. In: Vidimos AT, Ammirati CT, Poblete-Lopez C, Elston DM, editors. Dermatologic surgery: requisites in dermatology. New York: Saunders/Elsevier; 2009. p. 163–80.
3. Gladstone HB et al. An algorithm for the reconstruction of complex facial defects. Skin Therapy Lett. 2007;12(2):6–9.
4. Robinson JK. Segmental reconstruction of the face. Dermatol Surg. 2004;30(1):67–74.
5. Kouba DJ, Moy RL. Complications of reconstructive surgery. In: Nouri K, editor. Complications in dermatologic surgery. Philadelphia: Mosby/Elsevier; 2008. p. 65–90.
6. Brodland D. Complex closures. In: Ratz JL, Geronemus RG, Maloney ME, Goldman MP, Padilla RS, editors. Textbook of dermatologic surgery. Philadelphia: Lippincott-Raven; 1998. p. 183–200.

Prosthetic Rehabilitation

36

Glenn E. Turner and Jeffrey E. Rubenstein

Abstract

Loss of facial anatomy resulting from disfigurement secondary to trauma, surgical excision to eradicate benign or malignant lesion, or anatomical malformation resulting from congenital anomalies represents a loss of one's three-dimensional signature/identity. The psychological implications stemming from being different from the norm have significant impacts on ones' self-image. Since the focus of this text is management of malignancy of the facial structures, this chapter will limit itself to facial prosthetic rehabilitation associated with cancer management.

A variety of interventions for head and neck cancer management can be considered such as surgical excision/resection, radiotherapeutic management either as a single modality or in conjunction with surgery and/or chemotherapy in an adjuvant or concomitant approach. While Mohs surgical interventions attempt to address management of malignancy through chemo–surgical approaches for tissue preservation, the approach needed for addressing Maxillofacial Prosthodontic rehabilitation of lost/compromised facial anatomy calls for an entirely alternative approach. The mandate for such prosthodontic rehabilitative efforts calls for a stable tissue base to support and retain either an adhesive, mechanical, or implant retained craniofacial prosthesis. Appropriately addressing the tissue base is a key element for predictable and successful prosthodontic rehabilitation.

The information in this chapter represents an overview of the salient issues associated with craniofacial prosthetic rehabilitation. Four subcategories for the most commonly encountered treatments will be presented which are nasal, auricular, orbital, and multisite prostheses. One common thread for interventions of this type is coordination of care amongst the health-care providers that should include a Maxillofacial Prosthodontist at the time of the presurgical work-up.

G.E. Turner (✉)
Department of Prosthodontics, University of Florida College of Dentistry, Gainesville, FL, USA
e-mail: gturner@dental.ufl.edu

J.E. Rubenstein
Department of Restorative Dentistry, University of Washington School of Dentistry, Seattle, WA, USA

K. Nouri (ed.), *Mohs Micrographic Surgery*,
DOI 10.1007/978-1-4471-2152-7_36, © Springer-Verlag London Limited 2012

Keywords

Maxillofacial Prosthetics • Craniofacial • Nasal • Auricular • Orbital • Craniofacial implants • Moulage

Summary: Introduction

- A removable craniofacial prosthesis allows for easy access for inspection of the tissue bed to facilitate early detection of recurrent cancer.

36.1 Introduction

The treatment of cancer can no longer be undertaken unilaterally but instead must be multidisciplinary in nature. This basic rudiments of a "treatment team" includes a Surgeon, Radiation Oncologist, Medical Oncologist, Pathologist, and Maxillofacial Prosthodontist. In general, both the patient and the surgeon prefer surgical reconstruction. However, in partial or total rhinectomy, total or partial auriculectomy, and in orbital exenteration, a prostheses is the treatment of choice. A removable craniofacial prosthesis allows for easy access for inspection of the tissue bed to facilitate early detection of recurrent cancer.

The key to successful prosthetic reconstruction is coordinated planning between the Surgeon and the Prosthodontist [1]. The patient should be seen by the Prosthodontist prior to surgery to have impressions made and discuss the prosthodontic rehabilitation procedures that will be possible after surgery. Prior to surgery, a planning conference that includes the Surgeon and the Maxillofacial Prosthodontist is held to determine the anticipated extent of the resection.

Summary: Moulage Impression Procedure

- A moulage impression procedure is the technique for making a record of the facial anatomy, which can be obtained pre- and/or postoperatively.

36.2 Moulage Impression Procedure

The workhorse of craniofacial prosthetic intervention necessitates obtaining an accurate record of the area to be treated [2]. The impression material is applied first then backed with some material that can be incorporated into the impression material which is then captured with a "tray" usually fast set plaster to provide rigid support to prevent distortion when recovering the moulage impression. Commonly, alginate impression material offers a cost effective tool for recording a facial moulage. Usually, 50% more water than that which is used for intraoral impressions is used with this material when mixing it for recording of facial tissues. This ratio provides a smooth mix that does not apply much load, hence minimizing distortion of the tissues being recorded. Alternative materials commonly used today include low viscosity polyether or polyvinylsiloxane impression materials.

When recording a full facial moulage maintaining the airway is obviously an essential element in the preparation prior to recording the impression. This can be done via nasal or oral airways. Drinking straws fit to the nasal airway by incorporating soft wax around the straws fit into the nasal apertures, but done with care not to distort the nasal anatomy is important to accomplish prior to recording the impression.

It is also important to explain the procedures associated with the moulage impression to the patient. Most important is to determine whether or not the patient considers himself/herself to be claustrophobic. If so, a complete facial moulage may need to be obtained in sections so that the patient's anxiety is not exacerbated.

The latest evolving technology associated with obtaining records, planning and fabrication of facial prosthesis relates to 3-D digital imaging (e.g., 3-D MD, Atlanta, GA), and an evolving array of CAD/CAM approaches to computer generation of facial prostheses

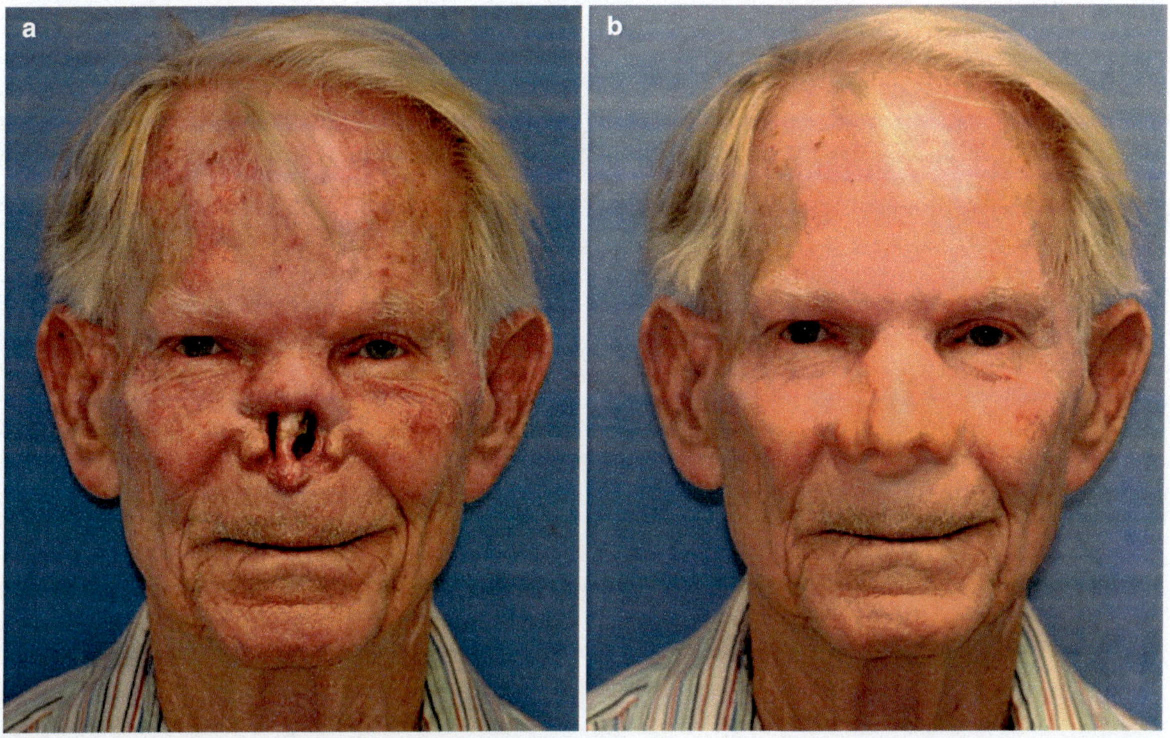

Fig. 36.1 Rhinectomy with alae and nasal septum remaining. (**a**) Full face showing defect. (**b**) Prosthesis is asymmetrical and too wide

anatomical contours. While this emerging technology is exciting in what it has to offer, it is in most circumstances self-limiting thus far in terms of being cost prohibitive. Nonetheless, the future offers some yet to be appreciated exciting opportunities to interface technological advances with craniofacial prosthodontic treatment.

Summary: Adhesive Retained Nasal Prosthesis

- Nasal prosthesis is a prosthesis that replaces all or part of the nasal anatomy.

36.3 Adhesive Retained Nasal Prosthesis

In the era of new age surgical reconstructive procedures via free flap tissue transfer the "fork of the road" for deciding whether to surgically reconstruct vs. proshodontically rehabilitate offers the respective clinicians a dichotomy or cross road that necessitates a mutually exclusive decision tree, i.e., tissue preservation or eradication. Too frequently, patients undergoing a partial or total rhinectomy are referred for prosthodontic rehabilitation with remnant tissue tags of residual ala or unsupported nasal anatomy remaining in place (see Fig. 36.1a, b). In doing so, the degree of difficulty of such situations exponentially complicates craniofacial prosthesis management/fabrication. It is very disconcerting to have to refer the patient back to the surgeon for further tissue revision after the patient has already undergone the trauma of losing facial anatomy only to be faced with yet another procedure to facilitate development of a more optimal base on which the prosthesis will sit. There have been occasions where this need arises, and the patient, in addition to surgical resection, has also undergone a full course of either pre- or postoperative radiotherapy making addressing the need for further surgery an indeterminate risk for possible healing compromise or development of soft tissue and/or osteoradionecrosis.

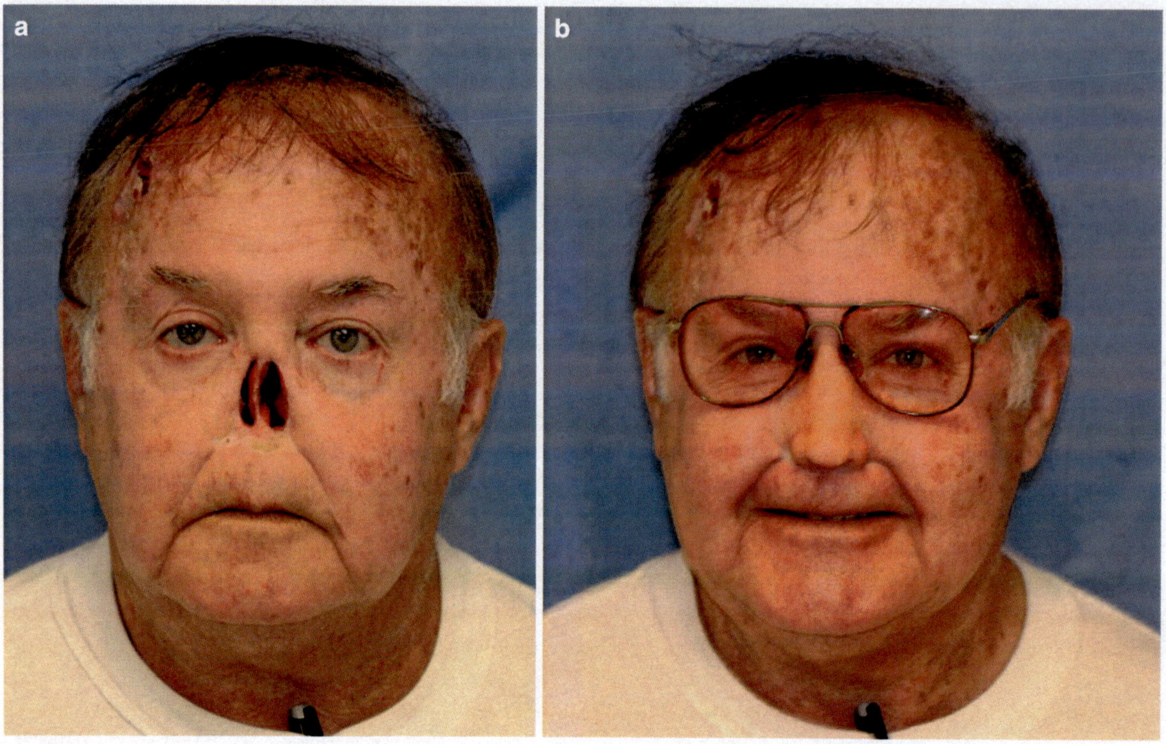

Fig. 36.2 Good tissue base (**a**) shows skin grafts at the margins and nasal septum resected. (**b**) Prosthesis with eyeglasses hiding some margins

If the patient pending a total rhinectomy procedure is able to consult with the Maxillofacial Prosthodontist prior to surgery, then the plan for the surgical resection can be better aligned with the development of a optimized site for placement of a nasal prosthesis. Ideally, the optimal foundation for a nasal prosthesis is comprised of the firm tissue base on which the prosthesis can rest. A split-thickness skin graft placed where possible on the borders of the resection with the underlying tissue, muscle, etc., (see Fig. 36.2a) debulked to the periosteum offers the best foundation on which the prosthesis can seat [3]. The most challenging marginal interface for a nasal prosthesis is the inferior margin because it, of necessity, rests on the superior aspect of the upper lip. This margin is a moving target for a statically configured prosthesis. Maintaining the nasal labial fold when possible (see Fig. 36.3a, b) affords a marginal adaptation for the lateral margins of the prosthesis that (see Fig. 36.4a, b) allows for camouflage/blending of the interface between the silicone margins with facial tissue. Moreover, for those individuals wearing eyeglasses, the eyeglass frames can provide an adjunctive role. Properly selected eyeglass frames can, in effect, become part of the prosthodontic management as they can cover the lateral marginal interface of the prosthesis (see Fig. 36.2b), thereby making it less obvious that anatomical loss has occurred when the prosthesis and eyeglasses are in place.

Summary: Adhesive Retained Auricular Prosthesis

- Auricular prosthesis replaces all or part of an ear.

36.4 Adhesive Retained Auricular Prosthesis

Loss of one or both ears represents a significant compromise from both a functional and esthetic perspective. The auricle is an essential anatomical element needed to funnel sound to the middle ear. As well, loss of an auricle can significantly impair ones' ability to wear eyeglasses. The much-needed support that results from missing the external pinna from one or both sides presents a significant rehabilitation challenge. Plastic surgeons will readily admit that the surgical reconstruction of an external pinna likely represents the

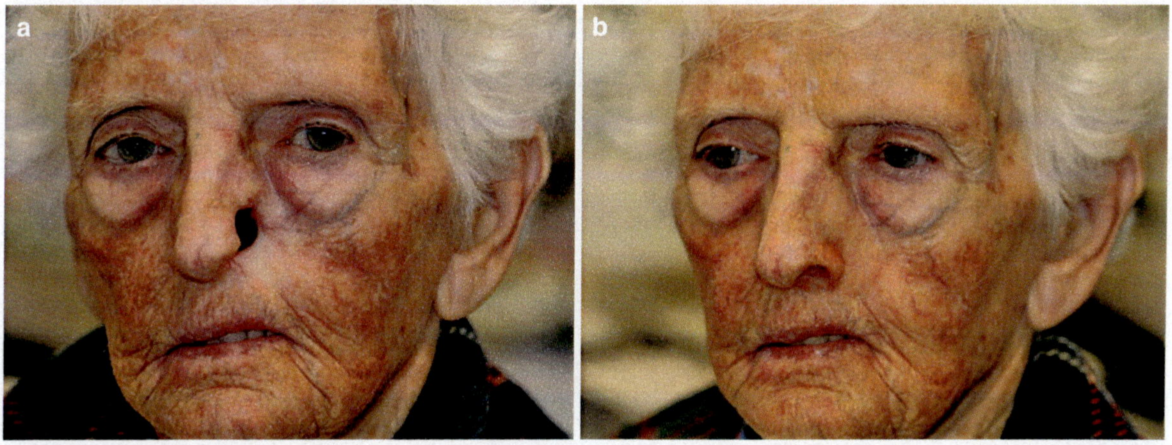

Fig. 36.3 Maintaining the nasolabial fold. (**a**) Defect. (**b**) Prosthesis

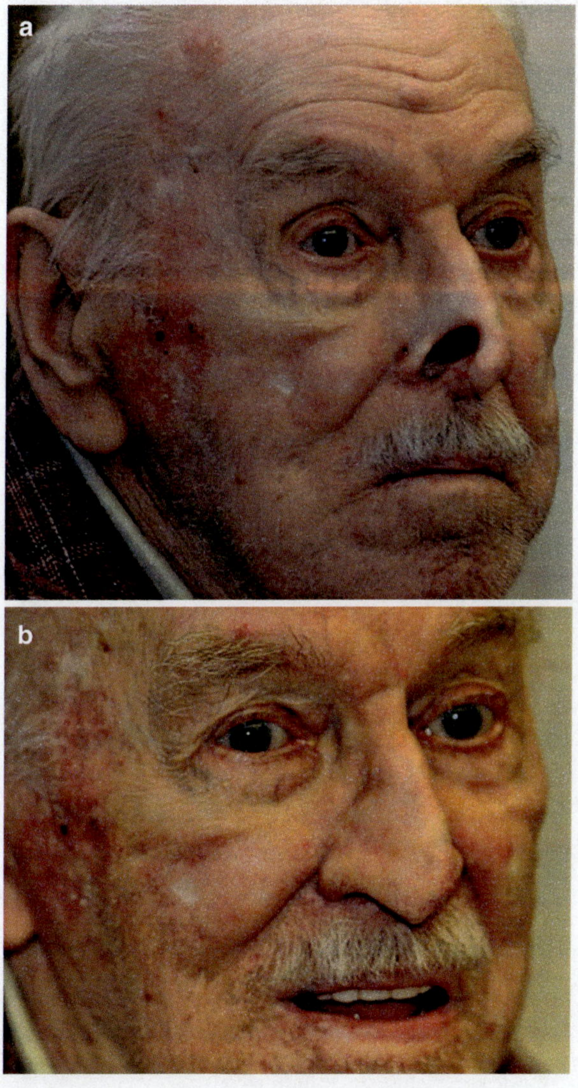

Fig. 36.4 Nasal defect to nasolabial fold. (**a**) Defect. (**b**) Prosthesis

most challenging surgical intervention with which they are confronted. As well, most plastic surgical colleagues will in most instances readily admit while the challenge of surgical reconstruction can be pursued via a multistaged procedure the end result cannot be equaled to the anatomical contours that can be developed with a prosthodontic approach. Clearly, surgical reconstruction offers the significant benefit of a good tissue color match and a procedure that, once done, leaves the patient with a lack of need to further ongoing prosthodontic maintenance, revisions, and remakes of the prosthesis. Again, the decision tree associated as to which path to follow is critical to determine prior to surgical eradication of a malignancy of the external pinna. In some circumstances, more tissue beyond the pinna is needed to be addressed, e.g., a temporal bone resection. In such circumstances the feasibility of surgical reconstruction is more muddled, and in many instances impractical (see Fig. 36.5).

As a counter point to the recommendation for a nasal prosthesis tissue bed to be devoid of remnant tissue tags, the auricular area actually can benefit by leaving the tragus, if feasible, in regard to tumor management. The rationale for this recommendation is that the anterior margin of an auricular prosthesis, generally speaking, is the most challenging to blend into surrounding tissues. By leaving the tragus, the anterior margin (see Fig. 36.6) of the prosthesis is broken up from its typical straight-line margin offering the benefit of achieving an improved outcome [4]. Another issue related to the anterior margin of an auricular prosthesis is to take note of the range of motion of the temporomandibular joint and the resultant change in the topography of the overlying tissue associated with

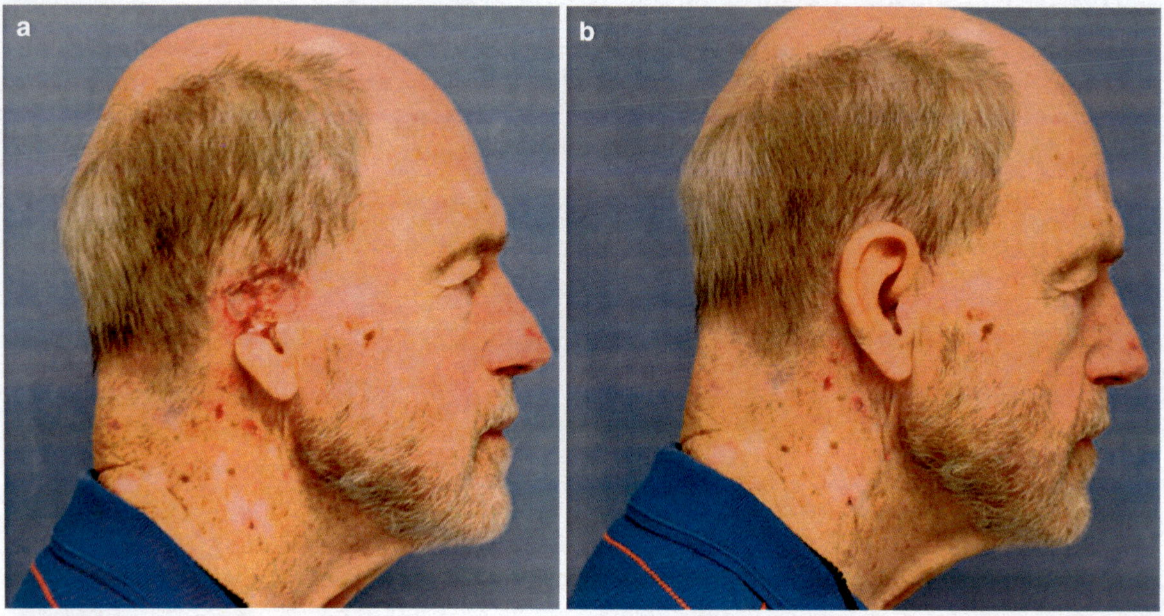

Fig. 36.5 Auricular defect involving the temporal bone. (**a**) Defect. (**b**) Prosthesis

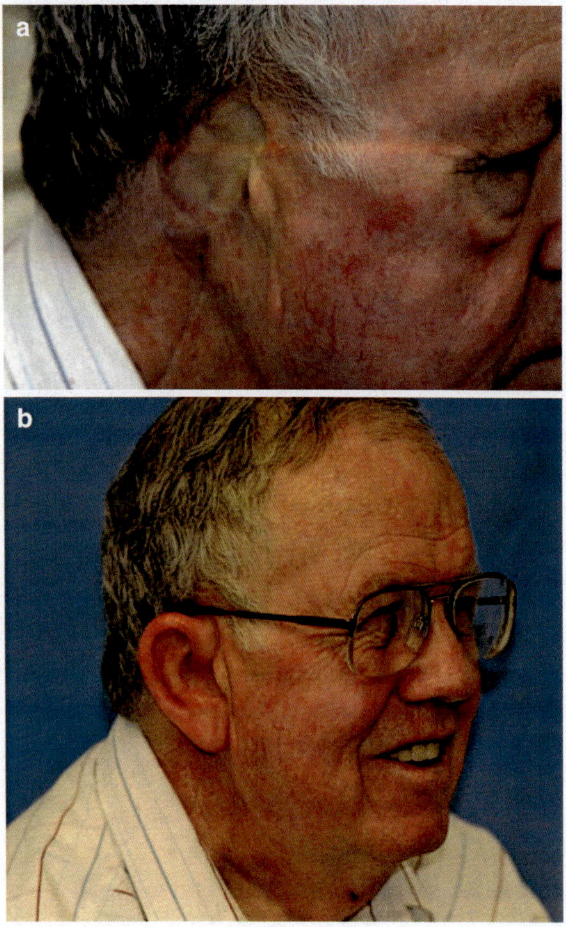

Fig. 36.6 Good skin graft leaving the tragus. (**a**) Healed surgical site. (**b**) Prosthesis

this movement. In some patients (much like variable tidal changes), this tissue topography can be quite dramatic and in others inconsequential. Nonetheless, aside from that already noted, a firm tissue base, i.e., a split-thickness (afollicular) skin graft (see Fig. 36.7) once again, is the order of the day for provision of an ideal base of support for an auricular prosthesis.

Preoperative moulage records are generally useful if the affected auricle is not significantly compromised anatomically by the progression of the malignancy. Even if so compromised, a preoperative record serves as a historical documentation that can never otherwise be obtained once the surgical resection is done.

Auricular impressions sometimes benefit by recording the ear canal along with the tissue base on which the prosthesis can rest. The impression of the canal can be performed with tempered compound (Green Stick Compound, Kerr Manufacturing Co. Romulus, MI) followed by a wash of an elastomeric impression material such as low viscosity polyether (Permadyne, 3M ESPE, St. Paul, MN).

Summary: Adhesive and/or Mechanically Retained Orbital Prosthesis

- Orbital prosthesis replaces globe, contents of the orbit, and surrounding tissue.

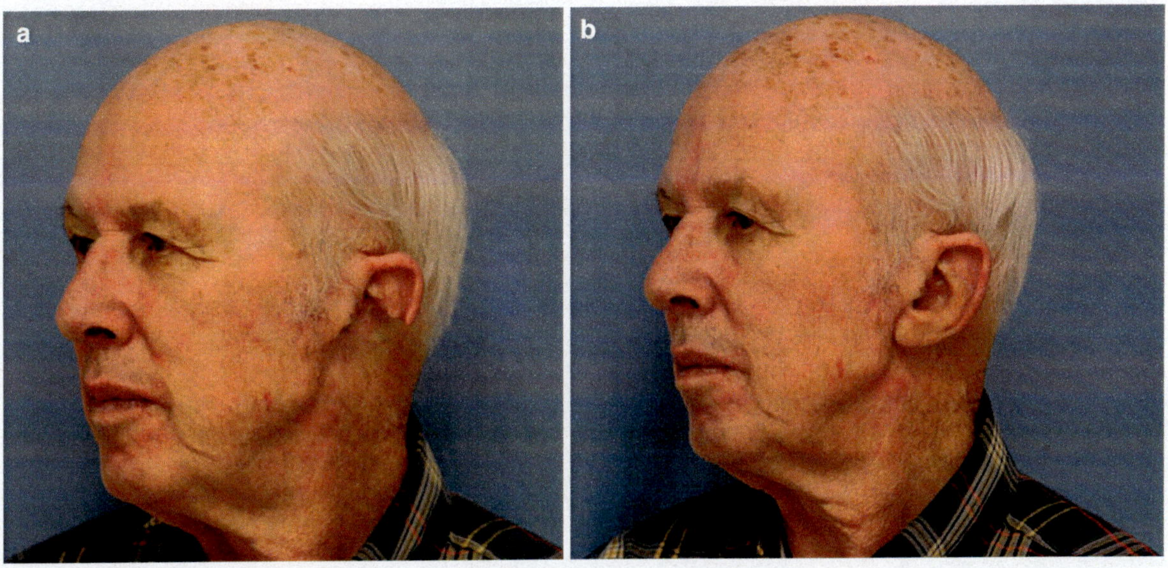

Fig. 36.7 Firm tissue base with split-thickness (a follicular) skin graft. (**a**) Healed surgical site. (**b**) Prosthesis

36.5 Adhesive and/or Mechanically Retained Orbital Prosthesis

The loss of the globe and surrounding contents of the orbit poses significant challenges as regards rehabilitation with an orbital prosthesis. This area in particular seems to be rife with confusion as to how to provide the best surgical management in regard to creating the ideal site for prosthetic management. Not infrequently, the patient having an orbital exenteration is seen by the Maxillofacial Prosthodontist only after tumor resection. The orbital defect is not uncommonly managed with free tissue transfer that obliterates the depth of the socket making it difficult if not impossible to place an orbital prosthesis that would represent restoration of symmetry and harmony to the facial contours. As previously noted, if the patient is afforded the opportunity to consult with the Prosthodontist prior to doing an orbital exenteration, this discussion could preclude the unfortunate circumstance of having to subject the patient to further surgical intervention or indicating that prosthodontic management is not possible.

From the prosthodontic perspective, lining the orbital socket with a split-thickness skin graft leaving a firm tissue base and deep, dry socket creates an ideal cavity for which an orbital prosthesis can be successfully provided [4] (see Fig. 36.8a). Sometimes, full-thickness coverage of the exenterated orbit is needed especially when post-op radiotherapy is planned.

There are occasions where orbital exenteration is combined with a maxillectomy for those tumors emanating from the maxillary sinus and eroding through the floor of the orbit. In general terms, the rehabilitation of such cases necessitates working from the inside out as the maxillary obturator or free flap reconstruction of the maxillectomy impacts the facial contours. This internal contouring of the facial anatomy needs to be established prior to developing the craniofacial prosthetic component of such patients' rehabilitation efforts.

Typically, the big departure between an ocular prosthesis for a patient missing the globe vs. that for an individual treated with an orbital exenteration is the requirement to have the ocular prosthesis for the latter be smaller and crescent-shaped for ease in placement and removal. Such a design/contour element of the ocular component of the silicone orbital prosthesis thereby prevents the prosthesis from becoming torn or damaged.

The major challenge for successful orbital rehabilitation is first and foremost to accurately orient the ocular component of the prosthesis to establish the appropriate "gaze." Given that the ocular component of an orbital prosthesis does not track, its three-dimensional spatial orientation needs to be precisely placed to afford symmetry in relation to the globe on the unaffected side. This cornerstone in fabrication is critical for arriving at a completed prosthesis that accurately represents restoration of normalized appearance (see Fig. 36.8b).

In some circumstances, the orbital cavity presents with undercuts posterior and superior to the superior orbital

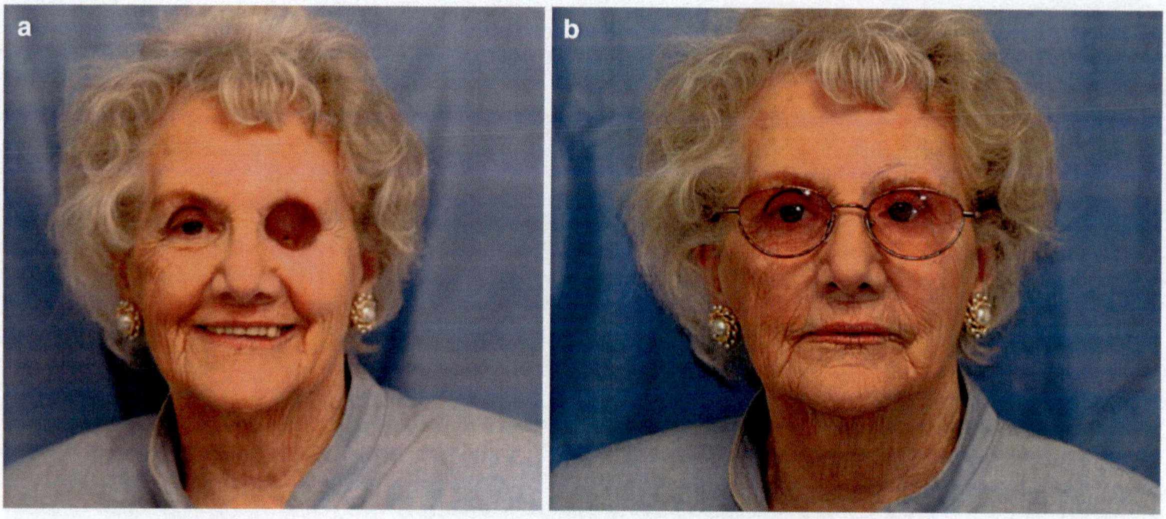

Fig. 36.8 Defect of orbital exenteration. (**a**) Split-thickness skin graft leaving a firm tissue base and deep dry socket. (**b**) Prosthesis with ocular properly aligned

rim and posterior and inferior to the infraorbital rim. Such a presentation can lend itself to the fabrication of a two-piece mechanically retained orbital prosthesis [5].

When implants are used to retain the orbital prosthesis, the space requirements needed for placement of the retaining elements for the prosthesis, be they independent or splinted, can challenge the positioning of the ocular component in its mandated and correct three-dimensional spatial orientation. This challenge can often result in the need for some creative engineering to accommodate and satisfy both form and retention requirements.

Summary: Midface/Multisite Craniofacial Prosthesis

- Facial prostheses that extend beyond one anatomic site.

36.6 Midface/Multisite Craniofacial Prosthesis

When facial anatomy compromise extends beyond one anatomic site, e.g., orbit/nose, orbit/cheek, nose/upper lip, etc., the need for craniofacial prosthetic rehabilitation becomes significantly more challenging and complex. Further, a combination intra/extra oral anatomical compromise such as that for an individual undergoing a maxillectomy and orbital exenteration, planning, and facilitation of such rehabilitation efforts extend beyond those of multi-facial site compromises [6]. Each of these situations tends to be unique and challenges the rehabilitation efforts and creativity of the individual providing such a service. Given the highly variable presentations of such treatment requirements makes it difficult to identify specific issues to address in this section. The necessity for combined intraoral/extraoral defect management to be planned and facilitated from inside out is an absolute requirement for this type of rehabilitation effort. Use of magnet retention is another technique for retaining prosthesis (see Fig. 36.9a–c).

For the combination craniofacial defects, the remaining anatomy must be viewed from the perspectives of where support, stability, and retention can be achieved by either engaging soft tissue undercuts (to do so is concerning for the radiated patient), use of adhesives, or possibly planning for use of craniofacial implants. The challenge for all craniofacial prosthetic rehabilitation efforts from the perspective of patients in need of such treatment, first and foremost, is the provision of a predictable retention system for prosthesis [7, 8]. The more anatomical compromise needing to be addressed, the more challenging it is to create an adequate retention system. Generally speaking, the larger facial anatomical malignancy mandates multimodality therapeutic interventions. Therefore, most of

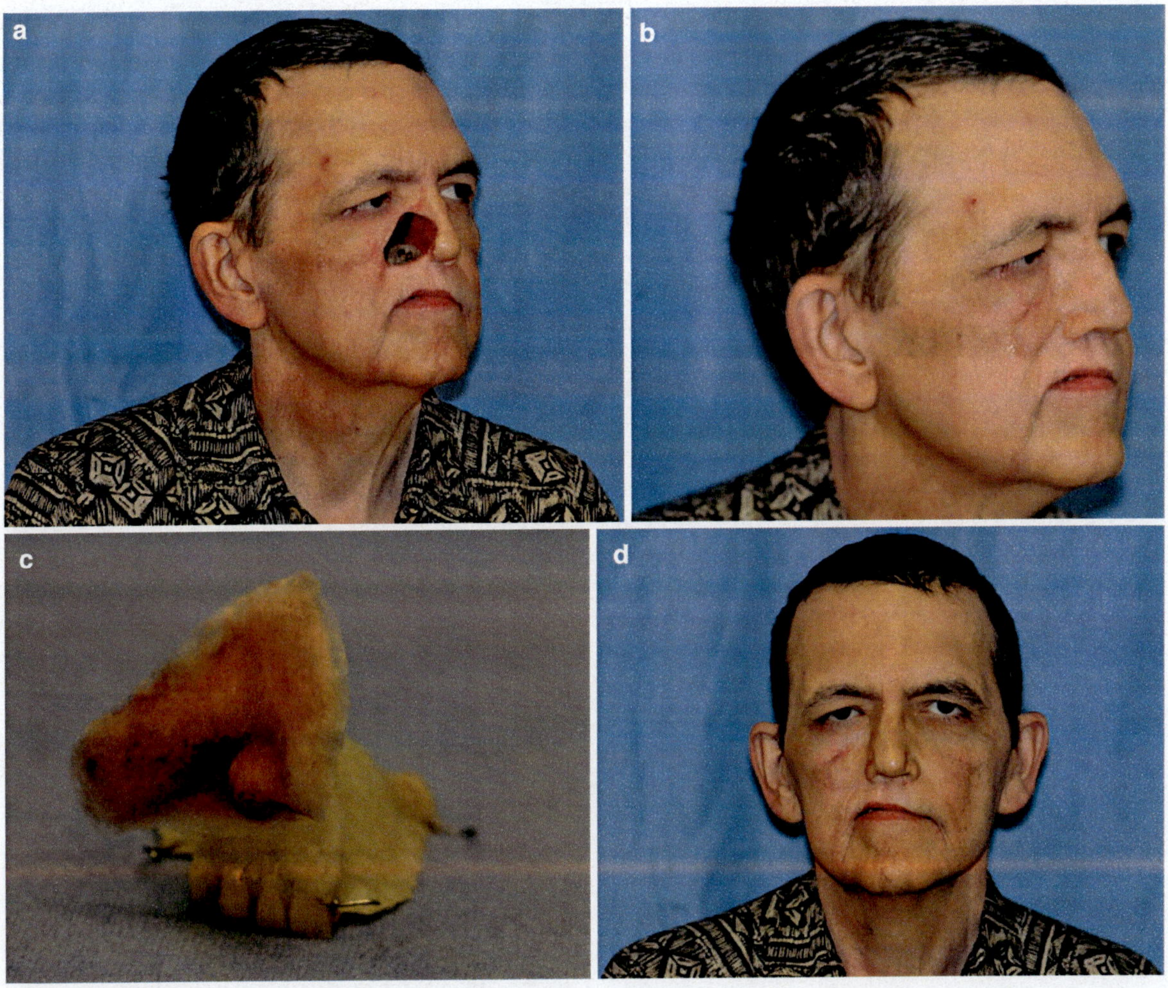

Fig. 36.9 Midface defect nasal, cheek and intraoral. (**a**) Defect with intraoral in place (note the magnet on intraoral). (**b**) Prosthesis lateral view. (**c**) Two-piece prosthesis with magnet. (**d**) Prosthesis frontal view

these patients have been treated with high doses of radiation with or without concomitant or adjunctive chemotherapeutic agents. Thus, the tissue base separate and apart from the surgical intervention is compromised and likely can be negatively impacted by daily use of adhesives to retain the prosthesis or pressure atrophy in sites where soft tissue undercuts are engaged by the prosthesis. Further, use of craniofacial implants can also be compromised in regard to either establishing a good bone/implant osseointegrated interface or over time become compromised by the latent long-term effects of radiotherapy on the tissue bed. All in all, achieving a suitable retention system for such situations, in and of itself, is challenging above and beyond creating a pleasing restoration of anatomical loss.

Summary: Considerations Regarding Implant Retained Craniofacial Prosthesis

- Osseointegrated implants are used for increasing the stability of craniofacial prostheses.

36.7 Considerations Regarding Implant Retained Craniofacial Prosthesis

Much like the requirements for adhesive retained facial prostheses, each treatment site for craniofacial implant retained prostheses has parameters for consideration in regard to optimizing implant placement and tissue base management. The common thread for implant retained facial prostheses is the need for a firm, thin, tissue interface in the peri-abutment region so as to minimize soft tissue complications [9, 10]. The need for good bone into which implants can be placed to obtain primary stability as with any implant intervention is critical to achieve successful osseointegration. The distribution and number of implants placed for retaining implant-based craniofacial prostheses has evolved over time. As well, the protocol for implant placement regarding one- versus two-stage surgery also presents the clinician with a choice on a case by case basis that needs to be factored into the treatment plan [11]. Success/survival rates of craniofacial implants suggest that in the auricular region (see Fig. 36.10a–c), one can expect implant success that is comparable to intraoral placement of implants in the anterior mandible [12]. The nasal region is the next site having implant integration being reasonably predictable. However, implant placement in the region of the orbit has the highest complication and failure rate. Controversy exists regarding the use of adjunctive pre- and post-craniofacial implant placement hyperbaric oxygen treatment. The data for success/survival rates for craniofacial implant placement does not clearly document for those data bases reported for implants placed in radiated treatment fields as to whether or not this adjunctive therapy was used [13–15].

Summary: Implant Retained Nasal Prosthesis

- Two or three osseointegrated implants are placed within the margins of the surgical defect.

36.8 Implant Retained Nasal Prosthesis

For implant retained nasal prostheses, placement of two implants in the lateral ala rims generally provides adequate support (see Fig. 36.11a–d). Not infrequently, the bone volume is adequate for use of conventional dental implants rather than shorter 3–4-mm craniofacial implants. By engaging the palatal bone implant, lengths up to 18 mm can be accommodated in some patients. Should additional implant support be needed, the nasal base midline can be considered as an alternate site for placement (see Fig. 36.12a–d). Consideration need be given to the apices of the maxillary anterior teeth if the patient is dentate in the anterior sextant so as not to amputate the root apices when preparing implant sites. Also, for the edentulous patient, consideration need be given to not encroach on the gingivobuccal sulcus which could impede the patient from being able to wear a maxillary complete denture. Reports of placing craniofacial implants in the region of the glabella have demonstrated 100% failure likely due to the fact that this region is a suture line between the cartilaginous make up of the vomer with that of the cranial bone of the forehead and adjacent frontal sinuses and cribriform plate [16, 17].

The peri-abutment region for implants placed in the nasal region is best managed with a split-thickness skin graft to afford the patient an ability to comfortably clean and maintain the peri-abutment tissue health. Despite the area being in the realm of ongoing mucous secretions and flow of particulate contaminants from the environment, anecdotally speaking, implants in the nasal region tend to do quite well over the long term.

Summary: Implant Retained Auricular Prosthesis

- Osseointegrated implants in the mastoid bone or temporal bones have the greatest long-term success.

36.9 Implant Retained Auricular Prosthesis

For craniofacial implant placement for patients missing one auricle or both auricles, the prior conventional wisdom was to place three or four craniofacial implants. In the recent past using two implants offers an adequate base of support to retain an implant retained auricular prosthesis. The placement of these implants is suggested as being approximately 18-20 mm posterior to the ear canal (if present) at approximately 1:00 and 3:00 o'clock on the patient's left side and 9:00 and 11:00 o'clock on the patient's right side. The bony architecture of mastoid region is replete with air cells, and as a result, it is sometimes difficult to ideally place implants exactly where prescribed by the implant surgical guide. In such cases, it is better to err by placing the implants further posterior so as not to encroach on the concha region of

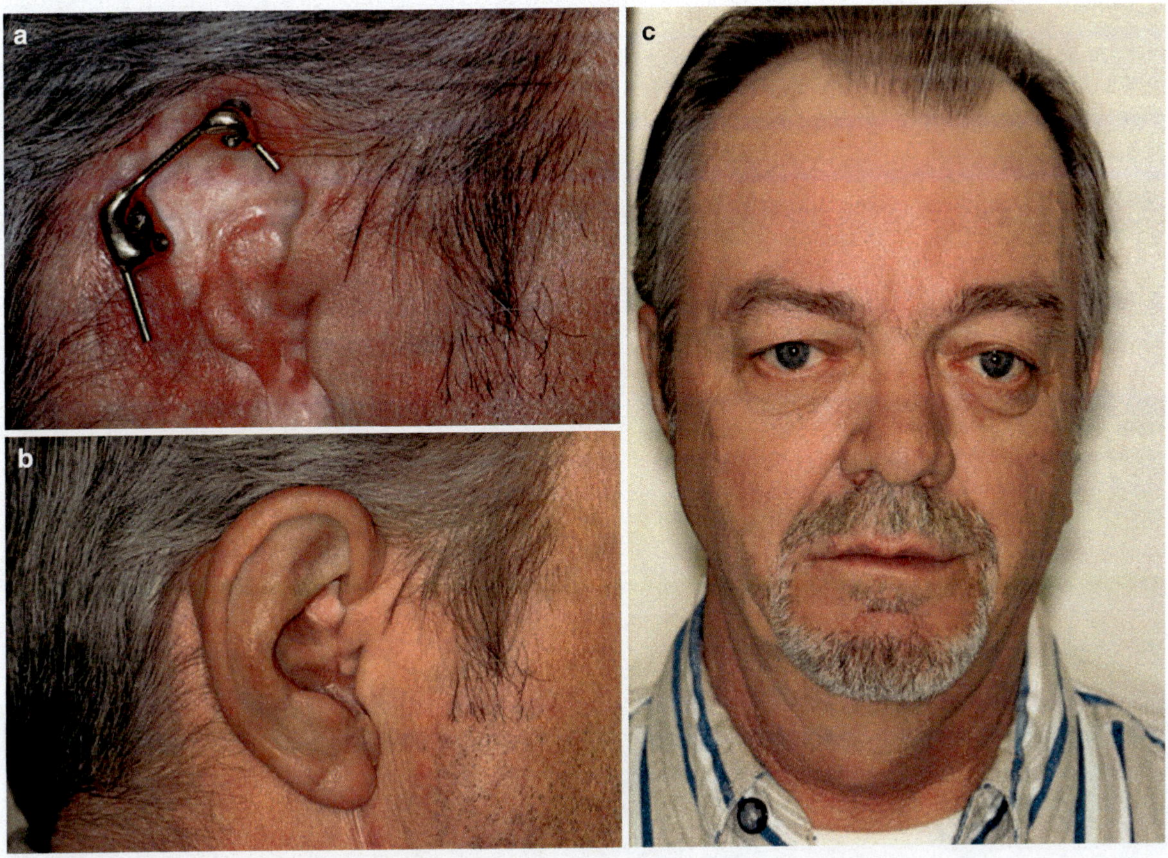

Fig. 36.10 Sixteen years status post right temporal bone resection and 6,000 CGy post-op radiation tx, pre- and post-craniofacial implant placement hyperbaric oxygen treatment. (**a**) Dolder Clip bar splinted to three craniofacial implants. (**b**) Silicone clip retained auricular prosthesis, lateral view. (**c**) Full face view with right silicone auricular clip retained implant prosthesis in place

the auricle that could result in an aberrant anatomical compromise of the prosthesis. The key is to have the implants situated under the planned tallest and thickest portion of the prosthesis so as to allow enough room for placement of the transmucosal abutments, retaining bar, attachments, attachment housings, acrylic substructure, and the overlying tissue skin tone matched silicone (see Fig. 36.13a–d).

The peri-abutment tissue in the auricular region can be addressed by either placing a split-thickness skin graft or undermining the tissue in this area at the time the abutments are placed. For patients who have been radiated, a staged procedure is generally advised so as to maximize the circulatory capacity during the healing period following implant placement surgery.

Another consideration for the prosthetic design is taking into account the movement of the temporomandibular joint. In some patients, the range of motion of the tissue overlying the temporomandibular joint is dramatic leading to the opening of a gap space between the anterior margins of the prosthesis during jaw movements [18]. This movement in the closing motion can sometimes dislodge the prosthesis from its retentive base. One approach to manage this for patients with an excess range of motion is to incorporate a magnet retainer on the inferior pole of the retaining bar allowing for disengagement and reengagement of the prosthesis so as to maintain a compatible retention mechanism for such situations.

Summary: Implant Retained Orbital Prosthesis

- Osseointegrated implants placed in the rim of an orbit have the least long term predictably.

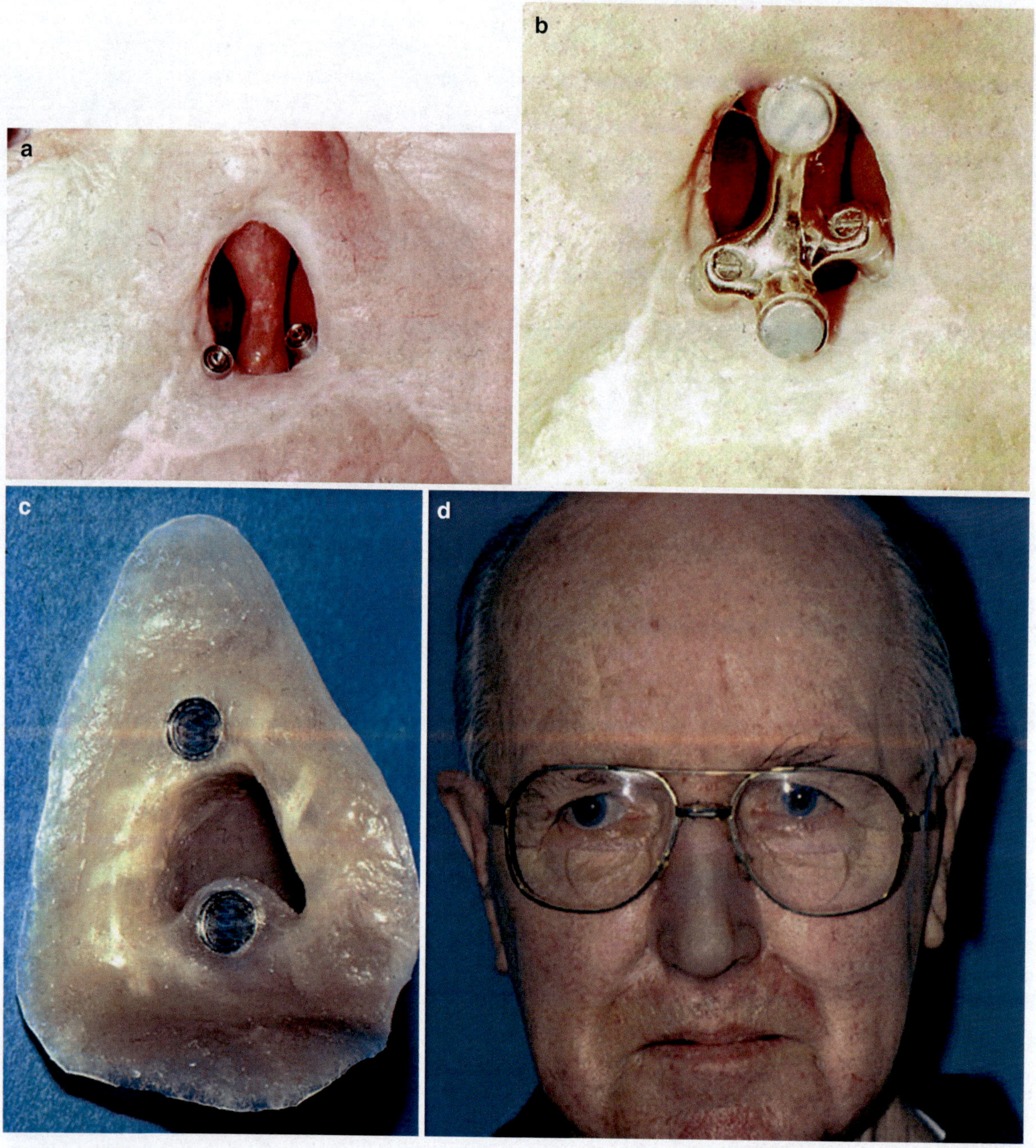

Fig. 36.11 Implant magnet retained nasal prosthesis. (**a**) Implants with transmucosal abutments in lateral ala region left and right. (**b**) Implant retention framework with two magnet keepers. (**c**) Tissue surface of silicone nasal prosthesis with two magnets (Technovent, Factor Two, Lakeside, AZ). (**d**) Magnet retained nasal prosthesis in place

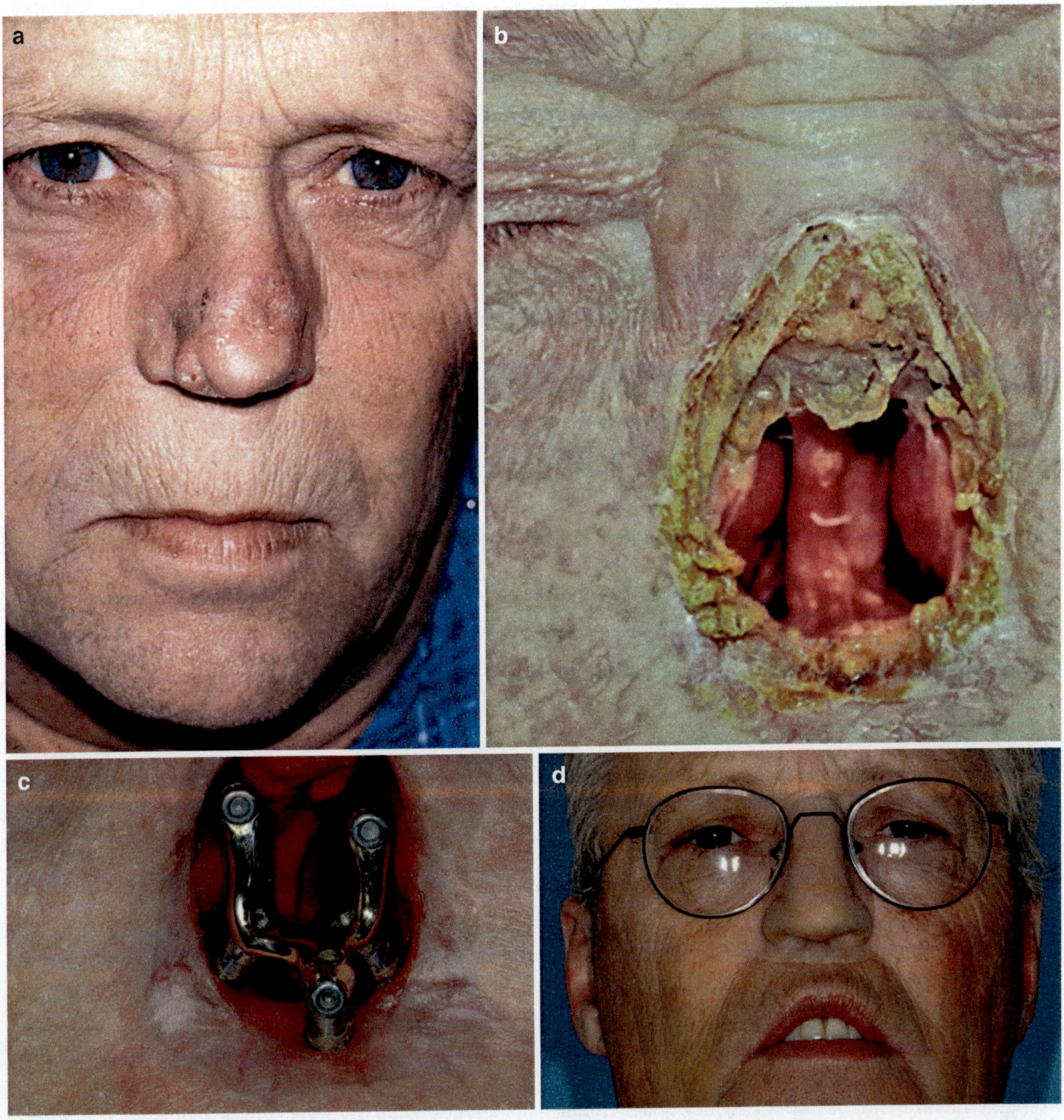

Fig. 36.12 Implant supported nasal prosthesis: (**a**) Pre-total rhinectomy for SCCA (*upper left*). (**b**) One week post-op (*upper right*). (**c**) Implant cast retaining structure with three resilient attachments (Locators, Zest Anchors LLC, Escondido, CA). (**d**) Implant retained silicone nasal prosthesis in place, full face view

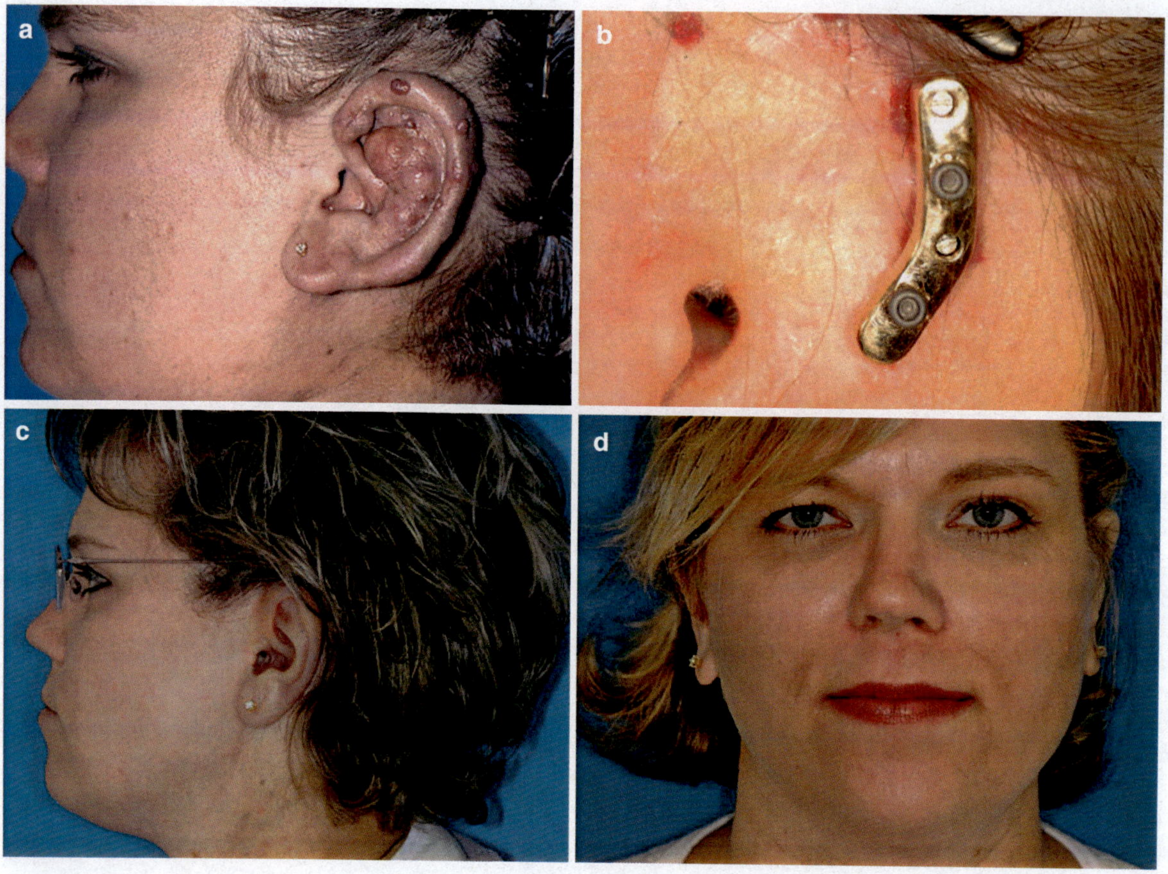

Fig. 36.13 (**a**) Aterio–venous (A/V) malformation right auricle (*upper left*). (**b**) Status post resection implant placement and retaining bar with two resilient attachments (Locator, Zest Anchors LLC, Escondido, CA). (**c**) Lateral view with silicone implant retained prosthesis in place. (**d**) Full face frontal view with silicone implant retained prosthesis in place

36.10 Implant Retained Orbital Prosthesis

Orbital implant placement considerations vary depending on the remaining boney architecture following orbital exenteration. If the floor of the orbit/infraorbital rim is left intact, then the goal for implant placement is to try to achieve a "milk stool" distribution of the implants that being an implant in the supraorbital rim, one in the lateral orbital rim and one in the infraorbital rim (see Fig. 36.14a–d). This distribution results in a tripod base of support for the orbital prosthesis. Given the lateral aspect of the frontal sinus frequently extends midway across the superior aspect of the orbit placement of an implant in the supraorbital rim is limited to where bone volume is and that does not encroach on invading the sinus.

From a prosthodontic perspective, the options for splinting vs. using independent retainers each offer their distinct challenges. Independent magnet retention using console abutments of varying angulations of the pod for placement of the magnet keeper not infrequently can create a problem with soft tissue management (Fig. 36.15a–d). With that said, a splinted bar construction can offer challenges as regards access for hygiene as well. It is difficult to achieve a firm tissue base in the peri-abutment region with either independent or splinted retention approaches. The path of placement for an orbital prosthesis unlike that for a nasal or auricular prosthesis is at 90° to the long axis of implants. While craniofacial prostheses do not have to contend with occlusal loading, their path of placement and removal might influence impact on the bone/implant interface. One can only speculate as to whether this difference, i.e., the nonaxial path of placement for an orbital prosthesis compared to auricular or nasal implant retained prostheses has an influence on the poorer success/survival rate [19–21].

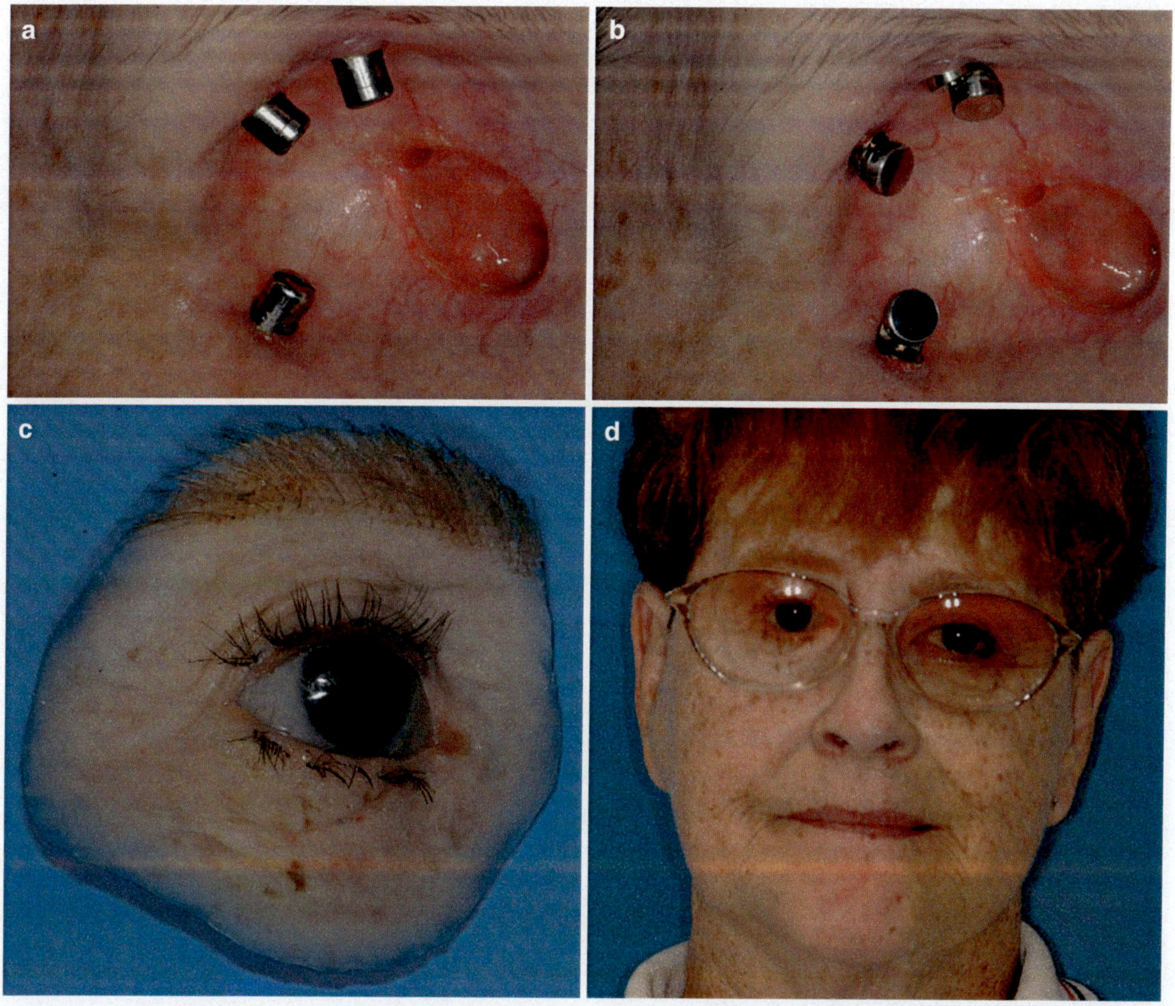

Fig. 36.14 Orbital exenteration to treat a melanoma. (**a**) Orbital defect status post-craniofacial implant placement in supraorbital, infraorbital, and lateral orbital rims with healing caps in place. (**b**) Implant with console abutments (Cochlear, Centennial, CO) with notable accumulation of secretions about the abutments. (**c**) Silicone orbital prosthesis. (**d**) Implant retained orbital prosthesis in place, full face view

Summary: Multisite Implant Retained Craniofacial Prosthesis

- Clearly this treatment modality requires an extensive level of experience and expertise.

36.11 Multisite Implant Retained Craniofacial Prosthesis

As regards multisite implant supported craniofacial prostheses, each case is so unique that it is not easy to identify specific recommendations as to implant sites, distribution, framework design, retention elements, etc. Clearly, this treatment modality is very challenging and requires an extensive level of experience and expertise. The lack of large numbers of patients requiring this type of treatment lends itself to representing uncharted territory. It is unlikely that this will change going forward as surgical interventions of this kind typically are deferred and relegated to patient's disease management with radiotherapy with or without chemotherapy largely to accommodate local control without intent for cure. The fact that large anatomical defects associated with the head and neck region give one pause to consider extensive surgical management and rehabilitation

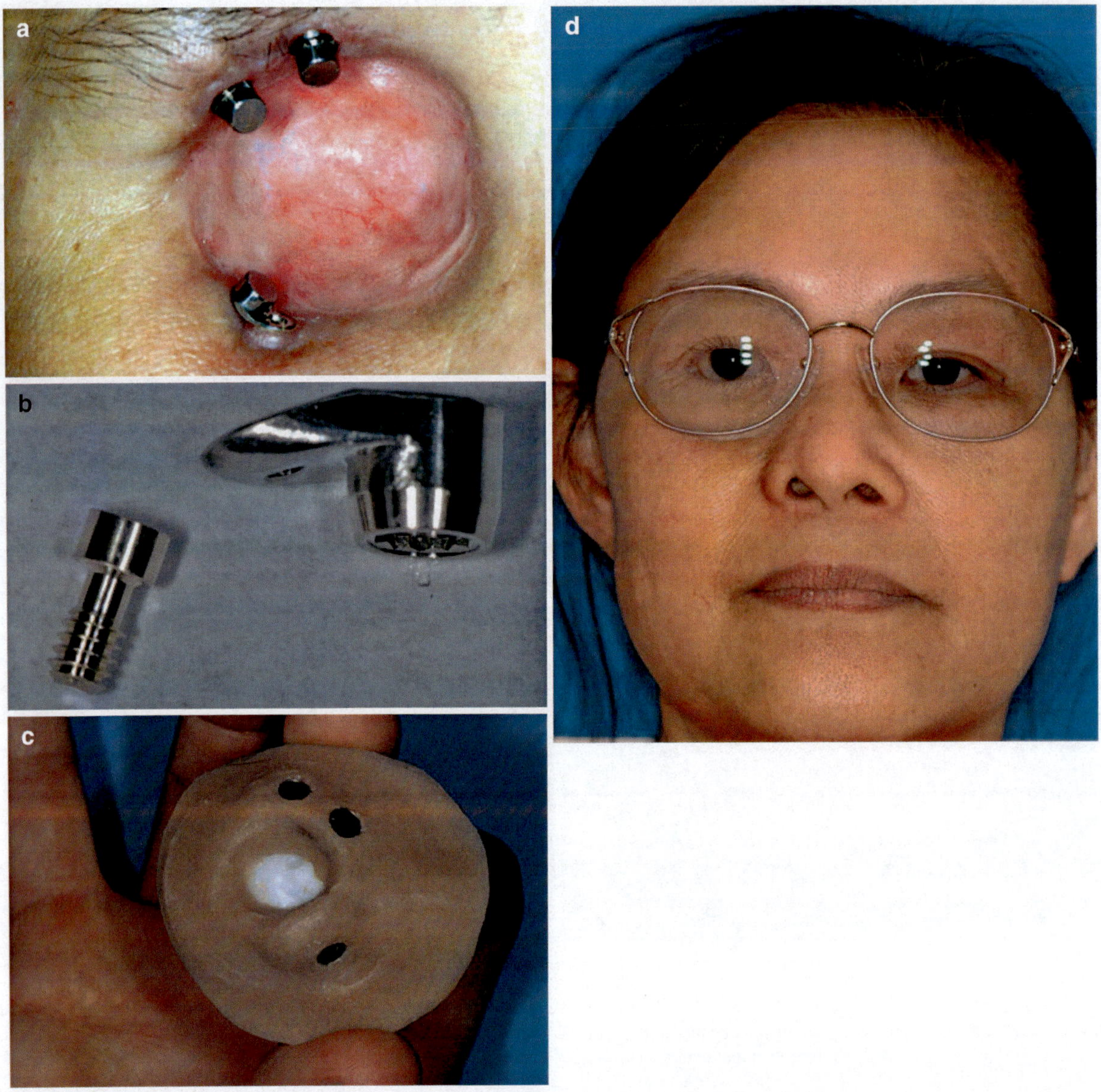

Fig. 36.15 Right orbital exenteration status post radiation treatment, pre- and post-craniofacial implant placement with adjunctive hyperbaric oxygen treatment. (**a**) Orbital craniofacial implants with console abutments in place on the implants. (**b**) Upper left, example of console abutment (Cochlear, Centennial, CO). (**c**) Tissue surface of the silicone orbital magnet retained prosthesis. (**d**) Full face view of the right silicone orbital prosthesis in place

with implant supported prostheses in that the overriding concern about recurrence and need for further management can create significant challenges for patient management, yet alone allow one to focus on their rehabilitation needs [22, 23].

Summary: Conclusion

- The best prosthetic results occur when the Surgeon Patient and Maxillofacial Prosthodontist meet prior to surgery.

36.12 Conclusion

Providing life like appearing craniofacial prostheses for head and neck cancer patients requires a team approach between the Surgeon, the Patient, and the Maxillofacial Prosthodontist. The patient should be referred to the Prosthodontist prior to surgery so that preop impressions can be made. The patient can be shown examples of similar prostheses available. The Surgeon and the Prosthodontist should meet prior to surgery to discuss creating a surgical base that can appropriately support the prosthesis.

Acknowledgements Appreciation and acknowledgement of the following individual whose efforts are associated with the fabrication of the prostheses in Figs. 36.1–36.9.

Robert Mann CDT CCA

University of Florida College of Dentistry, Maxillofacial Prosthetics.

Appreciation and acknowledgement of following individuals whose efforts are associated with the fabrication of the prostheses in Figs. 36.10–36.15. They are as follows:

Ruth Bourke CDT

Bud Perry CDT

William Desantis CDT

Calvin Cowan CDT

Sharron Haggerty MAMS CCA

University of Washington School of Dentistry, Maxillofacial Prosthetic Service

References

1. Milion R, Cassisi N. Management of head and neck cancer. In: Turner G, editor. Maxillofacial prosthetics. 2nd ed. Philadelphia: J B Lippincott; 1994. p. 169–83.
2. Taylor TD. Facial prosthesis fabrication. In: Andres C, Haug S, editors. Clinical maxillofacial prosthetics. Carol Stream: Quintessence; 2000. p. 223–36.
3. McKinstry RE. Fundamentals of facial prosthetics. In: Vergo T, editor. Nasal prostheses. Arlington: ABI Professional Publications; 1995. p. 137–8.
4. Beumer J et al. Restorations of facial deflects: maxillofacial rehabilitation. Tokyo: Ishaiyaku Euro-American, INC; 1996. p. 227–78, 399–433.
5. Barron J, Rubenstein J, Archibald D, et al. Two piece orbital prosthesis. J Prosthet Dent. 1983;49:386–8.
6. Reece G, Lemon J, Jacob R, et al. Total midface reconstruction after radical tumor resection. A case report and overview of the problem. Ann Plast Surg. 1996;36(5a):551–7.
7. Jani R, Schaaf N. An evaluation of facial prostheses. J Prosthet Dent. 1978;39:546–50.
8. Chen M-S, Udagama A, Drane J. Evaluation of facial prostheses for head and neck cancer patients. J Prosthet Dent. 1980;46:538–44.
9. Tjellström A, Yontchev E, Lindstöm J, Brånemark PI. Five years' experience with bone-anchored auricular prostheses. Otolaryngol Head Neck Surg. 1985;93(3):366–72.
10. Jacobsson M, Tjellström A, Fine L, Andersson H. A retrospective study of osseointegrated skin-penetrating titanium fixtures used for retaining facial prostheses. Int J Oral Maxillofac Implants. 1992;7(4):523–8.
11. Gitto CA, Plata WG, Schaaf NG. Evaluation of the peri-implant epithelial tissue of percutaneous implant abutments supporting maxillofacial prostheses. Int J Oral Maxillofac Implants. 1994;9(2):197–206.
12. Parel SM, Tjellström A. The United States and Swedish experience with osseointegration and facial prosthesis. Int J Oral Maxillofac Implants. 1991;6(1):75–9.
13. Wolfaardt JF, Wilkes GH, Parel SM, Tjellström A. Craniofacial osseointegration: the Canadian experience. Int J Oral Maxillofac Implants. 1993;8(2):197–204.
14. Granström G. Osseointegration in irradiated cancer patients: an analysis with respect to implant failures. J Oral Maxillofac Surg. 2005;63(5):579–85.
15. Tolman DE, Taylor PF. Bone-anchored craniofacial prosthesis study. Int J Oral Maxillofac Implants. 1996;11(2): 159–68.
16. Nishimura RD, Roumanas E, Moy PK, Sugai T. Nasal defects and osseointegrated implants: UCLA experience. J Prosthet Dent. 1996;76(6):597–602.
17. Lundgren S, Moy PK, Beumer 3rd J, Lewis S. Surgical consideration for endosseous implants in the craniofacial region: a 3-year report. Int J Oral Maxillofac Surg. 1993;22(5): 227–77.
18. Kubon TM, Anderson JD. An implant-retained auricular impression technique to minimize soft tissue distortion. J Prosthet Dent. 2003;89(1):97–101.
19. Toljanic JA, Eckert SE, Roumanas E, et al. Osseointegrated craniofacial implants in the rehabilitation of orbital defects: an update of a retrospective experience in the United States. J Prosthet Dent. 2005;94(2):177–82.
20. Nishimura RD, Roumanas E, Moy PK, Sugai T, Freymiller EG. Osseointegrated implants and orbital defects: U.C.L.A. experience. J Prosthet Dent. 1998;79(3):304–9.
21. Kosmidou L, Toljanic JA, Moran WJ, Panje WR. The use of percutaneous implants for the prosthetic rehabilitation of orbital defects in irradiated cancer patients: a report of clinical outcomes and complications. Int J Oral Maxillofac Implants. 1998;13(1):121–6.
22. Tolman DE, Desjardins RP, Jackson IT, Brånemark PI. Complex craniofacial reconstruction using an implant-supported prosthesis: case report with long-term follow-up. Int J Oral Maxillofac Implants. 1997;12(2):243–5.
23. Connor JN, Henry PJ, Wall CD. Osseointegration tissue prosthesis in the rehabilitation of maxillofacial defects. Aust Prosthodont Soc Bull. 1985;15:55–61.

Combination Therapy for the Nonsurgical Treatment of Skin Cancers: Latest Research at Mount Sinai

37

Ellen S. Marmur and Hooman Khorasani

Abstract

Nonmelanoma skin cancers have reached epidemic proportions. Not only is the incidence rising in younger patients and patients with darker skin types, there is also an increase of more aggressive forms of skin cancers. These advanced basal cell and squamous cell carcinomas are being treated by Mohs surgery. However, some cases are so advanced that they are not amenable to surgery and must be treated medically or with surgery plus adjuvant therapies. This chapter covers new treatments for aggressive nonmelanoma carcinomas, as well as new approaches for treating early skin cancers, field cancerization, and preventing recurrences after Mohs surgery.

Keywords

Imiquimod therapy • Radiation therapy • Sonic hedgehog pathway inhibitor • Photodynamic therapy • Adjuvant therapy with micrographic surgery

Summary: Adjuvant Treatment with Imiquimod

- Current evidence does not support neoadjuvant therapy with imiquimod before Mohs micrographic surgery. Micrographic surgery requires a tumor that is growing in continuous pattern; destructive neoadjuvant treatments may yield false-negative results with independent tumor islands remaining undetected.

E.S. Marmur (✉)
Division of Dermatologic & Cosmetic Surgery,
Department of Dermatology, The Mount Sinai Medical Center,
New York, NY, USA
e-mail: ellen.marmur@mssm.edu

H. Khorasani
Department of Dermatology, The Mount Sinai Medical Center,
New York, NY, USA

K. Nouri (ed.), *Mohs Micrographic Surgery*,
DOI 10.1007/978-1-4471-2152-7_37,

37.1 Adjuvant Treatment with Imiquimod

Neoadjuvant therapy prior to surgery has been utilized for a variety of cancers. This method reduces the tumor burden and hence facilitates excision of many cancers, in particular, colon, prostate, and breast [1–3]. The usefulness of neoadjuvant treatment of NMSC before Mohs micrographic surgery is controversial. Imiquimod has been utilized by some surgeons as a neoadjuvant therapy in order to reduce the size of the tumor and, thus, the number of stages necessary to clear the tumor margins with Mohs micrographic surgery [4].

Imiquimod, a synthetic imidazoquinoline, has become increasingly popular, and is FDA approved, for the treatment of nonfacial superficial BCC. More recently, it is being used off-label for the treatment of SCC in situ. Imiquimod acts as an immune response modifier targeting toll-like receptors 7 and 8. Studies indicate that imiquimod exerts its antitumor activity by inducing cytokines involved in the cell-mediated immune response such as interleukin (IL)-1, -6, -8, -10, and -12; interferon-alpha; and tumor necrosis factor gamma [5].

Butler and colleagues investigated the role of imiquimod 5% cream as adjunctive therapy for primary, solitary, nodular BCC before Mohs micrographic surgery. The objective of this double-blinded, vehicle-controlled study was to observe the effectiveness of imiquimod 5% cream in reducing the number of Mohs stages, defect size, cost of Mohs micrographic surgery, and reconstruction. Subjects applied the study medication for 6 weeks with occlusion followed by 4 weeks rest period before Mohs micrographic surgery was performed. At the end of this study, the authors did not observe any difference in the number of Mohs stages, defect size, or cost between the two groups. Only 42% of the patients in the treatment group were found histologically clear of tumor [6]. This is significantly less than the 82% imiquimod-induced histologic clearance of nonfacial superficial BCCs found previously [7].

This study's findings are similar to that of Eigentler and colleagues in patients with nodular BCC treated using imiquimod 5% cream for 8 weeks. In 36% of these patients treated with imiquimod 5% cream, Mohs micrographic surgery 8 weeks after the completion of treatment revealed persistent BCC. Interestingly, in almost 20% of the patients with clinical clearance, there was still histopathologic evidence of the tumor [8]. Thus, clinical clearance may not be indicative of a true, tumor-free field.

Current evidence does not support neoadjuvant therapy with imiquimod before Mohs micrographic surgery. In fact, some authors have suggested that any neoadjuvant treatment has a risk of creating skip lesions and interferes with the key principles of micrographic surgery [9]. Since the basic principle of micrographic surgery is excision of a tumor that is growing in continuous pattern, destructive neoadjuvant treatments may yield false-negative results with independent tumor islands remaining undetected.

However, there are authors that have described using adjuvant imiquimod therapy post-Mohs micrographic surgery [10]. Occasionally solid or aggressive types of BCC can also have histological superficial type of BCC at the border. Chasing these superficial tumors may cause large defects requiring reconstructions that may cause significant morbidity to the patient. In this situation, Mohs micrographic surgery is used to clear the solid or aggressive tumor, and imiquimod used as an adjuvant therapy for the remaining superficial tumor parts.

Summary: Adjuvant Treatment with Radiation

- Outcome data for high-risk SCC treated with adjuvant radiotherapy are sparse and inconclusive, even for perineural SCC. Radiotherapy may benefit some patients with high-risk SCC, particularly those with uncertain or positive surgical margins or with more advanced nerve involvement in particular cases involving the named nerves and nerves with a diameter of 0.1 mm or greater, or with clinical or radiologic evidence of nerve invasion.

37.2 Adjuvant Treatment with Radiation

Adjuvant radiotherapy (ART) has been recommended in certain patients with high-risk nonmelanoma skin cancers, particularly those with perineural invasion (PNI) [11–13]. ART is also occasionally considered in patients with SCC with multiple risk factors for recurrence and metastasis. These high-risk factors include size (>2 cm), depth of invasion (>4 mm), recurrent lesions, and in the setting of immunosuppression. Furthermore, SCCs near the parotid gland with lymphatic drainage to the periparotid lymph nodes such the ear, scalp, forehead, and lower lip are considered to be in high-risk locations [14].

The total dose and treatment regimen depends on many tumor factors including, size type, depth, and location. Radiation is usually administered over 20–30 sessions, so-called fractionations of total dosages, with cumulative doses ranging from 50 to 55 Gy. Therefore, RT is expensive and requires a significant time commitment from the patient. Radiation is not recommended in younger patients (under age of 50, because of the increased risk of radiodermatitis and scaring) or in patients with a previous history of radiation therapy [15]. Radiation is also contraindicated in patients with connective tissue diseases or genetic conditions predisposing to skin cancer (e.g., patients with Gorlin's syndrome or xeroderma pigmentosum).

Rakkit and colleagues surveyed 795 registered American College of Mohs surgery members in order to identify variable management practices of SCC of the skin that exhibit PNI. Among the 127 respondents, 122 (96.1%) use adjuvant radiation therapy in management of SCC with PNI, with most administering it between 75% and 100% of the time if such a tumor is encountered.

Although widely used, the utility of adjuvant radiation therapy in high-risk cases is still not established by evidence-based medicine. Additionally, ART has not been shown to lengthen survival or decrease morbidity. Therefore, the use of ART for high-risk SCC varies widely among clinicians, and the utility of adjuvant therapy in such cases is unknown.

Jambusaria and colleagues conducted a systematic review of the literature, reviewing 2,449 cases of high-risk SCC in which 91 were treated with ART and concluded that outcome data for high-risk SCC treated with ART are sparse and inconclusive, even for perineural SCC. The authors concluded that ART may benefit some patients with high-risk SCC, particularly those with uncertain or positive surgical margins or with more advanced nerve involvement in particular cases involving the named nerves and nerves with a diameter of 0.1 mm or greater, or with clinical or radiologic evidence of nerve invasion [16].

This study indicated that current data are insufficient to identify high-risk features or combinations of features associated with poor surgical outcomes in which ART may be beneficial.

A randomized double-blinded study is necessary to determine the extent of which ART reduces the risk of recurrence and metastasis in high-risk SCC. However, given the relatively low rate of recurrence of tumors with clear margins after Mohs, it may be difficult to design a study large enough to show a significant difference. It has been estimated that a study of 438 patients would be needed to detect a 10% decrease in risk of local recurrence with surgery and RT, assuming a 20% baseline risk with surgical monotherapy. Thus, further studies are needed to define the subset of patients who would benefit from ART [16].

At our institution selected patients are presented at the interdepartmental tumor board, and if deemed necessary, the patient is referred to the radiation oncologist for a consultation. Any patient with perineural, intraneural, dense perivascular, or intravascular tumor – regardless of the size of the nerve branch or vessel – is sent for an evaluation by radiation oncology but not necessarily to receive treatment. All tissue from these cases is thawed and sent for special immunostains to our senior dermatopathologists and presented at pathology conferences. Due to the lack of well-powered studies showing that there is no utility to adjuvant radiation therapy in such cases, we have a conservative approach and address each case from a collaborative view. Generally, a lowered threshold for adjuvant radiation is used in organ transplant patients with high-risk SCC.

Summary: Nonsurgical Treatment of Aggressive Basal Cell Carcinoma

- GDC-0449, a new promising chemotherapeutic oral agent that targets the hedgehog pathway, appears to have antitumor activity in locally advanced or metastatic basal cell carcinoma. The most common side effects include muscle cramping, hair loss, and dysgeusia.

37.3 Nonsurgical Treatment of Aggressive Basal Cell Carcinoma

A new and exciting chemotherapy that targets the Hedgehog signaling pathway (Hh) is being used for the treatment of basal cell carcinoma. The Hh pathway

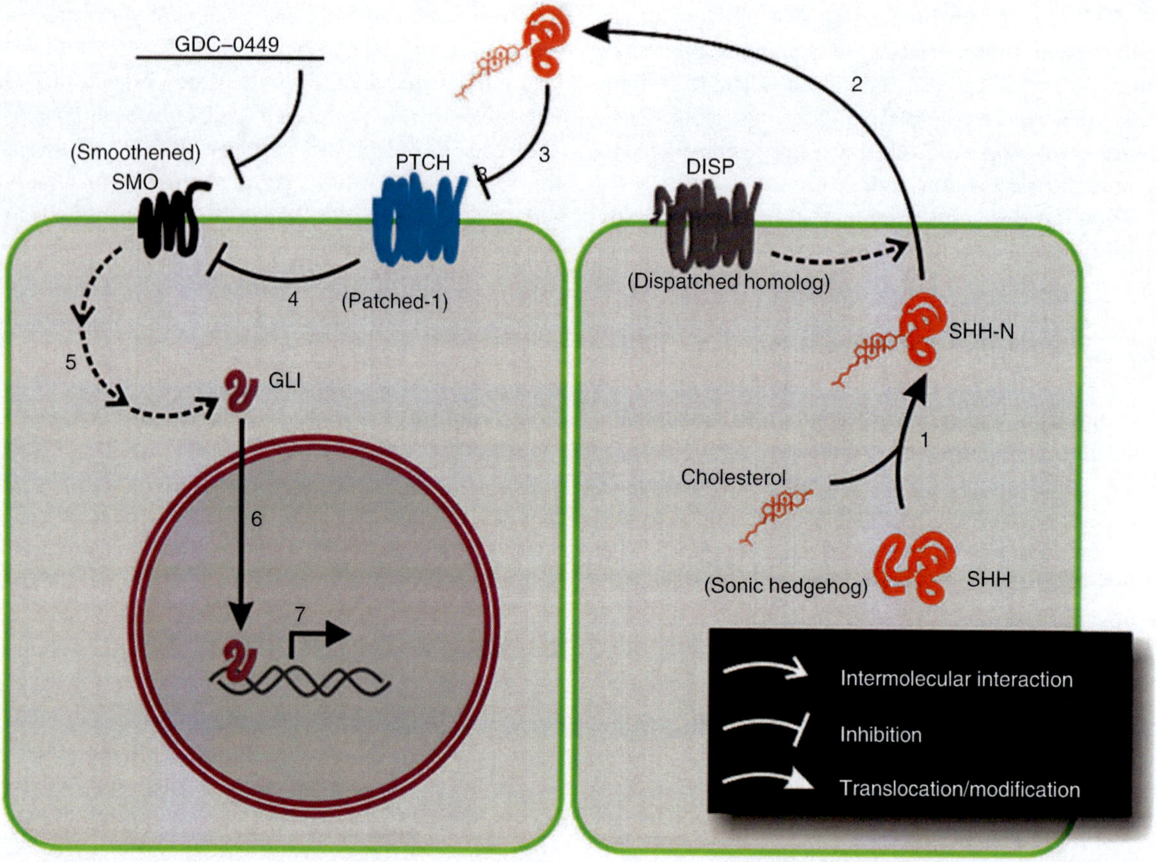

Fig. 37.1 Mechanism of action of GDC-0449. Hedgehog binding to PTCH1 relieves inhibition of SMO activation by PTCH1. In the absence of PTCH1, because of loss-of-PTCH1 mutations, SMO signaling occurs constitutively. GDC-0449 inhibits SMO signaling through direct interaction with SMO

activation has been implicated in several types of cancer such as Gorlin's syndrome or basal cell nevus syndrome and medulloblastomas, as well as rhabdomyosarcoma.

The active ingredient in cyclopamine was discovered in 1957 when a herd of female sheep in Idaho who had been grazing on wild corn lily gave birth to multiple one-eyed lambs with malformed brains. Medical experts at the US Department of Agriculture discovered that toxins in the corn lily are powerful teratogens that alter fetal development and named the toxin cyclopamine after the one-eyed sheep. Today, cyclopamine is the key ingredient in new cancer drugs, specifically because of its activity on Hedgehog signaling pathway.

This new medication, GDC-0449 drug, is a small molecule antagonist of the Hedgehog signaling pathway (Fig. 37.1). The molecular weight of GDC-0449 is 421.3 g per mole which binds to and inhibits SMOOTHENED, resulting in the blockage of the Hedgehog signaling pathway. GDC-0449 is effective in in vitro tumor models of mutated and ligand expressing tumors. A phase I study using the drug at various dosages was first published in the *New England Journal of Medicine* in September 2009. The authors of this chapter are investigators in the phase II study using GDC-0449 at 150 mg PO once daily on a continuous schedule for nonsurgical basal cell carcinoma, and more studies are planned as first line therapy for metastatic colorectal cancer, recurrent ovarian cancer, and both local and metastatic advanced basal cell carcinoma. The GDC-0449 patients in these studies have advanced solid malignancies that are refractory to standard therapy or for whom no standard therapy exists (Fig. 37.2). In summary, normal Hedgehog signaling pathway inhibits downstream cellular activity. In these solid tumors,

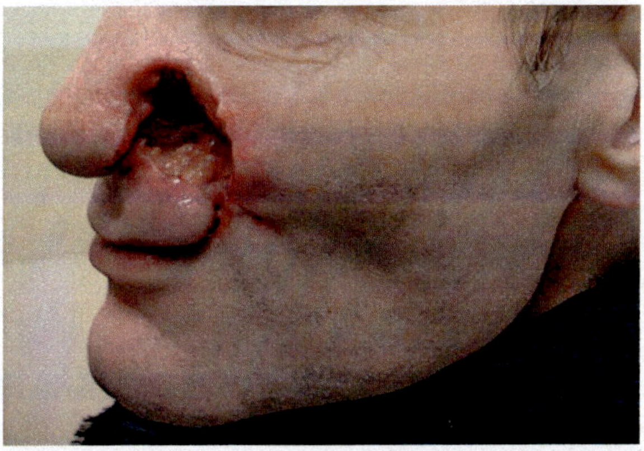

Fig. 37.2 Extensive basal cell carcinoma. This patient exemplifies an ideal candidate for treatment with GDC-0440

there is a ligand or genetic mutation of the Hedgehog signaling pathway, allowing cellular activity to be on, and therefore tumorigenesis. The drug effectively blocks the SMO portion of the pathway and thus blocks the downstream cellular activity thereby halting tumor genesis.

Dr. Daniel D. Von Hoff et al. published the original article entitled "*Inhibition of the Hedgehog Pathway in Advanced Basal-Cell Carcinoma*" [17]. This was a dosing and pharmacokinetic study of the drug GDC-0449 for metastatic or locally advanced basal cell carcinoma. Thirty-three patients with metastatic or locally advanced basal cell carcinoma were enrolled in the study and divided into three groups at three dosages. One group ($n = 17$) received 150 mg per day. The second group ($n = 15$) received 270 mg per day, and the third group ($n = 1$) received 540 mg per day. The tumor responses were assessed using the standard response, evaluation, criteria, and solid tumor (RECIST) and physical examination. The results showed that of the 33 patients, 18 had a significant response to the medication during the study period. The median duration of the study treatment was 9.8 months. In the study, imaging assessments showed improvement in 7 patients. Physical examination showed improvement in 10 patients. Both imaging and physical exam showed improvement in 1 patient. Of the 18 responders, 2 patients had complete response and 16 had partial response. Of the 15 patients who were nonresponders, 11 patients had stable disease but 4 patients progressed. In summary, 18 patients responded favorably, 11 stabilized, and 4 were treatment failures. Adverse events noted in this phase I study included fatigue, muscle spasm, atrial fibrillation, and hyponatremia. This study concluded that GDC-0449 appeared to have promising antitumor activity in basal cell carcinoma.

The phase II study, which is ongoing currently, is a pivotal, multicenter, single-arm, global trial evaluating the efficacy and safety of GDC-0449 in patients with advanced basal cell carcinoma.

We have 4 patients enrolled in this phase II study, 2 have progressive advanced local disease and 2 have metastatic disease. So far, we have observed both clinical and radiological clearance in some of the patients. However, each patient has experienced the side effects of muscle cramping, hair loss, and dysgeusia, which is loss of taste. The phase II study is a preliminary, unpublished, ongoing global study with full enrollment of 100 patients. Data for all patients will be coming out soon. As the incidence of basal cell carcinoma increases and aggressive and metastatic cases become more common, having a nonsurgical successful treatment will be very helpful.

Summary: PEP005 Topical Gel (3-Angel Oyl Ingenol) (Ingenol-3-Angelate)

- PEP005 is the latest of topical medications that cause local irritation and some type of immunostimulation that has been successful in treating actinic keratoses and superficial nonmelanoma skin cancers.

37.4 PEP005 Topical Gel (3-Angel Oyl Ingenol) (Ingenol-3-Angelate)

PEP005 is being developed for the topical treatment of actinic keratoses and nonmelanoma skin cancers and various medicinal uses [18]. It is an active compound in the sap from *Euphorbia peplus*, a noninvasive medicinal plant that has a long history of community use for the topical treatment of skin cancers. Its mechanism of action has been linked to macrocyclic diterpene of three different families of similar weeds. The mechanism of action is thought to be direct toxicity plus immunostimulation. In vitro and animal models have shown that PEP005 inhibits tumor cell line survival and has produced consistent drug induced inhibition of cell growth in human melanoma, prostate, and breast cancer cell lines. This growth inhibitory effect occurred with treatment times as short as 1-h application. Animal model dose regimen studies showed that the most effective topical dose was 10 μg applied overnight for 8 h, repeated daily for three consecutive days. PEP005 has limited skin penetration into systemic circulation after topical application and results in dermal irritation. No systemic toxicity has been observed in single or repeated doses in nonclinical studies of topical PEP005. PEP005 is an activator of protein kinase C, and other members of this pharmacological class have been found to have tumor promoting potential. However, no definitive studies have been conducted to evaluate the carcinogenic potential of PEP005. Because PEP005 may be severely irritating to the eye, precautions such as wearing gloves during application of the product and discarding those gloves immediately afterwards or using a clean Q-tip for application of the medication are important during patient instruction of this medication. Accidental ocular exposure could cause severe irritation to anything with which it comes into contact.

In three previous clinical trials, the safety and efficacy of PEP005 were impressive. In the early phase I/II trials, the final outcome of the treatment showed a complete clinical response rate of 66% for actinic keratoses, 57% for basal cell carcinomas (BCC), 50% for squamous cell carcinomas (SCC), and 81% for SCC in situ. In phase I trials, the most frequently observed adverse side effects were mild, local erythema (73%); scaling (27%); and scabbing (27%). In phase II trials, 71% of all lesions in the 0.05% PEP005 group were completely cleared compared to only 32% of lesions in the vehicle-controlled group.

On day 1 of the 3-day topical regimen, mild erythema was noted in all lesions and some of the surrounding skin. On day 4, after the three-dose regimen was completed, moderate erythema was noted of the entire area plus slight scabbing of each target lesion. On day 8, 5 days after the regimen was completed, the erythema persisted and adjacent areas begin to react. This may demonstrate local immunostimulation. On day 15, 12 days after the completion of the 3-day dose regimen, the erythema of the target area was subsiding, and the edges and area on the forehead showed persistent erythema. On day 29, the entire area was healed, and the target lesions were invisible. Six months posttreatment, the target area remained clear, and the adjacent areas also appeared to be cleared.

A robust response to the study drug was seen in one patient. This may indicate that there may be a cohort of patients who have extremely strong reactions to the medication. This patient developed mild erythema on day 1. On day 4, the patient had extreme erythema with ulceration and crusting. On day 8, the erythema and crusting persisted but were beginning to resolve. On day 15, the erythema was mild and the crusting was completely resolved. On day 29, the patient was healed with residual hyperpigmentation. Six months posttreatment, the area was completely clear, and the patient was very happy with the cosmetic result. PEP005 is the latest of topical medications that cause local irritation and some type of immunostimulation that has been successful in treating actinic keratoses and superficial nonmelanoma skin cancers.

Summary: Photodynamic Therapy

- Photodynamic therapy (PDT) consists of a chemical reaction activated by light energy that is used to selectively destroy tissue. PDT has proven to be effective for the treatment of actinic keratosis, basal cell carcinoma, and Bowen's disease. Intraoperative PDT after micrographic surgery is a new combination modality for patients with severe photo damage in order to prevent a neighboring secondary tumor.

37.5 Photodynamic Therapy

In our practice, we utilize photodynamic therapy (PDT) as a preventative and therapeutic measure for actinic keratoses [19]. We recommend a technique called enhanced-cyclic PDT three times a year for patients who have multiple actinic keratoses as the technique has been shown to reduce the tumor burden of patients in our clinic. Our treatment regimen is as follows:

Step I – microdermabrasion utilizing a mechanical, crystal-free microdermabrasion of the treatment area including the target lesions, for example, the entire face or arms or chest.

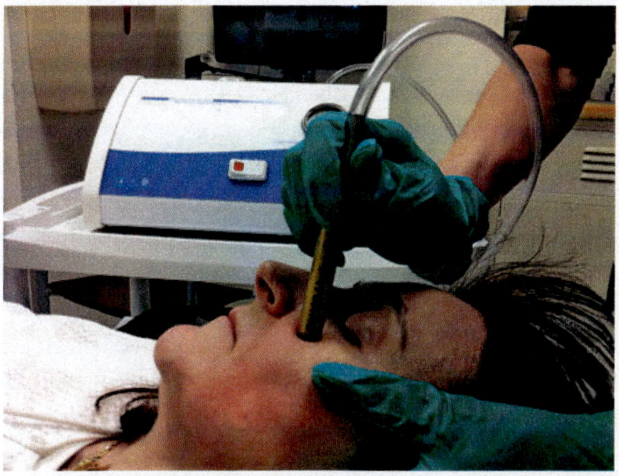

Fig. 37.3 Pre-PDT microdermabrasion. This technique uses two passes of a medium coarse wand, one horizontal pass, and one vertical pass using a diamond-studded hand piece with medium grit (100 μm particle)

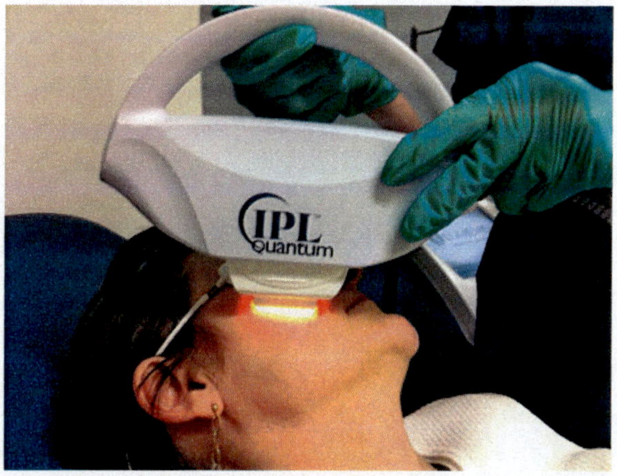

Fig. 37.4 ALA activation with IPL. Two passes of IPL using a 560 nm filter at 20 J/cm^2. Program one, 21 = 2.4 ms, 22 = 4.0 ms, with a 20 ms interpulse delay

Step II – is a 3-h incubation time of aminolevulinic acid (ALA). The ALA is applied in the provided stick to the entire area. Larger areas require multiple ALA Levulan® sticks to be utilized. The treatment time begins after the last medication has been applied. After 3 h, the ALA is washed off only if a lesser effect is desired. If the patient agrees to a stronger treatment, the ALA remains on the skin during treatment and is washed off after treatment. The standard illumination time of 16 min and 40 s is used with the BLU-U per treatment area. For example, if the scalp is treated for 16 min and 40 s and the next treatment area is the face, the ears and scalp are covered during the second illumination time so as not to expose the patient to a double treatment. In this way the arms, neck, back, legs, and any desired area can be treated. This procedure is repeated three times a year for 1–2 years until the patient and doctor agree the tumor burden has been decreased.

Variations on our enhanced-cyclic PDT regimen for those patients who have a robust reaction to the 3-h incubation time include 1-h incubation time, no microdermabrasion in advance, or microdermabrasion with 1-h incubation time illuminated with two passes of the intense pulsed light (IPL), and additionally BlU-U illumination of 16 min and 40 s. Figure 37.3 shows the microdermabrasion technique which uses two passes of a medium coarse wand, one horizontal pass, and one vertical pass using a diamond-studded hand piece with medium grit (100 μm particle). Figure 37.4 shows the IPL technique – two passes of IPL using a 560 nm filter at 20 J/cm^2. Program one, 21 = 2.4 ms, 22 = 4.0 ms, with a 20 ms interpulse delay.

Intraoperative PDT is a new combination modality for the treatment of SCC and BCC. Mohs surgery followed by PDT, either topical or injectable ALA, has been used in my practice in regions that have lesions, in areas of severe photodamage where I suspect a new secondary lesion will occur within a short amount of time. This combination modality may lower the recurrence rate of the surgically treated SCC and BCC, may treat early SCC and BCC that are not clinically evident in the area, may reduce the incidence of new SCC or BCC developing from actinic keratoses, may improve the healing process; may improve photodamaged skin, and ultimately, may be more convenient to patients by reducing the need for follow-up.

Summary: Off-Label Intraoperative PDT with Topical and Intralesional Aminolevulinic Acid on SCC of the Penis

- Micrographic surgery in combination with intraoperative PDT for nonmelanoma skin cancers of the penis has reduced the rate of penectomy at our institution.

37.6 Off-Label Intraoperative PDT with Topical and Intralesional Aminolevulinic Acid on SCC of the Penis

Squamous cell carcinoma in situ and stage T1 SCC of the glans penis have been indications for penectomy in the past. In our clinic, we collaborate with the Department of Urology to utilize Mohs surgery and intraoperative PDT plus cyclic PDT to treat patients with this disease in order to prevent penectomy. To date, this alternative has been extremely successful in a series of eight patients since 2005. Patients have ill-defined, macerated erythematous erosions on the glans and shaft of the penis. Surveillance biopsies are done of the outside margins for preoperative planning purposes. On the day of Mohs surgery, the most invasive lesions are removed using a bendable blade which allows for superficial planning of the skin. Our slides are reviewed by a dermatopathologist to evaluate for high-grade tumors and invasion into the dermal vasculature. The area is numbed with buffered 2% lidocaine with epinephrine 1:200,000 for surgery. Intralesional injection of ALA can be painful if the area is not anesthetized as the ALA does burn. Topical application of the ALA is done by using the Levulan Kerastick.

Topical PDT technique for penile SCC: The lesion itself plus the area surrounding the affected area is treated generously with ALA using the entire contents of the Kerastick. Overnight incubation is suggested for these cases. The patient returns to clinic in the morning and undergoes 16 min 40 s illumination with the BlU-U. The patient is instructed to rotate the area while under illumination in order to ensure thorough treatment of the area. Patients repeat overnight incubation PDT every 3 months and are instructed to use topical imiquimod three times a week for 16 weeks to any new or suspicious lesions. Side effects have included erythema and irritation for up to 1 week in the area. No infections have been seen and scarring from the Mohs surgery has been mild. No functional side effects have been reported including no strictures of the urethra and no phimosis has been reported.

Summary: Conclusion

- There are many adjunctive therapies available with Mohs micrographic surgery, including: immunomodulators, radiation, chemotherapeutic agents, and photodynamic therapy.

37.7 Conclusion

In conclusion, there are multiple options for adjunctive therapy with Mohs micrographic surgery. Current evidence does not support neoadjuvant therapy with imiquimod before Mohs micrographic surgery. Outcome data for high-risk SCC treated with adjuvant radiotherapy are sparse and inconclusive. Radiotherapy may benefit some patients with high-risk SCC, particularly those with uncertain or positive surgical margins or with more advanced nerve involvement. Aggressive BCC may have a chemotherapeutic option in the future. In addition, topical gel PEP005 for actinic keratoses has the benefit of a 3 day only treatment ensuring good compliance in addition to good success rates.

Finally, cyclic PDT and intraoperative PDT for nonmelanoma skin cancers and actinic keratoses may prevent tumor incidence in areas of field cancerization and may prove to be preventive medicine. Lastly, PDT with Mohs mircrographic surgery for superficially invasive penile carcinoma may prove to be an alternative to penectomy in selected patients.

References

1. Miller K, Lein M, Schostak M, Schrader M. Adjuvant and neoadjuvant drug therapy for prostate cancer. Urologe A. 2008;47(11):1460–4.
2. Kahan Z, Nikolenyi A, Uhercsak G, Thurzo L. Neoadjuvant systemic therapy in breast cancer. Orv Hetil. 2009;150(2): 65–71.
3. Yamashita F, Tanaka M, Yutani S, et al. Neoadjuvant chemotherapy of liver tumors metastasized by sigmoid colon cancer: a case report of CDDP/5-FU intraarterial infusion therapy followed by hepatectomy. Gan To Kagaku Ryoho. 1995;22(7):949–52.
4. Torres A, Niemeyer A, Berkes B, et al. 5% imiquimod cream and reflectance-mode confocal microscopy as adjunct modalities to Mohs micrographic surgery for treatment of basal cell carcinoma. Dermatol Surg. 2004;30(12 Pt 1): 1462–9.
5. Gupta AK, Browne M, Bluhm R. Imiquimod: a review. J Cutan Med Surg. 2002;6(6):554–60.
6. Butler DF, Parekh PK, Lenis A. Imiquimod 5% cream as adjunctive therapy for primary, solitary, nodular nasal basal cell carcinomas before Mohs micrographic surgery: a randomized, double-blind, vehicle-controlled study. Dermatol Surg. 2009;35(1):24–9.
7. Geisse J, Caro I, Lindholm J, Golitz L, Stampone P, Owens M. Imiquimod 5% cream for the treatment of superficial basal cell carcinoma: results from two phase III, randomized, vehicle-controlled studies. J Am Acad Dermatol. 2004;50(5): 722–33.

8. Eigentler TK, Kamin A, Weide BM, et al. A phase III, randomized, open label study to evaluate the safety and efficacy of imiquimod 5% cream applied thrice weekly for 8 and 12 weeks in the treatment of low-risk nodular basal cell carcinoma. J Am Acad Dermatol. 2007;57(4):616–21.
9. Moehrle M, Breuninger H, Schippert W, Hafner HM. Letter: imiquimod 5% cream as adjunctive therapy for primary, solitary, nodular basal cell carcinomas before Mohs micrographic surgery: a randomized, double-blind, vehicle-controlled study. Dermatol Surg. 2010;36(3):428–30.
10. Thissen MR, Kuijpers DI, Krekels GA. Local immune modulator (imiquimod 5% cream) as adjuvant treatment after incomplete Mohs micrographic surgery for large, mixed type basal cell carcinoma: a report of 3 cases. J Drugs Dermatol. 2006;5(5):461–4.
11. Miller SJ. The National Comprehensive Cancer Network (NCCN) guidelines of care for nonmelanoma skin cancers. Dermatol Surg. 2000;26(3):289–92.
12. Motley R, Kersey P, Lawrence C. Multiprofessional guidelines for the management of the patient with primary cutaneous squamous cell carcinoma. Br J Dermatol. 2002;146(1): 18–25.
13. Veness MJ. Treatment recommendations in patients diagnosed with high-risk cutaneous squamous cell carcinoma. Australas Radiol. 2005;49(5):365–76.
14. Veness MJ. High-risk cutaneous squamous cell carcinoma of the head and neck. J Biomed Biotechnol. 2007;3:80572.
15. Veness MJ, Palme CE, Morgan GJ. High-risk cutaneous squamous cell carcinoma of the head and neck: results from 266 treated patients with metastatic lymph node disease. Cancer. 2006;106(11):2389–96.
16. Jambusaria-Pahlajani A, Miller CJ, Quon H, Smith N, Klein RQ, Schmults CD. Surgical monotherapy versus surgery plus adjuvant radiotherapy in high-risk cutaneous squamous cell carcinoma: a systematic review of outcomes. Dermatol Surg. 2009;35(4):574–85.
17. Von Hoff DD, LoRusso PM, Rudin CM, et al. Inhibition of the hedgehog pathway in advanced basal-cell carcinoma. N Engl J Med. 2009;361(12):1164–72.
18. Siller G, Gebauer K, Welburn P, Katsamas J, Ogbourne SM. PEP005 (ingenol mebutate) gel, a novel agent for the treatment of actinic keratosis: results of a randomized, double-blind, vehicle-controlled, multicentre, phase IIa study. Australas J Dermatol. 2009;50(1):16–22.
19. Kuijpers DI, Smeets NW, Krekels GA, Thissen MR. Photodynamic therapy as adjuvant treatment of extensive basal cell carcinoma treated with Mohs micrographic surgery. Dermatol Surg. 2004;30(5):794–8.

38 Training and Regulation in Mohs Surgery

Suzanne M. Olbricht

Abstract

Initially the training of Mohs surgeons involved shadowing Dr. Frederic E. Mohs in Madison, WI, observing the *in vivo* fixative method and learning to heal the wounds by second intention. In 1967, Dr. Mohs founded the American College of Chemosurgery, now known as the American College of Mohs Surgery (ACMS), which sought to foster education in science and clinical practice. After the fresh frozen tissue method was introduced in the 1970's, the procedure achieved widespread acceptance by patients and physicians alike and the demand required a larger number of physicians to become trained in Dr. Mohs' technique. The ACMS established criteria for formal fellowships in order to promote a high quality of education with academic rigor and the first approved fellowships in the USA began in the early 1980s with international fellowships being approved approximately 10–12 years later. New Mohs surgeons were also trained in reconstructive techniques and developed many aesthetic procedures. By 2007, at least 77 approved fellowships existed worldwide. The ACMS transferred approval and oversight gradually to the ACGME beginning in 2010. By the spring of 2011, 39 programs were approved by the ACMS and 44 by the ACGME. This chapter details the evolution of the training and regulation of Mohs Micrographic Surgery.

Keywords

American College of Mohs Surgery (ACMS) • Site Inspection and Slide Review Board • LLC (SISRB) • Accreditation Council for Graduate Medical Education (ACGME) • Clinical Laboratory Improvement (CLIA) • Joint Commission on Accreditation of Healthcare Organizations (JCAHO) • College of American Pathologists (CAP)

S.M. Olbricht
Department of Dermatology, Lahey Clinic,
Burlington, MA, USA
e-mail: suzanne.m.olbricht@lahey.org

K. Nouri (ed.), *Mohs Micrographic Surgery*,
DOI 10.1007/978-1-4471-2152-7_38,

Dr. Frederic E. Mohs was always generous in welcoming interested dermatologists to his practice in Madison, WI, and teaching his technique [1]. Training was informal and consisted of shadowing Dr. Mohs in his office for a period of 3 days to several weeks. The emphasis of this training was to understand Dr. Mohs' approach to the patient with large or recurrent skin cancer, use of fixative in vivo, method of excision of tissue, technique of orientation and mapping of the specimens, and histologic diagnosis and correlation between the histopathologically involved margins and the tumor remaining in the patient at the edges of the wound. He also taught the concepts of wound care and the advantages of repair by second intention healing; other reconstructive procedures were not generally addressed. Several of the people who spent time with Dr. Mohs, including Dr. Perry Robins of New York and Dr. Philip Bailin of the Cleveland Clinic, taught the technique to their visitors and to residents in dermatology programs. The first international interest in Mohs surgery was initiated by Dr Robins' outreach through the International Society of Dermatologic Surgeons, and several individuals who learned the technique, including Dr. Gunter Burg of Germany and Dr. Antonio Picoto of Portugal, became important in Europe as trainers of a younger generation of Mohs surgeons, following the informal preceptorship model initiated by Dr. Mohs [2]. South American physicians studied in Spain with Dr. Francisco Camacho and Dr. Julian Sanchez Conejo Mir and took the technique back to their home countries.

In 1967, Dr. Mohs founded the American College of Chemosurgery (now called the American College of Mohs Surgery) to bring together those interested in the technique in order to foster mutual education and promote advances in science and practice. In a book published in 1970, Dr. Mohs wrote, "Facilities and personnel for the practice of chemosurgery eventually should be available in every large center of population. Presently, there are over fifty physicians who have been trained to use the method, but many sections of the country are still without this useful addition to our armamentarium against cutaneous cancer" [3]. The interest in performing the procedure at that time however was limited because of the difficulties for both patient and physician in the use of the in vivo chemofixation technique. Fortunately, in the 1970s, the procedure was modified to use fresh frozen tissue instead of in vivo fixed tissue for the histologic analysis of the tumor present in the margins of the wound. This major advance allowed the procedure to become mainstream since it was now practical and easy for both patients and physicians. It soon became apparent that extending the procedure to more patients would require more trained physicians.

In the late 1970s and early 1980s, the American College of Mohs Surgery (ACMS) with great foresight decided to foster the development of the technique and promote the highest quality of education, practice, and patient care by establishing criteria for formal fellowships and maintaining a process for certifying fellowships that met these criteria. The goal was to move the fellowships from the preceptor model to training programs with academic rigor. The Board created the Site Inspection and Slide Review Board LLC (SISRB) and charged it with setting standards, approving, and maintaining oversights for fellowships offered by ACMS members. The first approved fellowships began in the USA in the early 1980s. The first international fellowships were approved in 1996 with Dr. Alistair Carruthers in Canada and Dr. Robert Paver in Australia. Graduates of these programs could in turn become members of the ACMS and establish fellowships if so desired. The annual meeting of the ACMS changed to accept abstracts by fellows for oral or poster presentation, and the Tromovitch award became a highly coveted prize for the first ranked presentation. As programs evolved, more emphasis was placed on reconstruction so that graduating fellows were accomplished in not only the Mohs technique but also sophisticated repair techniques.

By 2007, there were 77 approved fellowships scattered about the United States and in Australia, Canada, Israel, and New Zealand. ACMS developed a core curriculum [4], policies for appropriate training [5], and a computer-based ranking process for approved fellowship positions in order to facilitate application and matching of applicant and program [6]. Table 38.1 defines the requirements of the ACMS for an approved program. Table 38.2 lists the requirements and responsibilities of the program director. SISRB annually reviews surgical logs and academic contributions of programs, directors, and fellows as well as written evaluations of the fellow's proficiency and the fellow's assessment of the educational value of the program. Site inspection and slide review of all programs are performed on a rotating basis as indicated by the approval process. Programs may be approved for 1–5 years.

Table 38.1 ACMS-approved fellowship program requirements

Duration	At least 1 year
Case material	500 cases with approved faculty for 1 year program/50 cases must be complex
	300 cases with approved faculty for each year of a 2-year program
	Hands-on experience (assistant or primary surgeon) required for fellow
Number of trainees allowed per program	Generally one. If more than one: one director/case material requirements/fellow
Support of fellow	Financial and benefit support sufficient that the fellow can spend time training
Association with area hospital	Detailed procedural plan for handling medical emergencies, patient needing hospitalization
Academic rigor	Journal club, evidence of ongoing teaching related to core curriculum, participation in Tumor Boards. Teaching plan must include most of fellow's time in Mohs surgery
Directors and surgical faculty	Director and associate director (Table 38.2). Surgical faculty approved by ACMS
Site inspection	Adequate space for patients, desk space for fellow, laboratory space for specimen processing. Appropriate surgical technique and histologic processes. References by physicians of other specialties. Evidence of compliance with regulations of OSHA and CLIA
Fellow selection	Compliance with rules of the match
Slide review	Slide preparation must be sufficient for accurate histologic diagnosis, and the surgeon must be proficient at reading the slides. Evaluation by both site surveyor and slide review committee

Table 38.2 Requirements and responsibilities of the program director

General	Licensed, ethical
Training	Graduate in good standing of ACMS-approved fellowship (some grandfathered directors)
Posttraining practice	Fellow of ACMS with at least 5 years experience
Academically based	Active contribution to the body of knowledge of Mohs surgery, cutaneous oncology, and related fields through papers, lectures, and attendance at ACMS annual meeting
Proficiency in surgery and pathology	300 cases per year

Because quality assurance is a matter of importance to the public, the Accreditation Council for Graduate Medical Education (ACGME) was established as a private, nonprofit organization responsible for the evaluation and accreditation of postgraduate medical education in the USA, overseeing residency and subspecialty programs. In 1998, the Residency Review Committee (RRC) for Dermatology asked the ACGME to accredit dermatology surgery fellowships. After much discussion, with comments from the public and from other medical and surgical specialties, the ACGME-approved program requirements in procedural dermatology in 2003 [7]. ACGME program requirements [8] are similar to the requirements already defined by the ACMS with some notable differences. The approved programs are approved by site, not director, although the director's qualifications remain intact. The fellow must be at least a PGY5, graduate of an ACGME-accredited dermatology residency program. Institutional oversight as required of other residency programs (e.g., a graduate medical office, grievance procedures, institutional evaluation) must be arranged. The curriculum for these fellowships is widened to include aesthetic procedures as well as those for the management of skin cancer. Of most concern to the ACMS is that the site inspector is an educator, not a Mohs surgeon, and cannot judge if the Mohs surgery is appropriately performed or the slides are of good quality and read accurately. Regardless, in 2007, the ACMS Board and the membership voted to move toward transitioning the approval and oversight of programs to the ACGME. Since July 2009, no new programs have been approved, and no existing programs have been renewed by the ACMS so that by 2014, ACMS will no longer have oversight for any programs in the USA. The ACMS however is committed to facilitating quality patient care and fellow education within programs and maintains the

SISRB program. In addition, the ACMS continues to approve and oversee international programs that are not eligible for ACGME accreditation. In the spring of 2011, there were 39 programs approved by the ACMS, 44 programs approved by the ACGME.

Not all dermatologists who perform Mohs surgery are fellowship trained. The American Society of Mohs Surgery administers a week-long didactic course in Mohs surgery and closures and maintains a preceptorship program of observation in a Mohs surgeon's office for three separate weeks over 2 years. A few dermatology residency programs allow the resident to obtain extensive experience in the Mohs procedure [9]. Some dermatologists work with the Mohs surgeon in their practice to develop expertise. As with any skill, repeated practice, especially practice under supervision, increases expertise. Patient groups tell their constituents to ask their doctor how many times they have performed the procedure. Certainly, for Mohs surgeons, improvement with more experience and a larger number of cases is apparent to the individual learner both in the surgical procedure itself as well as proficiency in reading the histology. A longitudinal study of one fellow's experience at a respected and busy Mohs practice documented that it required experience reading the histopathology of 1491 Mohs surgery cases in order to reduce the error rate to less than 1% [10].

Credentialing a physician to practice Mohs surgery at the current time depends on the site of practice, the insurance company paying for the service, and state regulations. Some institutions will only credential fellowship-trained Mohs surgeons while others will credential anyone of any specialty to do Mohs surgery depending on documentation of what the institution deems is adequate education and experience. The Mohs laboratory is subject to much greater regulation. In the USA, it requires at least a Clinical Laboratory Improvement Amendments (CLIA) certificate which is obtained with biannual site inspection by the state department of health and requires documentation of quality assurance programs and proficiency. Some institutions that are Joint Commission on Accreditation of Healthcare Organizations (JCAHO) approved require College of American Pathologists (CAP) approval for the Mohs laboratory. In many foreign countries, a pathologist must read the slides.

In the current regulatory environment, there is a general movement toward the concept that the public interest is best served by increasing accreditation and oversight of medical facilities and more focused credentialing and recredentialing of providers of care. In this milieu, it is possible that in the future, physicians will be held to a high standard of education and expertise to practice specialized procedures such as Mohs surgery and that they will need to maintain robust quality improvement programs. If Dr. Mohs were alive today, he might be surprised at the amount of regulation surrounding his innovative procedure, but he would doubtlessly be pleased that there is robust interest in teaching and learning the technique and in creating innovative modifications to stretch its indications and efficacy.

References

1. Trost LB, Bailin PL. History of Mohs surgery. Dermatol Clin. 2011;29:135–9.
2. Picoto A, Camacho F, Walker NPJ, Camps-Fresneda A. Mohs micrographic surgery: European experience. In: Roenigk RK, Roenigk HH, editors. Surgical dermatology. St Louis: Mosby Publishers; 1992. p. 125–31.
3. Mohs FE. Chemosurgery for the microscopically controlled excision of cutaneous cancer. In: Epstein E, editor. Skin surgery. Springfield: Charles C Thomas; 1970. p. 309.
4. http://www.mohscollege.org/sisrb/ACMSCoreCurriculum.pdf. Accessed June 7, 2011
5. http://www.mohscollege.org/sisrb/FTPPoliciesProcedures-Guidelines.pdf. Accessed June 7, 2011
6. http://www.sfmatch.org/. Accessed June 7, 2011
7. Nestler SP, Roenigk RK. Accreditation and certification in dermatologic surgery. Semin Cutan Med Surg. 2005;24:133–6.
8. http://www.acgme.org/acWebsite/downloads/RRC_progReq/081_procedural_derm_07012010_1-YR.pdf. Accessed June 7, 2011
9. Lee EH, Nehal KH, Dusza SW, et al. Procedural training during dermatology residency: a survey of third year dermatology residents. J Am Acad Dermatol. 2011;64L:475–83.
10. Murphy ME, Brodland DG, Zitelli JA. Errors in the interpretation of Mohs histopathology sections over a 1-year fellowship. Dermatol Surg. 2008;34:1637–41.

Establishing a Mohs Practice

39

Pearon G. Lang, Martin Braun III,
Carlette M. Geddis, and Jamie L. Benenhaley

Abstract
Setting up an office and establishing a Mohs surgery practice is a major undertaking and requires careful planning. There are many aspects that need to be addressed, including the design of the space, the setting up of the laboratory, the purchase of equipment and supplies, the hiring of personnel, medical record keeping, billing, marketing, the recruitment of referrals, regulatory issues, and the development of educational materials. Although one should be frugal, one should not skimp when it comes to equipment and supplies, setting up the laboratory, or hiring personnel.

Keywords
Equipment • Personnel • Laboratory • Billing • Marketing • Educational • Records

Summary: General Considerations

- One must decide whether to lease or build an office, as well as an ambulatory surgery center.
- The office should be large enough to allow for expansion.

39.1 General Considerations

When establishing a Mohs practice, there are a number of decisions to make. For example, should one purchase a space or lease with or without an option to buy? Also, should one have an ambulatory surgery facility? Many factors impact one's decision making, including the amount one must invest; the potential for appreciation; and whether or not there will be co-investors or if there is the potential for other physicians using the facility. Ambulatory surgery facilities can be a good source of income but carry with them the need for inspections, certification, rules, regulations, and record keeping.

Office space comes at a premium, and thus, one does not want to have excess space which may not be used for years. On the other hand, one should not be so intent on being frugal that they find within a short period of time that they have outgrown their space. If one feels compelled to "start slow," there should at least be the potential for expansion without relocating. Unless there is a large amount of unfurnished space, when one joins a preexisting practice, they may be limited in what they can design. However, there are certain minimum requirements, which must be satisfied if one is to have an efficient, patient-friendly practice.

P.G. Lang (✉) • C.M. Geddis • J.L. Benenhaley
Department of Dermatology Clinic, Charleston, SC, USA
e-mail: pearonlang@bellsouth.net

M. Braun III
Department of Dermatology Clinic, George Washington University, Washington, DC, USA

K. Nouri (ed.), *Mohs Micrographic Surgery*,
DOI 10.1007/978-1-4471-2152-7_39, © Springer-Verlag London Limited 2012

There can never be enough storage space for supplies, samples, etc. It will be amazing how quickly "excess" storage space becomes filled.

Summary: The Electronic Medical Record

- Check with colleagues and organizations before selecting a vendor for your electronic medical record (EMR).
- EMRs can do much more than record patient data.

39.2 The Electronic Medical Record

The electronic medical record (EMR) is here to stay and when one sets up an office, one should make provisions for this. Check with colleagues and organizations such as the AAD for tips and help. There are templates that can be created, which allows one to generate surgery notes with accompanying photographs and letters to referring physicians that saves time and the cost of transcription. Again, check with colleagues regarding programs they use. One advantage of the EMR is that it allows one to keep track of one's data, e.g., types of cancer treated, repairs, complications, etc. Thus, if one wants to look at their infection rate for a given time period, this can be easily generated. Although maintaining a complication log is not currently required, at some point in the future it could be. Therefore, it would be good to start accumulating this data from the beginning. If you have an ambulatory surgery facility, this would be required.

Summary: Credentials, Licensure, and Malpractice Insurance

- It is critical to start early getting credentialed and licensed, obtaining malpractice coverage, and getting signed up with third party carriers.

39.3 Credentials, Licensure, and Malpractice Insurance

Obtaining a license may require a considerable amount of time, and thus one needs to apply as soon as possible. This also applies to obtaining a DEA number and a state controlled substance number. Also make sure you have a valid NPI number.

When purchasing malpractice insurance, do not just look at cost but also consider the limits of coverage and whether or not you will need to purchase tail coverage when you close your practice.

Getting signed up with Medicare, Medicaid, and insurance companies may also require a considerable length of time. You will not get paid until you do and so, again you want to start working on this as soon as possible.

Summary: Quality Assurance

- A quality assurance (QA) program should be implemented from the very beginning.
- Colleagues can play a role in your QA program.

39.4 Quality Assurance

Although not currently required, it would be good to have a quality assurance program in place if there is another Mohs surgeon in the practice or there is another Mohs surgeon in the same community. Randomly selected slides can be reviewed in terms of quality and correctness of diagnosis. Any discordance in opinion could be resolved by an independent pathologist/dermatopathologist. In the future, organizations such as the American College of Mohs Surgery could offer such a service.

Summary: Cameras

- Cameras are essential for documentation and preparing manuscripts and presentations.

39.5 Cameras

Digital cameras are a must for documenting surgical procedures and biopsy sites. Ideally, there should be a camera in each room. The pictures can be incorporated into the Mohs surgery note or in the letter to the referring physician. They also can be incorporated into the EMR for later viewing. There are many "point and shoot" user-friendly digital cameras on the market. Again, check with colleagues for recommendations.

Summary: Care of Instruments
- Take care of your instruments. They are a significant investment and essential for your practice.

39.6 Care of Instruments

Space and equipment for sterilization of instruments should be available. For instruments requiring gas sterilization, a nearby hospital or surgery center that has this capability can be utilized.

A small room or area needs to be designated for soiled instruments. In this area, surgical trays can be broken down and dirty instruments can be cleaned in preparation for sterilization.

A place for the storage of clean and sterile instruments needs to be available. This can be in the form of cabinetry or a room where extra instruments, suture material, sterile packs, dressing materials, etc., are stored.

Summary: Work Rooms
- Work rooms can be useful for storage and handling messages.

39.7 Work Rooms

If possible, a small room, where nurses can take care of phone calls, is ideal since this ensures quietness and privacy. Such a room can also serve other purposes such as storage space for extra pamphlets and handouts or a secured area for controlled substances.

Summary: Microscopes
- A good microscope is essential for a Mohs practice.
- Do not economize.

39.8 Microscopes

If one plans to do general dermatology in addition to Mohs surgery, it would be best not to use their Mohs microscope for *KOHs*. The histotechnicians will need their own microscope for reviewing their sections and this can be used for *KOHs* as well. Since microscopic examination of the Mohs specimens is such an integral part of the procedure, this is not an area where one wants to "save money." When selecting the objectives of the scope, it is not necessary to have an oil immersion lens. A low-power, scanning lens is essential for viewing large specimens and precisely mapping areas positive for residual tumor. Olympus makes a super wide field objective for this purpose, but there may be other manufacturers that offer something similar. Another useful, but not necessarily essential, accessory is an ocular micrometer for measuring the depth of invasion of melanomas and squamous cell carcinomas. If one is not obtaining these measurements themselves, however, it is important to have access to a pathologist/dermatopathologist who will provide this information.

Another nice but nonessential accessory is a marking objective, which allows one to easily mark an area of concern, which a colleague can then review when another opinion is sought. If one anticipates publishing, one may also want to mount a digital camera on the scope. These are easy to use and yield high-quality photomicrographs.

If one anticipates teaching, a double-headed microscope is essential. A polarizer is a nice accessory, but one that is infrequently used.

The microscope for examining the Mohs specimens should be in close proximity to the Mohs lab. This provides for efficiency and ease of communication. One of the authors (PGL) has always preferred to have his microscope located in the laboratory.

Summary: Instrumentation
- To do surgery with ease and precision, one needs good instruments and high-quality ancillary supplies.

39.9 Instrumentation

Just as with the microscope, it is important to invest in high-quality instruments. Gold-handled instruments, which denote tungsten carbide, are of high quality and very desirable, but one needs to be selective since these tend to be expensive. For example, one would not purchase such scissors for cutting sutures, but it is well worth the extra money to have gold-handled Webster needle drivers.

The instruments used for Mohs surgery and repairs are basic and few in number. For a knife handle, the authors prefer a flat handle, which can be used for measuring and can accommodate #10, #11, and #15 surgical blades. Brown Adson tissue forceps are good for both Mohs surgery and for preparing a wound for repair and for excisions. Smooth (but serrated) Adson tissue forceps are useful for handling delicate tissues during Mohs surgery and for suture removal. Small, delicate toothed forceps are ideal for repairing wounds and can be used for obtaining tissue from delicate areas (e.g., the eyelid). These authors prefer single-pronged skin hooks, but others prefer double-pronged retractors. Supercut black-handled scissors are excellent tissue scissors and in the curved style are good for defatting full-thickness skin grafts.

If one is going to use large sutures with large needles, one needs to have on hand large needle carriers. Using regular size needle carriers to grab large needles will spring them, and they no longer will be useful when using small caliber sutures, e.g., 5-0, 6-0.

As regards needle carriers, do not purchase those with serrated jaws. Small caliber suture will slip through these. Also, they will fray the suture and cause it to break.

A useful instrument for helping to close large wounds, especially those of the scalp, is a towel clamp-like tissue approximator.

Unless one is planning to do full face dermabrasions, drywall sandpaper can be used for dermabrading small areas. For full-face dermabrasions or when large areas are being treated, we prefer motorized dermabraders with diamond fraizes.

If one is going to obtain bone specimens or decorticate the calvarium, one needs bone rongeurs and a hammer and chisel (osteotome).

For nail surgery, one needs nail splitters and nail elevators.

A periosteal elevator is essential when it is necessary to obtain periosteum for microscopic examination.

Chalazion clamps provide hemostasis and immobilize areas such as the eyelid and lip. When working in the ear canal, a right angle Beaver blade facilitates removing tissue.

It is important to have eye covers, eye chambers, eye pads, and saran wrap when dressing periocular Mohs wounds along with either a topical antibiotic or petrolatum-based lubricant. For the surgery itself, eyeshields may be needed. Plastic shields with short handles work well. If metal shields are used, they should be insulated since if they are touched with the electrocautery, this can damage the eye. The use of an eyeshield requires a topical anesthetic. When the shield is removed, the eye should be flushed with saline, and an antibiotic ointment or lubricant should be instilled.

When working on the penis and the tumor extends into the urethra, it may be necessary to insert a Foley catheter to ensure emptying of the bladder.

For open wounds, which want to ooze, hemostatic agents, such as Surgicel, may be helpful. This can also be wrapped around pedicles, which want to ooze. Xeroform gauze is also used to wrap pedicles and can be used for packing.

For large flap repairs, Penrose drains can be inserted to prevent hematomas and seromas.

Although everyone has their personal preferences for suture materials, we have found that chromic gut, Prolene, Monocryl, Vicryl, and silk suffice our everyday needs. A reversible cutting needle is preferable. A P-3 needle is used for most suturing, but a larger needle is used with larger suture. Chromic gut is desirable when one does not want to remove sutures, e.g., skin grafts, periocular area, ears, lips, and mucosa. Silk is useful around the eyes but is most commonly used on elderly patients who have such fragile skin that sutures such as Prolene tear through the skin.

Prolene sutures are ideal for running subcuticular suture. Prolene 3-0 is also useful for pulley stitches to help approximate the edges of large surgical defects.

For harvesting split thickness grafts, one can use a Padgett dermatome or a Weck knife (for small grafts). The donor site can be dressed with Opsite or Tegaderm, which can be left in place for a week. At that point, the patient can initiate wound care.

Summary: Regulations

- It is important to be knowledgeable about regulations.

39.10 Regulations

There are numerous regulations and regulatory bodies, which the physician and his staff need to be aware of, including HIPPA, CLIA, the Coding initiative, and the red flag rules. Unfortunately, ignorance of the law is not defensible. Organizations, such as the AAD, can serve as a resource for guidance regarding these regulations.

Summary: Reception Area

- To be efficient and patient friendly, an office needs to be well planned with adequate work and reception areas.

39.11 Reception Area

To facilitate patient flow and give some sense of privacy, it is important to have separate areas for patients to check in and check out. Although not always possible, it is ideal to have a small office, within the reception area, where bills and payment arrangements can be discussed in private.

A fax machine and a high-quality printer are essential items. There should be adequate phone lines so that the patient does not constantly get a busy signal.

A Rolodex with important and frequently called telephone numbers is also a must.

There should be two restrooms, one for the staff and a separate one for patients, which should be handicap accessible.

Summary: Waiting Area

- A sub-waiting room for Mohs patients is ideal.
- Recliners allow Mohs patients to wait in comfort.
- A television can help make waiting easier.
- A beverage center is appreciated by Mohs patients.

39.12 Waiting Area

Ideally, there should be two waiting areas, a larger general waiting area and a smaller sub-waiting area for Mohs surgery patients who are awaiting the results of the microscopic examination of their tissue. This sub-waiting area should have recliners and a beverage area, which has at least a coffeemaker and a source of water. Ideally, hot water should be available for those who prefer tea or hot chocolate. Soft drinks, juices, and snacks can be kept in a separate area and made available upon request. An extravagance but nice touch is a machine that dispenses hot water and also makes individual cups of different flavored coffees and teas. If the waiting area tends to be rather cold, blankets should be available. There is a blanket warmer, which can be used to heat the blankets and which also comes in handy for patients undergoing liposuction. A television can help entertain patients while they wait and can also be used for educational purposes.

Summary: Exam/Surgery Rooms

- There should be at least three surgery rooms.
- Tile floors are easier to maintain.
- Double surgical lights are ideal.
- There should be adequate cabinetry and surfaces on which to work.
- Power tables should be comfortable.
- Suction should be available.
- Consider having music in the rooms.
- A floor or wall-mounted buzzer system can allow one to easily call for assistance.

39.13 Exam/Surgery Rooms

At the very least, there should be three rooms available for patient care. Two of these should be set up for surgery so that while one patient is having surgery, another patient can be gotten ready for surgery. The third room can be used as a general exam room or for suture removals, etc. In anticipation of growth or the addition of a physician assistant (PA) who might assist with simple repairs, this third room should be of adequate size and designed similar to the surgery rooms so that very little needs to be done to convert this to a fully operational surgery suite. Although three rooms would suffice, we would suggest having four rooms, two of which are outfitted for surgery to allow for growth. Of course if one later added a PA or aesthetician or decided to use lasers, additional rooms would be required.

The exam/surgery rooms should have adequate cabinetry and counter space. A soap dispenser should be mounted over the sink, and by the door, there should be a dispenser with some type of soapless disinfectant for quickly disinfecting the hands before and after examining the patient.

Wall-mounted mirrors should be available for the patients to view themselves, and full-length mirrors are good if you are doing liposuction. Hand mirrors are a must for identifying the biopsy site, viewing the lesion preoperatively and viewing the Mohs defect. If the Mohs specimens are going to be color-coded and mapped in the operatory, a work area needs to be available where one keeps the dyes, Q-tips, cutting boards, and trays for transporting the tissue. Ideally, this needs to be a counter that is lower, so one can be seated while they process the tissue. If the counter/work space is of adequate size, a computer terminal can be located in this same area.

Music can be quite soothing and relaxing. However, there are times when either the patient or physician prefers to have it turned off. Each room can have a volume control, which allows this to be done.

During sterile procedures, the physician and his/her assistant may find that they need something or situations may arise where they need assistance with the patient. A floor switch, which activates a buzzer or light, is very useful at such times. A light or flag system is also essential to alert the physician to which room they need to go to next.

The surgical table needs to be capable of assuming multiple positions. Although tables, which can be programmed, are nice and efficient, they always seem to require reprogramming. The table needs to be well padded and comfortable. Patients often prefer tables with armrests. These need to be able to be moved out of the way when necessary. If one plans to sit and do surgery, one would opt for a narrower table and a dental chair-type headrest.

To have adequate lighting, we would suggest two overhead surgical lights, with handles, over which one can fit covers.

The electrosurgical machine should be capable of both cutting and coagulating. The cutting mode can be used to sculpt patients with rhinophyma and also can be used to debulk vascular tumors. A machine capable of bipolar cautery can be useful in patients with a pacemaker or deep brain stimulator. However, since this mode may be used infrequently, it is necessary to only have one such machine.

Each surgical room should have a kick bucket as well as large trash cans for hazardous and nonhazardous waste. A sharps box also needs to be available. Nonsurgical rooms also need to have containers for the disposal of waste and sharps.

Equipment for suction and the delivery of oxygen needs to be available. These can be portable sources, but if the cost is not prohibitive, wall-mounted sources are preferable. Cost would determine how many rooms were so outfitted. Chart racks need to be placed on the door or next to the door to each room. Coat hangers should be attached to the door for hanging clothes.

Although carpet looks nice, it is easily stained and can soon look shabby. We would suggest tile floors in the operating and exam rooms.

Summary: Physician Office

- The physician needs a private, quiet area for consultations, dictations, paper work, and phone calls.

39.14 Physician Office

The physician needs an office where he or she can dictate, do paper work, make and receive phone calls, read, and have private consultations with patients and families.

Summary: Nurses Work Station

- Nurses need a work area to make phone calls, access lab reports, and to carry out other required tasks

39.15 Nurses Work Station

The size and complexity of this area could vary from a simple counter to a larger area where meds could be drawn up or surgical trays could be prepared. At the very least, there should be adequate counter space for writing and computer terminals and for telephones. The station should be in close proximity to the surgery/exam rooms so that the nurses can monitor the rooms and patient flow and be readily available. Ideally, the nurses should also be able to see when charts are put in the "rack" so that they can get the patients back in a timely fashion. If this is not possible, a light system needs to be in place, which alerts the nurses when a chart is placed in the "rack."

Summary: Personnel

- Good personnel are essential to establish a practice that is efficient, productive, and patient friendly.
- Personnel should be well trained, efficient, show initiative, be team players, and be patient advocates.
- Personnel is not where one wants to economize.

39.16 Personnel

Personnel are a major expense, especially if one also provides benefits. Therefore, one does not want more help than they need; on the other hand, inadequate staffing can adversely affect employee morale, efficiency, and quality of care. It would be wise to consult with a management firm, which can assist in setting up your office and possibly with ongoing management, including accounting.

In addition to full-time employees, it is also desirable to have individuals who can work from time to time and fill in when needed. Cross-training is also helpful to ensure adequate coverage when there is an unexpected absence. As the practice grows, there will be an increased need for additional employees.

Although some physicians insist on having registered nurses (RN), they command a significant salary. Capable, well-trained medical assistants can perform as well as an RN and cost much less.

At a very minimum, one needs a receptionist, a nurse, a histotechnician, and a secretary/office manager/transcriptionist. However, once the Mohs surgeon becomes reasonably busy, they will need a second nurse and an office manager who oversees the practice and takes care of the billing. Obviously, as the practice grows, even more personnel will be required, including a second histotechnician.

Although an experienced, certified histotechnician may be more quickly trained, individuals with no background can be trained to be excellent histotechnicians.

All too often there is an attempt to save money when hiring a receptionist. This is the first person patients come in contact with, either in person or on the phone, and so it is important to have someone good. This is not the place to skimp.

Summary: The Laboratory

- A well-equipped and well-run laboratory is the cornerstone of a successful Mohs practice.
- The laboratory is a lifetime investment, and one should not try to economize.

39.17 The Laboratory

Good quality sections are essential if one is to properly perform Mohs surgery. Therefore, the Mohs lab needs to be equipped with the best equipment possible. This includes the cryostat, the microscope, and the stainer. When starting out, slides can be stained by hand, but once the Mohs surgeon becomes busy, especially if they only have one histotechnician, an automatic stainer will allow for faster turn around of the slides. The lab should be in close proximity to the operatories and to where the Mohs surgeon microscopically examines the slides. One of the authors (PGL) prefers to have the microscope located in the lab to facilitate communication with lab personnel. The size of the lab will be determined by what procedures are performed, i.e., only frozen sections or frozen sections plus permanent sections and/or immunostains. A used cryostat, for backup, is a good idea, but for many may be considered a luxury. However, when one has been in practice for a while, and is ready to replace their cryostat, the old cryostat, if still serviceable, should be kept for backup.

Good quality sections are essential if one is to properly perform Mohs surgery. Therefore, the Mohs lab needs to be equipped with the best equipment possible. This includes the cryostat, the microscope, and the stainer.

Summary: Space
- The lab needs to be large enough for two people.
- The lab needs to be kept cool.
- There should be adequate storage and work surfaces.
- The floor should be tile.
- A backup cryostat is ideal.

39.18 Space

The laboratory should be large enough to accommodate two workers. There should be an area to receive gross specimens. Always have the sink near the staining setup for easy access and connection to an automatic stainer.

It is very important that the laboratory be cool. Minimize the number of windows so that less heat is transmitted from outside. If possible, the lab should have its own air-conditioning system.

There should be adequate space for one or two cryostats (AC outlet), shelves, cabinets (including a cabinet for flammables), counter space (at least five feet) along one wall, a sink for staining, and a microscope to check slides while cutting. Bright overhead lighting and a magnification light are essential for the grossing area. Depending upon your state regulations, a fume hood over the staining setup may or may not be required, but is highly suggested. A separate counter space is needed for all paperwork, including a computer terminal. There should be space for a liquid nitrogen tank under one counter.

The floor should be linoleum or tile for easy cleanup.

Summary: Personal Protective Equipment
- Provide protective equipment

39.19 Personal Protective Equipment

Gloves, an impervious gown, and protective eyewear should be worn when processing fresh tissue because all tissue is considered to be a biohazard.

Summary: Mapping and Grossing the Tissue
- Either the Mohs surgeon or histotechnologist can gross, color-code, and map the specimens.

39.20 Mapping and Grossing the Tissue

The laboratory technician or the surgeon may gross, color-code, and map the specimens. This can be done in the operatory or in the laboratory. Precise orientation and mapping is essential. The tissue can be transported to the laboratory on a small metal tray or in a plastic gauze container. For the grossing of the tissue, one needs a cutting board with grooves on its borders where knife handles can be placed when not in use. A magnification light at the grossing station will aid in viewing the tissue samples more closely.

Marking dyes should be available in a variety of colors. A key should be on the map that indicates which colors are being used to color code the specimens. In addition to a key for color-coding, the map should also include the patient's name, the date, and the accession number. The type of tumor and its location can be written in if one map is used for multiple lesions, or there can be blank spaces for this if each tumor has its own map. The map should also include the preoperative size of the lesion and the size of the final surgical defect. There can also be blanks for the type of repair and the length of the suture line.

There are assorted forceps from which to choose depending on the height and size the laboratory technician prefers. One will need #15 and #10 surgical blades, and tissue scissors may also come in handy. A wide mouth thermos, without a lid, can be used to store liquid nitrogen in the cryostat and used in conjunction with sponge forceps when cutting fatty tissue.

Summary: Embedding Mohs Specimens [1]
- Embedding is critical to cutting good sections.
- There are a number of methods for embedding tissue.

39.21 Embedding Mohs Specimens [1]

Embedding refers to the process by which the fresh tissue specimen is prepared for cryostat sectioning. This is a crucial step to achieve slides of high caliber. The most commonly used embedding media includes O.C.T., Tissue Tek, TBS, and Richard Allen Neg. 50. There are many different embedding techniques, but it is best for the technician to find the method that works best for him or her and yields complete deep and peripheral margins.

Direct method – this method involves applying embedding medium to a metal disk or "chuck" on the freeze bar. After the embedding medium is partially frozen to a semisolid state, the specimen is applied to the chuck with the deep margin facing upward. The block face is then made smooth with a glass slide placed on top.

Glass slide technique – the specimen is placed on a glass slide with the deep margin face down. The epidermis is teased down onto the slide. Next, the glass slide containing the specimen is placed on the freeze bar to allow freezing of the specimen. The specimen is then coated with the embedding medium, which will turn opaque in color. Afterwards, a chuck is placed in the cryochamber and the embedding medium is applied. The chuck is then flipped upside down onto the glass slide containing the specimen. Once frozen together, one can use their thumb to separate the slide.

Freeze bar technique – this method involves placing the tissue sample, with the deep margin facing down, onto the freeze bar. The tissue is flattened, and the epidermis is teased down onto the freeze bar. The embedding medium is then applied on and around the specimen. The chuck is placed in the cryostat, and the embedding medium is applied, allowing a semisolid to form. The embedded specimen is then popped from the freeze bar and placed on the chuck with the deep margin facing upward.

Heat sink – this is a modified version of using a heat extractor. This device remains in the cryostat, and the deep margin of the inked tissue is flattened, and the epidermis is teased down onto the heat extractor. The coldness allows for easy manipulation of tissue that would otherwise be difficult to relax. Embedding medium is applied on and around the tissue, and a chuck to which embedding medium has been applied is placed in the cryostat. Once the embedded tissue has hardened, the heat extractor is inverted onto the chuck, allowing the two to freeze together. The heat extractor is subsequently separated.

CryoEmbedder – this device uses polished metal plates that have metal rails to guide and assure proper specimen orientation while embedding tissue and mounting it onto a chuck. It is time efficient, user-friendly, and can produce very high quality slides.

Summary: Devices to Aid Embedding

- There are a number of aids to assist with embedding.

39.22 Devices to Aid Embedding

Heat extractor – a pestal-like metal device with a cylindrical base that is usually housed inside the cryostat. It is used to flatten and promote freezing of the specimen.

Miami Special – a hand-held clamping device that helps flatten the specimen and promotes rapid freezing. This device has two opposing metal plates. One plate is used to hold the cryostat chuck onto which the specimen has been mounted in place, while the other plate clamps down on top of the specimen to flatten it. Once loaded, the device is placed in liquid nitrogen to allow the specimen to freeze. This device was designed by Dr. Henry Menn who was at the University of Miami.

CryoHist – this instrument is about the size of a cryostat and the latest invention that has attracted the attention of Mohs technicians due to its ability to orient, freeze, mount, and bring specimens to the proper cutting temperature with the use of liquid nitrogen. Its ability to handle delicate tissue or large specimens up to 5.5 cm is definitely an attractive feature. However, the main disadvantage is that the cryostat must have a pedestal object holder with a stem length of 20 mm and a stem diameter of 9.5 mm. If the object holders currently being used in your cryostat do not meet these measurement criteria, they will need to be re-machined.

Summary: Cryosectioning Tissue
- Buy a cryostat that can maintain low temperatures.
- The chuck holder should be a yoke type.
- Liquid nitrogen is an invaluable aid.

39.23 Cryosectioning Tissue

The cryostat, which is a microtome in a freezer, is the most important instrument in the Mohs laboratory. Therefore, it is best to know your needs before making this purchase. This instrument requires preventive maintenance service twice a year. There should be at least 6 in. of clearance on all sides to ensure adequate ventilation. Some technicians prefer to stand while cutting, while others prefer an adjustable stool.

When purchasing a cryostat, always ask for a demonstration for 30 days. Manufacturers will set up the cryostat in your lab. This will afford you the opportunity to see how it sections different types of tissue. Also ask your colleagues about their recommendations before deciding on a purchase.

The temperature inside the cryostat can range from −18° to −30° depending on the room temperature. Lower temperatures are essential for cutting fat. Cryostats vary in size and height. Special features may include a self-contained decontamination system, a vacuum to remove shavings, and the Peltier cooling mechanism. The object holder can be of two types – rectangular and the yoke. The rectangular type allows for only 180° of rotation of the block, whereas the yoke allows the block to be rotated 360°, which is preferable because it can be cut from any angle. Once the block is ready to be sectioned, it is placed in the object holder, which holds the block in place while the microtome advances the tissue toward the blade or knife. The knife holder may come with a detachable anti-roll plate, which allows sections to be cut without a lot of curling. We prefer this device, but others prefer using brushes or forceps. Disposable blades have largely replaced knives. These allow one to always have a sharp-cutting edge, whereas knives require periodic sharpening and realignment. A microscope in the lab allows the technician to check the completeness of the sections prior to staining them. This saves time for the technician and keeps the surgeon from having to ask for recuts.

A used cryostat, for backup, is a good idea, but for many may be considered a luxury. However, when one has been in practice for a while, and is ready to replace their cryostat, the old cryostat, if still serviceable, should be kept for backup.

Adhesive glass slides are used because the substance on the slide helps the tissue to adhere and remain intact throughout the staining process. They are kept outside of the cryostat because the sections adhere better to a warm slide. Clear communication should be given as to the order in which the tissue sections should be placed on the slides and how many sections are required. Depending on the size of the specimens, we like to have three sections on each slide, with the most superficial specimen being closest to the frosted end of the slide. The slides should have a frosted end to allow labeling with a special marking pen. A typical hand labeling system includes the patient's name, accession number, and site of surgery. Some laboratories apply computer-generated labels before the slides are filed. The blocks in the cryostat can be labeled by writing the patient's last name on the chuck or the accession number. The label can easily be removed by rinsing the chucks in alcohol once the specimen has been removed.

Summary: Staining
- Hematoxylin and eosin and toluidine blue are the most common stains used.
- An automatic stainer can improve efficiency and productivity.

39.24 Staining

Mohs laboratories employ a variety of fixatives, such as 10% neutral buffered formalin, alcoholic formalin, or alcohol as a fixative before staining slides. The most popular stain used for Mohs specimens is hematoxylin and eosin (H&E). However, there are some laboratories that prefer toluidine blue for staining basal cell carcinomas. In order to stain slides, one will need a fixative, water, stain (hematoxylin and eosin, or toluidine blue), alcohol (95% and 100%), and a clearing agent, such as xylene.

In the past, staining by hand was a common practice, but most people now have an automatic stainer for more consistent staining. This also frees up the technician so they can continue to embed and cut. There are several types of automatic stainers, some of which allow for only one slide to be loaded at a time and others that have a rack, which allows the continuous feeding of slides.

Summary: Coverslipping
- The mounting media and clearing agent must be miscible.

39.25 Coverslipping

Once the slides have been removed from the clearing agent, a drop of mounting media is carefully applied, along with a coverglass (24×60 mm), onto the slide. The mounting media and the clearing agent must be miscible. The back of the slides and the frosted edge are then wiped with a dry gauze. The slides are then placed on a tray, along with the map, and given to the surgeon for viewing.

Summary: At the End of the Day
- Disposal of tissue is strictly regulated.

39.26 At the End of the Day

Once each case becomes clear, place the slides on a tray to dry for 48 h.

According to who inspects your lab, there are different guidelines for saving tissue. For CAP, the thawed, wet tissue must be stored for 2 weeks after the report date in a fixative for frozen sections. For CLIA, the thawed tissue can be discarded in the lab's biohazard trash receptacle.

Summary: Permanent Sections and Immunostains
- For certain tumors, paraffin embedded sections or immunostains may be helpful.

39.27 Permanent Sections and Immunostains

Many Mohs surgeons still utilize paraffin embedded sections (permanent sections) when treating melanomas, as well as unusual and difficult tumors. The tissue from this so-called slow Mohs may be processed in the Mohs lab or in a pathology or dermatopathology lab. Due to the additional expense and space and personnel requirements, most Mohs surgeons do not process this tissue in their laboratory, but instead rely on their pathology/dermatopathology colleagues to provide this service.

39.27.1 Immunostains

In many instances, immunostains have replaced the need for "slow Mohs," especially when managing melanomas. They also may be useful when managing other difficult tumors such as perineural squamous cell carcinoma, extramammary Paget's disease and Merkel cell carcinoma.

However, like paraffin sections, they require additional space, equipment, and expense and will tie up a technician. The immunostains themselves are expensive and may have a limited shelf life. For a small lab, with one technician, doing immunostains may not be productive or cost-effective. Again, one could possibly utilize a colleague in pathology or dermatopathology to provide this service.

Summary: Training of Laboratory Technicians
- Your technician should be well trained.
- Consultants are available to assist with training and setting up a lab.
- Ask the American College of Mohs Surgery for help.

39.28 Training of Laboratory Technicians

He who can find a fully trained Mohs technician is indeed blessed. However, many Mohs surgeons must be either satisfied with a histopathology certified technician or someone who has no background whatsoever in the preparation of slides. Although fully trained histotechnicians may initially have an advantage, neophytes can mature into excellent Mohs technicians and demand a lesser salary. Although the Mohs surgeon may choose to train the technician, there are consultants who can assist in the establishment of a laboratory and the training of technicians. The American College of Mohs Surgery has, as a member service, designated trainers who can be of assistance in training a technician.

Acquiring and training a technician is a critical step in establishing a high-caliber Mohs practice. This is not where one wants to economize. A technician who is efficient and produces high-quality slides is worth their weight in gold. They will allow one's practice to be more productive, enjoyable, and more free of headaches.

Summary: Inspections and Regulations

- Learn the regulations regarding disposal of tissue, slide storage, and laboratory safety.

39.29 Inspections and Regulations

Depending on whether or not the laboratory is hospital based or in an outpatient setting, the laboratory will be subjected to periodic inspection by either CAP (College of American Pathologists) or CLIA (Clinical Laboratory Improvement Amendments). Outpatient laboratories cannot bill Medicare or Medicaid unless they are certified by CLIA. CLIA inspections are prearranged but CAP inspections may be unannounced. Certificates issued by these entities are good for 2 years.

In order to pass an inspection, it will be necessary to keep logs that chart such things as room temperature and humidity, refrigerator temperatures, and record the specimens handled in the lab and equipment maintenance. Methods used to assure quality will also be assessed. It is also necessary to develop a manual that describes in detail all procedures performed in the laboratory.

Since it is necessary to retain slides and pathology reports up to 10 years, it will be necessary to have a designated storage area.

For more information, one can visit these regulatory bodies' websites: www.cap.org and www.cms.hhs.gov/CLIA/downloads//CLIA.SA.pdf

There are also OSHA regulations that include having in place policies on dealing with chemicals, hazardous substances, and bloodborne pathogens. Personal protective equipment must be provided (gowns, gloves, masks, eyewear), and there must be an eyewash, fire extinguisher, shower, and a spill kit. Appropriate warning signs also need to be posted.

Summary: Marketing

- One can market their practice fairly inexpensively by making themselves known to the professional and lay community or can pay others considerable sums of money to market their practice.

39.30 Marketing

An endless amount can be spent on marketing, and thus, one must come up with a budget with which they can live. The Mohs College has developed a marketing kit, which is available to members and should be helpful.

There are many ways one can generate referrals inexpensively: (1) join the local hospital staff(s), go to their breakfasts and staff meetings, frequent the physician lounge, and offer to give presentations; (2) participate in free skin cancer screenings or have one in your office; (3) look for opportunities to speak to the public; (4) contact local media regarding your willingness to be interviewed; (5) visit potential referral sources, including those with whom you might interact, e.g., oculoplastic surgeons and head and neck surgeons; (6) send letters to potential referral sources introducing yourself; (7) participate in local and state dermatologic meetings and functions; (8) if there is a dermatology department, volunteer your services and attend conferences; and (9) consider having a open house and giving a presentation on Mohs surgery.

Make sure you get your name in the white pages and yellow pages as soon as you have picked a location for your practice.

Consider placing announcements in the local newspaper(s).

Create a website and link it to the Mohs College and Skin Cancer Foundation.

When you get a referral, make sure you write a thank you note and give the referring physician follow-ups at each visit. If the primary care physician is not the referring physician, make sure you copy the primary care physician on the letter to the referring physician and at each follow-up visit.

To let the referring physician know your level of expertise, it is nice if you can include pictures in your letter showing the lesion before Mohs surgery, the

Mohs defect, and the repair. These can be printed on the letter so that loose pictures do not need to be sent.

Summary: Preoperative Consultation

- The Mohs surgeon must decide which patients they need to see prior to surgery and how to best prepare the patients for surgery.

39.31 Preoperative Consultation

Whether or not the patient needs to be seen prior to Mohs surgery depends on a number of factors: (1) the Mohs surgeon's preference, (2) how difficult it is for the patient to come for the visit, (3) the complexity of the case, (4) whether imaging studies are necessary, and (5) whether or not other physicians will be involved in the patient's care.

For most cases, a separate preoperative consultation visit is not necessary. This can be handled over the phone by the Mohs surgeon or their assistant. However, it is ideal that some type of contact take place prior to the surgery to screen the patient in terms of medications and other health issues, as well as to educate them about Mohs surgery and what to expect.

In addition, it is ideal to have a brochure on Mohs surgery sent to the patient prior to the surgery in order to reinforce what to expect. The Mohs surgeon can prepare this, or the brochure from the Mohs College can be used. The brochure can also serve as a marketing tool.

Summary: Brochures and Handouts

- Brochures and handouts can be both educational and serve as marketing tools.

39.32 Brochures and Handouts

Brochures and handouts can be helpful for reinforcing verbal explanations and potentially could also serve as marketing tools. The brochures can be prepared by the Mohs surgeon or obtained from other sources, such as the Skin Cancer Foundation, the American Society for Dermatologic Surgery, or the American Academy of Dermatology.

Summary: Operative Consents

- Operative consents need to be specific and informative.

39.33 Operative Consents

Blanket consent forms should be avoided. Operative consents should be procedure specific and spell out all the potential complication. Avoid blanket statements such as "repair of the Mohs defect." Instead use phrases such as "repair of Mohs defect with a full-thickness skin graft from the right preauricular area."

Summary: Conclusion

- A well-planed office should be efficient; fully utilize all of the space, and allow for expansion.
- Purchase high-quality equipment.
- Personnel should be carefully selected and paid well.
- A well-equipped laboratory is essential to ensure high-quality sections.
- Billing, regulations, marketing, the development of educational materials, and electronic medical records are essential items that also require attention.

39.34 Conclusion

There are many things that go into setting up an office for and a practice in Mohs surgery. Much thought needs to go into the planning of the office in order to make sure it is designed properly for the best utilization of space and to make sure it will run efficiently. Future plans for expansion also need to be considered.

Equipment and instruments should be of good quality and considered a long-term investment. In the long run, equipment of high quality will save money, result in fewer headaches, and improve efficiency.

Paying a little extra for personnel will also pay off in terms of efficiency and fewer worries. Quality personnel can help enhance the reputation of the practice.

The laboratory is critical to the practice of Mohs surgery. High-quality sections are a must. To ensure quality, the equipment and personnel need to be top-notch. One should not skimp on cost in this area.

Although the above are probably the more important issues to address, other essentials also require consideration, such as billing, medical records, marketing, regulations, and the development of educational materials.

Reference

1. McColloch M, Geddis C, Hetzer MR, Beck C, Fisher SC. Embedding techniques. In: Fish FS, editor. Manual of frozen section processing for Mohs micrographic surgery. Milwaukee: American College of Mohs Surgery; 2008. p. 601–88.

International Perspective of Mohs Micrographic Surgery: South America

40

Luis Fernando F. Kopke and Gaston Nestor Galimberti

Abstract

The history of Mohs surgery in South America is not old. The influence of USA is naturally bigger than the European. Although it can be possible that Mohs surgery could be performed beyond these two countries in South America, the significant contribution in the field comes from Brazil and Argentina. In Brazil, it is remarkable that other methods of surgical margins control have been used. Both in Argentina and Brazil the number of Mohs surgeons is small in comparison with the population and size of the countries. Efforts have been made to change this situation, but there is still a long way to reach a good development, which could get more recognition for Mohs surgery in these countries.

Keywords

Ambulatory surgical procedures • Surgery • Mohs surgery • Skin neoplasms • History

Summary: The Brazilian Perspective

- Not only the original technique of Mohs surgery is performed in Brazil, but also some variations that are more known and used in Europe, mainly in Germany: the Munich method and the Tübingen Torte. The Brazilian Society of Dermatology recently has created a department of micrographic surgery, which put all techniques together, in a way to coordinate the growth of micrographic surgery in the country.

L.F.F. Kopke (✉)
Coordinator of the Department of Micrographic Surgery of the Brazilian Society of Dermatology,
President of the Brazilian Society of Dermatologic Surgery,
Florianopolis,
Santa Catarina, Brazil
e-mail: luiskopke@uol.com.br

G.N. Galimberti
Department of Dermatology,
School of Medicine Italian Hospital,
Buenos Aires, Argentina

K. Nouri (ed.), *Mohs Micrographic Surgery*,
DOI 10.1007/978-1-4471-2152-7_40, © Springer-Verlag London Limited 2012

40.1 The Brazilian Perspective

The history of the micrographic surgery in Brazil is quite new. At the beginning, individual but important contributions were essential to bring up the development that we have made over the years. Dr. Sebastião Sampaio, who was one the most important dermatologist in Brazil, should not be forgotten. Under his leadership in 1988 the Brazilian Society of Dermatologic Surgery (SBCD) was founded and since then the role of the surgical dermatology in Brazil has expanded enormously. The first Mohs surgery in Brazil was made in São Paulo in 1985 and in 1989 the first unit of Mohs micrographic surgery was created in the Clinical Hospital of the São Paulo University (HCUSP) [1]. Although at that time, this unit began to train some dermatologists in the field, with a 1 year duration fellowship, many of the new dermatologic surgeons in Brazil preferred to study about Mohs surgery abroad. The USA was the logical destination where the Brazilians went to and it still continues to be the main center today. In 1991, a Brazilian decided to take an alternative way to know about Mohs surgery: Germany. But he realized that what they called Mohs surgery over there was technically very different from the original method, so he proposed a new name for the procedure: *The Munich method* of micrographic surgery, which was used and called by Dr. Gunter Burg as *histographic surgery*, that means, *to control microscopically the surgical margins* without using the Mohs surgery [2, 3]. In the same context, Breuninger mentioned the *Tübinger Torte* just only in German literature, and many papers that he had published in English literature was interpreted as he had performed Mohs surgery, although it was not the real Mohs method [4]. Regarding this situation, only Rapini wrote clearly about it [5]. This is very important to understand how the micrographic surgery has grown in Brazil.

Despite the creation of the SBCD, the number of Mohs surgeons remained small for a big country like Brazil. The unit of HCUSP had formed only five surgeons, and since its creation fewer dermatologists have dedicated to micrographic surgery. Maybe the reasons lie in the current trend of cosmetic surgeries just at that time when the number of the Mohs surgeons was increasing. Our Public health care management also contributes with this. The procedure is not supported by the government or private health insurance groups. In order to change this situation, a small group of Mohs surgeons created the Brazilian Group of Mohs Surgery (GBMOHS), but again, the effects were still shy. Although the Mohs surgery is by large the mainly performed micrographic surgery in Brazil, other methods like The Munich and Tübingen methods are still used in the country. Therefore, it was recently created in the Brazilian Society of Dermatology (SBD), a department of micrographic surgery, which brought all kinds of microscopically controlled surgery together. The great step of this initiative was giving an official concern about the subject, nothing more as individual contributions, but as a goal of a dermatological society that recognizes the importance of microscopically controlled surgery in the field of cutaneous oncology. In Brazil, only few specialists besides the dermatologists know about Mohs surgery, and it would be important for the whole health system to spread out a concept that it can control better the threat of skin cancer. In its first year, the department has begun to discuss the basic formation of the Mohs surgeons, where and how they could be trained. With easier opportunities to travel abroad, we could already identify that many people are getting some knowledge in the field, but not in a trustworthy way. Therefore, in a recent survey we found out that in Brazil there are 29 surgeons that have some good experience with Mohs surgery or with another method, and maybe twice as much of dermatological surgeons that do not call themselves Mohs surgeons, although they have a good knowledge of the technique through the many trips to different centers in USA.

Today, there are only three dermatological residences services, where Mohs surgery can be done: Clinical Hospital of São Paulo University (HCUSP), Dermatologic Clinic of the ABC University, and Hospital Municipal de São Paulo (a Hospital of the City of São Paulo). Although other centers like Curitiba, Belo Horizonte and Rio de Janeiro are going to do the same soon, fellowship in Mohs surgery is only possible in São Paulo nowadays. The objective of the SBDs Department of micrographic surgery is to create conditions to increase the number of universities where Mohs Surgery or any other method of micrographic surgery could be learned and to standardize the way to teach this in our country. After that, maybe, other specialties could absorb the importance of micrographic surgery in cutaneous oncology. The seeds of Frederic Mohs are still alive in Brazil, and certainly it will improve.

Summary: The Argentinean Perspective

- Not only dermatologists do Mohs surgery in Argentine, but also some Head and Neck Surgeons, although most patients are treated by dermatologists. The insurance Companies pay the procedure, helping raising the number of patients that can be treated with the technique.

40.2 The Argentinean Perspective

The beginnings of Mohs micrographic surgery in Argentina are not linked to Dermatology.

Dr. Abel Gonzalez, Head and Neck Surgeon completed a period of time at Madison Wisconsin with Frederic Mohs and his chairman's Drs. Steve Snow and Paul Larson. In June, 1990 he introduced this technique at the Angel Roffo Oncology Hospital.

Dr. Gaston Galimberti has initiated his studies in skin cancer and Mohs micrographic surgery at Sagrat Cor, Barcelona Spain, where Dr. Pablo Umbert has been his mentor. He continued his research at Mount Sinai School of Medicine, Dermatology department (head of the Dermatology Department Dr. Mark Lebwohl) under the tutelage of Dr. James Spencer. In October, 2003 at Dermatology Department Hospital Italiano (head of the department Prof Ricardo Galimberti) Dr. Gaston Galimberti performed his first Mohs micrographic surgery.

There are a small numbers of private centers in Buenos Aires and other states that perform this technique.

Mohs micrographic surgery is linked directly to Dermatology; it is part of dermatology programs and residence. Nowadays there is only one dermatology residence where Mohs surgery can be performed: Hospital Italiano Buenos Aires, with more than 700 Mohs micrographic surgeries yearly it is a referral center to treat skin cancer. There is also an annual scholarship on Dermatology surgery and Mohs micrographic surgery whose chairman is Gaston Galimberti. The objective is to increase the number of Dermatology Surgeons that perform this important technique for the treatment of skin cancer.

The private insurance groups generally pay for this procedure and the social security does the same at Angel Roffo Oncology Hospital, free of charge.

In Argentina the incidence of skin cancer is growing up as well as other parts of the world. Lack of concern about the risk of sun exposure, in addition to skin phototype, genetics, and climatic changes, are the main factors.

The idea of treating skin cancer with this particular technique is not only good for our patients but also for Dermatology which will be more developed in the near future in Argentina.

Summary: Conclusion

- Mohs surgery practice in South America includes the original technique, as well as variations performed in Europe, especially in Germany.

40.3 Conclusion

In South America not only the original technique of Mohs surgery is performed, but also some variations that are more known and used in Europe, mainly in Germany: the Munich method and the Tübingen Torte.

References

1. Cernea SS. Experiência do grupo de cirurgia micrográfica de Mohs do HCFMUSP: dezembro/1989 a abril de 1993. An Bras Dermatol. 1994;69(5):365–73.
2. Kopke LFF, Konz B. Mikrographische chirurgie: eine methodische bestandsaufnahme. Hautarzt. 1995;46:607–14.
3. Burg G, Hirsch RD, Konz B, Braun-Falco O. Histographic surgery: accuracy of visual assessment of the margins of basal-cell epithelioma. J Dermatol Surg Oncol. 1975; 1:21–4.
4. Breuninger H, Dietz K. Prediction of subclinical tumor infiltration in basal cell carcinoma. J Dermatol Surg Oncol. 1991;17:574–8.
5. Rapini RP. On the definition of Mohs surgery and how it determines appropriate surgical margins. Arch Dermatol. 1992;128:673–8.

International Perspective of Mohs Micrographic Surgery: Europe

41

James A.A. Langtry

Abstract

Europe comprises a diverse group of sovereign nations, with a wide range of health service organisation in the public and private sectors. European authors have made a significant contribution to the evidence base for Mohs micrographic surgery (MMS) and to the debate about margin control in skin cancer surgery.

MMS has been an important influence in the development of dermatological surgery as a subspecialty of dermatology, in many European countries.

The continued development of MMS in Europe is likely to depend on a well trained body of practitioners committed to excellence in treatment outcomes for patients with skin cancer, high quality audit, outcome, cost analysis and clinical research.

MMS in Europe is likely to continue to flourish despite the manifold challenges that exist.

Keywords

Mohs micrographic surgery • Europe • Cutaneous oncology • Clinical research • Fellowship training

J.A.A. Langtry
Dermatology Department, Royal Victoria Infirmary,
Newcastle Upon Tyne, Tyne and Wear, UK
e-mail: james.langtry@nuth.nhs.uk

K. Nouri (ed.), *Mohs Micrographic Surgery*,
DOI 10.1007/978-1-4471-2152-7_41,

Mohs micrographic surgery (MMS) represents a paradigm shift in skin cancer excision technique. MMS is the brain child of Dr Frederic Mohs, who treated his first patient by the technique which now bears his name, in 1936 at Wisconsin General Hospital, Madison. The historical development of Mohs surgery is well documented [1], and progress in MMS has been hand in glove with the development of dermatologic surgery and skin surgical oncology. The legacy has been manifold and includes the establishment of a body of dermatologists who are specialists in skin cancer diagnosis and treatment and distinguished by the core skill of the Mohs micrographic excisional technique. MMS represents the gold standard in the treatment of skin cancers of the head and neck and those with a higher risk of local recurrence by non-Mohs techniques.

Mohs surgery has found wide acceptance by North American health care providers and patients. The American College of Mohs Surgery (ACMS) has a large membership with well-formed structures acting as advocates for the large well-trained body of ACMS Mohs surgeons practicing in North America. The ACMS has high standards of fellowship training and a strong annual scientific meeting focusing on new developments, research, and teaching components, as well as a parallel meeting of Mohs histotechnologists. Both the ACMS and the Mohs histotechnologists meetings attract an international audience, albeit a small fraction of the North American audience.

The ACMS website gives a geographical listing for members of the ACMS (www.mohscollege.org). The listing for the USA is by state and the total USA membership exceeds 600. The country outside the USA with most members listed is Australia with 22 and then Canada with 17. The only European countries listed are the UK with seven and Ireland with one. There are five ACMS members listed in Israel.

The history of MMS in Europe has been previously described [2]. Progress of MMS in Europe, by contrast with the USA, has generally been slow. MMS development has typically relied on the interest, insight, and energy of individuals to find training in MMS and develop a MMS service to a local population. The absence of a regional or national framework for MMS services or a critical mass of MMS practitioners forming a strong professional body with a common understanding and aim acting as the advocate for MMS training standards, practice standards, audit, and research has led to the slow and uncharted progress of MMS in Europe.

Mohs surgeons in Europe have acquired their training in a number of ways, including ACMS fellowships, visits to the Mohs centers in the USA, training in European countries which varies from within residency training (e.g., Holland), clinical attachments of up to 3 months duration (e.g., Portugal) and 1 year Mohs fellowship training programs (e.g., UK). It can be seen that training across Europe is diverse in

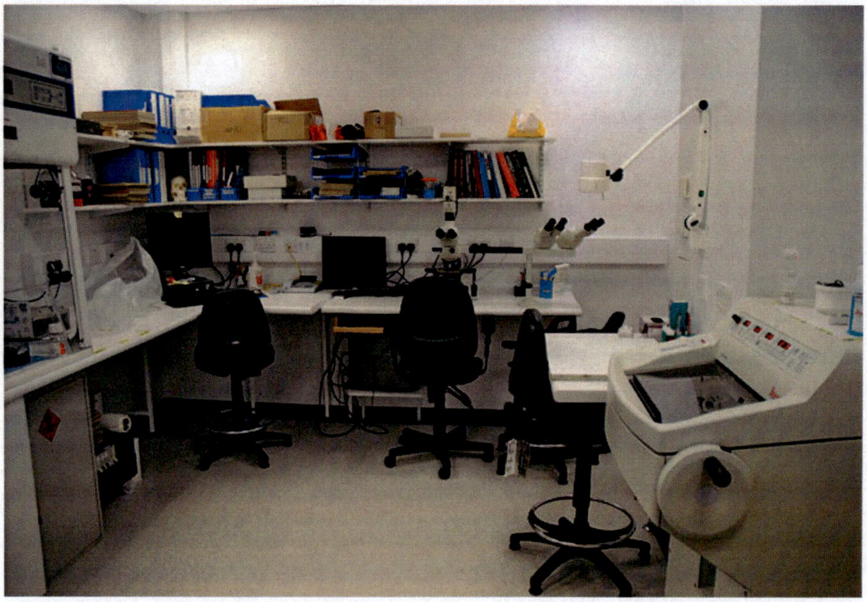

Fig. 41.1 Mohs laboratory at the dermatology surgery unit, Newcastle upon Tyne, UK

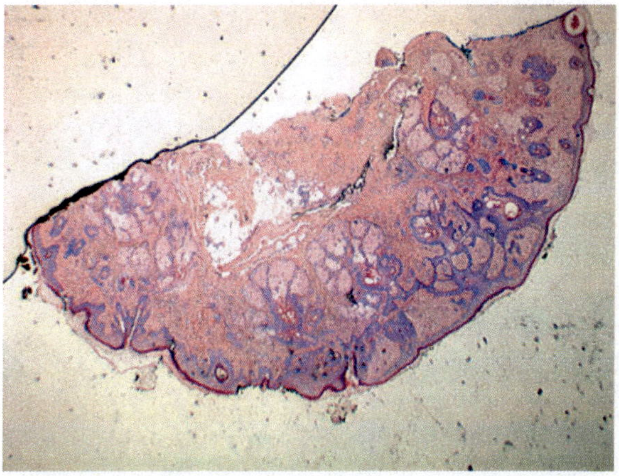

Fig. 41.2 Mohs section (H&E stain)

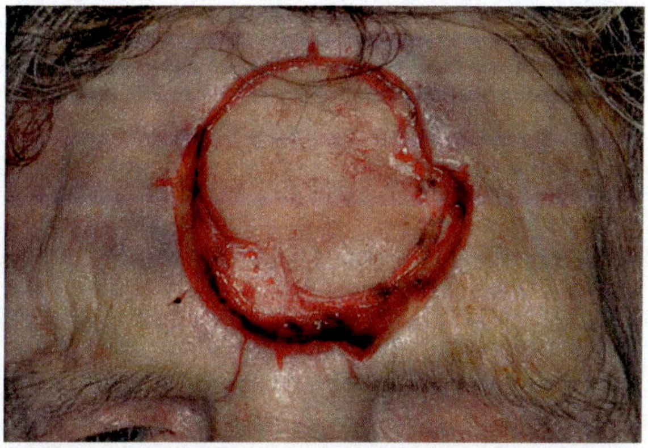

Fig. 41.4 Final Mohs wound microcystic adnexal carcinoma forehead after 4 stages and 15 blocks

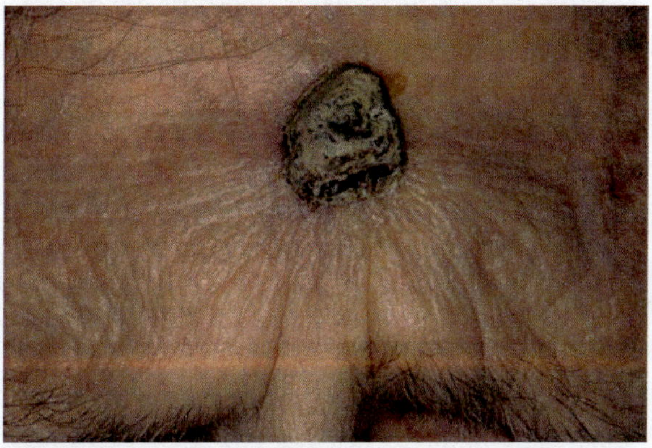

Fig. 41.3 Microcystic adnexal carcinoma of the forehead

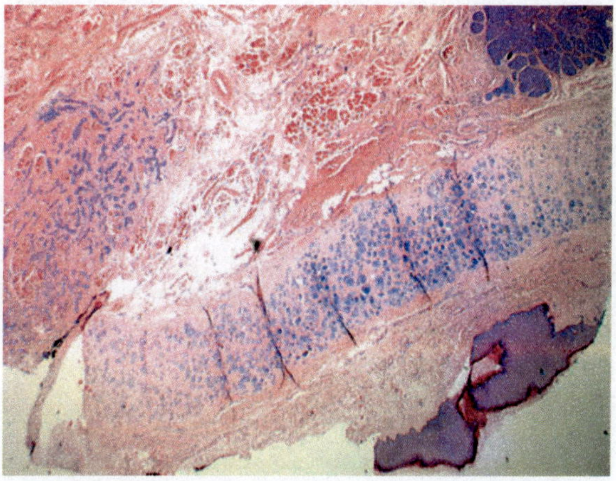

Fig. 41.5 Mohs section (H&E stain) of basal cell carcinoma nose showing mixed histological pattern of basal cell carcinoma and adjacent nasal cartilage

nature and even within countries Mohs practitioners training may have been from any of the sources described, vis-a-vis in residency, clinical attachment or fellowship.

Colleagues in Germany have developed a number of alternative margin control techniques which include the Munchner method, Tubinger tort, Muffin technique, La Galette method, and Wallgraben technique [3].

There are a number of well-established MMS services in Holland, Spain, Portugal, Sweden, UK, and Ireland. However a number of countries, including Denmark and Norway have no access to MMS.

Authors from European MMS units have made some important contributions to the literature, particularly in taking a critical approach to Mohs surgery where there exists a dearth of randomized controlled studies. Both extant prospective controlled studies are from European centers, one comparing Mohs surgery with standard excision [4] and one assessing the tissue-sparing outcome for small nodular basal cell carcinomas [5].

The European Society for Mohs Surgery (ESMS) was established several years ago (www.esme-mohs.eu) but has faced the challenges resulting from the diversity of Mohs across Europe. Unlike the USA where there is evidence of a well-attended body of MMS experts with a unified vision and direction, a coordinated approach is lacking within many European countries and maybe not surprisingly at European level.

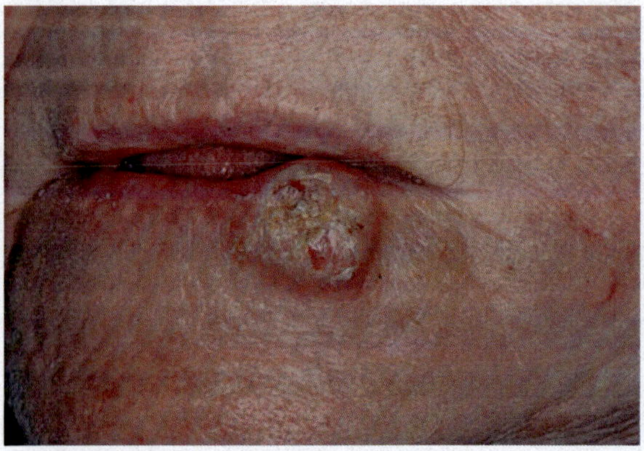

Fig. 41.6 Squamous cell carcinoma lower lip

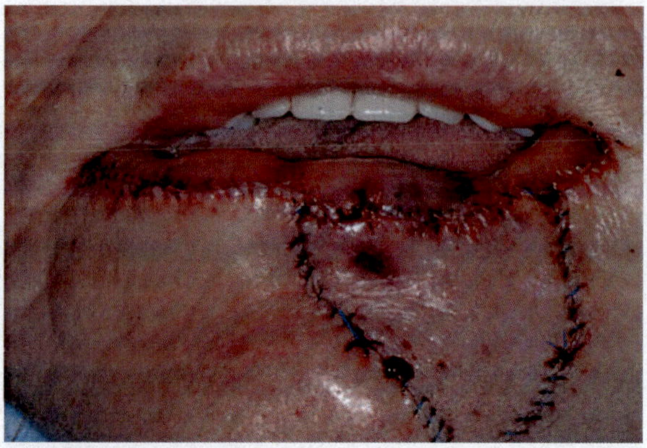

Fig. 41.8 Reconstruction lower lip with orbicularis muscle hinge flap, island pedicle flap and vermilion advancement

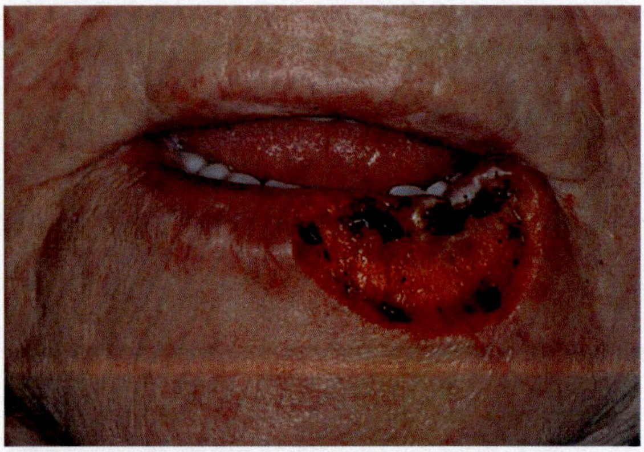

Fig. 41.7 Mohs defect squamous cell carcinoma lower lip after 1 stage and 4 blocks

The available evidence suggests an increasing incidence of skin cancer across Europe [6, 7] which is likely to continue to rise for several decades [8]. Along with changes in incidence of skin cancer there exist societal changes and an explosion in the availability of high quality information. The public at large is thus becoming an ever more sophisticated "consumer" of health services in general, and skin cancer treatment in particular. The demand for high-quality skin cancer treatment, and therefore MMS, is likely to continue to rise. Patients are increasingly consumers of healthcare rather than recipients, and are better placed than ever to understand the range of treatments available including MMS.

There is likely to be change in the direction of MMS, from large, neglected or recurrent tumors, toward the treatment of smaller tumors with resultant small Mohs wounds and the prospect of repair in a seamless manner.

In England and Wales, the National Health Service (NHS) 2006 Improving Outcomes Guidance [9], for skin cancer laid out a set of guidelines with recommendations for Mohs surgery as a desirable treatment outcome for defined indications, including basal cell carcinoma (BCC) greater than 2 cm diameter, BCC located in high-risk facial zones, recurrent BCC, and BCC with aggressive histological growth pattern. This has led to an increasing demand for Mohs surgeons in the UK.

The UK has a number of MMS units with good operating rooms and Mohs laboratory facilities, based mainly in teaching hospitals with annual MMS caseloads greater than 500 (including St John's Hospital, London, Cardiff, Manchester, Nottingham, and Newcastle upon Tyne). Recent years have seen the establishment of Mohs surgery fellowships in the UK, including those at St John's Hospital, London, Cardiff, Nottingham, and Newcastle upon Tyne.

The British Society for Dermatological Surgery (BSDS) has recently developed a dermatologic surgery fellowship curriculum (MMS training being central to this) as well as national guidelines ("MMS setting standards document") for MMS. The BSDS lists the MMS fellowships currently available in the UK on its website (www.bsds.org.uk) and in its newsletter. In recent years, the BSDS has seen an increasing number of MMS-related abstract submissions to the BSDS annual scientific meeting [10–12].

The development of a "British College of Mohs Surgery" has been a subject of discussion at various times in recent years.

Important agenda areas for MMS in Europe include, the development of information systems to record training, MMS practice, MMS outcomes, audits, cost and outcomes analysis, patient related outcomes, and high quality clinical research.

There remains much to be agreed and achieved in further developing MMS across Europe, but there is little doubt that MMS is having a significant impact in many countries despite the many challenges. MMS in Europe is likely to continue to develop and flourish.

Disclosures

Associate member of the ACMS since 1997.
ACMS Mohs fellowship 1996–1997, Vancouver, British Columbia, Canada.
President of the BSDS 2009–2011.
Chairperson of the North East England Cancer Network skin cancer TSSG (tumour specific sub-group).

References

1. Brodland DG, Amonette R, Hanke W, Robbins P. The history and evolution of Mohs micrographic surgery. Dermatol Surg. 2000;26:303–7.
2. Picoto A, Camacho C, Walker NPJ, Camps-Fresneda A. Mohs micrographic experience: European experience. In: Roenigk RK, Roenigk HH, editors. Surgical dermatology. Advances in current practice. London: Martin Dunitz; p. 125–129. Chap. 13.
3. Loser C, Romple R, Breuninger H, et al. Microscopically controlled surgery. JDDG. 2010;8(11):920–5.
4. Smeets NW, Krekels GA, Ostertag JU, et al. Surgical excision versus Mohs micrographic surgery for basal cell carcinoma of the face: randomised controlled trail. Lancet. 2004;364:1766–72.
5. Muller FM, Roberts SD, Moseley H, Fleming CJ. Randomised comparison of Mohs micrographic surgery and surgical excision for small nodular basal cell carcinoma: tissue sparing outcome. Dermatol Surg. 2009;35:1349–54.
6. Brewster DH, Bhatti LA, Inglis JH, Nairn ER, Doherty VR. Recent trends in incidence of non melanoma skin cancer in the East of Scotland. Br J Dermatol. 2007;156:1295–300.
7. Birch-Johansen F, Jensen A, Mortensen L, Olesen AB, Kjær SK. Trends in the incidence of non melanoma skin cancer in Denmark 1978–2007: rapid increase incidence among young Danish women. Int J Cancer. 2010;127:2190–8.
8. Diffey BL, Langtry JAA. Skin cancer incidence and the aging population. Br J Dermatol. 2005;153:679–80.
9. NICE. Guidance on cancer services: improving outcomes for people with skin tumors including melanoma: the manual. NICE. 2006. (www.nice.org.uk). Accessed date on 2006.
10. Rahim R, Langtry JAA. Mohs micrographic surgical excision for atypical fibroxanthoma at critical sites. Br J Dermatol. 2010;163 Suppl 1:109.
11. Foulkes A, Dunn S, Lawrence CM, Langtry JAA. Methicillin-resistant Staphylococcus aureus prevalence in a Mohs micrographic surgery service. Br J Dermatol. 2010;163 Suppl 1:110.
12. Tan WP, McKenna J, Robson A, Mallipeddi R. Mohs micrographic surgery for dermatofibrosarcoma protuberans: experience in a large regional center. Br J Dermatol. 2010;163 Suppl 1:110.

International Perspective of Mohs Micrographic Surgery: East Asia

42

Satoru Aoyagi

Abstract

Overall skin cancer rates are much lower in East Asian populations than in Caucasian populations. Pigmented basal cell carcinoma (BCC) is the most common type, and surgical excision with wide margins is the standard treatment for BCC in most East Asian countries. Due to differences among countries in insurance systems and surgical approaches, Mohs micrographic surgery (MMS) is an uncommon procedure in most Asian countries. Surgical excision is widely used in the major parts of East Asia because of its effectiveness and simplicity. MMS has been reported to be a successful treatment by particular institutions in Korea and Taiwan. However, MMS is not routinely available in most dermatologic units in East Asia. Intraoperative histological evaluation to control surgical margins is widely used instead of MMS for high-risk skin cancer. Complete histological margin control using a double-bladed scalpel may be easily applied to standard intraoperative frozen section evaluation in many institutions where MMS is difficult to perform. It is far less time-consuming and can be easily used by surgeons with existing systems, even in East Asian countries.

Keywords

Pigmented basal cell carcinoma • Surgical excision • Intraoperative histological evaluation • Double-bladed scalpel

Summary: Characteristics of Skin Cancers in East Asia

- Overall skin cancer rates are much lower in East Asian populations than in Caucasian populations.
- Pigmented basal cell carcinoma is the most common type of skin cancer, and squamous cell carcinoma has reportedly been on the rise on sun-exposed parts of the body during the past quarter century in Asians as well as Caucasians.

S. Aoyagi
Department of Dermatology,
Hokkaido University Graduate School of Medicine,
Sapporo, Japan
e-mail: saoyagi@med.hokudai.ac.jp

K. Nouri (ed.), *Mohs Micrographic Surgery*,
DOI 10.1007/978-1-4471-2152-7_42,

42.1 Characteristics of Skin Cancers in East Asia

Skin cancers are relatively rare in East Asia. In Japan, although the incidence of nonmelanoma skin cancer has not been estimated, the age-adjusted incidence rates are thought to be much lower than those in the USA. In Japan and other parts of East Asia, the incidence is estimated to equate to about one-tenth of that in the USA, resulting from differences in races and geographic distributions among East Asian and US individuals [1].

The high incidence of pigmentation in basal cell carcinoma (BCC) lesions is the most characteristic feature of BCCs in East Asian countries and Japan. Approximately 75% of the BCCs in the Japanese population show a brown to glossy black pigmentation, especially on their borders [2]. In Korea, approximately 69.2% of BCCs were found to be pigmented [3].

The prognostic significance of pigmented BCC has been discussed in previous studies. It was suggested that pigmented BCCs were more likely to be completely excised than were nonpigmented BCCs, and no pigmented BCCs recurred compared with a 20% recurrence rate in nonpigmented BCCs [4]. In another study, there was only one pigmented BCC (2.5%) with a positive margin compared with 17.7% positive margins in the nonpigmented BCCs [5]. It was proposed that dermal pigmentation of the lesion edges, or "shoulders," more clearly marks the tumor margins. Furthermore, we demonstrated that pigmented BCC, especially smaller tumors and the nonaggressive histologic subtype, requires a narrower surgical margin for complete tumor resection than does nonpigmented BCC [6]. The significance of these results is that the tumor borders in pigmented BCC are often more distinct because of the pigment and the fact that an infiltrative growth pattern is less common than in nonpigmented BCC. For these reasons, the local recurrence rate of surgical excision for BCC in East Asian populations is much lower than that in Caucasian populations [7].

Conversely, many squamous cell carcinomas (SCCs) that developed in injured or chronically diseased skin, including skin affected by long-standing ulcers and radiation dermatitis, could from then on be treated by wide excision followed by appropriate reconstructive procedures in Japan [1]. However, as in Caucasians, SCC has reportedly been on the rise on sun-exposed parts of the body during the past quarter century in Asians. This increase may be explained by the increasing proportion of elderly individuals with actinic keratosis-induced skin cancer.

Summary: Treatment of Skin Cancers in East Asia

- Due to differences among countries in insurance systems and surgical approaches, Mohs micrographic surgery is an uncommon procedure in most Asian countries.
- Surgical excision is widely used in the major parts of East Asia because of its effectiveness and simplicity.
- The studies of Mohs micrographic surgery from East Asia are very limited.
- Only a few recent instances of Mohs micrographic surgery have been reported to be a successful treatment by particular institutions in Korea and Taiwan.
- For institutions at which it is difficult to perform Mohs micrographic surgery, intraoperative frozen section evaluation is the treatment of choice.
- We introduced the double-bladed scalpel as a novel, simple method for complete histological margin control for improving the pathodiagnostic reliability of conventional intraoperative histological evaluation.

42.2 Treatment of Skin Cancers in East Asia

42.2.1 Standard Treatment of Skin Cancers

Of the treatment modalities employed, surgical resection for nonmelanoma skin cancer is widely used as a result of its effectiveness and simplicity in the major parts of East Asia.

For recurrent or histologically aggressive BCCs and SCCs, tumors with ill-defined clinical margins, and those located on high-risk anatomic sites, intraoperative frozen section evaluation is the treatment of choice. This evaluation is especially necessary before extensive reconstructive surgery is planned. It is frequently performed in many institutions where it is difficult to perform a complete Mohs micrographic surgery (MMS) procedure due to health insurance limitations and other reasons. In addition, it is especially commonly performed for surgeries under general anesthesia in which resection and reconstruction are completed simultaneously. However, in the conventional histological method of examining tumor margins, only certain slices perpendicular to the tumor are examined; therefore, an extension between the slices can be missed.

42.2.2 Present State of MMS in East Asia

Previous reports or studies of MMS from East Asia are very limited. Those that have been completed focused on extramammary Paget's disease (EMPD) [8], dermatofibrosarcoma protuberans (DFSP) [9], SCC of the lower lip [10], and some adnexal tumors [11, 12] reported by particular institutions in Korea and Taiwan.

Lee et al. [8] reported successful results of EMPD treatment. The local recurrence rate was 10% for MMS compared with 30% for wide excision. They concluded that MMS is superior to conventional wide excision for EMPD in Asians.

From the same institution, it was also reported that treatment of DFSP by MMS resulted in a low recurrence rate with possible benefits of smaller defects, as compared to wide local excision [9]. Additionally, MMS has been reported to be a successful treatment modality for rare types of skin tumors in East Asia, including squamoid eccrine ductal carcinoma [12] and syringo-cystadenocarcinoma papilliferum [11].

However, this technique is relatively specialized and is not routinely available in most dermatologic units because it is time-consuming, expensive, and requires the expertise of specially trained Mohs surgeons and technicians. In institutions in which MMS is unavailable, conventional excision with postoperative histological margin assessment remains the main form of surgical treatment. Therefore, in East Asia, where skin cancers are not as prevalent and where resources are limited, the feasibility and cost-effectiveness of setting up a Mohs unit are debatable. To save time and increase the accuracy of histological analysis of surgical margins, it is easier and more convenient to add a modified MMS technique to conventional intraoperative histological evaluation than to introduce a completely new MMS system. We recently reported a modified method of MMS for nonmelanoma skin cancers in Japan [13] (Fig. 42.1).

42.2.3 Modified MMS in Japan

Intraoperative histological evaluation by frozen section analysis is usually limited to suspicious areas. Therefore, the accuracy of such analysis of surgical margins of skin cancer is highly dependent on the methods used to obtain and analyze the margins. For institutions at which it is difficult to perform MMS, we introduced the double-bladed scalpel (DBS) as a novel, simple method for complete histological margin control [13]. A basic element of our procedure is resection of the whole tumor followed by excision of an additional outer layer for complete histological evaluation of the excision margins in three dimensions (Fig. 42.2a–f). This element involves performing the first two steps of MMS together by using permanent sections for histological evaluation of the tumor and using the frozen section only in re-excision of an additional outer layer from the tumor defect. This improves the pathodiagnostic reliability of conventional intraoperative histological evaluation.

Summary: Conclusion

- Complete histological margin control using a double-bladed scalpel may be easily applied to standard intraoperative frozen section evaluation in many institutions in East Asian countries where Mohs micrographic surgery is difficult to perform.

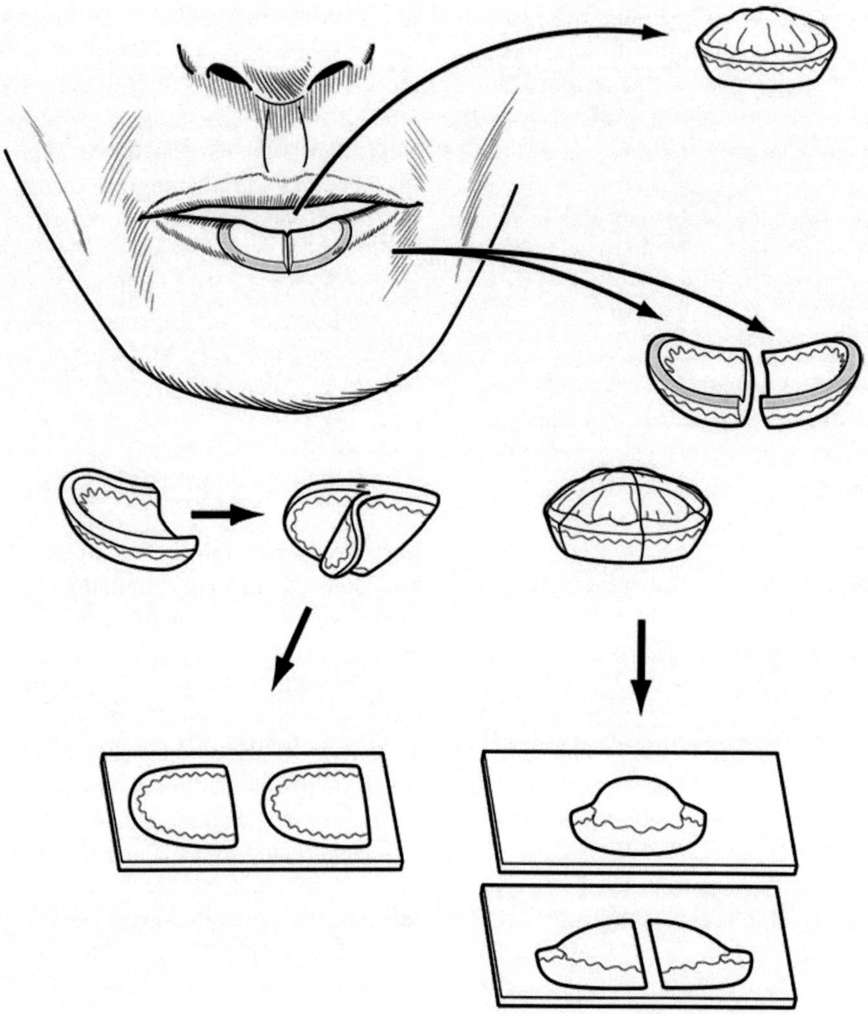

Fig. 42.1 Using the "double-blade method," parallel excisions are made and the gross tumor is excised in a bowl shape. An additional layer of tissue, along with 2-mm strips of the outer skin, is subsectioned into two to four regions and excised in a uniform width by scissors as in MMS. The excised tumor is then sent to the pathology lab and examined by breadloaf sectioning. Additional resected tissue is flattened and examined by *en face* frozen sectioning. If a tumor-positive margin in a re-excision specimen is obtained, additional layers of tissue are excised from the tumor-positive area. This procedure is repeated until negative margins are confirmed

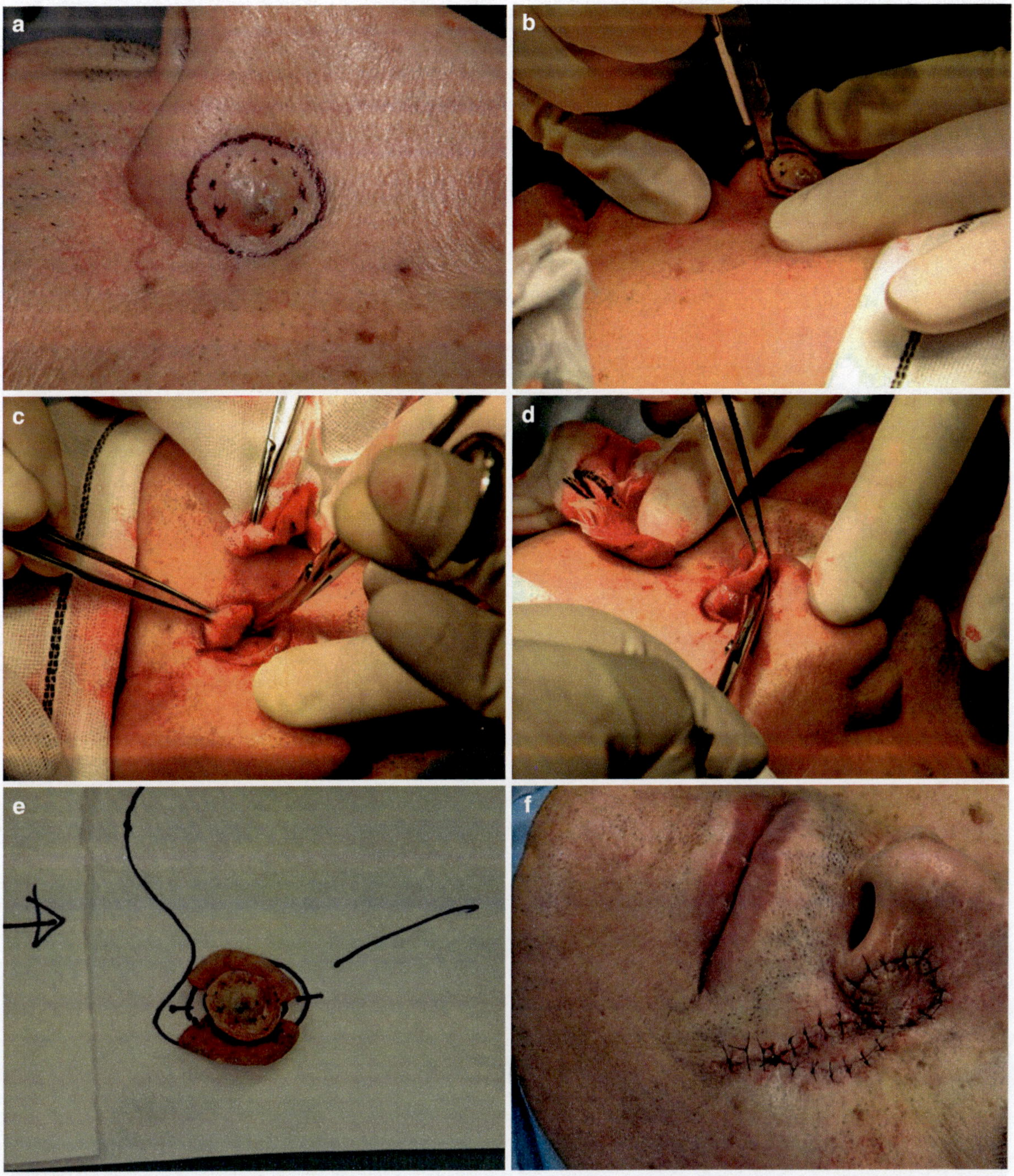

Fig. 42.2 Poorly defined nodule with a small amount of pigmentation on the left ala. (**a**) Initial surgical margin is 2 mm (*solid line*) from the clinical border (*dotted line*). (**b**) Using a DBS, parallel excisions are made around the tumor. (**c**) Gross tumor with initial surgical margins is excised in a bowl shape along the DBS inner excision. (**d**) Lateral margin specimen with 2-mm strips of outer skin is excised in a uniform width by scissors, taking great care to avoid tearing tissue. (**e**) Specimens from an additional layer are flattened, and sectioning is started from the true margin side. (**f**) Final defect after complete excision of tissue under histological evaluation by *en face* frozen section is reconstructed using a combined flap from the left cheek

42.3 Conclusion

Due to differences among countries in insurance systems and surgical approaches, MMS is still uncommon in most Asian countries. Surgical excision with wide margins is the standard treatment for low-risk nonmelanoma skin cancer. For high-risk skin cancer, intraoperative histological evaluation to control the surgical margins is widely used instead of MMS. Complete histological margin control using a DBS may be easily applied to standard intraoperative frozen section evaluation in many institutions where MMS is difficult to perform. It is far less time-consuming and can be easily used by surgeons with existing systems, even in East Asian countries.

References

1. Ohtsuka H, Nagamatsu S. Changing trends in the number of deaths from nonmelanoma skin cancer in Japan, 1955–2000. Dermatology. 2005;210(3):206–10.
2. Kikuchi A, Shimizu H, Nishikawa T. Clinical histopathological characteristics of basal cell carcinoma in Japanese patients. Arch Dermatol. 1996;132(3):320–4.
3. Cho S, Kim MH, Whang KK, Hahm JH. Clinical and histopathological characteristics of basal cell carcinoma in Korean patients. J Dermatol. 1999;26(8):494–501.
4. Hornblass A, Stefano JA. Pigmented basal cell carcinoma of the eyelids. Am J Ophthalmol. 1981;92(2):193–7.
5. Maloney ME, Jones DB, Sexton FM. Pigmented basal cell carcinoma: investigation of 70 cases. J Am Acad Dermatol. 1992;27(1):74–8.
6. Aoyagi S, Nouri K. Difference between pigmented and nonpigmented basal cell carcinoma treated with Mohs micrographic surgery. Dermatol Surg. 2006;32(11):1375–9.
7. Goh BK, Ang P, Wu YJ, Goh CL. Characteristics of basal cell carcinoma amongst Asians in Singapore and a comparison between completely and incompletely excised tumors. Int J Dermatol. 2006;45(5):561–4.
8. Lee KY, Roh MR, Chung WG, Chung KY. Comparison of Mohs micrographic surgery and wide excision for extramammary Paget's disease: Korean experience. Dermatol Surg. 2009;35(1):34–40.
9. Roh MR, Bae B, Chung KY. Mohs' micrographic surgery for dermatofibrosarcoma protuberans. Clin Exp Dermatol. 2010;35(8):849–52.
10. Whang KK, Do MO, Lee SM, Kim SH. W-modification of Abbe flap after Mohs surgery of squamous cell carcinoma on the lower lip. Dermatol Surg. 2007;33(4):485–7.
11. Chi CC, Tsai RY, Wang SH. Syringocystadenocarcinoma papilliferum: successfully treated with Mohs micrographic surgery. Dermatol Surg. 2004;30(3):468–71.
12. Kim YJ, Kim AR, Yu DS. Mohs micrographic surgery for squamoid eccrine ductal carcinoma. Dermatol Surg. 2005;31(11 Pt 1):1462–4.
13. Aoyagi S, Hata H, Homma E, Shimizu H. Controlling the histological margin for non-melanoma skin cancer conveniently using a double-bladed scalpel. J Surg Oncol. 2010;101(2):175–9.

International Perspective of Mohs Micrographic Surgery: Australia and New Zealand

43

Greg Julian Goodman, Vanessa A. Morgan, Tim J. Rutherford, Edward J. Upjohn, and Paul J.M. Salmon

Abstract

Mohs micrographic surgery (MMS) in Australia and New Zealand is of utmost importance given their extreme prevalence and incidence figures for skin cancer.

MMS is a rapidly growing subspecialty in Australia with surgeons exhibiting variable activity with the average number of cases per year being 201–300 of which 98% of tumors treated are located on head, neck, digits, or genitals.

The Mohs national database was established in 1993 to log the total number of cases performed in Australia and collected data on over 12,000 cases of Mohs surgery between 1993 and 1999.

Five-year follow-up studies have shown that 5-year recurrence rates for BCCs were 1.4% for primary and 4% for recurrent tumors. For SCCs, 5-year recurrence rates were 3.9% overall and 8% in those with perineural invasion. Perineural invasion was seen in 2.74% of BCCs and 5.95% of SCCs.

Mohs micrographic surgery and secondary intention wound healing of the nail apparatus for in situ and invasive SCC produce excellent wound healing and cure rate with retention of function.

New Zealand also has a very high rate of skin cancer, and MMS in New Zealand needs to be seen in the context of individuals with widespread sun-damaged skin. Multiple facial tumors in a patient are very common. A dysplastic field also influences repair options.

Keywords

Micrographic surgery • Nails • Australian Mohs database

G.J. Goodman, (✉)
Dermatology Institute of Victoria, South Yarra, VIC, Australia
e-mail: gg@div.net.au

V.A. Morgan • E.J. Upjohn
Skin and Cancer Foundation, Carlton, VIC, Australia

T.J. Rutherford
Victorian Dermatology & Surgery, Malnern, VIC, Australia

P.J.M. Salmon
Dermatologic Surgery, Skin Cancer Institute,
Tauranga Bay of Plenty, New Zealand

K. Nouri (ed.), *Mohs Micrographic Surgery*,
DOI 10.1007/978-1-4471-2152-7_43, © Springer-Verlag London Limited 2012

Summary: Introduction and Brief History of Mohs Micrographic Surgery in Australia and New Zealand

- Mohs micrographic surgery (MMS) in Australia and New Zealand is of utmost importance given the extreme prevalence and incidence figures for skin cancer seen in this part of the world.
- The Mohs national database has provided a fertile resource for important study of skin cancers and their outcomes.
- Repairs have been described in Australia for the very complex wounds created by surgical removal by MMS.

43.1 Introduction and Brief History of Mohs Micrographic Surgery in Australia and New Zealand

Skin cancer in Australia and New Zealand is at epidemic proportions with lifelong incidences of melanoma in certain parts of Australia and New Zealand approaching 6% and nonmelanoma skin cancer approaching 50%. Point prevalence figures show over 50% of over-40-year-olds harboring actinic keratoses and 3% nonmelanoma skin cancers [1, 2].

With these alarming figures, it is no surprise that micrographic surgery in Australia and New Zealand has a rich history with the beginnings in the 1970s but really reaching maturity with dermatologists training mainly in the USA in the 1980s. Coincident with this rise was the establishment of Skin and Cancer Foundations in Australia that fostered the growth of units devoted to the provision of skin cancer services in general and micrographic surgery in particular. With great foresight a centralized data collection for Australia was established and now houses enormous databases providing a rich resource for manuscripts on the provision of surgical techniques. Training facilities were first established first in the Skin and Cancer Foundation environment and then have spread to other facilities elsewhere in Australasia. One of the foundations has used a model of patient care and registrar training which encompasses a cooperative unit of dermatologists and plastic surgeons that has contributed to a textbook on flaps in cutaneous surgery.

Manuscripts have flowed from the database, in particular describing the behaviors of tumors according to tumor site (lips, scalp) [3, 4], type [basal-cell carcinoma (BCC)], in situ and invasive squamous cell carcinoma (SCC), basosquamous and microcystic adnexal carcinoma (MAC) [5–10], and pathologic behavior (perineural invasion in BCC and SCC) [11, 12], as well as by outcome of repair options or mixtures of these parameters with a heavy emphasis by one group studying the fate of periocular skin cancer [13–18]. Mapped serial excision for melanoma has also been studied using this database [19]. The sheer weight of this prospectively organized national database has been a major contribution to the literature and our understanding of disease behavior and the place of micrographic surgery in its management.

The database findings in relation to BCC and SCC will be further expanded in Sect. 43.3. The experience has been similar to that of other countries with very high cure rates in some smaller series [20–22] independent of the database findings.

Strange presentations of uncommon tumors and strange behaviors of tumors have been the subject of some literature from Australia and New Zealand [23–26]. The often-strange-shaped defects remaining after Mohs tumor clearances together with the confidence that these defects are likely tumor-free have fostered the development of novel methods of repair from many Mohs surgeons with Australasian practitioners being no exception. Flap designs have included repairs of simple and advanced nasal defects [27–31]. Flaps are the commonest method of MMS defects in Australia and represent some of the more challenging repairs. The use of the nasalis muscle to allow sliding-flap repair has been a commonly performed procedure in Australia and New Zealand for smaller repairs [28, 30]. For larger defects several variations of the nasolabial flap, either a modified 2-stage [29] or more recently a very novel single-stage flap repair, have emanated from this part of the world [27]. Termed the "tunneled and turned-over nasolabial flap for reconstruction of full thickness nasal ala defects," it describes an alternative to repairing full defects of the nasal ala without requiring a second-stage revision. In this repair a donor flap is harvested from the nasolabial fold and the cheek skin above. It is a flap, which is used when the lateral alar rim is left intact but there is a substantial full thickness ala defect. It is a single-stage competitor to a two-stage nasolabial or forehead flap repair. The flap is elevated and exists on a proximal pedicle near the top of the nasolabial groove and is then tunneled under the existing alar rim and folded back on itself to recreate the lining of the mucosa and the external shape. Clever use of redundancy in the flap design allows the re-formation of the alar bulk and projection.

Studied over time, there have been some changes in the practice of MMS in at least one major institution (Skin and Cancer Foundation of Australia). The major differences were a significant decrease in defect sizes and probably consequently a significant increase in the use of flap repair and side-to-side closures in 2007 as compared to more use of secondary intention wound healing and grafts being used in 1997 [32].

Summary: Work Practices of Australian Mohs Surgeons

- Rapidly growing subspecialty in Australia
- Wide range of annual number of Mohs cases performed, averaging 201–300 cases
- 98% of tumors treated located on head, neck, digits, or genitals
- 90% of surgical defects reconstructed by Mohs surgeons

43.2 Work Practices of Australian Mohs Surgeons

43.2.1 Background

In January 2010 a survey was conducted among Australian Mohs surgeons so as to record demographic data, methods of practice, and annual Mohs micrographic surgery caseloads. A web link was emailed to all those registered on the Australian Mohs surgeons email list, and respondents were asked to provide estimate on various aspects of their clinical practices. Of the 39 Mohs surgeons who were sent the survey, 33 (85%) responded, revealing the greatest proportion (37%) aged 40–44 years and 90% of Mohs surgeons as male. Seventy-six percent completed their Mohs training within Australia, and in keeping with Australia's population distribution, 88% work in an urban or suburban environment with the remaining 12% working in a rural setting.

43.2.2 Mohs Caseload

There is considerable variability in the number of Mohs cases performed annually in Australia, with 15% performing fewer than 100 cases per year and 12% performing greater than 500 cases (Fig. 43.1), which may be explained by the practice of most Australian Mohs surgeons of blending general dermatology and Mohs surgery. Additionally, the burden of skin cancer management is shared with several other specialties, and the Mohs technique is reserved for use on high-risk tumors that are located on the head and neck, digits, or genitals in 98% of cases (Fig. 43.2). Given this careful selection for high-complexity MMS cases, following tumor removal, flap reconstructions are required most often (48%), and then direct closure (25%) and skin grafts (17%) (Fig. 43.3). Accordingly, approximately half of Australian Mohs surgeons are skilled in more-complex reconstructions such as interpolation or tunneled flaps.

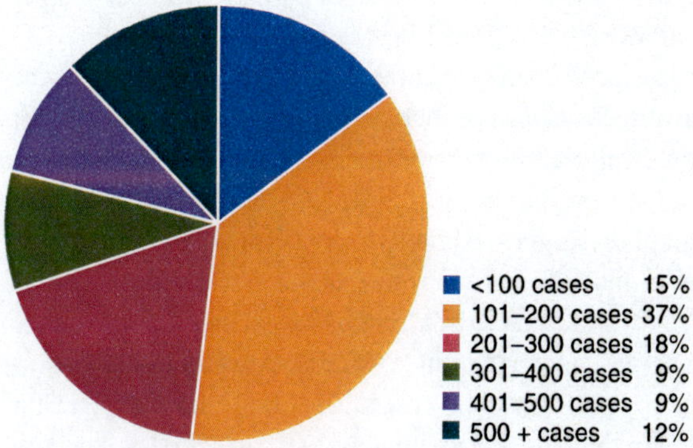

Fig. 43.1 Number of Mohs cases performed annually per practitioner

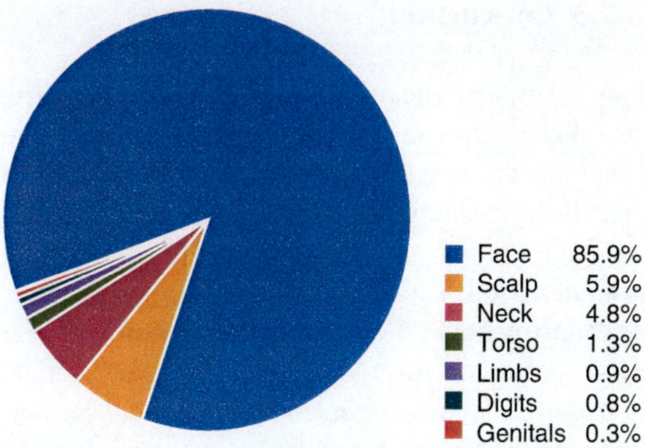

Fig. 43.2 Location of tumors treated with Mohs surgery

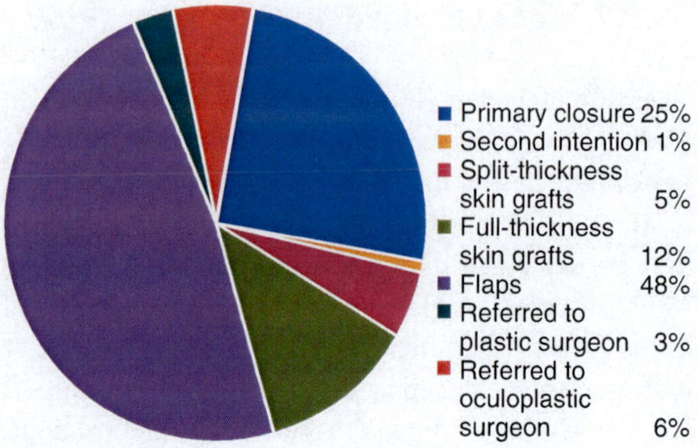

Fig. 43.3 Type of closures performed

Over the past decade there has been an increase in both the number of Mohs surgeons in practice and the annual caseload, with almost half of the current Australian Mohs surgeons having completed their Mohs fellowship during this period. Medicare statistics shows the total caseload having increased from 2268 Mohs cases in 1995 to 7757 cases in 2009, representing a per capita increase from 13 cases per 100,000 in 1995 to 35 cases per 100,000 in 2009. This increase may in part be a reflection on the increasing awareness among other medical practitioners of the technique, as evidenced by the largest number of referrals (37%) for Mohs micrographic surgery coming from dermatologists and the next most common from general practitioners (32%). Yet despite this increase in caseload and the high rates of skin cancer seen in Australia, Australian Mohs surgeons perform on average 201–300 cases per year, far fewer than the approximately 1,000 cases performed on average annually by Mohs surgeons in the USA [33].

43.2.3 Conclusion

Many Australian Mohs surgeons blend MMS into busy general and cosmetic dermatology practices, therefore explaining the range in number of cases performed annually in Australia. Given the technique is mostly reserved for tumors on higher-risk areas, it follows that Australian Mohs surgeons are highly skilled in surgical reconstructions. These data present a positive report on the health of Australian MMS with appropriate tumor selection, a strong interest among younger dermatologists and a significant level of experience among its constituents.

Summary: The Australian Mohs Database

- The Australian Mohs database collected data on over 12,000 cases of Mohs surgery between 1993 and 1999.
- Five-year follow-up studies have been published on SCC and BCC cases treated with Mohs surgery in Australia.
- For BCCs, 5-year recurrence rates were 1.4% for primary and 4% for previously recurrent tumors.
- For SCCs, 5-year recurrence rates were 3.9% overall and 8% in those with perineural invasion.
- Perineural invasion was seen in 2.74% of BCCs and 5.95% of SCCs.

43.3 The Australian Mohs Database

43.3.1 Introduction

The Australian Mohs database was established in 1992 and data were collected from January 1993 until 2002. The aim was to capture every Mohs micrographic surgery case performed in Australia, and data collection was centralized at the Skin and Cancer Foundation of Australia in Sydney. While data are no longer being collected, the database has been an unparalleled success and valuable resource for performing long-term follow-up for studies examining recurrence rates post Mohs surgery. The data collected continue to inform ongoing research and publications.

Recent publications based on such follow-up data include two long-term follow-up studies of BCCs and SCCs treated with Mohs surgery [5–7, 11, 12]. These papers reported on 11,127 patients treated for BCC and 1,263 patients treated for SCC. Key findings from these publications are outlined below:

43.3.2 Basal-Cell Carcinoma Treated with Mohs Surgery in Australia

A prospective follow-up study of patients enrolled in the Australian Mohs database included 3,370 patients (1,594 female and 1,776 male patients) at 5 years' follow-up out of 11,127 patients who underwent Mohs surgery for BCC [5]. Of 3,370 patients, 86 had a recurrence at follow-up. Of these 86 patients, 60 had originally been referred for Mohs surgery with a recurrent lesion. The 5-year follow-up study confirmed low 5-year recurrence rates in both primary (1.4%) and previously recurrent tumors (4%).

Perineural invasion (PNI) was examined in a separate article [11]. Of 10,035 patients who underwent MMS and had data recorded on the presence or absence of PNI, 283 showed PNI (2.74%). Of these, 61% were in male patients and 60.4% were previously recurrent tumors. Overall PNI was seen in 3.75% of recurrent BCCs and 1.94% of primary BCCs. Nose, cheek, and forehead were the most common sites. Histologically, 54.1% were infiltrating tumors and 24% were morphemic; the remainder were other types. Basosquamous tumors were also more likely than not to have PNI. Tumors with PNI took more stages to clear than those without PNI (mean of 2.5 vs. 1.72 stages) and were larger. A total of 3,020 patients with data on PNI were followed up at 5 years. Of these 78 had PNI and 6 of these tumors recurred by 5 years (7.7%) vs. 72 of those without PNI (2.4%). All 6 recurrent tumors had been previously recurrent prior to undergoing Mohs surgery and 83% were male.

43.3.3 Squamous Cell Carcinoma Treated with Mohs Micrographic Surgery in Australia

A total of 1263 patients were included over 10 years in the database of which 381 completed 5 years of follow-up; 15 showed recurrence of their tumors (3.9%) [7]. A subset of patients with PNI was also studied. Of the 1,177 patients for whom information invasion was available, 70 were diagnosed with PNI (5.95%). PNI was most common in the auricular area (18 cases, 25.7%), cheek and maxilla (15 cases, 21.4%), and forehead (13 cases, 18.6%), with significant association between forehead location and PNI ($p=0.05$) [12]. Of the 1,177 patients with SCC and data on PNI, 336 completed 5 years of follow-up. Of these 336 patients, 25 initially had PNI, and of these 2 had recurrence at 5 years. This recurrence rate of 8% was significantly higher than for those patients without PNI (3.7%) [12].

43.3.4 Conclusion

The initially small number of Mohs surgeons in Australia, all of whom knew each other, provided a unique opportunity to organize and pool data in a centralized database. This cooperative effort has been extremely useful and productive, and the landmark publications that have resulted have justified the existence and application of this surgical technique in the Australian context. The usefulness and cost effectiveness of Mohs surgery remain an ongoing controversy, and the quality publications that have their genesis in the Australian Mohs database provide a firm evidentiary foundation for what we do.

Summary: Some Useful Aspects of Secondary Intention Wound Healing

- Mohs micrographic surgery and secondary intention wound healing of the nail apparatus for in situ and invasive SCC appear to produce excellent wound healing and cure rate with retention of function.
- In the right patient, secondary intention wound healing of even broad areas of wounding remains a viable option.

43.4 Some Useful Aspects of Secondary Intention Wound Healing

Two instances of secondary intention wound healing will be highlighted: the use in MMS of the nail unit and for extensive scalp disease in a knowledgeable patient.

43.4.1 Mohs for Invasive SCC and SCC In Situ of the Nail Apparatus

Between the years 2000 and 2010, 16 patients (with 17 operated digits) at one institution (Skin and Cancer Foundation of Victoria) underwent MMS for histologically confirmed SCC either invasive (1) or in situ (14) on biopsy [34]. There were ten males and five females with an average age of 54. One patient had polydacty-

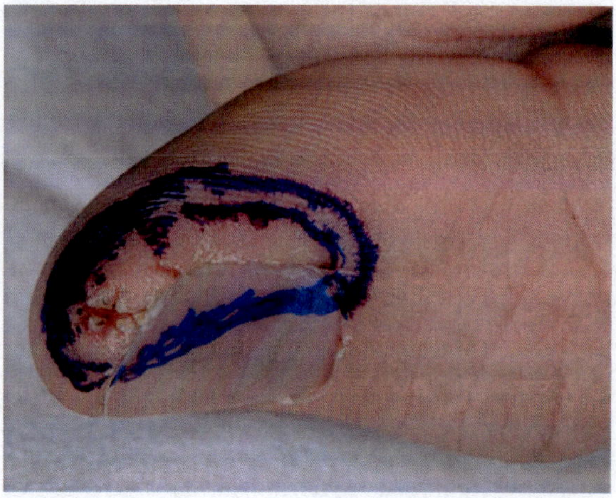

Fig. 43.4 Bowen's disease of R thumb marked for surgery

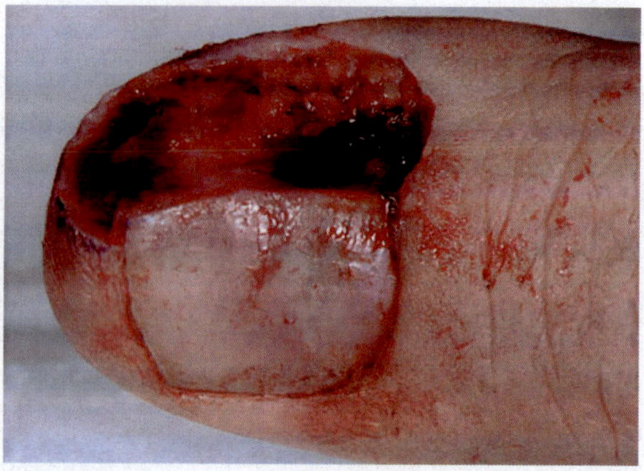

Fig. 43.5 Immediate post Mohs defect of R thumb

lous Bowen's disease and had two fingers operated on in different sessions. This patient also suffered SCC in situ on the foreskin of his penis and underwent circumcision and imiquimod therapy. One patient presented with a right second toe SCC in situ; in all others the fingers were affected (2 ring fingers, 4 middle, 4 index, 3 little, and 3 thumb). Of the fingers eight were on each of left and right sides.

Four patients had not had prior treatment; nine had recurrence after previous therapies. Two patients were uncertain. These therapies included excision (1 case), excision and grafting (1), imiquimod (6), photodynamic therapy (3), fluorouracil (1), topical steroids and antifungal creams (1), and cryotherapy (2).

Of the 17 operations, 8 underwent only 1 stage of micrographic surgery, 7 required 2 stages, and 2 required 3 stages.

Definitive repair was secondary intention in 15, primary closure in 1, and flap repair in 1. No complications were seen with any of the patients treated with secondary intention. Infection and subsequent distal phalanx amputation occurred in the distal flap repair patient. No further operations have been required in any patient, but follow-up on all patients is continuing and will be the subject of a future manuscript.

A typical instructive case is shown in Figs. 43.4–43.7 where a patient who appears to have lost the bulk of their nail apparatus has achieved a satisfactory result, the normal use of their thumb and some regrowth above what would be expected from their immediate

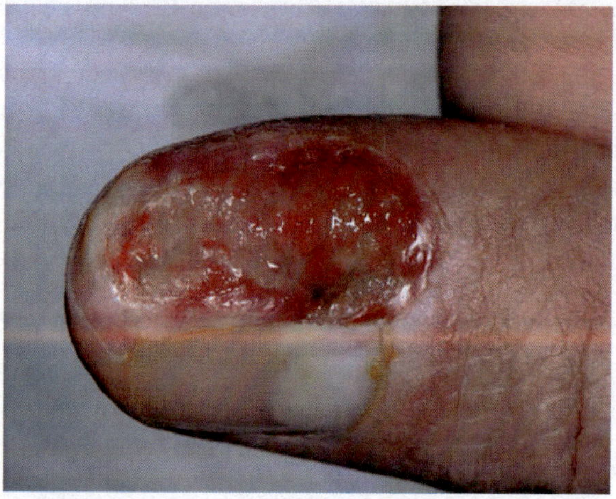

Fig. 43.6 Granulating secondary intention wound of R thumb

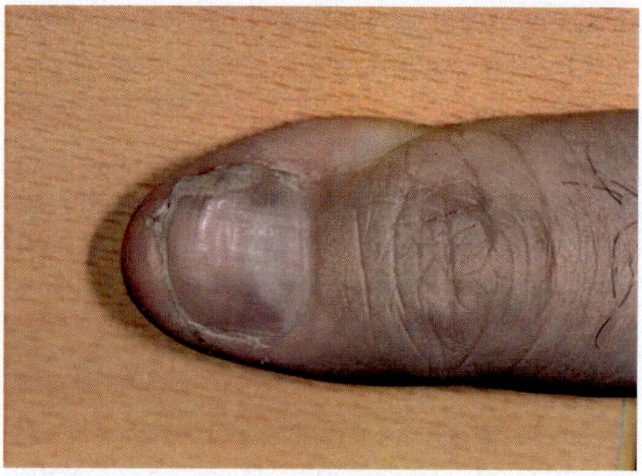

Fig. 43.7 Final result of R thumb showing minor residual onycholysis but with substantial regrowth of nail apparatus

postoperative result; in particular, note should be made of the apparent regrowth of the lunula and increase in width of the nail plate.

43.4.2 Extensive Use of Secondary Wound Healing in a Knowledgeable Patient

A veterinary surgeon underwent MMS for an extensive basal-cell carcinoma of the forehead in 1996. This was allowed to heal by secondary intention. Some 10 years later he represented with further similar tumor in his temple region. This was further treated and the defect again allowed to heal by secondary intention. Unfortunately, at a later date further tumor was identified on further staging biopsies in many disparate sites on the forehead, scalp, and L temple. It was decided to stage his MMS procedures with careful photography and allow incomplete margins along one healing edge, and to address these in further procedures, akin to a serial excision process. Eventually control was gained over his disease process. This approach was only really practical because of this man's broad experience with secondary intention in his treatment of race horse injuries, and in fact he was much more adept at promoting secondary intention wound healing than the Mohs team looking after him.

He continues disease-free after a further 2 years of follow-up (Figs. 43.8–43.13).

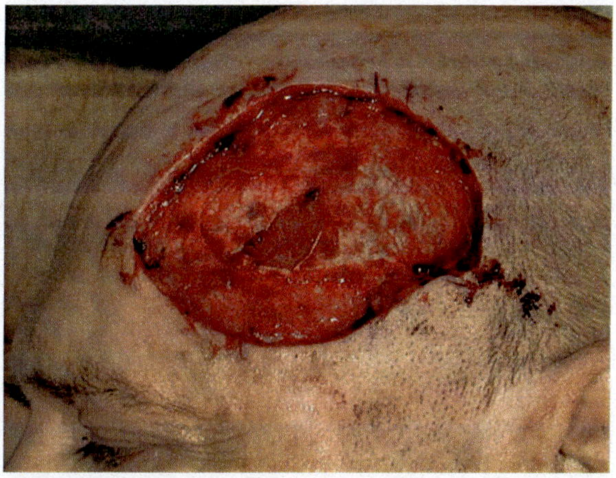

Fig. 43.9 Post Mohs defect of L forehead

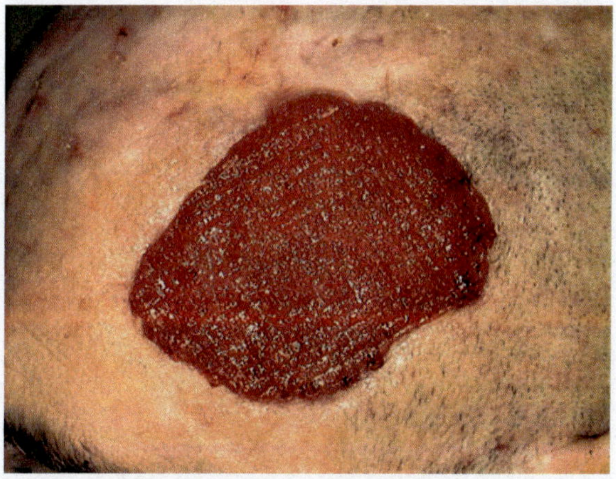

Fig. 43.10 Granulating wound of L forehead

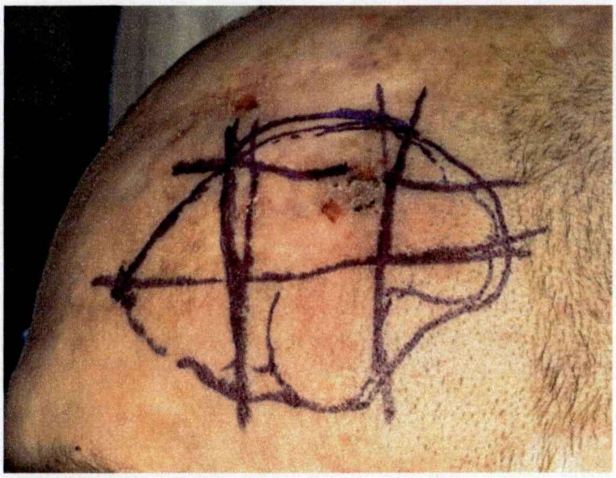

Fig. 43.8 Initial tumor marking of L forehead

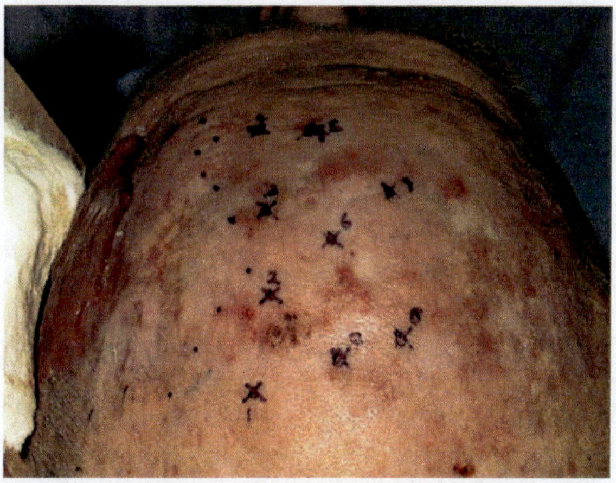

Fig. 43.11 Further tumor outlined center of forehead and scalp

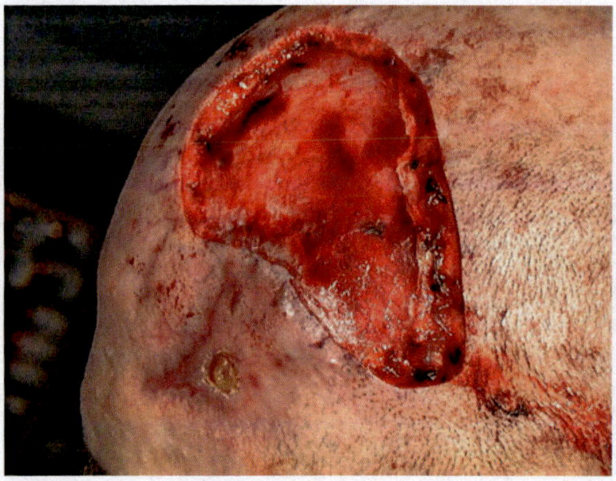

Fig. 43.12 Second excision of Mohs defect

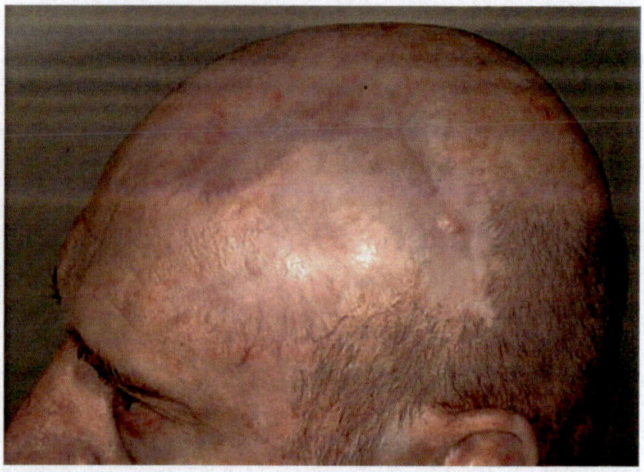

Fig. 43.13 Healing post secondary intention wound healing

Summary: Mohs Surgery in New Zealand

- New Zealand has a very high rate of skin cancer.
- MMS in New Zealand needs to be seen in the context of individuals with widespread sun-damaged skin.
- Multiple facial tumors in a patient are very common, and this and a dysplastic field influence repair options.
- Efficiencies in technique have been enacted to cope with the type of disease seen.

43.5 Mohs Surgery in New Zealand

Dr. Kevin McKerrow was the first New Zealander to complete a college fellowship (Don Grande). As at 2011, there were five college fellows and one ACMS-accredited fellowship training program (P Salmon, Tauranga). In Tauranga our Mohs surgery is related almost exclusively to tumors of the face and scalp (99.8%).

There are some challenges in practicing Mohs surgery in New Zealand. Our rate of skin cancer is similar to that of Queensland, Australia [35]. Happily, many of our family practitioners provide a very good basic skin cancer excision service. But for the Mohs surgeon practicing in New Zealand, certain problems are a unique part of daily practice. We routinely treat patients whose sun-exposed skin is a continuous field of dysplasia, and who present monthly with new tumors on the head and neck.

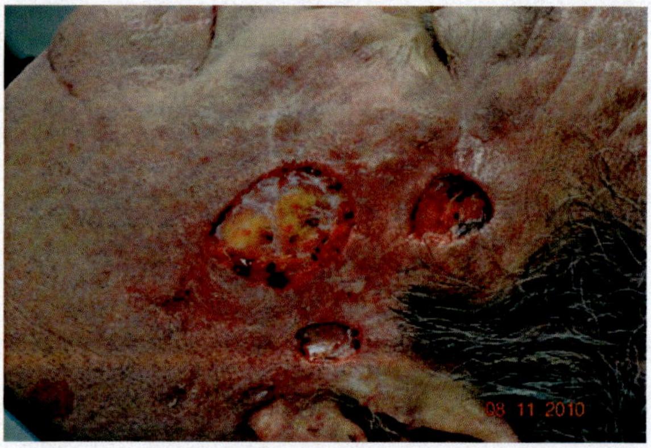

Fig. 43.14 Multiple tumor defects in the same cosmetic field with associated actinic keratosis

Patients presenting with multiple facial tumors are 21% of our Mohs caseload, and 12% have multiple tumors in the same cosmetic unit field (Fig. 43.14) providing challenges for aesthetic reconstruction.

Due to the high level of actinic damage, performing Mohs surgery in an area of field change of actinic keratosis is the norm rather than the exception. Curettage is often inappropriate as tumor surrounded by actinic keratosis may lead to an excessive and inappropriately large curette defect. This is especially a problem in older patients with more-fragile skin. This difficulty means curettage is undertaken cautiously and in a minority of our patients.

Because of the level of actinic damage, it is not uncommon to find additional unexpected tumors in the surgical field during microscopic examination of the processed tissue. There may also be difficulty in interpreting clearance of tumor when excising Bowen's disease, microinvasive SCC, and sometimes superficial basal-cell carcinoma, in patients with extensive actinic dysplasia (field change of solar keratosis, including Bowenoid keratosis and sometimes with areas of more-frank in situ SCC disease).

Rosacea is seen in 78% of patients presenting for Mohs surgery, and does add extra difficulty to the dogmatic exclusion of small amounts of tumor that could be hidden by perifollicular inflammation.

As there is no remunerative incentive related to the number of sections taken during a stage, efficiency has promoted the use of single-section stages and modification of equipment to allow large sections (technician skills in handling large specimens, oversize slides, large chucks, modification of automated stainers, 1.25× microscope objectives). Ninety-four percent of first stages are managed as a single section. Eight percent of stages utilize large format slides (38 mm × 76 mm).

Treatment of lentigo maligna melanoma is generally not undertaken with Mohs surgery in New Zealand because of the difficulty in pinpointing where the lesion finishes and the patient's normal atypical melanocyte population starts. Even with contralateral biopsy, the endpoint can be difficult to pinpoint with authority. Similarly, the risk of false positivity in MEL 5 staining from adjacent pigmented actinic keratoses in the field is a common issue. Reconstruction of defects often presents a compromise between good tissue match with an adjacent local flap or the choice of a less-camouflaged but better-quality full-thickness graft from a sun-protected area. Often the decision in choosing which local flap is preferred will hinge on the likelihood of subclinical unrelated cancer in adjacent tissue.

In summary, practicing Mohs surgery in New Zealand provides many technical challenges.

Summary: Conclusions

- MMS has provided an excellent modality for the treatment of a sun-damaged population prone to difficult skin tumors.
- Most closures are repaired by the operating Mohs surgeon.
- MMS continues to grow as a specialty within Australia and New Zealand and offers a very high cure rate even in awkward areas such as tumors of the nail apparatus.

43.6 Conclusions

Mohs surgery in Australia and New Zealand has had a rich heritage with the Mohs database providing some of the most important data on the procedure, its utility, and long-term success in treating a variety of skin tumors and tumor behaviors. We have a particularly sun-damaged population with many patients exhibiting multiple tumors at initial diagnosis and a sun-damaged field making it difficult both for repair and for judging recurrence.

Excellent and innovative flap repairs have emanated from Australia and New Zealand and would be expected to continue to evolve.

MMS is a rapidly growing subspecialty in Australia with 98% of tumors treated located on head, neck, digits, or genitals and 90% of surgical defects reconstructed by the operating Mohs surgeon.

Mohs micrographic surgery and secondary intention wound healing of the nail apparatus for in situ and invasive SCC appear to produce excellent wound healing and cure rate with retention of function, and in the right patient, secondary intention wound healing of even broad areas of wounding remains a viable option.

References

1. Marks R, Ponsford MW, Selwood TS, Goodman G, Mason G. Non-melanotic skin cancer and solar keratoses in Victoria. Med J Aust. 1983;2(12):619–22.
2. Marks R, Foley P, Goodman G, Hage BH, Selwood TS. Spontaneous remission of solar keratoses: the case for conservative management. Br J Dermatol. 1986;115(6):649–55.
3. Leibovitch I, Huilgol SC, Richards S, Paver R, Selva D. Scalp tumors treated with Mohs micrographic surgery: clinical features and surgical outcome. Dermatol Surg. 2006;32(11):1369–74.
4. Leibovitch I, Huilgol SC, Selva D, Paver R, Richards S. Cutaneous lip tumours treated with Mohs micrographic surgery: clinical features and surgical outcome. Br J Dermatol. 2005;153(6):1147–52.
5. Leibovitch I, Huilgol SC, Selva D, Richards S, Paver R. Basal cell carcinoma treated with Mohs surgery in Australia II. Outcome at 5-year follow-up. J Am Acad Dermatol. 2005;53(3):452–7.
6. Leibovitch I, Huilgol SC, Selva D, Richards S, Paver R. Basal cell carcinoma treated with Mohs surgery in Australia I. Experience over 10 years. J Am Acad Dermatol. 2005;53(3):445–51.
7. Leibovitch I, Huilgol SC, Selva D, Hill D, Richards S, Paver R. Cutaneous squamous cell carcinoma treated with Mohs micrographic surgery in Australia I. Experience over 10 years. J Am Acad Dermatol. 2005;53(2):253–60.

8. Leibovitch I, Huilgol SC, Selva D, Richards S, Paver R. Basosquamous carcinoma: treatment with Mohs micrographic surgery. Cancer. 2005;104(1):170–5.
9. Leibovitch I, Huilgol SC, Selva D, Richards S, Paver R. Cutaneous squamous carcinoma in situ (Bowen's disease): treatment with Mohs micrographic surgery. J Am Acad Dermatol. 2005;52(6):997–1002.
10. Leibovitch I, Huilgol SC, Selva D, Lun K, Richards S, Paver R. Microcystic adnexal carcinoma: treatment with Mohs micrographic surgery. J Am Acad Dermatol. 2005;52(2): 295–300.
11. Leibovitch I, Huilgol SC, Selva D, Richards S, Paver R. Basal cell carcinoma treated with Mohs surgery in Australia III. Perineural invasion. J Am Acad Dermatol. 2005;53(3): 458–63.
12. Leibovitch I, Huilgol SC, Selva D, Hill D, Richards S, Paver R. Cutaneous squamous cell carcinoma treated with Mohs micrographic surgery in Australia II. Perineural invasion. J Am Acad Dermatol. 2005;53(2):261–6.
13. Malhotra R, James CL, Selva D, Huynh N, Huilgol SC. The Australian Mohs database: periocular squamous intraepidermal carcinoma. Ophthalmology. 2004;111(10):1925–9.
14. Leibovitch I, Huilgol SC, Hsuan JD, Selva D. Incidence of host site complications in periocular full thickness skin grafts. Br J Ophthalmol. 2005;89(2):219–22.
15. Leibovitch I, Huilgol SC, Richards S, Paver R, Selva D. Periocular microcystic adnexal carcinoma: management and outcome with Mohs' micrographic surgery. Ophthalmologica. 2006;220(2):109–13.
16. Malhotra R, Huilgol SC, Huynh NT, Selva D. The Australian Mohs database: periocular squamous cell carcinoma. Ophthalmology. 2004;111(4):617–23.
17. Malhotra R, Huilgol SC, Huynh NT, Selva D. The Australian Mohs database, part I: periocular basal cell carcinoma experience over 7 years. Ophthalmology. 2004;111(4):624–30.
18. Malhotra R, Huilgol SC, Huynh NT, Selva D. The Australian Mohs database, part II: periocular basal cell carcinoma outcome at 5-year follow-up. Ophthalmology. 2004;111(4): 631–6.
19. Huilgol SC, Selva D, Chen C, Hill DC, James CL, Gramp A, et al. Surgical margins for lentigo maligna and lentigo maligna melanoma: the technique of mapped serial excision. Arch Dermatol. 2004;140(9):1087–92.
20. Kumar B, Roden D, Vinciullo C, Elliott T. A review of 24 cases of Mohs surgery and ophthalmic plastic reconstruction. Aust N Z J Ophthalmol. 1997;25(4):289–93.
21. Limawararut V, Leibovitch I, Sullivan T, Selva D. Periocular squamous cell carcinoma. Clin Experiment Ophthalmol. 2007;35(2):174–85.
22. Chan FM, O'Donnell BA, Whitehead K, Ryman W, Sullivan TJ. Treatment and outcomes of malignant melanoma of the eyelid: a review of 29 cases in Australia. Ophthalmology. 2007;114(1):187–92. Epub November 30, 2006.
23. Ooi CG, James CL, Huilgol SC. Metastatic Bowen carcinoma. Australas J Dermatol. 2006;47(4):277–80.
24. Leibovitch I, Selva D, Huilgol S, Davis G, Dodd T, James CL. Intraepithelial sebaceous carcinoma of the eyelid misdiagnosed as Bowen's disease. J Cutan Pathol. 2006;33(4): 303–8.
25. Ly H, Selva D, James CL, Huilgol SC. Superficial malignant fibrous histiocytoma presenting as recurrent atypical fibroxanthoma. Australas J Dermatol. 2004;45(2):106–9.
26. Lai TF, Huilgol SC, Selva D, James CL. Eyelid sebaceous carcinoma masquerading as in situ squamous cell carcinoma. Dermatol Surg. 2004;30(2 Pt 1):222–5.
27. Kearney C, Sheridan A, Vinciullo C, Elliott T. A tunneled and turned-over nasolabial flap for reconstruction of full thickness nasal ala defects. Dermatol Surg. 2010;36(8):1319–24. Epub June 24, 2010.
28. Salmon P, Stanway A. Nasalis flap and graft repair provides reliable closure for denuded defects of the nose. Dermatol Surg. 2005;31(6):692–6.
29. Smith H, Elliot T, Vinciullo C. Repair of nasal tip and alar defects using cheek-based 2-stage flaps: an alternative to the median forehead flap. Arch Dermatol. 2003;139(8):1033–6.
30. Salmon PJ, Mortimer NJ, Hill SE. Muscular hinge flaps: utility and technique in facial reconstructive surgery. Dermatol Surg. 2010;36(2):227–34.
31. Tan E, Mortimer NJ, Hussain W, Salmon PJ. The nasal sidewall rotation flap: a workhorse flap for small defects of the distal nose. Dermatol Surg. 2010;36(10):1563–7.
32. Lim P, Paver R, Peñas PF. Mohs micrographic surgery at the Skin and Cancer Foundation Australia, 10 years later (1997 vs. 2007). J Am Acad Dermatol. 2010;63(5):832–5.
33. Campbell RM, Perlis CS, Mohsin K, et al. Characteristics of Mohs practices in the United States: a recall survey of ACMS surgeons. Dermatol Surg. 2007;33:1413–8.
34. Goodman GJ, Tuxen AJ. Mohs micrographic surgery and subsequent secondary intention wound healing for squamous cell carcinoma and Bowen's disease of the nail unit. In preparation.
35. Salmon PJM et al. Extremely high levels of melanoma in Tauranga, New Zealand: possible causes and comparisons with Australia and the northern hemisphere. Australas J Dermatol. 2007;48(4):208–16.

44 Information for Patients and Safety Considerations

Ilya Reyter, Abel Torres, and Neda Mehr

Abstract

The proper execution of Mohs surgery requires proper planning. Both patient and physician alike must be adequately prepared for the procedure in order to optimize outcomes and enhance safety. For the Mohs surgeon, this entails maximizing the preoperative visit, where the patient can be properly assessed for any conditions or comorbidities that may pose a real or potential risk to the patient during or after the procedure. The Mohs surgeon should be well versed on safety issues commonly encountered in skin cancer patients, such as cardiovascular complications, antibiotic prophylaxis for infections, anticoagulation issues, and anesthesia safety. Patients should also be educated about the procedure as well as their role in postoperative care. Staff must also be informed about office safety protocols and should be trained on how to respond to potential office emergencies.

Keywords

Mohs • Surgical complications • Patient safety • Patient information • Preoperative evaluation • Preoperative planning • Staff safety

Summary: Introduction

- Preparation is critical for success in surgery.

44.1 Introduction

Proper planning is central to the success of any endeavor. Mohs surgery is no exception and requires planning by both the physician and the patient to optimize outcomes. The physician must take proper measures to educate his patients and staff about the potential pitfalls of Mohs surgery, so as to insure the safety of the patient and staff alike. For everyone involved with surgery, an old adage holds true: To be forewarned is to be forearmed.

I. Reyter • A. Torres (✉) • N. Mehr
Department of Dermatology,
Loma Linda University School of Medicine,
Loma Linda, CA, USA
e-mail: abelt@aol.com; cmorrill@llu.edu

K. Nouri (ed.), *Mohs Micrographic Surgery*,
DOI 10.1007/978-1-4471-2152-7_44, © Springer-Verlag London Limited 2012

Summary: Patient Safety Considerations
- The preoperative evaluation is an important part of Mohs surgery.
- Key parts of the medical record are best verified for accuracy prior to surgery.
- A detailed preoperative history and physical exam can uncover important patient safety issues.

44.2 Patient Safety Considerations

The first step of ensuring patient safety during Mohs surgery is the preoperative evaluation. The preoperative visit provides an ideal venue for the physician to evaluate a patient's overall health status, screen for any conditions that pose a threat to safe execution of the surgery or recovery from the procedure, and educate the patient about his or her role in Mohs surgery. By establishing rapport during this visit, the Mohs surgeon can bring the patient into the "team" thereby helping to enhance outcomes and simultaneously screen for any comorbidities that pose safety issues before, during, or after surgery.

44.2.1 The Preoperative Visit

In a busy Mohs surgical practice, it is tempting to view the preoperative visit as a mere formality and rush through it on the way to more "important" or lucrative work. However, this would not be advisable, as, by doing so, one could miss a critical first step in planning for a successful outcome. In the authors' experience, mistakes occur when assumptions are not verified. Here, it is best to follow the proverb made famous by President Ronald Reagan: "Trust but verify."

For instance, physicians, staff, and patients typically assume that prior medical records are correct and complete. However, it is not uncommon for seasoned Mohs surgeons to tell of multiple instances of inconsistencies in patients' accompanying medical records, such as conflicting information on the anatomic site of the cancer or the type of cancer itself.

Whether the Mohs surgeon is dealing with a preexisting patient or a referral from a colleague, it is a good habit to assemble the prior records prior to surgery and assess them for accuracy and consistency. In Mohs surgery, a prior biopsy has almost always been done. It is very helpful if the pathology report is present at the preoperative visit, and, if so, the date of biopsy and site of biopsy should be verified with the patient. Again, it is best to trust the report, but nonetheless verify with the patient the most pertinent facts. The authors find it useful to hand the patient a mirror and ask the patient to point out where the biopsy was performed. This spot is marked and matched against the spot indicated on the pathology report and any chart notes or photographs. This step helps in identifying and correcting possible errors in previous charting. If an error is located or a patient indicates a site different from that supported by the records, additional information is often requested from the referring physician and the inconsistency cleared before proceeding. By adhering to these principles whenever possible, the authors have identified and corrected charting and lab errors that could have potentially resulted in wrong-site and wrong-diagnosis surgery.

44.2.2 Past Medical History and Physical Exam

Another key step in the preoperative evaluation is taking a detailed history and physical exam. Granted, Mohs surgery has a very low incidence of complications. In fact, a recent evaluation by Cook and Perone reported the incidence of complications associated with Mohs to be 1.64% [1]. However, as anyone doing Mohs can attest, it is definitely not risk-free. In the process of performing a thorough history and physical, the surgeon can identify factors that pose real or potential safety issues. For instance, patients may have sensitivities to local anesthetics, have conditions that inhibit proper wound healing, have risk factors for infection, or be on medications that predispose them to bleeding or inhibit appropriate immune responses.

These, and other topics, frequently come up in the course of discussing a detailed past medical history. Patients are then given information and specific recommendations to help plan for a successful surgical outcome. The following is information useful to patient education and surgical planning.

Summary: Information for Patients

- While Mohs surgery has a very low rate of complications, there are still some important safety considerations for patients to consider preoperatively.
- Cardiovascular complications can be related to discontinuation of anticoagulants as well as use of electrosurgery in the presence of implanted cardiac devices.
- Antibiotic prophylaxis is important for select patients, but is likely unnecessary for routine use in all patients.
- Local anesthesia surgery has many advantages, but physicians and patients should be aware of its limitations.

44.3 Information for Patients

44.3.1 Cardiovascular Complications

Mohs micrographic surgery is an inherently safe procedure with few major complications or cardiovascular events. While there have been reported thrombotic events during or immediately after Mohs surgery, these are often associated with *discontinuation* of anticoagulant medications [2, 3]. Such medications include warfarin (Coumadin), heparin, aspirin, and clopidogrel (Plavix). Commonly, patients inquire about stopping their anticoagulation medications prior to surgery, as they may assume that these medications predispose them to bleeding complications during surgery. However, patients should be informed that the decision to stop anticoagulant medications must not be taken lightly, as this discontinuation may predispose them to thromboembolic complications. Recommendations concerning anticoagulants in dermatologic surgery have been published, and they are summarized later in the chapter.

Additional cardiovascular issues involve pacemakers and implantable cardiac devices (ICD), and these are also useful to share with patients. These devices are becoming increasingly common in the treatment of cardiac disease. It is not uncommon to encounter patients with these devices needing electrosurgery at the time of Mohs surgery. Although technological improvements have made the implantable devices more resistant to electromagnetic interference, there still is a risk of potentially serious consequences [4–7]. Electrosurgery can cause implanted cardiac units to malfunction through several different mechanisms, including reprogramming, battery depletion, or direct damage to the device [8, 9]. Likewise, electrosurgery can stimulate other implanted electrical devices, such as central nervous system (CNS) devices.

It is a good habit to screen for the presence of an implanted cardiac (or neurological) device during the preoperative history and physical. If a pacemaker, ICD, or nerve stimulator is in fact present, a Mohs surgeon can follow recommended precautions that have appeared in the dermatologic literature [4]. In selected patients with cardiac disease, these precautions can include obtaining a baseline electrocardiographic study prior to surgery. Such testing can screen for pacemaker-dependent patients, who may be unable to tolerate unit malfunction from electromagnetic interference. Additional recommendations include the use of bipolar forceps, which may cause minimal interference, and/or electrocautery (heat cautery), which causes no interference [8, 10–12]. If the latter options are not available, another recommendation is to avoid the use of electrosurgery within 15 cm of the device, using short bursts of electricity, placing grounding plates as far from the device as possible, using minimal power, and avoiding cutting current, which is more likely to cause interference [4]. A final option is that the device in question can be turned off for the procedure and then reactivated after the procedure is completed. In the authors' experience, the latter approach is not as effective for nerve stimulators, as it can lead to uncontrolled muscle tremors.

Published recommendations regarding cardiac devices include the suggestion that patients have preoperative and postoperative cardiology evaluation if electrosurgery is used, while others have suggested that such evaluation is made unnecessary by using only electrocautery (heat cautery) or bipolar forceps for hemostasis during the procedure [4, 8, 10–12]. If the surgeon has any doubt about the status of the implanted device during surgery or should the patient have any cardiac related symptoms, postoperative interrogation of the unit can help rule out damage to the device.

In any case, as with most patient safety issues, it is wise to have a protocol in place should a patient with an implanted cardiac or neurological unit need surgical care. Such protocols may help identify patients who

Table 44.1 Antibiotic prophylaxis – high- and low-risk conditions

High-risk conditions	Low-risk conditions
For infective endocarditis:	For infective endocarditis:
• Prosthetic heart valve	• Pacemaker
• History of bacterial endocarditis	• Vascular stents (peripheral or coronary)
• Congenital cardiac malformation	• Vascular grafts
• Unrepaired cyanotic malformations	
• Completely repaired congenital defects using prosthetic device, in the first 6 months postprocedure	
• Repaired congenital defect with residual deficits	
• Heart transplant recipients who subsequently develop valve disease	
For hematogenous joint infection:	
• First 2 years after joint replacement	
• Prior history of prosthetic joint infection	
• Immunocompromised or immunosuppressed patients	
• HIV	
• Malignancy	
• Malnutrition	
• Insulin-dependent diabetes	
• Hemophilia	
For surgical site infections:	
• Leg	
• Groin	
• Skin graft	
• Skin flap on nose	
• Wedge excision of the ear or lip	
• Inflammatory skin disease (extensive)	

Data compiled from references [15, 17]

need to obtain cardiology or neurological consultations and can ensure that the office has the requisite equipment to facilitate patient safety during the surgery day. For such situations, the authors find it helpful to always have ready-to-use bipolar forceps and cords as well as new, disposable electrocautery (heat cautery) units.

44.3.2 Antibiotic Prophylaxis

Mohs surgery is best considered to be a clean or clean-contaminated procedure rather than a sterile procedure [13, 14]. After all, during Mohs surgery, patients undergo serial rounds of excisions and bandaging and often leave the surgical area while the tissue is being processed. This is very different from traditional sterile technique in the operating room. Frequently questions arise from patients about the need for antibiotics. Therefore, during the preoperative visit, it is helpful to inform patients about the low infection rates of Mohs surgery. It may be useful to discuss studies like the one performed by Maragh and Brown, which prospectively evaluated 1,000 consecutive patients undergoing Mohs surgery without postoperative antibiotics [15]. That study reported a surgical site infection rate of 0.7%. This low rate of infection is excellent and is more consistent with "clean" procedures, in which a 1–3% infection rate is acceptable [16].

Simultaneously, in the preoperative visit, the surgeon can screen for any conditions that may warrant the use of antibiotics. A recent advisory statement regarding indications for antibiotic prophylaxis in dermatologic surgery was published by Wright et al. in the Journal of the American Academy of Dermatology in 2008 [17]. It was based on the updated guidelines of the American Heart Association, the American Dental Association, with the American Academy of Orthopaedic Surgeons. It details antibiotic prophylaxis for the prevention of infective endocarditis, hematogenous total joint infection, and surgical site infection

Table 44.2 Antibiotic recommendations for prophylaxis of endocarditis and hematogenous total joint infection in dermatologic surgery

Site	Antibiotic	Dose[a]
Skin	Cephalexin	2 g PO
	Dicloxicillin	2 g PO
	Clindamycin[b]	600 mg PO
	Azithromycin/ clarithromycin[b]	500 mg PO
Oral lesions and nasal mucosa	Amoxicillin	2 g PO
	Clindamycin[b]	600 mg PO
	Azithromycin/ clarithromycin[b]	500 mg PO

Data adapted from reference [17]
[a]All are single dose, given 30–60 min preoperatively
[b]Alternate medication for penicillin allergic patients

Table 44.3 Antibiotic recommendations for prophylaxis of surgical site infection

Surgical site	Antibiotic	Dose[a]
Wedge excision (lip or ear); any skin graft; flaps on nose	Cephalexin	2 g PO
	Dicloxicillin	2 g PO
	Clindamycin[b]	600 mg PO
	Azithromycin/ clarithromycin[b]	500 mg PO
Groin and lower extremity lesions	Cephalexin	2 g PO
	TMP-SMX-DS[b]	1 tablet PO
	Levofloxacin[b]	500 mg PO

Data adapted from reference [17]
[a]All are single dose, given 30–60 min preoperatively. However, may consider extended course of antibiotic treatment (e.g., 1 week, in addition to preoperative dose) for patients at high risk
[b]Alternate medication for penicillin-allergic patients

for patients with an increased risk for developing these infections. Drawing on recent evidence, the authors outline the types of patients and procedures that would benefit from antibiotic prophylaxis (summarized as part of Tables 44.1–44.3). While this publication indicates that routine, prophylactic administration of antibiotics for all skin surgery is likely unnecessary, it is also just a guideline, and the Mohs surgeon should take the unique characteristics of each case into account when making antibiotic prophylaxis decisions.

44.3.3 Anticoagulation

Patients taking some form of blood-thinning agent, either as a prescribed medication or an herbal supplement, are common to dermatology surgery practices (Table 44.4). In a careful history and physical, the surgeon can uncover use of these agents. Patients often inherently understand that blood thinners predispose them to some degree of prolonged bleeding, and can express concern about the use of these medications during surgery. Also, given the choice, many surgeons would likely prefer to work on patients with normal blood clotting functions. So there may be temptation by physicians and patients alike to temporarily discontinue the anticoagulant medication(s).

Table 44.4 Anticoagulant medications

Medically necessary/prescription	Herbal/nonprescription
Warfarin (Coumadin)	Vitamin E
Asprin	Fish oil
Clopidogrel (Plavix)	Feverfew
Heparin	Garlic
Low molecular weight heparin	Ginko
	Ginseng
	Ginger
	Green tea extract
	Alcohol

Data adapted from reference [3]

However, the decision to stop any medically necessary anticoagulants should not be taken lightly. As mentioned previously, it is very helpful to inform patients that stopping their anticoagulants is not a riskless endeavor. Kovich and Otley investigated thrombotic complications related to discontinuation of warfarin and aspirin therapy for dermatologic surgery procedures. They uncovered thrombotic events and even deaths related to simply the cessation of aspirin, and found them to be comparable to the adverse events related to the cessation of warfarin [18]. This finding was particularly interesting and contradicted the previous reports that suggested that stopping aspirin was not associated with the complications of stopping warfarin [19]. Additionally, for cutaneous surgery such as Mohs, ample evidence indicates that there is no significant increased frequency and or severity of bleeding complications in patients taking blood thinners [20–24].

Taken together, this information suggests that the risks of routine discontinuation of medically necessary blood thinners for dermatologic surgery likely exceed any potential benefits. This is especially true with Mohs surgery, and patients should be counseled preoperatively on this subject. Many patients taking these medications are older, and may still recall prior, outdated recommendations regarding blood thinners and surgery. As a potential thrombotic complication can be a far greater patient safety hazard than a post-operative bleeding complication, any counseling is time well spent with the patient. After all, most intra-operative and postoperative cutaneous bleeding complications can be managed with pressure, cautery, and/or vessel ligation. The risk of blood loss severe enough to cause significant morbidity or mortality during Mohs surgery is remote.

However, a patient's care should be individualized. If a patient's unique circumstances necessitate the discontinuation of medically necessary blood thinners, it is preferable to work with the prescribing physician to stop and restart the anticoagulants. For non-medically necessary blood-thinning agents, such as herbs (ginko, garlic, etc.), supplements (fish oil, vitamin E, etc.), or aspirin taken purely for preventative purposes, the dermatologic surgeon may choose to recommend that the patient forgo taking them 10–14 days prior to the procedure and then 5–7 days postoperatively [25].

44.3.4 Anesthesia

Mohs surgery and subsequent reconstruction are commonly performed using only local anesthesia, and patients are usually informed of this at the preoperative visit. Patients have become accustomed to the idea of surgery under local anesthesia, and in fact, often express relief that they will not need general anesthesia. However, there are patients who may not be comfortable with the idea of being awake for any type of surgery. The surgeon would be wise to advise patients of the risks and benefits of local as well as general anesthesia, emphasizing the outstanding safety record of procedures using local anesthesia only.

The safety of office-based surgery under local anesthesia has been the focus of much recent interest and study. Florida and other states have instituted mandatory reporting of office surgery deaths and injuries, and the generated data further supports the superior safety of office-based, local anesthesia surgery [26]. In fact, the complication rate for office-based procedures commonly performed by a dermatologist is reported to be <0.5% [27]. After citing the safety data to patients, the authors find that patients prefer the local anesthesia option.

The typical local anesthetic employed for most dermatologic surgery, including Mohs, is 0.5–2% lidocaine with epinephrine. For nontumescent anesthesia procedures, such as Mohs surgery, the recommended maximum dosage of lidocaine in adults is 4.5 mg/kg without epinephrine and 7.0 mg/kg with epinephrine. In tumescent anesthesia used for liposuction, the maximum recommended dosage is 35–55 mg/kg [25]. Symptoms of lidocaine toxicity are directly related to the serum lidocaine level, and include, at the early stages, circumoral paresthesia, tinnitus, visual disturbances, slurred speech, and muscle twitching. Finally, seizure, coma, and cardiac arrest occur at high levels of lidocaine overdose [28, 29].

Lidocaine toxicity is a concern during Mohs surgery, especially for larger tumors requiring prolonged procedures. Addressing this issue, Alam et al. prospectively evaluated the serum lidocaine concentration of patients undergoing Mohs surgery [30]. The patients required from 5 to 48 mL of lidocaine 1% with 1:200,000 epinephrine for the procedures. The study patients underwent serial blood draws over a span of up to 8 h to measure peak serum lidocaine concentrations. The highest serum lidocaine level detected at any time for any patient was 0.3 μg/mL. This was far below the threshold for objective signs of lidocaine toxicity such as tinnitus, paresthesias, and muscle twitching, which occurs at about 5 μg/mL, or roughly 16 times the peak levels observed in the study [31]. Seizures, coma, and respiratory arrest typically require even greater serum lidocaine concentrations, typically exceeding 9 μg/mL [28, 29].

If a patient has a history of anxiety surrounding surgical procedures, it is helpful to have an anxiolytic medication, such as lorazepam, available at time of local anesthesia surgery, and to inform patients of this option. Should the anxiolytic be necessary, the patient would generally be advised to avoid operating a motor vehicle and would need to arrange alternative means of transportation.

44.3.5 Allergies

It is very useful to elicit a careful medication allergy history from the patient. The physician must also differentiate from true allergic reactions to medications, such as a rash from penicillin, and sensitivity or adverse reactions to compounds. It is not uncommon for patients and healthcare workers alike to confuse adverse reactions, such as nausea from opiates or palpitations from epinephrine with a true type I (immediate) or type IV (delayed) hypersensitivity reaction to medication.

Summary: Planning for the Surgical Day

- Even minor procedures can incite patient anxiety.
- Preparing the patient for what to expect on the day of surgery and during the postoperative course can help reduce potential stress surrounding Mohs surgery.

44.4 Planning for the Surgical Day

Patients typically appreciate information on what to expect the day of surgery, as this greatly allays their anxiety about the procedure. In addition to providing them the aforementioned information during the preoperative visit, patients are informed that Mohs surgery can be a lengthy procedure, and they should plan on being in the office for at least a few hours. They are asked to shower either the day of surgery or the day prior, and they are instructed to eat a normal meal before surgery and to bring snacks and reading materials with them to the office.

If the surgical site is around the eyes where a postoperative bandage can interfere with vision, the patient is then told to avoid driving themselves home from the procedure and to arrange alternate transportation. Similarly, as stated previously, if the patient requires an anxiolytic medication on the day of surgery, such as lorazepam (Ativan) or diazepam (Valium), or any other medication that can impair cognition, they will be instructed to avoid driving until the effects of the medications wear off.

Postoperative wound care is typically straightforward. However, if a patient lives alone or is elderly and it is suspected that he may have difficulty complying with wound care instructions, it is usually best to have the patient enlist the help of a friend or family member after surgery.

Summary: Office Safety Considerations

- Planning for emergencies helps ensure appropriate responses in stressful situations.
- The Mohs surgeon is well served by playing an active role in ensuring the safety of patients as well as staff.

44.5 Office Safety Considerations

It is most useful to have an office prepared to handle serious patient and staff complications. Just as it is important to prepare for fire with fire extinguisher and evacuation plan, it is good practice to prepare for patient and staff emergencies.

44.5.1 Patient Emergencies

Although state laws may vary on the need for the availability of crash carts and personnel trained in ACLS (advanced cardiac life support), it is of great benefit to nonetheless prepare for emergencies that may arise. At the minimum, personnel should be familiar with BLS (basic life support). Appropriate algorithms should be in place to stabilize a patient until paramedics can arrive and transport the patient to the emergency room, if necessary. Staff should be encouraged to rehearse the steps for an emergency patient situation, and duties may be assigned ahead of time to help prevent confusion and disorder at the time of an emergency.

From managing anaphylactic reactions to cardiac events, proper stock of emergency supplies is important. Newer generation automatic external cardiac defibrillator units (AEDs) can even be operated by the lay public, and, at minimum, such devices are very useful to have in the office or surgical center to handle cardiac emergencies. Staff should be familiarized with location and use of the devices. Emergency medications, such as epinephrine for anaphylaxis and benzodiazepines for seizure, can be helpful and, if made available, should be reviewed regularly. Periodic mock drills may be helpful in reinforcing core concepts and helping physicians and staff alike to anticipate and properly manage emergency situations.

44.5.2 Staff Safety

Medical personnel regularly work around potentially infectious as well as toxic agents. State and federal workplace regulations provide guidelines for medical staff safety, and the adoption of universal precautions has done much to reinforce the concept that prevention of exposure is paramount. However, errors and accidents do occur, and it is wise to include personnel exposure algorithms to any office emergency procedures.

Medical staff should be aware of risk of exposure to bacterial and viral pathogens, as well as postexposure protocols, including information on decontamination and up-to-date recommendations about prophylactic medication use. For instance, personnel should have information about proper protective equipment and sharps handling, as well as whom to contact in the event of accidental exposure, such as a needle stick. Also, they should be aware that use of postexposure prophylaxis against HIV is most effective if initiated without delay [32].

The United States Department of Labor Occupational Safety and Health Administration (OSHA) provides many guidelines and federal regulations concerning medical office personnel safety. Much of this information can now be found online (www.osha.gov).

44.5.3 Mohs Lab Safety

Ensuring the safety of those working to section and stain tissue in a Mohs lab is an important task. If the Mohs physician owns the practice, this responsibility ultimately rests on him. There are multiple state and federal regulations that apply to Mohs labs, such as those issues by OSHA and Clinical Laboratory Improvement Amendments (CLIA). An entire chapter, if not a whole textbook, can easily be devoted to these dictates, which cover everything from storage of staining reagents to maintaining adequate ventilation to providing staff with appropriate protective equipment.

Updated CLIA information can be found through state health service agencies or from the federal department of Health and Human Services (available online at http://www.cms.gov/clia). Additional information may be obtained from the American Academy of Dermatology and the American College of Mohs Surgery.

Summary: Conclusion

- Mohs surgery has an excellent safety record, but complications can still occur.
- A Mohs surgeon can optimize surgical outcomes through adequate preparation, planning, and patient screening.

44.6 Conclusion

Skin cancer surgery, like any surgical procedure, has inherent risks, and complications can occur. However, many of the risks can be mitigated by proper patient selection, adequate planning, and careful surgical technique. Physicians who take measures to educate themselves, their staff, and their patients on up-to-date recommendations and safety information are usually rewarded with fewer surprises and superior results.

References

1. Cook JL, Perone JB. A prospective evaluation of the incidence of complications associated with Mohs micrographic surgery. Arch Dermatol. 2003;139:143–52.
2. Kouba DJ, Moy RL. Complications and pitfalls of skin cancer surgery/Mohs micrographic surgery. In: Nouri K, editor. Complications in dermatologic surgery. Philadelphia: Mosby Elsevier; 2008. p. 37–63.
3. Otley CC. Continuation of medically necessary aspirin and warfarin during cutaneous surgery. Mayo Clin Proc. 2003;78:1392–6.
4. Matzke TJ, Christenson LJ, Christenson SD, Atanashova N, Otley CC. Pacemakers and implantable cardiac defibrillators in dermatologic surgery. Dermatol Surg. 2006;32:1155–62.
5. Aggarwal A, Farber NE, Kotter GS, Dhamee MS. Electrosurgery-induced ventricular fibrillation during pacemaker replacement: a unique mechanism. J Clin Monit. 1996;12:339–42.
6. Kellow NH. Pacemaker failure during transurethral resection of the prostate. Anaesthesia. 1993;48:136–8.
7. Krull EA, Pickard SD, Hall JC. Effects of electrosurgery on cardiac pacemakers. J Dermatol Surg. 1975;1:43–5.
8. El-Gamal HM, Dufresne RG, Saddler K. Electrosurgery, pacemaker and ICDs: a survey of precautions and complications experienced by cutaneous surgeons. Dermatol Surg. 2001;27:385–90.
9. Hayes DL, Vliestra RE. Pacemaker malfunction. Ann Intern Med. 1993;119:828–35.
10. Fader DJ, Johnson TM. Medical issues and emergencies in the dermatology office. J Am Acad Dermatol. 1997;36:1–16.

11. Epsein MR, Mayer Jr JE, Duncan BW. Use of an ultrasonic scalpel as an alternative to electrocautery in patients with pacemakers. Ann Thorac Surg. 1998;65:1802–4.
12. Stenquist BC, Holt PJ, Motley RJ. Computerized bipolar diathermy with scissors and forceps in cutaneous surgery. Dermatol Surg. 2002;28:601–2.
13. Rhinehart BM, Murphy ME, Farley MF, Albertini JG. Sterile versus nonsterile gloves during Mohs micrographic surgery: infection rate is not affected. Dermatol Surg. 2006;32:170–6.
14. Whitaker DC, Grande DJ, Johnson SS. Wound infection rates in dermatologic surgery. J Dermatol Surg Oncol. 1988;14:525–8.
15. Maragh S, Brown M. Prospective evaluation of surgical site infection rate among patients with Mohs micrographic surgery without the use of prophylactic antibiotics. J Am Acad Dermatol. 2008;59:275–8.
16. Dineen P. Prevention and treatment of deep wound infections. In: The surgical wound. Media: Lea & Febiger; 1981. p. 146–9.
17. Wright TI, Baddour LM, Berbari EF, et al. Antibiotic prophylaxis in dermatologic surgery: advisory statement 2008. J Am Acad Dermatol. 2008;59:464–73.
18. Kovich O, Otley CC. Thrombotic complications related to discontinuation of warfarin and aspirin therapy perioperatively for cutaneous operation. J Am Acad Dermatol. 2003;48:233–7.
19. Goldsmith SM, Leshin B, Owen J. Management of patients taking anticoagulants and platelet inhibitors prior to dermatologic surgery. J Dermatol Surg Oncol. 1993;19:578–81.
20. Otley CC, Fewkes JL, Frank W, Olbrich SM. Complications of cutaneous surgery in patients who are taking warfarin, aspirin, or nonsteroidal anti-inflammatory drugs. Arch Dermatol. 1996;132:161–6.
21. Billingsley EM, Maloney ME. Intraoperative and postoperative bleeding problems in patients taking warfarin, aspirin, and nonsteroidal anti-inflammatory agents: a prospective study. Dermatol Surg. 1997;23:381–3.
22. Bartlett GR. Does aspirin affect the outcome of minor cutaneous surgery? Br J Plast Surg. 1999;52:214–6.
23. Lawrence C, Sakuntabhai A, Tiling-Grosse S. Effect of aspirin and nonsteroidal anti-inflammatory drug therapy on bleeding complications in dermatologic surgical patients. J Am Acad Dermatol. 1994;31:988–92.
24. Alcalay J. Cutaneous surgery in patients receiving warfarin therapy. Dermatol Surg. 2001;27:756–8.
25. Ostad A, Kageyama N, Moy RL. Tumescent anesthesia with a lidocaine dose of 55 mg/kg is safe for liposuction. Dermatol Surg. 1996;22:921–7.
26. Venkat AP, Coldiron B, Balkrishnan R, Camacho F, Hancox JG, Fleischer Jr AB, et al. Lower adverse event and mortality rates in physician offices compared with ambulatory surgery centers: a reappraisal of Florida adverse event data. Dermatol Surg. 2004;30(12 pt 1):1444–51.
27. Elston DM, Taylor JS, Coldiron B, Hood AF, Read SI, Resneck JS, et al. Patient safety. Part I. Patient safety and the dermatologist. J Am Acad Dermatol. 2009;61(2):179–90.
28. Becker DE, Reed KL. Essentials of local anesthetic pharmacology. Anesth Prog. 2006;53:98–109.
29. Foldes FF, Molloy R, McNall PG, Koukal LR. Comparison of toxicity of intravenously given local anesthesia agents in man. JAMA. 1960;172:1493–8.
30. Alam M, Ricci D, Havey J, Rademaker A, Witherspoon J, West DP. Safety of peak serum lidocaine concentration after Mohs micrographic surgery: a prospective cohort study. J Am Acad Dermatol. 2010;63:87–92.
31. Butterwick KJ, Goldman MP, Sriprachya-Anunt S. Lidocaine levels during the first two hours of infiltration of dilute anesthetic solution for tumescent liposuction: rapid versus slow delivery. Dermatol Surg. 1999;25:681–90.
32. Tolle MA, Schwarzwald HL. Postexposure prophylaxis against human immunodeficiency virus. Am Fam Physician. 2010;82(2):161–6.

45 Ethical Issues Related to Mohs Skin Cancer Surgery

David J. Goldberg

Abstract

Although legal considerations can arise in the performance of any aspect of a dermatology practice, they are more likely to occur in the areas of diagnosis and treatment of skin cancers. Although there is no substantiated data about dermatologic skin cancer litigation, and specifically Mohs surgery, there are anecdotal suggestions that such malpractice claims have increased. Mohs surgeons, often performing some of the most complex skin cancer treatments, are clearly at risk for both ethical and legal issues related to their treatment. This chapter will look at the interplay between legal and ethical issues with an emphasis on those issues that specifically can arise in the practice of Mohs surgery.

Keywords

Mohs • Ethics • Legal issues • Malpractice • Non-physicians • Skin cancer

Summary: Introduction

- Elements of negligence
- Hypothetical cases
- Ethics in Mohs surgery

45.1 Introduction

In the most simplistic terms, the definition of ethics often relates to knowing and doing the right thing as compared to the wrong thing. Because of this, most ethical issues in medicine ultimately become legal issues. This chapter will look at legal considerations as they arise in Mohs surgery and will ultimately focus on two examples of ethical issues that can lead to legal issues. Although legal considerations can arise in the performance of any aspect of a dermatology practice, they are more likely to occur in the areas of diagnosis and treatment of skin cancers. Although there is no

D.J. Goldberg
Department of Dermatology,
Mount Sinai School of Medicine, New York, NY, USA
e-mail: drdavidgoldberg@skinandlasers.com

K. Nouri (ed.), *Mohs Micrographic Surgery*,
DOI 10.1007/978-1-4471-2152-7_45, © Springer-Verlag London Limited 2012

substantiated data about dermatologic skin cancer litigation, and specifically Mohs surgery, there are anecdotal suggestions that such malpractice claims have increased. Mohs surgeons, often performing some of the most complex skin cancer treatments, are clearly at risk for both ethical and legal issues related to their treatment. A full textbook on health care ethics and law is an appropriate reading to comprehensively cover all the legal aspects as they relate to Mohs skin cancer surgery. Issues that arise include negligence, billing fraud, and privacy concerns. Since the most likely cause of a legal mishap in current-day Mohs skin cancer dermatology involves negligence, it will be discussed first in this chapter.

Initially, the first part of the chapter will discuss the elements of negligence and the evolution of a medical malpractice cause of action involving the diagnosis and treatment of skin cancer with Mohs surgery. This will then be followed by a description of two hypothetical cases and the likelihood of a successful malpractice case evolving from such a scenario. The final portion of the chapter will look at the ethical issues surrounding the hypothetical treatment of actinic keratoses with Mohs surgery and the ethical and legal issues of using extenders to perform Mohs surgery.

Summary: The Four Elements
- Duty
- Breach of duty
- Causation
- Damages

45.2 The Four Elements

Any analysis of physician negligence must first begin with a legal description of the four required elements for a cause of action in negligence: duty, breach of duty, causation, and damages. The suing plaintiff must show the presence of all four elements to be successful in his or her claim [1].

The duty of a physician evaluating and treating skin cancers is to perform that surgery in accordance with the standard of care. Although the elements of a cause of action in negligence are derived from formal legal textbooks, the standard of care is not necessarily derived from some well-known textbooks. It is also not articulated by any judge. The standard of care is defined by some, as whatever an expert witness says it is, and what a jury will believe. In a case against any Mohs surgeon, the specialist must have the knowledge and skills ordinarily possessed by a specialist in that field, and have used the care and skill ordinarily possessed by a specialist in that field in the same or similar locality under similar circumstances. A dermatologist, plastic surgeon, otolaryngologist, or any practitioner purportedly evaluating and treating with the Mohs technique will be held to an equal standard. A failure to fulfill such a duty may lead to loss of a lawsuit by the physician. If the jury accepts the suggestion that the doctor mismanaged the case and that the negligence led to damage of the patient, then the physician will be liable. In the case of skin cancer, misdiagnosis and/or mistreatment may both lead to damages and physician liability. Conversely, if the jury believes an expert who testifies for the defendant doctor, then the standard of care, in that particular case, has been met. In this view, the standard of care is a pragmatic concept, decided case by case, and based on the testimony of an expert physician. The dermatologist, or any other physician using the Mohs technique, is expected to evaluate skin cancers in a manner of a reasonable Mohs surgeon. He need not be the best in his field; he need only perform the procedure in a manner that is considered reasonable by an objective standard. Perhaps missing the diagnosis of amelanotic melanoma might not be considered a breach in the standard of care because a reasonable physician might miss this diagnosis. Using the Mohs technique for amelanotic melanoma may be debatable.

It is important to note that where there are two or more recognized methods of diagnosing or treating the same condition, a physician does not fall below the standard of care by using any of the acceptable methods even if one method turns out to be less effective than the other. Finally, in many jurisdictions, an unfavorable result due to an "error in judgment" by a physician is not in and of itself a violation of the standard of care if the physician acted appropriately prior to exercising his or her professional judgment.

Summary: Standard of Care
- Standard of care is an objective standard.
- National standards exist.
- Standard of care of ten suggested by an expert.

45.3 Standard of Care

Evidence of the standard of care in a specific malpractice case includes laws, regulations, and guidelines for practice, which represent a consensus among professionals on a topic involving diagnosis or treatment, and the medical literature including peer-reviewed articles and authoritative texts. In addition, obviously, the view of an expert is crucial. Although the standard of care may vary from state to state, it is typically defined as a national standard by and for Mohs skin cancer surgeons.

Most commonly for litigation purposes, expert witnesses articulate the standard of care. The basis of the expert witness's testimony, and therefore the origin of the standard of care, is grounded in the following:

1. The witness's personal practice
2. The practice of others that he has observed in his experience
3. Medical literature in recognized publications
4. Statutes and/or legislative rules
5. Courses where the subject is discussed and taught in a well-defined manner

The standard of care is the way in which the majority of the physicians in a similar medical community would practice. If, in fact, the expert herself does not practice like the majority of other physicians, then the expert will have a difficult time explaining why the majority of the medical community does not practice according to her ways. The use of extracts to treat skin cancer, a method used by homeopathic experts, may not be in accordance with the standard of care as opined by a dermatology expert. It certainly would not be considered the standard of care by a fellowship trained Mohs surgeon. Such treatment might be considered both unethical and illegal. Malpractice issues may arise. In addition, there may be state medical board issues raised. Finally, such unethical treatments may lead the Mohs surgeon to be questioned by ethics organizations of the various societies to which he/she is a member.

It would seem then that in the perfect world, the standard of care of both ethical and legal practice in every case would be a clearly definable level of care agreed upon by all physicians and patients. Unfortunately, in the typical situation, the standard of care is an ephemeral concept resulting from differences and inconsistencies among the medical profession, the legal system, and the public.

At one polar extreme, the medical profession is dominant in determining the standard of care in the practice of medicine. In such a situation, recommendations, guidelines, and policies regarding varying treatment modalities for different clinical situations published by nationally recognized boards, societies, and commissions establish the appropriate standard of care. Even in some of these cases, however, factual disputes may arise because more than one such organization will publish conflicting standards concerning the same medical condition. Adding to the confusion, local societies may publish their own rules applicable to a particular claim of malpractice.

Thus, in most situations, the standard of care is neither clearly definable nor consistently defined. It is a legal fiction to suggest that a generally accepted standard of care exists for any area of practice. At best there are parameters within which experts will testify. The Mohs skin cancer physician's best defense that he is acting in accordance with the standard of care is to document appropriate risk assessment of the patient, to provide appropriate medical record documentation and informed consent, and finally to utilize appropriate diagnostic and treatment approaches.

In recent years, American physicians have put forth substantial efforts toward setting standards and specifying treatment approaches to various conditions. Clinical practice guidelines have been developed by specialty societies such as the American Academy of Dermatology and the American College of Mohs Micrographic Surgery and Cutaneous Oncology. The Institute of Medicine has defined such clinical guidelines as "systemically developed statements to assist practitioner and patient decisions about appropriate health care for specific clinical circumstances." Such guidelines represent standardized specifications for performing a procedure or managing a particular clinical problem.

Summary: Clinical Guidelines
- Guidelines are not "law."
- Guidelines are offered at testimony as piece of evidence.
- Guidelines are often determined by national societies.

45.4 Clinical Guidelines

Clinical guidelines raise thorny legal issues [2]. They have the potential to offer an authoritative and settled statement of what the standard of care should be for a given skin cancer. A court would have several options when such guidelines are offered as evidence. Such a guideline might be evidence of the customary practice in the medical profession. A doctor acting in accordance with the guidelines would be shielded from liability to the same extent as one who can establish that she or he followed professional customs. The guidelines could play the role of an authoritative expert witness or a well-accepted review article. Using guidelines as evidence of professional custom, however, is problematic if they are ahead of prevailing medical practice.

Clinical guidelines have already had an effect on settlement, according to surveys of malpractice lawyers. A widely accepted clinical standard may be presumptive evidence of due care, but expert testimony will still be required to introduce the standard and establish its sources and its relevancy.

Professional societies often attach disclaimers to their guidelines, thereby undercutting their defensive use in litigation. The American Medical Association, for example, calls its guidelines "parameters" instead of protocols intended to significantly impact physician discretion. The AMA further suggests that all such guidelines contain disclaimers stating that they are not intended to displace physician discretion. Such guidelines, in such a situation, could not be treated as conclusive.

Summary: Legal Relevance
- Negligence may also be established by:
  - An admission by the defendant that he or she was negligent
  - Common knowledge standard

45.5 Legal Relevance

Plaintiffs usually will use their own expert, as opposed to the physician's expert, to define the standard of care. Although such a plaintiff's expert may also refer to clinical practice guidelines, the physician's negligence can be established in other manners as well. These methods include: (1) examination of the physician defendant's expert witness; (2) an admission by the defendant that he or she was negligent; (3) testimony by the plaintiff, in a rare case where she is a medical expert qualified to evaluate the allegedly negligent physician's conduct; and (4) common knowledge in situations where a layperson could understand the negligence without the assistance of an expert [3, 4].

It is clear then that in order for the plaintiff to win her negligence cause of action against a Mohs surgeon, she must establish that her physician had a duty of reasonable care in treating her and had in fact breached that duty. However, that breach must also lead to some form of damages. A mere inconvenience to the plaintiff, even in the setting of a physician's breach, will usually not lead to physician liability in a cause of action for negligence.

It is often difficult to predict, in any given malpractice cause of action, what the ultimate outcome will be. The following teaching hypotheticals are designed to be suggestive of potential malpractice cases and the likely results. Any connection between these scenarios and actual malpractice cases is fortuitous.

Summary: Case Example 1
- Negligence after Mohs surgery is not established solely:
  - Recurrence of skin cancer
  - Metastatic disease
  - Death of patient for the patient from the skin cancer treated with the Mohs technique

45.6 Case Example 1

DS is a 48-year-old man with a multiple squamous cell carcinoma and a history of immunosuppression. He was seen every 6 months for skin evaluations. His cancerous lesions were treated with a variety of methods including electrical destruction, topical agents, and Mohs surgery.

Some of the Mohs-treated lesions recurred. Ultimately, DS develops metastatic disease from a recurrent lesion. He dies leaving behind multiple family members. The plaintiff's estate sues the Mohs surgeon. They contend that there must have been a breach of duty for the skin cancer to return. Perhaps more frequent office visits and/or more aggressive treatments would have prevented the unfortunate death of their family member.

Did the Mohs surgeon breach the standard of care? If so, will he be liable for negligence? The patient records are evaluated by an expert for the suing plaintiff's estate. The records all appear to be reasonable. The plaintiff's expert refuses to testify because there is no evidence of malpractice by the defendant Mohs surgeon. The plaintiff's expert testifies that Mohs slides were all clear of malignancy. Six-month evaluations were considered to be reasonable. There is no evidence to suggest that monthly visits would have stopped metastatic spread in this immunosuppressed individual. Recurrence of skin cancer, metastatic disease, and even death are not evidence of de facto negligence. The case will likely be lost by the plaintiff.

Summary: Case Example 2
- Permanent damage is not evidence of negligence.
- Verbal consent is legally acceptable.
- Written consent is easier to prove than verbal consent.

45.7 Case Example 2

A well-known dermatologist treats in excess of 600 Mohs patients each year. He treats a large number of basal cell carcinoma and squamous cell carcinoma patients. A referred patient has a large recurrent ulcerative basal cell carcinoma of the cheek. In consultation, the patient is told, by way of informed consent, that the facial nerve may be damaged during the proposed Mohs surgery. The patient is also told the consequences of such nerve damage. After the third stage of Mohs surgery, it is quite evident that the tumor involves a significant portion of the parotid gland. In removing the remaining tumor, the facial nerve is partially severed with a resultant unilateral lower facial paralysis. The patient sues the Mohs surgeon.

Is the Mohs surgeon liable? It is clear that there is permanent damage to patient. Reconstructive surgery can improve the situation but may never return to the patient's full use of the nerve. The Mohs surgeon did provide informed consent to the patient. Although verbal consent legally is enough, the written consent provides documentation that the Mohs surgeon performed his legal duty. It is unlikely that the Mohs surgeon will lose this case. The surgeon is advised that legible chart documentation, and documented signed consent, will only help him at trial.

Skin cancers continue to increase in number. There are, as described in this book, numerous accepted techniques for the removal of many skin cancers. By the nature of any treatment, complications may arise. It is imperative that physicians be aware of their duty of reasonable care. Should they breach that duty, they may be found liable in a medical malpractice cause of action in the diagnosis of and treatment for skin cancer.

Summary: Ethical Relevance
- Actinic keratoses (AKs) may become squamous cell carcinoma (SCC).
- Mohs surgery is an acceptable, ethical approach to treat SCC.
- There are many acceptable approaches to treat AK.
- Mohs surgery is not an ethical technique to sue in the treatment of AK.

45.8 Ethical Relevance

45.8.1 Actinic Keratoses

There are no ethical issues surrounding the use of the Mohs technique for designated basal cell and squamous cell carcinoma. Numerous other cutaneous malignancies can also be successfully treated with this technique. What about actinic keratoses? With all the techniques available, there are many good options for the treatment of AKs. From a statistical point of view, no approach should give a higher cure rate than Mohs surgery for the treatment of AKs. It has been suggested that Mohs surgery has been overused. In no scenario has the ethical misuse for this technique been more blatant than with those physicians who contend that all actinic keratoses (AKs) are, in fact, squamous cell carcinoma and should be treated with the Mohs technique. This approach raises thorny ethical issues.

Patients with actinic keratoses (AKs), as all Mohs surgeons know, have rough, keratotic, white, 1–2-mm papules and larger plaques that are typically found on the sun-exposed areas of the body, especially seen on the hands, arms, and faces of middle-aged individuals. These patients invariable have sustained a significant amount of sun damage and account for the second most common diagnosis given for seeking dermatologic care. There is clearly a wide array of AK treatment options that can be used to fit a patient's needs [5].

The recognition of actinic keratoses is important because of their association with squamous cell carcinoma (SCC), an invasive cancer with the capacity to metastasize and result in significant morbidly and even mortality. With few exceptions, like thermal burn scars, chronic leg or decubitus ulcers, and smoking, the generally accepted theory is that AKs represent a precursor to squamous cell carcinomas resulting from chronic sun exposure.

The explanation given for treating AKs is that they represent precursors to SCCs [6]. Epidemiological data from the National Ambulatory Medical Care Survey (NAMCS) estimates that in 1993–94, there were 7.2 million office visits with the ICD-9 code diagnosis of AKs. The incidence of non-melanoma skin cancers (NMSCs) is strongly associated with age. If AKs are precursors to NMSC, then a similar age distribution should also exist for them as well. In fact, NAMCS data has shown that there were 6.3 million visits for NMSCs during that same time period. Similar results have also been shown in previously published studies. At least one high-profile article has been published in which the author makes the argument that AKs are the earliest form of SCC that can be identified and should be treated as such, not as a preventative measure. If they represent SCC, then a variety of techniques (perhaps including the Mohs technique) can be considered as treatment options.

If one takes the counterposition that AKs are only precursor lesions to SCCs, then some estimate must be made as to the rate of the progression from AK to NMSC. Otherwise, it would be logical to treat all AKs as soon as they are diagnosed in order to prevent the subsequent development of SCCs [7]. Estimates of the progression from AK to SCC have varied widely from a low of only 0.025% to as much as 16% per year. Clinical experience has shown that some AKs do not evolve into cancer at all, or that evolution occurs so slowly that treatment can be delayed or postponed indefinitely, since some of these lesions may even disappear without treatment. What are the treatment options one might consider?

45.8.1.1 Invasive Techniques

Cryosurgery

Cryosurgery, using liquid nitrogen in a spray or contact technique with cotton tip applicators or solid metal probes, remains the most common form of treatment used today. Multiple lesions can be treated quickly, and the cure rate is high.

Curettage and Electrodessication

Other invasive techniques have also been used in the treatment of AKs. One of the oldest techniques, curettage and electrodessication, is used when the lesion is large, has indistinct margins, or there is concern about the depth of the growth.

Dermabrasion and Chemical Peels

When a multitude of AKs involve large areas of the face or scalp, cryosurgery or curettage and electrodessication are usually inappropriate treatment options. In these situations, dermabrasion or chemical peels using topically applied trichloroacetic acid (TCA) or phenol can be considered. It must be remembered that complications can be expected when dermabrasion or chemical peels are used to treat AKs on the thinner skin of the hands and where there are limited numbers of skin appendages, like hair follicles or eccrine sweat ducts, from which reepithelialization can occur.

Carbon Dioxide or Erbium:YAG Laser Ablation

Over the past 10 years, several short-pulsed lasers, like the carbon dioxide and erbium:YAG, have been successfully used for skin rejuvenation due to their limited collateral thermal effects. These same devices can simultaneously be used to remove AKs as well.

45.8.1.2 Non-invasive Techniques

Topical Chemotherapy

When patients have large numbers of AKs and do not want to undergo treatment with one of the invasive techniques, several different topical agents have shown to have beneficial results. The oldest technique consists of the topical application of a chemotherapeutic agent, 5-fluorouracil (5-FU), for 4–6 weeks. This drug works by inhibiting thymidylate synthetase to deplete thymidine and reduce DNA synthesis by active proliferating cells. There can be a severe reaction to this agent with swelling, erythema, dryness, crusting, and burning pain that may cause some patients to become non-compliant and not complete the full course of therapy. However, when used as directed topical 5-FU can be very effective. Use of topical retinoic acid has also been shown to be effective in treating AKs, but typically requires long treatment schedules of many months duration. Due to its rejuvenation effects, many patients may tolerate this form of therapy better than a shorter course of treatment using 5-FU.

A newer form of topical chemotherapy that is well tolerated in the treatment of AKs consists of the application of one of the non-steroidal anti-inflammatory drugs, diclofenac. This drug selectively inhibits COX-II and after 3 months of therapy has reduced the number of AKs without significant side effects. Although less effective than 5-FU, it may provide a treatment alternative to patients who cannot tolerate the irritation of other treatments.

Photodynamic Therapy (PDT)

PDT can be used to treat AKs using topically applied delta-aminolevulinic acid (ALA) as the photosensitizer and a variety of non-laser lights for the activator. While the treatments were painful and resulted in crusting and erythema in some patients, it produced relatively high cure rates.

Topical Immune Response Modifier Therapy

A non-specific method to activate an enhanced local immune response has recently been developed to treat AKs. One of these agents, imiquimod, stimulates the production of interferons and natural killer cells that clear the AKs with less swelling, redness, and crusting than seen with topical 5-FU.

When selecting the proper form of treatment for AKs, the patient must play an important role in choosing what is right for their particular circumstances. The patient should always be allowed to make an informed decision as to what type of treatment they wish to receive. A younger patient working with the public may choose a procedure or therapeutic method that has little risk of scarring or hypopigmentation and the best chance for a good cosmetic outcome. A physically active patient may choose a technique that produces the least restriction on their activities. An elderly patient may choose a form of treatment that would reduce the number of return visits to their physicians' offices. All of this is as it should be, for that is the art of medicine – helping the patient to make the best decision as to their health care options. With all of these highly successful available methods, there would seem to be no ethical justification for the treatment of AKs with Mohs surgery.

45.8.2 Non-Physician Performance of Mohs Surgery

Medicare Part B pays for services that are billed by physicians but are performed by non-physicians. These services often are called "incident to" services, or services provided under the "incident to" rule. "Incident to" services in theory may be vulnerable to overutilization and may place patients at risk of receiving treatment that does not meet professionally recognized standards of care. In a recent Officer of Inspector General (OIG) from Department of Health and Human Services analysis, a random selection of 250 "physician day" treatments were analyzed. Physicians were asked to submit relevant credentials for the non-physician-provided services [8]. Part of the analysis looked at whether such non-physicians were qualified to render the particular services. In making these determinations, the nurse reviewers considered any relevant Medicare requirements, state laws and regulations, and the evaluating nurse's own professional judgment as to whether the provided services generally fell within the standard competencies of the particular non-physician provider who rendered the services. In the evaluation, particular focus was placed on physicians who billed for more than 24 h worth of service in a day. It was determined that physicians performed about half of these services. Non-physicians performed the remaining half of the services in which physicians billed as "incident to" services. In the 3-month OIG evaluation period, Medicare allowed $105 million for approximately 934,000 services that physicians personally performed and approximately $85 million for 990,000 that non-physicians performed during this time period. Of note, non-physicians performed almost 2/3 of the invasive procedures that Medicare allowed the physicians. Of these procedures, Medicare allowed $12.6 million for approximately 210,000 services performed by unqualified non-physicians. These non-physicians did not possess the necessary licenses or certifications, had no verifiable credentials, or lacked the training to perform the service. Non-physicians with inappropriate qualifications performed 7% of the invasive procedures that physicians did not perform. It should be noted that guidelines used for analysis included those considered "relevant Medicare requirements, state laws and regulations." Guidelines of relevant medical societies such as those of the American Academy of Dermatology and the American College for Mohs Micrographic Surgery and Cutaneous Oncology were not used.

If Mohs surgery is being provided by some of the above-identified poorly trained non-physicians, such treatments may or may not be legal – they certainly are unethical.

References

1. Furrow BF, Greaney TL, Johnson SH, Jost TS, Schwartz RL. Liability in health care Law. 3rd ed. St. Paul: West Publishing Co; 1997.
2. Hyams AL, Shapiro DW, Brennan TA. Medical practice guidelines in malpractice litigation: an early retrospective. J Health Polit Policy Law. 1996;21:289–313.
3. *Lamont v. Brookwood Health Service, Inc.*, 446 So.2d 1018 (Ala.1983)
4. *Gannon v. Elliot*, 19 Cal.App.4th 1 (1993)
5. Frost CA, Green AC. Epidemiology of solar keratoses. Br J Dermatol. 1994;131:455–64.
6. Ackerman AB. Solar keratosis is squamous cell carcinoma. Arch Dermatol. 2003;139:1216–7.
7. Glogau RG. The risk of progression to invasive disease. J Am Acad Dermatol. 2000;43:S23–4.
8. Prevalence and Qualifications of Non-Physicians Who Performed Medicare Physician Services. OIG Report, OEI-09-06-00430, August 2009.

46 Medicolegal Issues Regarding Mohs Micrographic Surgery

Ilya Reyter, Tanya Nino, and Abel Torres

Abstract

Almost two thirds of US physicians can expect to be sued at least once during their career. The key, however, is not to wait until that time to start learning about medicolegal issues. A physician with preemptive knowledge about the legal system can incorporate such information into a Mohs practice, thereby enhancing patient safety while minimizing malpractice risk. Physicians armed with legal information can also be better prepared to properly respond to adverse events, such as those that can occur in Mohs surgery. Not all adverse events, however, need to proceed to litigation. When an adverse event occurs, there is much a physician can do to enhance patient well-being, restore trust, and hopefully keep the issue out of court. Should the matter in fact proceed to a lawsuit, a physician with legal knowledge can be in a better position to prevent typical missteps and mount an aggressive defense.

Keywords

Medicolegal • Medical malpractice • Informed consent • Medical records • Duty • Breach of duty • Causation • Damages

Summary: Introduction

- It is important for physicians to be aware of their legal responsibilities and to gain a foundation in medical-legal perspectives.

46.1 Introduction

Over the course of a career in dermatology, a physician will encounter the legal system in many ways. Thus, it is important for a doctor to preemptively become aware of his or her legal responsibilities and develop a framework for understanding critical legal issues in medicine. Unfortunately, this information is typically not covered in most medical school curriculums, and physicians are tasked with learning the information on their own, often in no formal or organized manner. Occasionally, confusion over legal issues and responsibilities leads to fear

I. Reyter • T. Nino • A. Torres (✉)
Department of Dermatology,
Loma Linda University School of Medicine,
Loma Linda, CA, USA
e-mail: abelt@aol.com; cmorrill@llu.edu

K. Nouri (ed.), *Mohs Micrographic Surgery*,
DOI 10.1007/978-1-4471-2152-7_46, © Springer-Verlag London Limited 2012

of lawsuits, which, in turn, causes doctors to limit the level of treatment offered to patients [1, 2]. Furthermore, the increasing demand for documentation is forcing providers to devote more time and attention to what is recorded in the chart, reducing the time available for patient care [1, 2].

While the natural response to all this is to practice defensive medicine, a more practical approach is to gain a better understanding of the medical-legal issues, learn how to minimize malpractice exposure, and simultaneously provide patient care unhindered by the fear of litigation.

This chapter will provide a foundation in medical-legal issues and help to clarify some difficult concepts. It is important to highlight the fact that federal and state laws govern the duties of both patients and physicians and that some laws vary from state to state. Therefore, physicians should not make assumptions about a given law and should always check to see what the laws and regulations of their jurisdiction require. In addition, this chapter should not substitute for an attorney's advice should an actual medical-legal issue arise.

Summary: Medical Malpractice

- Understanding negligence is necessary when approaching medical malpractice cases.
- Negligence has four essential elements.
- Both physicians and patients can be negligent.

46.2 Medical Malpractice

Medical liability costs are rising in the United States. Those costs are then passed along to physicians in the form of increased malpractice insurance premiums and to society, at large, as an increase in the expense of practicing defensive medicine [3]. For dermatologists, surgical procedures and skin cancer management are at the root of many legal claims [4]. As Mohs surgeons deal mainly with skin cancer, it is of particular interest that an analysis of almost 100 skin cancer lawsuits between 1986 and 2001 found that the most common allegation was failure to diagnose [3]. In almost half of those cases, the claim was that a biopsy should have been (but was not) performed. Other allegations involved misdiagnosis, failure to refer, failure to obtain informed consent, and surgical and medical complications [3]. These are summarized in Fig. 46.1 [1].

Addressing a malpractice claim requires a significant amount of a physician's time and resources, regardless of the validity of the claim. Even if a physician is ultimately exonerated of any wrongdoing, the amount of time spent dealing with the allegations usually translates to significant amounts of lost time and income. Also, the stress of the proceedings does no favors for the physician's physical or mental well-being. Therefore, it behooves a physician to become familiar with the basic principles of malpractice law, and thereby, hopefully minimize stress and missteps in the event of a lawsuit.

Central to any discussion of malpractice law is the Tort Law of Negligence, which addresses unreasonable actions of a person that result in physical or mental injuries to another person [4]. The following four elements constitute negligence [1, 4]:

- Duty
- Breach of duty
- Causation
- Damages

46.2.1 Duty

Once the physician-patient relationship is established, a physician owes a duty of care to the patient. Of note, the establishment of duty does not necessarily require an office setting or even physical contact with the patient [5–7]. For example, a dermatopathologist who reads a biopsy slide and diagnoses a basal cell carcinoma may establish a duty without ever seeing the patient. What is required is that there be a reasonable reliance by the patient on the actions or lack of action by the physician. In some circumstances, courts have ruled that the act of scheduling a patient appointment may imply a relationship if the appointment is for a specific medical condition [8]. Even if the patient misses the appointment, it can be claimed that a relationship has been established. The logic in such cases has usually been that the patient reasonably relied on that appointment for their care. This is more likely to be held to be the case when the physician is a specialist and provides a level of care that is not easily accessed. In other words, if the physician is closer to the only game in town, the more likely that reliance on the appointment by the patient is likely to be considered

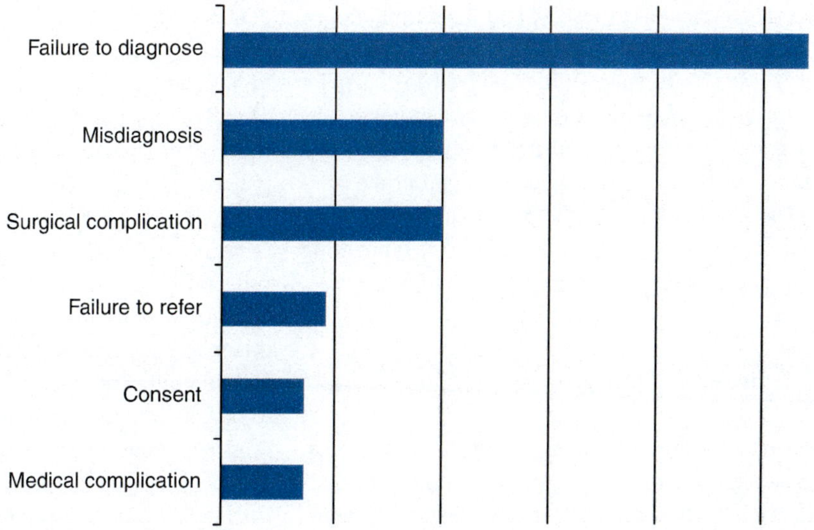

Fig. 46.1 A bar graph is shown depicting the proportion of skin cancer lawsuits by allegation (Copyright Elsevier [1]. Used with permission)

reasonable. In the case of Mohs surgeons, this is especially important since it is not uncommon to find that there are a limited number of well-qualified/trained Mohs surgeons in many communities. In other words, the Mohs surgeon may be the only option in town. Therefore, it is prudent to correspond with patients regarding missed appointments, particularly when the dermatologist is one of a few physicians capable of providing the specific service [1].

Duty can also be established in non-traditional settings. Almost all dermatologists, at one point or another, have been in a situation where they are asked to give advice or to evaluate a lesion outside of the clinical setting. Consider the following scenario:

> A dermatologist at a social function is approached by an acquaintance who asks for advice about a basal cell carcinoma that was surgically removed years ago, but now a small flat brown spot appeared just adjacent to it. She wants to make sure that it is just a sun spot and nothing to worry about.

If a physician were to give advice or provide a service in the above social setting, a relationship and duty to the patient can be established, even if there was no fee charged for the encounter [1]. Rather than avoiding communication with anyone seeking advice or opinions at social functions for fear of unnecessarily establishing duty, the dermatologist should be prepared to give an appropriate response to such requests. For example, an appropriate response in the above situation would be to explain, in general terms, about the ABCDEs of melanoma and skin cancer as they relate to all patients. As far as specific diagnosis and recommendations about the lesion in question, the physician can offer an opinion but should make sure that there is no reasonable reliance on an opinion offered in a suboptimal setting. Thus, it would be prudent to assert that this individual should seek evaluation in a more appropriate setting, such as his office, or by another physician, where proper lighting and methods for documentation are available. The natural impulse may be to diagnose the lesion and to give advice on the spot, but doing so can result in the physician having no documentation to help defend him in the event of legal action. Being prepared to respond appropriately in such a situation can help the dermatologist manage social obligations without unnecessarily exposing the physician to additional risk.

The scope of a physician's duty is to act with the knowledge, care, and skill exercised by reasonable and prudent practitioners under similar circumstances [9]. This means that the dermatologist is held to the standard of other practitioners in his or her community. With advances in technology, communication, and integration of practice of medicine globally, the physician's community is expanding [10]. Furthermore, if a physician performs a procedure that is usually performed by a specialist, it is likely that the physician will be held to the standard of care of the specialist [11]. For example, if a dermatologist experienced in surgery performs an eyelid or lip reconstruction and encounters a complication, it is conceivable that the defense in a lawsuit will call on a surgeon who specializes in ocular or oral reconstruction to testify, and the dermatologist may be held to the standard of the surgical specialist. Nevertheless, Mohs surgery has evolved to the point where there are many experienced dermatologic surgeons with extensive reconstruction experience, and the authors believe this should be the appropriate standard. The key point is that the physician should make sure he or she has adequate training before embarking on these types of complex repairs.

46.2.2 Breach of Duty

Breach of duty usually requires a physician to fail to meet the standard of care [4, 9, 10]. In medical malpractice cases, the standard of care is not predetermined by a judge or textbook, but, rather, is usually defined through expert testimony by another physician. The expert witness, by virtue of his or her education, skill, and experience, must have specialized and practiced in a similar situation as the case in question. Given the constant evolution of therapies and evidence-based medicine, it will serve the dermatologist well to keep current with continuing medical education as it changes. Of note, when regarding specialty care such as dermatology, the standard of care applies not only to dermatologists but also to any nurse practitioner, physician assistant, or even an internist undertaking a dermatologic procedure such as Mohs surgery or reconstruction [12].

A standard of care issue that can arise in dermatology proceedings is the extent of the skin exam. Is it always necessary to perform a full skin exam, or should the exam focus on only the lesion in question? If a full exam is done, should it be done to screen patients on initial visits, on follow-up visits, or only when a patient's condition justifies the examination? While some dermatologists advocate that a full skin exam helps to better advise the patient on a lesion in light of the comprehensive clinical picture, others will argue that performing a complete skin exam on each patient is not needed and imposes an unnecessary economic burden on the medical system, as a full skin exam takes longer to perform and document, and therefore may be coded at a higher level than a simple, problem-oriented evaluation.

On one hand, performing a complete skin exam avoids the possibility of missing a concealed malignancy, such as an asymptomatic melanoma on the plantar aspect of the foot. Conversely, can a wider impact be achieved by utilizing the time with patients to, instead, educate them on self-skin exams, ABCDEs of melanoma, and sun protection? Clearly, there can be more than one valid use of a physician's time with patients. However, the physician needs to consider the repercussions of a patient having a melanoma on the unexamined skin. If the community standard is to offer full body exams, and the physician chose instead to educate the patient on self exams to be done at home, this may be argued as a failure to meet the standard of care in court. Yet, many factors, as noted above, need to be considered before it can be said that there was a failure to meet the standard of care. Of particular note, for Mohs surgeons, often the patient is being referred for a specific lesion rather than for a general evaluation. Thus, if the patient is a referred patient for Mohs, a full skin exam should only be necessary as needed by the surgeon to provide the surgical service.

In the courtroom setting, it is up to the testifying experts to aid the judge and jury in determining the applicable standard of care, and usually the most persuasive expert will prevail. *Ultimately, the most important component to satisfying the standard of care is to act within the patient's best interest.*

An exception to the need for expert testimony is the doctrine of Res Ipsa Loquitur, which translates to "The Thing Speaks for Itself." Three elements must be present for this doctrine to be satisfied [4]:

1. The occurrence does not ordinarily happen unless someone has been negligent.
2. The instrumentality that caused the injury must have been within the defendant's (the physician's) exclusive control.
3. The injury must not have been caused by the plaintiff (the patient).

Common examples of this doctrine include situations in which the physician left surgical instruments or supplies inside a patient's body or operated on the wrong part of the patient's body. Such examples usually demonstrate obvious negligence. Thus, if Res Ipsa Loquitur is applied, there is no requirement for expert testimony to prove a breach in the duty to uphold the standard of care. Although Res Ipsa Loquitur is not accepted in all of the states, dermatologists need to be aware of its applicability for their state and its implication that negligence can be demonstrated without the need for an expert witness to prove a departure from the standard of care.

46.2.3 Causation

This element of medical negligence holds that the patient-plaintiff must establish that he or she was actually injured by the physician-defendant's breach of duty and that there was a foreseeable and causal relationship between that departure from the standard of care and the harm that came to the patient as a result [4, 13]. This is the idea behind the proximate cause of medical malpractice liability, which requires that the breach of duty must have directly caused the patient's injury and also that the injury could have been foreseen and prevented had the physician upheld the standard of care [7].

46.2.4 Damages

Even if the above three elements have been satisfied, a physician cannot be held liable for medical malpractice unless the patient-plaintiff can prove that the physician's action caused harm. Consider the following example:

> One week after excision of a basal cell carcinoma of the back, your patient presents to you with erythema, tenderness, and yellow discharge from the operative site. You obtain a wound culture and empirically prescribe dicloxicillin for a wound infection, overlooking the patient's documented allergy to penicillin. You notice your mistake the next day and call the patient immediately. She confirms the information, but states that the reported allergic reaction happened only once, when she was an infant. She has already started taking the antibiotic and reports no current problems or allergic reactions. You immediately switch the medication to doxycycline while awaiting the wound culture and sensitivity. The patient experiences no adverse events during follow up care and the infection clears.

In this example, the physician has established a duty, there was a breach of duty, and potential causation, but the patient has suffered no harm/damages from the oversight. Thus, it is unlikely that the physician can be held liable for medical malpractice.

However, it is not necessary that the damage be physical, such as a scar or severe allergic reaction. Rather, the damage can be psychological or emotional, such as anxiety or depression. Many patients view surgery and post-operative complications with fear and misunderstanding, and it is up to the dermatologist to facilitate communication while addressing any patient anxiety. This approach not only advocates responsible patient care but also preempts potential legal damages for psychological or emotional reasons [1].

In some cases, a patient's own negligence may contribute to injury. For example, in dermatologic surgery, it is highly important for patients to perform proper post-operative wound care in order to achieve optical cosmetic and functional results [14]. A *lack* of appropriate action by the patient may constitute negligence on the patient's part, such as failing to show up to a post-operative wound check or failing to follow post-operative instructions. By failing to follow instructions or notify their physician of a problem, a patient may be held accountable for his or her own non-compliance. In a case of patient-plaintiff negligence, a court judgment of medical negligence against a physician-defendant may be reduced or nullified. In most jurisdictions, juries may weigh in the amount of negligence a patient has contributed to his or her own damage in order to offset malpractice liability [1].

Thus, it is important to educate patients on proper wound care techniques to improve outcome and patient satisfaction [14]. Dermatologists should make themselves or a knowledgeable staff member readily accessible to patients for any pre- or post-operative questions or concerns and should also monitor patients' progress throughout both medical and surgical treatment. This not only promotes good patient care but also ensures patients' responsibility for their own actions, minimizing legal liability.

Summary: Consent/Refusal for Treatment

- Consent can be implied, verbal, or written.
- Informed consent is an involved process where physicians and patients work together towards a medical decision.

46.3 Consent/Refusal for Treatment

Obtaining consent from a patient is usually more than just obtaining a signature on a legal document. It is a process by which patients take part in their own medical decision making. Failure by the physician to obtain informed consent could lead to legal allegations of an intentional tort, breach of contract, or negligence [15].

Assault is an intentional tort characterized as an act intended to cause harmful or offensive apprehension of contact with a battery being the actual occurrence of that harmful or offensive touching/contact [4]. Performing a

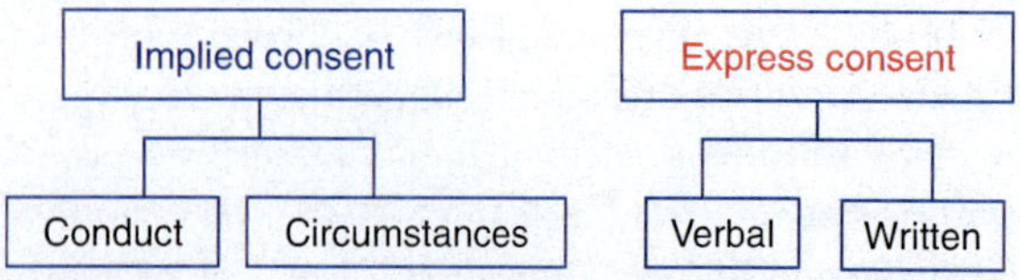

Fig. 46.2 Consent can fall into the categories of implied consent and express consent (Copyright Elsevier [1]. Used with permission)

treatment without a patient's consent leaves the physician susceptible to a claim of assault and/or battery that may not be covered by malpractice insurance [16]. It may also constitute a criminal offense in select circumstances.

It is of paramount importance that physicians understand the intricacies of obtaining proper consent for skin cancer treatment. Consent can fall into the various categories shown in Fig. 46.2 [1].

46.3.1 Implied Consent

Consent may be implied from a patient's conduct or from the surrounding circumstances. If a patient's conduct indicates awareness and understanding of the planned treatment, then implied consent may exist [17]. Also, if it is probable that a patient would reasonably consent to treatment, even if the patient is unable to express consent, then consent is implied. For example, implied consent may be sufficient to proceed in a simple situation such as performing a straightforward physical examination in the clinic. In more complex situations, relying on implied consent can be risky since the burden will generally rest on the physician to prove that the patient's conduct implied consent. For example, consider a patient who complains of possible lesions on the arms, and the physician performs a breast exam as part of the evaluation. If such an exam was unwarranted under the circumstances, this may constitute a lack of implied consent. Thus, relying on implied consent can be risky, and a physician is best advised to obtain express consent whenever possible.

46.3.2 Express Consent

Physicians should obtain express consent, written or oral, in most situations or treatments which present an appreciable risk to the patient. All consent requires is that patients are able to clearly communicate their desires for medical treatment with their physician. Verbal consent is as valid as written consent. However, verbal consent may be problematic, as it is usually not documented in writing, and therefore it is subject to the burden of proof that consent was actually obtained. Further complicating the concept of verbal consent is that patients often fail to recall details of a procedure they previously approved. In fact, it has been documented that patients only remember 35–55% of the information told to them after 1 week [3]. Patients may even change their minds or later take the position that they did not authorize a particular procedure. Furthermore, witnesses to informed consent are more likely to be unavailable the longer the elapsed time between when the consent was obtained and when the consent is called into question. For these reasons, it is prudent to obtain written consent, not only to ensure a framework for addressing pertinent information but also to serve as a record in the patient's chart for documentation [3]. Such written consent can be in the manner of a formal consent form, or it can be as a written note in the patient's chart. The problem with the latter is that it may not have a patient's signature or initials to indicate that the patient participated in the consent process. Nevertheless, a properly prepared note can serve as documentation.

46.3.3 Informed Consent

Physicians may avoid legal action regarding skin cancer treatment by properly performing the informed consent process [18]. In general, complete informed consent includes the following elements:

- Nature of the procedure
- Risks
- Benefits
- Alternatives
- Assessment of patient understanding
- Acceptance of the intervention by the patient

This communication process constitutes an ethical and legal obligation prior to performing a procedure, using a device, or even prescribing a medical treatment. Informed consent allows patients to be active decision makers in their own treatment, deciding with their physicians what is in their best interest [19]. A competent patient who makes an informed decision to forego a recommended test or treatment has made an informed refusal [1].

In judging whether disclosure is adequate, a physician can use the following two standards that the courts use as a guide:

46.3.3.1 Reasonable Doctor Standard/Professional Standard

This standard promotes that a physician reveal the same information that other physicians would disclose in the same or similar circumstances [20].

46.3.3.2 Reasonable Patient Standard/Legal Standard

This standard holds that a physician reveal the information that a reasonable person would consider material in deciding whether to undergo or forego treatment [21].

The standard used by the courts varies according to the laws of each state. Dermatologists should acquaint themselves with the standard used in their jurisdiction to ensure that their disclosure is both medically and legally adequate.

Both informed consent and refusal take on important roles in the treatment of skin cancer because many different treatment options exist. It is important to discuss with patients their diagnosis, its progression if left untreated, the recommended treatment along with potential risks and benefits, and viable alternatives including their respective risks and benefits [22]. Viable alternatives is an important concept in that a physician does not need to disclose a diagnostic or treatment option he or she does not believe is viable. Yet, physicians should be careful to make sure that they have solid reasoning when they decide an option is not viable.

The best way for physicians to avoid problems with informed consent and informed refusal issues is to communicate fully and document as well as possible. This process should not be rushed, and patients should be given the opportunity to ask questions and express any concerns. In addition, it is important for patients to verbalize understanding of the procedure or the possible consequences of refusal of treatment.

Summary: Medical Records

- Medical records are extremely important when a medicolegal situation arises.
- Medical records should be complete and tailored to the individual patient's case.

- A discussion of risks, benefits, and alternatives should be documented in the medical record prior to any surgical procedure.

46.4 Medical Records

It is difficult to overemphasize the importance of the medical record. After all, the medical record is the central repository of all patient-related medical information and is vital for planning, delivering, and chronicling medical care. In the event of a legal situation, the contents of this record may often be the only available credible evidence [23]. Thus, it is of utmost importance to both patient care and malpractice defense that a physician takes care to insure the accuracy and completeness of the medical record.

When contemplating the types of information that should be recorded in a medical record, a physician should keep in mind that most objective patient information, such as positive or negative findings which are essential to care or are customarily recorded, should be included [24]. Discussions with patients or relevant third parties, whether conducted in or out of the office, should also be documented whenever possible [24]. Additionally, the entire informed consent process should be recorded, including signed forms, treatment plans, and warnings given to patients [24]. Finally, any adverse events or complications should be included [24].

The following is a checklist for keeping medical records:

- *Avoid disapproving comments* or statements that are self-serving. Document from a patient care perspective.
- Record should be *complete* and, preferably, *concise.*
- Records should be *consistent.* Avoid lengthy chart entries as methods of risk management if the typical note for such an encounter is brief. This type of deviation in record keeping can invite unwanted suspicion.
- *Do not alter medical records*, unless it is *essential* for patient care. If a correction to the record is necessary, it is preferable to line out the item and initial and date the correction. It is also acceptable to enter a new note or addendum referencing the correction or addition. Avoid attempts to hide, make illegible, or delete the initial entry without indicating that you have done so.

- Make sure that *HIPAA* guidelines are followed in the preservation and distribution of medical records. Avoid releasing a patient's medical record unless proper authorization is obtained.

One option is to utilize preprinted informed consent forms. The authors prefer to maximize the patient's medical record for patient care purposes by recording a brief note in the chart reflecting a broad description stating that the risks, benefits, and alternatives (R,B,A) were discussed with the patient and that consent to treatment was obtained. It is preferable to avoid the implication that this is a perfunctory note or chart entry. Criticism of such a note by some attorneys is that if it is too generic, it may be challenged as to its validity of documenting informed consent. To minimize this issue, the authors make it a point to document at least one sentence that indicates an issue that would have been important to the specific patient's decision. An example of such a note is: "The R,B,A were discussed with the patient with emphasis on risk of temporal nerve damage and the patient agreed to proceed." In another instance, if a patient with Fitzpatrick type V skin was having an excision performed, it could be of value to indicate the following: "The risks, benefits and alternatives of the procedure were discussed with the patient, with emphasis on the patient's high risk of pigmentation changes and scarring." On occasion, such as when the issue may be a very critical one, the authors may ask the patient to read and initial the note to acknowledge that informed consent was obtained.

Summary: Complications in Skin Cancer Treatment

- The more experienced a Mohs surgeon, the higher the likelihood of encountering a complication in his or her career.

46.5 Complications in Skin Cancer Treatment

In the course of a career treating skin cancers, it is inevitable that a complication may occur. However, the existence of a complication may not necessarily lead to an adverse event, subsequent patient dissatisfaction, and, ultimately, litigation [25]. The physician is not powerless and can do much to restore the desired initial outcome by approaching the event in a compassionate, sympathetic manner, working to ensure the best interests of the patient. These efforts can simultaneously increase patient physical and/or psychological well-being and curb initiation of the legal process.

While it may seem that the antidote to lawsuits is greater experience and skill, the evidence speaks to the contrary. It has been shown that the probability of malpractice suits does not decrease as the surgeon's experience increases. Quite the opposite, studies show that the more experienced the Mohs surgeon, the higher the overall likelihood of him being sued for malpractice [14]. This likely is the result of the greater number of procedures such an experienced surgeon will have performed over the course of a long career.

Mohs surgeons would rightly assume that the most litigious site for complications regarding skin cancer excision and reconstruction is a patient's face. In fact, in a lawsuit analysis, this assumption was confirmed, with the face having roughly three times the rate of malpractice lawsuits (45%) as the next most litigious site (ear/scalp 18%) [3].

Summary: Rectifying Adverse Events: Key Steps

- Trust building is integral to the physician-patient relationship.
- The physician must take an active role, particularly listening to the patient's concerns.
- It is important to be available to the patient while dealing with an adverse event.
- Should litigation arise, the physician should contact the malpractice carrier for guidance.

46.6 Rectifying Adverse Events: Key Steps

46.6.1 Build Trust

A common sense but nonetheless critical element in dealing with adverse events is to strengthen the trust between the physician and the patient. Obviously, this is easier if the trust has been strengthened prior to the occurrence of the adverse event. If an adverse event has occurred, it would be unwise for the physician to erode the trust in the relationship by denying the existence of the problem and minimizing its significance. A physician would be well served to address it with honesty and integrity. If the adverse result was caused by a mistake, a prudent physician will communicate honestly with the patient, making sure to reconcile the facts of the situation. Patients have been shown to prefer such honest communication by their physicians, even if the mistake was minor [26]. However, physicians should be forewarned that the same patient survey showed that even when a physician admits to a mistake in an open, honest communication with patients, there is still a measure of trust lost in the physician-patient relationship. Yet, far greater trust was lost in the survey's hypothetical scenario where the physician did not disclose the mistake, and the patient uncovered it on his or her own.

46.6.2 Take an Active Role

The physician is usually best served by taking an active role to minimize the impact of the adverse event on the desired clinical outcome. The doctor can begin by actively listening to the patient's complaints, no matter how trivial, and making sure that he acknowledges the patient's complaint and communicates his concern for the patient. In discussing the problem with the patient or others, the physician should stay away from offering opinions and discuss only the facts. This is because opinions may often be based on premature conclusions without adequate facts.

If the patient pursues litigation, it is also advantageous for the physician to take an active role and meet regularly with his attorney and malpractice carrier. One of the first steps of the malpractice suit is the deposition. There is much a physician can do to prepare for the deposition, and taking an active role in the preparation can be extremely valuable. The following guidelines can be used while navigating the deposition portion of a lawsuit [27]:

- The deposition is where many cases are won or lost.
- Preparation is crucial.
- Be familiar with the medical records.
- When asked a question, do not rush to answer. Take a deep breath, collect your thoughts, answer slowly, and give your attorney time to object, if necessary.
- Resist the urge to justify rationale; keep your answers simple and brief.
- Opposing counsel will use a variety of tactics and questions to get you, the physician, to say an incriminating statement or admit to something that may look like incompetence.

46.6.3 Help the Patient

The next step a physician should take is to mitigate any injury to the patient. This action can simultaneously aid the patient's well-being and potentially mitigate legal damages. It is important that the physician takes positive measures that help the patient and stays away from negative actions such as blaming others, if not warranted. Likewise, a physician should accept responsibility for taking care of the complications but should be careful not to acknowledge a premature liability until all the facts are clear. As the physician deals with the adverse event, he or she needs to make sure that nothing is assumed and the facts are carefully investigated. Remember that perceptions may vary from the patient to the staff to the physician, and the perceptions and assumptions have to be separated from the facts. Clarify any misperceptions before they become false facts.

46.6.4 Enlist Help from Others

During this time, it is helpful for both the patient and physician to consult other health care providers, as needed, to provide the optimum care for the patient. In this regard, it is best for a physician to have a pre-existing contact list with the names of trusted providers that will put the patient's interests above any other agenda (e.g., turf battles, etc.). Similarly, the physician may be stressed by the situation, and it can be tempting to blame others. Nevertheless, the preferred course of action is to avoid criticizing or pointing fingers prematurely. A good piece of business advice that is applicable to risk management is to "praise in public and criticize in private." This does not imply that anything should be hidden, but, instead, that criticizing in public or prematurely merely creates an environment that is not conducive to finding out the truth or addressing the patient's needs.

Additionally, if litigation is pursued, the stress on the physician is real and can be immense. This is sometimes referred to as Medical Malpractice Stress Syndrome [27]. Attorneys typically tell physicians not to discuss details of the case with anyone other than the malpractice carrier and their own lawyer. This is prudent advice, as any details of these discussions may have to be recounted at a later date under oath. However, this may lead a physician to feel further isolated, thereby adding to the level of stress. To help mitigate the stress and isolation, it would be wise for a physician to share his feelings with a spouse or appropriate person while, of course, avoiding discussion of case details.

The following are symptoms of Medical Malpractice Stress Syndrome (MMSS) [27]:

- Sense of shame, bitterness, low self-esteem
- Depression, anxiety, insomnia
- Gastrointestinal symptoms, angina, myocardial infarction
- Sporadic outbursts against others

46.6.5 Be Available

Throughout this period, it is important that the patient have easy access to the physician or someone he or she designates as the contact person. This promotes good patient care and avoids the patient seeking comfort from others that may have different goals or agendas. This easy access reassures the patient and allows for any problems to be addressed in a timely manner before the issues can become more difficult. Having a designated contact person other than the physician is also very helpful. It can prevent misperceptions such as can occur if a misinformed staff member, unaware of the facts, makes a comment that creates undue anxiety for a patient. It goes without saying that honesty is the cornerstone to handling an adverse event, and all communication must be honest.

46.6.6 Contact the Malpractice Carrier

If the situation warrants, the physician should contact his or her malpractice carrier for guidance. This is prudent not only because the carrier may have valuable resources to offer but also because some carriers may have a contractual clause that limits their liability to the physician if they are not informed of an adverse event in a timely manner. Besides contacting his or her carrier, a physician may also organize a meeting with the patient's significant others. This helps to minimize misunderstandings and often recruits an ally to assist the patient. Of course, federal laws and privacy rules must be observed, and contact of significant others should take place with the patient's consent.

46.6.7 Preserve Evidence

If the adverse event involves a device such as an electrocautery machine, that device should be evidence that needs to be preserved in its original state until the physician's investigation of the incident is complete. Preservation of this evidence is important not only because a defective device may pose a future patient care danger but also because the device may be subject to product liability rules, and this can mitigate the liability for the physician.

46.6.8 Document the Facts of the Event

Finally, it is important that the adverse event is documented appropriately. The emphasis should be on documentation for patient care and not for risk management. Thus, it is crucial to avoid premature conclusions, and it is usually better to stick to the facts of what has happened so that a more accurate record is preserved for patent care. Likewise, the records are best left unaltered and should only be altered if essential for patient care. Furthermore, if an alteration is done, any alteration should be carefully documented preferably by lining out the item, initializing, and dating the change. This will prevent any misinterpretation that the records are being tampered with for personal rather than patient care reasons.

Unfortunately, when an adverse event occurs, it is usually accompanied by much stress and anxiety on both the part of the physician as well as the patient. Hopefully, the physician will have read this chapter and follow the steps outlined above to maximize patient care while minimizing legal risk. However, it is likely that the physician will need to refer back to this chapter, from time to time, as a refresher. In the meantime, the following tables may help the physician approach the situation.

The following is the AAA MNEMONIC for handling adverse events:

- A – **A**cknowledge the complaint.
- A – **A**ccessibility – Be accessible at all times.
- A – **A**lter not. (Do *not* alter records!)

The following guidelines can be used while navigating a malpractice lawsuit [27]:

- Two thirds of US physicians are sued at least one time in their career.

- Lawsuit process takes 3–5 years. Dig in and be in honest communication with your attorney.
- Do contact your malpractice carrier early and, if no response in few days, send a certified letter since many carriers require prompt notification. Also, there is a time limit to responding to complaints, and certain states can move to a default judgment if you wait too long.
- Do not change the medical record, speak to the plaintiff's attorney, or discuss details of the case with others, including your colleagues.
- Malpractice carrier will likely ask you to choose from a panel of pre-selected lawyers. The carrier may also honor choice of an alternate attorney.
- Choose an attorney by word of mouth or hospital list ahead of time. Assess the attorney's willingness to listen to you.
- Options for a malpractice case: (1) case is dropped plaintiff, (2) case goes to trial, (3) case is settled using indemnity funds, (4) plaintiff's attorney is reimbursed for costs, without using indemnity funds. (Indemnity funds, like adverse judgments, are reportable.)
- If consent clause is present in your malpractice policy (check your policy now), the malpractice carrier cannot settle out of court without your approval.

Summary: Conclusion

- It is important to understand the components of medical malpractice and take measures to mitigate risk, acting with the best interest of the patient in mind.

46.7 Conclusion

It goes without saying that this chapter can only chip away at what is a very important part of a Mohs surgery practice. If a lawsuit is initiated against a physician, the best action a physician can take is to consult with his attorney and malpractice carrier. This chapter is not intended to provide a substitute for guidance or advice in that regard. Nevertheless, knowledge is power, and understanding the process and issues presented here can help the physician through this difficult ordeal. It is information that is at once, important, interesting, tedious, frustrating, and anxiety provoking, but can also be reassuring. Much of its value will depend on how the practitioner approaches it. Regardless, what is critical is that the information be addressed before any legal action occurs. Hopefully, the lessons therein will be incorporated into a Mohs surgery practice to help both patients and physicians alike.

References

1. Torres A, Chiang M, Cockerell C, Strahan J, Nino T. Medical and legal aspects of skin cancer patients. In: Rigel D, editor. Cancer of the skin. 2nd ed. China: Elsevier Saunders; 2010.
2. Eisenberg D, Siegger M. The doctor won't see you now. Time Mag. 2003;161:46–62.
3. Lydiatt D. Medical malpractice and cancer of the skin. Am J Surg. 2004;187(6):688–94.
4. Prosser L, Owen DG, Keeton RE. Prosser and Keeton on the Law on Torts. 5th ed. St Paul: West Publishing Co; 1984.
5. Hiser v Randolph, 617 P.2d 774 (Ariz 1980).
6. Hamil v Bashline, 305 A2d 57 (1973).
7. Ratushny V, Allen HB. The effect of medical malpractice on dermatology and related specialties. J Med Sci Res. 2007; 30(1):15–20.
8. Lyons v Grether, 239 SE 2d 103 (1977).
9. Fiscina FS. Medical law for the attending physician. Carbondale: Southern Illinois Press; 1982.
10. Sills H. What is the law? Dent Clin North Am. 1982;26: 256.
11. Rapp JA, Rapp RT. Medical malpractice: a guide for the health sciences. St. Louis: CV Mosby Co; 1988.
12. Goldberg D. Legal issues in laser operation. Clin Dermatol. 2006;24:56–9.
13. Flamm MB. Medical malpractice: physician as defendant. In: Falk KH, ACLM, editors. Legal medicine: legal dynamics of medical encounters. 2nd ed. St Louis: CV Mosby; 1991. p. 525–34.
14. Perlis C et al. Incidence of and risk factors for medical malpractice lawsuits among mohs surgeons. Dermatol Surg. 2006;32:79–83.
15. Meisel A, Kabnick L. Informed consent to medical treatment: an analysis of recent legislation. Univ Pittsbq Law Rev. 1980;407:410.
16. Bommareddy v Superior Court, 222 Cal.App. 3d 1017 (1990).
17. Flannery FT et al. Consent to treatment, legal medicine: legal dynamics of medical encounters. St. Louis: CV Mosby Company; 1988.
18. Waltz JR, Sheuneman TW. Informed consent to therapy. Nw UL Rev. 1970;64(5):628.
19. Cobbs v Grant, 8 Cal 3d.229, 502 P.2d 1, (1972).
20. Redden EM, Baker BC. Medicolegal problems in the management of patients with skin cancer. In: Friedman RJ, Rigel DS, Kopf AW, et al., editors. Cancer of the Skin. Philadelphia: WB Saunders; 1991. p. 603–10.

21. Natanson v Kline, 350 P2d 1093 (1960).
22. Logan v Greenwich Hosp. Ass'n, 191 Conn. 282 (1983).
23. Holder AR. The importance of medical records. JAMA. 1974;228:118–9.
24. Tennehouse J, Kasher MP. Risk prevention skills. San Rafael: Tennenhouse Professional Publications; 1988. p. 69.
25. Keyes C, ed. Responding to adverse events. Forum: Risk Management Foundation of the Harvard Medical Institutions Inc., Adverse Events. 1997;18(1):2–5.
26. Wiman A, Park D, Hardin S. How do patients want physicians to handle mistakes? A survey of internal medicine patients in an academic setting. Arch Intern Med. 1996; 156:2565–9.
27. Schwartz SK. Malpractice: navigating a lawsuit. Physicians Pract. 2008;18(15):1–3.

Psychological Issues Regarding Mohs Micrographic Surgery

47

Misha M. Heller, Tina Bhutani, Eric S. Lee, and John Koo

Abstract

Mohs surgery can have profound psychological impact on patients. Considered the treatment of choice for the excision of cosmetically sensitive, treatment-resistant cutaneous tumors, Mohs surgery can offer many potential beneficial effects. For a majority of patients, Mohs surgery provides good cosmetic outcomes and a feeling of relief that their cancer has been eradicated. Patients may even demonstrate improvements in quality of life and sun-protection behavior. However, for a significant group of patients, Mohs surgery can cause serious psychological problems because of the disfigurement that has resulted from surgery. Disfigurement, especially that of the face, can have detrimental effects on a patient's psyche. Patients with disfigurement suffer from negative self-image and are often confronted with stigmatization in social interactions. Consequently, patients with disfigurement may develop secondary psychiatric disorders, including social phobia, generalized anxiety, or depression. Understanding how to best diagnose and manage patients with such psychiatric sequelae is extremely important aspect of patient care in dermatological surgery practice.

Keywords

Mohs micrographic surgery • Disfigurement • Social phobia • Generalized anxiety disorder • Depression

Summary: Introduction

- It is essential to recognize that Mohs surgery can have positive or negative psychological effects on patients.

47.1 Introduction

Understanding the psychological impact of Mohs surgery is a crucial aspect of managing patient care. Unfortunately, however, this topic has been largely neglected in the literature. As far as we are aware, there are only two published studies that specifically examine the psychosocial issues of Mohs surgery [1, 2]. Both of these studies seem to focus only on the psychological benefits of Mohs surgery. While it is important to recognize how patients undergoing Mohs surgery can improve overall quality of life, it is just as

M.M. Heller (✉) • T. Bhutani • E.S. Lee • J. Koo
Department of Dermatology,
UCSF Psoriasis and Skin Treatment Center,
San Francisco, CA, USA
e-mail: misha.max.heller@gmail.com

K. Nouri (ed.), *Mohs Micrographic Surgery*,
DOI 10.1007/978-1-4471-2152-7_47, © Springer-Verlag London Limited 2012

important to acknowledge the potential for severe psychological problems because of disfigurement. Significant disfigurement is a possible outcome following treatment of cutaneous neoplasms with Mohs surgery. Consequently, patients are at risk of developing significant psychiatric morbidity secondary to the postsurgical disfigurement. This may manifest, for example, as social phobia, generalized anxiety, or depression.

It is essential to identify patients who have psychiatric problems as a result of surgical disfigurement, since many of these patients can be helped by seeking professional help. Unlike patients with chronic psychiatric disorders, many of these patients have reasonable premorbid psychological adaptation levels. If treatment is provided through the crisis period, these patients can overcome the many difficulties of disfigurement and become fully functional in society once again.

In the following discussion, we will elaborate on the psychological benefit, as well as detrimental psychological impact of patients following Mohs surgery. We will explain how Mohs surgery can result in significant disfigurement and why such disfigurement can cause severe psychiatric problems. Finally, we hope to provide the Mohs surgeon with practical guidelines to help diagnose and manage these patients.

Summary: The Psychological Benefits of Mohs Surgery

- It seems almost intuitive to assume that Mohs surgery can offer many beneficial psychosocial effects. Mohs surgery has long been considered the gold standard for the excision of cutaneous tumors because it can maximize cure rates and minimize the loss of normal surrounding tissue. Mohs surgery is typically performed for tumor resection in aesthetically important anatomic locations [3, 4]. Such locations include the ears, periauricular region, temporal region, periocular region, nasal tip, nasal ala, melolabial sulcus, and upper lip (also known as, the "H-zone" of the face) [5]. Surgical excision scars following Mohs surgery are generally small, can be inconspicuous, and are often hidden in natural facial creases. Thus, Mohs surgery is considered to be a superior surgical technique in its abilities to offer definitive tumor excision and cure rate, with minimal functional disability and good cosmetic outcomes [6–10].
- In general, patients are satisfied with the cosmetic results following Mohs surgery and are left with an added sense of relief that their cancer has been successfully resected. In the following section, potential areas of psychological and behavioral benefits experienced by patients following Mohs surgery will be discussed.

47.2 The Psychological Benefits of Mohs Surgery

47.2.1 Improvement in Quality of Life and Sun-Protection Behavior

The two published studies that investigated the impact of Mohs surgery found that post-Mohs surgery patients appear to improve quality-of-life outcomes [1] and change-sun protection behavior [2]. To be specific, the study by Chren et al. [1] examined quality-of-life outcomes following treatment for cutaneous basal cell carcinoma and squamous cell carcinoma. A prospective cohort study was performed, consisting of 633 consecutive patients with non-melanoma skin cancer, who were followed for 2 years after treatment. Tumor-related quality-of-life scores 1–2 years after treatment were determined using the 16-item version of Skindex, a validated measuring index. Skindex quality-of-life scores ranged from 0 (best) to 100 (worst) and were assessed in three domains: Symptoms, Emotions, and Functioning. Treatment options included electrodessication and curettage (ED&C) in 21% (136 patients), surgical excision in 40% (251 patients), and Mohs surgery in 39% (246 patients). The study found that patients treated with Mohs surgery were more likely, than those treated with ED&C or surgical excision, to report worse emotional quality of life prior to therapy. However, after therapy, patients treated with surgical excision or Mohs surgery showed statistically significant improvements in all three quality-of-life domains ($p<0.05$).

There was no change in tumor-related quality-of-life domains following ED&C. For Mohs surgery, the mean-adjusted quality-of-life score for symptoms, emotions, and functioning improved by 10.2 points (95% CI: 7.4, 12.9), 21.7 points (95% CI: 18.1, 25.3), and 5.0 points (95% CI: 2.4, 7.6), respectively. There were also no differences in the amount of improvement on any of the quality-of-life domains between surgical excision and Mohs surgery [1].

The study by Maser et al. [2] attempted to determine changes in patient perception and behavior post-Mohs surgery. A mailed questionnaire was sent to 260 patients treated with Mohs surgery. Patients were asked questions regarding sun-protection behavior (i.e., sunscreen use, self-exam for abnormal moles, and exams performed by physicians). The study showed that patients treated with Mohs surgery appear to take preventative measure to avoid skin cancer. Of the patients who reported no sunscreen use before Mohs surgery, 70.1% of these patients began using sunscreen post Mohs surgery. Of the patients who reported using sunscreen before Mohs surgery, 40.7% of these patients increased the SPF by an average of 14.9 post-Mohs surgery. About half of the patients (53.3%) started to perform more self-exam for abnormal moles, and over a quarter of patients (28%) had a physician examine their moles more frequently [2].

Summary: The Potential Detrimental Impact of Mohs Surgery

- While Mohs surgery can offer many psychological and perhaps behavioral benefits, it can also result in adverse psychological consequences for a significant number of the patients. Mohs surgery is often reserved for excision of large, histologically aggressive tumors, with poorly delineated clinical borders that are likely to recur or even metastasize [4, 9]. Consequently, excision of these tumors can result in large surgical defects and complex reconstructive procedures, usually in highly visible anatomic locations (i.e., the face) [11]. Thus, disfigurement, particularly facial disfigurement, can result following Mohs surgery. Disfigurement of any type can have serious psychological consequences. But, facial disfigurement is especially concerning. In the subsequent sections, a discussion is given on the significance of surgical disfigurement, particularly facial disfigurement, and how disfigurement can lead to a negative self-image, difficulties in social interactions, and serious psychological distress [12].

47.3 The Potential Detrimental Impact of Mohs Surgery

47.3.1 Acquired Surgical Disfigurement

Mohs surgery can result in serious acquired surgical disfigurement. Studies have illustrated that surgical defects following Mohs surgery can be extensive in size and require complex reconstructive procedures. For instance, the study by Kimyai-Asadi et al. [11] examined 3,937 patients undergoing Mohs surgery. Of these patients, 86% had tumors located on the head and neck regions. The study found that the average tumor measured 1.1 cm × 1.0 cm, and resulted in an average surgical defect of 2.4 cm × 1.8 cm. Linear closures, skin flaps, skin grafts, and secondary-intention healing were employed in 69%, 14%, 6%, and 11% of defects, respectively [11].

Any of the above-mentioned reconstructive procedures have the potential consequence of significant disfigurement [7, 13, 14]. For example, primary closure of oval defects can frequently result in "dog ear" deformities, or redundant skin folds from closure of unfavorably shaped defects. Further correction of "dog ear" deformities may require additional incisions with necessary increases in wound length. Split-thickness skin grafts (e.g., grafts harvested from the pre- or retroauricular areas and grafted to repair nasal tip defects) can often differ in coloration and texture from the surrounding skin [7]. In addition, skin retraction following graft placement can commonly occur [13].

Composite grafts (i.e., grafts consisting of both skin and cartilage) are also frequently used to correct full-thickness defects following tumor excision. For example, composite auricular grafts can be used to repair small nasal alar rim defects. However, composite grafts pose the added concern for inadequate replacement of nasal lining and supporting structures, as well as poor restoration of nasal contour. Finally, delayed reconstruction of the surgical defect is another real possibility following tumor excision. Patients having tumors with questionable bone invasion, or with a high likelihood of recurrence, often have delayed reconstruction 1–2 years later. In such cases, immediate reconstruction is not possible because it would hinder early detection of tumor recurrence or mask tumor invasion. Consequently, these patients may have to wear obvious external prostheses, either temporarily or permanently [7].

47.3.2 Significance of the Face

Having extensive facial disfigurement can have profound emotional impact on the patient's psyche because of the tremendous significance of the face itself. The face is the most visible and, arguably, the most important part of the body. The face functions as the organ of communication with the outside world. We use our facial gestures to express symbolic messages of our internal feelings and motivations. The face is the window by which others can peer into our innermost self. It is how others come to know who we are. The face provides information regarding gender, age, ethnicity, and identity. As social beings, the face is crucial to successful interpersonal relationships and is, therefore, vital to our overall health and wellbeing [12, 15–17].

47.3.3 "View from Inside" vs. "View from Outside"

The psychological impact of facial disfigurement is very much dependent upon both intrapsychic (internal) and external factors. This two-sided perspective is often termed the "view from inside", vs. the "view from outside," respectively. The "view from inside" is how appearance affects one's self-perception (i.e., body image). The "view from outside" is how appearance affects social interactions with other people. Consequently, a change in appearance can alter not only an individual's self-image, but also social relationships with family, friends, and the outside world. These alterations in self-image and social relationships ultimately influence the extent to which patients with disfigurement experience psychological difficulties [18]. Thus, it is not the disfigurement itself that has the profound impact on those affected. Instead, it is how the patients and others respond to the disfigurement [19].

47.3.4 Negative Self-Image

To understand how disfigurement can alter body image, one must first have a good understanding of what body image is. The classic definition of body image, written by Paul Schilder in his 1935 book, is "the picture of our body which we form in our mind, that is to say the way in which our body appears to ourselves" [20]. Body image is dynamic, continually changing over time. It can change gradually over a lifetime, or it can change suddenly in response to short-term alterations (such as, changes in mood, clothing, or acute trauma). Bob Price [21] developed one of the most comprehensive descriptions of body image. Price created a three-component model of body image, consisting of body reality, body ideal, and body presentation. Body reality is the way our body really is. Body ideal is how we want our body to look. Body presentation is the manner in which we dress and act toward those around us. Based on this model, these three related components are continually being weighed against one another. When these components are held in state of balance, an individual is able to maintain a healthy body image [19].

However, changes in body reality (e.g., from acquired surgical disfigurement) can disrupt the delicate balance between body reality and body ideal. The individual may attempt to cope with such deficiencies in body reality, with compensatory changes in both body presentation and body ideal. In instances of acquired surgical disfigurement, the individual may change body presentation by wearing make-up or clothing that can conceal this disfigurement. The individual may also invoke good coping strategies and adequate social support to help develop a revised concept of what constitutes their body ideal [19, 22–24].

Most patients make reasonable psychological adjustment to disfigurement, regardless of the cause or severity. West et al. [25] studied 152 patients with facial disfigurement following treatment of extensive head and neck cancer. An astonishing 82.6% of these patients adapted well to their disfigurement [25].

For many patients, however, disfigurement can have serious negative effects on self-esteem, self-confidence, and self-image. These patients are regrettably unable to compensate for the changes in body reality as a result of surgical disfigurement. This is understandable in light of the fact that people, especially those in Western societies, tend to hold very narrow standards of physical beauty. Faces that are round, symmetrical, and without blemishes are considered more attractive [26]. So, despite a patient's best efforts, attempting to fit a cosmetic defect within the rigid framework of one's body ideal may not be possible.

47.3.5 Psychological Distress As a Result of Difficulties in Social Interactions

Surgical disfigurement has been demonstrated to be related to high levels of psychological distress [27]. In general, psychological distress secondary to surgical disfigurement can be grouped into two broad categories: (1) those that are distressing to the patient, but not severe enough to meet the Diagnostic and Statistical Manual of Mental Disorders, 4th edition text revision (DSM-IV-TR) [28] criteria for mental illness, and (2) those that are distressing enough to meet psychiatric diagnostic criteria. In this section, difficulties from social interactions that are not severe enough to be diagnosed as a psychiatric condition will be discussed.

One of the predominant concerns for patients with disfigurement, especially facial disfigurement, is learning how to cope with the stigma of the disfigurement. Stigma is a mark of disgrace that devalues persons who are seen as different. Here disfigurement becomes the focus of a person's social identity. It discredits all other attributes that the person possesses and labels the person to be different from the norm [12, 29].

Frances Macgregor [30], in her extensive work on facial disfigurement, explains that people with visible disfigurement are victims of much social inequities, including blatant stares and hurtful comments.

> In their efforts to go about their daily affairs they are subjected to visual and verbal assaults and a level of familiarity from strangers (not) otherwise dared: naked stares, startle reactions, "double-takes," whispering remarks, furtive looks, curiosity, personal questions, advice, manifestations of pity or aversion, laughter, ridicule, and outright avoidance. Whatever form the behaviors may take, they generate feeling of shame, impotence, anger, and humiliation in their victims [30].

Individuals with disfigurement report significant difficulties in social interactions (e.g., meeting new people, forming long-term friendships, etc.) [18, 31–33]. As briefly mentioned in Macgregor's quote, people go out of their way, either consciously or subconsciously, to avoid those with disfigurement [30]. Studies have shown that people generally sit further away [34] and offer less help to those with facial disfigurement [35]. It is also well established that people hold stereotypes against those with disfigurement. Studies have found that individuals with abnormal facial appearances are presumed to be less honest, less employable, less capable, and less intelligent than individuals with normal facial appearances [36].

For many patients with disfigurement, these continual negative encounters in social situations may eventually result in social withdrawal. Many will limit their social contacts to only immediate family members or close friends. In the extreme circumstances, social withdrawal can result in complete social isolation, or as Macgregor termed "social death" [23, 37]. The severity of social difficulties may not just present itself as social isolation, but also as coexisting feelings of anxiety in any social setting.

Thus, the social difficulties experienced by those with facial disfigurements might be secondary to phobic anxiety in social situations. The study by Moolenburgh et al. [38] compared 30 patients with partial or total nasal amputation following radical tumor resection, majority of which were being treated for BCC or SCC, against 99 control participants. Based on the Social Avoidance and Distress Scale, the study found that patients reported significantly higher levels of social anxiety and avoidance [38]. For most patients, the psychological distress from social interactions is not severe enough to be considered a psychiatric disorder. However, for some, this may develop into genuine social phobia (discussed in detail in Sect. 47.4.1).

47.3.6 Location, Age, Gender, and Severity as They Relate to the Psychological Distress of Disfigurement

Studies suggest that location of disfigurement, and possibly even age or gender, are correlated with extent of psychological impairment. Disfigurement on visible locations, especially the face, is intuitively and clinically related to greater difficulties [27]. The study by Gardiner et al. [39] found cosmetic defects on the young and female to be associated with greater impact than those on the old and male. Defects of the central face may also hold greater relevance than those found more peripherally [39].

Recent studies have attempted to examine this relationship between objective severity of disfigurement and degree of distress. It may seem logical to expect that more severe disfigurement would be correlated to greater levels of psychological distress. For example, a person with a scar over 25% of their face may have significantly more difficulties than a similar person with a scar covering only 5% of their face [40].

The study by Tebble et al. [19] found that objective measures of disfigurement severity are related to psychosocial adjustment. Specifically, the study recruited 63 patients with minor, yet visible, facial lacerations over 1.5 cm in size. The study found that those with larger scar size (4 cm or above) reported significantly higher levels of self-consciousness and anxiety [19].

However, the study by Moss [41] suggested that subjective measures of disfigurement severity (or, patient-rated measures of disfigurement severity) are better correlated with levels of psychological distress, than objective measures of disfigurement severity. Specifically, the study analyzed 400 patients with a wide array of physical differences in appearance. Patients rated subjective severity of disfigurement, whereas physicians rated objective severity of disfigurement. The study determined subjective severity to be linearly correlated to psychological adjustment, with increased subjective ratings of severity to be associated with worse adjustment. Objective severity demonstrated a complex, rather than linear, relationship to adjustment for visible anatomic locations, but not for non-visible anatomic locations. Objective severity rated as "mild" or "severe" was associated with better adjustment than "moderate" severity. In other words, the data indicated that patients with objective severity rated as "moderate" disfigurement actually faired worse than those with objective severity rated as "severe" disfigurement [41]. This illustrates how severity of disfigurement does not necessarily predict level of distress.

From a scientific, evidence-based perspective, it may seem rational to assume that objective measures of disfigurement severity hold greater significance. However, in regards to assessment of the disfigurement severity, it is generally the case that subjective measures, not objective measures, are correlated with psychosocial adjustment and quality-of-life impact. In fact, even minor disfigurement can be profoundly disturbing [40]. Body image is clearly subjective. If a patient with minor disfigurement places significant weight on physical appearance, that patient may have as great, if not greater, psychological distress as someone with major disfigurement who is less focused on physical appearance [23].

Furthermore, Frances Macgregor [37] made the counterintuitive argument that people with more extensive disfigurement often fair better overall than people with lesser disfigurement. Based on this argument, those with obvious disfigurement have an easier time adapting to social interactions because they can reliably predict the social response to their facial appearance. But, those with less noticeable disfigurement struggle with a constant sense of uncertainty in social settings. They are in, what can be described as, a state of "limbo," which may inevitably lead to greater levels of anxiety and social distress [23].

Summary: Psychiatric Disorders Secondary to Disfigurement

- It is important to realize that patient with disfigurement, regardless of the location, age, gender, or severity, may experience psychological distress following Mohs surgery. Depending on the severity of distress, patients may meet DSM-IV-TR criteria for psychiatric illness. In the following sections, the most common psychiatric conditions resulting from disfigurement (i.e., social phobia, generalized anxiety, and depression) are discussed, along with a description of the diagnostic criteria and appropriate management of these conditions.

47.4 Psychiatric Disorders Secondary to Disfigurement

47.4.1 Social Phobia

Patients with disfigurement are at risk of developing social anxiety that is distressing enough to meet DSM-IV-TR diagnostic criteria of social phobia. The study by Newell et al. [42] compared 112 facially disfigured patients with 66 patients with social phobia and 68 patients with agoraphobia. The study suggested that facially disfigured patients resembled patients with social phobia, as they had similar scores on the anxiety and depression subscales of the Fear Questionnaire [42].

According to the DSM-IV-TR [28], social phobia refers to a condition in which the patient develops a persistent fear of social situations where he or she is likely to be scrutinized by others. If the patient is under the age of 18 years, the duration must be at least

6 months. Once social phobia has begun, it gradually becomes worse because of two factors. First, anticipatory anxiety gradually develops whenever the person is confronted with the necessity to enter a social gathering. Second, the patient's social performance becomes impaired by this underlying anxiety, resulting in the development of a vicious cycle. Exposure to the feared social situation will almost invariably provoke an immediate anxiety response. Some patients with social phobia will try to avoid social situations, while others will try to force themselves to endure the social situation despite their intense anxiety. Eventually, this progression toward complete social isolation will cause the patient to suffer serious social or occupational impairment. Patients with social phobia usually retain the insight to recognize that their fears are excessive or unreasonable, even in view of their disfigurement. Therefore, these patients tend to be receptive to the suggestion that they should obtain professional help from a psychiatrist or other mental health professionals [28].

There are three general types of therapies available for the treatment of social phobia. The first approach is a behavioral therapy technique involving "exposure" or "flooding." In exposure, patients are presented with increasingly anxiety-provoking social situations, initially in the form of imagery and later as real-life encounters. At each stage of exposure, care should be taken to make sure that the patient's anxiety level does not go out of control. Through this process known as systematic desensitization, the patient gradually learns not to fear the social situation [43]. In flooding (also termed, "implosion"), the patient is exposed to an enormous volume of phobic material in an attempt to overwhelm the phobic response. This technique can also be used in either imagery or real-life situations.

The second approach involves psychotherapy, in which the patient explores different psychological issues with the therapist. This approach can take many different forms, depending on the particular orientation of the therapist. Some therapists favor psychodynamic therapy (i.e., emphasizing the use of Freudian principles), while others favor a cognitive approach (i.e., actively trying to change the patient's thinking habits by challenging existing semiautomatic or automatic thought patterns).

The third approach is the use of pharmacotherapy. Antianxiety drugs (discussed in detail in Sect. 47.4.2) are used to treat anxiety symptoms, whereas antidepressants (discussed in greater detail in Sect. 47.4.3) are used to treat phobic symptoms. Several serotonin selective receptor inhibitors (SSRIs) and one serotonin norepinephrine receptor inhibitor (SNRI) are approved by the US Food and Drug Administration (FDA) as medications for social phobia. These include fluvoxamine extended release (Luvox CR) (100-300 mg/day), paroxetine (Paxil) (20 mg/day), paroxetine extended release (Paxil CR) (12.5-37.5 mg/day), sertraline (Zoloft) (50-200 mg/day) and venlafaxine extended release (Effexor XR) (75 mg/day), respectively. [44].

47.4.2 Generalized Anxiety Disorder

The anxiety experienced by patients with disfigurement may extend beyond just anxiety in social situations. Patient may experience more generalized forms of anxiety and even depression [19, 45–47]. The study by Rumsey et al. [46] evaluated 220 patients with disfiguring conditions as a result of burns, skin conditions, or head and neck cancer. The study found that patients displayed increased levels of anxiety, depression, and social anxiety/avoidance [46].

To be diagnosed with Generalized Anxiety Disorder (GAD), a patient must have excessive anxiety and worry about everyday events and activities for at least 6 months. The patient finds it difficult to control worrying. The anxiety is associated with at least three of the following symptoms: restlessness, fatigue, difficulty concentrating, irritability, muscle tension, or sleep disturbance. The focus of the anxiety is generalized in nature. It is not focused to any given stressor or social situation. This anxiety will inevitably cause impairments in social, occupational, or other important areas of functioning. Most patients with GAD do not initially seek psychiatric help. Instead, patients will often go to a medical specialist in hopes of alleviating the physical complaints that accompany this disorder (i.e., muscle tension or fatigue) [28].

The most effective treatment approach for GAD is the combination of psychotherapy and pharmacotherapy. Patient should be made aware of the chronic nature of the condition and the tendency of symptom severity to vary over time. Behavior therapy may be useful in teaching a patient how to control anxiety. Relaxation training, including breathing exercises and progressive muscle relaxation, may also be of benefit [44].

As far as medication, there are several drugs approved by the FDA for the treatment of GAD. These include the SSRIs paroxetine (20 mg/day) and excitalopram (Lexapro) (10 mg/day), the SNRI venlafaxine extended release (Effexor XR) (75-225 mg/day), and the non-benzodiazepine anxiolytic buspirone (BuSpar) (20-30 mg/day) [44].

Buspirone is a non-sedating, nonaddictive anti-anxiety medication that is slow in onset of action. This medication must be taken on a regular basis (2 to 3 times per day) because it is not effective on an "as needed" basis. It takes up to 4 weeks or more for the clinical effects of buspirone to become evident, and therefore it is ideal for patients with a chronic anxiety disorder 20 to 30 mg per day (divided dose 2 or 3 times per day). The oral dosage of buspirone ranges from However, this must be individualized for each patient, beginning with the lowest dosage and titrating upward until the optimal dosage is achieved. The side effects of buspirone include dizziness, nausea, headache, nervousness, lightheadedness, and excitement.

Benzodiazepines such as alprazolam (Xanax) (0.75-1.5 mg/day, divided dose 3 times per day), lorazepam (Ativan) (2-4 mg/day, divided dose 2 or 3 times per day), and clonazepam (Klonopin) (0.5-1.5 mg/day, divided dose 2 or 3 times per day) are highly effective anti-anxiety medications. They are rapid acting, but can be highly sedating and potentially addictive. The major difference between these medications is the half-life. Medications with a shorter half-life carry a greater the risk of rebound anxiety and addiction. Alprazolam has the shortest half-life, whereas clonazepam has the longest half-life. The authors generally favor the above newer benzodiazepinas over the older benzodiazepines, such as diazepam (Valium) and chlordiazepoxide (Librium), because they have many active metabolites that can accumulate in the body and can compromise mental functioning when used long-term.

The optimal usage of benzodiazepines involves careful titration of the dosage beginning with a low starting dose. Once the anxiety is well controlled, the dosage should be gradually tapered. Abrupt discontinuation should be avoided, as it carries the risk of seizures, as well as recurrence or exacerbation of anxiety. Benzodiazepines should be reserved for short-term use only to help overcome acute episodes of severe anxiety. A psychiatrist should be consulted if usage is required beyond 2 to 4 weeks. Patients should be counseled regarding the risk of abuse or dependence with this class of medications [48, 49].

47.4.3 Depression

Patients with acquired surgical disfigurement, especially those with facial disfigurement, have a higher risk of developing clinical depression [18, 23, 46]. One of the challenges, however, is being able to distinguish clinical depression from other conditions that may mimic depression. These include normative sadness, depressant effects of certain medications (e.g., benzodiazepines), or comorbid medical conditions (e.g., hypothyroidism), just to name a few.

Patients with depression are less likely to comply with medical recommendations for wound care management. They are, therefore, more likely to have poor wound healing and potentially greater disfigurement. Even more significantly, patients with depression are at an increased risk of attempting suicide [23]. Thus, it is essential that patients with depression be identified early and provided with the necessary treatment intervention(s).

To diagnose major depressive disorder, the following DSM-IV-TR criteria apply. A major depressive episode is defined as having at least five of the following symptoms for at least a 2-week period: depressed mood, anhedonia (loss of interest or pleasure), change in appetite or body weight, insomnia or hypersomnia, psychomotor agitation or retardation, fatigue or loss of energy, feelings of worthlessness or excessive guilt, difficulty in concentration, and recurrent thoughts of death or suicide. At least one of these symptoms must include either depressed mood or anhedonia. Patients must have no history of a manic or hypomanic episode. The depression must cause significant social or occupational impairment [28].

There are many treatment approaches for depression. Psychotherapy can be used alone, or in combination with pharmacotherapy. Psychotherapy options include behavior therapy, cognitive therapy, supportive psychotherapy, dynamic psychotherapy, and family therapy. Hospitalization may be indicated if patients are at risk of suicide, homicide, or are unable to care for themselves [44].

Pharmacologic treatment of depression consists of SSRIs, TCAs, and MAOIs. SSRIs, such as fluoxetine (Prozac) (20-80 mg/day), sertraline (Zoloft) (50-200 mg/day), paroxetine (Paxil) (20-50 mg/day), citalopram (Celexa) (20-60 mg/day), and escitalopram

(Lexapro) (10-20 mg/day), are generally safe and better tolerated than other classes of antidepressants. SSRIs are considered to be first-line pharmacologic therapy for depression. Headache and gastrointestinal (GI) disturbances, such as nausea and diarrhea, are the most common adverse effects. Giving the medication with food often helps prevent nausea, which is usually transient. Some SSRIs, namely sertraline, paroxetine, and citalopram, can be sedating. If sedating, the medication should be given at bedtime. In contrast, SSRIs like fluoxetine and escitalopram, can be activating. If activating, the medication should be taken in the morning. SSRIs can also be associated with sexual dysfunction and, therefore, patients should be educated about this side effect prior to starting therapy [50].

Initial therapeutic effects of SSRIs may be seen in about 2-3 weeks, but optimal therapeutic effects may take up to 4-6 weeks. When SSRIs are abruptly discontinued, patients may experience headaches, GI upset, dizziness, lethargy, insomnia, nightmares, irritability, agitation, anxiety, dysphoria, confusion, and emotional instability (known as, discontinuation syndrome). So, taper the dose gradually over several weeks to help prevent such symptoms.

The TCAs doxepin (100 mg/day), amitriptyline (Elavil) (50-150 mg/day), desipramine (Norpramin) (100-200 mg/day), and clomipramine (Anafranil) (150-250 mg/day) are all effective antidepressants but can be lethal in overdose. Therefore, if there is potential for suicidality, it is best to avoid TCAs or, at the very least, limit the quantity of TCAs dispensed per visit. Common side effects include sedation, weight gain, orthostatic hypotension, and anticholingeric effects (i.e. constipation, urinary hesitation, tachycardia, blurred vision, and dry mouth). TCAs can also cause cardiac conduction disturbance (i.e. prolongation of the QT interval), especially in elderly patients. So, consider checking an ECG at baseline and then periodically, especially when high-dosages are used. Today, TCAs are rarely used as an antidepressant since they have more risks than SSRIs. When discontinuing TCAs, taper the dose gradually. Abrupt cessation of TCAs can cause withdrawal symptoms including nausea, vomiting, diarrhea headache, sleep disturbances, dizziness, malaise, hyperthermia, irritability, akathisia [51], [52].

MAOIs, such as phenelzine (Nardil) and translcypromine (Parnate), are virtually never used nowadays, since they have less favorable risk-to-benefit ratio as compared to the other treatment options as described above. However, they have been used in treating depressed patients whose symptoms do not respond to the other antidepressants (also known as, refractory depression). MAOIs should be prescribed with caution because of the potentially dangerous side effects. Common side effects include orthostatic hypotension, drowsiness, weight gain, sexual dysfunction, dry mouth, and sleep dysfunction. MAOIs should not be used in combination with TCAs or SSRIs due to the risk of serotonin syndrome, a potentially life-threatening adverse drug reaction. In addition, MAOIs have an increased risk of hypertensive crisis if taken with sympathomimetics or tyramine-rich foods, like wines and cheeses. Because of these serious risks, MAOIs are rarely used today and when prescribed are preferably used as monotherapy [44].

Electroconvulsive therapy (ECT) may be indicated if symptoms are unresponsive to pharmacotherapy, or if the patient cannot tolerate pharmacotherapy. ECT is considered to be a safe and effective form of treatment for depression. ECT can be used alone, or in combination with pharmacotherapy. About eight treatments are typically administered over a 2–3-week period. But, patients often report significant improvement after the first treatment. Because ECT can help rapidly reduce depressive symptoms, it may be useful in treating patients who are at risk of attempting suicide. The most common side effect is retrograde amnesia, which usually disappears within 6 months [44].

Summary: Conclusion

- Mohs surgery can have tremendous psychological affects on patients. In the ideal situation, patients will experience the benefits of Mohs surgery, including a sense of relief that their cancer has been resected and improvements in quality of life. Unfortunately, however, the excision of the large, aggressive tumors on highly visible anatomical locations can result in surgical disfigurement. Patients with surgical disfigurement are at risk of developing secondary psychiatric disorders, including social phobia, generalized anxiety, and depression. It is, therefore, important that Mohs surgeons can appropriately diagnose and manage these debilitating, potentially life-ruining psychiatric disorders.

47.5 Conclusion

Many psychological issues may develop following treatment of skin cancer with Mohs surgery because of surgically induced disfigurement. The basic diagnostic criteria and treatment modalities have been described in detail. The information provided here should serve as a useful tool in identifying and managing patients with psychological difficulties secondary to disfigurement. Mohs surgeons, however, should not be expected to treat patients with psychiatric problems on a regular basis. Whenever feasible, these patients should be referred to a board-certified psychiatrist. If the patient refuses such a referral, as is frequently the case, the treating physician should not be discouraged. It may still be possible to obtain a consultation from a psychiatrist or other mental health professional if the referral is presented to the patient as an extra assistance above and beyond the continuing dermatological care, thereby allaying any patient fear of abandonment. Ultimately, it is our sincere hope this discussion helps the Mohs surgeon to more effectively handle the psychological problems that may arise in the clinical setting.

References

1. Chren MM, Sahay AP, Bertenthal DS, Sen S, Landefeld CS. Quality-of-life outcomes of treatments for cutaneous basal cell carcinoma and squamous cell carcinoma. J Invest Dermatol. 2007;127(6):1351–7.
2. Maser E, Berg D, Solish N. Changes in patient perception and behavior following Mohs micrographic surgery. J Cutan Med Surg. 2001;5(1):14–7.
3. Neville JA, Welch E, Leffell DJ. Management of nonmelanoma skin cancer in 2007. Nat Clin Pract Oncol. 2007;4(8): 462–9.
4. Cumberland L, Dana A, Liegeois N. Mohs micrographic surgery for the management of nonmelanoma skin cancers. Facial Plast Surg Clin North Am. 2009;17(3):325–35.
5. Vuyk HD, Lohuis PJ. Mohs micrographic surgery for facial skin cancer. Clin Otolaryngol Allied Sci. 2001;26(4):265–73.
6. Downes RN, Walker NP, Collin JR. Micrographic (MOHS) surgery in the management of periocular basal cell epitheliomas. Eye (Lond). 1990;4(Pt 1):160–8.
7. Dobke MK, Miller SH. Tissue repair after Mohs surgery. A plastic surgeon's view. Dermatol Surg. 1997;23(11): 1061–6.
8. Inkster C, Ashworth J, Murdoch JR, Montgomery P, Telfer NR, Leatherbarrow B. Oculoplastic reconstruction following Mohs surgery. Eye (Lond). 1998;12(Pt 2):214–8.
9. Garcia C, Holman J, Poletti E. Mohs surgery: commentaries and controversies. Int J Dermatol. 2005;44(11):893–905.
10. Moul DK, Chern PL, Shumaker PR, Zelac DE, Greenway HT. Mohs micrographic surgery for eyelid and periorbital skin cancer. Int Ophthalmol Clin. 2009;49(4):111–27.
11. Kimyai-Asadi A, Goldberg LH, Peterson SR, Silapint S, Jih MH. The incidence of major complications from Mohs micrographic surgery performed in office-based and hospital-based settings. J Am Acad Dermatol. 2005;53(4):628–34.
12. Furr LA, Wiggins O, Cunningham M, Vasilic D, Brown CS, Banis Jr JC, et al. Psychosocial implications of disfigurement and the future of human face transplantation. Plast Reconstr Surg. 2007;120(2):559–65.
13. Ge NN, McGuire JF, Dyson S, Chark D. Nonmelanoma skin cancer of the head and neck II: surgical treatment and reconstruction. Am J Otolaryngol. 2009;30(3):181–92.
14. Kikkawa DO, Korn BS, Annunziata CC. Reconstruction of large and complex periorbital defects from cutaneous cancer. Int Ophthalmol Clin. 2009;49(4):237–45.
15. Adsett CA. Emotional reactions to disfigurement from cancer therapy. Can Med Assoc J. 1963;89:385–91.
16. Bowers B. Providing effective support for patients facing disfiguring surgery. Br J Nurs. 2008;17(2):94–8.
17. Soni CV, Barker JH, Pushpakumar SB, Furr LA, Cunningham M, Banis Jr JC, et al. Psychosocial considerations in facial transplantation. Burns. 2010;36(7):959–64.
18. Thompson A, Kent G. Adjusting to disfigurement: processes involved in dealing with being visibly different. Clin Psychol Rev. 2001;21(5):663–82.
19. Tebble NJ, Thomas DW, Price P. Anxiety and self-consciousness in patients with minor facial lacerations. J Adv Nurs. 2004;47(4):417–26.
20. Schilder P. The image and appearance of the human body: studies in the constructive energies of the psyche. London: K. Paul, Trench, Trubner & Co. Ltd; 1935.
21. Price B. Body image: nursing concepts and care. New York: Prentice Hall; 1990.
22. Newell RJ. Altered body image: a fear-avoidance model of psycho-social difficulties following disfigurement. J Adv Nurs. 1999;30(5):1230–8.
23. Sarwer DB, Pruzinsky T. Psychological aspects of reconstructive and cosmetic plastic surgery: clinical, empirical, and ethical perspectives. Philadelphia: Lippincott Williams & Wilkins; 2006.
24. Sainsbury DC. Body image and facial burns. Adv Skin Wound Care. 2009;22(1):39–44.
25. West DW. Social adaptation patterns among cancer patients with facial disfigurements resulting from surgery. Arch Phys Med Rehabil. 1977;58(11):473–9.
26. Hill-Beuf A, Porter JD. Children coping with impaired appearance: social and psychologic influences. Gen Hosp Psychiatry. 1984;6(4):294–301.
27. Cash TF, Pruzinsky T. Body image: a handbook of theory, research, and clinical practice. New York: Guilford Press; 2002.
28. American Psychiatric Association. Diagnostic and statistical manual of mental disorders, Text Revision. 4th ed. Washington: American Psychiatric Publishing, Inc.; 2000.
29. Bonanno A, Esmaeli B, Fingeret MC, Nelson DV, Weber RS. Social challenges of cancer patients with orbitofacial disfigurement. Ophthal Plast Reconstr Surg. 2010;26(1):18–22.
30. Macgregor FC. Facial disfigurement: problems and management of social interaction and implications for mental health.

Aesthetic Plast Surg. 1990;14(4):249–57. Reprinted with kind permission from Springer Science+Business Media.
31. Jowett S, Ryan T. Skin disease and handicap: an analysis of the impact of skin conditions. Soc Sci Med. 1985;20(4):425–9.
32. Lanigan SW, Cotterill JA. Psychological disabilities amongst patients with port wine stains. Br J Dermatol. 1989;121(2): 209–15.
33. Porter JR, Beuf AH, Lerner AB, Nordlund JJ. The effect of vitiligo on sexual relationships. J Am Acad Dermatol. 1990; 22(2 Pt 1):221–2.
34. Houston V, Bull A. Do people avoid sitting next to someone who is facially disfigured? Eur J Soc Psychol. 1994;24:279–84.
35. Piliavin I, Piliavin J, Rodin L. Costs, diffusion and the stigmatised victim. J Pers Soc Psychol. 1976;32:429–38.
36. Rankin M, Borah GL. Perceived functional impact of abnormal facial appearance. Plast Reconstr Surg. 2003;111(7):2140–8.
37. Macgregor FC. After plastic surgery: adaptation and adjustment. New York: New York Times Book Company; 1979.
38. Moolenburgh SE, Mureau MA, Versnel SL, Duivenvoorden HJ, Hofer SO. The impact of nasal reconstruction following tumour resection on psychosocial functioning, a clinical-empirical exploration. Psychooncology. 2009;18(7):747–52.
39. Gardiner MD, Topps A, Richardson G, Sacker A, Clarke A, Butler PE. Differential judgements about disfigurement: the role of location, age and gender in decisions made by observers. J Plast Reconstr Aesthet Surg. 2010;63(1):73–7.
40. Rumsey N, Clarke A, Musa M. Altered body image: the psychosocial needs of patients. Br J Community Nurs. 2002; 7(11):563–6.
41. Moss TP. The relationships between objective and subjective ratings of disfigurement severity, and psychological adjustment. Body Image. 2005;2(2):151–9.
42. Newell R, Marks I. Phobic nature of social difficulty in facially disfigured people. Br J Psychiatry. 2000;176:177–81.
43. Cassell WA. Desensitization therapy for body image anxiety. Can Psychiatr Assoc J. 1977;22(5):239–42.
44. Andreasen N, Black D. Introductory textbook of psychiatry. 4th ed. Washington: American Psychiatric Publishing, Inc.; 2006.
45. Sen P, Ross N, Rogers S. Recovering maxillofacial trauma patients: the hidden problems. J Wound Care. 2001;10(3): 53–7.
46. Rumsey N, Clarke A, White P. Exploring the psychosocial concerns of outpatients with disfiguring conditions. J Wound Care. 2003;12(7):247–52.
47. Tebble NJ, Adams R, Thomas DW, Price P. Anxiety and self-consciousness in patients with facial lacerations one week and six months later. Br J Oral Maxillofac Surg. 2006;44(6):520–5.
48. Fawcett J, Edwards JH, Kravitz HM, Jeffriess H. Alprazolam: an antidepressant? Alprazolam, desipramine, and an alprazolam-desipramine combination in the treatment of adult depressed outpatients. J Clin Psychopharmacol. 1987;7(5): 295–310.
49. Feighner JP, Boyer WF, Tyler DL, Neborsky RJ. Adverse consequences of fluoxetine-MAOI combination therapy. J Clin Psychiatry. 1990;51(6):222–5.
50. Physician's Desk Reference. 45th ed. Oradell: Medical Economics; 1991.
51. Schatzberg A, Cole J. Handbook of clinical psychopharmacology. Washington: American Psychiatric Press; 1986.
52. Cole JO. The drug treatment of anxiety and depression. Med Clin North Am. 1988;72(4):815–30.
W

Index

K. Nouri (ed.), *Mohs Micrographic Surgery*,
DOI 10.1007/978-1-4471-2152-7, © Springer-Verlag London Limited 2012